Histology

Histology

A TEXT AND ATLAS

Johannes A. G. Rhodin, M.D., Ph.D.

NEW YORK MEDICAL COLLEGE

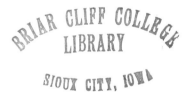
NEW YORK · OXFORD UNIVERSITY PRESS · LONDON TORONTO 1974

COVER
Electron micrograph of numerous myelinated
nerve processes
in cross-sectioned optic
nerve of the rat. X 2650.

This book is dedicated to my sons
ANDERS and ERIK—students of
medicine and architecture

Preface

This book has been created for college and medical students placed in an informal learning environment of a contemporary curriculum. The author does intend this volume to replace elaborate standard texts and atlases in the hope of assisting overburdened science students. The text is an up-to-date brief account of the structure, ultrastructure, and function of mammalian tissues, cells, and organelles. The photographs are carefully selected and organized to show sequential magnifications of the same field from light microscopy to low magnification electron microscopy as well as medium and high magnification electron microscopy. The numerous electron micrographs shown at magnifications ranging from 600× to 2000× are unique in their detailed and crisp outlining of organs, tissues, and cells. These illustrations will prove to be of particularly great value in helping the student bridge the difficult gap between light microscopy and high magnification electron microscopy.

The illustrations are found on the right hand page, the text and figure captions on the left. Thus, the book combines the concise and complete wording of a text with the descriptive legends and illustrations of an atlas, saving the student the time and effort involved in studying both a textbook and an atlas. Numerals are used to identify structures in the illustrations. The student will, therefore, easily find a specific item in the picture, and the micrographs can readily be used by the student and the teacher for testing purposes.

In the textual material, lengthy introductions were avoided on the assumption that at this level students have acquired some knowledge of the gross appearance and position of organs. Emphasis has been placed on present knowledge of structural architecture rather than on introductory historical background and accounts of the many special techniques utilized in arriving at a certain item of information. The author's experience in teaching has convinced him that histology should be presented in terms of the structural appearance of tissues as observed by both the light and the electron microscopes. Therefore, the text combines the light and electron microscope descriptions of organs, tissues, and cells.

The collection of illustrations is prepared by the author especially for this book. It includes analyses of many organs which have not previously been described adequately in the literature. The chapters on human blood cells and hemopoiesis represent the first comprehensive account of this topic, and the thorough analyses of the ultrastructure of the spleen, lymphopoiesis, and blood vessels present many new functional aspects of these organs and their components. The chapter on the cell and cell organelles summarizes current knowledge in this field, and establishes a firm base for extended studies in cytochemistry, cell biology, and physiology. The light microscope preparations are almost exclusively taken from human or monkey tissues. The electron microscope preparations are taken for the most part from rats and cats. Human tissues were used in instances in which they differ considerably from those of lower mammals.

To achieve superior resolution numerous illustrations are taken from electron micrographs even though a similar magnification could have been achieved by the light microscope. The panoramic low magnification electron micrographs are intended to replace many of the drawings and composite diagrams of standard histology textbooks. The author does not believe that teaching histology should aim primarily at the "reading" of routine slides. Instead, it should enable the student to form some concrete visualization of structures and locations involved in the life processes. The cytologically informative and clearly delineated preparations reproduced in this book should provide the student with correspondingly clear concepts of biological structure.

New York
November 1973   Johannes A. G. Rhodin

Acknowledgments

The author is greatly indebted to his research associates, Miss Shirley Lim Sue and Mrs. Carin Silversmith, for their very skillful assistance in preparing the material through vascular perfusion, embedding, sectioning, electron microscopy, photographic printing, final mounting, and labeling of the illustrations. Without their willingness to tackle these chores, their cheerful encouragement and incredible endurance, the illustrations would not have materialized.

Dr. Yen Fen Pei, M.D., secured the material necessary to illustrate the chapter on the eye. Her knowledge of ophthalmology contributed invaluably to the careful selection and proper preservation of the specimens. Her unselfish technical assistance and suggestions for the text on the eye are gratefully acknowledged.

The maintenance of the electron microscopes by Mr. Eugene W. Minner throughout the several years of specimen preparation was of immeasurable help.

Special appreciation is extended to my wife Gunvor Rhodin for preparing the drawings, as well as for her never failing readiness to assist in whatever crises developed during the making of this book.

Mrs. Betsey Stiepock, Administrative Assistant of the Department of Anatomy, was most helpful in typing and proofreading the manuscript. Her constant willingness to take on additional duties in the department, particularly during the final year of intense work on this text is indeed greatly appreciated.

Dr. Louis L. Bergmann, M.D., gave freely of his time in critically reading parts of the manuscript, and his corrections and suggestions greatly improved the text.

Figures 2-22, 2-23, and 31-22 are reprinted by permission of National Tuberculosis and Respiratory Diseases Association; figures 4-25, 23-8, 23-9, and 16-32 by permission of Academic Press; figures 16-35, 16-38 and 16-41 by permission of Harper and Row; and figure 32-5 is redrawn and modified by permission of Dr. L. C. Junqueira and Dr. J. Carneiro.

The cooperation and enthusiasm of Mr. William C. Halpin, Vice-President, and of his staff at Oxford University Press throughout the preparation of the text are deeply and sincerely appreciated.

Contents

1 Introduction

WHAT IS HISTOLOGY?

Histology deals with the normal microscopical appearance of the body. It is the basis for the understanding of physiological and pathological processes. The light microscope is used to observe an organ, either *in vivo* or after its removal from the body. *In vivo* observations are restricted to observing the general, coarse texture of the component parts, as well as the pattern of blood flow. After the removal of an organ, it can be examined with both the light microscope and the electron microscope following preservation by fixative solutions, dehydration, embedding, sectioning, and staining. This results in the light microscopical slides used routinely in the histological laboratory and surgical pathology. Entire organs or parts thereof can be sectioned. (Fig. 1-1) For electron microscopy, only small pieces can be preserved at a time, and the sections must be extremely thin (100 Å– 1000 Å).

Light microscopy relies on the staining of the sections to bring out variations in color. This is desirable since the resolving power of the light microscope is in the order of 0.2 μ (2000 Å), and differences in optical density of various organ components are enchanced by the dye, aiding in the discrimination of one component from another. The electron microscope also relies on the staining of the sections, although to a´lesser degree. The theoretical limit of the resolving power of the electron microscope is in the order of 2 Å. The practical limit of resolution in ultra-thin sections is about 10 Å; in thin sections about 25 Å; and in thick sections about 50–100 Å. The resolving power (resolution) is dependent, therefore, on the thickness of the section and the wave length of the source of radiation. It is a linear measure of the smallest distance at which two structures can still be distinguished from each other. The following is a table for measuring structures in histology:

1 mm = 1000 microns (μ)
1 μ = 10,000 Angstrom units (Å)
In some texts, micron (μ) is often expressed as micrometer (μm) 1 μ = 1 μm.
Average diameter of a red blood cell = 7 μ
Average diameter of a ribosome = 200 Å

ORGAN COMPONENTS

Based on light and electron microscope observations, it has been established that organs consist of four primary tissues: epithelium, connective tissue, muscle tissue, and nervous tissue. Each tissue in turn consists of **cells** and **extracellular components**. Each cell consists of a cell mem-

Fig. 1-1. Section of entire organ. Kidney. Rabbit. L.M. X 15.5. This demonstrates the considerable amount of structural information which can be obtained at low magnification in the light microscope, if the tissue section is of proper thickness and the colored dyes carefully selected to show differences in optical density of different structures. **1.** Capsule. **2.** Cortex. **3.** Medulla. **4.** Pyramid. **5.** Papilla. **6.** Renal pelvis. **7.** Adipose tissue in renal sinus. **8.** Ureter. This section is enlarged further in Fig. 32-2 (p. 649).

Fig. 1-2. Proximal convoluted tubule of the nephron. Cross section. Enlargement of area similar to circle in Fig. 1-1. Kidney. Rabbit. L.M. × 1100. This demonstrates the practical limit of light microscopical resolution in a routinely prepared histological specimen. The preparation included formalin fixation, paraffin emebdding, and staining with hematoxylin and eosin. **1.** Lumen. **2.** Brush border zone. **3.** Nuclei.

Fig. 1-3. Proximal convoluted tubule of the nephron. Kidney. Rat. E.M. X 1100 (as in Fig. 1-2). This demonstrates the superiority of the preparation techniques and resolving power of the electron microscope. The tissue was fixed by intravascular perfusion of glutaraldehyde followed by intravascular perfusion of osmium tetroxide, embedding in epoxy resin, thin-sectioning, and staining with lead citrate. **1.** Lumen. **2.** Microvilli. **3.** Apical vacuoles (not present in Fig. 1-2). **4.** Nucleus. **5.** Cytoplasmic granules (mitochondria and secondary lysosomes). **6.** Peritubular capillary. Section of a similar area is enlarged further in Fig. 32-13 (p. 657).

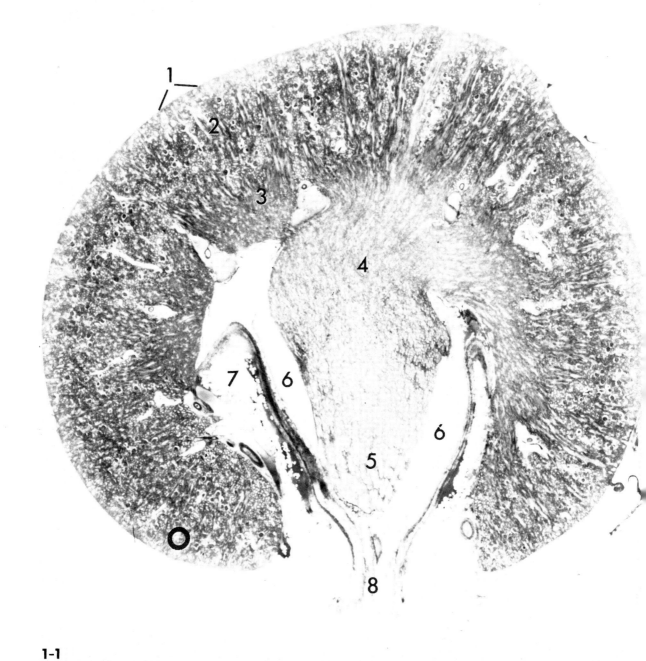

1-1

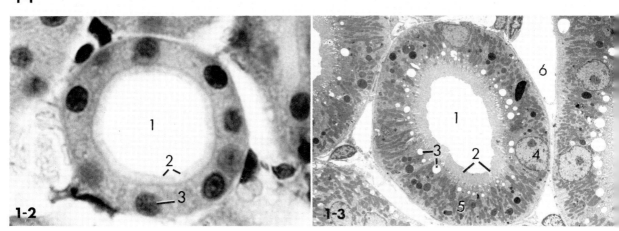

1-2

1-3

brane, the nucleus, organelles, and inclusions. All organs, tissues, cells, and cell organelles of the mammalian body are described in subsequent chapters.

Knowledge of the structural architecture of living substance and its components is only one aspect of understanding the intricate mechanisms involved in the functions of organs, tissues, cells, and organelles. Many techniques are now available to identify biochemically the many varied components. During the last two decades, a combination of light microscopy, electron microscopy, histochemistry, radioautography, cell fractionation, differential centrifugation, and cytochemistry has contributed greatly to a better understanding of structural and functional interrelationships. It is considered beyond the scope of this book to describe these techniques which are accounted for in detail in standard textbooks of research methods in cell biology.

GUIDE TO ILLUSTRATIONS

The illustrations in this book were obtained by photographing sectioned specimens under light and electron microscopes. In order to bring out differences in density between organs, tissues and cellular components, stains were applied to enhance the inherent light and electron density of a given structure.

In **light microscopy** the sections are stained with a variety of colored dyes, the most common being a combination of eosin and hematoxylin. The proteins of cells and extracellular components take on a red or pink color with eosin, whereas nucleic acids of the nuclei and certain components of the cytoplasm take on a deep blue color with hematoxylin. In **electron microscopy,** a solution of osmium tetroxide is used both as a general fixative and as an electron stain. In addition, salt solutions of heavy metals (lead, phosphotungstic acid) are used to enhance the electron density of tissue components. It should be kept in mind that these metals are not bound specifically to cellular or tissue components, although a **linear arrangement** of structures enhanced by the electron stain is generally accepted to indicate the location of membranes or filaments, whereas a **granular** configuration is believed to reflect a particulate arrangement of molecules. (Fig. 1-4)

The importance of staining a light microscope section by a variation of colored dyes is often overemphasized in the study of histological and pathological slides. Since the electron microscope cannot reproduce colors but depends entirely on differences in electron density of the tissue components, the light micrographs in this book are presented in black and white to facilitate the transition from light microscopy to electron microscopy. (Figs. 1-2, 1-3)

The adjectives **ultrastructural, submicroscopic,** and **fine structural** often used in contemporary textbooks of histology and cell biology express the details resolved by the electron microscope which lie beyond the resolving power of the light microscope.

Fig. 1-4. Detail of parenchymal cell. Liver. Rat. E.M. × 160,000. This demonstrates the resolving power of the electron microscope and the enhancement of the electron density of linear and granular components of the cell by osmium tetroxide fixation and staining of the section with lead citrate. **1.** Mitochondria. **2.** Mitochondrial external envelope, total thickness 200 Å. Each dense linear component of this envelope is 60 Å thick and consists of three subunits, each averaging 20 Å in thickness. The resolution achieved in this electron micrograph is therefore approximately 20 Å. **3.** Mitochondrial cristae, each originating from the inner membranous component of the mitochondrial external envelope. **4.** Membrane of granular endoplasmic reticulum, 60 Å thick. This membrane also consists of three subunits, each 20 Å thick. **5.** Ribosomes, particles averaging 200 Å in diameter.

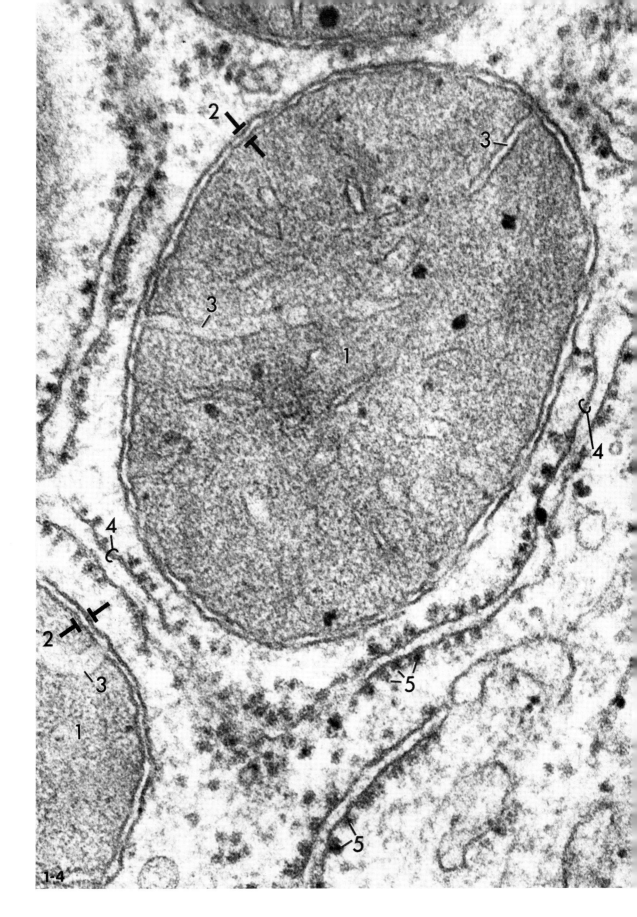

References

Hollenberg, M. J. and Erickson, A. M. The scanning
electron microscope: potential usefulness to biolo-
gists. A review. J. Histochem. Cytochem. *21*: 109–130
(1973).

Kay, D. H. Techniques for Electron Microscopy. F. A.
Davis Co., Philadelphia, 1965.

Pearse, A. G. E. Histochemistry, Theoretical and Applied.
Third Edition, Little, Brown, Boston, 1968.

Pease, D. C. Histological Techniques for Electron Microscopy. Second Edition. Academic Press, New York,
1965.

Rogers, A. W. Techniques of Autoradiography. American Elsevier, New York, 1967.

Sjöstrand, F. S. Electron Microscopy of Cells and Tissues.
Vol. I. Instrumentation and Techniques. Academic
Press, New York, 1967.

Wied, G. L. (Ed.). Introduction to Quantitative Cytochemistry. Academic Press, New York, 1966.

2 Cells and organelles

GENERAL CONSIDERATIONS

The cell is the functional unit of the mammalian body. It consists of protoplasm, bounded by a delicate cell membrane. The protoplasm consists of the nucleus (karyoplasm) and the cytoplasm. The cytoplasm contains a matrix (hyaloplasm), cell organelles, and inclusion bodies. The size, shape, and function of mammalian cells vary considerably and the study of cells and tissues deals with precisely these parameters. In general terms, the **protoplasm** is a heterogeneous aqueous phase which contains many biochemical components required for the varied metabolic processes that underlie and represent life. In addition, the protoplasm contains genetic material which determines the character of the cell in processes of cell multiplication and growth.

In mammalian cells the cytoplasm contains the biochemical components of the protoplasm, whereas the genetic material in the form of nucleic acids is concentrated largely in the karyoplasm (nucleus). The **cytoplasm** contains water (75%), salts (1%), proteins (20%), lipids (3%), carbohydrates (1%), and nucleic acids. The percentages indicated are approximate; they vary considerably from cell type to cell type. Some of the cellular **water** is present as bound water and held loosely by protein molecules, whereas most exists as free water, available for metabolic processes. Of the **salts,** cations are represented by sodium, potassium, calcium, magnesium, and minute concentrations of several other ions. Major concentrations of anions are phosphate, bicarbonate, and chloride. The concentrations of the various salts in the cell and in the extracellular milieu, and the transport back and forth across the cell membrane of these salts as a result of changes in membrane permeability, are vital for the maintenance and normal functioning of the cell.

Proteins and **lipids** are present as highly ordered arrays of molecules, forming **membranes,** both as part of the cell membrane and the membranes surrounding and constituting an essential part of the many varied subunits of the cell, referred to as cell organelles. Proteins also exist in the cytoplasmic matrix (hyaloplasm) in soluble form, and lipids can be stored as droplets. **Carbohydrates** may occur as glycogen, as small particles which are not membrane-bound, and represent a high polymer of the monosaccharide glucose. Carbohydrates are also conjugated with proteins to form mucopolysaccharides.

Cell **organelles** are structural subunits of the cytoplasm, each characterized by its specific enzymatic content, ultrastructure, and function. Considered as organelles (Fig. 2-1) are the ribosomes and polysomes, granular and agranular endoplasmic reticulum, Golgi apparatus, annulate lamellae, mitochondria, lysosomes and related particles, centrioles, microtubules, and filaments. Pinocytotic vesicles are intracellular derivatives of the cell membrane, and as such should be included among the organelles. The cell organelles are closely integrated with, and vital for, the metabolic processes of the cell. Structures not included among organelles were, in the past, referred to as **inclusion bodies.** Among these were such structures as pigment granules, stored lipids, and carbohydrates (glycogen), secretory granules, and crystals. Many of the inclusion bodies were considered non-living components of the cell and of little importance in maintaining cell life. Recent investigations seem to indicate that these structures,

Fig. 2-1. Macrophage. This connective tissue cell contains a fair representation of the many varied components of a mammalian cell. Interstitial tissue. Testis. Rat. E.M. X 22,000. **1.** Nuclear euchromatin. **2.** Nuclear heterochromatin. **3.** Nuclear envelope. **4.** Cell membrane. **5.** Microvilli or sheet-like cell processes. **6.** Pinocytic vesicles. **7.** Phagocytic vacuoles **8.** Phagosomes. **9.** Granular endoplasmic reticulum. **10.** Golgi apparatus. **11.** Mitochondria. **12.** Condensing vacuoles. **13.** Primary lysosomes. **14.** Secondary lysosomes. **15.** Extracellular collagenous fibrils.

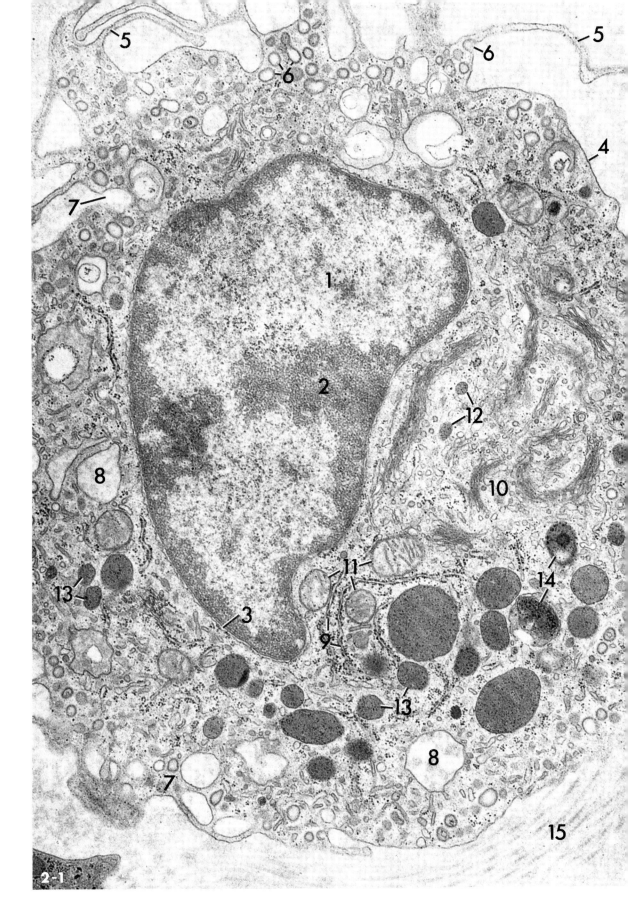

with only few exceptions, are just as vital for the proper function of those cells where they occur as the ordinary cell organelles.

CELL MEMBRANE

The cell membrane, as seen in conventional, transmission electron microscope preparations, emerges as a 90 Å-thick, **trilaminar** structure, the outer surface of which is covered by a finely filamentous layer, the **glycocalyx** or cell coat. Its thickness varies from 75 Å to 2000 Å. The three leaflets of the trilaminar cell membrane vary in electron density. Two highly electron-dense leaflets, each about 25 Å thick, enclose a central electron-lucent layer, approximately 30 Å thick. (Figs. 2-2 and 2-3) This complex is often referred to as the **unit membrane.** Cell membranes preserved in a less conventional way seem to consist of particulate components with a range of dimensions from below 40 Å to 100 Å in diameter. Functional experiments indicate that the cell membrane may contain minute **pores** used by lipid-insoluble substances such as water and urea molecules. Their diameter would be 2–10 Å, but actual channels of this size have not been resolved with the electron microscope.

From correlated chemical and structural studies, it is known that the cell membrane, as well as other intracellular membranes, consists of lipids (phospholipids and cholesterol) and proteins. Small amounts of polysaccharides are also present in the cell membrane. On a weight basis, there are one to four times as much protein as lipid. However, since lipid molecules are smaller than protein molecules, there are many more lipid than protein molecules present.

It is presently not fully established how the lipid and protein molecules interrelate structurally. According to the concept presented by Danielli and Davson in the early 1930s, the backbone of the membrane is formed of a continuous bilayer of phospholipid molecules. The hydrophobic tails of the lipid molecules appose each other within the bilayer, the hydrophilic polar heads point outward, and globular protein molecules cover the lipid molecules on either side. In the conventional electron microscope image of the cell membrane, the central electron-lucent layer would be made up of the hydrophobic tails of the lipid molecules, and the two electron-dense layers would be formed by the hydrophilic polar heads and the globular proteins. In the unit membrane, as proposed by Robertson in the late 1950s, the electron-dense outer leaflets might correspond to flattened protein molecules, and the electron-lucent center to the bilayer of lipid molecules. In a more recent proposal, Sjöstrand suggested in 1968–69 that the mitochondrial membranes, and perhaps also the cell membrane, are composed of non-lamellar globular or polygonal lipo-protein complexes. The protein molecules are thought to project across the membrane in a repetitive fashion at a period of about 100 Å or less, separated by septa approximately 10 Å thick. In an attempt to reconcile the several proposals, it has been suggested that the cell membrane does indeed consist of phospholipids, arranged in a continuous bilayer formation with the polar lipid heads facing out toward either of the surfaces of the bilayer formation. Globular or irregularly shaped proteins may project at inter-

Fig. 2-2. Epithelial cell. Longitudinal section. Large intestine. Rat. E.M. X 211,000.
   1. Lumen of gut. **2.** Finely filamentous glycoprotein coating (glycocalyx). **3.** Cell membrane. **4.** Microvillus. **5.** Tight junction (zonula occludens). **6.** Punctate contacts of fusion marked by **arrows.**
Fig. 2-3. Cross-sectioned microvilli. Epithelial cell. Large intestine. Rat. E.M. X 440,000. (1 mm=22 Å). **1.** Center of microvillus with core filaments, 45 Å in diameter. **2.** Trilaminar cell membrane, 90 Å. **3.** Electron-dense leaflet, 25 Å in diameter. **4.** Electron-lucent middle layer, 35 Å in diameter. **5.** Dotted line indicates approximate height of glycoprotein surface layer (glycocalyx), 75 Å.

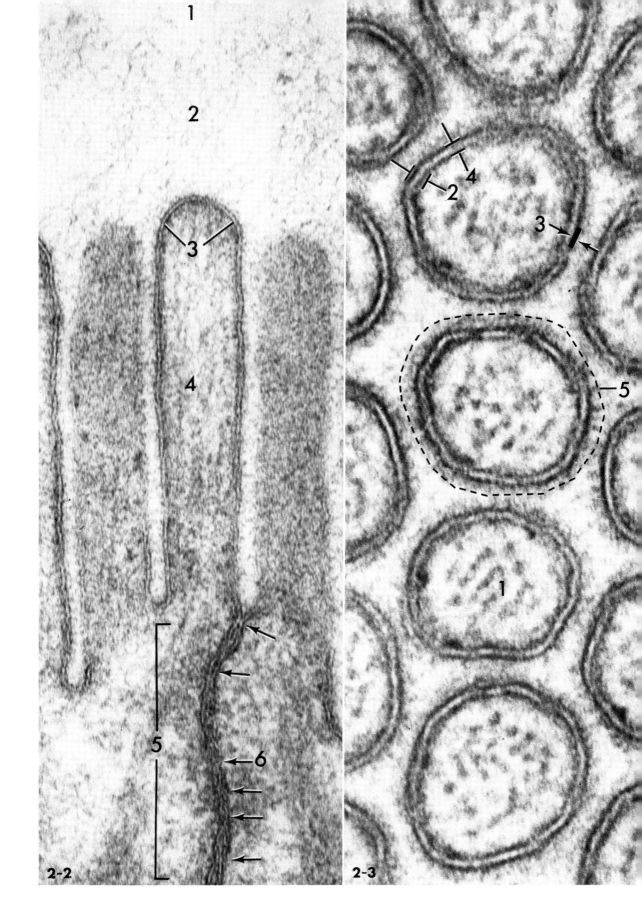

vals, across the phospholipids, probably representing areas for certain special functions, perhaps related to membrane permeability, and sometimes referred to as "protein pores."

Among the main **functions** of the cell membrane are the maintenance of the integrity of the cytoplasm and the control and influence on active and passive transport of materials across the membrane, both into and out of the cell. Enzymes form an essential part of the cell membrane, and participate both as building blocks and functionally active factors in the transport mechanisms across the membrane. One enzyme, ATP-ase, is present in many cell membranes, and is believed to participate in the transport of sodium ions across the cell membrane. The surface mucopolysaccharides provide attachment sites in intercellular relationships and contact, providing the basis for the "stickiness" of normal cells. They participate in mediating normal activities of cells, particularly those related to water-soluble materials. They also serve as recognition sites, acting as antigenic determinants which render the cell surface its immunochemical characteristics.

SPECIALIZATIONS OF CELL SURFACE

The cell membrane and the cell surface of mammalian cells can be highly specialized and modified, depending on functional demands and relationship to neighboring cells. Among such specializations are: 1) cellular attachment devices; 2) invaginations; 3) microvilli; and 4) cilia.

Attachment devices. Cells of epithelia, muscle, and nervous tissues are held together by specializations of the cell membrane. These specializations are often arranged as pairs of specialized regions of apposed cell membranes. A combination of different types of attachment devices is often referred to as **junctional complexes, terminal bars**, and **intercalated disks** (p. 236). Among the attachment devices are recognized the following categories: a) tight junctions; b) gap-junctions; c) inter-

mediate junctions; d) desmosomes. In the **tight junction** (zonula occludens) the cell coat (glycocalyx) is not present, the outer leaflets of the apposing cell membranes have fused and become a single leaflet with a thickness equal to that of one outer leaflet. (Figs. 2-4, 2-5) Focal splittings of the fused leaflets with punctate contacts occur quite often. (Fig. 2-2) This type of

Fig. 2-4. Attachment devices of surface epithelial cells. Stomach. Rat. E.M. X 90,000. **1.** Trilaminar cell membrane. **2.** Tight junction (zonula occludens). **3.** Intermediate junction (zonula adhaerens).

Fig. 2-5. Junctional complex of surface epithelial cells. Large intestine. Rat. E.M. X 155,000. **1.** Tight junction. **2.** Intermediate junction. **3.** Desmosome (macula adhaerens).

Fig. 2-6. Gap-junction. Parenchymal cells. Liver. Rat. E.M. X 124,000. **1.** Lumen of bile canaliculus. **2.** Gap-junction (nexus). **3.** Intermediate junction. **4.** Agranular endoplasmic reticulum. **5.** Intercellular space of regular width.

Fig. 2-7. Gap-junction. Blood capillary. Cardiac muscle. Rat. E.M. X 128,000. **1.** Lumen of capillary. **2.** Endothelial cell cytoplasm. **3.** Gap-junction. **4.** Possible punctate fusion of apposed cell membranes. **5.** Thin basal lamina.

Fig. 2-8. Surface epithelial cells, cross-sectioned at a slight angle. This demonstrates the distribution of the junctional complex in the "horizontal" plane. Jejunum. Rat. E.M. X 40,000. **1.** Base of microvilli. **2.** Core filaments. **3.** Tight junction between **arrows**. **4.** Intermediate junction with parajunctional filamentous network. **5.** Desmosome.

Fig. 2-9. Desmosome (macula adhaerens). Epidermis. Human. E.M. × 114,000. **1.** Cell A. **2.** Cell B. **3.** Intercellular space. **4.** Trilaminar cell membrane. **5.** Intercellular laminar density. **6.** Plate-like paradesmosomal material. **7.** Area of anchorage for cytoplasmic filaments.

Fig. 2-10. Stratified squamous epithelium, non-keratinized. Soft palate. Kitten. E.M. X 116,000. **1.** Cytoplasm of cell, detached in preparation for sloughing. **2.** Intercellular space. **3.** Cytoplasmic filaments (tonofilaments). **4.** Half desmosome. **5.** Inner leaflet of trilaminar cell membrane is thicker in this epithelial cell than in other cells, averaging 80 Å. **6.** Outer leaflet of cell membrane with filamentous glycocalyx.

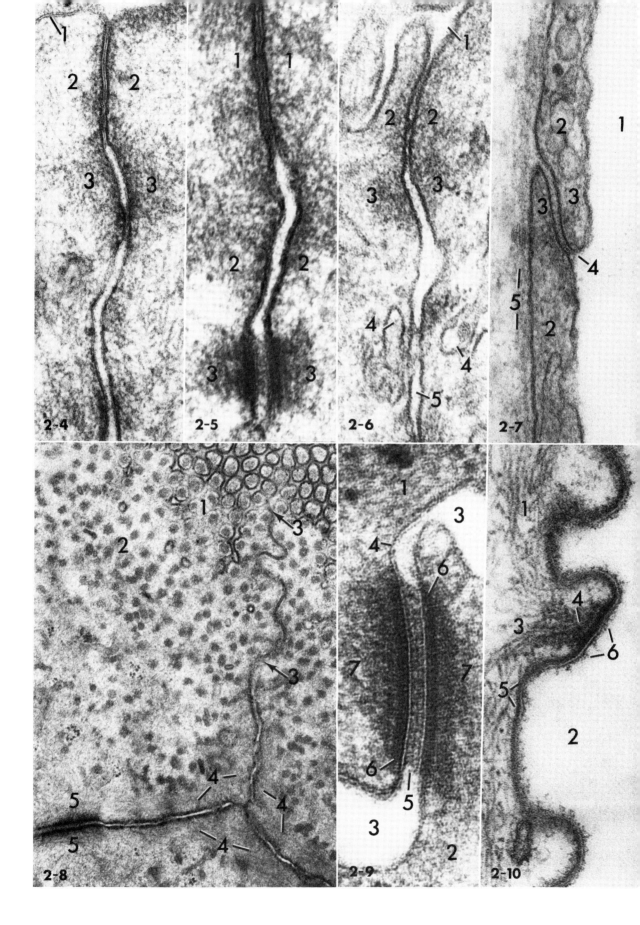

specialization of the cell membrane is common in interendothelial contacts of brain tissue capillaries, and in epithelia of the gastrointestinal tract. It is believed that the tight junctions represent barriers to large molecular substances which try to cross epithelia via the intercellular route. They probably also participate in intercellular interactions such as ionic and metabolic coupling in addition to firm cell adhesion.

In the **gap-junction** (nexus) the outer leaflets of apposing cell membranes are separated by a distance of about 20 Å. (Fig. 2-6) There are hexagonal arrays of minute, polygonal subunits in this intercellular space and within each apposed cell membrane. In permanganate-fixed specimens, the intercellular distance is completely obliterated, which first led to the erroneous conclusion that the nexus also represents a tight junction. The gap-junctions occur in epithelia, muscle, and nervous tissues. They are regions of low electrical resistance for cell-to-cell propagation of excitation-contraction impulses, and they are also preferential crossing-over points for molecules being transported from one cell to the next.

In the **intermediate junction** (zonula adhaerens and fascia adhaerens) the intercellular space is larger than normal, averaging about 200 Å. (Fig. 2-5) It is filled with medium electron-dense amorphous material, in which occasionally is present a central faint layer of somewhat higher electron density. The nature of this material is not known, although it is assumed to represent glycoprotein. At the level of the intermediate junction, the adjacent cytoplasm is filled with minute filaments which form part of the terminal web in some epithelia (p. 558 intestine). Plate-like densifications may occur parallel to the cell membrane within this parajunctional fibrillar cytoplasm. The intermediate junctions are quite extensive in the intercalated disks of the cardiac muscle cells, and they are there referred to as fasciae adhaerentes. The **desmosomes** (maculae adhaerentes)

are distinct plaques at the cell surface. (Fig. 2-9) In most instances they occur as paired, button-like structures, but sometimes so-called **half-desmosomes** (Fig. 2-10) occur toward the basal lamina of the epithelium. The intercellular space of the desmosome is about 250 Å. It is filled with electron-dense material, often containing several laminar densities. The paradesmosomal cytoplasm displays plate-like structures, and the cytoplasm here offers an area of anchorage for converging cytoplasmic filaments. The desmosomes are points of firm intercellular adhesion and are particularly numerous in the stratified epithelia of the skin, mouth, esophagus, and vagina. Based on the limited resolu-

Fig. 2-11. Part of late erythroblast. Bone marrow. Human. E.M. X 128,000. **1.** Cell membrane (trilaminar structure not resolved). **2.** Different stages of **endocytosis.** Cytoplasmic aspect of pinocytic membrane is smooth, but a faint coating appears at the bottom of the invaginations. Ferritin particles appear as small, distinct dots within the coating. **3.** Hemoglobin.

Fig. 2-12. Part of cell process. Fibroblast. Urethra. Kitten. E.M. X 128,000. **1.** Cell membrane. **2.** Micropinocytic uncoated vesicles with trilaminar membranes. **3.** Collagenous fibril.

Fig. 2-13. Surface of macrophage. Interstitial tissue. Testis. E.M. X 165,000. **1.** Connective tissue space. **2.** Microvilli. **3.** Cell membrane. **4.** Coated pinocytic invagination. **5.** Coated pinocytic vesicles.

Fig. 2-14. Coated pinocytic vesicle. Macrophage. Interstitial tissue. Testis. Rat. E.M. X 240,000. **1.** External coating of spines or bristles. **2.** Boundary membrane, seen in a phase where the molecules of the membrane are rearranging from a trilaminar (a) to a unilaminar (b) structure. **3.** Internal lining of flocculent material.

Fig. 2-15. Surface of osteoblast. Diaphysis of radius. Two-day-old rat. E.M. X 66,000. **1.** Golgi zones (dictyosomes). **2.** Cisternae of granular endoplasmic reticulum. **3.** Small coated vesicles. **4.** Coated vesicles fusing with the cell membrane in a process of **exocytosis. 5.** Discharge of materials almost completed. **6.** Periosteoblastic connective tissue space.

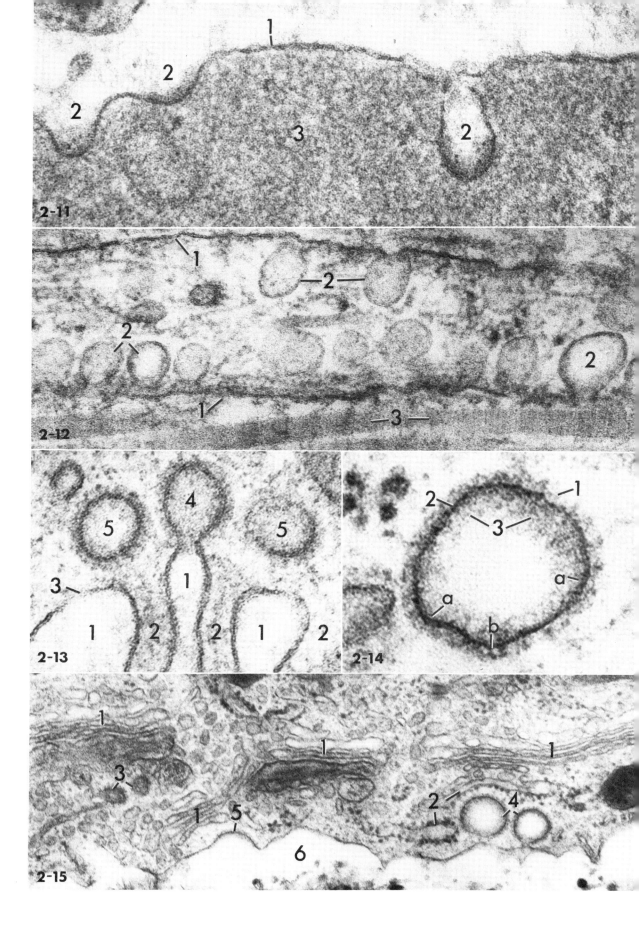

tion of the light microscope, they were erroneously considered to represent intercellular bridges.

INVAGINATIONS OF THE CELL MEMBRANE

The cell membrane displays at least two major types of invagination: 1) vesicular pits and 2) infoldings.

The **vesicular pits** occur as pinocytic vesicles, tubular invaginations, and vacuoles. **Pinocytic vesicles** (synonyms: micropinocytotic vesicles; caveolae) are droplike invaginations of the trilaminar cell membrane. They average 500 Å in diameter and occur both as coated and uncoated (smooth) vesicles. Larger vesicles are referred to as **phagocytic vacuoles.** Pinocytosis means "cell drinking" and phagocytosis "cell eating," terms that were first used to describe activities in tissue-culture cells and the amoeba. The **coated vesicles** (synonyms: spiny or bristle-coated vesicles; acanthosomes) have an internal lining of flocculent material, and are studded externally with spines about 150 Å long. (Fig. 2-14) The **uncoated vesicles** are filled with finely granular material of low electron density, and the cytoplasmic aspect of the trilaminar membrane is smooth. (Fig. 2-12) Phagocytic vacuoles are not coated.

The pinocytic vesicles participate in an uptake of extracellular material, **endocytosis,** as well as in a segregation or discharge of intracellular material, **exocytosis.** The mechanisms and factors which regulate these processes, and the reasons for the presence or absence of coating, are not entirely known. Uncoated smooth vesicles predominate in endothelial, mesothelial, and smooth muscle cells. They are most likely involved in a bulk transport of proteins and other molecules across these membranes. In erythroblasts, uncoated vesicles are engaged in the uptake of ferritin. (Fig. 2-11) Coated vesicles occur abundantly in macrophages (Fig. 2-13), hepatic cells, proximal tubule cells of the kidney, intestinal absorptive cells, and epithelial cells of ductus deferens. Here they are engaged in ingestion of proteins, metabolic end-products, foreign particles, and bacteria. Pinocytic and phagocytic invaginations which engulfed fluid and/or materials break off from the cell membrane and are referred to as **phagosomes.** As the vesicles and vacuoles engulf the material and move away from the cell surface, the boundary membrane becomes thinner. They subsequently merge with primary lysosomes, acquire lysosomal hydrolases, and become secondary lysosomes (p. 36). Coated as well as uncoated vesicles also occur in fibroblasts (Fig. 2-12), chondrocytes, osteoblasts (Fig. 2-15), and odontoblasts. In these instances, it is believed that they are engaged in processes of exocytosis (reversed pinocytosis), secreting or segregating proteins, tropocollagen units, and/or carbohydrate components to the interstitial space of the connective and hard tissues. The origin of coated and uncoated vesicles which ultimately end up fusing with the cell membrane in a process of exocytosis is most likely the Golgi zone, which abounds with both types of vesicle. Smooth vesicles also

Fig. 2-16. Stereocilia. Epididymis. Rat. E.M. X 9000. **1.** Stereocilia, 10-15 μ long. **2.** Cores of filaments in apical cell cytoplasm.

Fig. 2-17. Brush border. Proximal tubule cell. Kidney. Rat. E.M. X 11,000. **1.** Lumen of tubule. **2.** Microvilli, 3 μ long. **3.** Pinocytic invaginations and vesicles. **4.** Enlarged pinocytic vesicle (apical vacuole).

Fig. 2-18. Striated border. Epithelial surface cell. Large intestine. Rat. E.M. X 92,000. **1.** Filaments of glycocalyx projecting into the gut lumen. **2.** Microvilli: length 0.6 μ; width 0.1 μ **3.** Core of filaments. **4.** Terminal web.

Fig. 2-19. Epithelial cells of distal tubule. Kidney. Rat. E.M. X 33,000. **1.** Lumen of tubule. **2.** Short microvilli. **3.** Cell with electron-lucent cytoplasm. **4.** Cell with electron-dense cytoplasm. **5.** Invagination of basal cell surface. **6.** Cytoplasmic lamellae of dark and light cells interdigitate. **7.** Basal lamina.

Fig. 2-20. Short microvillus. Epithelial surface cell. Stomach. Rat. E.M. X 189,000. **1.** Lumen of stomach. **2.** Glycocalyx. **3.** Trilaminar cell membrane. **4.** Microvillus; length 0.1 μ; width 0.1 μ. **5.** Core filaments.

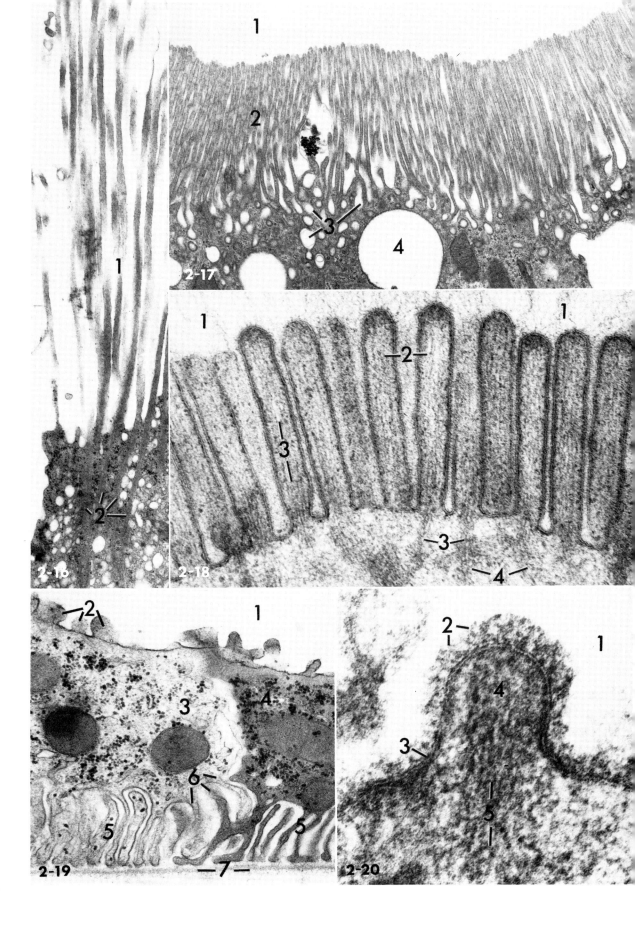

occur in the parietal cells of gastric glands and cells in the distal convoluted tubules of the kidney. It has been suggested that these vesicles actively transport chloride ions as part of the formation of hydrochloric acid by these cells.

The **infoldings** of the cell membrane greatly increase the surface of the cell, although they vary in depth. They are present mostly in epithelial cells such as the proximal and distal tubule cells of the kidney (Fig. 2-19), the striated ducts of some salivary glands, and the ciliary body of the eye. These cells are engaged in active and passive transport of fluid and ions across the epithelium, and the enlarged surface of the cell serves as interface for enzymatic processes and transport across the cell membrane.

MICROVILLI

From the surface of most cells in the mammalian body project a varied number of differently shaped cellular extensions, collectively referred to as microvilli. They are covered by the trilaminal cell membrane and are devoid of cell organelles except for a varied number of straight filaments which form a central core in most microvilli. The microvilli serve the purpose of increasing the cell surface area available for exchange processes. In movable cells the microvilli also facilitate movements and passage in between other cells and interstitial components.

A highly organized array of straight and equally sized cellular extensions characterizes the luminal surface of the absorptive cells of the intestinal epithelium, referred to as **striated border.** (Fig. 2-18) The cell membrane of these microvilli is covered by a 75–200 Å thick layer of delicate filaments, the external coat of glycocalyx. They have a central core of about 40 filaments, averaging 45 Å in diameter. The apical surface of the proximal tubule cells of the kidney has a less orderly arrangement of long and densely packed microvilli of varied dimensions called the **brush border.** (Fig. 2-17) Their glycocalyx averages 75 Å in thickness, equaling the glycoprotein coat associated with most cell membranes. Long and slender microvilli of variable length unevenly distributed at the apical cell surface are called **stereocilia.** (Fig. 2-16) They also have a core of irregularly arranged straight filaments. This type of microvillus is associated with the epithelial cells of the epididymis and vas deferens, as well as with the supporting cells of the olfactory epithelium, and the receptor cells of the taste buds, cochlear and vestibular cells. They are nonmotile processes and do not possess the ultrastructure and motility of ordinary cilia. **Short microvilli** are associated with most epithelial cells, connective tissue cells, and leukocytes. The cell processes of neurons are not categorized as microvilli. Short microvilli usually do not exceed 0.2 μ in length. They are less numerous than other types of microvilli but generally contain 5–10 core filaments. (Fig. 2-20)

Microvilli probably do not maintain a constant length and diameter. However,

Fig. 2-21. Cilia. Epithelial cell. Oviduct. Rat. E.M. X 6200. **1.** Lumen. **2.** Cilia; length 6 μ; width 0.3 μ. **3.** Microvilli. **4.** Basal bodies, some with spurs. **5.** Mitochondria.

Fig. 2-22. Cross-sectioned cilia. Epithelial cell. Trachea. Human. E.M. X 144,000. **1.** Cell membrane. **2.** Central pair of microtubules. **3.** Peripheral doublets of microtubules. **4.** Arms. **5.** Faint radial spokes. **6.** Triplets of microtubules. **7.** Spur. **A, B, C, D,** and **E** correspond to levels of cilium indicated in Figs. 2-23, 2-24, and 2-25.

Fig. 2-23. Three-dimensional diagram of microtubular disposition in cilium and basal body. From Rhodin, Am. Rev. Respir. Dis. 93: 1 (1966). **A.** Tip of cilium. **B.** Tapering part of cilium. **C.** Middle part of cilium. **D.** Transitional, narrowed segment between cilium and basal body. **E.** Basal body.

Fig. 2-24. Longitudinally sectioned cilium. Respiratory nasal epithelium. Cat. E.M. X 68,000. **1.** Cell membrane. **2.** Central microtubules. **3.** Peripheral microtubules. **4.** Basal body. **5.** Rootlets. **6.** Spur.

Fig. 2-25. Tip of cilium. Trachea. Human. E.M. X 78,000. **1.** Cell membrane. **2.** Central microtubules. **3.** Peripheral microtubules.

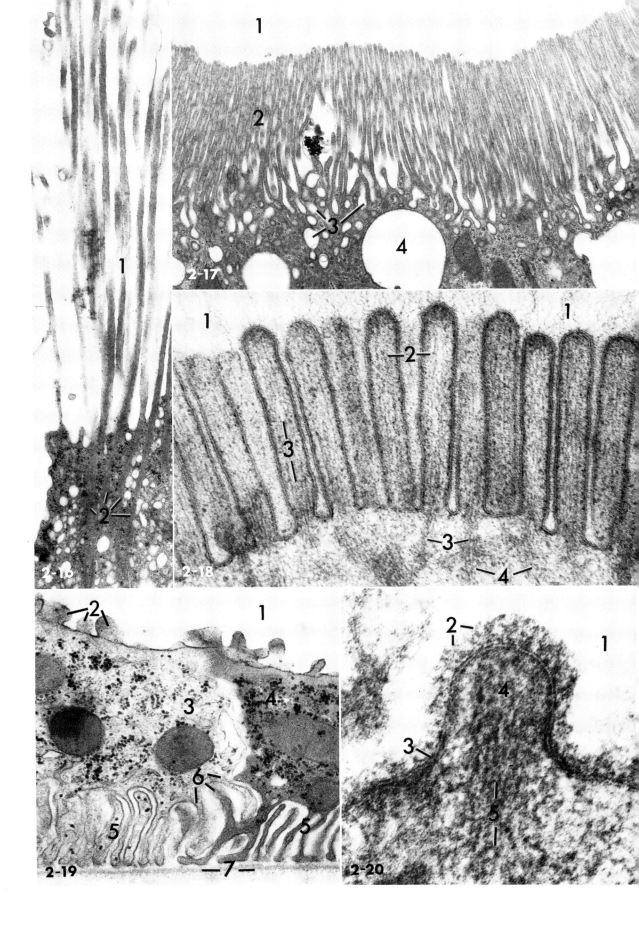

occur in the parietal cells of gastric glands and cells in the distal convoluted tubules of the kidney. It has been suggested that these vesicles actively transport chloride ions as part of the formation of hydrochloric acid by these cells.

The **infoldings** of the cell membrane greatly increase the surface of the cell, although they vary in depth. They are present mostly in epithelial cells such as the proximal and distal tubule cells of the kidney (Fig. 2-19), the striated ducts of some salivary glands, and the ciliary body of the eye. These cells are engaged in active and passive transport of fluid and ions across the epithelium, and the enlarged surface of the cell serves as interface for enzymatic processes and transport across the cell membrane.

MICROVILLI

From the surface of most cells in the mammalian body project a varied number of differently shaped cellular extensions, collectively referred to as microvilli. They are covered by the trilaminal cell membrane and are devoid of cell organelles except for a varied number of straight filaments which form a central core in most microvilli. The microvilli serve the purpose of increasing the cell surface area available for exchange processes. In movable cells the microvilli also facilitate movements and passage in between other cells and interstitial components.

A highly organized array of straight and equally sized cellular extensions characterizes the luminal surface of the absorptive cells of the intestinal epithelium, referred to as **striated border.** (Fig. 2-18) The cell membrane of these microvilli is covered by a 75–200 Å thick layer of delicate filaments, the external coat of glycocalyx. They have a central core of about 40 filaments, averaging 45 Å in diameter. The apical surface of the proximal tubule cells of the kidney has a less orderly arrangement of long and densely packed microvilli of varied dimensions called the **brush border.** (Fig. 2-17) Their glycocalyx averages 75 Å in thickness, equaling the glycoprotein coat associated with most cell membranes. Long and slender microvilli of variable length unevenly distributed at the apical cell surface are called **stereocilia.** (Fig. 2-16) They also have a core of irregularly arranged straight filaments. This type of microvillus is associated with the epithelial cells of the epididymis and vas deferens, as well as with the supporting cells of the olfactory epithelium, and the receptor cells of the taste buds, cochlear and vestibular cells. They are nonmotile processes and do not possess the ultrastructure and motility of ordinary cilia. **Short microvilli** are associated with most epithelial cells, connective tissue cells, and leukocytes. The cell processes of neurons are not categorized as microvilli. Short microvilli usually do not exceed 0.2 μ in length. They are less numerous than other types of microvilli but generally contain 5–10 core filaments. (Fig. 2-20)

Microvilli probably do not maintain a constant length and diameter. However,

Fig. 2-21. Cilia. Epithelial cell. Oviduct. Rat. E.M. $\times$ 6200. **1.** Lumen. **2.** Cilia; length 6 μ; width 0.3 μ. **3.** Microvilli. **4.** Basal bodies, some with spurs. **5.** Mitochondria.

Fig. 2-22. Cross-sectioned cilia. Epithelial cell. Trachea. Human. E.M. $\times$ 144,000. **1.** Cell membrane. **2.** Central pair of microtubules. **3.** Peripheral doublets of microtubules. **4.** Arms. **5.** Faint radial spokes. **6.** Triplets of microtubules. **7.** Spur. **A, B, C, D,** and **E** correspond to levels of cilium indicated in Figs. 2-23, 2-24, and 2-25.

Fig. 2-23. Three-dimensional diagram of microtubular disposition in cilium and basal body. From Rhodin, Am. Rev. Respir. Dis. 93: 1 (1966). **A.** Tip of cilium. **B.** Tapering part of cilium. **C.** Middle part of cilium. **D.** Transitional, narrowed segment between cilium and basal body. **E.** Basal body.

Fig. 2-24. Longitudinally sectioned cilium. Respiratory nasal epithelium. Cat. E.M. $\times$ 68,000. **1.** Cell membrane. **2.** Central microtubules. **3.** Peripheral microtubules. **4.** Basal body. **5.** Rootlets. **6.** Spur.

Fig. 2-25. Tip of cilium. Trachea. Human. E.M. $\times$ 78,000. **1.** Cell membrane. **2.** Central microtubules. **3.** Peripheral microtubules.

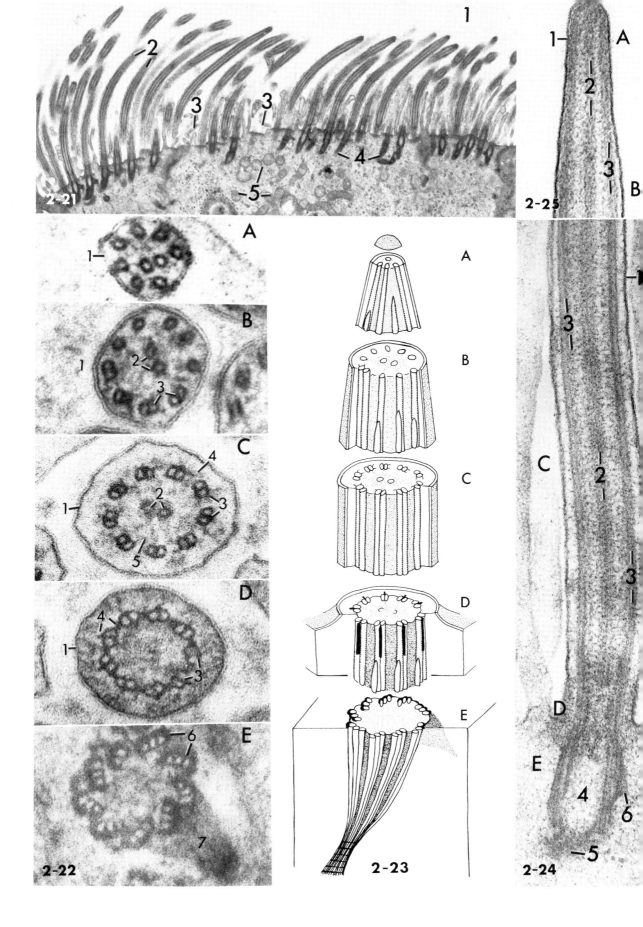

2-21

2-25

A

B

2-22

A

B

C

D

E

2-23

A

B

C

D

E

2-24

this question is largely unexplored. Microvilli generally are thought to participate in absorptive processes, and in the intestine and proximal tubules of the kidney their cell membranes contain enzymes which hydrolyze various carbohydrates and other molecules. The filamentous core probably aids the transport of absorbed materials in addition to its obvious cytoskeletal (supportive) function. The microvilli of wandering cells (macrophages, lymphocytes, granular leukocytes) are very likely instrumental in cellular movements, detection of antigens, toxins, and uptake of foreign materials such as viruses and bacteria.

CILIA

The cilia are motile projections mostly from epithelial cell surfaces, keeping a film of superficial moisture moving. They are numerous in relation to the epithelia of the upper respiratory tract and in specific parts of the male and female reproductive tracts. (Fig. 2-21) Ependymal cells of the ventricles of the brain are provided with a small number of cilia, and most cell types of the mammalian body are provided with a single cilium at one time or another during the life span of the cell. The tail of the spermatozoon is made up of a flagellum which, essentially, is a long cilium with some modifications of its ultrastructural architecture. (Fig. 33-20)

With the exception of the tail of the spermatozoon, all other cilia are 5–10 μ long and about 0.5 μ wide. There is an average of 250 cilia per cell in the upper respiratory tract. Each cilium is covered by the trilaminar cell membrane and consists of a long shaft, a tapered tip, and a basal body, the last located in the apical cytoplasm beneath the cell surface. (Fig. 2-24) The ciliary cytoplasm contains a core of regularly arranged **microtubules** (axial "filament" complex). There are nine evenly spaced pairs of microtubules, arranged to form a long cylindrical core, and two single microtubules in a central position. (Fig. 2-22) The two microtubules

which make up each cylinder (submicrotubules A and B) share a portion of the adjoining microtubular walls. Each microtubule is, in turn, made up of 13 beaded microfilaments, 45 Å thick and arranged helically. Short arms extend in some species from submicrotubule A halfway toward submicrotubule B. In the tip of the cilium, the peripheral double microtubules become single, and even reduced in number. (Fig. 2-25) In the **basal body** the peripheral double microtubules are joined by a third microtubule to make up a pattern very similar to that which characterizes the centrioles. (Fig. 2-61) The central, single microtubules do not descend into the basal body but terminate at the level of the cell surface. The triplet microtubules of the basal body descend as **rootlets** and gradually taper off in the apical cytoplasm. In some species these rootlets are provided with cross-bandings, and sometimes the basal body has a "spur" of rootlets deviating at right angles from the other rootlets. Faint radial spokes of dense cytoplasm extend from the inner microtubules toward the outer doublets throughout the shaft. (Fig. 2-23)

The motility of the cilia is characterized by a rapid forward beat (effective stroke), and a slow return (recovery) stroke. The movements of the cilia are synchronized, producing metachronal waves which pass over the epithelial surface, thereby moving the film or "blanket" of moisture in one particular direction. The origin and nature of the ciliary stroke are

Fig. 2-26. Endoplasmic reticulum. Parenchymal cell. Liver. Rat. E.M. X 64,000. **1.** Cisternae of granular endoplasmic reticulum. **2.** Tubules of agranular endoplasmic reticulum. **3.** Free ribosomes. **4.** Mitochondria. **5.** Microbody. **6.** Glycogen particles. **7.** Surface microvilli projecting into space of Disse.

Fig. 2-27. Ribosomes. Epithelial cell of proximal tubule. Kidney. Rat. E.M. X 192,000. **1.** Free ribosomes, averaging 175 Å in diameter. **2.** Groups of ribosomes (polysomes).

Fig. 2-28. Ribosomes. Parenchymal cell. Liver. E.M. X 182,000. **1.** Free ribosomes. **2.** Groups of ribosomes (polysomes).

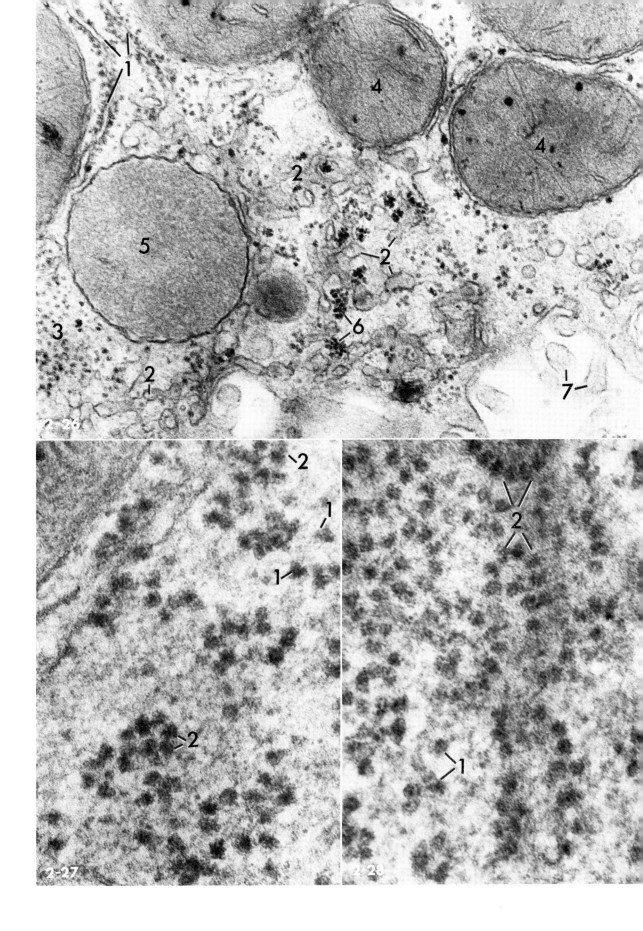

poorly understood. In some way, the basal body seems to control, and perhaps initiate, the stroke. The pairs of microtubules do not contract during the bending phases of the stroke. They seem rather to slide in relation to their neighbors, perhaps aided by the arms of the microtubules which contain the enzyme ATPase, acting in a fashion similar to what occurs in muscular contraction, when myofilaments slide past each other (p. 232) .

ENDOPLASMIC RETICULUM AND RIBOSOMES

The endoplasmic reticulum is a submicroscopic organelle, consisting of a network of **paired membranes,** vesicles, vacuoles, tubules, and flattened cisternae. (Fig. 2-26) Many of these profiles are in direct continuity with each other. The membranes are trilaminar, but they are thinner than the cell membrane, averaging 60 Å in diameter. Associated with the cytoplasmic aspect of some membranes of the endoplasmic reticulum are **ribosomes,** minute granular structures. Based on the presence or absence of attached ribosomes, the endoplasmic reticulum is divided into **granular** (rough surfaced) endoplasmic reticulum, and **agranular** (smooth surfaced) endoplasmic reticulum. There is structural continuity between the membranes and cavities of the two types of endoplasmic reticulum, and both types can be present in the same cell. Although the endoplasmic reticulum is present in most cell types, there are some exceptions.

The two types of endoplasmic reticulum and the ribosomes are engaged in a great variety of functions, among which are primarily protein and steroid synthesis.

Ribosomes. The ribosomes are minute, angular particles with a diameter ranging between 150 Å and 250 Å. (Figs. 2-27, 2-28) Mammalian ribosomes consist of at least two subunits, 40S and 60S. They are classified as 40S and 60S according to their sedimentation rates in the ultracentrifuge (S = Svedberg unit of sedimentation rate). The whole ribosome, consisting of a 40S

subunit and 60S subunit, itself has a sedimentation rate of 80S. Note that this is not the sum of the sedimentation rates of the subunits, since the Svedburg unit is based on particle shape and density, as well as molecular weight. Each subunit, in turn, can be fractionated, and its components will sediment at different rates.

Ribosomes occur singly (monoribosomes) or in clusters as rosettes, spirals, or helices (polyribosomes; polysomes). Either category may also occur freely in the cytoplasm or attached to the membranes of the endoplasmic reticulum. (Fig. 2-30) The ribosomes of **polysomes** are attached to, and strung along, a 15 Å-thick filament, the messenger RNA. The number of ribosomes varies according ot the specific synthetic action of the polysome. (Fig. 2-32)

The ribosomes contain ribonucleic acid (ribosomal nucleic acid; r-RNA) and protein, the weight ratio being 1:1. Ribosomes are present in all cells except the

Fig. 2-29. Granular endoplasmic reticulum. Acinar cell. Pancreas. Mouse. E.M. X 35,000. **1.** Membranes and cisternae in parallel arrays, sectioned in a plane perpendicular to the membranes. **2.** Membranes sectioned tangentially. **3.** Mitochondria.

Fig. 2-30. Granular endoplasmic reticulum. Enlargement of area similar to rectangle (A) in Fig. 2-29. Parenchymal cell. Liver. E.M. X 173,000 (1 mm= 60 Å). **1.** Membranes of the granular endoplasmic reticulum, 60 Å in diameter. A trilaminar substructure is seen at arrows. **2.** Cisterna. **3.** Attached ribosomes. **4.** Free ribosomes. **5.** Circle: glycogen particles (alpha type). **6.** Cross-sectioned tubule of agranular endoplasmic reticulum.

Fig. 2-31. Tangentially sectioned membranes of granular endoplasmic reticulum. Enlargement of area similar to rectangle (B) in Fig. 2-29. Fibroblast. Urethra. Kitten. Rat. E.M. X 124,000. **1.** Ribosomes. **2.** Polysomes. **3.** Area of cisterna.

Fig. 2-32. Polysomes. Kupffer cell. Sinusoid. Liver. Rat. E.M. X 124,000. **1.** Free ribosomes. **2.** Polysome; 11 ribosomes seem to make up this particular polysome. The thin strand of connecting messenger RNA can be resolved only after cell fractionation and negative staining.

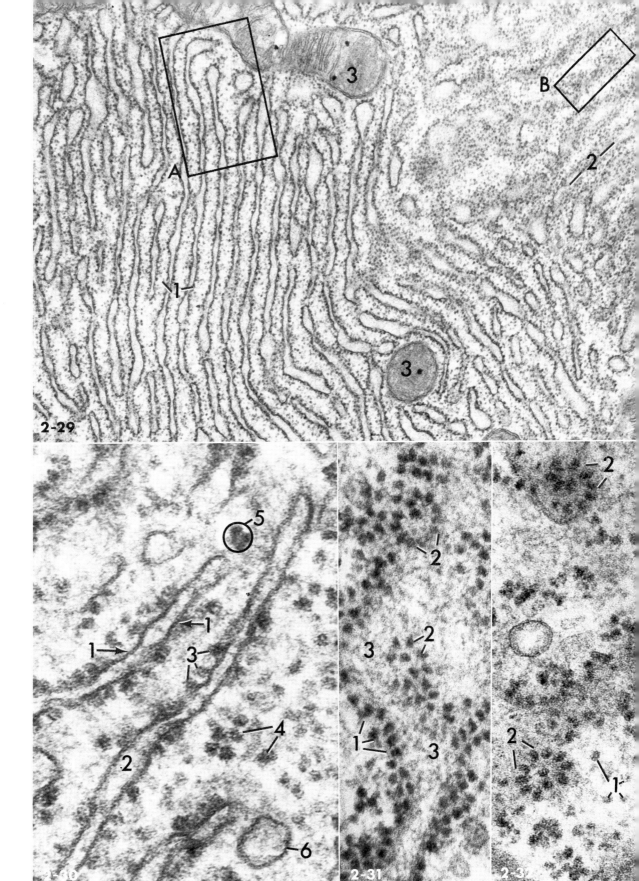

mature erythrocyte, and represent the sites where amino acids are incorporated into peptides and protein molecules. The ribosomes are responsible for the cytoplasmic basophilia observed in light microscope preparations. The basophilia is diffuse in lymphocytes and early erythroblasts, appears patchy in neurons (Nissl bodies), and has a dense dissemination in the exocrine acinar cells of the pancreas and salivary glands. Free polysomes synthesize proteins for intracellular consumption during cell division and growth, and as replacement for regular turnover of membranous and hyaloplasmic proteins. Polysomes attached to the membranes of the endoplasmic reticulum produce proteins for extracellular usage as part of secretory (enzymes, hormones) and segregational (tropocollagen units, antibodies) processes.

The **ribosomal RNA** (r-RNA) is synthesized in the nucleolus and transported to the ribosomes. The **messenger RNA** (m-RNA) is produced in the nucleus and moves to the cytoplasm where it forms the 15 Å-thick filament which links the ribosomes in the polysome. Ribosomes receive instructions from the m-RNA which transcribes (decodes) the genetic code of the **transfer RNA** (t-RNA or s-RNA; s for soluble). The t-RNA is formed in the nucleus and is specific for a single nucleic acid, which is picked up by the t-RNA and delivered to the m-RNA of the polysome. As a result of the decoding of the t-RNA by the m-RNA, the proper amino acids are brought to the condensing sites of the ribosomes in specific sequence, and as a result, the appropriate peptides and protein molecules are synthesized.

Ribosomes are thought to move along the m-RNA filament as they receive instruction from the m-RNA. Ribosomes unattached to an m-RNA filament are presumably unable to synthesize proteins. The number of ribosomes in a polysome determines the length of the protein molecule to be synthesized: the longer the poly-

peptide chain, the larger the number of ribosomes.

Granular endoplasmic reticulum. This organelle corresponds to the chromidial substance and the ergastoplasm of early light microscopical descriptions. It consists of paired membranes, 60 Å thick, which form vesicles, vacuoles, and flattened cisternae. The cytoplasmic aspect of the membranes is studded with ribosomes and polysomes. The larger subunit (60S) of the ribosome is attached to the membrane.

The membranous patterns of the granular endoplasmic reticulum vary from profiles of one or two flat cisternae in most cells, to many and widely distended cisternae in plasma cells and epithelial cells of the thyroid gland, to stacks of widely distributed, parallel flat membranes and cisternae in acinar cells of the pancreas. (Fig. 2-29) The electron density of the cisternae also varies and a flocculent, evenly distributed content may alternate with accumulations of spherical densities. The profiles of the granular endoplasmic re-

Fig. 2-33. Agranular endoplasmic reticulum. Parenchymal cell. Liver. Rat. E.M. X 166,000. **1.** Lumina of agranular, smooth tubules; average width 500 Å. **2.** Membrane of agranular endoplasmic reticulum; 60 Å in diameter. **3.** Indication of a trilaminar substructure at arrows. **4.** Glycogen particles (alpha type). **5.** Glycogen particles (beta type).

Fig. 2-34. Continuity of granular and agranular endoplasmic reticulum. Parenchyma cell. Liver. Rat. E.M. X 152,000. **1.** Cisterna and membranes of granular endoplasmic reticulum with attached ribosomes. **2.** Tubular profiles of agranular endoplasmic reticulum. **3.** Point of continuity between the two types of endoplasmic reticulum. **4.** Glycogen particles (alpha type).

Fig. 2-35. Relationship of agranular endoplasmic reticulum to other cytoplasmic components. Epithelial cell. Adrenal cortex. Zona fasciculata. Rat. E.M. X 98,000. **1.** Tubules and vesicles of agranular endoplasmic reticulum. **2.** Mitochondrial external envelope. **3.** Interface: cytoplasm/lipid droplet. **4.** Lipid droplet. **5.** Mitochondrial matrix. **6.** Vesicular cristae. **7.** Glycogen particles (beta type).

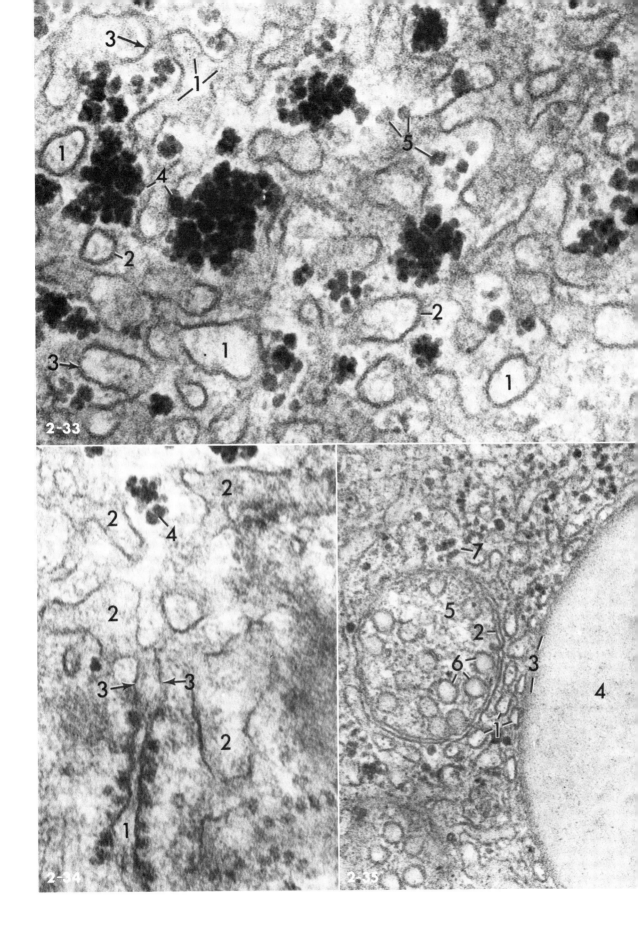

ticulum are sometimes continuous with those of the agranular endoplasmic reticulum (Fig. 2-34), the Golgi zone, and the nuclear membrane. Vesicles appear to break away from the ends of the cisternae, and are referred to as **transfer vesicles** (p. 86). The term **microsome** appears often in the literature in relation to the granular endoplasmic reticulum. A microsome is a small, membrane-bound sphere, the outside of which is studded with ribosomes. Microsomes are not present as discrete structures in the cell, but are broken up pieces of granular endoplasmic reticulum derived from the damage caused to cells as they are minced and subjected to differential centrifugation.

Based on a combination of biochemical, histochemical, autoradiographic, and electron microscopical investigations, it can be concluded that the granular endoplasmic reticulum is a dynamic system of membranes and ribosomes involved in protein synthesis. The ribosomes which are attached to the membranes of the granular endoplasmic reticulum (Fig. 2-30) are thought to contain a central canal (not resolved by electron microscopy) which connects the interior of the large subunit 60S with the lumen of the cisterna across the cisternal boundary membrane. Hypothetically, this canal is used to release the newly synthesized peptide chains into the cisterna, where they are further assembled into larger protein molecules. As indicated, the cisternal space varies in size and electron density, perhaps depending upon the amount and type of protein material assembled. The protein molecules are stored temporarily in the cisternae, and then transported to the Golgi zone via transfer vesicles for further synthesis and, in some cases, conjugation with carbohydrates, as well as packaging and condensation (see p. 86).

Agranular endoplasmic reticulum. This organelle consists of vesicles and/or irregularly shaped, interconnected tubules. (Fig. 2-33) The tubule wall averages 60 Å in thickness, and the tubular lumen about 500 Å. The agranular endoplasmic reticulum lacks ribosomes.

The tubules are often connected with the components of the Golgi zone. The membranes of the agranular endoplasmic reticulum contain a variety of enzymes required in lipid and carbohydrate metabolism. Glycogen particles are often situated in the intertubular cytoplasm. (Fig. 2-33) The tubules also invest closely the boundary membranes of mitochondria and lipid droplets. (Fig. 2-35)

The agranular endoplasmic reticulum is involved in a multiplicity of functions other than protein synthesis. It probably serves a major role in several steps of steroid hormone synthesis, as indicated by its abundance in the cells of the adrenal cortex, interstitial cells of testis, and the cells of the corpora lutea. In liver cells the agranular endoplasmic reticulum is involved in glycogen formation, cholesterol synthesis, and detoxification processes. In the parietal cells of the stomach, it may participate in the formation of hydrochloric acid. In the skeletal muscle cell, it forms an extensive system of sarcotubules related to the binding and release

Fig. 2-36. Golgi apparatus. Epithelial cell. Prostate gland. Rat. E.M. X 9000. **1.** Golgi zones (dictyosomes). **2.** Dilated cisternae of granular endoplasmic reticulum. **3.** Nucleus. **4.** Nucleolus. **5.** Lysosome. **6.** Base of cell. **7.** Basal lamina. **8.** Mitochondria. **9.** Cell membranes. **10.** Junctional complex. **11.** Lumen of gland.

Fig. 2-37. Golgi apparatus. Fibroblast during active synthesis of tropocollagen. Dermis. Human. E.M. X 31,000. **1.** Golgi zones (dictyosomes). **2.** Condensing vacuoles. **3.** Coated vacuoles. **4.** Granular endoplasmic reticulum. **5.** Mitochondria. **6.** Cell membrane. **7.** Nucleus.

Fig. 2-38. Golgi apparatus. Macrophage. Interstitial tissue. Testis. Rat. E.M. X 120,000. **1.** Part of mitochondrion. **2.** Cisterna and membrane of granular endoplasmic reticulum. **3.** Forming, convex, face. **4.** Maturing, concave, face. **5.** Saccules. **6.** Vesicles "budding off" from saccule. **7.** Uncoated vesicles. **8.** Coated vesicles. **9.** Distended saccule.

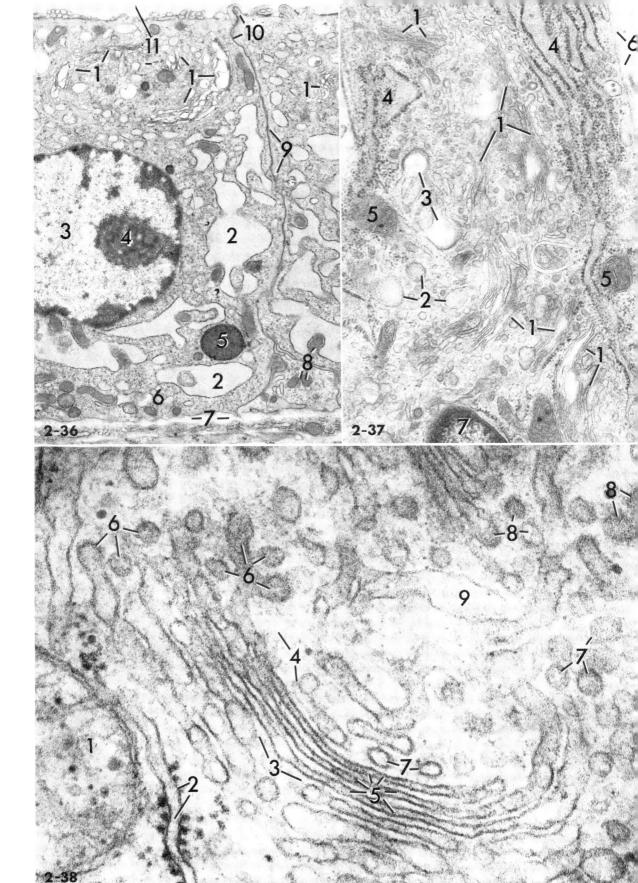

of calcium ions for contraction-relaxation processes. In megakaryocytes, it delineates platelet zones in preparation for the release of thrombocytes, and it probably forms the nuclear membrane in the telophase of mitosis.

GOLGI APPARATUS

The Golgi apparatus (synonyms: Golgi zone, region, body, complex, substance; dictyosome) is a heterogeneous cell organelle, especially large and prominent in cells secreting either protein or complex polysaccharides, and present in almost all mammalian cells. In silver-impregnated light microscope preparations it appears as a reticular network or system of canals and vacuoles. In some cells (plasma cells, epithelial cells of the ductus deferens), the Golgi apparatus stands out as a pale-staining area (negative image) against the surrounding dark-staining ribosome-rich cytoplasm (ergastoplasm). In most cells the Golgi apparatus is located around or in the vicinity of the nucleus. (Fig. 2-37) In exocrine cells it is always found between the nucleus and the apical surface (Fig. 2-36), whereas in large neurons such as the spinal ganglion cells, it is broken up into smaller areas scattered throughout the cytoplasm.

As resolved by electron microscopy, the Golgi apparatus consists of three principal components: 1) saccules, 2) vesicles, and 3) vacuoles. The three-dimensional distribution of the components is bowl-shaped and curved. The convex side is referred to as the **forming** outer face (immature or proximal pole), whereas the concave side is called the **maturing** inner face (secreting or distal pole). (Fig. 2-38)

The saccules (or cisternae) are flattened structures, consisting of 3–12 paired, smooth-surfaced, curved membranes, stacked in parallel and separated from each other by a distance of 200 Å–300 Å. Ribosomes are not attached to these membranes. The saccular cavities may contain a medium electron-dense material. The term **dictyosome** is now often used to describe a small number of closely associated Golgi saccules which occur either singly throughout the cell without apparent structural continuity, or in groups of saccules arranged to form a large Golgi zone. Originally, dictyosome referred to Golgi-like bodies found in invertebrate and plant cells. The membranes of the saccules average 60 Å in thickness at the outer face which borders on the membranous components of the endoplasmic reticulum. The saccular membranes near the inner face of the Golgi apparatus average 80 Å in diameter.

The Golgi **vesicles** range from 400 Å to 800 Å in diameter, and the cytoplasmic aspect of their 60 Å boundary membrane can be either coated or uncoated as in pinocytic vesicles (p. 16). The vesicles are grouped near the ends of the saccules but also occur near the outer and inner faces of the Golgi apparatus.

The large Golgi **vacuoles** are bounded by a 80 Å smooth trilaminar membrane. They vary in diameter from 0.1 μ to 0.5 μ, and occur near the dilated, bulbous ends of the saccules. The larger vacuoles are referred to as **condensing** vacuoles and occur mostly near the inner, secretory face of the Golgi apparatus. Illustrations of the Golgi apparatus in other cell types are seen in Figs. 4-17, 7-29, 20-12, 24-7, 33-15.

Fig. 2-39. Mitochondrion. Epithelial cell of proximal tubule. Kidney. Mouse. E.M. X 82,000. **1.** External envelope. **2.** Membranous, flat cristae. **3.** Matrix. **4.** Matrix granules.

Fig. 2-40. Mitochondrion. Muscle cell. Myocardium. Rat. E.M. X 93,000. **1.** Delicate external envelope. **2.** Densely packed membranous cristae. **3.** Sparse matrix. **4.** Matrix granule. **5.** Myofilaments.

Fig. 2-41. Mitochondrion. Parenchymal cell. Liver. Rat. E.M. X 114,000. **1.** External envelope. **2.** Small number of cristae, mostly membranous. **3.** Matrix abundant. **4.** Matrix granules. **5.** Mitochondrial crista originates from inner membranous component of external envelope. **6.** Profiles of granular endoplasmic reticulum.

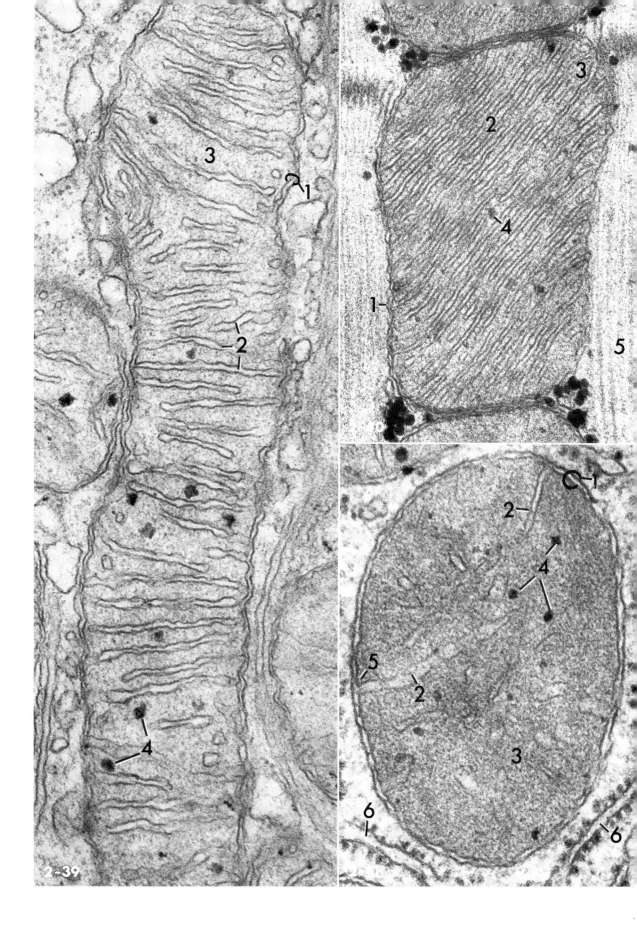

2-39

Functions. It has been postulated that there is a movement of membranes and components within the Golgi apparatus. Transfer vesicles from the endoplasmic reticulum fuse continuously with the outer surface, and condensing vacuoles leave from the inner face and the ends of the saccules. It is also possible that the saccules near the outer face gradually move toward the inner face in a continuous process of maturation. This hypothesis is supported by the fact that the diameters of the membranes gradually increase from the outer to the inner surface.

The Golgi apparatus accumulates and concentrates protein-rich secretory products brought to its outer surface from the endoplasmic reticulum via transfer vesicles, and packages the secretory products (digestive enzymes, for instance) in its condensing vacuoles. As part of a secretion process, these are discharged at the cell surface as secretory granules and droplets (p. 86). Certain hydrolytic enzymes are similarly packaged by the Golgi apparatus, but remain in the cell to form the primary lysosomes of macrophages and leukocytes. The enzyme hyaluronidase is concentrated within a Golgi saccule of the spermatocyte. The saccule and the enzyme later form the headcap and acrosome of the mature sperm (p. 684). Sugars are added to proteins in the Golgi apparatus during the synthesis of glycoproteins and mucopolysaccharides in processes of mucus production and formation of the carbohydrate component of the cell surface (glycocalyx). Carbohydrates are also sulfated in the Golgi zone as part of matrix formation in cartilage tissues.

ANNULATE LAMELLAE

In rapidly dividing and proliferating cells such as embryonic and neoplastic cells, as well as in male and female germ cells occurs a membranous system near the nucleus which is called annulate lamellae. It consists of 3–10 pairs of parallel smooth membranes, each pair containing a varied number of regularly spaced pores, similar to those present in the nuclear membrane. (Fig. 2-82) They are considered to represent a specialized form of endoplasmic reticulum, but their specific function is not known. Hypothetically, they could transfer genetic material from the nucleus to the cytoplasm.

MITOCHONDRIA

Mitochondria are small, membrane-bound granular, enzyme-containing organelles, self-replicating and representing the major source of cellular energy. They are visible in light microscope preparations only after supravital staining with Janus Green B, or staining of the sections with iron hematoxylin. Through electron microscopical analyses, it became obvious that mitochondria can be rod-shaped, spherical, and ovoid, averaging $0.5\ \mu$ in width and ranging between $2\ \mu$ to $5\ \mu$ in length. (Fig. 2-39) There is a scarcity of mitochondria in undifferentiated cells, lymphocytes, and cells of the epidermis. Fibroblasts and secretory cells have an average number of mitochondria, whereas they

Fig. 2-42. Mitochondrion. Epithelial cell. Adrenal cortex. Zona reticularis. Rat. E.M. X 58,000. **1.** Delicate external envelope. **2.** Cross-sectioned tubular cristae. **3.** Longitudinally sectioned, interconnected tubular cristae. **4.** Sparse matrix.

Fig. 2-43. Mitochondrion. Epithelial cell. Adrenal cortex. Zona fasciculata. Rat. E.M. X 204,000. **1.** External envelope. **2.** Vesicular cristae. Their limiting membrane shows a trilaminar substructure. **3.** Cross-sectioned tubular cristae. **4.** Sparse matrix. **5.** Membrane of vesicular crista in continuity with inner membranous component of external envelope.

Fig. 2-44. Mitochondrial replication. Parenchymal cell. Liver. Rat. E.M. X 65,000. **1.** External envelope. **2.** Mitochondrial "bud." **3.** Constriction precedes separation of bud from maternal mitochondrion. **4.** Membranous cristae form separation plate.

Fig. 2-45. Mitochondrial replication. Parenchymal cell. Liver. Rat. E.M. X 96,000. **1.** Constriction and separation almost completed. **2.** Membranous cristae in continuity with inner membranous component of external envelope.

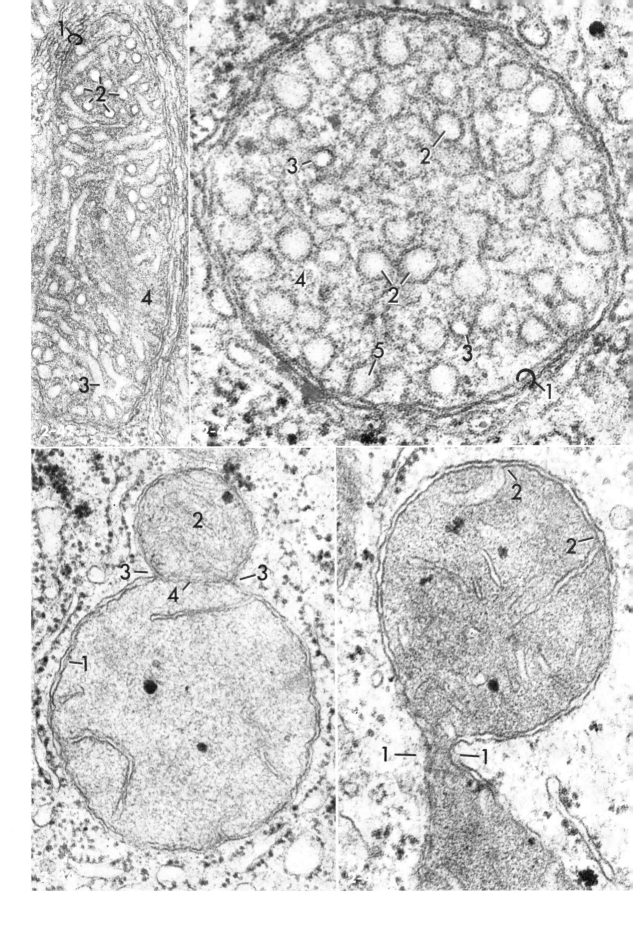

are extremely numerous in liver parenchymal cells, parietal cells of the gastric glands, proximal tubule cells of the kidney, and the cells of the adrenal cortex.

Each mitochondrion has an external envelope and an inner matrix. The **external envelope** (boundary membrane) is smooth. (Fig. 2-41) It consists of an outer and an inner electron-dense membranous component, each about 60 Å thick. They are separated by an 80 Å electron-lucent layer. The inner membranous component has a varied number of extensions or projections inward to the matrix. (Fig. 2-39) These are called **cristae** and can be membranous (flat), tubular, or vesicular. Closely packed membranous cristae (Figs. 2-39, 2-40) characterize mitochondria in cells with a high rate of oxidative metabolism (skeletal muscle, proximal and distal tubules of the kidney) whereas tubular and vesicular cristae (Figs. 2-42, 2-43) are present in cells which synthesize steroid hormones (adrenal cortex, interstitial cells of testis). On the matrix side the cristae are coated with minute particles with a 90 Å spherical head and a 50 Å-long and 30 Å-thick stalk, attached to the surface of the crista. These are **elementary particles** (synonym: electron transport particles) which are resolved only after the application of special preparation procedures (cell fractionation and differential centrifugation; negative staining) quite different from those used to obtain conventional electron microscope specimens.

The **matrix** of the mitochondrion is an amorphous or finely granular substance which contains delicate strands of DNA, some RNA, and possibly ribosomes. In the matrix of many mitochondria occur highly electron-dense intramitochondrial **matrix granules.** (Fig. 2-41) They average 500 Å in diameter and may represent binding sites for calcium ions, since crystal formation has been observed to start in these granules during pathological calcification of some cell types. Mitochondrial inclusions such as protein crystals, glycogen particles, and myelin (lipid) figures can

also be present in some mitochondria. The myelin figures often arise in conjunction with oxygen deprivation and postmortem changes of the tissue, and are probably artifacts.

Functions. Mitochondria are self-replicating organelles, probably because of their supply of genetic information (DNA and RNA) and their ability to synthesize protein through the mitochondrial ribosomes. The replication occurs through budding or division. (Figs. 2-44, 2-45)

Mitochondria are the chief energy source of the cell and the principal site

Fig. 2-46. Primary lysosome (0.1 μ wide). Kupffer cell. Liver. Rat. E.M. X 228,000. **1.** Boundary membrane, 60 Å in diameter. **2.** Condensing matrix.

Fig. 2-47. Phagosome. Kupffer cell. Liver. Rat. E.M. X 168,000. **1.** Boundary membrane of pinocytic vesicle appears single, except at **arrow** where it is trilaminar. **2.** Engulfed material.

Fig. 2-48. Primary lysosome (0.3 μ wide). Kupffer cell. Liver. Rat. E.M. X 140,000. **1.** Boundary membrane, 60 Å in diameter. **2.** Matrix.

Fig. 2-49. Fusion of pinocytic vesicle and primary lysosome, resulting in a secondary lysosome. Kupffer cell. Liver. Rat. E.M. X 156,000. **1.** Pinocytic, uncoated vesicle. **2.** Matrix of primary lysosome. **3.** Boundary membrane. **4.** Point of continuity between pinocytic vesicle and primary lysosome. *Note:* The possibility exists that this is a fusion between a small primary lysosome (1) and a secondary lysosome (2) at the moment when the latter receives an additional "shot" of hydrolytic enzymes.

Fig. 2-50. Lysosomes. Macrophage. Interstitial tissue. Testis. Rat. E.M. X 120,000. **1.** Primary lysosome. **2.** Secondary lysosome with lipoprotein material being hydrolyzed. **3.** Boundary membrane, 60 Å in diameter.

Fig. 2-51. Secondary lysosome (residual body). Kupffer cell. Liver. Rat. E.M. X 84,000. **1.** Boundary membrane, 60 Å in diameter. **2.** Matrix. **3.** Lipid droplets. **4.** Vesicles.

Fig. 2-52. Lipofuscin granule. Odoriferous sweat gland. Axilla. Human. E.M. X 60,000. **1.** Boundary membrane (difficult to resolve because of dense granule content). **2.** Lipid droplets. **3.** Minute, highly electron-dense particles of unknown nature. **4.** Matrix.

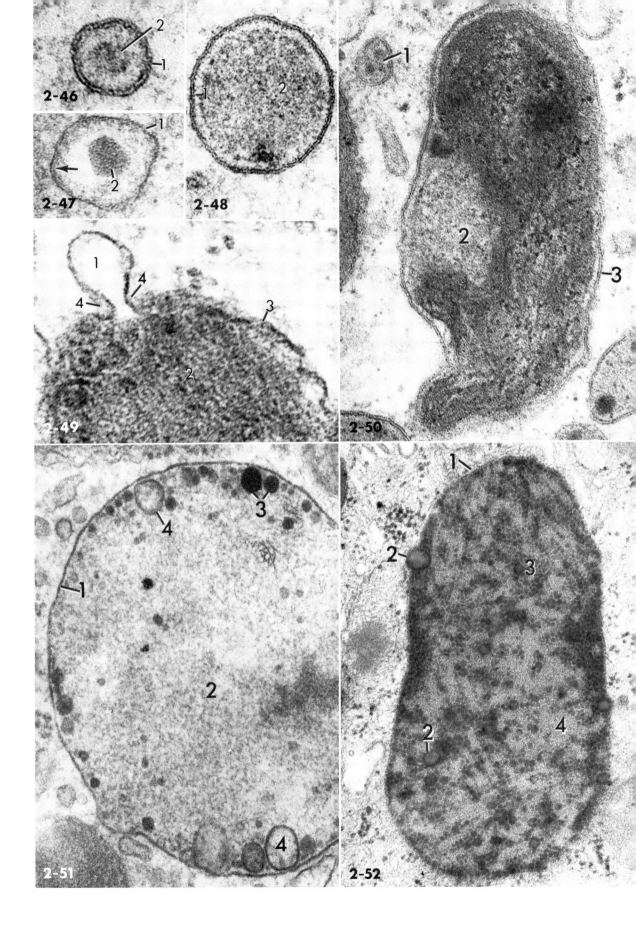

2-46

2-47

2-48

2-49

2-50

2-51

2-52

of several enzyme systems, among which are those necessary for the Krebs citric acid cycle, as well as those for the oxidative phosphorylation processes. The mitochondrial **matrix** contains the enzymes required for the **citric acid cycle** which deals with the final breakdown of carbohydrates, fatty acids, and some amino acids. The hydrogen liberated through the enzymatic processes of the Krebs cycle is delivered to an intricate chain of flavoproteins and cytochromes, the so-called respiratory chain or electron transport system. Electron transport is an essential factor in **oxidative phosphorylation,** and it is believed that most of the oxidative enzymes (dehydrogenases) are contained in the elementary particles at the surface of the **mitochondrial cristae,** or reside in the lipoprotein framework of the membranous, tubular, or vesicular cristae. Through the oxidative phosphorylation, adenosinediphosphate (ADP) is converted to adenosinetriphosphate (ATP). The ATP is extremely rich in energy. It is stored for energy-demanding cellular processes such as muscle contraction, active transport, and protein synthesis. By splitting the terminal phosphate of ATP, energy is released for these processes when required.

LYSOSOMES

Lysosomes are minute granular, membrane-bound organelles which contain lytic enzymes for intracellular digestion. The lysosomes represent an essential part of the cellular defense and transport systems, and these organelles abound in macrophages, polymorphonuclear leukocytes, hepatic parenchymal cells, and proximal tubule cells of the kidney. Structurally and functionally, lysosomes are divided into two categories: 1) primary lysosomes and 2) secondary lysosomes. It is presently held that primary lysosomes are organelles which have not yet become engaged in enzymatic activity, whereas secondary lysosomes are, or have been, involved in enzymatic digestive activities, and there-

fore contain a collection of membranous and granular structures missing in the primary lysosomes. Consequently, the following structures can be classified as secondary lysosomes: multivesicular bodies, autosomes, residual bodies, and lipofuscin granules.

Lysosomes are spherical or ovoid organelles which range in size from 250 Å to 0.8 μ. They are present in almost all cell types. They were first identified through a combination of cell fractionation, differential centrifugation, and biochemical analysis. In tissue sections, they can be identified histochemically both in light microscopy and electron microscopy because of a positive reaction for acid phosphatase, which is one of the lysosomal enzymes. Ultrastructurally, lysosomes have an outer limiting membrane averaging 60 Å in diameter, and a finely granular matrix which contains a multitude of varied membranous and granular structures in secondary lysosomes.

Primary lysosomes. The smallest pri-

Fig. 2-53. Multivesicular body. Kupffer cell. Liver. Rat. E.M. X 96,000. **1.** Boundary membrane, 60 Å in diameter. **2.** Electron-lucent matrix. **3.** Vesicles of varied diameters. **4.** Mitochondrion. **5.** Filaments.

Fig. 2-54. Autosome (autophagic vacuole). Macrophage. Interstitial tissue. Testis. Rat. E.M. X 105,000. **1.** Boundary membrane consists of two trilaminar membranes, total diameter 270 Å. **2.** Matrix density similar to that of surrounding cytoplasm. **3.** Vesicles and membranes. **4.** Part of secondary lysosome.

Fig. 2-55. Microbody (peroxisome). Parenchymal cell. Liver. Rat. E.M. X 135,000. **1.** Boundary membrane, 60 Å in diameter. **2.** Matrix. **3.** Area of crystalloid (no substructure resolved in this illustration). **4.** Profile of granular endoplasmic reticulum. **5.** Profile of agranular endoplasmic reticulum.

Fig. 2-56. Specific endothelial granules. Pulmonary vein. Rat. E.M. X 108,000. **1.** Boundary membrane, 40 Å in diameter. **2.** Matrix.

Fig. 2-57. Specific endothelial granule. Renal vein. Rat. E.M. X 268,000. **1.** Boundary membrane. **2.** Component tubules, cross-sectioned, averaging 200 Å in diameter.

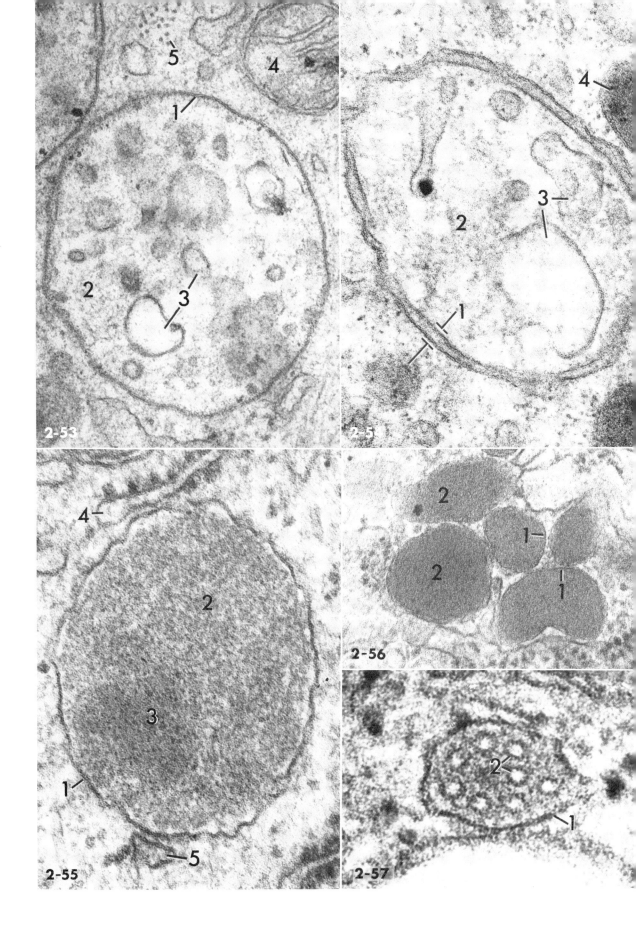

2-53

2-54

2-55

2-56

2-57

mary lysosomes are identical with Golgi vesicles, ranging in size between 250 Å and 500 Å. These vesicles can be of the coated variety, reminiscent of coated pinocytic vesicles (p. 16). Other primary lysosomes are uncoated and vary greatly in size, and contain a matrix of medium to high electron density. Their boundary membrane is trilaminar and 60 Å thick. (Fig. 2-48) It is postulated that the enzymes of the lysosomes are synthesized at ribosomes of the granular endoplasmic reticulum, shed into the cisternae, and transferred to the Golgi zone of the cell. The primary lysosomes then arise from the Golgi apparatus (or possibly the granular endoplasmic reticulum) as small vesicles which gradually increase in size. They contain a large number of hydrolytic enzymes (12 or more) which can break down proteins, carbohydrates, fats, and nucleic acids. The exact number and kinds of enzymes are highly variable from tissue to tissue.

The primary lysosomes function as digestive organelles during pinocytosis, phagocytosis, and autophagy (self-phagocytosis). Pinocytic and phagocytic invaginations which have engulfed fluid and/or materials break off from the cell membrane and are referred to as **phagosomes**. (Fig. 2-47) The boundary membrane of the primary lysosome then fuses with the phagosome membrane (Fig. 2-49) and the content of the phagosome becomes exposed to the hydrolytic enzymes of the primary lysosome. The merged organelles are referred to as secondary lysosomes. During autophagy (self-phagocytosis), part of the cytoplasm becomes sequestered by a confluence of vesicular or flat paired membranes, so-called isolation membrane, derived either from the Golgi apparatus or the agranular endoplasmic reticulum. Primary lysosomes are added to this structure to form a secondary lysosome, referred to as an autosome.

Secondary lysosomes. To this group of organelles belong structures of varied names: multivesicular bodies, residual bodies, autosomes, hemosiderin granules,

and lipofuscin granules. They all arise through a fusion of a primary lysosome and a vacuole of varied nature and origin. The **multivesicular bodies** are membrane-bound vacuoles, 0.2–0.3 μ wide, which contain small vesicles and a matrix which gives positive histochemical reaction for acid phosphatase. (Fig. 2-53) Small coated vesicles have been seen to fuse with the vacuole to form the multivesicular body. Little is known of the origin, fate, and specific function of these bodies. **Autosomes** (synonyms: autosomal bodies, cytolysosomes, autophagic vacuoles) are large secondary lysosomes bordered by two trilaminar membranes. They may contain ribosomes, mitochondria, profiles of the endoplasmic reticulum, glycogen particles, microbodies, lipid droplets, and pieces of membranes. (Fig. 2-54) Autosomes are the result of cellular action to dispose of and digest damaged, unwanted, or aged components of the cytoplasm. Soluble products of the hydrolysis taking place in the autosomes (as well as in other types of secondary lysosomes) diffuse into the cytoplasm and is there utilized for the synthesis of cellular components. Autophagy probably also takes place in some cells

Fig. 2-58. Two centrioles (one diplosome). Macrophage. Spleen. Rat. E.M. X 54,000. **1.** Longitudinally sectioned centriole. **2.** Obliquely sectioned centriole. **3.** Golgi zones (dictyosomes).

Fig. 2-59. Macrophage. Spleen. Rat. E.M. X 38,000. **1.** Centriole. **2.** Pericentriolar satellites (centrosphere). **3.** Microtubules. **4.** Primary lysosomes. **5.** Secondary lysosomes. **6.** Golgi apparatus. **7.** Mitochondria. **8.** Lobe of nucleus.

Fig. 2-60. Longitudinally sectioned centriole. Myelocyte. Bone marrow. Human. E.M. X 94,000. **1.** Peripheral microtubules. **2.** Location of spiral filament (not resolved unequivocally). **3.** Pericentriolar satellites (centrosphere). **4.** Golgi apparatus.

Fig. 2-61. Cross-sectioned centriole. Epithelial surface cell. Large intestine. Rat. E.M. X 245,000. **1.** Triplets of fused microtubules. **2.** Faint indication of spiral filament and "cartwheel" configuration. **3.** Centrosphere.

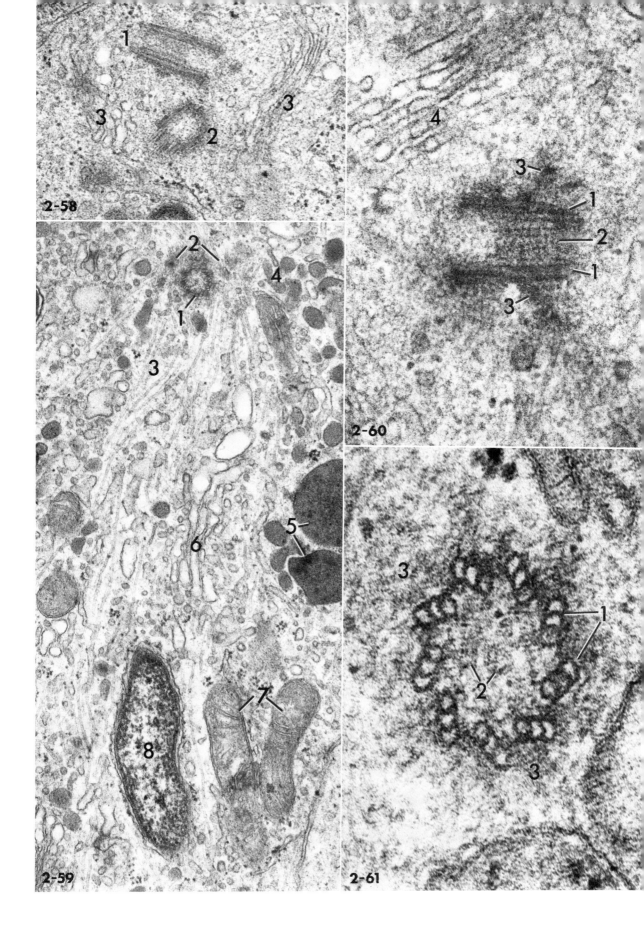

during starvation to aid in the survival of the cell. **Residual bodies** is a collective name for secondary lysosomes which contain indigestible residue after any lysosomal action, be this phagocytic or autophagic. (Fig. 2-51) The residual bodies may contain sequestered silica or asbestos particles in pulmonary macrophages, dye particles as a result of a tattoo process in dermal macrophages, or surplus cholesterol in the form of crystals in normal adrenal cortex cells (Fig. 2-76), as well as in pathologically changed vascular smooth muscle cells during atherosclerosis. **Lipofuscin granules** represent secondary lysosomes which accumulate in aging cells, particularly in the central nervous system and the myocardium. They contain a variety of lipid droplets, vacuoles, and highly electron-dense granules of unknown nature (Fig. 2-52), rendering the cells a brownish-yellow color.

The digestive enzymes are normally confined to the lysosome by its boundary membrane. If this membrane is ruptured, or its permeability changed for whatever reason, the lytic enzymes gain access to the cytoplasm, which may result in cellular lysis and **cell death.** Many polymorphonuclear leukocytes are killed by this process during phagocytosis of bacteria. Although not completely understood, a similar mechanism of cell death may occur during the development of the embryo, since many cells are known to succumb during remodeling of organs and tissues.

MICROBODIES

Microbodies (synonym: peroxisomes) constitute a distinct class of membrane-bound, granular organelles which, in mammals, occur in parenchymal cells of the liver, tubule cells of the kidney, nonciliated cells of pulmonary bronchioles, and in odontoblasts. The microbodies are spherical, ovoid, or angular and range between 0.3–0.5 μ in diameter. A trilaminar limiting membrane, averaging 60 Å in diameter, surrounds a finely granular matrix (Fig. 2-55) which, in liver cells and odontoblasts, contains a dense structure (core; crystalloid; nucleoid) not present in kidney microbodies. The crystalloid consists of sheets of parallel rods or cylinders with a center-to-center spacing of about 120 Å. The microbodies are probably formed from the granular endoplasmic reticulum.

The microbodies contain catalase and several oxidative enzymes such as urate oxidase, amino acid oxidase, and isocitrate dehydrogenase. Acid hydrolases, typical for lysosomes have not been demonstrated in microbodies. This is important since it is often difficult to differentiate between microbodies and primary lysosomes on an ultrastructural basis alone, at least when the crystalloid is not seen. The oxidases produce hydrogen peroxide and the catalase destroys it. It is believed that the presence of peroxisomes in the kidney and the liver is of importance to prevent

Fig. 2-62. Microtubules. Endothelial cell. Peritubular capillary. Kidney. Rat. E.M. X 70,000. **1.** Lumen of capillary. **2.** Bundle of parallel microtubules in endothelial cytoplasm.

Fig. 2-63. Microtubules. Kupffer cell. Liver. Rat. E.M. X 137,000. **1.** Microtubules, average width 250 Å.

Fig. 2-64. Parenchymal cell. Liver. Rat. E.M. X 161,000. **1.** Microtubule; width between T-bars: 270 Å. **2.** Glycogen particles (alpha type). **3.** Glycogen particles (beta type).

Fig. 2-65. Parenchymal cell. Liver. Rat. E.M. X 178,000. **1.** Cross-sectioned microtubule. **2.** Cross-sectioned tubule of agranular endoplasmic reticulum. **3.** Mitochondrial external envelope.

Fig. 2-66. Part of mitotic spindle. Metaphase of dividing membrana granulosa cell. Follicle. Ovary. Rat. E.M. X 17,000. **1.** Two centrioles (at right angles to each other). **2.** Spindle microtubules. **3.** Chromosomes in equatorial plate. **4.** Kinetochore regions. **5.** Vesicular profiles of endoplasmic reticulum.

Fig. 2-67. Metaphase. Dividing membrana granulosa cell. Follicle. Ovary. Rat. E.M. X 75,000. **1.** Centriole with central "cartwheel" configuration. **2.** Centrosphere (pericentriolar satellites). **3.** Spindle microtubules. **4.** Kinetochore region. **5.** Chromosomal material. **6.** Ribosomes.

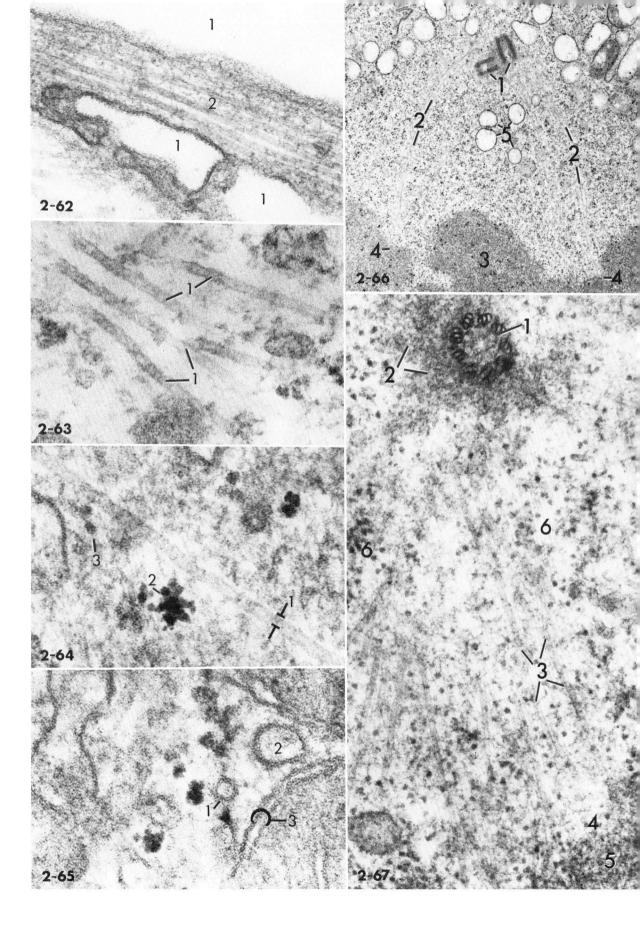

2-62

2-63

2-64

2-65

2-66

2-67

harmful effects of excessive hydrogen per-oxide production, and that they also may participate in converting fat to carbohy-drate (gluconeogenesis).

SPECIFIC ENDOTHELIAL GRANULES

In the endocardium and endothelial cells of some mammalian blood vessels (aorta, pulmonary arteries and veins, renal veins, dermal veins, and venules) occur mem-brane-bound granular structures which in size and ultrastructure are reminiscent of microbodies. (Fig. 2-56) They have a sin-gle limiting membrane, averaging 40 Å in diameter, and a finely granular matrix which sometimes contains a limited num-ber of microtubules arranged in parallel rows. (Fig. 2-57)

The function of the specific endothelial granules is not known, although it has been suggested that the granules may con-tain a procoagulative substance which be-comes discharged into the vascular lumen in response to high plasma concentrations of epinephrine.

CENTRIOLES

Centrioles are short, fibrous, rod-shaped organelles. In the intermitotic cell, there are usually two centrioles, collectively re-ferred to as the **diplosome**. (Fig. 2-58) They are located near the resting inter-phasic nucleus in the center of the cell, surrounded by the Golgi zone if this orga-nelle is present. (Fig. 2-60)

Each centriole is a short cylinder made up of 9 sets of 3 microtubules, arranged equidistantly to form the wall of the cylin-der. In each set, the triple microtubules are fused and parallel with the long axis of the cylinder. (Fig. 2-61) Each centriole is about 0.4μ long and 0.15μ wide, and the two centrioles are, in most instances, oriented perpendicularly to each other. The microtubules are embedded in a medium electron-dense, amorphous sub-stance which extends radially into the sur-rounding cytoplasm as so-called **pericen-triolar satellites** or **centrosphere**. The two centrioles and the surrounding centro-sphere are referred to as the **centrosome.** The center of the centrioles may contain a spirally arranged filament, and near the one end can be seen, at times, a "cartwheel" structure. (Fig. 2-61) This structural polar-ity may be of importance when the centri-ole assumes the position of a basal ciliary body, since ciliary microtubules apparently grow out at the pole opposite the "cart-wheel" structure of the centrioles. Radi-ating out from the centrosphere of the centriole during cell division are the micro-tubules of the spindle fibers in the aster. (Figs. 2-66, 2-67)

The centrioles are self-replicating orga-nelles. The pericentriolar satellites may be the material which gives rise to new centrioles. **Procentrioles** arise *de novo*

Fig. 2-68. Tonofilaments. Superficial cell of stratified squamous, non-keratinized epithelium. Soft palate. Kitten. E.M. X 84,000. **1.** Filaments, averaging 75 Å in diameter. **2.** Fibrils (= bundle of filaments).

Fig. 2-69. Cytoplasmic filaments. Endothelial cell. Aorta. Squirrel monkey. E.M. X 93,000. **1.** Lumen of aorta. **2.** Cell membrane. **3.** Pinocytic invaginations. **4.** Specific endothelial granule. **5.** Cytoplasmic filaments, averaging 80 Å in diameter, some with a minute, electron-lucent core.

Fig. 2-70. Myofilaments. Skeletal muscle. Rat. E.M. X 66,000. **1.** Thin actin filaments, 50 Å in diameter. **2.** Zone of thin filament attachment (Z-line). **3.** Glycogen particles (beta type). **4.** Zone of interdigitating thin and thick filaments (A-band). **5.** Thick myosin filaments. **6.** Zone of laterally interconnected thick filaments (M-band).

Fig. 2-71. Myofilaments. Cross-sectioned. Skeletal muscle. Rat. E.M. X 132,000. **1.** Thin filaments. **2.** Thick filaments.

Fig. 2-72. Microtubules and filaments. Tail of spermatozoon. Cross-sectioned. Testis. Rat. E.M. X 104,000. **1.** Central pair of microtubules. **2.** Peripheral 9 doublets of fused microtubules, one of which has an electron-dense core, and therefore could be classified as filament. **3.** Minute longitudinal filaments. **4.** Longitudinal fibrous columns. **5.** Rib of fibrous sheath. **6.** Cell membrane.

Fig. 2-73. Neurofilaments. Axon of sciatic nerve fiber. Rat. E.M. X 93,000. **1.** Neurofilaments, 55 Å in diameter. **2.** Microtubules, 225 Å in diameter.

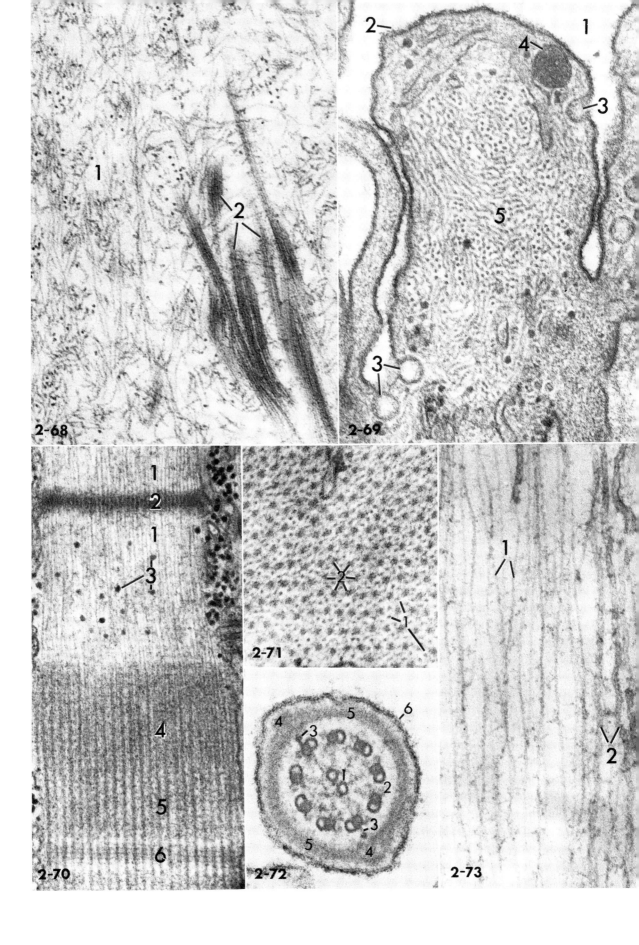

within this region, appearing first as small centrioles, but structurally similar to the "old" centriole. The centrioles organize and perhaps give rise to the microtubules of the mitotic spindle. They determine the polarity of the cell during late prophase and metaphase of cell division, when they become located at the opposite poles of the spindle. The nature of their organizing capacity is not known. The centrioles can also move to a position beneath the cell membrane and there, through replication, give rise to basal bodies, cilia, and flagellae.

MICROTUBULES

Microtubules are straight or slightly curved, delicate cylindrical organelles, present in almost every cell type, both dividing and non-dividing. The microtubules occur: 1) singly, scattered throughout the cytoplasm; 2) in groups arranged in parallel; and 3) fused to form doublets and triplets.

Microtubules occurring singly average 250 Å in diameter (Figs. 2-63, 2-64); their length is indeterminate. The electron-lucent core is about 150 Å wide, and the wall averages 50 Å in diameter (Fig. 2-65), consisting of 13 longitudinal beaded filaments, arranged helically and resolved only after cell fractionation and negative staining of the specimen. In doublets and triplets of microtubules the same general ultrastructural pattern prevails, with the exceptions that the fused microtubules share part of the microtubule wall, and that the entire core of some microtubules may be occupied by an electron-dense structure rather than by an electron-lucent substance. (Fig. 2-72) Short arms may extend across from one microtubule to the adjacent one. In microtubules of nerve cells, a delicate filament is situated in the center of the core, parallel to the long axis of the microtubule. The microtubules are made up of a protein, the amino acid of which is very similar to the muscle protein actin.

Microtubules serve several basic cellular functions. They maintain cell shape in a **cytoskeletal** capacity as, for instance, in platelets where they are arranged in a circular band beneath the surface at the edge of these disk-shaped blood elements. They participate in **intracellular movements** by changing the shape of cells and the position of cell components during cell division and cell maturation. This is indicated by their prominent role in forming the mitotic spindle and moving the chromosomes (Fig. 2-66), as well as by the reshaping of the nucleus of the spermatid through a collection of microtubules, referred to as manchette. The nature of these microtubular activities is not known, but it could be related to the action of microtubules in cilia and flagella, where movement of these cell surface projections is thought to be brought about through a sliding mechanism of microtubules in relation to their neighbors, possibly aided

Fig. 2-74. Lipid droplets. Epithelial cell. Adrenal cortex. Zona fasciculata. Rat. E.M. X 100,000. **1.** Large lipid droplet. **2.** Developing lipid droplets. **3.** Casing of merging tubules of agranular endoplasmic reticulum. **4.** Interface membrane; cytoplasm/lipid droplet. **5.** Mitochondrion. **6.** Part of nucleus.

Fig. 2-75. Proteinaceous secretory granule. Serous gland. Tongue. Rat. E.M. X 108,000. **1.** Secretory granule. **2.** Boundary membrane.

Fig. 2-76. Cholesterol crystal in lysosome. Epithelial cell. Adrenal cortex. Zona fasciculata. Rat. E.M. X 180,000. **1.** Cholesterol crystal (dissolved). **2.** Boundary membrane (trilaminar) of lysosome. **3.** Matrix of lysosome. **4.** Vesicular mitochondrial cristae. **5.** Glycogen particles (beta type).

Fig. 2-77. Lipoprotein crystal in lysosome. Eosinophilic leukocyte. Mouse. E.M. X 134,000. **1.** Boundary membrane of lysosome (specific eosinophilic granule). **2.** Matrix. **3.** Lipoprotein crystal.

Fig. 2-78. Glycogen particles. Parenchymal cell. Liver. Rat. E.M. X 166,000. **1.** Alpha particles. **2.** Beta particles. **3.** Tubules of agranular endoplasmic reticulum.

Fig. 2-79. Pigment granules (melanosomes). Epidermal cell. Skin. Squirrel monkey. E.M. X 90,000. **1.** Delicate boundary membrane (mostly obscured). **2.** Dense core of melanosome. **3.** Filaments.

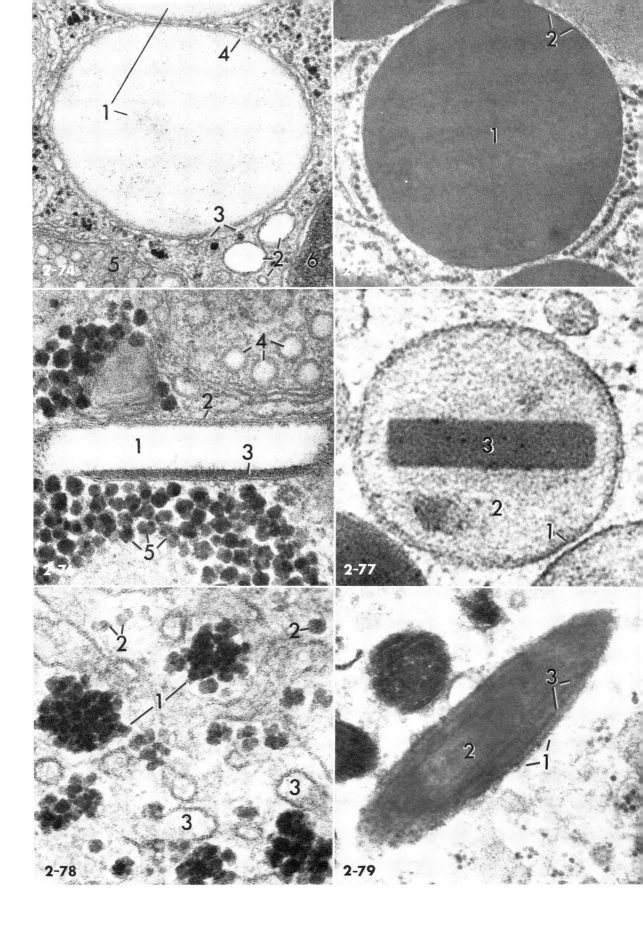

by the minute side arms. Recently, it has been proposed that microtubules aid in intracellular transport by serving as diffusion channels for water and metabolites. This may explain their relative abundance in axons and dendrites of nerve cells, podocytes of renal glomeruli, and endothelial cells of most blood vessels (Fig. 2-62), and smooth muscle cells. In melanophores of fishes, it is known that groups of microtubules form channels which facilitate the rapid movement of pigments back and forth.

It is not known how microtubules form in the cytoplasm, except that the centriolar and ciliary basal body triplets of microtubules are instrumental in forming ciliary microtubules. The centrosphere (pericentriolar satellites) supposedly is the site of origin for the mitotic spindle microtubules. (Fig. 2-67) The drug colchicin blocks the formation of these microtubules, since it becomes bound to specific sites of the protein molecules which otherwise would form the microtubules.

FILAMENTS

Filaments are organelles present in almost all kinds of cells. They are particularly abundant in muscle cells, neurons, and glial cells, and in the cells of stratified squamous epithelia. The filaments range in diameter from 50 Å to 150 Å, and may have an electron-lucent core. Their length is indeterminate. Filaments are aggregates of elongated molecules of many different proteins, depending upon function. **Intracellular** fibrous elements are subdivided into 1) filaments, 2) fibrils, and 3) fibers. **Filament** is a submicroscopical structure ranging in size from 50 Å to 150 Å. **Fibril** can be seen in light microscope preparations under oil immersion. It is a bundle of filaments, and ranges from 0.2 μ to about 1 μ, the upper limit not being very exact. **Fiber** is a bundle of fibrils and can be seen in light microscope preparations even at low magnifications.

The intracellular filaments can be subdivided according to their function: 1)

cytoskeletal filaments, 2) myofilaments, and 3) neurofilaments. The cytoskeletal filaments are most abundant in the cells of stratified squamous epithelia, where they are referred to as **tonofilaments.** (Fig. 2-68) They provide these cells with rigidity, as well as tensile strength and resilience. They also participate in forming the keratin filaments of the keratinized cells (p. 000). Other epithelial cells, including vascular endothelial cells (Fig. 2-69), as well as fibroblasts and fibrous astrocytes (glial cells), contain a loose network of cytoskeletal filaments. In epithelial cells with microvilli at their apical surface, the filaments form a zone of densely and irregularly arranged filaments at the base of the microvilli, the **terminal web** (Fig. 2-71), and they also form a core of filaments in the microvilli.

The **myofilaments** contain contractile proteins and represent a very important functional part of muscle cells. Striated muscle cells contain thick myofilaments, which average 100 Å in diameter, containing the protein myosin, as well as thin filaments which average 50 Å in diameter and contain actin. (Figs. 2-70, 2-71) Smooth muscle cells contain three sets of fila-

Fig. 2-80. Interphase (intermitotic) nucleus. Acinar cell. Pancreas. Rat. E.M. X 24,000. **1.** Electron-lucent euchromatin. **2.** Electron-dense heterochromatin (karyosome). **3.** Marginated heterochromatin. **4.** Nucleolus. **5.** Nucleolus-associated chromatin. **6.** Nuclear pore. **7.** Nuclear envelope. **8.** Granular endoplasmic reticulum. **9.** Mitochondria.

Fig. 2-81. Nuclear margin. Enlargement of area similar to rectangle in Fig. 2-80. Parenchymal cell. Liver. Rat. E.M. X 184,000. **1.** Euchromatin. **2.** Chromatin particles of marginated dense heterochromatin. **3.** Inner nuclear membrane. **4.** Perinuclear cisterna. **5.** Outer nuclear membrane. **6.** Nuclear pore with diffuse plug-like substance. **7.** Ribosomes attached to outer nuclear membrane. **8.** Cytoplasm.

Fig. 2-82. Tangential section of nuclear envelope. Spermatocyte Testis. Mouse. E.M. X 51,000. **1.** Chromatin particles of nucleus. **2.** Annuli of nuclear pores. **3.** Ribosomes of cytoplasm.

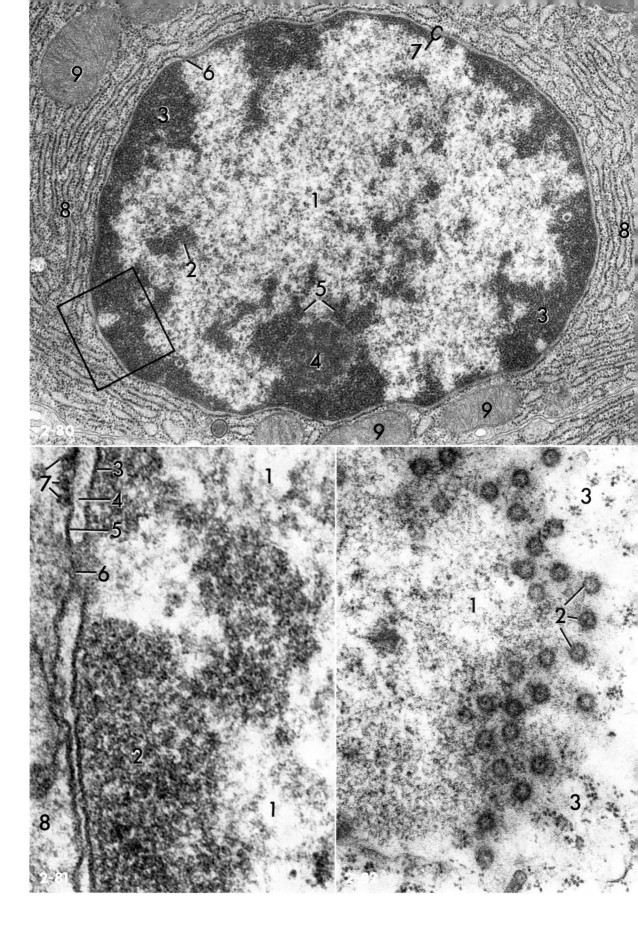

ments, averaging 150 Å, 100 Å, and 50 Å respectively (p. 248). It is presently believed that the cytoplasmic filaments of endothelial cells in capillaries and other blood vessels (Fig. 2-69) may have contractile properties in addition to their assumed cytoskeletal function.

The **neurofilaments** which are present in axons and dendrites of most neurons range in size between 50 and 100 Å. (Fig. 2-73) They may be involved in intracellular transport of ions and metabolites in addition to their possible cytoskeletal function.

STORED MATERIALS AND PRODUCTS

In the form of granules and droplets, cells store food materials as well as products resulting from their synthesizing processes. These are protein, fat, and carbohydrate, and have by tradition, been referred to as **cytoplasmic inclusions,** that is, they were not considered essential for the maintenance of cell life. It is now known that many of these components participate to a large extent in the metabolism and normal functions of the cell, in addition to their being stored temporarily in the cell.

Fat. Fat is segregated from the rest of the cytoplasm in the shape of small **vacuoles** and **droplets,** containing fatty acids, triglycerides, cholesterol, and cholesterol esters. In their nascent stage the droplets arise within Golgi vesicles or vesicular profiles of the agranular endoplasmic reticulum, and are bordered by a 60 Å-thick membrane. With increasing size the boundary membrane of the lipid droplets becomes thinner, and in many instances remains only as an interfacial surface between lipid droplet and cytoplasm. Lipid droplets occur abundantly in fat cells and cells of the adrenal cortex (Fig. 2-74), but are present in almost all cell types to a limited degree. Under normal conditions, cholesterol **crystals** occur within the lysosomes of the cells of the adrenal cortex. (Fig. 2-76)

Protein. As a result of secretory processes, protein is segregated and stored

temporarily in **secretory granules** (Fig. 2-75) and primary **lysosomes** (Fig. 2-77), separated from the cytoplasm by a 60–80 Å-thick membrane. Proteinaceous **crystals** (or crystalloids) are another form of storage, in which macromolecular spherical units of protein are arranged in an orderly fashion. In the Sertoli and interstitial cells of the testis, the protein crystals (of Reincke) are not surrounded by a membrane. In other instances, protein crystalloids are situated in the cisternae of the granular endoplasmic reticulum (salamander liver cells), mitochondrial cristae (oocytes), or lysosomes (granules of eosinophilic leukocytes). (Fig. 2-77)

Carbohydrate. Stored carbohydrates can be preserved and stained for electron microscopy, and are then resolved as small particles representing glycogen, a polymer formed from glucose. The **glycogen particles** occur freely in the cytoplasm. They are not surrounded by a limiting membrane, and they are unattached to membranes, although they often occur in the intertubular spaces near the membranes of the agranular endoplasmic reticulum. (Fig. 2-78) The particles occur in essentially two forms: β- and α-particles. The β-particles are round and average 300 Å in diameter. The α-particles are complexes of several smaller particles, appearing as blackberries, and averaging 900 Å in diameter. Glycogen particles are abundant in liver cells, muscle cells, and cells of the adrenal cortex, but they occur sparingly in most cell types.

PIGMENTS

Pigments (synonyms: melanin granules; melanosomes) are membrane-bound gran-

Fig. 2-83. Nucleolus. Primary oocyte. Ovary. Rat. E.M. × 22,000.

Fig. 2-84. Nucleolus. Enlargement of Fig. 2-83. E.M. × 90,000. **1.** Nucleolar-associated heterochromatin. **2.** Euchromatin. **3.** Pars amorpha of nucleolus. **4.** Filamentous part of nucleolonema. **5.** Nucleolar ribosomes of nucleolonema; particles averaging 110 Å in diameter.

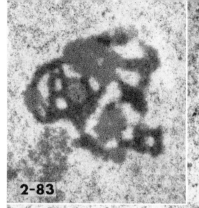

2-83

2

3

4

5

4

3

3

5

4

1

2

2-84

ular structures which are present only in certain cells (melanocytes, epidermal cells, and pigment epithelial cells of iris and retina). They arise from Golgi vesicles in a process called melanogenesis. The vesicles increase in size and accumulate an electron-lucent matrix and filaments, which are oriented parallel to each other. (Fig. 2-79) The filaments increase gradually in electron density by a deposition of melanin often with a helical, striated periodicity. The process involves the conversion of the amino acid tyrosine to melanin by tyrosinase. The mature melanin granule has little or no visible substructure.

NUCLEUS

General considerations. The nucleus is a distinct feature of all cells except erythrocytes and platelets. It contains genetic information and has a decisive influence on the metabolic activities of the cytoplasm. It is essential for sustaining the life of the cell, since protein synthesis of the cytoplasm ceases in cells which have lost their nucleus. When a cell divides, the genetic information is distributed equally to the two resulting cells. The nucleus goes through several phases in preparation for the cell division. The non-dividing nucleus is said to be in interphase or rest, and most somatic cells are preserved in the interphase stage in routine preparations for light and electron microscopy. The stages directly involved in cell division (prophase, metaphase, anaphase, telophase) can also be preserved and analyzed and are described on p. 56.

The nucleus stains dark blue with basic dyes because of its content of deoxyribonucleoprotein, the coded genetic material. The shape of nuclei varies from spherical in most cells to ovoid, rod-shaped, and cup-shaped in others. They also occur with one or several indentations, and in some instances, the nucleus is lobated with one or more lobes (leukocytes). The size of the nucleus ranges between 3μ and 25μ. The largest nucleus of the human

body is in the ovum. Most cells have only one nucleus, whereas some cells are binucleate (neurons, liver parenchymal cells, cardiac cells). In a few instances there are many nuclei in the same cell (skeletal muscle, osteoclasts of bone tissue).

In the interphase nucleus the following major components can be seen in both light and electron microscope (Fig. 2-80) preparations: 1) nuclear envelope (membrane); 2) chromatin material; 3) nucleolus; and 4) nuclear sap. The term **karyoplasm** is used for the entire nucleus when considered in relation to the surrounding **cytoplasm** of the cell. The karyoplasm and the cytoplasm form the **protoplasm** of the cell.

Nuclear envelope. The nuclear envelope (often also referred to as nuclear membrane) is a membranous sac, consisting of: 1) outer nuclear membrane; 2) inner nuclear membrane; 3) perinuclear cisterna; and 4) nuclear pores. (Fig. 2-81) The outer and inner nuclear membranes each average 80 Å in diameter, and have a trilaminar structure. The cytoplasmic aspect of the **outer membrane** is studded with ribosomes in most cells, and in some nuclei, the karyoplasmic aspect of the **inner membrane** is lined by an electron-dense, fibrous lamina, averaging 250 Å in diameter. The **perinuclear cisterna** is electron-lucent and about 200–500 Å wide. It communicates

Fig. 2-85. Early prophase nucleus. Membrana granulosa cell. Follicle. Ovary. Rat. E.M. X 15,000. **1.** Euchromatin (less electron-dense than cytoplasm). **2.** Contracting (condensing) areas of heterochromatin (= chromosomes). Nuclear DNA has now replicated. **3.** Nucleolus beginning to disperse. **4.** Nuclear enveope still intact. **5.** Cell membrane.

Fig. 2-86. Late prophase nucleus. Membrana granulosa cell. Follicle. Ovary. Rat. E.M. X 15,000. **1.** Euchromatin (now same electron density as cytoplasm). **2.** Chromosomes. **3.** Nucleolus further dispersed (compared to Fig. 2-85). **4.** Nuclear envelope starts to disintegrate. **5.** Centriole. **6.** Spindle microtubules. **7.** Elements of endoplasmic reticulum. **8.** Cell membrane.

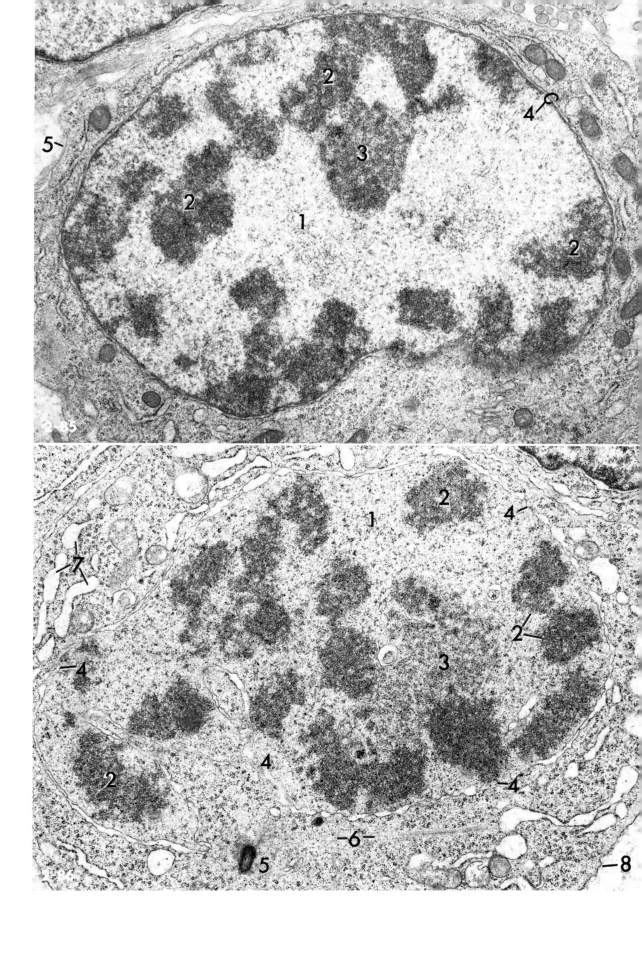

occasionally with the cisternae of the endoplasmic reticulum of the cytoplasm, and it may at times contain some electron-dense granular material. The **nuclear pores** are about 500–700 Å wide, spaced at relatively equal distances, and occupying as much as 25 per cent of the nuclear envelope in some cells. The outer and inner nuclear membranes are continuous at the nuclear pore, forming the **annulus** (ring) of the pore. (Fig. 2-82) A thin, diffuse diaphragm and/or plug-like structure stretches across or fills the pore.

The nuclear envelope is too thin to be seen in light microscope preparations. However, since nuclear chromatin material often is attached to the karyoplasmic aspect of the inner nuclear membrane as marginated chromatin, the level of the cytoplasmic/karyoplasmic interface can be identified. The nuclear envelope is believed to represent a membranous barrier between karyoplasm and cytoplasm. The nuclear pores and associated annuli are considered potential channels for exchange and interaction between karyoplasm and cytoplasm. The mechanisms of movement are not known.

Chromatin material. It must be recognized that present preparation techniques for light microscopy and electron microscopy are inadequate for the proper preservation of the genetic substance of the nucleus which, collectively, is referred to as chromatin material. In the living cell, the karyoplasm is optically homogeneous except for the nucleolus. After fixation and other tissue preparation procedures for light microscopy and electron microscopy, the karyoplasm appears divided into irregular dense, coarsely granular areas (heterochromatin) and optically light areas (euchromatin). This image of the round nucleus is reminiscent of early survey photographs of the moon. In many ways, the structure of the chromatin is as unexplored as the moon was then.

The **heterochromatin** material forms a network of electron-dense **chromatin granules** (synonym: karyosomes), ranging from 0.1 μ to 1 μ in diameter. The karyosomes are not membrane-bound. The dense chromatin material is often marginated at the nuclear envelope, usually leaving the nuclear pore-areas free. Some dense heterochromatin is attached to the nucleolus, referred to as nucleolar-associated chromatin. Nuclei of some cell types (undifferentiated mesenchymal cells, hemocytoblasts, nerve cells) contain a finely dispersed heterochromatin material, whereas others have a heavily concentrated heterochromatin (spermatocytes;

Figs. 2-87 through 2-94. Some of the more obvious stages of **mitotic division** have been selected from dividing membrana granulosa cells of the rat ovary. They have been arranged to facilitate the study of nuclear, chromosomal, and cytoplasmic changes during division of a mammalian cell. Centrioles are not seen in most of the illustrations, since these organelles are not always in the plane of section. In contrast to some plant and vertebrate cells which are anastral, centrioles are always present during cell division in mammalian cells. The cells are not shown at the same magnifications since eight dividing cells would not fit into the space allotted. The purpose of this display is to give a quick overview of mitosis as it appears with the resolving power of the electron microscope. Membrana granulosa cells. Follicle. Ovary. Rat.

Fig. 2-87. Early prophase. Enlarged in Fig. 2-85. E.M X 5600.

Fig. 2-88. Late prophase. Enlarged in Fig. 2-86. E.M. X 5600.

Fig. 2-89. Metaphase. Chromosomes lined up in the equatorial plate. Similar cell enlarged further in Fig. 2-95. E.M. X 4500.

Fig. 2-90. Late anaphase. Chromosomes have separated and almost arrived at opposite cell poles. E.M. X 5500.

Fig. 2-91. Early telophase. Cytoplasmic furrow starts to appear. E.M. X 4400.

Fig. 2-92. Early telophase. Cytoplasmic furrow deepens. E.M. X 4500.

Fig. 2-93. Mid-telophase. Nuclear envelope reappears. Cytoplasmic cleavage furrow quite deep. Enlarged further in Fig. 2-97. E.M. X 3600.

Fig. 2-94. Late telophase. Mid-body present. Enlarged further in Figs. 2-98 and 2-99. E.M. X 5200.

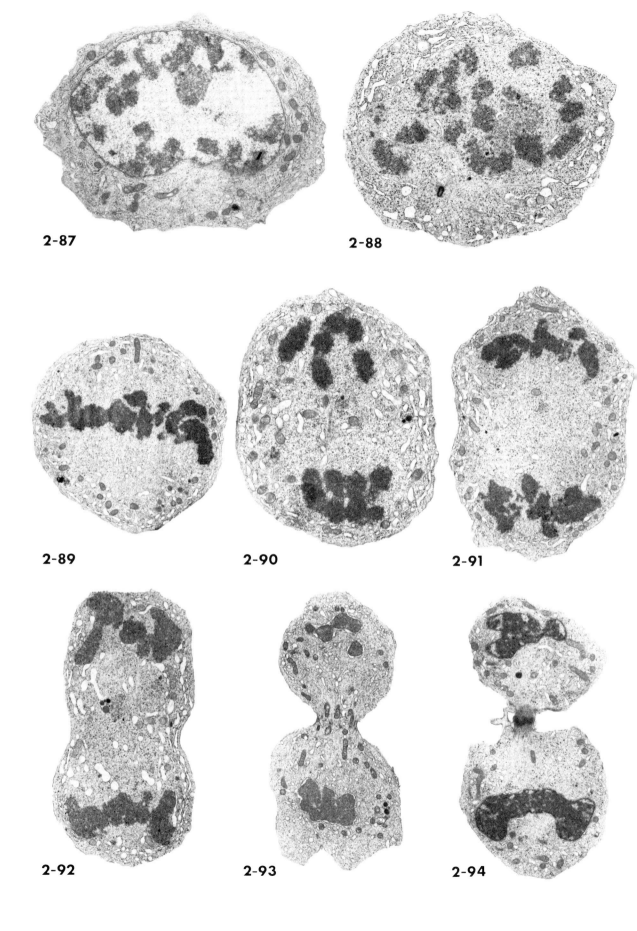

2-87

2-88

2-89

2-90

2-91

2-92

2-93

2-94

neutrophil polymorphonuclear leuko-cytes). Late erythroblasts, preparing for nuclear extrusion, and dying cells have nuclei with extremely dense heterochro-matin, a stage referred to as pyknosis.

With present-day, conventional prepa-ration procedures in electron microscopy, the heterochromatin material is seen to consist of numerous **chromatin particles,** averaging 50–100 Å in diameter (Fig. 2-81), and coiled, thin **filaments.** Many investi-gators believe that the particles and fila-ments are artifacts, and that they do not represent the true structure of the genetic material. In the interphase, as well as the mitotic nucleus, the genetic material is present in the form of **chromosomes** which are long and very slender, thread-like structural complexes of deoxyribonucleic acids, and basic and acidic proteins, seen at their best advantage during cell divi-sion. This is discussed further on p. 56. It is presently believed that the hetero-chromatic part of the interphasic nucleus represents the contracted (coiled; non-dispersed) part of the chromosomes.

The **euchromatin** material is repre-sented by the electron-lucent areas of the nucleus. (Fig. 2-81) They do not contain chromatin particles, and they do not stain with basic dyes. It is assumed that they contain the extended (synonyms: un-coiled; dispersed) part of the chromo-somes, in addition to occasional small particles, averaging 150 Å in diameter, which probably represent nucleolar ribo-somes in transit from the nucleolus to the cytoplasm. The light, euchromatic areas of the nucleus are also believed to have a relatively high proportion of nuclear sap, the fluid component of the karyoplasm.

Nucleolus. The interphase nucleus con-tains one or several nucleoli. These are discrete, round or ovoid, strongly baso-philic bodies which are not delineated by a membrane. The nucleoli disappear dur-ing cell division. They occur freely in the karyoplasm, or are attached to the inner nuclear membrane. Nucleoli are particu-larly large and prominent in rapidly grow-ing cells, and in cells with a high rate of protein synthesis (undifferentiated mesen-chymal cells, pancreatic acinar cells, nerve cells).

In the light microscope, the nucleolus is seen to consist of 1) a dense, coiled fibril, the nucleolonema (synonym: pars densa); 2) an amorphous, less dense part, the pars amorpha (synonym: pars fibrosa); and 3) patches of chromatin attached to its pe-riphery, the condensed boundary (syno-nym: nucleolar-associated chromatin). As seen by electron microscopy (Figs. 2-83, 2-84), the **nucleolonema** is composed of small particles, 100–150 Å in diameter, and short, delicate filaments, 50–70 Å in diameter. The particles are believed to contain nucleolar RNA and the filaments non-ribosomal nucleolar proteins. The **pars amorpha** of the nucleolus occupies irregular and spherical spaces within the coiled nucleolonema, and contains a me-dium electron-dense, finely filamentous substance and some chromatin particles. The **condensed boundary** of the nucleolus contains so-called nucleolus-associated chromatin which also may be present in the pars amorpha. The material is very likely of DNA-histone nature. The con-fusing nomenclature describing the dif-ferent parts of the nucleolus reflects the variation in appearance of these compo-nents after different preparation proce-

Fig. 2-95. Metaphase. Membrana granulosa cell. Follicle. Ovary. Rat. E.M. X 15,000.
  1. Centriole with dense centrosphere.
  2. Pericentriolar satellites (centrosphere).
  3. Mitotic spindle microtubules.
  4. Chromosomes in equatorial plate.
  5. Mitochondria. **6.** Vacuolar and tubular profiles of endoplasmic reticulum.
  7. Lysosomes. **8.** Cell membrane. **9.** Nuclei of neighboring cells of membrana granulosa.

Fig. 2-96. Kinetochore. Enlargement of area similar to rectangle in Fig. 2-95. **Metaphase.** Membrana granulosa cell. Follicle. Ovary. Rat. E.M. X 58,000. **1.** Ribosomes. **2.** Microtubules of mitotic spindle, averaging 250 Å in width. **3.** Particulate structure of chromosomes. **4.** Amorphous structures of kinetochore. **5.** Insertion and/or penetration of mitotic spindle microtubules.

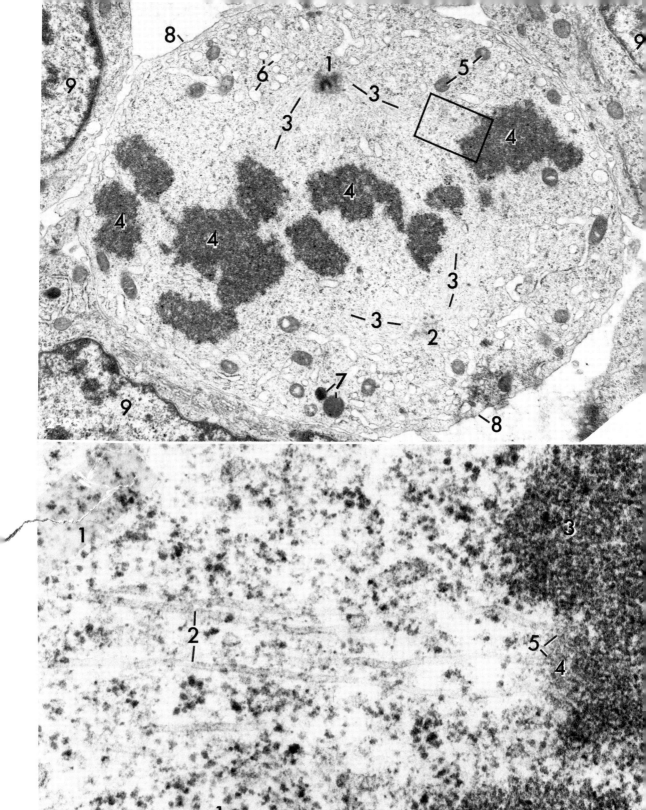

dures. It also reflects the present uncertainty with regard to the biochemical composition and functions of the several components of the nucleolus.

The following is a brief outline of the major function of the nucleolus as it relates to the control over cytoplasmic protein synthesis. Under the control of the self-replicating nuclear deoxyribonucleic acid (DNA), probably the nucleolus-associated chromatin, the nucleoli synthesize actively ribonucleic acid (RNA) and serve as a source for cytoplasmic ribosomal RNA, messenger RNA, and transfer RNA. **Ribosomal RNA** (r-RNA) is synthesized and assembled in the nucleolus by the nucleolar ribosomes. Subsequently, it moves out to the cytoplasm through the nuclear pores and forms with proteins the cytoplasmic ribosomes. A different, low molecular nucleolar RNA moves to the cytoplasm as **transfer RNA** (t-RNA). The t-RNA is also referred to as **soluble RNA** (s-RNA). The t-RNA recognizes, picks up, and transfers amino acids from the cytoplasmic pool to the polyribosomes. **Messenger RNA** (m-RNA) of high molecular weight also originates in the nucleolus. It becomes coded by the chromosomal DNA in a complementary fashion, moves out from the nucleolus to the cytoplasm, where it forms the 15 Å filament of the polysomes. A more detailed description of these events is found above under ribosomes (p. 22).

Nuclear sap. The nuclear sap is a more or less fluid component of the nucleus in which the chromatin material and the nucleolus are suspended. It contains dissolved or suspended substances such as soluble RNA, glycoproteins, and others in transit from the nucleus to the cytoplasm.

CHROMOSOMES

The nucleus contains the genetic information, the hereditary characteristics, in the form of deoxyribonucleic acid (DNA) molecules. The DNA molecule is a double helix, 20 Å in diameter. With basic proteins (histones) added, the deoxyribo-

nucleoprotein (DNP) has a diameter of about 50 Å. Strands of DNP are in turn coiled to form units averaging 250 Å in width, and up to 22,000 μ in length, collectively referred to as **chromosomes.** It is beyond the scope of this book to discuss the light microscopical, biochemical, and functional details of chromosomes. However, it must be pointed out that the chromosomes consist of a series of genes. A **gene** is a complex of DNA in which the bases adenosine, thymine, guanine, and cytosine are arranged in pairs between two helical chains of deoxyribose and phosphoric acid molecules. The genetic information related to cellular and species characteristics is provided by permutations in the succession and position of the four bases along the chromosomes.

In the **interphase** (intermitotic) nucleus, segments of the coiled strands of DNP are believed to exist as highly elongated and thin chromosomal threads, a stage, referred to as **dispersed** or uncoiled, corresponding to the light euchromatin areas of the interphase nucleus. Other parts of the chromosomes are less dispersed or contracted, appearing as dense heterochromatin.

In the **mitotic nucleus**, chromosomal material is markedly contracted, the chromosomal threads highly coiled and shortened, assuming the shape of cords or rods of varying length, the chromosomes. All somatic cells contain 23 homologous (identical) pairs of chromosomes (46, diploid or double number of chromosomes). In man, one pair of chromosomes may not be identical (homologous). These are the sex chromosomes. In the female, they are identical, each termed an X chromosome.

Fig. 2-97. Mid-telophase. Membrana granulosa cell. Follicle. Ovary. Rat. E.M. × 11,500.
1. Deep cytoplasmic cleavage furrow.
2. Mitochondria. **3.** Profiles of endoplasmic reticulum. **4.** Remaining spindle microtubules.
5. Formation of nuclear envelope.
6. Chromosomes. **7.** Some imperfections in nuclear envelope. **8.** Cell membrane. **9.** Nuclei of neighboring cells of membrana granulosa.

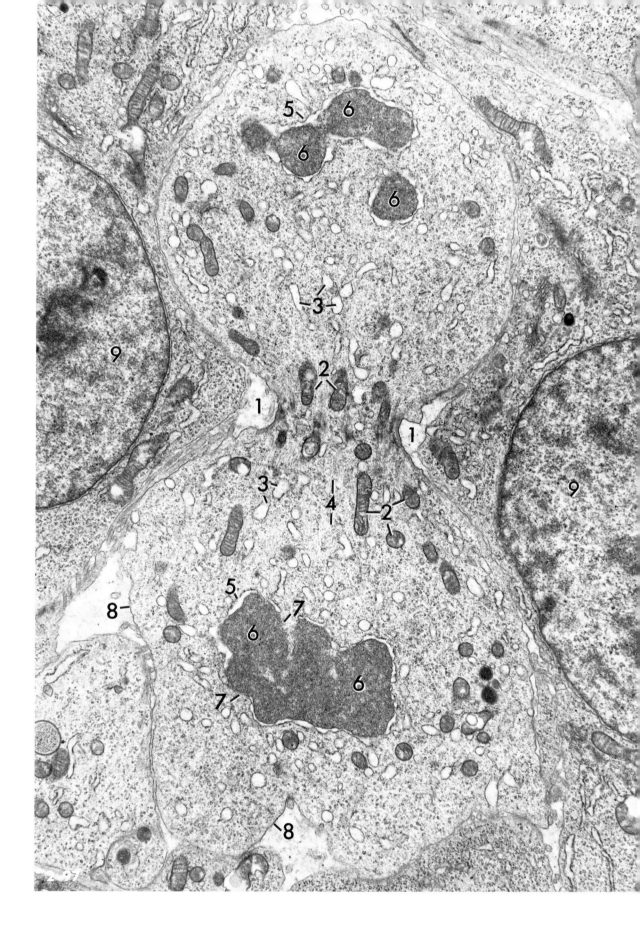

In the male, there is one X and one Y chromosome. The other pairs of chromosomes can be identified individually, depending on length, site of constrictions, and general configuration. The analysis and identification of chromosomes are used in diagnosing chromosomal aberrations. For a detailed discussion of chromosome patterns consult genetics textbooks.

In preparation for cell division during late interphase, there is a replication (doubling) of the amount of DNA present in the chromosomes. Although not entirely correct, one can visualize the result of this replication as follows: After DNA replication, each chromosome appears to consist of two halves, each half termed a **chromatid.** The two chromatids are united at the primary constriction of the chromosome by a structure called **kinetochore.** Therefore, prior to mitosis the amount of DNA present in each chromosome has doubled, and each chromosome consists of two chromatids.

CELL DIVISION

Cell division entails a doubling of a genetic material (DNA) and an equal separation of chromosomal material, cytoplasm, and cell organelles to be distributed among the resulting two cells. All somatic cells undergo a cell division which is called **mitosis,** whereas gametes (spermatocytes and oocytes) undergo a cell division referred to as **meiosis.** Briefly stated, there is a distribution of an identical (diploid) number of chromosomes and a double amount of DNA to the daughter cells during mitosis; whereas in meiosis, the daughter cells end up with only the haploid (half) number of chromosomes and half the amount of DNA compared to the parental cell. This will be further explained below.

MITOSIS

This type of cell division occurs in all somatic cells. It can be subdivided into the following stages: interphase, prophase, metaphase, anaphase, and telophase. It should be recognized that cell division is continuous and that the habit of naming the different stages is merely for the convenience of description.

Interphase. This is the so-called resting phase in which most nuclei exist during the major part of the cell's life span. Toward the end of interphase, and in preparation for cell division, there is a replication of nuclear DNA, and the cell now contains twice the normal content of genetic material. This can be expressed symbolically as follows. The resting somatic cell nucleus contains genetic material in the amount of 2DNA which is doubled to 4DNA in preparation for mitosis. However, the chromosome number is still diploid, 2×23 (46).

Prophase. The chromosomes shorten and thicken during this phase to the extent that they now can be recognized as structural entities under the light microscope. (Figs. 2-84, 2-86) Each chromosome appears split longitudinally into two precisely equal halves, each half a **chromatid,** but united at the primary constriction by the **kinetochore.** The kinetochore is an amorphous, plate- or ring-like structure firmly attached to the chromosome/chromatid. (Fig. 2-96) The two centrioles of the cell duplicate, separate, and each set of two new centrioles moves to opposite poles of the cell. Microtubules appear

Fig. 2-98. Late telophase (immediately preceding cell separation). Membrana granulosa cell. Follicle. Ovary. Rat. E.M. X 15,000.
1. Cleavage furrow extremely deep. **2.** Midbody. **3.** Nuclear membrane completely surrounding the chromosomes.
4. Chromosomes start to become dispersed (uncoiled) and areas of electron-lucent euchromatin reappear. **5.** Remnants of spindle microtubules. **6.** Mitochondria. **7.** Endoplasmic reticulum. **8.** Cell membrane. **9.** Nuclei of neighboring cells of membrana granulosa.
Fig. 2-99. Mid-body (intermediate body). Late telophase. Membrana granulosa cell. Follicle. Ovary. Rat. E.M. X 60,000. **1.** Mitotic spindle microtubules. **2.** Electron-dense material associated with microtubules. **3.** Cell membrane.

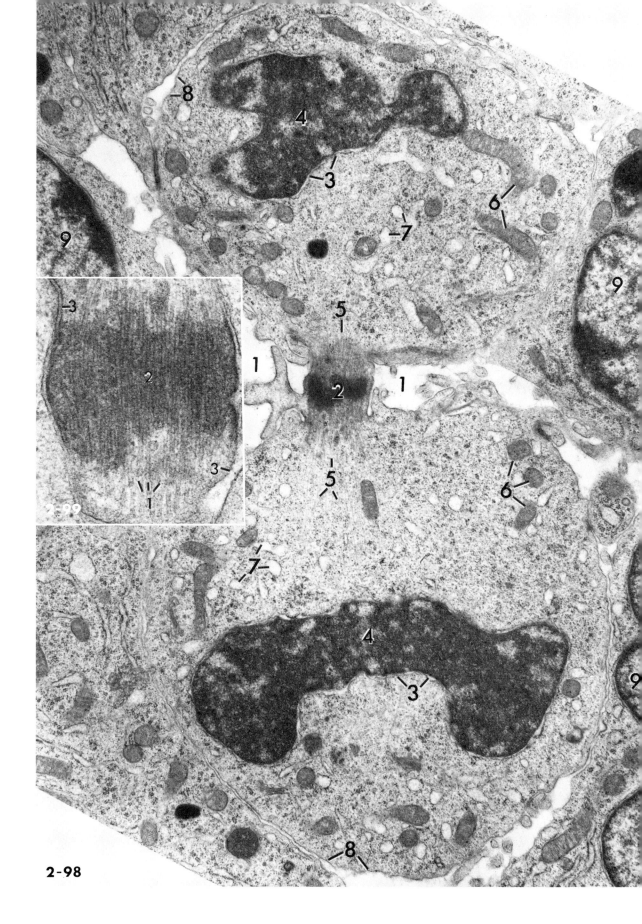

between the opposed sets of centrioles and form the **mitotic spindle.** The nucleolus disappears, since its content is distributed and attached to the chromatids as **nucleolar organizing material.** Finally, the nuclear envelope disintegrates (Fig. 2-86), breaking up into small vacuoles, and the chromosomes are released into the cytoplasm.

Metaphase. The spindle microtubules which are strung between opposing sets of centrioles move into the central region of the cell. The kinetochores double in number, and the spindle microtubules become attached to or pierce the kinetochores. (Fig. 2-96) The kinetochores divide, making it possible for each chromosome to split completely. Each half chromosome, the chromatid, now becomes a daughter chromosome. At this point, there is a tetraploid number of chromosomes, 4×23 (92). The 92 chromosomes migrate to the center of the mitotic spindle, and are arranged as the **equatorial plate.** (Figs. 2-89, 2-95).

Anaphase. By a sliding interaction with other microtubules, the kinetochores with attached daughter chromosomes (chromatids) are moved to opposite poles of the mitotic spindle (Fig. 2-90), resulting in a diploid number of chromosomes, 2×23 (46), at opposite poles. A cytoplasmic cleavage furrow appears midway between the poles (Fig. 2-91), and cytoplasm and cell organelles are divided equally.

Telophase. The daughter chromosomes, grouped at opposite poles, begin to elongate (disperse) and become less distinct. (Fig. 2-92) The nucleoli and the nuclear envelope reappear, and the cytoplasmic furrow deepens. (Fig. 2-93) The last link between the two daughter cells remains temporarily as the **intermediate** (mid) **body** (Fig. 2-94) before the final break occurs. The mid-body contains densely packed microtubules. (Fig. 2-99)

MEIOSIS

The meiotic division occurs in spermatocytes and oocytes. The basic principle in-

volved is that the number of chromosomes and the amount of genetic material are halved, so that when the sperm and the oocyte unite, the fertilized ovum will have the normal, diploid number of chromosomes and the diploid amount of DNA (rather than the tetraploid number and amount). During meiosis there are two rapid divisions in succession: meiotic division I and meiotic division II.

First meiotic division. Prior to the first meiotic division, DNA is replicated, and the chromosomal material contains twice the normal content of DNA (4DNA). The **prophase** of this division is a rather prolonged and complicated phase which has five stages: lepotene, zygotene, pachytene, diplotene, and diakinesis. From an ultrastructural point of view, the stages are not well defined, and it is beyond the scope of this book to describe the cytomorphological and functional details. Briefly, during this prolonged prophase, homologous chromosomes lie together closely, paired gene for gene in what is called **synapsis.** Toward the end of prophase, each of the 46 (2×23) chromosomes is separated (except at the kinetochore) into two chromatids, as in somatic cells.

During **metaphase,** one chromosome (consisting of two united chromatids) of each homologous pair moves to opposite poles, but the component two chromatids remain together. This ensures that homologous chromosomes separate, distributing to the daughter cells either an X or a Y sex chromosome. The anaphase and telophase of meiosis do not differ from those described under mitosis. By this first meiotic division, the number of chromosomes given to each daughter cell is half (haploid), 1×23, of that possessed by the parent cell 2×23 (46), since the chromosomes did not divide into their component chromatids. The DNA is reduced to the diploid value (2DNA), having been tetraploid (4DNA) before the completion of the first meiotic division.

Second meiotic division. This division is similar to a mitotic division. There is no pairing of chromosomes, since there exists in each cell only a haploid number of chromosomes (1×23). During the metaphase of the second meiotic division, the chromatids separate completely from each other. Each chromatid becomes a daughter chromosome, and migrates to the opposite poles of the new daughter cells. Thereby, the number of chromosomes is maintained at the haploid number (1×23) and the diploid amount of DNA in the parent cell (2DNA) is reduced to half the amount (1DNA) in each daughter cell.

References

GENERAL

Brown, W. V. and Bertke, E. M. Textbook of Cytology. C. V. Mosby, St. Louis, 1969.

Burke, J. D. Cell Biology. Williams and Wilkins, Baltimore, 1970.

De Robertis, E. D. P., Nowinski, W. W. and Saez, F. A. Cell Biology, 5th ed. W. B. Saunders, Philadelphia, 1970.

DuPraw, E. J. Cell and Molecular Biology. Academic Press, New York, 1968.

Fawcett, D. W. An Atlas of Fine Structure. The Cell. Its Organelles and Inclusions. W. B. Saunders, Philadelphia, 1966.

Fell, D. H. and Brachet, J. L. (Eds.). A discussion on cytoplasmic organelles. Proc. Royal Soc. (London) *173*: 1–111 (1969).

Finean, J. B. Biological ultrastructure. *In* Biological Ultrastructure (Eds. A. Engström and J. B. Finean). Academic Press, New York, 1967.

Matthews, J. L. and Martin, J. H. Atlas of Human Histology and Ultrastructure. Lea & Febiger, Philadelphia, 1971.

Novikoff, A. B. and Holtzman, E. Cells and Organelles. Holt, Rinehart and Winston, New York, 1970.

Oberling, C. The structure of the cytoplasm. Int. Rev. Cytol. *8*: 1–32 (1959).

Porter, K. R. and Boneville, M. A. Fine Structure of Cells and Tissues. Lea & Febiger, Philadelphia, 1968.

Rhodin, J. A. G. An Atlas of Ultrastructure. W. B. Saunders, Philadelphia, 1963.

Sandborn, E. B. Cells and Tissues by Light and Electron Microscopy. Academic Press, New York, 1970.

Sjöstrand, F. S. The ultrastructure of cells as revealed by the electron microscope. Int. Rev. Cytol. *5*: 455–533 (1956).

Sjöstrand, F. S. Electron Microscopy of Cells and Tissues. Academic Press, New York, 1967.

Toner, P. G. and Carr, K. E. Cell Structure. Williams and Wilkins, Baltimore, 1968.

Threadgold, L. T. The Ultrastructure of the Animal Cell. Pergamon, Oxford, 1967.

CELL MEMBRANE

Benedetti, E. L. and Emmelot, P. Studies on plasma membranes. IV. The ultrastructural localization and content of sialic acid in plasma membranes isolated from rat liver and hepatoma. J. Cell Sci. *2*: 499–512 (1967).

Bretscher, M. S. Membrane structure: some general principles. Science *181*: 622–629 (1973).

Brunser, O. and Luft, J. H. Fine structure of the apex of absorptive cells from rat small intestine. J. Ultrastruct. Res. *31*: 291–311 (1970).

Fawcett, D. W. Surface specializations of absorbing cells. J. Histochem. Cytochem. *13*: 75–91 (1965).

Fishman, A. P. (Ed.). Symposium on the plasma membrane (New York Heart Association). Circulation *26*: Suppl. 983–1232 (1962).

Gesner, B. M. Cell surface sugars as sites of cellular reactions: possible role in physiological processes. Ann. N.Y. Acad. Sci. *129*: 758–766 (1966).

Groniowski, J., Biczyskowa, W. and Walski, M. Electron microscope studies on the surface coat of the nephron. J. Cell Biol. *40*: 585–601 (1969).

Hendler, R. W. Biological membrane ultrastructure. Physiol. Rev. *51*: 66–97 (1971).

Higgins, J. A., Florendo, N. T. and Barrnett, R. J. Localization of cholesterol in membranes of erythrocyte ghosts. J. Ultrastruct. Res. *42*: 66–81 (1973).

Ito, S. The enteric surface coat on cat intestinal microvilli. J. Cell Biol. *27*: 475–491 (1965).

Ito, S. Structure and function of the glycocalyx. Fed. Proc. *28*: 12–25 (1969).

Korn, E. D. Structure of biological membranes. Science *153*: 1491–1498 (1966).

Loewenstein, W. R. Permeability of membrane junctions Ann. N.Y. Acad. Sci. *137*: 441–472 (1966).

Porter, K. R., Kenyon, K. and Badenhausen, S. Specializations of the unit membrane. Protoplasma *63*: 262–274 (1967).

Rambourg, A. and Leblond, C. P. Electron microscope observations on the carbohydrate-rich cell coat present at the surface of cells in the rat. J. Cell Biol. *32*: 27–53 (1967).

Robertson, J. D. The unit membrane. *In* Electron Microscopy in Anatomy (Eds. J. D. Boyd and J. D. Lever). Arnold, London, 1961.

Robertson, J. D. The structure of biological membranes. Arch. Intern. Med. *129*: 202–228 (1972).

Sjöstrand, F. S. The ultrastructure of the plasma membrane of columnar epithelium cells of the mouse intestine. J. Ultrastruc. Res. *8*: 517–541 (1963).

Stoeckenius, W. and Engelman, D. M. Current models for the structure of biological membranes. J. Cell Biol. *42*: 613–646 (1969).

Weiss, L. The cell periphery. Int. Rev. Cytol. *26*: 63–105 (1969).

VESICLES

Bodian, D. An electron microscopic characterization of classes of synaptic vesicles by means of controlled aldehyde fixation. J. Cell Biol. *44*: 115–124 (1970).

Casley-Smith, J. R. The dimensions and numbers of small vesicles in cells, endothelial and mesothelial and the significances of these for endothelial permeability. J. Microscopy *90*: 251–269 (1969).

Friend, D. and Farquhar, M. G. Functions of coated vesicles during protein absorption in the rat vas deferens. J. Cell Biol. *35*: 357–376 (1967).

Holter, H. Pinocytosis. Int. Rev. Cytol. *8*: 481–505 (1959).

Kanaseki, T. and Kadota, K. The "vesicle in a basket." A morphological study of the coated vesicle isolated from the nerve endings of the guinea pig brain, with special reference to the mechanism of membrane movements. J. Cell Biol. *42*: 202–220 (1969).

Palade, G. E. and Bruns, R. R. Structural modulations of plasmalemmal vesicles. J. Cell Biol. *37*: 633–649 (1968).

Zucker-Franklin, D. and Hirsch, J. G. Electron microscope studies on the degranulation of rabbit peritoneal leukocytes during phagocytosis. J. Exp. Med. *120*: 569–576 (1964).

CELL JUNCTIONS

Brightman, M. W. and Reese, T. S. Junctions between intimately apposed cell membranes in the vertebrate brain. J. Cell Biol. *40*: 648–677 (1969).

Bullivant, S. and Loewenstein, W. R. Structure of coupled and uncoupled cell junctions. J. Cell Biol. *37*: 621–632 (1968).

Cobb, J. L. S. and Bennett, T. A study of nexuses in visceral smooth muscle. J. Cell Biol. *41*: 287–297 (1969).

Dewey, M. M. and Barr, L. A study of the structure and distribution of the nexus. J. Cell Biol. *23*: 553–585 (1964).

Farquhar, M. G. and Palade, G. E. Junctional complexes in various epithelia. J. Cell Biol. *17*: 375–412 (1963).

Flickinger, C. J. Extracellular specializations associated with hemidesmosomes in the fetal rat urogenital sinus. Anat. Rec. *168*: 195–202 (1970).

Friend, D. S. and Giluda, N. B. Variations in tight and gap junctions in mammalian tissues. J. Cell Biol. *53*: 758–776 (1972).

Goodenough, D. A. and Revel, J. P. A fine structural analysis of intercellular junctions in the mouse liver. J. Cell Biol. *45*: 272–290 (1970).

Kelly, D. E. Fine structure of desmosomes, hemidesmosomes, and an adepidermal globular layer in developing new epidermis. J. Cell Biol. *28*: 51–72 (1966).

McNutt, N. S. and Weinstein, R. S. The ultrastructure of the nexus. A correlated thin-sectioning and freeze-cleave study. J. Cell Biol. *47*: 666–688 (1970).

Reese, T. S. and Karnovsky, M. J. Fine structural localization of a blood-brain barrier to exogenous peroxidase. J. Cell Biol. *34*: 207–217 (1967).

Revel, J. P. and Karnovsky, M. J. Hexagonal array of subunits in intercellular junctions of the mouse heart and liver. J. Cell Biol. *33*: C7–C12 (1967).

Steere, R. L. and Sommer, J. R. Stereo ultrastructure of nexus faces exposed by freeze-fracturing. J. Microscopie *15*: 205–218 (1972).

MICROVILLI AND CILIA

Crane, R. K. Structural and functional organization of an epithelial cell brush border. Symp. Int. Soc. Cell Biol. *5*: 71–102 (1966).

Fawcett, D. W. Cilia and flagella. *In* The Cell (Eds. J. Brachet and A. E. Mirsky), *2*: 217–297. Academic Press, New York, 1961.

Frisch, D. and Farbman, A. I. Development of order during ciliogenesis. Anat. Rec. *162*: 221–232 (1968).

Gibbons, I. R. The structure and composition of cilia. Symp. Int. Soc. Cell Biol. *6*: 99–114 (1967).

Grimstone, A. V. Observations on the substructure of flagellar fibres. J. Cell Sci. *1*: 351–362 (1966).

Hopkins, J. M. Subsidiary components of the flagella of *Chlamydomonas Reinhardii*. J. Cell Sci. *7*: 823–839 (1970).

Kalnins, V. I. and Porter, K. R. Centriole replication during ciliogenesis in the chick tracheal epithelium. Z. Zellforsch. *100*: 1–30 (1969).

Millecchia, L. L. and Rudzinska, M. A. Basal body replication and ciliogenesis in a suctorian, *Tokophrya infusionum*. J. Cell Biol. *46*: 553–563 (1970).

Parducz, B. Ciliary movement and coordination in ciliates. Int. Rev. Cytol. *21*: 91–128 (1967).

Satir, P. Studies on cilia. II. Examination of the distal region of the ciliary shaft and the role of the filaments in motility. J. Cell Biol. *26*: 805–834 (1965).

Satir, P. Studies on cilia. III. Further studies on the cilium tip and a "sliding filament" model of ciliary motility. J. Cell Biol. *39*: 77–94 (1968).

Steinman, R. M. An electron microscopic study of ciliogenesis in developing epidermis and trachea in the embryo of *Xenopus laevis*. Am. J. Anat. *122*: 19–56 (1968).

GRANULAR ENDOPLASMIC RETICULUM

Dallner, G., Siekevitz, P. and Palade, G. E. Biogenesis of endoplasmic reticulum membranes. J. Cell Biol. *30*: 73–96 (1966).

Garrett, R. A. and Wittmann, H.-G. Structure and function of the ribosome. Endeavour *32*: 8–14 (1973).

Haguenau, F. The ergastoplasm: its history, ultrastructure and biochemistry. Int. Rev. Cytol. *7*: 425–483 (1958).

Palade, G. E. A small particulate component of the cytoplasm. J. Biophys. Biochem. Cytol. *1*: 59–68 (1955).

Palade, G. E. and Porter, K. R. Studies on the endoplasmic reticulum. I. Its identification in cells in situ. J. Exp. Med. *100*: 641–656 (1956).

Palade, G. E. and Siekevitz, P. Pancreatic microsomes. J. Biophys. Biochem. Cytol. *2*: 671–690 (1956).

Rich, A. Polyribosomes. Sci. American *209*: 44–53 (1963).

Sjöstrand, F. S. Endoplasmic reticulum *In* Cytology and Cell Physiology (Ed. G. H. Bourne), pp. 311–376 Academic Press, New York, 1964.

Spirin, A. S. and Gavrilova, L. P. The Ribosome. Springer-Verlag, New York, 1969.

AGRANULAR ENDOPLASMIC RETICULUM

Christensen, A. K. Fine structure of testicular interstitial cells in the guinea pig. J. Cell Biol. *26*: 911–935 (1965).

Emans, J. B. and Jones, A. L. Hypertrophy of liver cell smooth surfaced reticulum following progesterone administration. J. Histochem. Cytochem. *16*: 561–570 (1968).

Jones, A. L. and Fawcett, D. W. Hypertrophy of the agranular endoplasmic reticulum in hamster liver induced by phenobarbital. J. Histochem. Cytochem. *14*: 215–232 (1966).

Ito, S. The endoplasmic reticulum of gastric parietal cells. J. Biophys. Biochem. Cytol. *11*: 333–347 (1961).

Porter, K. R. The sarcoplasmic reticulum: Its recent history and present status. J. Biophys. Biochem. Cytol. *10*: 211–226 (1961).

GOLGI APPARATUS

Beams, H. W. and Kessel, R. G. The Golgi apparatus: structure and function. Int. Rev. Cytol. *23*: 209–276 (1968).

Jamieson, J. D. and Palade, G. E. Intracellular transport of secretory proteins in the pancreatic exocrine cell. I. Role of the peripheral elements of the Golgi complex. J. Cell Biol. *34*: 577–596 (1967).

Neutra, M. and Leblond, C. P. The Golgi apparatus. Sci. American *220*: 100–107 (1969).

Northcote, D. H. The Golgi apparatus. Endeavour *30*: 26–33 (1971).

Novikoff, A., Essner, E. and Quintana, N. Golgi apparatus and lysosomes. Fed. Proc. *23*: 1010–1022 (1964).

Thiéry, J.-P. Role de l'appareil de Golgi dans la synthèse des mucopolysaccharides. Etude cytochimique. I. Mise en évidence de mucopolysaccharides dans les vésicules de transition entre l'ergastoplasme et l'appareil de Golgi. J. Microsc. *8*: 689–708 (1969).

Zeigel, R. F. and Dalton, A. J. Speculations based on the morphology of the Golgi systems in several types of protein-secreting cells. J. Cell Biol. *15*: 45–54 (1962).

ANNULATE LAMELLAE

Kessel, R. G. Annulate lamellae. J. Ultrastruct. Res. Suppl. *10*: 1–82 (1968).

Maul, G. G. Ultrastructure of pore complexes of annulate lamellae. J. Cell Biol. *46*: 604–610 (1970).

Wischnitzer, S. The annulate lamellae. Int. Rev. Cytol. *27*: 65–100 (1970).

MITOCHONDRIA

Barnard T. and Afzelius, B. A. The matrix granules of mitochondria: a review. Sub-Cell. Biochem. *1*: 375–389 (1972).

Butler, W. H. and Judah, J. D. Preparation of isolated rat liver mitochondria for electron microscopy. J. Cell Biol. *44*: 278–289 (1970).

Green, D. E. The mitochondrion. Sci. American *210*: 67–74 (1964).

Hackenbrock, C. R. Ultrastructural bases for metabolically linked mechanical activity in mitochondria. II. Electron transport-linked ultrastructural transformations in mitochondria. J. Cell Biol. *37*: 345–369 (1968).

Lehninger, A. L. The Mitochondrion. Benjamin, New York, 1965.

Malhotra, S. K. and Eakin, R. T. A study of mitochondrial membranes in relation to elementary particles. J. Cell Sci. *2*: 205–212 (1967).

Palade, G. An electron microscope study of mitochondrial structure. J. Histochem. Cytochem. *1*: 188–211 (1953).

Sjöstrand, F. S. Electron microscopy of mitochondria and cytoplasmic double membranes. Nature *171*: 30–32 (1953).

Sjöstrand, F. S. and Barajas, L. A new model for mitochondrial membranes based on biochemical information. J. Ultrastruct. Res. *32*: 293–306 (1970).

Tandler, B., Erlandson, R. A., Smith, A. L. and Wynder, E. L. Riboflavin and mouse hepatic cell structure and function. II. Division of mitochondria during recovery from simple deficiency. J. Cell Biol. *41*: 477–493 (1969).

Weber, N. E. Ultrastructural studies of beef heart mitochondria. III. The inequality of gross morphological change and oxidative phosphorylation. J. Cell Biol. *55*: 457–470 (1972).

LYSOSOMES AND RELATED BODIES

Arstila, A. U., Jauregui, H. O., Chang, J. and Trump, B. F. Studies on cellular autophagocytosis. Relationship between heterophagy and autophagy in HeLa cells. Lab. Investig. *24*: 162–174 (1971).

Björkerud, S. The isolation of lipofuscin granules from bovine cardiac muscle with observations on the properties of the isolated granules on the light and electron microscopic levels. J. Ultrastruct. Res. Suppl. *5*: 1–47 (1963).

DeDuve, C. and Wattiaux, R. Functions of lysosomes. Ann. Rev. Physiol. *28*: 435–492 (1966).

Friend, D. S. Cytochemical staining of multivesicular body and Golgi vesicles. J. Cell Biol. *41*: 269–279 (1969).

Gahan, P. B. Histochemistry of lysosomes. Int. Rev. Cytol. *21*: 1–63 (1967).

Goldfischer, S. and Bernstein, J. Lipofuscin (aging) pigment granules of the newborn human liver. J. Cell Biol. *42*: 253–261 (1969).

Goldfischer, S., Novikoff, A. B., Albala, A. and Biempica, L. Hemoglobin uptake by rat hepatocytes and its breakdown within lysosomes. J. Cell Biol. *44*: 513–529 (1970).

Ma, M. H. and Biempica, L. The normal human liver cell (emphasis on lysosomes). Am. J. Path. *62*: 353–376 (1971).

Malkoff, D. and Strehler, B. The ultrastructure of isolated and in situ human cardiac age pigment. J. Cell Biol. *16*: 611–616 (1963).

Marshall, J. and Ansell, P. L. Membranous inclusions in the retinal pigment epithelium: phagosomes and myeloid bodies. J. Anat. *110*: 91–104 (1971).

Martin, B. J. and Spicer, S. S. Multivesicular bodies and related structures of the syncytiotrophoblast of human term placenta. Anat. Rec. *175*: 15–36 (1973).

Novikoff, A. B. Lysosomes in nerve cells. In The Neuron (Ed., H. Hydén). Elsevier, Amsterdam 1967.

Nunez, E. A. and Becker, D. V. Secretory processes in follicular cells of the bat thyroid. I. Ultrastructural changes during the pre-, early and mid-hibernation periods with some comments on the origin of autophagic vacuoles. Am. J. Anat. *129*: 369–397 (1970).

René, A. A. Darden, J. H. and Parker, J. L. Radiation-induced ultrastructural and biochemical changes in lysosomes. Lab. Investig. *25*: 230–239 (1971).

Samorajski, T., Ordy, J. M. and Rady-Reimer, P. Lipofuscin pigment accumulation in the nervous system of aging mice. Anat. Rec. *160*: 555–574 (1968).

Weissmann, G. Lysosomes (analytical review). Blood *24*: 594–606 (1964).

MICROBODIES

DeDuve, C. and Baudhuin, P. Peroxisomes (microbodies and related particles). Physiol. Rev. *46*: 323–357 (1966).

Essner, E. Endoplasmic reticulum and the origin of microbodies in the fetal mouse liver. Lab. Investig. *17*:71–87 (1967).

Fahimi, H. D. Cytochemical localization of peroxidatic activity of catalase in rat hepatic microbodies (peroxisomes). J. Cell Biol. *43*: 275–288 (1969).

Hruban, Z., Vigil, E. L., Slesers, A. and Hopkins, E. Microbodies. Constituent organelles of animal cells. Lab. Investig. *27*: 184–191 (1972).

Novikoff, A. B. and Goldfischer, S. Visualization of microbodies for light and electron microscopy. J. Histochem. Cytochem. *16*: 507 (1968).

Novikoff, P. M. and Novikoff, A. B. Peroxisomes in absorptive cells of mammalian small intestine. J. Cell Biol. *53*: 532–560 (1972).

Svoboda, D., Grady, H. and Azarnoff, D. Microbodies in experimentally altered cells. J. Cell Biol. *35*: 127–152 (1967).

Tsukada, H. Mochizuki, Y. and Konishi, T. Morphogenesis and development of microbodies of hepatocytes of rats during pre- and postnatal growth. J. Cell Biol. *37*: 231–243 (1968).

FILAMENTS AND MICROTUBULES

Behnke, O. and Forer, A. Evidence for four classes of microtubules in individual cells. J. Cell Sci. *2*: 169–192 (1967).

Brody, I. The ultrastructure of the tonofibrils in the keratinization process of normal human epidermis. J. Ultrastruct. Res. *4*: 264–297 (1960).

Carr, I. The fine structure of microfibrils and microtubules in macrophages and other lymphoreticular cells in relation to cytoplasmic movement. J. Anat. *112*: 383–389 (1972).

Gall, J. G. Microtubule fine structure. J. Cell Biol. *31*: 639–643 (1966).

Olson, L. W. and Heath, I. B. Observations on the ultrastructure of microtubules. Z. Zellforsch. *115*: 388–395 (1971).

Peters, A. and Vaughn, J. E. Microtubules and filaments in the axons and astrocytes of early post-natal rat optic nerves. J. Cell Biol. *32*: 113–119 (1967).

Wessells, N. K. How living cells change shape. Sci. American *225*: 77–82 (1971).

Wikswo, M. A. and Novales, R. R. Effect of colchicine on microtubules in the melanophores of *Fundulus heteroclitus*. J. Ultrastruct. Res. *41*: 189–201 (1972).

CENTRIOLES

Perkins, F. O. Formation of centriole and centriole-like structures during meiosis and mitosis in *Labyrinthula* Sp. (Rhizopodea Labyrinhulida). J. Cell Sci. *6*: 629–653 (1970).

Sorokin, S. P. Reconstruction of centriole formation and ciliogenesis in mammalian lungs. J. Cell Sci. *3*: 207–230 (1970).

Szollosi, D. Centrioles, centriolar satellites and spindle fibers. Anat. Rec. *148*: 343 (1964).

STORED PRODUCTS

Caro, L. G. and Palade, G. E. Protein synthesis, storage, and discharge in the pancreatic exocrine cell. J. Cell Biol. *20*: 473–495 (1964).

de Bruijn, W. C. Glycogen, its chemistry and morphologic appearance in the electron microscope. J. Ultrastruct. Res. *42*: 29–50 (1973).

Napolitano, L. The differentiation of white adipose cells. J. Cell Biol. *18*: 663–679 (1963).

Revel, J. P. Electron microscopy of glycogen. J. Histochem. Cytochem. *12*: 104–114 (1964).

PIGMENTS

Barnicot, N. A. and Birbeck, M. S. C. The electron microscopy of human melanocytes and melanin granules. *In*: The Biology of Hair Growth. (Eds. W. Montagna and R. A. Ellis). Academic Press, New York, 1958.

Drochmans, P. Melanin granules. Their fine structure, formation and degradation in normal and pathological tissues. Int. Rev. Exp. Path. *2*: 357–422 (1963).

Hearing, V. J., Phillips, P. and Lutzner, M. A. The fine structure of melanogenesis in coat color mutants of the mouse. J. Ultrastruct. Res. *43*: 88–106 (1973).

Hu, F., Endo, H. and Alexander, N. J. Morphological variations of pigment granules in eyes of the rhesus monkey. Am. J. Anat. *136*: 167–182 (1973).

NUCLEUS AND NUCLEOLUS

Abelson, H. T. and Smith, G. H. Nuclear pores: the pore-annulus relationship in thin section. J. Ultrastruct. Res. *30*: 558–588 (1970).

Busch, H. and Smetana, K. The Nucleolus. Academic Press, New York, 1970.

Dalton, A. J. and Haguenau, F. (Eds.). The Nucleus. Academic Press, New York, 1968.

Everid, A. C., Small, J. V. and Davies, H. G. Electron-microscope observations on the structure of condensed chromatin: evidence for orderly arrays of unit threads on the surface of chicken erythrocyte nuclei. J. Cell Sci. *7*: 35–48 (1970).

Fawcett, D. W. On the occurrence of a fibrous lamina on the inner aspect of the nuclear envelope in certain cells of vertebrates. Am. J. Anat. *119*: 129–146 (1966).

Hardin, J. H. and Spicer, S. S. Ultrastructure of neuronal nucleoli or rat trigeminal ganglia: comparison of routine with pyroantimonate-osmium tetroxide fixation. J. Ultrastruct. Res. *31*: 16–36 (1970).

Mitchison, J. M. Some functions of the nucleus. Int. Rev. Cytol. *19*: 97–110 (1966).

Patrizi, G. and Poger, M. The ultrastructure of the nuclear periphery. The zonula nucleum limitans. J. Ultrastruct. Res. *17*: 127–136 (1967).

Recher, L. Fine structural changes in the nucleus induced by adenosine. J. Ultrastruct. Res. *32*: 212–225 (1970).

Recher, L., Whitescarver, J. and Briggs, L. The fine structure of a nucleolar constituent. J. Ultrastruct. Res. *29*: 1–14 (1969).

Sadowski, P. D. and Steiner, J. W. Electron microscopic and biochemical characteristics of nuclei and nucleoli isolated from rat liver. J. Cell Biol. *37*: 147–161 (1968).

Shinozuka, H. Intranucleolar dense particles in rat hepatic cell nucleoli. J. Ultrastruct. Res. *32*: 430–442 (1970).

Sidebottom, E. and Harris, H. The role of the nucleolus in the transfer of RNA from nucleus to cytoplasm. J. Cell Sci. *5*: 351–364 (1969).

Wiener, J., Spiro, D. and Loewenstein, W. R. Ultrastructure and permeability of nuclear membranes. J. Cell Biol. *27*: 107–117 (1965).

MITOSIS AND MEIOSIS

Baker, T. G. and Franchi, L. L. The fine structure of oogonia and oocytes in human ovaries. J. Cell Sci. *2*: 213–224 (1967).

Brinkley, B. R. and Stubblefield, E. Ultrastructure and interaction of the kinetochore and centriole in mitosis and meiosis. *In* Advances in Cell Biology, Vol. 1 (Eds. D. M. Prescott, L. Goldstein and E. McConkey). Appleton-Century-Crofts, New York, 1971.

deHarven, E. The centriole and the mitotic spindle. *In* The Nucleus (Eds. A. J. Dalton and F. Haguenau), pp. 197–227. Academic Press, New York, 1968.

Ford, E. H. R., Thurley, K. and Woollam, D. H. M. Electron-microscopic observations on whole human mitotic chromosomes. J. Anat. *103*: 143–150 (1968).

Friedländer, M. and Wahrman, J. The spindle as a basal body distributor: a study in the meiosis of the male silkworm moth, *Bombyx mori*. J. Cell Sci. 7: 65–89 (1970).

Hepler, P. K. and Jackson, W. T. Isopropyl N-phenyl-carbamate affects spindle microtubule orientation in dividing endosperm cells of *Haemanthus Katherinae Baker*. J. Cell Sci. 5: 727–743 (1969).

Hepler, P. K., McIntosh, J. R. and Cleland, S. Intermicrotubule bridges in mitotic spindle apparatus. J. Cell Biol. *45*: 438–444 (1970).

Jokelainen, P. T. The ultrastructure and spatial organization of the metaphase kinetochore in mitotic rat cells. J. Ultrastruct. Res. *19*: 19–44 (1967).

Journey, L. J. and Whaley, A. Kinetochore ultrastructure in vincristine-treated mammalian cells. J. Cell Sci. 7: 49–54 (1970).

Mazia, D. How cells divide. Sci. American *205*: 100–120 (1961).

McIntosh, J. R. and Landis, S. C. The distribution of spindle microtubules during mitosis in cultured human cells. J. Cell Biol. *49*: 468–497 (1971).

Reith, E. J. and Jokelainen, P. T. Cytokinesis in the stratum intermedium of the rat molar enamel organ. J. Ultrastruct. Res. *42*: 51–64 (1973).

Robbins, E. and Gonatas, N. K. The ultrastructure of a mammalian cell during the mitotic cycle. J. Cell Biol. *21*: 429–263 (1964).

Robbins, E. and Jentzsch, G. Ultrastructural changes in the mitotic apparatus at the metaphase-to-anaphase transition. J. Cell Biol. *40*: 678–691 (1969).

Roos, U.-P. Light and electron microscopy of rat kangoroo cells in mitosis. Chromosma *40*: 43–82 (1973).

3 Epithelia

GENERAL CONSIDERATIONS

The outer surfaces of the body and the inner surfaces of body cavities, tubes, and sacs are covered and lined by cells derived from ectoderm and endoderm and are collectively referred to as **epithelial cells.** The component cells of the epithelia of the body are arranged differently in different parts of the body. This chapter gives an overview of the organization of the several types of epithelium. Cells with special function, secretory cells, may occur within the epithelium, or may form evaginations of and accumulations beneath the epithelial surface as distinct organs or glands. This type of epithelial specialization is described on p. 78 in Chapter 4 on glands.

The epithelium is an avascular tissue which consists of one or several layers of cells. A **basement membrane** forms a support for the epithelium and connects it to the underlying connective tissue. The epithelial cells are geometrically quite regular, having the shape of flat polygons, cubes, or polygonal cylinders. Epithelial cells are held together by the stickiness characteristic of all cells, and by cohesive forces between the parallel surfaces of adjacent cells. In addition, the cell membrane has areas of specialization which provide for firm attachment between neighboring epithelial cells.

The epithelial cells which border on the free surface of epithelia are modified according to the local functional demands. Dry surfaces of the body are generally provided with flat, cornified (keratinized) cells which can resist abrasion and protect the epithelial surface. The keratinization process is described on p. 482. Moist surfaces of the mouth and esophagus also have flat cells, but they are usually not cornified. Surfaces of the respiratory passages have cilia, motile hair-like processes which keep a superficial film of moisture and mucus moving. Absorptive and secretory surfaces of the intestinal and reproductive tracts are provided with numerous minute cell processes, the microvilli, which increase the cell surface and participate in exchange processes across the epithelium. The ultrastructure of microvilli and cilia is described on p. 18.

From a functional point of view, epithelia serve as protection of the body against damaging factors such as abrasion, microorganisms, and excessive loss of heat and moisture. Epithelia also participate in exchange processes between the outside world and the inner tissue environment. In the case of the cardiovascular system,

Fig. 3-1. Simple *squamous* epithelium (flat face). Mesothelium of mesentary. Silver impregnation. Rat. L.M. × 1100. **1.** Nuclei of mesothelial cells. **2.** Cell borders, enhanced by silver salts. **3.** Nucleus of connective tissue cell underneath the mesothelium.

Fig. 3-2. Simple *squamous* and *cuboidal* epithelia. Cross section of nephrons in outer medullary zone of rat kidney. The magnification is too low to show subtle differences between the two types of epithelia. It does show the difference in height of cells which line the various tubules. Kidney. Rat. E.M. × 620. **1.** Squamous epithelium. **2.** Low cuboidal epithelium. **3.** Cuboidal epithelium.

Fig. 3-3. Simple *squamous* epithelium. Parietal layer of Bowman's capsule. Renal corpuscle. Kidney. Rat. E.M. × 2100. **1.** Nuclei of squamous epithelial cells. **2.** Urinary space of Bowman's capsule. **3.** Lumina of glomerular blood capillaries. **4.** Nuclei of podocytes.

Fig. 3-4. *Squamous* epithelial cell (endothelium). Venous sinus (lacuna). Corpus cavernosum penis. Rat. E.M. × 10,000. **1.** Lumen of sinus. **2.** Nucleus. **3.** Centriole. **4.** Mitochondrion. **5.** Gap-junctions. **6.** Basal lamina.

Fig. 3-5. Transition between *low squamous* and *high squamous* simple epithelium. Hairpin turn of Henle's loop. Entire turn shown in Fig. 32-18. Nephron. Kidney. Rat. E.M. × 1300. **1.** Lumen of tubule. **2.** Nuclei of low squamous epithelial cells. **3.** Nuclei of cells changing from low to high squamous shape. **4.** Nuclei of high squamous cells. **5.** Arrows indicate approximate points of interdigitation between adjacent cells.

Fig. 3-6. *Low cuboidal* cell of simple cuboidal epithelium. Cortical collecting tubule. Kidney. Rat. E.M. × 4700. **1.** Nucleus. **2.** Cell borders. **3.** Lumen of tubule.

Fig. 3-7. *Cuboidal* cells of simple cuboidal epithelium. Bile ductule. Liver. Rat. E.M. × 10,000. **1.** Lumen of ductule. **2.** Nuclei of cuboidal cells. **3.** Cell bodies. **4.** Basal lamina.

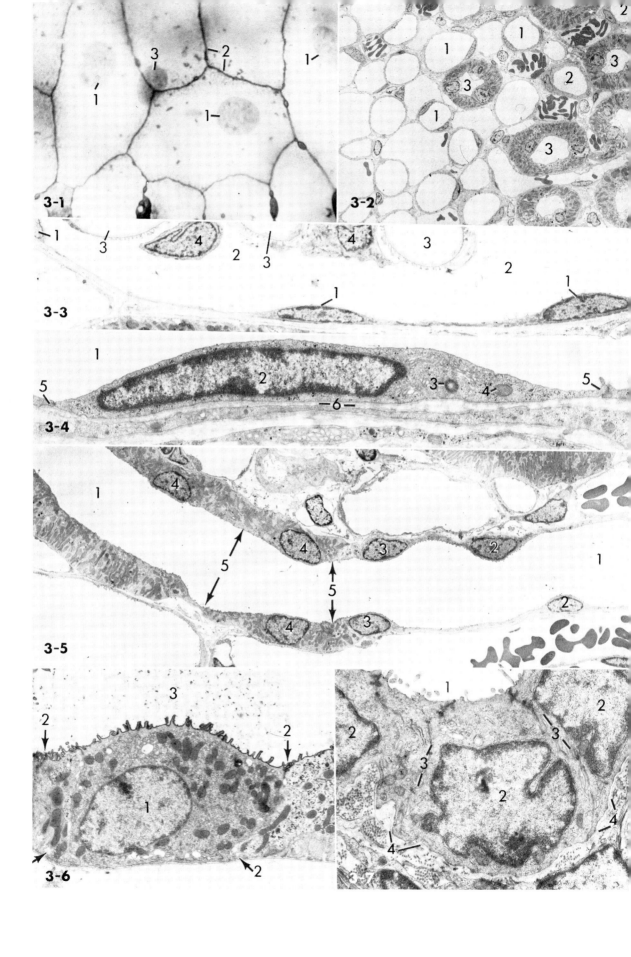

it participates in the exchange between the blood of the vascular channels and the surrounding tissue, at times creating a barrier (central nervous system), at other times providing for an easy exchange (liver sinusoids).

TYPES OF EPITHELIA

The epithelia of the human body can be classified according to several criteria: 1) number of cell layers; 2) shape of outermost cells; 3) type of cell processes of outermost cells; and 4) physicochemical properties of outermost cells. This classification is helpful to the student at the beginning of his studies of cells and tissues. However, the varied structures and functions of epithelia will become meaningful only when they are studied in their specific environment and in relation to the different functional systems of the body. Because of this, the description of the several types of epithelia is kept short.

NUMBER OF CELL LAYERS

A **simple** epithelium consists of one layer of cells in which all cells contact the basement membrane. A **stratified** epithelium consists of two or more layers of cells in which only the cells of the basal layer contact the basement membrane. In a **pseudostratified** epithelium, all cells contact the basement membrane, but all do not reach the surface of the epithelium.

SHAPE OF OUTERMOST CELLS

The shape of the cells in a simple epithelium or the shape of the cells in the outermost cell layer in a stratified epithelium gives the name to the epithelium. A **squamous** epithelium consists of cells which are flat with irregular or multiangular shape. A **cuboidal** epithelium has cells which are as wide as they are high, whereas in a **columnar** epithelium, the cells are higher than they are wide. There are also all kinds of intermediate sizes and shapes, such as thin or thick squamous, low or high cuboidal, and low or high columnar.

TYPE OF CELL PROCESSES

The presence or absence of cilia on the free surface of the outermost cells determines the further classification of epithelia into **ciliated** and **non-ciliated** types.

PROPERTIES OF OUTERMOST CELLS

This pertains only to stratified squamous epithelia, which can be subdivided into **keratinized** and **non-keratinized** types. The outermost cells of these epithelia may, or may not, be keratinized. The keratinization process entails, among other things, the replacement of the nucleus and almost all cell organelles with densely packed keratin filaments.

SIMPLE SQUAMOUS EPITHELIUM

The component cells are thin and flat with only the centrally placed nucleus causing a slight cellular bulge toward the free surface. The cells are irregularly diamond-shaped and held together by junctional complexes. The apposed cell membranes can be made visible in light microscope preparations by silver impreg-

Fig. 3-8. Simple *columnar* epithelium (height 19 μ). Collecting duct. Kidney. Rat. E.M. X 5000. **1.** Lumen of tubule. **2.** Short microvilli. **3.** Junctional complexes. **4.** Nuclei of columnar epithelial cells. **5.** Intercellular space. **6.** Basal lamina.

Fig. 3-9. Simple *columnar* epithelium (height 55 μ). Absorptive epithelial cells. Small intestine. Rat. E.M. X 2300. **1.** Gut lumen. **2.** Striate border (long microvilli). **3.** Junctional complexes. **4.** Nuclei of tall columnar epithelial cels. **5.** Intercellular spaces. **6.** Basal lamina.

Fig. 3-10. Simple *columnar* ciliated epithelium (height 28 μ including cilia). Tertiary bronchus. Lung. Rat. E.M. X 3200. **1.** Lumen of bronchus. **2.** Cilia. **3.** Nuclei of ciliated columnar cells. **4.** Nuclei of mucous cells. **5.** Basal lamina. **6.** Nuclei of fibroblasts in subepithelial connective tissue.

Fig. 3-11. *Pseudostratified columnar* epithelium (height 45 μ). Duct of epididymis. Rat. E.M. X 2200. **1.** Lumen of duct. **2.** Stereocilia. **3.** Junctional complexes. **4.** Large Golgi zones. **5.** Nuclei of columnar cells. **6.** Nuclei of basal cells. **7.** Basal lamina. **8.** Nuclei of connective tissue cells.

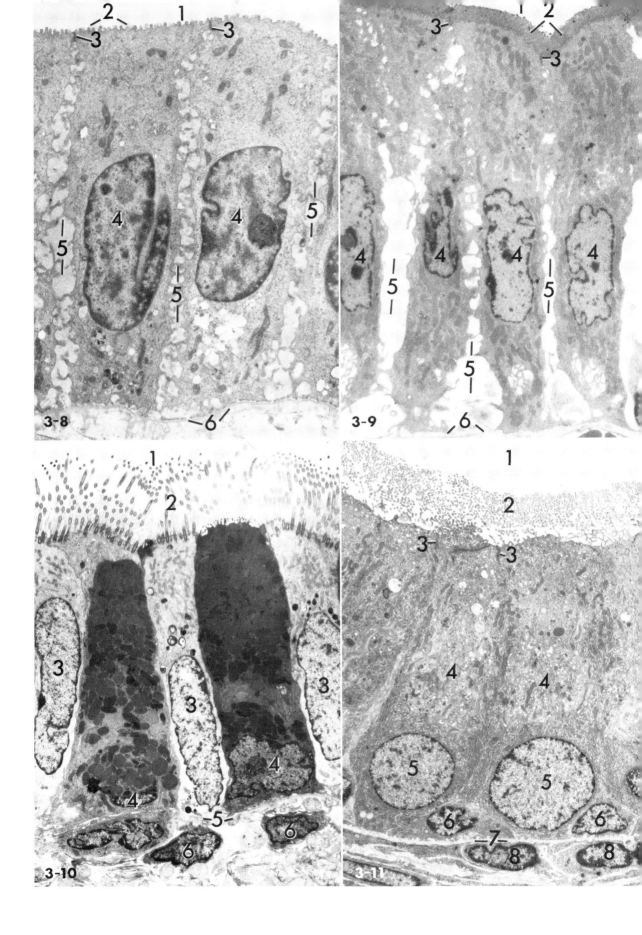

nation. (Fig. 3-1) This type of epithelium occurs in some parts of the nephron (glomerular capsule, Fig. 3-3; and thin segment of Henle's loop, Fig. 3-2). It lines the walls of blood vessels and the heart chambers under the name of **endothelium** (Fig. 3-4), and the peritoneal, pleural and pericardial cavities as **mesothelium.** (Fig. 3-1) A very special type of epithelium consists of high squamous cells. This epithelium is encountered in the proximal and distal tubules of the nephron. (Fig. 3-5) Lateral cell borders are difficult to resolve in light microscope preparations, since the sides of adjacent cells interlock closely in a complicated system of grooves and ridges, revealed only by electron microscopy. All simple squamous epithelia are non-ciliated.

SIMPLE CUBOIDAL EPITHELIUM

The component cells are usually polyhedrons held together by junctional complexes near the epithelial surface. The nucleus is round and placed centrally in the cell. Short microvilli are usually present at the free surface. **Non-ciliated** simple cuboidal epithelium occurs in the collecting tubules of the kidney (Fig. 3-6), in some parts of ducts of salivary glands, in the choroid plexus, in the thyroid follicles, in the terminal respiratory bronchioles, in the bile ducts (Fig. 3-7), and on the surface of the ovary. **Ciliated** cuboidal cells occur in the terminal bronchioles and in the ependymal lining of the ventricular system of the brain. Most secretory cells of endocrine glands and liver (being of epithelial origin) often have a polyhedral shape, but are mentioned here only in passing since they do not form a simple epithelium in the majority of glands; they are dealt with separately in the chapter on glands (p. 78).

SIMPLE COLUMNAR EPITHELIUM

The cells of this kind of epithelium are prismatic, tall multiangular or round columns, held together by junctional complexes near the epithelial surface. The

nucleus is oval and usually located in the basal one-third of the cell. Many of the cells of simple columnar epithelium are provided with numerous, long microvilli, stereocilia, or cilia. **Non-ciliated** simple columnar epithelium is the prevalent type in the stomach and the intestines. (Fig. 3-9) It also occurs in the large collecting ducts of the kidney (Fig. 3-8), in the striated ducts of the salivary glands, and in the gallbladder. Some cells are glandular in nature, forming the secretory surface epithelium of the stomach or the secretory acini of salivary glands and the pancreas, in the latter cases assuming a pyramidal rather than a columnar shape. **Ciliated** simple columnar epithelium occurs in the tertiary bronchi (Fig. 3-10), the oviducts, and the uterus.

PSEUDOSTRATIFIED COLUMNAR EPITHELIUM

This type of epithelium is characterized by tall cells with oval nuclei. The basal

Fig. 3-12. *Stratified squamous non-keratinized* epithelium. Esophagus. Cat. L.M. X 200. **1.** Lumen of esophagus. **2.** Stratified squamous epithelium. **3.** Lamina propria. **4.** Connective tissue papillae.

Fig. 3-13. Stratified squamous non-keratinized epithelia. Enlargement of area similar to rectangle in Fig. 3-12. Esophagus. Cat. E.M. X 1600. **1.** Lumen. **2.** Superficial squamous cell being sloughed. **3.** Nuclei of squamous cells. **4.** Nucleus of cell changing from polyhedral to squamous shape. **5.** Nucleus of polyhedral cell. **6.** Nucleus of cuboidal basal cell. **7.** Basal lamina.

Fig. 3-14. *Stratified squamous keratinized* epithelium. Epidermis. Human (Negro). E.M. X 640. **1.** Skin surface. **2.** Stratified squamous epithelium **3.** Dermis.

Fig. 3-15. Stratified squamous keratinized. epithelium. Enlargement of area similar to rectangle in Fig. 3-14. Skin. Human (Negro). E.M. X 1800. **1.** Surface of skin. **2.** Stratum corneum: keratinized squamous cells. **3.** Thin stratum granulosum. **4.** Nucleus of squamous non-keratinized cell. **5.** Intercellular space with cell processes attached by desmosomes. **6.** Nuclei of polyhedral cells in stratum spinosum. **7.** Cuboidal basal cells. **8.** Basal lamina. **9.** Melanosomes (pigment granules.).

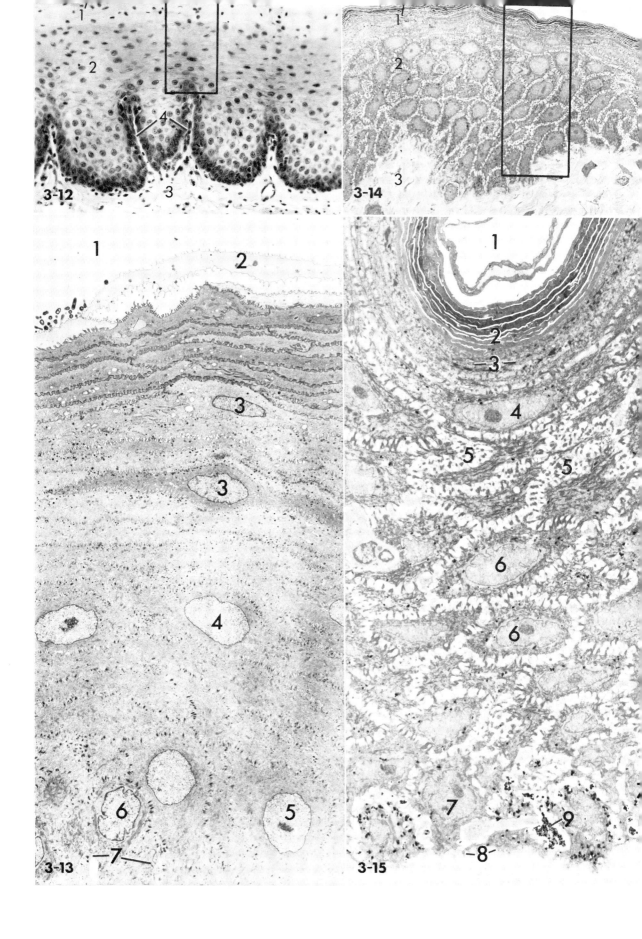

3-12

3-14

3-13

3-15

part of the cell tapers off as it approaches its contact with the basement membrane. The apical surface is provided with microvilli, stereocilia, or cilia. Between the basal ends of the columnar cells occur small polyhedral or conical cells with round nuclei. The basal cells rest against the basement membrane. **Non-ciliated** pseudostratified columnar epithelium occurs in parts of the male urethra, excretory ducts of many glands, the ductus epididymis (Fig. 3-11), and the ductus deferens. In the latter two examples, stereocilia are prominent. **Ciliated** pseudostratified columnar epithelium occurs in the nasal cavity, trachea, primary and secondary bronchi.

STRATIFIED SQUAMOUS EPITHELIUM

In the stratified squamous epithelia, there are three or more cell layers, of which the most superficial layer consists of cells which are squamous. The cells of the basal layer are columnar or polyhedral, and the intermediate layers consist of polyhedral cells. Numerous desmosomes establish firm attachment points between cells of the basal and intermediate cell layers. The cells of the superficial layers of non-keratinized stratified squamous epithelium are not as firmly attached, the number of desmosomes decreases, cells become detached and are sloughed. The cells of the superficial layers of keratinized, stratified squamous epithelium become filled with keratin filaments which obscure or replace other cell organelles and the nucleus. The attachment of the keratinized cells is secured not only by desmosomes but also by an intercellular, proteinaceous material, and an increase in the diameter of the cell membrane. The number of keratinized cell layers varies greatly, depending on location and presence or absence of abrasive forces.

Non-keratinized squamous stratified epithelia occur in the cornea, epiglottis, vocal folds, parts of the mouth, esophagus (Figs. 3-12 and 3-13), intermediate zone of the anal canal, vagina, female urethra,

and fossa navicularis of the male urethra. The keratinized type prevails in the epidermis (Figs. 3-14, 3-15), but occurs also in certain parts of the mouth (hard palate, filiform papillae of the tongue).

STRATIFIED CUBOIDAL EPITHELIUM

This is a rare type of epithelium in which the superficial layer of cells consists of cuboidal cells which are mostly non-ciliated. The number of cell layers, all consisting of polyhedral cells, varies from 3 to 10. The stratified cuboidal epithelium occurs in the ducts of sweat glands, sebaceous glands, pars cavernosa of the male urethra (Fig. 3-18), and the seminiferous tubules of the testis. (Fig. 3-17)

STRATIFIED COLUMNAR EPITHELIUM

This is also a rare type of epithelium. The cells of the superficial layer are columnar, often provided with cilia. The underlying layers consist of polyhedral (cuboidal) cells. The stratified columnar epithelium occurs in some parts of the ducts of salivary (Fig. 3-16) and mammary glands, pharynx, larynx, and male urethra. As a rule the stratified cuboidal or columnar epithelia are present where simple columnar and pseudostratified columnar epithelia border on a stratified squamous epithelium.

Fig. 3-16. *Stratified columnar* epithelium. Interlobular duct. Sublingual salivary gland. Monkey. L.M. X 665. **1.** Lumen of duct. **2.** Microvilli. **3.** Surface layer of columnar cells. **4.** Middle layer of cuboidal cells. **5.** Layer of basal cuboidal cells. **6.** Basement membrane.
Fig. 3-17. *Stratified cuboidal* epithelium. Seminiferous tubule. Testis. Rat. E.M. X 680. **1.** Lumen. **2.** Layer of early spermatids. **3.** Layers of primary spermatocytes. **4.** Layer of spermatogonia. **5.** Basal lamina.
Fig. 3-18. *Stratified cuboidal* epithelium. Urethra. Rat. E.M. X 5000. **1.** Lumen of urethra. **2.** Short microvilli. **3.** Nuclei of low cuboidal surface cells. **4.** Nuclei in several layers of cuboidal cells. **5.** Basal lamina. **6.** Nuclei of fibroblasts in subepithelial connective tissue.

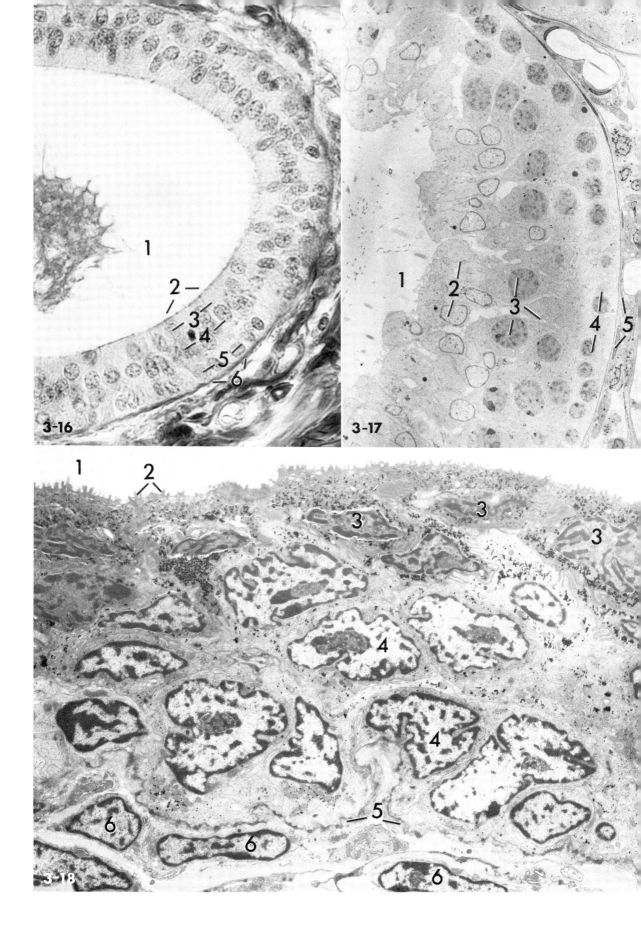

3-16

3-17

3-18

TRANSITIONAL EPITHELIUM

This epithelium lines the ureter (Fig. 3-20), the urinary bladder (Fig. 3-19), and certain restricted parts of the male and female urethra. It is a stratified epithelium in which the superficial cells are either cuboidal or flat, very much depending on the degree of distention of the cavity or tube lined by the epithelium. The superficial cells are always non-ciliated. There are only 2–3 cell layers in the distended epithelium, but 5–10 in the non-distended or collapsed transitional epithelium. The cells of the basal and intermediate cell layers are always poly-hedral with a round nucleus, whereas the superficial cells contain numerous discoid vesicles.

RENEWAL OF EPITHELIAL CELLS

In **simple** epithelia where there is only one layer of cells, replacement and renewal of epithelial cells take place through mitotic activity among the component cells. (Fig. 3-21) In **stratified** epithelia, where there are several cell layers, the cells of the basal layer serve as "stem" cells. By mitotic activity, newly formed cells move to the cell layers above, and undergo maturation as they change in shape, composition of cellular structures, and function. The oldest and most mature cells are therefore those which form the superficial cell layer. It is also from this layer that cells are lost as a result of sloughing, wear and tear, or simply because they reached the end of their life span.

INTERCELLULAR ATTACHMENT

Cells of simple epithelia are held together near the apical surface by **junctional complexes,** in many earlier textbooks referred to as **terminal bars.** They consist of specialized regions of the cell membrane, in which apposing cell membranes have either fused (**tight junction**) or are separated by a 20 Å intercellular gap (**gap-junction**) or by a 200 Å-gap filled with glycoprotein material (**intermediate junc-**

tion). Cells of stratified epithelia may also be provided with similar junctional complexes. However, more often, the attachment is secured by multiple point junctions (**desmosomes**) in which apposing cell membranes are reinforced by intercellular fibrillar material, and the intercellular gap is filled with lamellar material, probably glycoprotein. A more detailed description of the several specializations of the cell membrane is given on p. 12.

BASEMENT MEMBRANE

Epithelia rest on a basement membrane which also represents the line of separation between the epithelium and underlying connective tissue. There is no basement membrane under the ependymal lining of the ventricular system of the brain. The basement membrane consists of a thin **basal lamina,** about 300–700 Å in diameter, and a network of **reticular fibrils,** the fibrils averaging 300 Å in diameter. The network occupies a space of about 0.1–2 μ, and blends with other connective tissue fibrils of larger diameter. The basal lamina is rich in mucopolysaccharides and amino acids, similar in com-

Fig. 3-19. *Transitional* epithelium. Collapsed urinary bladder. Human. L.M. X 640.
1. Lumen. **2.** Superficial cells. **3.** Intermediate cell layers. **4.** Basal cell layer. **5.** Level of basement membrane. **6.** Subepithelial connective tissue.

Fig. 3-20. *Transitional* epithelium. Ureter. Rat. E.M. X 20,000. **1.** Lumen. **2.** Nucleus of large umbrella-like surface cell. Cytoplasm is filled with a multiude of flat, discoid vesicles. **3.** Nuclei of cuboidal cells of intermediate cell layers. **4.** Cuboidal basal cells. **5.** Level of basal lamina. **6.** Blood capillaries in subepithelial connective tissue.

Fig. 3-21. Renewal of cells in simple squamous epithelium (endothelium) during vascular growth. Postcapillary venule. Uterus. Rat. E.M. X 4000. **1.** Lumen of venule. **2.** Erythrocyte. **3.** Nuclei of endothelial cells. **4.** Nucleus of pericyte. **5.** Nucleus of fibroblast. **6.** Endothelial cell in late anaphase of mitotic division. **7.** Chromosomes. **8.** Centrioles. **9.** Cleavage furrow.

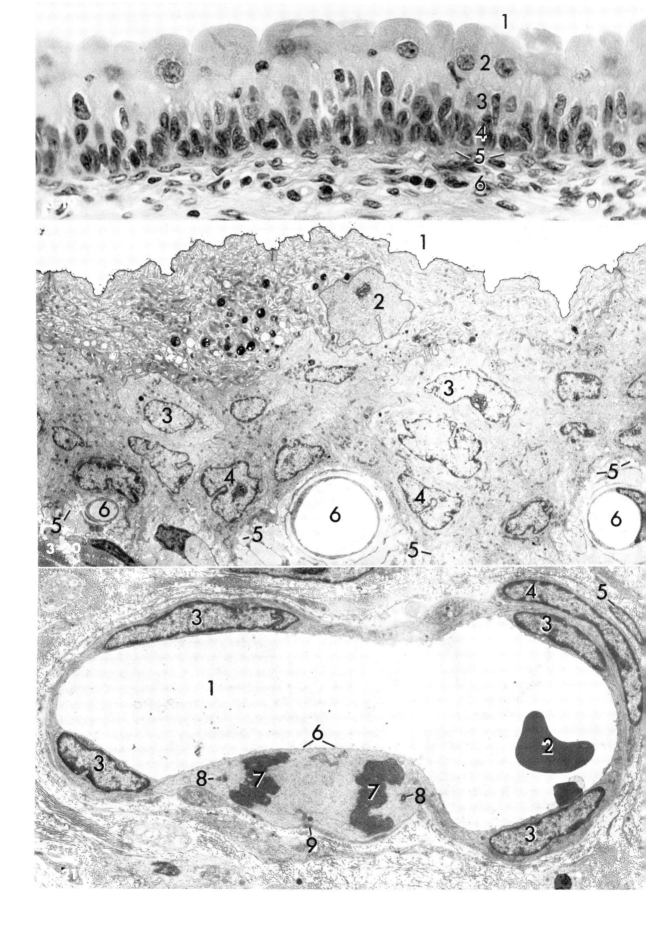

position to that of collagen. The reticular fibrils are essentially delicate collagenous fibrils. It is very likely that the basal lamina is formed by the basal epithelial cells, and that the reticular fibrils are formed by the fibroblasts of the connective tissue underneath the basement membrane.

A more complete description of the basement membrane and its functions appears on p. 178.

References

Adams, D. R. Olfactory and non-olfactory epithelia in the nasal cavity of the mouse. Am. J. Anat. *133*: 37–50 (1972).

Baradi, A. F. and Hope, J. Observations on ultrastructure of rabbit mesothelium. Expt. Cell Res. *34*: 33–44 (1964).

Bertalanffy, F. D. and Nagy, K. P. Mitotic activity and renewal rate of the epithelial cells of human duodenum. Acta. Anat. *45*: 362–370 (1961).

Clermont, Y. The cycle of the seminiferous epithelium in man. Am. J. Anat. *112*: 35–52 (1963).

Clyman, M. J. Electron microscopy of the human fallopian tube. Fertil. & Steril. *17*: 281–301 (1966).

Kurtz, S. M. The fine structure of the lamina densa. Lab. Investig. *10*: 1189–1208 (1961).

Leblond, C. P., Greulich, R. C. and Pereira, J. P. M. Relationship of cell formation and cell migration in the renewal of stratified squamous epithelia. *In* Advances in the Biology of the Skin. (Eds. W. Montagna and R. E. Billingham). Vol. *5*: 39–67. Pergamon Press, New York 1964.

Lipkin, M., Sherlock, P. and Bell, B. Cell proliferation kinetics in the gastrointestinal tract of man. Gastroenterology *45*: 721–729 (1963).

Monis, B. and Zambrano, D. Transitional epithelium of urinary tract in normal and dehydrated rats. Z. Zellforsch. *85*: 165–182 (1968).

Niemi, M. The fine structure and histochemistry of the epithelial cells of the rat vas deferens. Acta Anat. *60*: 207–219 (1965).

Parakkal, P. F. An electron microscopic study of esophageal epithelium in the newborn and adult mouse. Am. J. Anat. *121*: 175–196 (1967).

Pierce, G. B., Jr., Midgley, A. R. and Sri Ram, J. The histogenesis of basement membranes, J. Expt. Med. *117*: 339–348 (1963).

Piezzi, R. S., Santolaya, R. S. and Bertini, F. The fine structure of endothelial cells of toad arteries. Anat. Rec. *165*: 229–236 (1969).

Rhodin, J. A. G. Ultrastructure and function of the human tracheal mucosa. Am. Rev. Resp. Dis. *93*: 1–15 (1966).

Smith, B. G. and Brunner, E. K. The structure of the human vaginal mucosa in relation to the menstrual cycle and to pregnancy. Am. J. Anat. *54*: 27–86 (1934).

Zelickson, A. S. (ed.) Ultrastructure of Normal and Abnormal Skin. Lea & Febiger, Philadelphia, 1967.

4 Glands

Glands are derivatives and invaginations of epithelial surfaces of the body. In the broad sense, glands can be characterized as **one or several** epithelial cells which are engaged in synthesis, storage, and discharge of secretory products. From a functional point of view, glands are divided into two categories: 1) endocrine glands and 2) exocrine glands. The **endocrine** glands do not have a duct system. Their secretory products (hormones) are delivered to the interstitial fluid, and from there diffuse into lymphatics and blood capillaries. The hormones are chemical substances which are carried by the bloodstream to other parts of the body where they influence the activities of various cells. The **exocrine** glands do have a duct system, and the secretory products (for instance, enzymes, mucus, bile, sweat, sebum) emerge onto a body surface. The secretory products of the exocrine glands participate in a great variety of body functions such as digestion, water-salt balance, and protection of internal and external body surfaces. The various endocrine and exocrine glands are described separately in detail elsewhere in this book. The following is a discussion of some general and some specific characteristics of glands and the secretory processes.

Varieties of Glands

ENDOCRINE GLANDS

In some instances, **single cells** with endocrine functions are present in various areas of the body. Examples are the several types of enterochromaffin and argyrophil cells in the mucous membrane and glands of the stomach (Fig. 38-20), the intestines (Fig. 29-16), the paraganglia (p. 464), the parafollicular cells of the thyroid gland (Fig. 21-6), and the epithelial cells of the placentar villi.

Most endocrine glands are **reticular** in nature. They consist of polyhedral cells which form clumps, cords, and plates supported by delicate collagenous fibrils and permeated by a rich capillary network.

To this group belong the pituitary (p. 428), pineal body (p. 468), parathyroid glands (p. 450), pancreatic islets of Langerhans (p. 600), adrenal glands (p.456), corpora lutea of the ovary (p. 712), and the interstitial cells of Leydig in the testis (p. 676).

There are two instances where the endocrine glands are **follicular** in nature: the thyroid gland (p. 442) and the ovarian follicles (p. 706). Here, the endocrine cells form rounded vesicular groups of cells. The secretory products are temporarily collected in the central cavity of each follicle. The secretions are subsequently transported to the perifollicular capillaries across the same endocrine cells that were responsible for their synthesis in the first place.

A **special kind** of endocrine secretion takes place in neurons and their derivatives. This aspect of neuronal activity has been explored and elucidated only recently. The medullary cells of the adrenal glands (p. 462) are modified nerve cells with pronounced endocrine activity. Hypothalamic neurons synthesize secretory granules which are passed along their

Fig. 4-1. *Unicellular* exocrine mucous gland. Goblet cell. Large intestine. Rat. E.M. X 6000. **1.** Connective tissue of lamina propria. **2.** Basal lamina. **3.** Tapered base of goblet cell. **4.** Intercellular space. **5.** Nucleus of mucous (goblet) cell. **6.** Nucleus of absorptive epithelial cell. **7.** Golgi zone. **8.** Goblet (apical part of cell) filled with mucigen droplets. **9.** Apex of mucous cell. **10.** Microvilli of absorptive cell. **11.** Lumen of gut. Areas similar to rectangles (A) and (B) are enlarged in Figs. 4-21 and 4-22.

Fig. 4-2. *Simple tubular* straight, non-branching multicellular gland. Crypt of Lieberkühn. Jejunum. Rat. E.M. X 1300. **1.** Lumen of intestinal gland. **2.** Nuclei of mucous cells. **3.** Intracellular accumulation of mucigen droplets. **4.** Nucleus of Paneth cell with secretory granules (proteinaceous secretion). **5.** Nuclei of undifferentiated cells. **6.** Nuclei of apparent absorptive cells. **7.** Undifferentiated cells in varied stages of mitosis. **8.** Connective tissue of lamina propria. **9.** Lumen of capillaries.

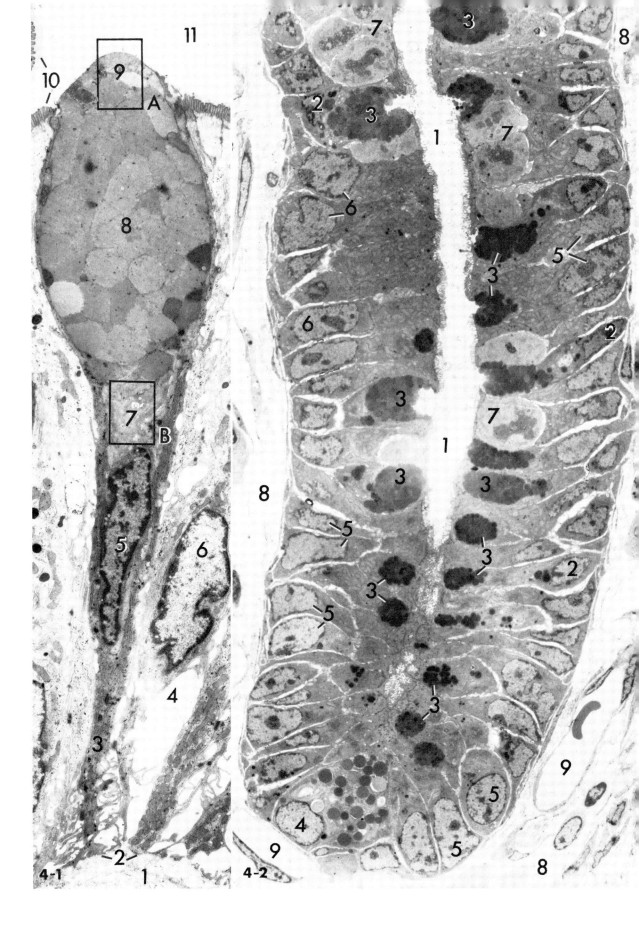

axons and released in the neurohypophysis (p. 000), a process referred to as neurosecretion. All other neurons synthesize and release neurotransmitter substances, either along their axons or at the nerve endings. In the classical sense, these examples of secretion do not belong among glands. However, it is undeniable that these cells synthesize, store, and release products which have endocrine functions.

EXOCRINE GLANDS

Exocrine glands can be divided into 1) unicellular glands and 2) multicellular glands.

Unicellular glands. Single cells with exocrine function are represented by the mucus-producing goblet cells (Fig. 4-1), which occur throughout the epithelial lining of the respiratory (p. 620) and digestive (p. 556) tracts. In several other instances, mucus-producing cells occur side by side within the epithelium, either in small groups (oviduct, p. 720) or as large epithelial sheets (stomach, p. 538).

Multicellular glands. Multicellular exocrine glands are the most numerous type in the mammalian body. They consist of a varied number of secretory cells all of which are located beneath the epithelial lining from which they are derived, and with which they remain in contact via a system of ducts. The multicellular glands vary greatly in size, shape, and cellular composition. For the sake of simplification, and to facilitate memorization—but certainly not based on functional considerations—the following subdivision is found useful by some students: 1) simple multicellular glands; 2) compound multicellular glands.

The **simple multicellular glands** have one non-branching duct and secretory end-pieces that are either tubular or acinar (synonyms: alveolar, shaped like a grape). The simple **tubular** glands can be straight (intestinal crypts of Lieberkühn, Fig. 4-2), coiled (sweat glands, Fig. 4-6), and branched (uterine glands, p. 722; gastric glands, p. 540). The simple **acinar**

glands may be unbranched (seminal vesicle, Fig. 4-3) or branched (sebaceous glands, p. 494). The acini are dilated in the two examples given, and the glands are therefore usually referred to as **saccular.**

The **compound multicellular glands** generally have one main excretory duct which gives rise to several generations of branches. The secretory end-pieces are numerous and can be either tubular, acinar, or a combination of the two, tubulo-

Fig. 4-3. *Simple saccular* coiled, non-branching multicellular gland. Seminal vesicle. Monkey. L.M. X 27. **1.** Main lumen of gland. **2.** Saccular dilatations. **3.** Diverticuli. **4.** Ridges covered by secretory epithelium. **5.** Connective tissue.

Fig. 4-4. *Compound saccular,* multicellular gland. Lactating mammary gland. Human. L.M. X 280. **1.** Branch of terminal duct. **2.** Saccules (distended acini; alveoli). **3.** Simple cuboidal secretory epithelium. **4.** Intralobular connective tissue. **5.** Blood capillary.

Fig. 4-5. Small *compound tubulo-acinar* multicellular gland. Mucous salivary gland. Soft palate. Monkey. L.M. X 92. **1.** Lumen of secretory tubules. **2.** Acinar end-pieces. **3.** Nuclei of mucous cells, flattened against base of cells. **4.** Intralobular connective tissue. **5.** Interlobular connective tissue.

Fig. 4-6. *Simple tubular* coiled, non-branching multicellular gland. Cross section. Odoriferous sweat gland. Human. E.M. X 600. **1.** Lumen. **2.** Simple columnar epithelium, consisting of secretory cells. **3.** Nuclei of secretory cells. **4.** Accumulations of electron-dense granules representing lysosomes (lipofuscin granules). They are not secretory granules in the classical sense. **5.** Cross-sectioned myoepithelial cells appear as regularly spaced, electron-dense profiles at the base of the epithelium. **6.** Peritubular connective tissues. This gland is enlarged further in Figs. 25-58, 25-59, and 25-60.

Fig. 4-7. Simple columnar secretory epithelium in *simple branched tubular* gland. Mucous gland. Cervix of uterus. Human. E.M. X 1800. **1.** Connective tissue elements. **2.** Nuclei of mucous cells. **3.** Mucigen droplets are most numerous in apical part of cell, but also occur below the nucleus. **4.** Lumen of tubule.

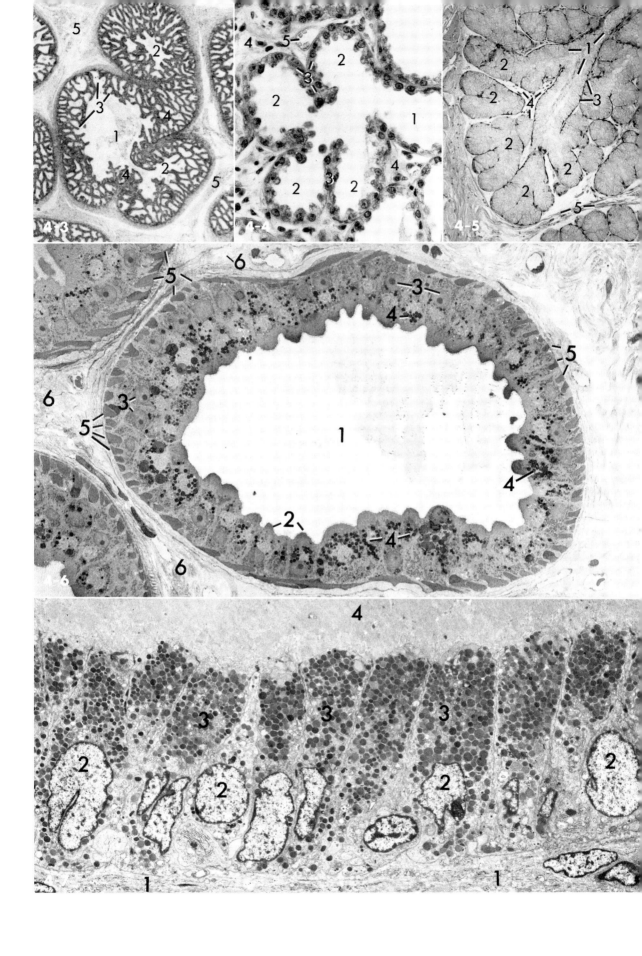

acinar. Examples of compound **tubular** glands are the testis (p. 678) and the kidney (p. 652). Compound **acinar** glands are represented by some of the simple glands of the passages of the respiratory tract (p. 622). A gland with **saccular** end-pieces (dilated acini) is represented by the mammary gland. (Fig. 4-4) **Tubulo-acinar** glands are very common. The terminal parts of the duct system connect with secretory tubules, which in turn, have acinar end-pieces. Examples of this type are the salivary glands (Fig. 4-5 and 4-9), pancreas (p. 596), lacrimal glands, and the large glands of the esophagus and the respiratory tract.

The largest exocrine gland of the body, the liver, develops as a compound tubular gland. It later undergoes a drastic remodeling, and the final arrangement of the secretory epithelial cells does not make it possible to classify the liver either as an acinar or tubular gland.

Organization of Compound Glands

STROMA

Compound glands have a varied amount of connective tissue cells and extracellular fibrils, collectively referred to as **stroma.** Compound exocrine glands are surrounded by a connective tissue **capsule** of varied thickness and fiber density. Extending into the glandular **parenchyma** (collective name for secretory epithelial cells and duct cells) are connective tissue **trabeculae** and **septa** which divide the parenchyma of the larger glands into units called **lobes.** (Fig. 4-8) More delicate connective tissue septa subdivide the lobes into **lobules.** (Fig. 4-9) The lobules are made up of a varied number of secretory tubules and acini which are partly separated from neighboring tubules and acini by a thin **basal** (external) **lamina** and a network of delicate collagenous and reticular fibrils. In small glands, the lobulation is less distinct and the connective tissue septa more delicate.

DUCTS

The **main** duct of compound exocrine glands undergoes multiple dichotomous branching, giving rise to several classes or generations of ducts which vary in length and diameter from gland to gland. The larger ducts travel in the connective tissue septa of the gland, and depending on location, are referred to as either **lobar** (synonym: interlobar), **interlobular,** or **intralobular.** The secretory lumina of the tubules and acini are connected to the intralobular ducts by the smallest segment of the glandular duct system, the **intercalated** ducts. (Fig. 4-13) There is some variation in the height of the epithelial cells which line the different segments of the duct system. In the larger ducts (main duct; lobar ducts; interlobular ducts), the epithelial cells are columnar and arranged in a stratified or pseudostratified fashion. (Figs. 4-11 and 4-15) In the medium-size ducts (end of interlobular ducts; intralobular ducts), the duct epithelium is of the sim-

Fig. 4-8. Large *compound tubulo-acinar* gland. Sublingual salivary (mixed) gland. Human. L.M. X 22. **1.** Connective tissue capsule with some adipose tissue. **2.** Interlobar connective tissue septum. **3.** Lobar (interlobar) arteries. **4.** Interlobular connective tissue septum. **5.** Interlobular ducts. **6.** Dashed line indicates approximate limits of one lobule. **7.** Intralobular ducts.

Fig. 4-9. *Compound tubulo-acinar* gland. Enlargement of area similar to rectangle in Fig. 4-8. Sublingual salivary (mixed) gland. Rat. E.M. X 600. **1.** Lumen of secretory tubule. **2.** Lumen of acinar end-piece. **3.** Serous demilunes. **4.** Lumen of intercalated ducts at point of connection with secretory tubule. **5.** Interlobular connective tissue septum, slightly distended by tissue preparation. **6.** Delicate interacinar connective tissue septa.

Fig. 4-10. Acinar *end-piece*. Enlargement of area similar to rectangle in Fig. 4-9. Sublingual salivary (mixed) gland. Rat. E.M. X 1800. **1.** Acinar lumina. **2.** Accumulation of mucigen droplets. **3.** Nucleus of mucous cells. **4.** Nuclei of serous cells in demilunes. **5.** Secretory granules. **6.** Nucleus of myoepithelial cells. **7.** Interacinar connective tissue septa. **8.** Lumen of blood capillary.

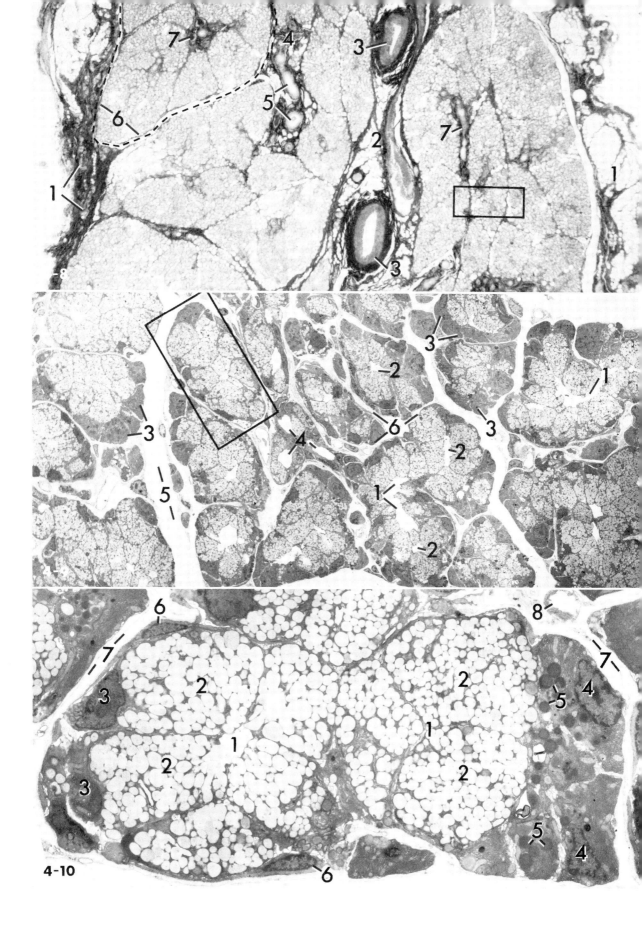

ple columnar or cuboidal types. (Fig. 4-12) In the submandibular and parotid glands (p. 524), the distal parts of the intralobular ducts are referred to as **striated** ducts. (Fig. 4-14) The base of the high columnar duct cells contains striations, oriented perpendicularly to the basal lamina. They are caused by elongated mitochondria and deep infoldings of the basal cell membrane. The intercalated ducts are lined by a low, simple cuboidal epithelium.

SECRETORY END-PIECES

The secretory end-pieces of compound exocrine glands are made up of cells which synthesize a variety of secretions. All exocrine secretory cells have a structural and functional polarity which is not apparent in most endocrine glands. The secretory droplets or granules are always accumulated in the apical part of the cell and discharged at the luminal surface. In the digestive and respiratory tracts, the end-pieces contain cells which synthesize and discharge a mucinous and/or serous solution. Accordingly, some acini may be **mucous,** some **serous** (synonyms: albuminous, zymogenic), and others a mixture of the two, seromucous or **mixed.** In the last case, the serous cells often lie at one end of the acinus as a serous **demilune** (crescent; half-moon) between the mucous cells and the basal lamina. (Fig. 4-10) The serous secretion must then pass in narrow intercellular canaliculi past the mucous cells to reach the lumen of the acinus. In the acinar periphery of some compound glands, myoepithelial cells are interposed between the secretory cells and the basal lamina. These are flat, smooth muscle cells with many long cytoplasmic extensions embracing the acinus. (Figs. 4-10 and 4-13)

Cytology of Secretion

Traditionally, secretory cells are divided according to the physicochemical proper-

ties of their secretory products. Thus, one has classified the secretory cells as mucous, and as cells with other kinds of secretion, including those which occur in endocrine glands, sebaceous glands, and mammary glands. Another way of classifying secretory cells and secretion is according to the means of secretion expulsion, including such categories as merocrine, apocrine, and holocrine secretion.

With improved techniques in biochemistry and cytology, including cytochemistry, histochemistry, radioautography, electron microscopy, and fractionated centrifugation, a better understanding of the synthesis, storage, and release of secretory products has made it possible to simplify the description of the secretory

Fig. 4-11. Lobar (interlobar) duct. Sublingual salivary gland. Human. L.M. × 315. **1.** Lumen with some secretory material. **2.** Stratified columnar epithelium. **3.** Connective tissue of interlobar septum.

Fig. 4-12. Parotid (serous salivary) gland. Human. L.M. × 200. **1.** Interlobular duct with pseudostratified columnar epithelium. **2.** Arteriole. **3.** Interlobular connective tissue with low cuboidal epithelium. **4.** Intralobular duct. **5.** Intercalated duct. **6.** Serous acini. **7.** Fat cells (lipid content dissolved).

Fig. 4-13. Junction between secretory tubule and intercalated duct. Sublingual salivary (mixed) gland. Rat. E.M. × 4800. **1.** Lumen of duct. **2.** Nuclei of cuboidal duct cells. **3.** Mucigen droplets of secretory acinar cells. **4.** Nucleus of myoepithelial cell. **5.** Cytoplasmic processes of myoepithelial cell. **6.** Location of basal lamina (not resolved). **7.** Lumen of blood capillary.

Fig. 4-14. Striated (intralobular) duct. Sublingual salivary (mixed) gland. Rat. E.M. × 1600. **1.** Lumen of duct. **2.** Nuclei of columnar duct cells. **3.** Basal striations (mitochondria and infoldings of cell membrane). **4.** Location of basal lamina (not resolved). **5.** Lumen of capillary.

Fig. 4-15. Interlobular duct. Stratified cuboidal epithelium. Sublingual gland. Rat. E.M. × 1900. **1.** Lumen of duct. **2.** Nucleus of cuboidal surface cells. **3.** Nuclei of cells in intermediate epithelial layer. **4.** Nuclei of basal cells. **5.** Location of basal lamina (not resolved). **6.** Connective tissue of interlobular septum.

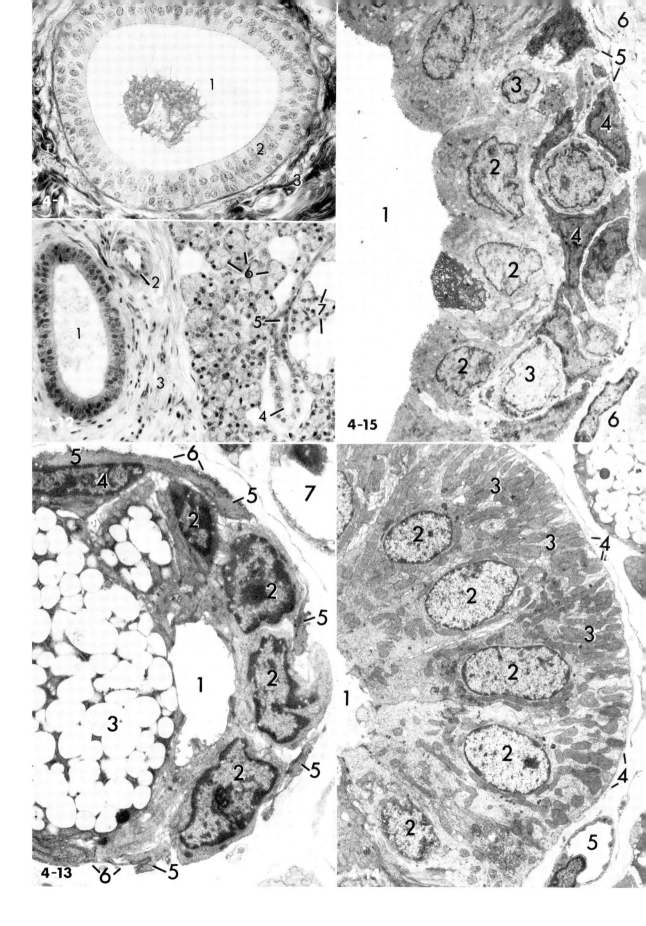

processes, as they take place in a large variety of both exocrine and endocrine glands. The following is an attempt to summarize the present knowledge of the secretory processes according to biochemical, ultrastructural, and radioautographical information.

PROTEINACEOUS SECRETION

Cells which synthesize secretory products of high protein and amino acid content are present both in exocrine and endocrine glands. Examples of exocrine glands are the serous acini of the digestive and respiratory tracts, prostate, seminal vesicle, and mammary glands. Endocrine glands include the pituitary, thyroid gland, parathyroids, pancreatic islets, adrenal medulla, and argentaffin cells of the intestinal tract.

With minor variations, the synthesis, storage, and release of the secretory products engage the following cell structures and processes: polyribosomes, granular endoplasmic reticulum, Golgi zone, secretory granules, and exocytosis. The **granular endoplasmic reticulum** is invariably abundant in the cells of these glands. (Fig. 4-16) The most active sites of amino acid incorporation are the **polyribosomes,** which are ribosomes held together by a thin strand of messenger RNA. The newly formed protein material is freed from the ribosomes and aggregated in the cisternae of the granular endoplasmic reticulum. From the cavities of the cisternae, the protein is transported via **transfer vesicles** to the Golgi zone. These vesicles are formed and pinched off from the cisternae of the granular endoplasmic reticulum. Upon reaching the Golgi zone, the vesicles fuse with the Golgi saccules at the outer, immature (forming) face of the Golgi zone. The content of the vesicles is released into the Golgi saccules. **Condensing vacuoles** and **presecretory granules** are formed from the Golgi saccules by an accumulation of material with increasingly higher electron density (Fig. 4-19), and the formation and separation of these vacuoles from the ends

of the saccules. (Fig. 4-17) Initially, the presecretory granules are less electron dense and more mottled in texture than the mature secretory granules, perhaps because of a higher fluid content.

The mature secretory granules accumulate in the apical portion of exocrine cells, but are present throughout the cytoplasm of most endocrine cells. The discharge of the secretory droplets, containing proteins, protein-rich enzymes, and hormones, occurs through a process of **exocytosis** (synonyms: emiocytosis; **merocrine** secretion). The boundary membrane of the secretory granule fuses with the cell membrane, and the content of the granule is discharged

Fig. 4-16. Proteinaceous secretion. Exocrine gland. Acinar cell. Pancreas. Rat. E.M. X 13,000. **1.** External (basal) lamina. **2.** Granular endoplasmic reticulum. Cisternae are both saccular and vesicular. **3.** Mitochondria. **4.** Nucleus. **5.** Golgi zone. **6.** Condensing vacuoles and presecretory granules. **7.** Mature secretory granule. **8.** Acinar lumen with expelled secretory material. **9.** Cytoplasm of centroacinar cell.

Fig. 4-17. Golgi zone. Enlargement of area similar to rectangle (A) in Fig. 4-16. Acinar cell. Pancreas. Rat. E.M. X 66,000. **1.** Spherical cisterna of granular endoplasmic reticulum with attached ribosomes. **2.** Transfer vesicles. **3.** Golgi saccules. **4.** Bulbous ends of Golgi saccules with medium electron-dense material. **5.** Condensing vacuoles and/or presecretory granules bounded by a distinct membrane. **6.** Mature secretory granules with highly electron-dense material.

Fig. 4-18. Discharge of exocrine secretory granule. *Merocrine* secretion. Apical part of serous acinar cell. Enlargement of area similar to rectangle (B) in Fig. 4-16. Lingual salivary (mixed) gland. Rat. E.M. X 96,000. **1.** Mature secretory granules. **2.** Secretory granule at the moment of discharge through the process of *exocytosis.* Matrix of granule is now less electron-dense than in the unexpelled mature granules. **3.** Boundary membrane of discharging granule. **4.** Lumen of acinus. **5.** Points of fusion between surface cell membrane and granule boundary membrane. **6.** Junctional area of apposed acinar cell membranes.

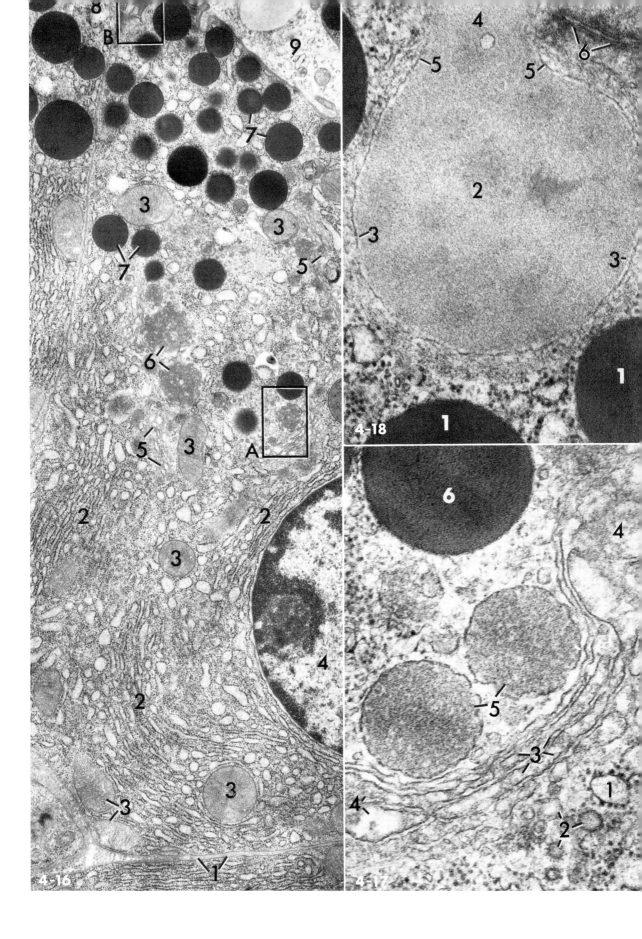

4-16

4-18

4-17

either into the lumen of the acinus (exocrine glands, Fig. 4-18), the cavity of the follicle (thyroid gland), or the interstitial space (most endocrine glands). (Fig. 4-20)

MUCOID SECRETION

Cells which secrete mucins are present in the digestive, respiratory, and reproductive systems. They occur singly as goblet cells, in groups and sheets (stomach, uterus), and as mucous tubules and acini (large intestine, sublingual gland).

Generally, mucus contains a mixture of proteins and sugars (glycoproteins). There is some variation in the chemical composion and reaction of mucins, depending on the location of the cells which produce them. A sulfomucin is produced by the sublingual glands and a sialomucin by the submandibular glands. The surface mucous cells of the stomach contain largely neutral polysaccharides, whereas the mucous neck cells of the gastric glands are characterized by the presence of acid mucopolysaccharides. The secretory products of Brunner's glands in the duodenum and the non-ciliated cells of the oviducts are rich in proteins, which makes them intermediate between mucous and serous secretory cells. The secretory cells of the uterine glands, on the other hand, synthesize a highly viscous product, extremely rich in glycogen. Finally, the mucus produced by the endocervical glands of the uterus is alkaline.

The synthesis and storage of mucigens engage ribosomes, granular endoplasmic reticulum, Golgi zone, and secretory droplets. The **protein moiety** of mucous glycoproteins is synthesized by the ribosomes and the granular endoplasmic reticulum, organelles present in relatively large amounts in the basal region of most mucous cells. The protein material is transported to the Golgi zone as indicated for proteinaceous secretions on p. 86. The **carbohydrate moiety** of mucous glycoproteins is produced within the Golgi zone and linked to the protein there. Presecretory mucigen droplets are formed by the

Golgi saccules (Fig. 4-21) and subsequently separated from this zone. The mucigen droplets gradually increase in size (Fig. 4-21), and they coalesce in most mucous cells as their boundary membrane disintegrates in places. In typical goblet cells the apical part is filled with coalescing mucigen droplets. (Fig. 4-22) In other mucous cells, as for instance the surface cells of the stomach, the mucigen droplets do not coalesce.

The discharge of mucigen droplets occurs in the majority of cases through a process of exocytosis, similar to that which occurs in proteinaceous secretion. The gastric surface cells are exceptions to this rule, since their mucigen droplets have not been seen in a position of being expelled.

Fig. 4-19. Proteinaceous secretion. Endocrine gland. Gonadotroph cell. Adenohypophysis. Rat. E.M. X 51,000. **1.** Mitochondria. **2.** Ribosomes. **3.** Cisternae of granular endoplasmic reticulum. **4.** Golgi zone. **5.** Condensing presecretory material within Golgi saccules. **6.** Mature secretory granules with boundary membrane.

Fig. 4-20. Discharge of endocrine secretory granules. Gonadotroph cell. Adenohypophysis. Rat. E.M. X 93,000. **1.** Mature secretory granules. **2.** Discharging secretory granules. **3.** Points of fusion between boundary membrane of secretory granule and cell membrane. **4.** Cell membrane. **5.** External (basal) lamina of endocrine cell cords. **6.** Basal (external) lamina of blood capillary. **7.** Capillary (sinusoidal) endothelium. **8.** Fenestrations closed by a thin diaphragm. **9.** Capillary lumen.

Fig. 4-21. Mucoid secretion. Mucous (goblet) cell. Enlargement of area similar to rectangle (B) in Fig. 4-1. Tracheal epithelium. Human. E.M. X 33,000. **1.** Golgi zone with saccules. **2.** Transfer vesicles. **3.** Condensing vacuoles. **4.** Presecretory mucigen droplets. **5.** Mucigen droplets. **6.** Mature mucigen droplet with disintegrating boundary membrane.

Fig. 4-22. Discharge of mucoid secretion. Mucous (goblet) cell. Enlargement of area similar to rectangle (A) in Fig. 4-1. Tracheal epithelium. Human. E.M. X 33,000. **1.** Merging mucigen droplets. **2.** Disintegrating boundary membranes. **3.** Surface cell membrane of goblet cell. **4.** Lumen of trachea.

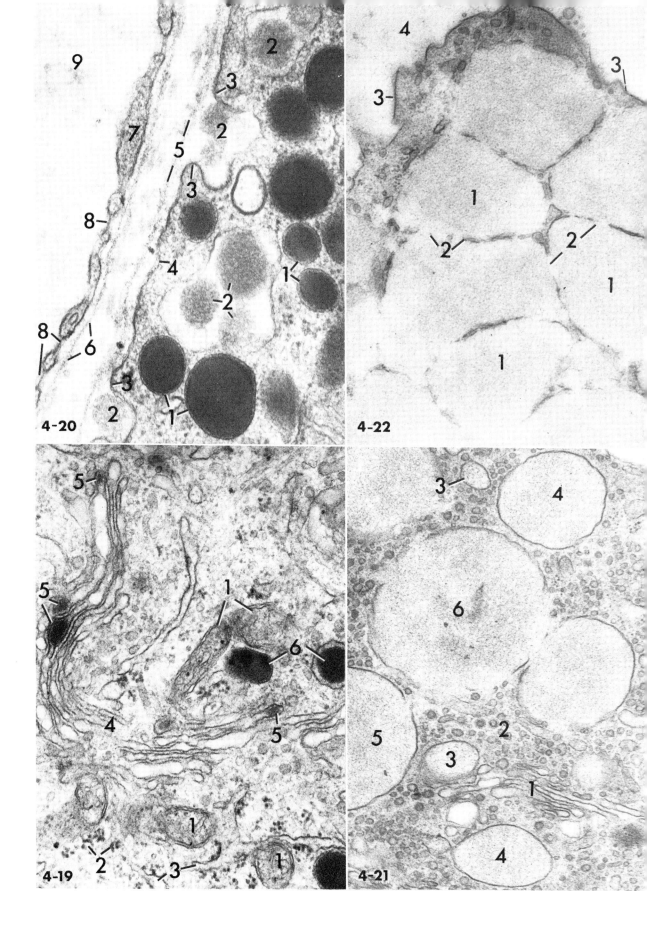

4-20

4-22

4-19

4-21

LIPID SECRETION

The term "lipid secretion" is used here broadly to identify secretory processes which involve the synthesis and storage of fatty acids, triglycerides, cholesterol, and cholesterol esters. Glandular cells involved in lipid secretion are present in mammary glands, sebaceous glands, adrenal cortex, corpora lutea, and interstitial cells of Leydig in the testes.

The synthesis and storage of the secretory products engage the Golgi zone, mitochondria, and the agranular endoplasmic reticulum. Classical secretory granules do not occur, but a varied number of lipid droplets are present.

The initial lipid product appears within Golgi vesicles which enlarge and take the shape of increasingly larger lipid droplets. (Fig. 23-6) Each droplet has a very thin boundary (interface) membrane. As the lipid droplets grow in size, they become surrounded by short profiles of the agranular endoplasmic reticulum. With further enlargement of the lipid droplets, they become closely surrounded by a membranous casing of merging profiles of smooth endoplasmic reticulum. This arrangement of the agranular endoplasmic reticulum in relation to the lipid droplets is typically seen in cells of endocrine glands which synthesize steroid hormones (adrenal cortex, Fig. 23-7, interstitial cells of testis), in sebaceous glands, but only to a limited degree in mammary glands. Interestingly, it is quite prominent in ordinary fat cells during the formation of lipid droplets in these connective tissue cells. (Fig. 7-42)

It is presently not known whether steroid hormones are present in the lipid droplets or in the surrounding agranular endoplasmic reticulum. It is definitely known that the fatty component of the milk is represented by the lipid droplets, and that the secretion of the sebaceous glands, the sebum, consists to a large extent, of merging lipid droplets.

The release of the lipid droplets of the sebaceous gland cells occurs through a process referred to as **holocrine** secretion.

The cells become filled with large lipid droplets. Other cell organelles, including the nucleus, disintegrate, changing the entire cell to a huge drop of sebum which is extruded *in toto*. (Fig. 4-23)

The lipid droplets of the mammary gland cells are discharged at the apical cell surface by a mechanism referred to as **apocrine** secretion. The lipid droplet lifts the cell surface together with a rim of sur-

Fig. 4-23. *Holocrine* secretion. Sebaceous gland. Monkey. E.M. X 5000. **1.** Nucleus of secretory cell, highly compressed. **2.** Irregularly shaped and densely packed sebaceous lipid droplets. **3.** Narrow strands of cytoplasm. This cell is ready to be expelled by a process of holocrine excretion. The entire cell represents a small drop of sebum.

Fig. 4-24. *Apocrine* secretion. Discharge of lipid droplet. Lactating mammary gland. Mouse. E.M. X 10,000. **1.** Nucleus of secretory cell. **2.** Mitochondria. **3.** Granular endoplasmic reticulum. **4.** Small intracellular lipid droplet. **5.** Large lipid droplet at the moment of apocrine discharge. **6.** Thin rim of cell membrane and cytoplasm surrounds the lipid droplet. **7.** Discharged lipid droplet. **8.** Milk protein particles. These are discharged from the secretory cells by a process of merocrine secretion (exocytosis). **9.** Lumen of saccular acinus with finely granular proteinaceous secretion.

Fig. 4-25. *Endoplasmocrine* secretion. Cells of zona fasciculata. Adrenal cortex. Rat. The sequence A–D is arranged to simulate an assumed mechanism of lipid droplet discharge concurrent with steroid hormone release under normal and experimental conditions. (From: Rhodin J. Ultrastruct. Res. 34:23-71 (1971).) Magnifications: A) X 42,000; B) X 62,000; C) X 68,000; D) X 64,000. **1.** Lipid droplet. **2.** Interface membrane: lipid droplet/cytoplasm. **3.** Membranous casing of merging tubules of agranular endoplasmic reticulum. **4.** Cell membrane. **5.** Extracellular (interstitial) space. **6.** Fusion of cell membrane and peripheral lamina of agranular endoplasmic reticulum casing. **7.** Content of lipid droplet has disappeared, leaving behind a membranous ghost. **8.** Membranous ghost enters extracellular space, leaving behind a pit-like invagination of the cell surface. Stages similar to Fig. 4-25 B and C are seen in figs. 23-8 and 23-9 at higher magnification.

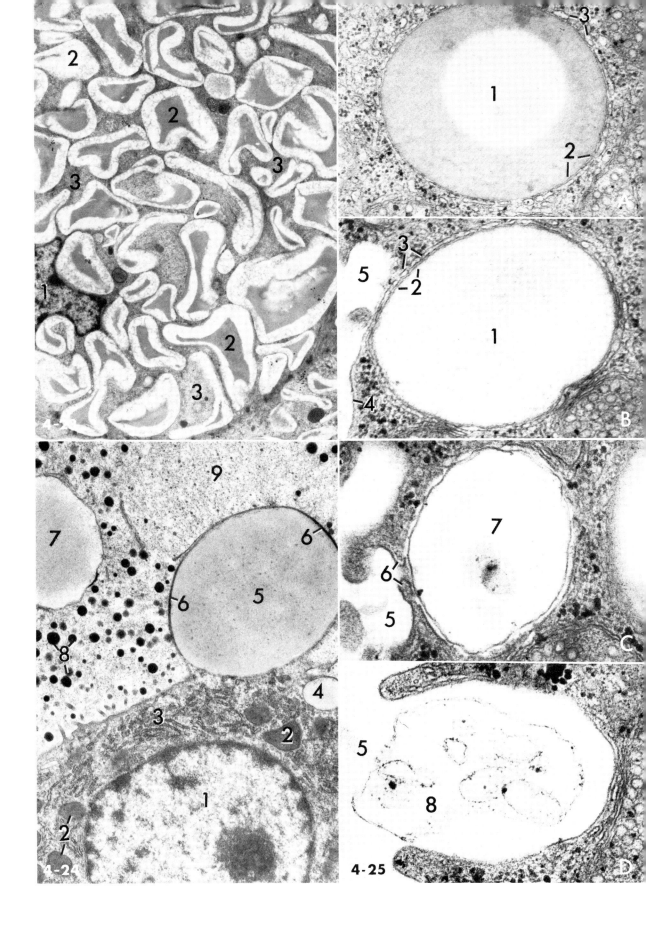

rounding cytoplasm. (Fig. 4-24) At the moment of release, the droplet, the cytoplasmic rim, and the cell membrane break away from the cell surface. The temporarily ruptured cell membrane closes again behind the discharged package.

The lipid droplets of the adrenal cortex cells gradually reach the surface cell membrane. The outer lamina of the casing of the granular endoplasmic reticulum then merges with the cell membrane. Through the opening thus established, the content of the lipid droplet is discharged into the extracellular space. Subsequently, the boundary membrane of the lipid droplet and the inner lamina of the endoplasmic casing are released. The surface of the cell remains invaginated for a short period after the discharge of the lipid droplet. This discharge mechanism seems to represent a compromise between merocrine and apocrine secretions, and has been termed **endoplasmocrine** secretion. (Fig. 4-25)

PHASES OF SECRETION

Most secretory cells are said to go through phases (cycles) of activity and rest. These divisions may be somewhat artificial since they were introduced at a time when glandular activity was measured in terms of number of secretory droplets accumulating in the cell. It is now known that a pronounced cellular activity of protein synthesis precedes the appearance of secretory droplets and granules in the cells which produces a proteinaceous secretion. However, in response to nervous, chemical, and hormonal stimulation, secretory cells will speed up the synthesis and release of their products with a shortening of the time these products are stored in the cell.

References

Freeman, J. A. Goblet cell fine structure. Anat. Rec. *154*: 121–148 (1966).

Hand, A. R. The fine structure of von Ebner's gland of the rat. J. Cell Biol. *44*: 340–353 (1970).

Hokin, L. E. Dynamic aspects of phospholipids during protein secretion. Int. Rev. Cytol. *23*: 187–208 (1968).

Kurosumi, K. Electron microscopic analysis of the secretion mechanism. Int. Rev. Cytol. *XI*: 1–124 (1961).

Moe, H. On goblet cells, especially of the intestine of some mammalian species. Int. Rev. Cytol. *IV*: 299–334 (1955).

Neutra, M. and Leblond, C. P. Synthesis of the carbohydrate of mucus in the Golgi complex as shown by electron microscope radioautography of goblet cells from rats injected with glucose-H^3. J. Cell Biol. *30*: 119–136 (1966).

Palay, S. The morphology of secretion. *In* Frontiers in Cytology (Ed. S. Palay), pp. 305–342, Yale University Press, New Haven, 1958.

Peterson, M. and Leblond, C. Synthesis of complex carbohydrates in the Golgi region, as shown by radioautography after injection of labeled glucose. J. Cell Biol. *21*: 964–974 (1959).

Rhodin, J. A. G. The ultrastructure of the adrenal cortex of the rat under normal and experimental conditions. J. Ultrastruct. Res. *34*: 23–71 (1971).

5 Blood and lymph

GENERAL CONSIDERATIONS

Blood is composed of: 1) freely floating red blood cells (erythrocytes) and white blood cells (granular and non-granular leukocytes); 2) blood platelets (thrombocytes); and 3) plasma. (Fig. 5-1) **Lymph** consists of freely floating cells (lymphocytes) and plasma.

Blood is often regarded as a fluid tissue in which cells are entirely separated from each other by plasma under normal conditions. The blood volume in a healthy male weighing 70 kg amounts to about 5–6 liters. The formed elements constitute 46% of this volume, and the fluid 54%. The proportion of formed elements is used in routine blood tests and is called **hematocrit**. Therefore, the hematocrit in a healthy subject should be 46. The redness of the blood is due to the hemoglobin content of the erythrocytes.

Blood transports oxygen, water, food materials, and products of body metabolism and internal secretion. Blood circulates constantly through the cardiovascular system, and by this circulation the constancy of the internal environment is maintained. The blood is separated from the cells of the body by the wall of the blood vessels. In the capillaries this wall is extremely thin and of variable permeability. Of the formed elements, red blood cells and platelets (Fig. 5-2), do not normally leave the vascular channels except in the splenic pulp. The white blood cells, as a rule, leave the vascular system by traversing the walls of postcapillary venules. Granular leukocytes (Fig. 5-3) can do this in any tissue and organ. Non-granular leukocytes (lymphocytes) do this in lymph nodes (Fig. 5-4) and Peyer's patches of the intestines as part of a constant recirculation of lymphocytes (see p. 392). Monocytes (Fig. 5-6) may leave the lumen of a blood vessel at any time to become macrophages in the interstitial tissue.

PLASMA

Blood **plasma** contains 91% water and 9% solids, among which are found the proteins globulin and albumin, inorganic salts, and organic compounds. In the plasma are dissolved nutritive substances, metabolic waste products, secretions from endocrine cells, enzymes, and antibodies. Blood **serum** is blood plasma freed of one of its proteins, the fibrinogen which participates in the clotting mechanism. The final step in the clotting is the precipitation of fibrin filaments from the precursor, fibrinogen.

LYMPH

Lymph is an intercellular tissue fluid which is drained by lymph capillaries, filtrated through lymph nodes and delivered by lymph vessels to the venous system. Lymph consists of freely floating cells and plasma. The cells consist largely of lymphocytes which average 14,000 per cubic millimeter as compared to 2000 in the same volume of blood. Of the lymphocytes, most are small and about 10% are medium-sized. (Fig. 5-5) Polymorphonu-

Fig. 5-1. Smear preparation of circulating blood cells. Human. L.M. X 350. **1.** Erythrocytes. **2.** Polymorphonuclear leukocytes (neutrophils). **3.** Small lymphocyte. **4.** Monocyte. **5.** Platelets.

Fig. 5-2. Sectioned blood cells in the lumen of blood vessel. Rabbit. E.M. X 4500. **1.** Erythrocytes (biconcave disks, 7 μ in diameter). **2.** Thrombocytes (platelets). **3.** Blood plasma (finely precipitated).

Fig. 5-3. Polymorphonuclear leukocyte (neutrophil, 9 μ in diameter. Bone marrow. Human. E.M. X 9000. **1.** Lobated nucleus. **2.** Specific and azurophilic granules. This neutrophil is further enlarged in Fig. 5-10.

Fig. 5-4. Small lymphocyte (4 μ in diameter) in medullary sinus of lymph node. Cat. E.M. X 10,500. **1.** Nucleolus. **2.** Nucleus. **3.** Cytoplasm. This lymphocyte is further enlarged in Fig. 5-16.

Fig. 5-5. Medium-sized lymphocyte (5.5 μ in diameter) in medullary sinus of lymph node. Cat. E.M. X 10,500. **1.** Nucleoli. **2.** Nucleus. **3.** Cytoplasm. This lymphocyte is enlarged further in Fig. 17-24.

Fig. 5-6. Monocyte (8 μ in diameter). Bone marrow. Human. E.M. X 10,000. **1.** Nucleus. **2.** Nucleolus. **3.** Cytoplasm. **4.** Azurophilic granules. **5.** Mitochondria.

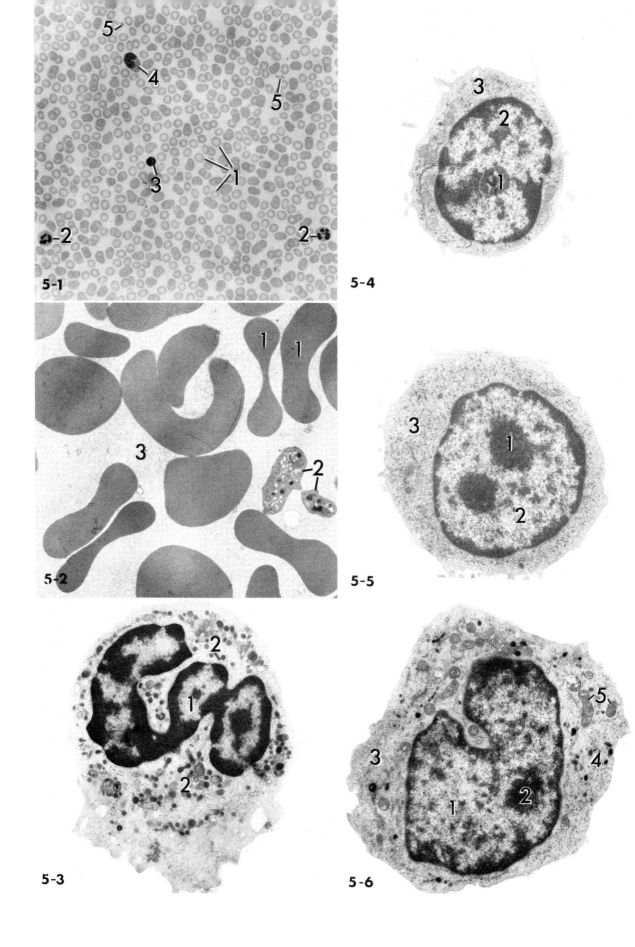

5-1

5-2

5-3

5-4

5-5

5-6

clear leukocytes and erythrocytes are occasionally present, whereas monocytes and macrophages are more frequently found. The content of the lymph plasma varies according to body region. There is more protein and fat in the lymph from the abdomen than in lymph from the extremities. The proteins are the same as in blood plasma but only half the amount.

FORMED ELEMENTS

To this category belong red blood cells (erythrocytes and reticulocytes), white blood cells (granular leukocytes, lymphocytes, monocytes), and platelets (thrombocytes).

Erythrocytes. There are about 5.4 million erythrocytes per cubic millimeter in the adult male and 4.8 million in the adult female. By comparison, there are about 5000 white blood cells in the same volume of blood. **Erythron** is the total number of erythrocytes in the body. There are 27×10^{12} in males and 18×10^{12} in females. The erythrocyte is a cell without a nucleus which has the shape of a biconcave disk with a diameter of about 7μ. (Fig. 5-7) The red blood cell is very pliable and, by folding and assuming a bell shape, squeezes through narrow blood capillaries with a luminal diameter of $3-4 \mu$.

The erythrocyte is surrounded by a 70 Å-thick cell membrane. It is likely that the antigens which make it possible to identify the major blood groups (O, A, B, AB) are built into this membrane. Functionally important enzymatic systems are also located in this membrane. The interior of the erythrocyte is filled with a lipid-protein complex, **hemoglobin,** which is the carrier of oxygen and carbon dioxide. The amount of hemoglobin present in 100 ml of blood is $16 \text{ g} \pm 2$ in males, and $14 \text{ g} \pm 2$ in females. When one observes erythrocytes in a blood smear, a pale area is present in the center. This is caused by the thinness of the hemoglobin layer in the center of the biconcave disk. The nucleus as well as cell organelles are missing in the erythrocyte, since they are

extruded during the final stages of red blood cell maturation. If water leaves the erythrocyte, as it does in hypertonic solutions, the red cell shrinks and turns into a spiny round, **crenated** corpuscle. Under normal circumstances, however, the red cell surface is smooth and pseudopodia are not present. In hypotonic solutions, water enters the red cell, changing it from a biconcave disk to a sphere, possibly also rupturing the cell membrane. Simultaneously, hemoglobin leaves the erythrocyte, resulting in essentially a colorless membranous sac or red cell **ghost.** This process is called **hemolysis.** Erythrocytes are not actively motile as are leukocytes, although red cells can be moved passively across a vascular wall, a phenomenon referred to as **diapedesis.** While within the vascular channels, erythrocytes may adhere to one another in a **rouleaux** formation, the cause of which is unknown. These stacks of red cells can easily break up again, but an **agglutination** (clumping) of erythrocytes represents a pathological phenomenon as part of thrombosis formation and cannot be reversed. The life span of an erythrocyte is about 120 days. Toward the end the elasticity of the erythrocyte decreases, and it is believed that this contributes to the termination of its usefulness. While trying to pass through the interstices of the splenic pulp, the old erythrocytes are caught and devoured by

Fig. 5-7. Sectioned blood cells in lumen of blood vessel. Rabbit. E.M. X 21,000.
1. Erythrocytes sectioned perpendicularly to equatorial plane. 2. Erthrocyte sectioned through equatorial plane. 3. Cell membrane of erythrocyte. 4. Part of small lymphocyte. 5. Platelet. 6. Blood plasma.
Fig. 5-8. Reticulocyte. Bone marrow. Human. E.M. X 24,000. 1. Mitochondria. 2. Pinocytotic invaginations. 3. Vesicles. 4. Siderosomes. 5. Part of macrophage.
Fig. 5-9. Enlargement of rectangle in Fig. 5-8. E.M. X 60,000. 1. Mitochondrion. 2. Siderosome, containing ferritin particles. 3. Membranous sacs of Golgi zone. 4. Polyribosomes.

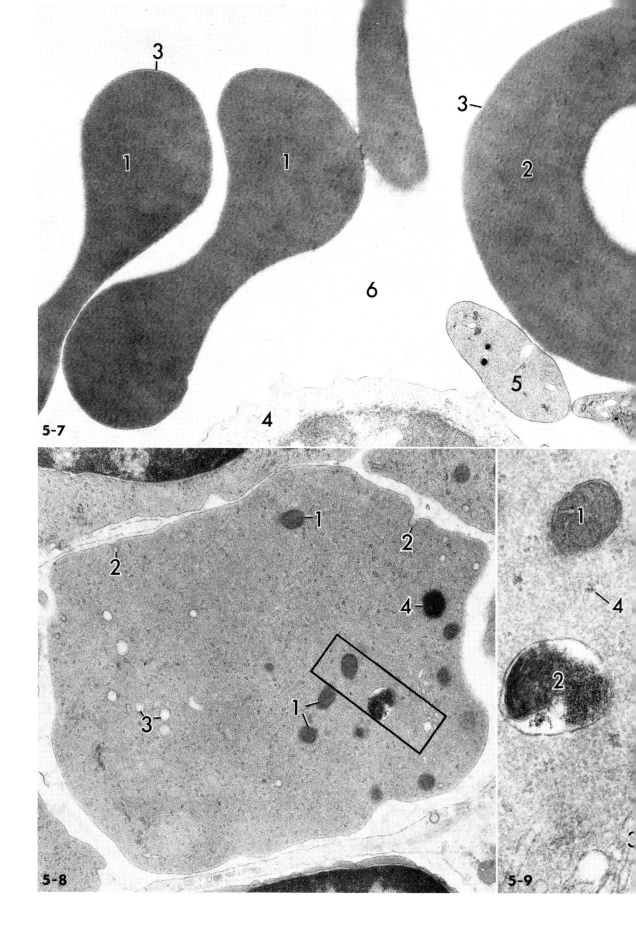

5-7

5-8

5-9

the numerous macrophages or reticular cells of the spleen. As a result the hemoglobin is broken down into its constituents, iron and protein. The iron is stored in the macrophage and is reutilized in the formation of hemoglobin during erythropoiesis.

Reticulocytes. A reticulocyte is a nearly mature erythrocyte which is present in the bone marrow. Normally about 1% of the circulating erythrocytes are reticulocytes. The size of the reticulocyte is similar to that of the mature erythrocyte. The shape is irregular (Fig. 5-8) when the reticulocyte is lodged in the bone marrow, but upon reaching the circulating blood, it assumes the approximate shape of the mature erythrocyte. There is less hemoglobin in the reticulocyte than in the mature erythrocyte, but a small number of cell organelles such as mitochondria, Golgi vesicles and polysomes are present. These structures give the cytoplasm a slight basophilic reaction when stained supravitally and appear as a net-like (reticular) formation from which stems the term "reticulocyte." In addition, the cell membrane of the reticulocyte shows an active uptake of ferritin via micropinocytotic vesicles as an indication that hemoglobin synthesis is not completed, and there are still hemosiderin storage granules, **siderosomes,** present in the cytoplasm. (Fig. 5-9) An increase in the number of reticulocytes in the blood usually indicates an increased rate in red blood cell formation in the bone marrow in response to an increased rate of erythrocyte destruction or loss by bleeding. The reticulocyte retains its reticulum for about 24 hours in the circulating blood before it becomes a mature erythrocyte.

White blood cells (leukocytes). All white blood cells (leukocytes) are nucleated cells and possess ameboid properties. There are about 5000 leukocytes per cubic millimeter of human blood. For descriptive convenience leukocytes are divided into those which have numerous large, distinct cytoplasmic granules and a markedly lobulated nucleus, **granular leukocytes (granulocytes).** To this category belong the neutrophil polymorphonuclear leukocytes (polymorphs), the eosinophil leukocytes, and the basophil leukocytes. This subdivision is based on the staining properties of the cytoplasmic granules. Those leukocytes in which cytoplasmic granules cannot readily be detected by light microscopy are called **non-granular (mononuclear) leukocytes.** To this category belong the lymphocytes and the monocytes. The granular leukocytes are generally concerned with protective functions against infective organisms and toxic absorption. The monocytes are believed to represent precursors of macrophages, since they show phagocytic properties, particularly upon leaving the circulating blood. The lymphocytes play an important role in the immunological defense system of the body.

Neutrophil polymorphs. Neutrophil polymorphs are migratory and phagocytic. They make up 50–80% of the total number of white blood cells, the wide range depending upon the health condition of the individual. A slight infection increases the number of polymorphs. They remain in the circulating blood only for a few days. The average width of the cell is about 10–12 μ. The shape of the polymorph is spherical (Fig. 5-10) in the circu-

Fig. 5-10. Polymorphonuclear leukocyte (neutrophil). Bone marrow. Human. E.M. X 24,000. **1.** Heterochromatin of lobated nucleus. **2.** Euchromatin. **3.** Nuclear membrane. **4.** Short profile of granular endoplasmic reticulum. **5.** Azurophilic (primary) granules. **6.** Specific (secondary) granules. **7.** Cytoplasm with free monoribosomes and glycogen particles. **8.** Hyaloplasm of pseudopod. **9.** Phagocytic vacuoles. **10.** Cell membrane.

Fig. 5-11. Detail of neutrophil polymorphonuclear leukocyte. Bone marrow. Human. E.M. X 90,000. **1.** Azurophilic (primary) granules. **2.** Specific (secondary) granules. **3.** Granules with extracted core ("degranulated"). **4.** Particulate glycogen (beta-particles).

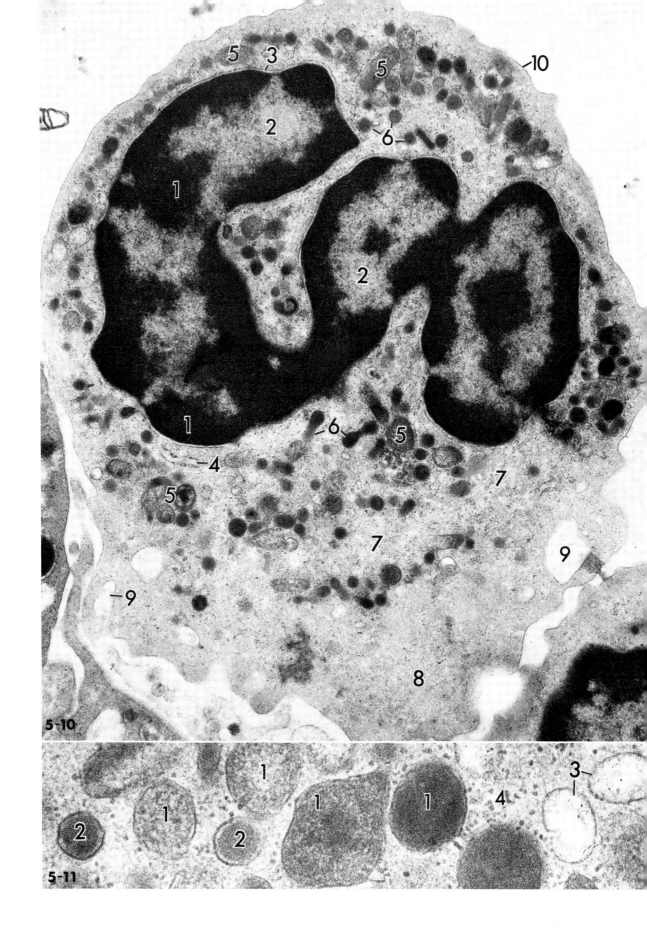

5-10

5-11

lating blood, where the polymorphs have a tendency to travel near the walls of the blood vessel at a slower speed than the erythrocytes, particularly in the postcapillary venules and muscular venules. The polymorphs change shape as they go through the wall of the venule to reach the extravascular space. The cytoplasm extends long pseudopodia in ameboid movements. The foot-like processes are temporarily devoid of cell organelles and this part of the cytoplasm is then referred to as **hyaloplasm.** (Fig. 5-10) The nucleus is multilobated in older cells. In younger forms the segmentation is less pronounced. The many shapes of the nucleus have contributed to the term "polymorph" for the neutrophil granulocytes. The lobes are connected by a narrow strand of nucleoplasm. Heavy masses of dense heterochromatin are distributed against the nuclear membrane, and the loosely arranged euchromatin is found mostly in the center. A well-delineated nucleolus is generally not present. There are fewer nuclear pores than in the bone marrow precursors of the polymorphs.

The cell surface of the circulating polymorphs is provided with a small number of short narrow microvilli. The cytoplasm contains a large number of small membrane-bound granules (Fig. 5-11), which are present in mainly two categories: azurophilic granules and specific granules in the ratio of 1:2. The larger **azurophilic (primary) granules** represent primary lysosomes and contain peroxidase and several acid hydrolases concerned with antibacterial and digestive functions. They occur in two different forms, rounded and football-shaped. These granules are very active in phagocytosis and can be stained specifically with methylene azure. The more numerous **specific (secondary) granules** are small, spherical or elongated, and lack lysosomal enzymes. They can be stained with neutral dyes, thus the name neutrophilic. They contain alkaline phosphatase and an antibacterial substance, phagocytin.

The cytoplasm of the polymorph contains a large number of glycogen particles but other organelles are scarce. The Golgi apparatus is rudimentary, centrioles are found only with difficulty, and mitochondria are few in number and rod-shaped.

The **prime function** of the neutrophil polymorphs is phagocytosis and inactivation (digestion) of the phagocytosed material. As a result of phagocytosis, the polymorphs become degranulated. Bacteria are killed and digested but in the process, the polymorphs often die in large numbers, giving rise to an accumulation of dead polymorphs referred to as pus.

Eosinophils. The eosinophils normally make up about 1–2% of the circulating leukocytes. (Fig. 5-12) They are slightly larger than the neutrophils, averaging 10–15 μ in diameter. These cells circulate for about 8 days and leave the venules by very slow ameboid movements via a route similar to that taken by the neutrophils. Eosinophils are quite common in the loose connective tissue of the lamina propria of the intestinal tract and the respiratory system. The cells are fragile and rupture easily when spread in a blood smear preparation.

The nucleus is typically bilobed and the cytoplasm is packed with large **specific granules** which are eosinophilic and have a high refractive index. The granules have a diameter of about 1 μ. (Fig. 5-13) They are membrane-bound and contain a matrix in which is located a central angular dense bar or crystalloid. The specific

Fig. 5-12. Eosinophil polymorphonuclear leukocyte. Bone marrow. Human. E.M. X 24,000. **1.** Heterochromatin of bilobed nucleus. **2.** Euchromatin. **3.** Mitochondria. **4.** Specific granules. **5.** Phagocytic vacuoles. **6.** Cell membrane.

Fig. 5-13. Detail of eosinophil polymorphonuclear leukocyte. Bone marrow. Human. E.M. X 60,000. **1.** Boundary membrane of specific granules. **2.** Fine granular matrix of specific granules. **3.** Crystalloids.

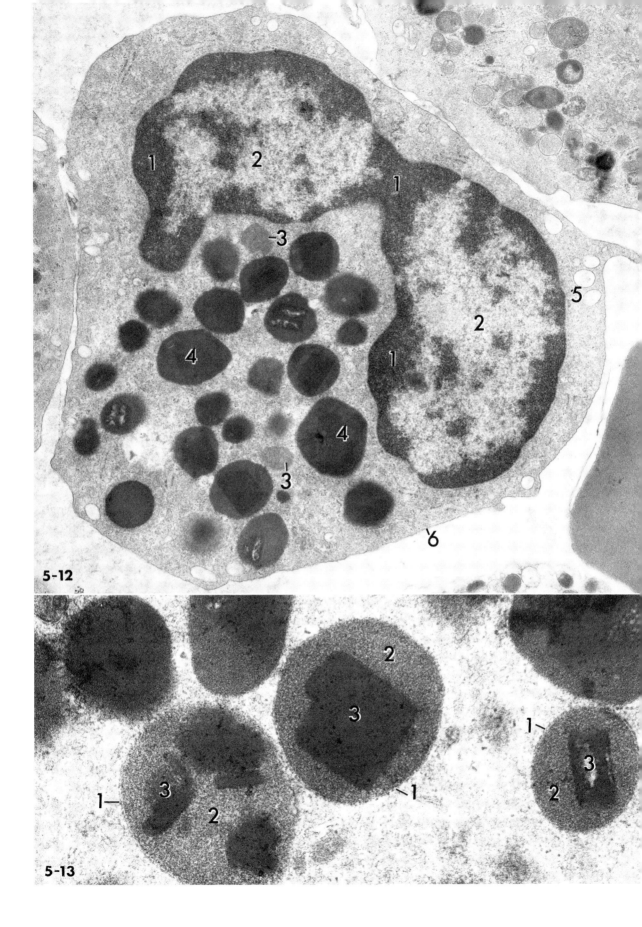

5-12

5-13

granules represent lysosomes and the matrix contains peroxidase as well as hydrolytic enzymes. The content and the role of the crystalloid bar is not known. Mitochondria are more numerous and larger than those of neutrophils. The Golgi zone is well developed, and ribosomes, glycogen particles, as well as profiles of both granular and agranular endoplasmic reticulum, are generally present.

The eosinophilic leukocyte is a phagocyte with preference for antigen-antibody complexes. Soluble antigens or antibodies alone do not seem to be taken up. The discharge of the lytic enzymes occurs intracellularly into phagocytic vacuoles as in neutrophils, and can be recorded as a degranulation of the cell. Eosinophils become more numerous in blood during parasitic infestations and allergic diseases where hypersensitivity reactions occur. However, little is really known about the normal function of eosinophils. It has been suggested that they liberate or absorb histamine, a substance which generally is released both under normal and allergic conditions.

Basophils. The basophils are the most rare of the polymorphonuclear leukocytes, constituting about 0.5% of all leukocytes in the circulating blood. The cell is slightly larger than the neutrophil with a diameter of about 8–10 μ. (Fig. 5-14) After leaving the bone marrow compartment, the basophils circulate for 12–15 days, but their ultimate fate is unknown. Cells of similar appearance, the mast cells, occur extravascularly, and it was earlier believed that they represented basophils which had left the circulation. However, the fine structure of the mast cell is different from that of the basophil, and the transformation hypothesis has been abandoned.

The nucleus is bilobed or kidney-shaped. The cytoplasm contains numerous large round, oval, or angular **granules** which are stainable with basic dyes and have a low refractive index. The granules, which average 1 μ in width, are highly water soluble and are therefore difficult

to preserve. (Fig. 5-15) Each granule is surrounded by a membrane and is partially or completely filled with small particles of fairly uniform size, measuring about 150 Å. The granules contain histamine and heparin and are not generally recognized as lysosomes. The remainder of the cytoplasm of the basophil shows a variable number of ribosomes, some profiles of granular endoplasmic reticulum, several mitochondria, and a fairly well-developed Golgi zone. The cytoplasm also contains an abundance of small, 250–300 Å, particles which are believed to be glycogen, although they may also represent the heparin precursor, heparin monosulfuric ester.

The basophils display ameboid motion. They do not appear to be highly phagocytic, although in the presence of complement, the cells have been shown to engulf sensitized erythrocytes and zymosan particles. The **prime function** of the basophil is to synthesize heparin and histamine which are aggregated in the granules and discharged at the cell surface by a process of exocytosis (reversed pinocytosis). As a result, a degranulation of the basophil occurs. A degranulation occurs in hypotonic shock, freezing, and thawing and can be brought about by emulsifiers, com-

Fig. 5-14. Slightly immature basophilic polymorphonuclear leukocyte (late basophilic metamyelocyte). Bone marrow. Human. E.M. X 15,000. Since basophilic leukocytes are rare in normal human blood and marrow, and difficult to preserve adequately, a late basophilic metamyelocyte is included here. **1.** Nucleus. **2.** Granules with dense core (probably immature). **3.** Granules with light core (probably mature). **4.** Profiles of granular endoplasmic reticulum. **5.** Short dilated cisternae of granular endoplasmic reticulum. **6.** Mitochondria. **7.** Cell membrane.

Fig. 5-15. Detail of mature basophilic polymorphonuclear leukocyte. Bone marrow. Human. E.M. X 60,000. **1.** Boundary membrane of granule. **2.** Core of 150 Å particles. **3.** Short profile of granular endoplasmic reticulum. **4.** Free monoribosomes. **5.** Particulate glycogen (beta particles). **6.** Cell membrane.

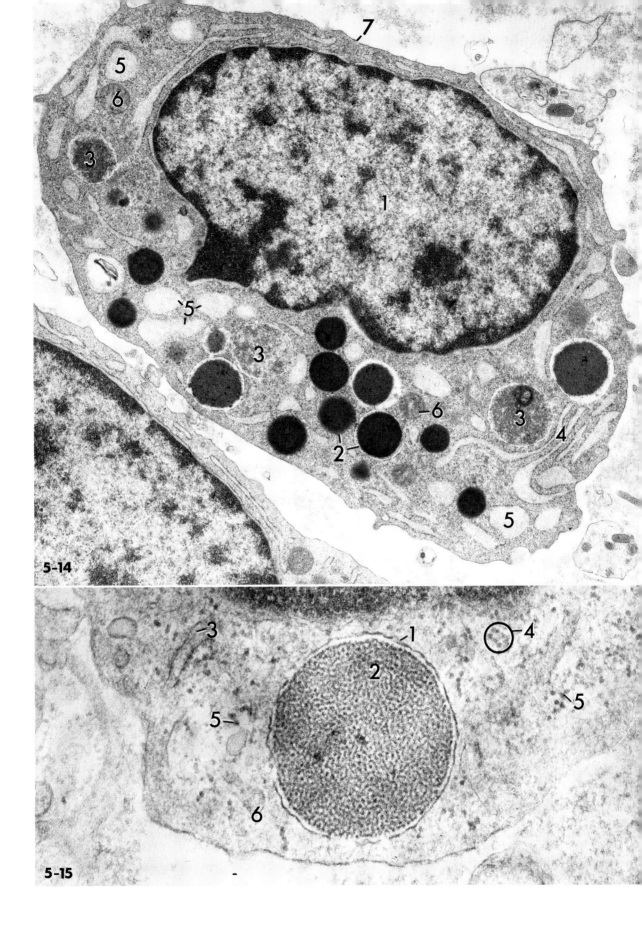

5-14

5-15

pound 48/80 (a histamine liberator), eosinophilic peroxidase, and a variety of immune reactions involving antigen, antibody, and complement.

Lymphocytes. Lymphocytes belong to the category referred to as non-granular leukocytes, although some lymphocytes may contain a limited number of small azurophilic granules. About 25% of the circulating leukocytes are lymphocytes. The lymphocytes are all spherical in the blood and lymph streams, but vary slightly in size. The majority are **small lymphocytes** with an average width of 8 μ. About 10% are **medium-sized lymphocytes,** averaging 12 μ in width. In the germinal centers of lymph nodes and spleen occurs an even larger type of lymphocyte which is called **large lymphocyte** or **lymphoblast.** It averages 18 μ in width but does not normally circulate in the blood or lymph. The main structural difference between small and medium-sized lymphocytes relates to the amount of cytoplasm, which in the small lymphocyte is only slightly larger than the nucleus, whereas in the medium-sized lymphocyte, the cytoplasm occupies a zone 2–3 μ wide around the nucleus. The following description refers largely to the small lymphocytes. (Fig. 5-16) For further details on medium-sized and large lymphocytes, see p. 388.

The nucleus is round with a slight indentation. The chromatin is relatively condensed. It stains darkly in routine blood smear preparations and obscures the nucleoli which are visible only with electron microscopy. The cell surface is provided with a small number of short microvilli. The cytoplasm is very sparse, occupying a thin rim around the nucleus. It is strongly basophilic because of a relatively large number of free ribosomes. Profiles of granular endoplasmic reticulum are few in number. The Golgi region is quite small, and centrioles are usually present together with a small number of spherical mitochondria. A limited number of small **azurophilic granules** occur in about 10% of all circulating lymphocytes.

As to their **function,** lymphocytes are antigen-reactive cells involved in the immunological defense system of the body. There are known to exist several functionally different lymphocytes in the circulating blood, although structural differences have not been detected. At the moment, the functions of the lymphocytes and the relationships of small, medium-sized, and large lymphocytes are being subjected to extensive investigations. It is generally accepted that the medium-sized lymphocyte represents either an intermediate developmental stage of a small lymphocyte differentiating into plasma cells, or is the result of a division of large lymphocytes. This is discussed further on p. 384.

The lymphocytes which develop in the thymus seem to have a life span of only a few days, whereas those which develop in lymph nodes, spleen, Peyer's patches, and bone marrow may have a life span of weeks and months, and some may last throughout the life of the individual. The lymphocytes stay less than a day in the bloodstream, migrating across the wall of the postcapillary venules at any place in the body. They do this routinely in the lymph nodes as part of a recirculation mechanism between blood and lymph streams. They also leave the bloodstream and become lodged in the loose connective tissue of the lamina propria of the digestive tract as well as the respiratory and urinary systems. A more complete discussion of the functions of lymphocytes is found on p. 386.

Monocytes. Monocytes normally make up about 5% of all white cells in the

Fig. 5-16. Small lymphocyte in medullary sinus of lymph node. Cat. E.M. X 40,000.
1. Heterochromatin of nucleus.
2. Euchromatin. 3. Nucleolus. 4. Nuclear pore areas. 5. Nuclear membrane.
6. Mitochondria. 7. Profile of granular endoplasmic reticulum. 8. Free monoribosomes.
9. Small (azurophilic) granule. 10. Microvilli.
11. Cell (surface) membrane.

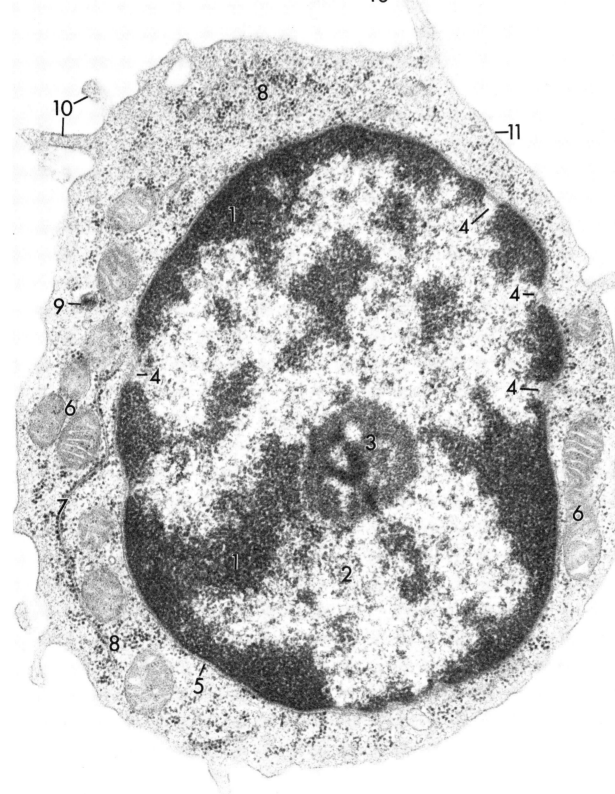

blood. They are the largest of the circulating leukocytes, averaging 15 μ in width. Monocytes develop in the bone marrow but may finish their maturation in the circulating blood where they stay an average of 2–3 days before migrating across the walls of postcapillary venules to become wandering macrophages in the connective tissue space. The cell is oval in the circulating blood but changes shape constantly as it migrates with ameboid movements through the connective tissue spaces.

The nucleus is kidney- or horseshoe-shaped and placed eccentrically in the cell. The heterochromatin forms a delicate lacy skein and stains less intensely than in lymphocytes. Nucleoli can be seen in routine preparations for light microscopy. In electron microscope preparations the cell surface displays irregular microvilli and pseudopodia as well as several vacuoles just beneath the cell membrane. The cytoplasm is more abundant than in lymphocytes. It has a clear appearance and is less basophilic because of a smaller number of free ribosomes. Short profiles of the granular endoplasmic reticulum and small round mitochondria are quite abundant. The Golgi apparatus is prominent with centrioles, vacuoles, and vesicles in close proximity. There is a single population of small round membrane-bound **azurophilic granules.** (Fig. 5-18) They are more numerous but smaller and more refractive than those in lymphocytes. The granules have a dense homogeneous center containing hydrolytic enzymes and peroxidase. They represent primary lysosomes and merge with phagocytic vacuoles during phagocytosis.

The prime **function** of the monocytes is to serve as precursor cells to macrophages, and they differentiate into phagocytes once the extravascular space is reached. As macrophages, they are indistinguishable from other connective tissue histiocytes and become highly phagocytic of larger particles, protozoal parasites, and cells. In acute inflammation, polymorphonuclear leukocytes arrive first on the scene, whereas monocytes come late. The polymorphs usually reach the end of their life span once they leave the bloodstream, but monocytes are capable of continued enzyme synthesis in the tissue and may live up to two months.

Thrombocytes (platelets). The platelets, or thrombocytes, are small, oval biconvex disks, 2–4 μ in diameter. (Fig. 5-19) They are enucleate fragments which become detached from megakaryocytes in the bone marrow. There are about 300,000 platelets in one cubic millimeter of blood. The platelets remain in the circulation for an average of 7 days, and are removed from it by the spleen and lungs. They form an important part of the clotting reaction of the blood.

As indicated, the platelets do not have a nucleus. They are surrounded by an 80 Å-thick cell membrane which has an external fuzzy coat of mucopolysaccharides averaging 500 Å in thickness. Based on light microscopical observations, the platelet was divided into a central **granulomere** which seemed to contain most of the organelles and inclusions, and a clear peripheral **hyalomere** free of these structures. After fixation for electron microscopy this subdivision is less valid since organelles are found throughout the platelet. The cytoplasm contains several small mitochondria, a limited number of ribosomes, and some particulate glycogen. It is pervaded by a **system of smooth in-**

Fig. 5-17. Monocyte. Bone marrow. Human. E.M. X 18,000. **1.** Euchromatin of nucleus. **2.** Heterochromatin. **3.** Nucleolus. **4.** Mitochondria. **5.** Golgi zone. **6.** Short profiles of granular endoplasmic reticulum. **7.** Azurophilic granules. **8.** Cell membrane.

Fig. 5-18. Detail of monocyte. Bone marrow. Human. E.M. X 60,000. **1.** Golgi sacs. **2.** Golgi vesicles, probably precursors of azurophilic granules. **3.** Mitochondria. **4.** Cisternae of granular endoplasmic reticulum. **5.** Free monoribosomes. **6.** Boundary membrane of azurophilic granules. **7.** Finely stippled core of azurophilic granules.

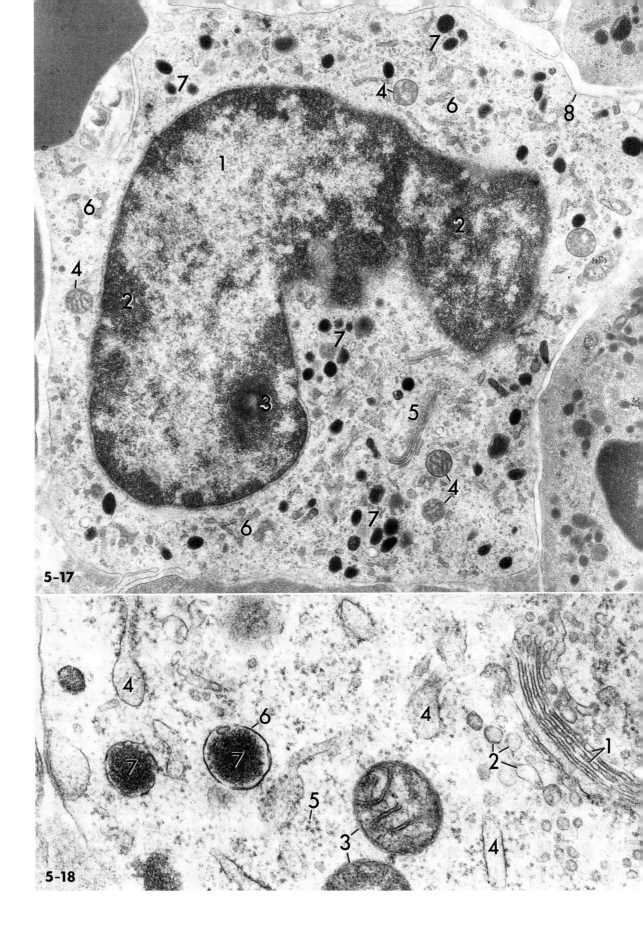

5-17

5-18

terconnected **tubules** which also is connected with the cell membrane. The tubules contain an amorphous substance which is light in some tubules, in other tubules dense. A bundle of **microtubules** encircles the platelet beneath the longest circumference. Microfilaments traverse the cytoplasm. Vesicles and vacuoles occur in an arrangement reminiscent of a small Golgi zone. There is an abundance of round or oval membrane-bound granules, **alpha granules,** which average $0.2\,\mu$ in diameter. (Fig. 5-20) They have a finely granular core. A second type, referred to as **very dense granules,** is rare in human blood platelets. They each contain a small, extremely dense, and eccentrically located core. (Fig. 5-21)

The platelets contain several factors which are functionally important in triggering the clotting reaction, but the specific contents of various organelles and inclusions have not been clearly established. Platelets readily adhere to one another even in the flowing blood, and it is believed that the surface coat forms bridges during platelet aggregation. A contractile protein, **thrombosthenin,** is very likely bound to the microfilaments. This protein changes the shape of the platelet, and when released upon platelet disintegration, it participates in clot retraction. Several factors (presently at least 10 are known) are required to bring about clot formation. Of these, **platelet factor 3,** a phospholipid, is probably located in the alpha granules. This factor participates in the formation of **thromboplastin,** an enzyme which transforms **prothrombin** to **thrombin,** but the exact location of thromboplastin in the platelet is not known. Platelets are slightly phagocytic, and one cannot exclude that some of the factors required for blood clotting are absorbed and carried by the platelet to the site of blood coagulation. **Serotonin** and **ATP** occur in platelets, probably located in the very dense granules. Serotonin makes vascular smooth muscle contract, which is important when the vascular

wall has been severed; and **ATP** is needed for the action of thrombosthenin. In the final phases of the clotting reaction, thrombin converts **fibrinogen** to **fibrin.** A mixture of fibrin, platelets, and erythrocytes is called a **thrombus.**

References

Anderson, D. R. Ultrastructure of normal and leukemic leukocytes in human peripheral blood. J. Ultrastruct. Res. Suppl. *9:* 5–42 (1966).

Behnke, O. Electron microscopic observations on the membrane systems of the rat blood platelet. Anat. Rec. *158:* 121–137 (1967).

Behnke, O. Electron microscopical observations on the surface coating of human blood platelets. J. Ultrastruct. Res. *24:* 51–69 (1968).

Born, G. V. R. The functional physiology of blood platelets. Symp. Zool. Soc. Lond. *27:* 75–89 (1970).

Cohn, Z. A. The structure and function of monocytes and macrophages. Adv. Immunol. *9:* 163–214 (1968).

Daems, W. Th. On the fine structure of human neutrophilic leukocyte granules. J. Ultrastruct. Res. *24:* 343–348 (1968).

David-Ferreira, J. F. The blood platelet: electron microscopic studies. Int. Rev. Cytol. *17:* 99–148 (1964).

Fedorko, M. E. and Hirsch, J. G. Structure of monocytes and macrophages. Seminars in Hematology *7:* 109–124 (1970).

Gardner, H. A., Simon, G. and Silver, M. D. The fine structure of rabbit platelets fixed in acetaldehyde. Anat. Rec. *163:* 509–516 (1969).

Lowenstein, L. M. The mammalian reticulocyte. Int. Rev. Cytol. *8:* 136–174 (1959).

Miller, F., deHarven, E. and Palade, G. E. The structure of eosinophil leukocyte granules in rodents and in man. J. Cell. Biol. *31:* 349–362 (1966).

Scott, R. E. and Horn, R. G. Ultrastructural aspects of

Fig. 5-19. Platelets (thrombocytes) from lumen of artery. Mouse. E.M. X 30,000. **1.** Platelet sectioned through equatorial plane. **2.** Biconvex platelets, cross-sectioned. **3.** Surface membrane. **4.** Fuzzy coat. **5.** Mitochondria. **6.** Alpha granules. **7.** System of smooth interconnected tubules. **8.** Glycogen particles.
Fig. 5-20. Thrombocyte. Mouse. E.M. X 47,000. **1.** Surface membrane. **2.** Fuzzy coat. **3.** Mitochondria. **4.** Alpha granules. **5.** Golgi complex. **6.** Smooth tubules. **7.** Smooth tubules connected to surface membrane.
Fig. 5-21. Thrombocyte. Rabbit. E.M. X 45,000. **1.** Surface membrane. **2.** Smooth tubules. **3.** Alpha granules. **4.** Very dense granules with small eccentrically placed, extremely dense core.

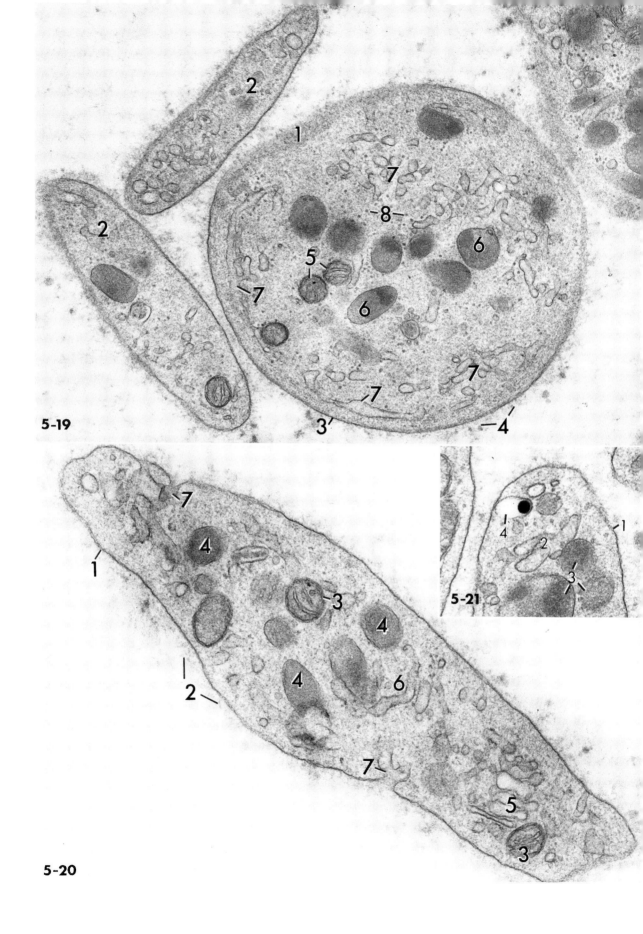

5-19

5-20

5-21

neutrophil granulocyte development in humans. Lab. Investig. *23*: 202–215 (1970).

Silver, M. D. and Gardner, H. A. The very dense granule in rabbit platelets. J. Ultrastruct. Res. *23*: 366–377 (1968).

Spicer, S. S. and Hardin, J. H. Ultrastructure, cytochemistry and function of neutrophil leukocyte granules. A review. Lab. Investig. *20*: 488–497 (1969).

White, J. G. Interaction of membrane systems in blood platelets. Am. J. Path. *66*: 295–312 (1972).

Wivel, N. A., Mandel, M. A. and Asofsky, R. M. Ultrastructural study of thoracic duct lymphocytes of mice. Am. J. Anat. *128*: 57–72 (1970).

Zucker-Franklin, D. The ultrastructure of cells in human thoracic duct lymph. J. Ultrastruct. Res. *9*: 325–339 (1963).

Zucker-Franklin, D. Electron microscopic study of human basophils. Blood *29*: 878–890 (1967).

Zucker-Franklin, D. Electron microscopic studies of human granulocytes: structural variations related to function. Seminars in Hematology *5*: 109–133 (1968).

Zucker-Franklin, D. and Hirsch, J. G. Electron microscope studies on the degranulation of rabbit peritoneal leukocytes during phagocytosis. J. Expt. Med. *120*: 569–576 (1964).

6 Blood cell formation

GENERAL CONSIDERATIONS

Blood-forming organs in the human adult body are represented by 1) bone marrow; 2) lymph nodes; and 3) spleen. In the fetus, hemopoiesis first occurs in the so-called blood islands of the mesenchyme. Subsequently it takes place within blood vessels, liver, and spleen. Blood cells are formed in the loose connective tissue of these organs, and it is only upon reaching maturation that the blood cells enter the blood circulation under normal conditions by traversing the walls of capillaries and postcapillary venules of these organs.

In the adult human, the **red blood cells** (erythrocytes) are formed exclusively in the bone marrow. (Fig. 6-1) The **granular leukocytes** (neutrophils, eosinophils, basophils) are similarly formed in the bone marrow. (Fig. 6-3) The **non-granular leukocytes** (lymphocytes, monocytes) are formed in the lymph nodes and the spleen, and perhaps to some extent, in the bone marrow. The **megakaryocytes** and the **thrombocytes** are formed in the bone marrow. Exceptions to these rules are found in certain pathological conditions in man. Erythrocytes and megakaryocytes are generally also formed in the spleen of lower mammals such as the rat and the bat.

Uncertainty still exists as to the details of the formation of blood cells, be they in bone marrow, lymph nodes, or spleen. (Fig. 6-4) Generally, there are three schools of thought concerning the origin of blood cells. The **polyphyletic theory** holds that there is a stem cell for each of the mature blood cells. The **dualistic** theory maintains that there are two stem cells, one for the myeloid cells (granular leukocytes, erythrocytes) and one for the lymphoid cells (non-granular leukocytes). The **monophyletic** (unitarian) theory claims that all blood cells originate from a common stem cell, generally referred to as **hemocytoblast** or **reticular cell**. For more than seven decades a great many investigators have researched extensively the area of hemopoiesis, and strong evidence for the

correctness of one or the other of these theories has been put forth from time to time. It is beyond the scope of this book to elaborate in depth on these theories. However, within the last several years new techniques have shed additional light on the problem of the hemopoietic stem cell. Based on some recent work involving radioisotope marking followed by radioautography as well as X-irradiation of the bone marrow with subsequent injection of bone marrow cells, there is now strong evidence for the existence of a **free stem cell** in the bone marrow. This stem cell can give rise to all the different blood cell lines, including lymphocytes and monocytes. This is the pluripotent hemopoietic precursor cell, the **hemocytoblast.** However, it is not entirely clear from whence this cell takes its origin. Several possibilities have been suggested but it seems that only three are worth mentioning here.

One possibility is that cells which are

Fig. 6-1. Section of red bone marrow. Human. L.M. X 150. **1.** Bone trabecula. **2.** Fat cells. **3.** Myeloid tissue (individual cell types cannot be identified at this magnification). **4.** Arteriole. **5.** Circle: sinusoidal capillary filled with blood cells. **6.** Megakaryocyte.

Fig. 6-2. Smear-preparation of bone marrow cells. Human. L.M. X 380. At this magnification some cells can easily be identified. Other cells cannot, particularly since this is a black and white illustration. **1.** Myeloblast. **2.** Promyelocyte. **3.** Neutrophil myelocyte. **4.** Eosinophil myelocyte. **5.** Neutrophil metamyelocyte. **6.** Neutrophil metamyelocyte (band cell). **7.** Neutrophil polymorph. **8.** Basophil erythroblast. **9.** Polychromatic erythroblast. **10.** Orthochromatic erythroblast. **11.** Erythrocyte.

Fig. 6-3. Section of red bone marrow fixed in situ. Human. E.M. X 1900. At this magnification most cells can be identified with accuracy. **1.** Hemocytoblast or very early myeloblast. **2.** Late promyelocyte. **3.** Myelocyte. **4.** Metamyelocyte. **5.** Neutrophil polymorph. **6.** Eosinophil metamyelocyte. **7.** Late proerythroblast. **8.** Basophil erythroblast. **9.** Erythrocyte. **10.** Promonocyte. **11.** Small lymphocyte. **12.** Nucleus of promegakaryocyte.

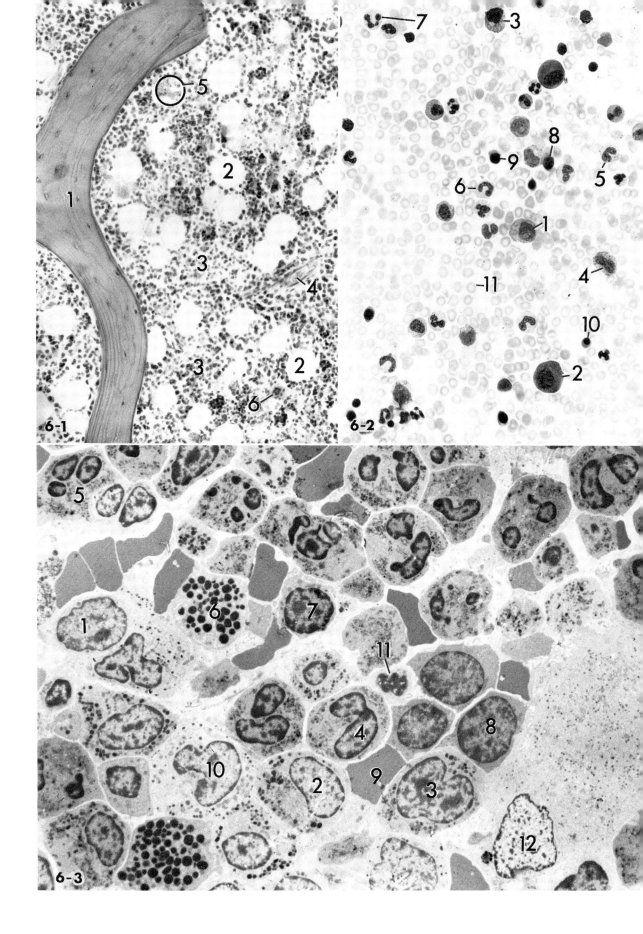

structurally similar to small or medium-sized lymphocytes are carried from lymphoid organs to the bone marrow, where they settle down and persist throughout life as stem cells for blood cells. However, this possibility has largely been ruled out by recent experiments which showed that cells obtained from lymphatic tissue will not repopulate a bone marrow which has been depleted of its myeloid elements through X-irradiation. The second possibility is that the **reticular cell** of the bone marrow represents the precursor cell, since it is usually considered to be a poorly differentiated primitive mesenchymal cell wherever it occurs in the body. During mitosis, this cell would round up, detach from the network of reticular fibrils associated with it, and become a free cell, the blood progenitor, now recognized as **hemocytoblast.** The third possibility is that the hemocytoblasts develop early from the mesenchyme in the bone marrow and are maintained there throughout life by mitotic activity. It has been established that such free stem cells would constitute only about 0.3 to 5% of the marrow cells. Upon division, the hemocytoblasts give rise to both new stem cells and cells which differentiate along mainly two lines. On the one hand, they give rise to **myeloid elements** which develop within the bone marrow. On the other hand, they also give rise to **lymphoid elements,** represented by bone marrow lymphocytes (**B cells**) and their precursors. According to the discussion on p. 394, the B cells settle down temporarily in the thymus where an induction occurs. After this they are called thymic lymphocytes (**T cells**) and migrate to spleen, lymph nodes, and Peyer's patches to become progenitors of immunologically competent lymphocytes.

Bone Marrow

Before describing the development of the white and red blood cells in the bone marrow, it is helpful to outline briefly the

Fig. 6-4. Blood cells, their precursors in myeloid and lymphoid tissues, and some closely related cells have been selected and arranged to facilitate the study of nuclear and cytoplasmic ratios, shapes, sizes, and other characteristics. With few exceptions, the cells are presented at approximately the same magnification. Most cells or parts thereof have been further magnified for detailed study on subsequent pages or elsewhere in this book. Human (except as indicated). E.M. X 4500 (except as indicated).

Neutrophilic leukocyte series
1. Late hemocytoblast or early myeloblast. See Fig. 6-9.
2. Early promyelocyte. See Fig. 6-10.
3. Late promyelocyte. X 4000. See Fig. 6-11.
4. Late myelocyte. See Fig. 6-12.
5. Metamyelocyte (band cell). See Fig. 6-13.
6. Neutrophil polymorph. See Fig. 5-10.

Erythrocytic series
7. Late hemocytoblast or early proerythroblast. See Fig. 6-21.
8. Basophilic erythroblast. See Fig. 6-24.
9. Polychromatic erythroblast. See Fig. 6-23.
10. Orthochromatic erythroblast. See Fig. 6-26.
11. Reticulocyte. See Fig. 5-8.
12. Erythrocyte. Rabbit. See Fig. 5-7.

Plasma cell
13. Plasma cell. Bone marrow. See Fig. 7-29.

Monocytic series
14. Late monoblast. See Fig. 6-18.
15. Promonocyte. See Fig. 6-19.
16. Monocyte. See Fig. 5-17.

Basophilic polymorph
17. Basophilic polymorph. X 3500. See Fig. 5-14.

Eosinophilic polymorph
18. Eosinophilic polymorph. See Fig. 5-12.

Megakaryocytic series
19. Promegakaryocyte. X 1500. See Fig. 6-28.
20. Megakaryocyte. Spleen. Rat. X 930. See Fig. 6-31.
21. Thrombocytes/platelets. Mouse. See Fig. 5-19.

Lymphocytic series
22. Lymphoblast/large lymphocyte. Spleen. Rat. X 3500. See Fig. 17-26.
23. Medium-sized lymphocyte. Lymph node. Rat. See Fig. 17-24.
24. Small lymphocyte. Lymph node. Rat. See Fig. 5-16.

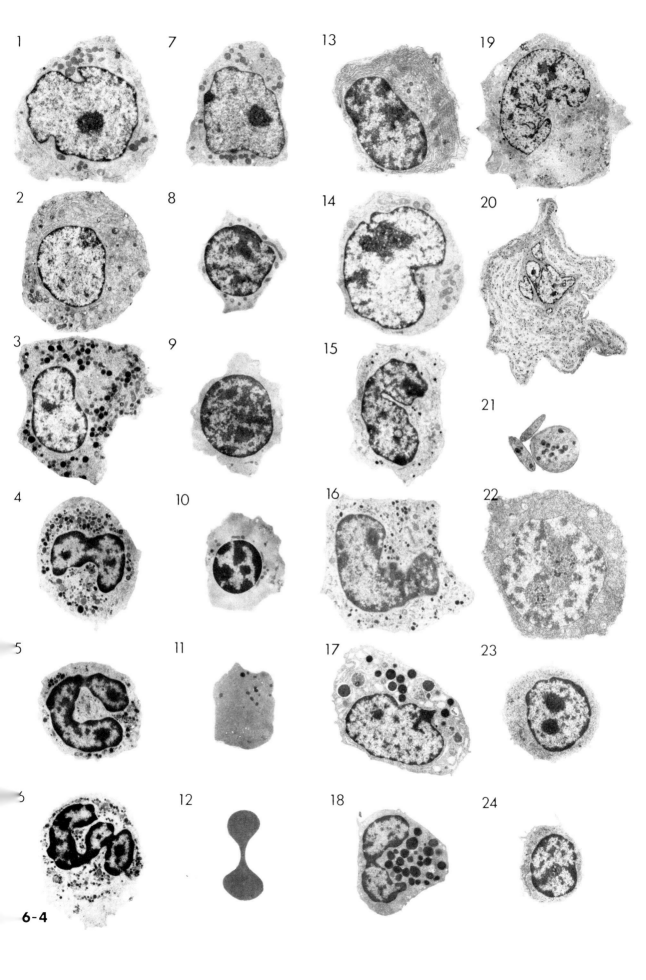

general architecture and constituents of the bone marrow (Fig. 6-5) since this is the hemopoietic tissue for most cells circulating in the blood.

The bone marrow is located in the cavity of the shaft of long bones and in the interspicular spaces of spongy bones. In early childhood, the marrow is exclusively a **red bone marrow** because of the large amount of **myeloid** elements (marrow cells) and the active part the marrow takes in the formation of the marrow cells. Later in life, the red marrow is gradually replaced by **yellow bone marrow.** This is done through an infiltration of fat cells, predominantly in the shaft of long bones and indicates a reduction of myeloid elements. However, yellow bone marrow can be replaced by red marrow and vice versa depending on the need.

The **red bone marrow** consists of a **loose stroma** made up of a wide meshwork of delicate reticular **fibrils** and **reticular cells.** The reticular cells are supporting elements (Fig. 6-7) and may have phagocytic properties. They may also represent undifferentiated mesenchymal stem cells. Free **macrophages** are present in the reticular meshes. The vascular tree of the bone marrow receives its blood from the nutrient arteries of the bone which break up into arterioles feeding into the vast system of large thin-walled **sinusoidal capillaries** lined by littoral endothelial cells. Some **fibroblasts, mast cells,** and **plasma cells** usually accompany the blood vessels. The large **extravascular tissue** consists of a great variety of developing and mature blood cells. These free cells comprise, in the white blood cells series, **myeloblasts, myelocytes,** and **polymorphonuclear leukocytes** (neutrophils, eosinophils, basophils). Representatives of the red blood cell series are **erythroblasts** (basophilic, polychromatic, orthochromatic), **reticulocytes,** and **erythrocytes.** Present are also **monoblasts, promonocytes,** and **monocytes,** as well as **megakaryoblasts, megakaryocytes, thrombocytes** (platelets), and **small** and **medium-sized lymphocytes.** It

has not been established whether **large** lymphocytes occur, since their appearance would be identical to that of myeloblasts, proerythroblasts, and monoblasts. Indeed, the last four types of cells may also be referred to as **hemocytoblasts** since they cannot be readily separated ultrastructurally from each other, although from a functional point of view they each represent potential stem cells for four different cell lines. Where the marrow cells are in contact with the spicules of the spongy bone are also found potential **osteoblasts** and **osteoclasts.** Finally, **fat cells** are intermingled with the myeloid elements, although they are less frequent in the red bone marrow than in the yellow bone marrow.

Each of the above cell types will now be described. The description of the developing white and red blood cells in this chapter is based largely on electron microscopical analyses of human bone marrow fixed *in situ.* The difference in appearance between cells in bone marrow

Fig. 6-5. Section of red bone marrow fixed by arterial perfusion *in situ.* Cells are slightly separated, probably because of too high perfusion pressure, but this phenomenon facilitates the study of the reticular cells of the marrow. Newborn rat. Femur. E.M. X 1800. **1.** Lumen of sinusoidal capillary. **2.** Endothelium. **3.** Pericapillary cells. **4.** Reticular cells. **5.** Hemocytoblasts or myeloblasts. **6.** Small lymphocytes. **7.** Myelocyte. **8.** Free macrophage. **9.** Polymorphs.

Fig. 6-6. Section of red bone marrow fixed *in situ.* Human. E.M. X 4200. **1.** Nucleus of reticular cell. This cell is also a fixed macrophage since its cytoplasm contains lysosomes. **2.** Nucleus of late neutrophil promyelocyte. **3.** Nucleus of late neutrophil myelocyte. **4.** Band cells. **5.** Polychromatic erythroblast. **6.** Nucleus of small lymphocyte.

Fig. 6-7. Bone marrow. Same preparation as in Fig. 6-5. Femur. Newborn rat. E.M. X 23,000. **1.** Nucleus of reticular cell. **2.** Mitochondria. **3.** Granular endoplasmic reticulum. **4.** Particulate glycogen. **5.** Slender cytoplasmic extensions give this cell a stellate shape. **6.** Fine reticular fibrils.

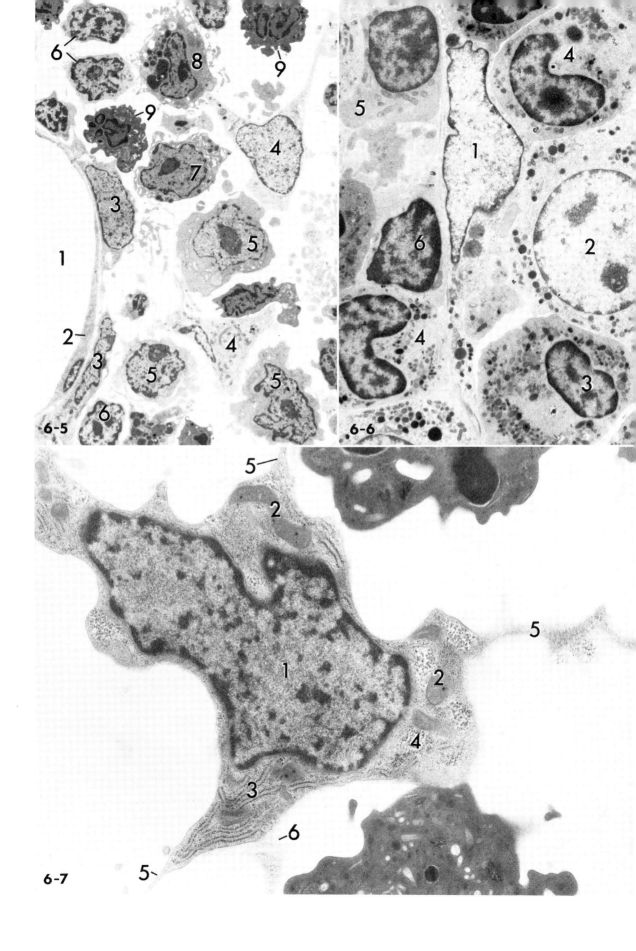

6-5

6-6

6-7

smears and in marrow cells fixed *in situ* refers mainly to size and distribution. In the smear, cells become flattened out and their diameter increases. Furthermore, their topographic relationship to each other and their distribution in the marrow is lost.

RETICULAR CELLS

Reticular cells are present in both lymphoid and myeloid tissues. They form a wider meshwork in the bone marrow (Fig. 6-7) than they do in the spleen and lymph nodes. They are sometimes attached to the tissue aspect of the wall of the sinusoidal capillaries and are then recognized as pericapillary cells. Delicate bundles of reticular fibrils are found near the surface of the reticular cells, but they are not embraced by the cytoplasm of the reticular cells as intimately as in the spleen (Fig. 18-15) and lymph nodes (Fig. 17-21) The shape of the reticular cell of the bone marrow varies considerably from angular-stellate to flattened or spindle-shaped. The size of the cell averages to that of a fibroblast in loose connective tissue. The nucleus is large, ovoid or kidney-shaped but can also be slender and elongated. It is rather pale staining since it contains a large amount of euchromatin and only a narrow rim of heterochromatin near the nuclear membrane. At least one nucleolus is always present.

The cytoplasm is drawn out into many irregular extensions which are both blunt and narrow. In ordinary hematoxylin and eosin preparations, the cytoplasm stains faintly, and the outline of the cell is therefore difficult to see. There are a fair number of free ribosomes, some profiles of the granular endoplasmic reticulum, a few mitochondria and particulate glycogen granules. The Golgi apparatus varies in size but is always present. Secretory granules do not occur. Lysosomes may be present as an indication of phagocytic activity by the reticular cell. However, the reticular cells of the bone marrow are less prone to become fixed macrophages than

their counterparts in the spleen and lymph nodes.

The **function** of the reticular cells is to support the myeloid elements and if stimulated, to become phagocytic. Their postulated role as undifferentiated mesenchymal cells and precursors of hemocytoblasts during hemopoiesis has been questioned lately. However, one cannot rule out the possibility that the reticular cells can serve as stem cells in case the free hemocytoblasts fail to fulfill this function.

HEMOCYTOBLASTS

There are many ways of defining these cells but, based on several recent investigations, it is generally assumed that there exist free hemopoietic stem cells which permanently reside in the reticular meshwork of the bone marrow. The hemocytoblasts may assume a number of shapes to conform to their surroundings and they may even look like reticular cells, but they definitely represent free ameboid cells. In contrast to the fixed reticular cells, the hemocytoblasts have a relatively smooth cell membrane which only rarely displays projections longer than 0.1 μ. (Fig. 6-8) The diameter averages 12 μ. The nucleus is large, round or ovoid, and stains poorly since the nuclear chromatin is fine with only some peripheral condensation of heterochromatin. There are one or more prominent nucleoli. The cytoplasm forms

Fig. 6-8. Hemocytoblast. Although not identified by radioautography, but based on its ultrastructural characteristics, this cell could very well represent a free hemopoietic stem cell. Bone marrow. Human. E.M. X 21,000.
1. Nucleus. **2.** Mitochondria. **3.** Ribosomes. **4.** Granular endoplasmic reticulum. **5.** Blunt cytoplasmic extensions give this cell an angular shape. **6.** Cytoplasm of myelocytes.
Fig. 6-9. Early myeloblast or late hemocytoblast. Bone marrow. Human. E.M. X 18,000.
1. Abundant euchromatin. **2.** Nucleolus. **3.** Narrow rim of heterochromatin. **4.** Nuclear membrane. **5.** Mitochondria. **6.** Ribosomes. **7.** Granular endoplasmic reticulum. **8.** Smooth surface gives this cell a rounded shape.

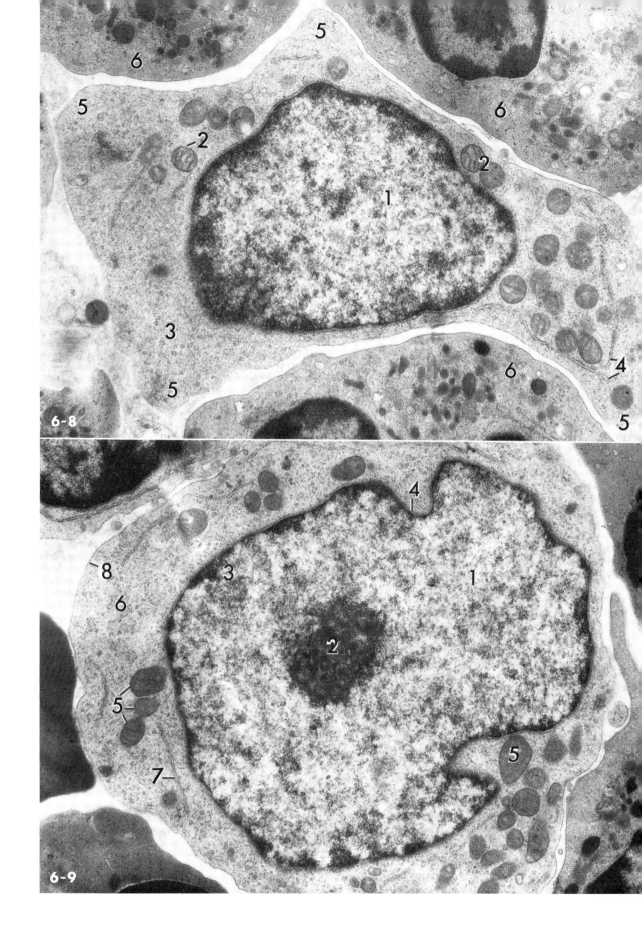

a narrow rim around the nucleus and is relatively basophilic because of a large number of free monoribosomes and a few profiles of granular endoplasmic reticulum. There is a moderate number of small and spherical mitochondria and a Golgi region with adjoining centrioles. Lipid droplets, lysosomes, and other types of membrane-bound granules are absent.

The hemocytoblasts are actively mitotic and give rise to new stem cells as well as to cells which differentiate into myeloblasts, proerythroblasts, megakaryoblasts, monoblasts, and lymphoblasts. This differentiation entails first a rounding up of the cytoplasm and the nucleus before signs of specific nuclear and cytoplasmic differentiation appear. Presently, it is not clear what determines the differentiation of the hemocytoblast. It has been suggested that the hemocytoblastic stem cell, in its cell cycle, progresses through differing phases of humoral receptivity, and that a combination of stem cell maturity and environmental factors influences its differentiation into one or the other cell line.

ORIGIN OF GRANULAR LEUKOCYTES

The granular leukocytes take their origin from **myeloblasts** which develop to **promyelocytes, myelocytes,** and **metamyelocytes** before they finally mature into polymorphonuclear leukocytes. Presently, little is known of the early stages of differentiation into lines of eosinophils and basophils, and the following description deals only with the development of the neutrophils. It should be recognized that the number of leukocytes and their precursors in the bone marrow exceeds that of the erythrocyte series.

Myeloblasts. The earliest cell of the neutrophilic series is the myeloblast which makes up about 2% of all nucleated blood cells in the bone marrow. It is a round cell, averaging 10 μ in diameter. (Fig. 6-9) The nucleus is large and round with shallow indentations. It occupies a major part of the cell and stains faintly because of an abundance of euchromatin. A thin edge of the nucleus is occupied by dense heterochromatin. One or two prominent nucleoli are present. The cytoplasm is scant and devoid of membrane-bound granules but contains abundant free polyribosomes and monoribosomes in addition to a few short profiles of the granular endoplasmic reticulum. Small spherical mitochondria abound.

There are few structural features that make this cell differ from the hemocytoblast described on p. 118 except the round shape and round nucleus. In fact, some investigators claim that the hemocytoblast and the myeloblast cannot be told apart from an ultrastructural point of view. Furthermore, the myeloblast may very well also be identical to the early proerythroblast, except that the cytoplasm of the latter shows an increased accumulation of free ribosomes as compared to the myeloblast.

Promyelocytes. Promyelocytes are among the largest of the immature neutrophil leukocytes. About 5 per cent of all nucleated blood cells in the bone marrow are promyelocytes. They arise from myeloblasts through differentiation and growth and average 15 μ in diameter as late promyelocytes. In the early promyelocytes (Fig. 6-10) the nucleus is large, round, and

Fig. 6-10. Early neutrophilic promyelocyte. Bone marrow. Human. E.M. X 21,000. **1.** Round nucleus with abundant euchromatin. **2.** Heterochromatin. **3.** Centriole. **4.** Golgi zone. **5.** Mitochondrion. **6.** Granular endoplasmic reticulum. **7.** Dilated cisternae of granular endoplasmic reticulum. **8.** Early light azurophilic (primary) granules. **9.** Ribosomes. **10.** Cell membrane. Enlarged detail of this cell in Fig. 6-14.

Fig. 6-11. Late neutrophilic promyelocyte. Bone marrow. Human. E.M. X 18,000. **1.** Slightly indented, oval nucleus with decreasing amounts of euchromatin. **2.** Heterochromatin. Nucleolus not in plane of section. **3.** Centriole. **4.** Golgi zone. **5.** Mitochondria. **6.** Granular endoplasmic reticulum. **7.** Late dense azurophilic (primary) granules. **8.** Cell membrane. Enlarged detail of this cell in Fig. 6-15.

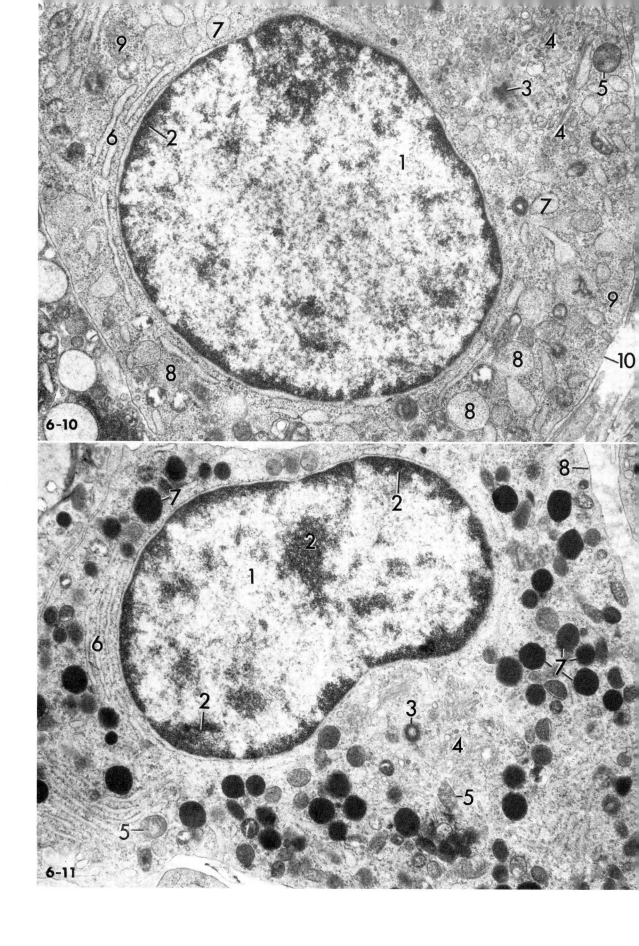

pale staining since it is dominated by the light euchromatin; the dense heterochromatin is concentrated near the nuclear membrane. In mid-promyelocytes and late promyelocytes (Fig. 6-11) the nucleus changes from oval to crescentic or kidney-shaped. Nucleoli are present, although they are not always easily recognized in routine light microscope preparations. The cytoplasm is abundant and contains numerous free monoribosomes which contribute to its strong basophilic reaction. There is a large Golgi region with associated centrioles. Mitochondria are fairly numerous in the early promyelocytes but are drastically reduced in number in the late promyelocytes. The granular endoplasmic reticulum is rather extensive and the cisternae often change from the ordinary flat shape to distended and even round vesicular forms. They contain a flocculent material which is reactive to peroxidase.

The maturation of the promyelocytes is characterized particularly by the appearance and development of primary, large dense **azurophilic granules** which represent a special type of primary lysosomes containing peroxidase and lysosomal digestive enzymes. Enzymes and chemical substances, which are to be included in the primary granules, are transported from the granular endoplasmic reticulum via transfer vesicles to the Golgi complex. From the concave inner face of the Golgi apparatus arise enlarging vesicles and condensing saccules which transform into the primary, azurophilic granules. These granules vary in size and shape. The predominant form is round with a flocculent content (Fig. 6-14) that later condenses as the granule matures. (Fig. 6-15) Football-shaped forms are less common. They often contain a central crystal-like inclusion.

Promyelocytes divide and give rise to other promyelocytes which differentiate into myelocytes. However, the majority of mitoses seen among immature neutrophil leukocytes occurs at the myelocytic stage.

From a light microscopical point of view, a promyelocyte changes to a myelocyte when the cytoplasmic granules take on such size, shape, and color that one can tell that they are neutrophils, eosinophils, or basophils. Under the electron microscope, the development of a second type of cytoplasmic granule makes it quite possible to separate neutrophilic promyelocytes from myelocytes.

Myelocytes. The myelocyte is smaller than the late promyelocyte, averaging 10 μ in diameter. (Fig. 6-12) About 12% of all nucleated blood cells in the bone marrow are myelocytes. They arise from late promyelocytes by a continued differentiation that started in the early promyelocyte. The nucleus is kidney-shaped and indented. There is a marked increase in the amount of heterochromatin, and in the late myelocytes, nucleoli are rarely seen. The cytoplasm is relatively abundant but the number of free ribosomes and profiles of granular endoplasmic reticulum is greatly reduced which is reflected in the gradual disappearance of a basophilic staining reaction. There is a gradual increase in particulate glycogen, whereas the number of mitochondria is further reduced compared to the late promyelocyte. Those present are rod-shaped rather than spherical. The Golgi

Fig. 6-12. Late neutrophilic myelocyte. Bone marrow. Human. E.M. X 24,000.
1. Kidney-shaped nucleus with small amounts of euchromatin. **2.** Greatly increased amounts of heterochromatin. **3.** Golgi zone (mostly out of plane of section). **4.** Mitochondrion. **5.** Azurophilic (primary) granules. **6.** Specific (secondary) granules. Enlarged detail of this cell in Fig. 6-16.
Fig. 6-13. Late neutrophilic metamyelocyte (band cell). Bone marrow. Human. E.M. X 24,000. **1.** Horse-shoe shaped nucleus with small amounts of euchromatin. **2.** Heterochromatin. **3.** Centriole. **4.** Golgi zone. **5.** Granular endoplasmic reticulum. **6.** Mitochondria. **7.** Azurophilic (primary) granules. **8.** Specific (secondary) granules. **9.** Cell membrane. Enlarged detail of this cell in Fig. 6-17.

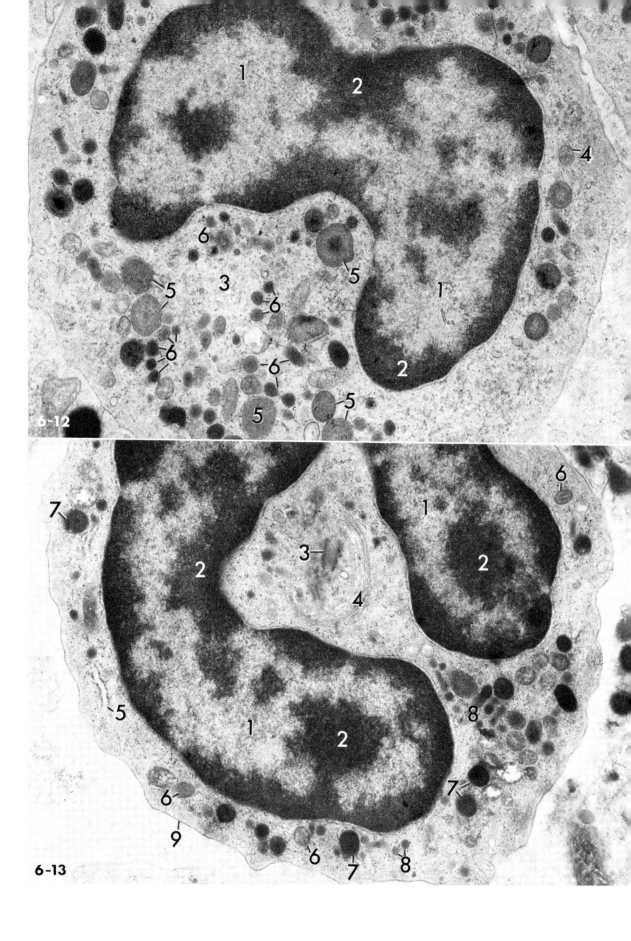

6-12

6-13

region is extensive and the outer (distal or convex) lamellae of its component parts are actively engaged in the production of cytoplasmic granules which are peroxidase negative.

The appearance of a second population of cytoplasmic granules, the secondary **specific granules,** marks the transition of promyelocytes to myelocytes. The secondary granules contain alkaline phosphatase but lack lysosomal enzymes and peroxidase. They vary in shape but typically occur as membrane-bound spheres or rods, the latter often dumbbell-shaped. (Fig. 6-16) Their size is relatively uniform. The core is homogeneously dense with a light peripheral submembranous halo. The existence of a true tertiary granule population has not been convincingly established in man but has been demonstrated in the rabbit.

Mitoses occur during the early and mid-myelocytic phases, but cease toward the late myelocyte and early metamyelocyte phases. These cell divisions provide for a subsequent large population of metamyelocytes. As a result of the mitotic activity, the primary azurophilic granules are reduced by roughly 50%, whereas the active production of secondary specific granules results in a late myelocyte where the specific granules outnumber the azurophilic two to one.

Metamyelocytes. The metamyelocytes are slightly smaller than the myelocytes. They constitute about 22% of all nucleated blood cells of the bone marrow. They are easily recognized because of the typical shape of the nucleus which progresses from a kidney shape through a horseshoe shape to a lobed or segmented configuration as the metamyelocyte matures into a polymorphonuclear neutrophilic leukocyte. The late metamyelocyte is the smallest of all metamyelocytes and is called **band cell** (staff or stab cell) because of the typical curved, horseshoe shape of its nucleus. (Fig. 6-13) In general, the nucleus of the metamyelocytes has a large amount of heterochromatin and nucleoli

are absent. The cytoplasm generally becomes less abundant with metamyelocyte maturation and contains a small number of free ribosomes and a few short profiles of granular endoplasmic reticulum. The Golgi zone becomes small and inactive, since the production of specific granules gradually ceases. Mitochondria are sparse and rod-shaped. **Glycogen particles** increase greatly in number and there is an increase in the opacity of the cytoplasmic matrix (ground substance). The significance of this increase may relate to the initiation of active ameboid movements and Brownian motion near the end stage of the developing neutrophil as it becomes ready to enter the circulating blood.

There is a mixed granule population in metamyelocytes. The primary **azurophilic granules** make up about half the number. They are somewhat smaller and more oval as compared to their appearance in the myelocyte. The secondary **specific granules** are numerous and retain their original size and oval or dumbbell-shaped configuration. (Fig. 6-17)

Fig. 6-14. Detail of early neutrophilic promyelocyte. Bone marrow. Human. E.M. X 60,000. **1.** Cisternae of granular endoplasmic reticulum. **2.** Ribosomes. **3.** Early azurophilic (primary) granules. These develop from small Golgi vesicles (a), enlarge and accumulate a flocculent material (b) which gradually is condensed (c & d). **4.** Boundary membrane of azurophilic granule.

Fig. 6-15. Detail of late neutrophilic promyelocyte. Bone marrow. Human. E.M. X 60,000. **1.** This stage is characterized by an increase in number and core density of the azurophilic (primary) granules. **2.** Ribosomes. **3.** Circle: Glycogen particles.

Fig. 6-16. Detail of neutrophilic myelocyte. Bone marrow. Human. E.M. X 60,000. **1.** Azurophilic (primary) granules. **2.** Specific secondary) granules. **3.** Extracted ("degranulated") granule. **4.** Circle: glycogen particles.

Fig. 6-17. Detail of neutrophilic metamyelocyte. Bone marrow. Human. E.M. X 60,000. **1.** Azurophilic (primary) granules. **2.** Specific (secondary) granules. **3.** Extracted ("degranulated") granules. **4.** Glycogen particles.

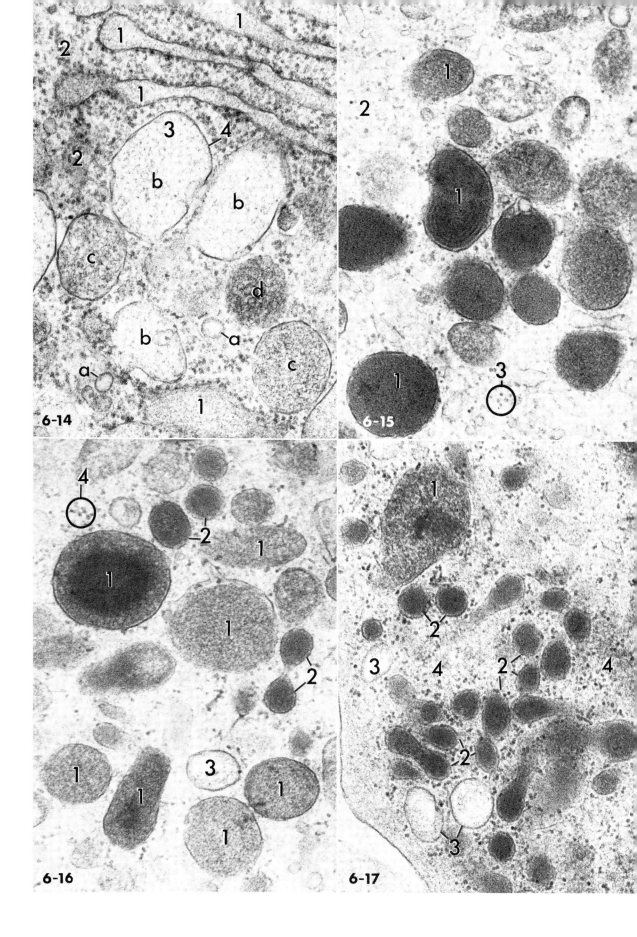

6-14

6-15

6-16

6-17

The metamyelocytes do not undergo cell division. They gradually mature into segmented, polymorphonuclear neutrophils before they leave the bone marrow compartment and enter the circulation by diapedesis across the walls of the sinusoidal blood capillaries of the marrow. Late metamyelocytes (band cells) normally occur to about 2 per cent in the peripheral blood and even early metamyelocytes may appear there under normal circumstances. The time required for a myeloblast to develop into a mature polymorphonuclear leukocyte in the bone marrow averages 14 days, of which about 7.5 days are needed for the promyelocyte and myelocyte stages, and about 6.5 days for the final maturation of the metamyelocyte into a polymorphonuclear neutrophilic leukocyte.

Neutrophil polymorphs. A detailed description of these cells is given on p. 98.

ORIGIN OF LYMPHOCYTES

A detailed description and discussion of the development of lymphocytes as it has been analyzed in the germinal centers of lymph nodules is found on p. 388.

ORIGIN OF MONOCYTES

The origin of monocytes has only recently become more fully understood. In the past, it was believed that medium-sized or large lymphocytes represented precursors of monocytes. It had also been suggested that monocytes could arise from reticular cells of lymphatic tissue. Clear evidence is now at hand that monocytes are formed in the bone marrow, and that they originate from the same pool of stem cells which gives rise to both myeloid and lymphoid elements. The evidence is based on radioautography, chromosome marker techniques, and electron microscope analyses. The earliest precursor cells recognized are the **monoblasts** which differentiate into **promonocytes** and mature monocytes.

Monoblasts. These cells are very similar to myeloblasts, both in size, shape, and

major ultrastructural features such as numerous polyribosomes, small round mitochondria, and a limited number of short profiles of granular endoplasmic reticulum. One can justify calling the cell a monoblast only if, simultaneously, the two first signs of differentiation into a promonocyte have appeared. One criterion is a slight indentation of the nucleus, changing its shape from round or oval to slightly kidney-shaped. (Fig. 6-18) The second criterion is the appearance of small azurophilic granules emerging from a relatively large Golgi zone, lodged in the nuclear indentation.

Promonocytes. The promonocyte is an oval or irregularly shaped cell which varies greatly in size, ranging from 7 to 15 μ. It is easily recognized in the light microscope because of its irregularly shaped nucleus and lightly stained cytoplasm. A marked indentation of the nucleus is the first sign of differentiation from a monoblast to a promonocyte. (Fig. 6-19) The indentations become more numerous and progressively deeper as the promonocyte matures. There is a fine network of heterochromatin in the younger promonocytes but it becomes somewhat denser in the late promonocytes. Two or several

Fig. 6-18. Early monoblast. Bone marrow. Human. E.M. X 18,000. **1.** Large indented nucleus with large amounts of euchromatin. **2.** Small amounts of heterochromatin. **3.** Nucleolus. **4.** Small Golgi zone. **5.** Granular endoplasmic reticulum. **6.** Mitochondria. **7.** Ribosomes. **8.** Small azurophilic granules. **9.** Cell membrane.

Fig. 6-19. Promonocyte. Bone marrow. Human. E.M. X 25,000. **1.** Deeply indented nucleus with relatively large amounts of euchromatin. **2.** Heterochromatin. **3.** Cytoplasmic indentation, sectioned longitudinally. **4.** Cytoplasmic indentation, cross-sectioned. **5.** Golgi zone. **6.** Mitochondria. **7.** Granular endoplasmic reticulum. **8.** Azurophilic granules. **9.** Ribosomes. **10.** Cell membrane.

Fig. 6-20. Detail of promonocyte. Bone marrow. Human. E.M. X 62,000. **1.** Mitochondrion. **2.** Boundary membrane of azurophilic granules. **3.** Dense core. **4.** Ribosomes.

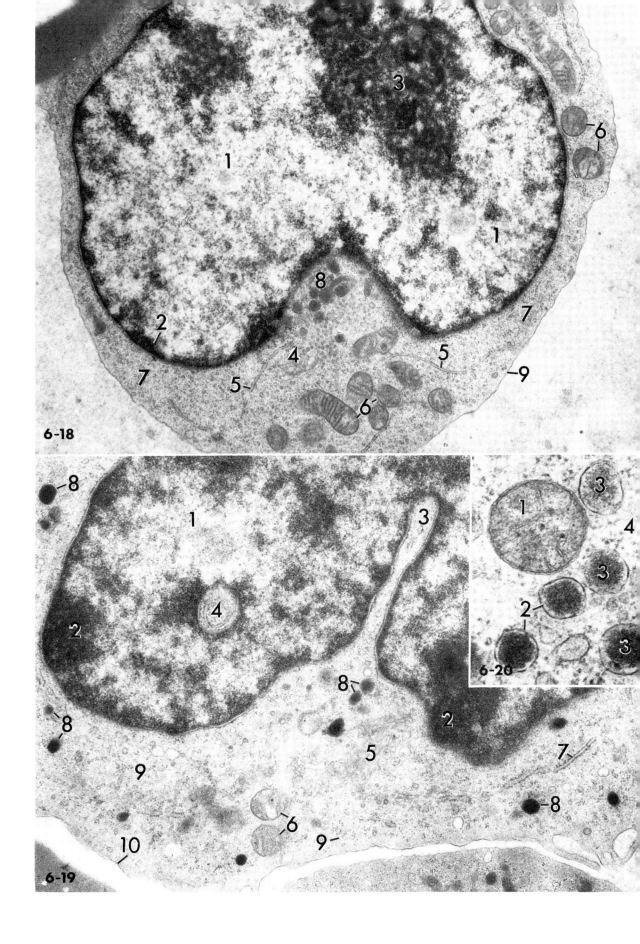

nucleoli are present. The cytoplasm is abundant and lightly basophilic because of a moderate number of polyribosomes, monoribosomes, and short profiles of granular endoplasmic reticulum. Mitochondria are spherical but scarce. Glycogen particles do not occur. The Golgi region is located at the concave side of the nucleus. It consists largely of vesicular components and some membranous cisternae. From the Golgi region arise many small vesicles and vacuoles containing a flocculent, light core which gradually condenses as the vacuoles increase in size. These vacuoles are precursors of the small round, membrane-bound **azurophilic granules** which accumulate in the cytoplasm with the maturation of the promonocyte. (Fig. 6-20) It should be remembered that this maturation can take place both in the bone marrow and in the circulating blood. The azurophilic granules of the promonocyte represent primary lysosomes since it has been demonstrated that they contain hydrolytic enzymes, dehydrogenases, esterases, and peroxidase, as do the primary azurophilic granules of the neutrophil polymorphs. The promonocytes do not develop a second population of granules.

Promonocytes are occasionally seen in mitosis in the bone marrow. They gradually mature to monocytes, a process which entails a slight decrease in nuclear size and number of free polyribosomes, whereas the azurophilic granules become more numerous, larger, and their cores more uniformly dense and homogeneous. The mature monocyte is phagocytic and becomes a macrophage when it reaches the connective tissue space after its short sojourn in the peripheral blood.

Monocytes. A detailed description of these cells is given on p. 104.

ORIGIN OF ERYTHROCYTES

The red blood cells take their origin from **proerythroblasts** which develop to **erythroblasts** and **reticulocytes** before they mature into **erythrocytes**. The developing and mature red blood cells represent a minority of the blood cells present in the bone marrow. Furthermore, the early stages of the erythrocyte series are often seen together, forming "nests" or colonies (clones) of erythroid elements, usually gathered around a free macrophage. (Fig. 6-22) The development of the red blood cell precursor is characterized by a gradual reduction in size of the cell and the nucleus, a gradual condensation of the nuclear chromatin followed by an extrusion of the nucleus and loss of organelles, and a gradual acquisition of hemoglobin in the cytoplasm, the latter phenomenon reflected in a change from a basophilic to an eosinophilic cytoplasm. The development of the mature erythrocyte takes about 3 days. However, reticulocytes may become discharged into the peripheral circulation, in which case they usually mature to erythrocytes within 24 hours. There are many names applied to the cells of the erythroid series. The most common will be mentioned in parentheses after the name preferred by the author of this textbook.

The **proerythroblast** (rubriblast; pronormoblast) is the earliest cell of the erythrocytic series. In the very earliest forms it is indistinguishable from the myeloblast. (Fig. 6-21) The proerythrocyte is the largest cell in the series. Both the cell and the

Fig. 6-21. Early proerythroblast or late hemocytoblast. Bone marrow. Human. E.M. X 21,000. **1.** Abundant euchromatin. **2.** Nucleolus. **3.** Narrow rim of heterochromatin. **4.** Nuclear membrane. **5.** Mitochondria. **6.** Ribosomes. **7.** Cell membrane.

Fig. 6-22. Colony of erythroid elements. Bone marrow. Human. E.M. X 4500. **1.** Nucleus of macrophage. **2.** Cytoplasm containing a variety of secondary lysosomes. **3.** Nucleus of proerythroblast. **4.** Nucleus of basophilic erythroblast. **5.** Basophilic erythroblast in mitosis. **6.** Nuclei of polychromatic erythroblasts. **7.** Area where cytoplasmic extensions of erythroblast make contact with the macrophage. Similar area is enlarged in Fig. 6-24. **8.** Neutrophilic myelocyte. **9.** Neutrophilic metamyelocyte.

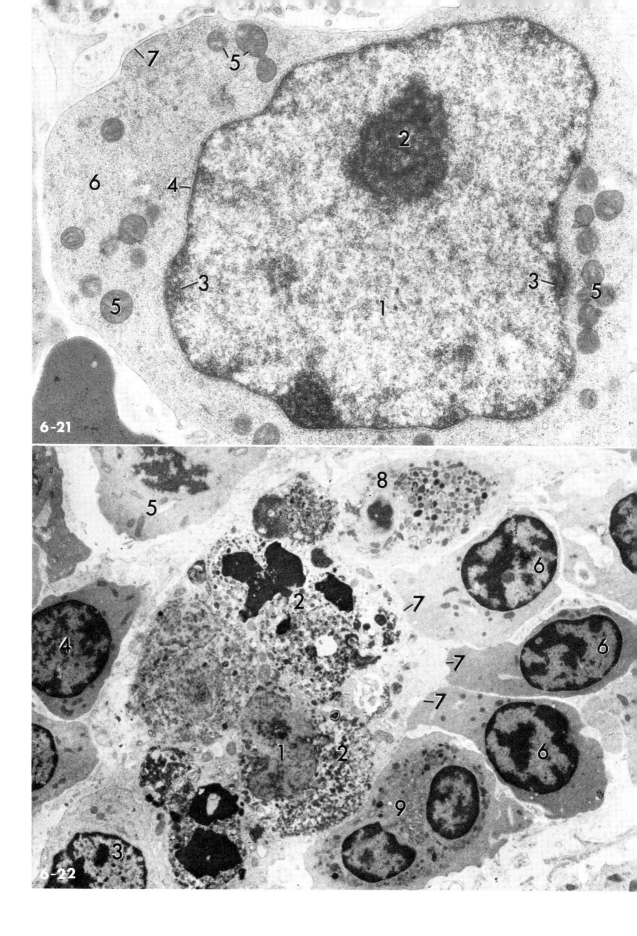

nucleus are slightly angular. The nuclear chromatin is made up largely of light euchromatin with a marginal rim of dense heterochromatin. The nucleolus is well developed, reaching its maximum size at this stage. The first indication that this cell represents a proerythroblast and not a myeloblast is the faint increase in number of polyribosomes and monoribosomes observed in the light microscope as an increase in the basophilia of the cytoplasm when compared to the myeloblast. Mitochondria are scarce, small, oval or round. In addition, there are only traces of granular endoplasmic reticulum, and the size of the Golgi zone, particularly in human proerythroblasts, is small. Secretory granules do not occur. The proerythroblasts gradually differentiate into basophilic erythroblasts through nuclear and cytoplasmic changes.

Basophilic erythroblasts (prorubricytes; basophilic normoblasts; early erythroblasts) are slightly smaller than the proerythrocytes, averaging 10 μ in diameter. The cell is less angular than the proerythroblast and the nucleus is oval or smoothly round. There is an increase in large and small masses of dense heterochromatin in the nucleus, forming a coarse network. The nucleolus is difficult to find at this stage. The cytoplasm is relatively sparse. It often forms long broad extensions toward a near-by free macrophage, and basophilic erythroblasts are often lined up side by side around the macrophage. There are a few small mitochondria and some vesicular elements in a cytoplasm otherwise devoid of most other organelles. The basophilia of the cytoplasm is caused by the large number of **polyribosomes** (Fig. 6-24) and monoribosomes which are involved in the production of **hemoglobin.**

Although it has not been possible to identify the factor that stimulates the development of the granular leukocytes, it is known that **erythropoietin** is instrumental in initiating and governing the rate of hemoglobin synthesis, thereby stimulating the development of erythroid elements and affecting the size of the red blood cells and their release to the circulating blood. Erythropoietin is a humoral factor, a glycoprotein hormone containing sialic acid, which probably is synthesized in the juxtaglomerular cells of the afferent arterioles of the kidney glomeruli. The synthesis of the hemoglobin involves several steps, but it is beyond the scope of this book to give a detailed account of these steps. In brief, hemoglobin is formed from heme, globin, and iron. **Heme** is a porphyrin, and the human **globin** consists of two complex polypeptide chains. **Iron** occurs as ferritin and hemosiderin. Large quantities of **micellar iron** are incorporated into **ferritin** which is an electron-dense molecule with an average width of about 80 Å. Some of the ferritin is bound to **transferrin**, a plasma globulin, whereas the majority of ferritin is stored either as ferritin or **hemosiderin** in macrophages,

Fig. 6-23. Polychromatic erythroblast. Bone marrow. Human. E.M. X 24,000. **1.** Round nucleus with reduced amount of euchromatin. **2.** Heterochromatin. **3.** Mitochondria. **4.** Micropinocytotic invaginations of cell membrane. **5.** Micropinocytotic vesicles. **6.** Polyribosomes.

Fig. 6-24. Detail of contact between macrophage and basophilic erythroblast. Bone marrow. Human. E.M. X 90,000. **1.** Cytoplasm of macrophage with numerous 80 Å ferritin particles. **2.** Invagination of macrophage cell membrane. The direction of membrane movement can be either inward (pinocytosis) or outward (exocytosis). **3.** Cell membrane of basophilic erythroblast. **4.** Micropinocytotic invagination of cell membrane containing some ferritin particles. **5.** Micropinocytotic vesicles with ferritin particles. **6.** Monoribosomes. **7.** Polyribosomes. **8.** The low background density of the cytoplasm is caused by a small concentration of hemoglobin.

Fig. 6-25. Detail of orthochromatic erythroblast. Bone marrow. Human. E.M. X 90,000. **1.** Mitochondrion. **2.** Siderosome, packed with ferritin particles. **3.** Micropinocytotic vesicles with ferritin particles. **4.** Polyribosomes. **5.** The high background density is caused by a large concentration of hemoglobin.

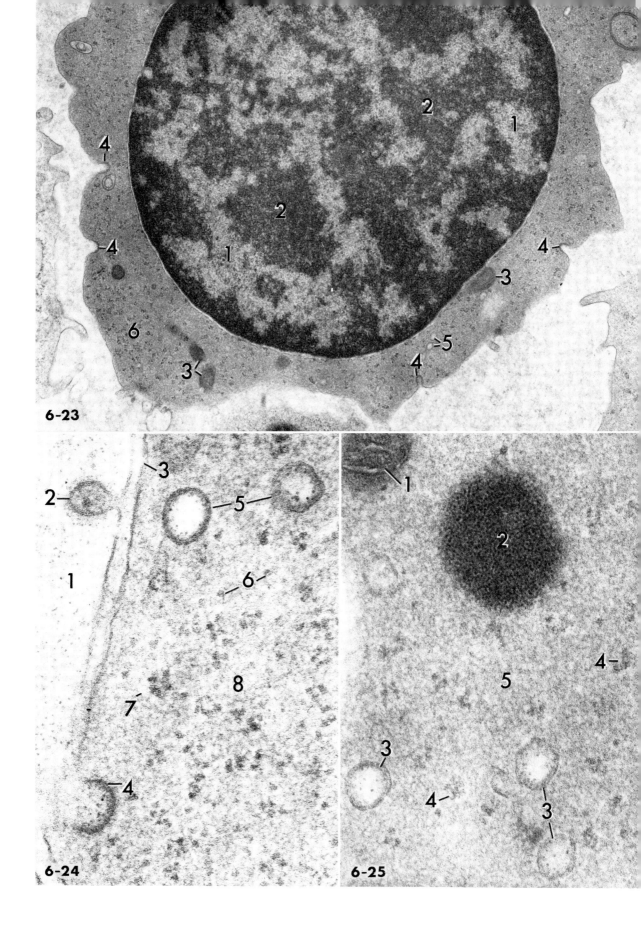

erythroblasts, and reticulocytes as **sidero-somes.** (Fig. 6-25) About two-thirds of the iron that circulates in the blood as trans-ferrin comes from the destruction of old erythrocytes, and one-third is taken from the ferritin stored in macrophages, Kupffer cells, or liver cells. A very small quantity is taken up from the food by the intestine. The stored ferritin is returned to the circulation by a process of exocytosis of these cells, and it is probably taken up by the erythroblasts by a process of pinocytosis as indicated by the many pinocytotic vesicles at the surface of these cells. (Fig. 6-24) The synthesis of hemoglobin in the continued development of erythroid elements requires vitamin B_{12}, ascorbic acid, and the intrinsic factor of the stomach. The last-named is needed for the proper absorption of vitamin B_{12}. The basophilic erythroblasts undergo numerous **mitotic divisions,** producing a large number of polychromatic erythroblasts.

Polychromatic erythroblasts (rubricytes; intermediate erythroblasts; polychromatic normoblasts) are smaller than the basophilic erythroblasts. The nucleus is usually round, and the heterochromatin occupies a larger part than in the basophilic erythroblasts. (Fig. 6-23) There is no nucleolus. The cytoplasm is purplish blue to lilac or gray in routine marrow smears because of increasing amounts of pink-staining hemoglobin and the remaining polyribosomes, although they gradually decrease in number. The polychromatic erythroblasts go through numerous mitotic divisions and seem to give rise to two populations of cells. One forms a reservoir of polychromatic erythroblasts, the other differentiates into orthochromatic erythroblasts.

Orthochromatic erythroblasts (metarubricytes; late erythroblasts; normoblast) are slightly smaller than the polychromatic erythroblasts, but the nucleus has decreased considerably in size with its heterochromatin arranged in a dense "pyknotic" pattern with only a small amount of euchromatin mixed in. (Fig.

6-26) The cytoplasm is largely acidophilic because of the increased amount of hemoglobin and decrease in number of polyribosomes. Accumulations of ferritin particles often occur as siderosomes either with or without a boundary membrane. (Fig. 6-25) The orthochromatic erythroblasts do not show mitotic activity. The nucleus gradually moves toward the cell surface and **becomes extruded** together with a thin coat of cytoplasm. (Fig. 6-27) The extruded nucleus is picked up and digested by macrophages of the bone marrow. As a result of the nuclear extrusion, a reticulocyte emerges.

Reticulocytes. A detailed description of these cells is given on p. 98.

Erythrocytes. A detailed description of these cells is given on p. 96.

ORIGIN OF THROMBOCYTES
The thrombocytes (platelets) are detached fragments of the **megakaryocytes** and appear as free elements in the circulating blood. These fragments do not have a nucleus but contain at least two kinds of membrane-bound granules in addition to organelles such as mitochondria, ribosomes, and a system of interconnected smooth tubules. In man the megakaryocytes reside in the bone marrow alone, but in mammals such as the rat and rabbit they also occur in the spleen. The megakaryocytes originate from **megakaryoblasts,** and as discussed on p. 116, these megakaryoblasts are very likely derived from the free hemocytoblasts of the bone

Fig. 6-26. Orthochromatic erythroblast. Bone marrow. Human. E.M. X 28,000. **1.** Small, round nucleus with greatly reduced amount of euchromatin. **2.** Heterochromatin. **3.** Areas of nuclear pores. **4.** Mitochondria. **5.** Siderosomes. **6.** Micropinocytotic vesicles. **7.** Ribosomes. **8.** Cell membrane. **9.** Macrophage cytoplasm.

Fig. 6-27. Nuclear extrusion in orthochromatic erythroblast. Bone marrow. Human. E.M. X 15,000. **1.** Nucleus. **2.** Thin rim of cytoplasm. **3.** Incumbent reticulocyte. **4.** Mitochondria. **5.** Siderosome.

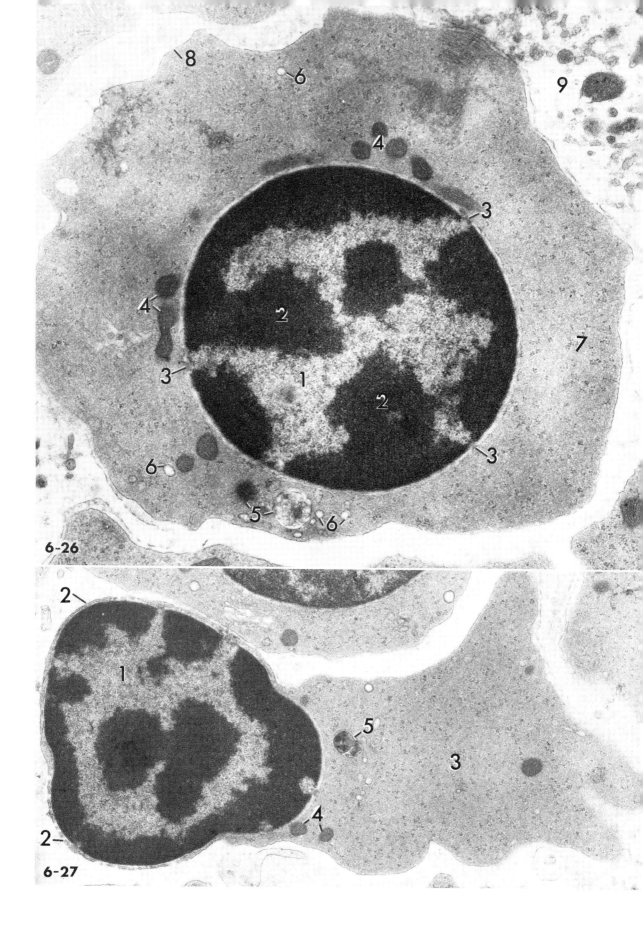

6-26

6-27

marrow. The megakaryoblasts differentiate via **promegakaryocyte** to megakaryocytes.

Megakaryoblasts. The early megakaryoblasts are indistinguishable from myeloblasts, proerythroblasts, and monoblasts. However, an early sign of differentiation toward the megakaryocytic series is seen in the nucleus.

The nucleus, which is round or oval, gradually enlarges and stands out among all nuclei of the bone marrow as the largest. Its surface becomes indented in numerous places and the heterochromatin becomes denser and coarser than in the hemocytoblasts or the myeloblasts. Several nucleoli are present, sometimes as many as five or six. The cytoplasm is quite sparse and is slightly basophilic because of a fair number of free ribosomes. The Golgi zone is relatively large, whereas the mitochondria are small and round. Membrane-bound granules appear in small numbers in the late megakaryoblast. Gradually the late megakaryoblast differentiates into a promegakaryocyte.

Promegakaryocytes. The size of the promegakaryocytes gradually increases from about 15 μ to about 40 μ. There is a marked lobulation of the nucleus (Fig. 6-28) and a tremendous increase in the amount of cytoplasm. It is assumed that the nuclei of the megakaryoblasts and promegakaryocytes go through mitoses, but that neither the daughter nuclei nor the cytoplasm separate. This would explain the giant nuclei and their intricate lobulations as well as the vast cytoplasm. The cytoplasm is distinctly basophilic, particularly near the nucleus, because of the large amount of free ribosomes and the profiles of granular endoplasmic reticulum. The Golgi apparatus is divided into several zones of stacked membranes and vesicles. Mitochondria are small and spherical and distributed evenly throughout the cytoplasm. (Fig. 6-29) Particulate glycogen is present in fair numbers. Small **azurophilic granules** abound. They originate from the Golgi vesicles

which gradually enlarge and accumulate a content of finely granular material, which in man has a central irregularly dense core. This type of granule is referred to as **alpha granule.** (Fig. 6-30) In rabbit promegakaryocytes, a second type of granule is formed called **very dense granule,** in which the finely granular content is absent but in which is present a small, round, and very dense core, placed eccentrically; it is much smaller than the boundary membrane of the granule itself. The major part of the cytoplasm, particularly its peripheral portion, is pervaded by a system of **vesicles, tubules,** and elongated, flat **membranous sacs,** collectively referred to as **platelet demarcation membranes and channels.** The membranes that bind these structures are smooth. Many of the tubules are interconnected. (Fig. 6-30) The cell surface is relatively smooth with only occasional short pseudopods or microvilli.

Megakaryocytes. These giant cells can attain a diameter of up to 100 μ, probably by continued mitotic activity and differentiation. However, the actual life cycle of the megakaryocyte has not been worked out. The megakaryocytes are usually located near, or border on, the sinusoidal capillaries of the bone marrow, or as in

Fig. 6-28. Promegakaryocyte. Bone marrow. Human. E.M. X 6000. **1.** Nucleus. **2.** Nucleoli. **3.** Deep indentations of nuclear surface. **4.** Golgi zone. **5.** Central cytoplasm. **6.** Peripheral cytoplasm. **7.** Cell membrane.

Fig. 6-29. Promegakaryocyte. Enlargement of rectangle in Fig. 6-28. Bone marrow. Human. E.M. X 21,000. **1.** Nucleus **2.** Golgi zones. **3.** Mitochondria. **4.** Granular endoplasmic reticulum. **5.** Alpha granules. **6.** Lysosome. **7.** System of interconnected vesicles, tubules and flat membranous sacs referred to as platelet demarcation membranes and channels.

Fig. 6-30. Detail of promegakaryocyte. Bone marrow. Human. E.M. X 41,000. **1.** Ribosomes. **2.** Alpha granules. **3.** Vesicles. **4.** Tubules. **5.** Interconnected flat membranous sacs.

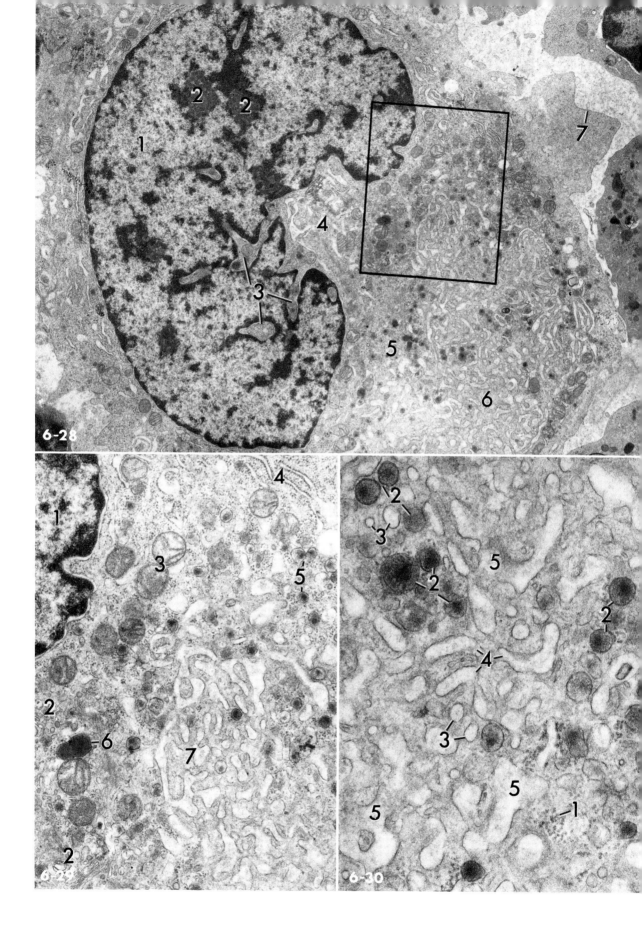

6-28

6-29

6-30

the spleen, the venous sinusoids. (Fig. 6-31) The nucleus is highly lobulated with dense heterochromatin distributed largely along the nuclear membrane. Several nucleoli may be present. The cytoplasm has increased in volume to enormous dimensions. Its component parts are similar in distribution to that of the promegakaryocyte, only that there is now a larger number. The azurophilic granules, the majority of which are referred to as **alpha granules,** have become relatively more numerous. (Fig. 6-32)

The periphery of the megakaryocyte is highly irregular with both large and small pseudopods. Some of these processes protrude across the sinusoidal wall into the circulating blood. It is believed that the cytoplasmic system of interconnected vesicles and membranes of the megakaryocyte by a gradual confluence is largely responsible for the detachment of pieces of the peripheral cytoplasm of the megakaryocyte which thereby become **thrombocytes** and can circulate freely in the blood. Once the megakaryocyte is deprived of most of its cytoplasm, it undergoes degenerative changes and is ultimately digested by macrophages of the bone marrow.

Thrombocytes (platelets). A detailed description of these cell fragments is given on p. 106.

References

Ackerman, G. A. Ultrastructure and cytochemistry of the developing neutrophil. Lab. Investig. *19:* 290–302 (1968).

Ackerman, G. A. The human neutrophilic promyelocyte. Z. Zellforsch. *118:* 467–481 (1971).

Ackerman, G. A. The human neutrophilic myelocyte. Z. Zellforsch. *121:* 153–170 (1971).

Bainton, D. F. and Farquhar, M. G. Segregation and packaging of granule enzymes in eosinophilic leukocytes. J. Cell Biol. 45: 54–73 (1970).

Bainton, D. F., Ullyot, J. L. and Farquhar, M. G. The development of neutrophilic polymorphonuclear leukocytes in human bone marrow. J. Exp. Med. *134:* 907–934 (1971).

Dekkum, D. W. van, Noord, M. J. van, Maat, B. and Dicke, K. A. Attempts at identification of hemopoietic stem cell in mouse. Blood *38:* 547–558 (1971).

Berman, I. The ultrastructure of erythroblastic islands

and reticular cells in mouse bone marrow. J. Ultrastruct. Res. *17:* 291–313 (1967).

Bessis, M. and Thiery, J. Electron microscopy of human white blood cells and their stem cells. Int. Rev. Cytol. *12:* 199–214 (1961).

Caffrey, R. W., Everett, N. B. and Rieke, W. O. Radioautographic studies of reticular and blast cells in the hemopoietic tissues of the rat. Anat. Rec. *155:* 41–58 (1966).

Capone, R. J., Weinreb, E. L. and Chapman, G. B. Electron microscopic studies on normal human myeloid elements. Blood *23:* 300–320 (1964).

Fedorko, M. Formation of cytoplasmic granules in human eosinophilic myelocytes: an electron microscopic autoradiographic study. Blood *31:* 188–194 (1968).

Hardin, J. H. and Spicer, S. S. An ultrastructural study of human eosinophil granules: maturation stages and pyroantimonate reactive cation. Am. J. Anat. *128:* 283–310 (1970).

Hesseldahl, H. and Falck-Larsen, J. Hemopoiesis and blood vessels in human yolk sac. Acta Anat. *78:* 274–294 (1971).

King, J. E. and Ackerman, G. A. Erythropoiesis in the bone marrow of the fetal rabbit. Anat. Rec. *157:* 589–606 (1967).

Lennert, K. Bildung und Differenzierung der Blutzellen, insbesondere der Lymphocyten. Verh. deutsch. Ges. Pathol. *50:* 163–213 (1966).

Marks, P. A. and Rifkind, R. A. Protein synthesis: its control in erythropoiesis. Science *175:* 955–961 (1972).

Murphy, M. J., Bertles, J. R. and Gordon, A. S. Identifying characteristics of the hematopoietic precursor cell. J. Cell Sci. *9:* 23–47 (1971).

Nichols, B. A., Bainton, D. F. and Farquhar, M. G. Differentiation of monocytes. Origin, nature, and fate of their azurophilic granules. J. Cell Biol. *50:* 498–515 (1971).

Nowell, P. C. and Wilson, D. B. Lymphocytes and hemic stem cells. Am. J. Pathol. *65:* 641–652 (1971).

Orlic, D. Ultrastructural analysis of erythropoiesis. *In* Regulation of Hematopoiesis. (Ed. A. S. Gordon), Vol. *1:* 271–296. Appleton-Century-Crofts, New York, 1970.

Orlic D., Gordon, A. S. and Rhodin, J. A. G. An ultrastructural study of erythropoietin-induced red cell formation in mouse spleen. J. Ultrastruct. Res. *13:* 516–542 (1965).

Fig. 6-31. Megakaryocyte. Diameter about 35 μ. Spleen. Rat. E.M. X 3600. **1.** Lobulated nucleus. **2.** Central cytoplasm. **3.** Peripheral cytoplasm with numerous azurophilic granules. **4.** Pseudopod protruding into the lumen of splenic venous sinus.

Fig. 6-32. Enlargement of megakaryocyte pseudopod seen in Fig. 6-31. Spleen. Rat. E.M. X 15,000. **1.** Lumen of venous sinus. **2.** Cytoplasm of lining (littoral) cells. **3.** Stoma (opening) between lining cells, penetrated by megakaryocyte pseudopod. **4.** Alpha granules (azurophilic). **5.** Cytoplasm rich in glycogen particles. **6.** Platelet demarcation channels and membranes. **7.** Free platelet (thrombocyte). **8.** Reticulocyte.

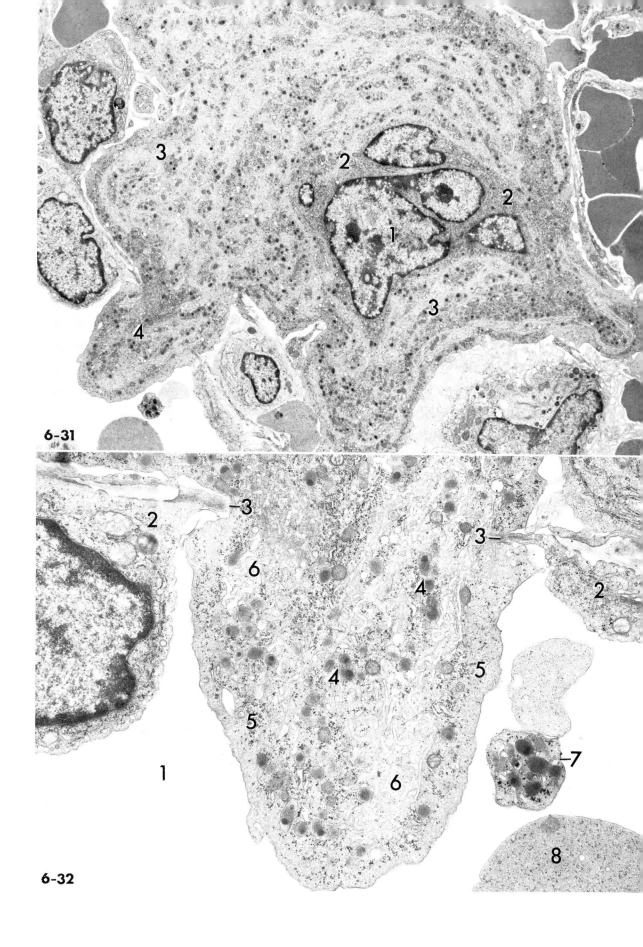

6-31

6-32

Orlic, D., Gordon, A. S. and Rhodin, J. A. G. Ultrastructural and autoradiographic studies of erythropoietin-induced red cell production. Ann. N.Y. Acad. Sci. *149*: 198–216 (1968).

Pease, D. C. An electron microscope study of red bone marrow. Blood *11*: 501–526 (1956).

Richter, G. W. A study of hemosiderosis with the aid of electron microscopy, with observations on the relationship between hemosiderin and ferritin. J. Exp. Med. *106*: 203–217 (1957).

Rifkind, R. A., Danon, D. and Marks, P. A. Alterations in polyribosomes during erythroid cell maturation. J. Cell Biol. *22*:599–611 (1964).

Scott, R. E. and Horn, R. G. Fine structural features of eosinophile granulocyte development in human bone marrow. J. Ultrastruct. Res. *33*: 16–28 (1970).

Simpson, C. F. and Kling, J. M. The mechanism of denucleation in circulating erythroblasts. J. Cell Biol. *35*: 237–245 (1967).

Simpson, C. F. and Kling, J. M. The mechanism of mitochondrial extrusion from phenylhydrazine-induced reticulocytes in the circulating blood. J. Cell Biol. *36*: 103–109 (1968).

Skutelsky, E. and Danon, D. An electron microscope study of nuclear elimination from the late erythroblast. J. Cell Biol. *33*: 625–635 (1967).

Yamada, E. The fine structure of the megakaryocyte in the mouse spleen. Acta Anat. *29*: 267–290 (1957).

Zucker-Franklin, D. The ultrastructure of megakaryocytes and platelets. *In* Regulation of Hematopoiesis. (Ed. A. S. Gordon), Vol. *2*: 1533–1586. Appleton-Century-Crofts, New York, 1970.

7 Connective tissue

GENERAL CONSIDERATIONS

The connective tissues of the mammalian body serve the purpose of supporting and binding together groups of cells which have aggregated to form special tissues and organs because of similarity in function and structure. There are essentially three kinds of connective tissue: 1) connective tissue proper; 2) cartilage; and 3) bone. This chapter deals only with connective tissue proper. Cartilage is discussed in Chapter 8 (p. 174) and bone in Chapter 9 (p. 186). All connective tissues have certain factors in common which consist of cells and extracellular components. The **specific cells** of the connective tissues are the **fibroblasts** (connective tissue proper), the **chondrocytes** (cartilage), and the **osteocytes** (bone). The **extracellular components** are represented by **fibers** (collagenous, reticular, elastic), **ground substance** (jelly-like consistency in connective tissue proper; solid without calcium crystals in cartilage; hard with calcium crystals in bone), and **extracellular fluid.**

There is great variation in relative amount and number of the specific cells and the extracellular components, largely depending on the functional demand and local conditions. The **primary function** of the connective tissue is supportive. A small number of fibers, arranged in a loose network, gives limited support but great flexibility, mobility, and elasticity as in **loose** connective tissue (intestinal lamina propria, connective tissue framework of the lungs). A large number of fibers, densely arranged either in an interwoven network or in parallel, gives great tensile strength but limited flexibility and motion to the parts as in **dense** connective tissue (tendons, ligaments, fasciae, capsules). An even greater supportive strength is achieved by a polymerization of the ground substance, as in cartilage, or by an infiltration and crystallization of calcium salts in the ground substance, as in bone.

Depending on location of the connective tissue proper and its relationship to the specific cells of individual organ and tissue, the connective tissue serves other, **secondary functions.** It serves as a transport medium for the diffusion of metabolites from the vascular system to the specific organ cells as well as a temporary storage area for lipids (fat cells, adipose tissue), electrolytes, and water. In addition, the connective tissue proper represents a compartment with great potential to serve as a protective medium against foreign proteins (antigens, bacteria, viruses) because of the several blood-borne cell types which have left the vascular system and settled down more or less temporarily in the loose connective tissue: neutrophilic polymorphs, eosinophils, monocytes, and lymphocytes.

The precursor of adult connective tissue is the **embryonal connective tissue.** In the fetus and the infant, this exists in essentially two forms, the mesenchymal connective tissue and the mucous connective tissue. The **mesenchymal connective tissue** is a loose, spongy tissue filling in the spaces between the developing organs of the embryo. (Fig. 7-1) It consists of numerous mesenchymal cells, some extracellular fibers, and a fluid ground substance. The mesenchymal cells (Fig. 7-2) are stellate or fusiform with long and slender extensions which adhere to those of neighboring cells, often by means of gap-junctions.

Fig. 7-1. Mesenchymal connective tissue. Hindleg. Rat fetus; 14th day of gestation. E.M. X 620. **1.** Epidermis. **2.** Ground substance of mesenchyme. **3.** Undifferentiated mesenchymal cells. **4.** Small blood vessels. **5.** Small nerve bundle.

Fig. 7-2. Mesenchymal cell. Enlargement of area similar to rectangle in Fig. 7-1. Rat fetus. E.M. X 9000. **1.** Nucleoli. **2.** Mixture of dense heterochromatin and light euchromatin. **3.** Cytoplasmic processes. **4.** Ground substance (semifluid). **5.** Thin fiber bundles. **6.** Granular endoplasmic reticulum. **7.** Mitochondria. **8.** Golgi zone. **9.** Lipid droplet.

Fig. 7-3. Fiber bundle. Enlargement of rectangle in Fig. 7-2. E.M. X 62,000. The individual fibrils average 250 Å in width. Axial banding is not clearly seen in this preparation.

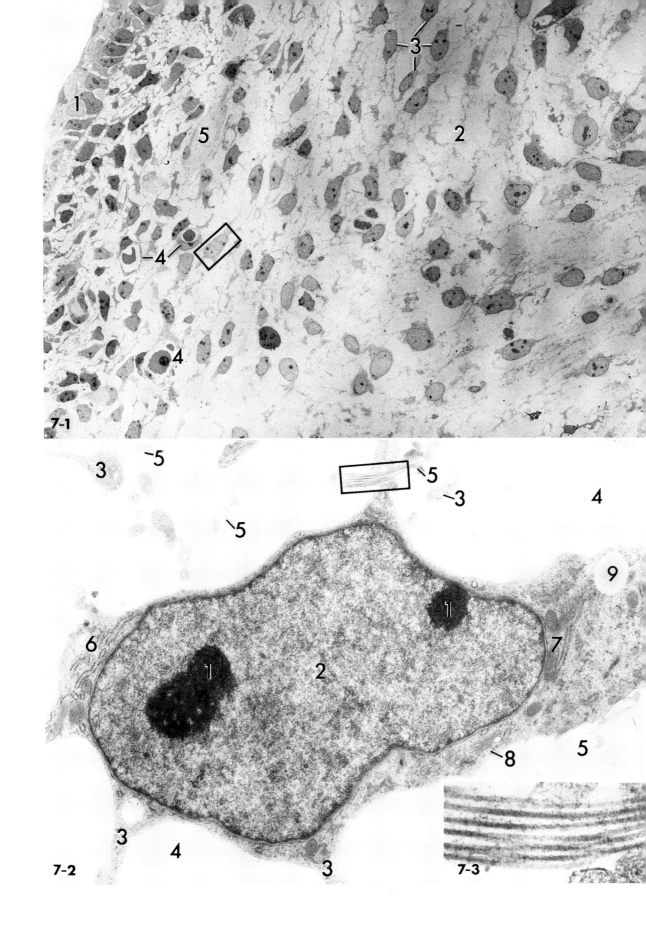

7-1

7-2

7-3

The nucleus is large with several distinct nucleoli. There is an equal amount of euchromatin and heterochromatin distributed throughout the nucleus. The cytoplasm occupies a small zone around the nucleus. Ribosomes abound, whereas profiles of granular endoplasmic reticulum and mitochondria occur in small number. The Golgi zone is small. The **extracellular fibers** are thin and form a very wide meshwork, often without special relationship to the mesenchymal cells. Each fiber is composed of several small fibrils (Fig. 7-3), each averaging about 400 Å in width, and with an axial banding of 250 Å periodicity. In adult connective tissue, these fibrils would be referred to as reticular fibrils (p. 148). The **ground substance** is very scanty and is usually dissolved with present electron microscopical fixation techniques.

The mesenchymal cell is multipotential, and it can develop into many kinds of connective tissue cells including fibroblasts, chondroblasts, osteoblasts, and fat cells. It also gives rise to smooth and striated muscle cells, blood cells, and vascular cells such as endothelium and pericytes.

The **mucous connective tissue** is structurally very similar to mesenchymal tissue. It makes up the umbilical cord (p. 731) and consists of a small number of mesenchymal fibroblasts and large amounts of fine collagenous fibrils, some elastic fibers, and a highly mucoid ground substance which gives it a gelatinous consistency (Wharton's jelly).

Characteristics of Adult Connective Tissue Proper

The connective tissue proper consists of 1) fibers; 2) ground substance; and 3) cells.

FIBERS

There exists essentially three categories of fibers: 1) collagenous; 2) elastic; and 3) reticular. These may occur singly or together in quite varied proportions depending on functional demands. The term **fiber** is used to describe fibrous structures which can readily be resolved with the light microscope, whereas **fibril** is a term reserved for structural units that can be resolved only with the electron microscope. Few investigators distinguish between fibril and filament. However, in our opinion, the term **filament** should be used only for straight, thread-like ultrastructural units which range between 40 Å and 150 Å in diameter. Many times a filament and a microtubule (see p. 44) may have the same diameter, and it is in this general area that one has to employ biochemical and biophysical techniques to be able to separate functionally these minute thread-like intracellular and extracellular structures.

Collagenous fibers. The collagenous (white) fibers vary in width from 1 μ to 20 μ. (Fig. 7-4) Their length has not been

Fig. 7-4. Collagenous fibers of dense fibrous connective tissue. Ligament. Knee joint. Rat. E.M. X 9000. **1.** Cross-sectioned collagenous fibers. **2.** Longitudinally sectioned collagenous fiber. Width averages 1.6 μ. Individual collagenous fibrils appear as small dots. **3.** Ground substance. Note absence of fibroblasts.

Fig. 7-5. Collagenous fibrils sectioned longitudinally. Enlargement of area similar to rectangle in Fig. 7-4. Tunica albuginea testis. Rat. E.M. X 62,000. **1.** Width of individual fibril averages 650 Å. **2.** Spacing between arrows averages 600 Å.

Fig. 7-6. Single collagenous fibril. Enlargement of area similar to rectangle in Fig. 7-5. Sclera. Mouse. E.M. X 200,000. **1.** Width: 600 Å. **2.** Axial periodicity: 500 Å.

Fig. 7-7. Chorda tendinea. Cross section. Heart. Rat. E.M. X 51,000. **1.** Narrow cytoplasmic process of fibroblast. **2.** Mitochondrion. **3.** Collagenous fibrils, average width 500 Å. **4.** Amorphous substance of elastic fiber. **5.** Microfibrils of elastic fiber. **6.** Microfibrils unassociated with elastic amorphous substance.

Fig. 7-8. Cross-sectioned collagenous fibrils. Ligament. Knee joint. Rat. E.M. X 50,000. In this part of the ligament, the collagenous fibrils vary greatly in width. **1.** Width 1000 Å. **2.** Width: 600 Å. **3.** Width: 400 Å.

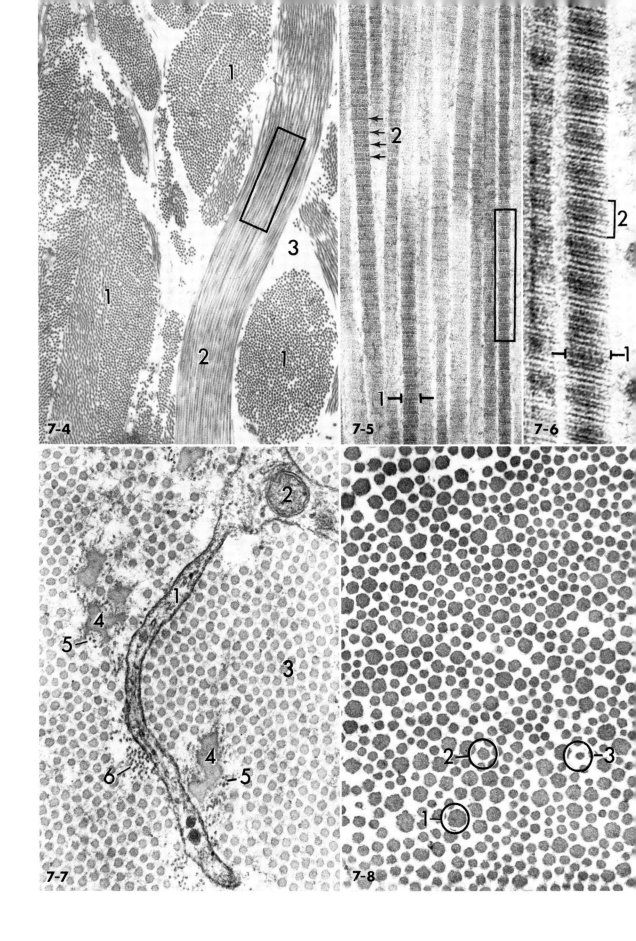

7-4

7-5

7-6

7-7

7-8

determined but it is assumed that they extend for distances well over several hundred millimeters. Some fibers are situated close to fibroblasts but others run independently and seemingly without relating to fibroblasts. Their course may be straight (tendon), undulating (loose connective tissue), in parallel (tendon), or they may cross each other (aponeurons, ligaments) and the fibers may be densely packed or loosely arranged, all depending on location and functional demands. Each fiber is made up of numerous **collagenous fibrils** which average 650 Å in width. (Figs. 7-5, 7-6) Their length has not been determined. Newly formed collagenous fibrils have a diameter of about 200 Å, and it is generally accepted that the width of the fibril increases with age. On the other hand, in some areas of the body, the collagenous fibers are made up solely of 500 Å-wide fibrils throughout life, whereas other fibers contain both large (1000 Å) and small (300 Å) fibrils. (Figs. 7-7, 7-8) Whether large or small, the fibrils are made up of numerous **tropocollagen units** (also called protofibrils), arranged in parallel, end-to-end, and in a staggered array, held together by side bonds, all of which renders the collagenous fibril a cross-banded periodicity of 640 Å. The collagen is rich in hydroxyproline and hydroxylysine in addition to proline and glycin. These amino acids form three helical polypeptide chains which in turn are twisted around each other to form a larger spiral, the **tropocollagen macromolecule,** measuring 14 Å in width and 2800 Å in length. The characteristic cross-banding of the collagenous fibril is due to a 25% overlap of the length of the tropocollagen units. Collagen is excreted by the fibroblasts into the extracellular space as a monomere and is polymerized extracellularly (see p. 152).

The collagenous fibers have a high tensile strength and are only slightly elastic. The fibers may give the appearance of being branched, but are merely small bundles of fibrils which deviate. Individual fibrils as well as smaller bundles of fibrils are bound together by small amounts of interfibrillar substance.

Elastic fibers. The adult elastic (yellow) fibers vary in width from 1 μ to 10 μ. (Fig. 7–9) They branch and anastomose as they course straight through loose or dense, irregular connective tissue where they are quite abundant. The elastic fibers may also fuse to form extensive fenestrated membranous sheets, particularly in making up the walls of blood vessels. The elastic fibers and the elastic membranes consist of two components: 1) microfibrils and 2) amorphous substance. The **microfibrils** constitute the predominant structure of developing elastic fibers and grad-

Fig. 7-9. Elastic and collagenous fibers. Tunica albuginea testis. Rat. E.M. X 32,000. **1.** Elastic fiber, sectioned longitudinally; width 0.5 μ; central amorphous substance. **2.** Collagenous fibrils. **3.** Peripheral microfibrils of elastic fiber. **4.** Cytoplasmic strands of fibroblasts.

Fig. 7-10. Part of fibroblast and collagenous fibrils. Chorda tendinea. Heart. Rat. E.M. X 120,000. **1.** Cisternae of granular endoplasmic reticulum. **2.** Ribosomes. **3.** Cell membrane of fibroblast. **4.** Cross-sectioned collagenous fibrils; width 600 Å. **5.** Ground substance of connective tissue contains some minute filaments which average 80 Å in width. They may represent double-beaded collagenous filaments or immature collagenous fibrils.

Fig. 7-11. Cross-sectioned elastic fiber (width 0.5 μ). Chorda tendinea. Heart. Rat. E.M. X 120,000. **1.** Central amorphous substance. **2.** Peripheral mantle of microfibrils; width of microfibrils averages 130 Å. **3.** Some microfibrils within amorphous substance.

Fig. 7-12. Part of fibroblast and longitudinally sectioned elastic fiber. Tunica albuginea testis. E.M. X 120,000. **1.** Cytoplasmic matrix of fibroblast. **2.** Ribosomes. **3.** Cisternae of granular endoplasmic reticulum. **4.** Central cavity of smooth surfaced micropinocytotic invaginations. **5.** Trilaminar cell membrane. **6.** Microfibrils. **7.** Amorphous substance.

Fig. 7-13. Periphery of elastic fiber sectioned longitudinally. Tunica albuginea testis. E.M. X 120,000. **1.** Arrows point to peripheral microfibrils of elastic fiber. **2.** Parts of central amorphous substance of elastic fiber.

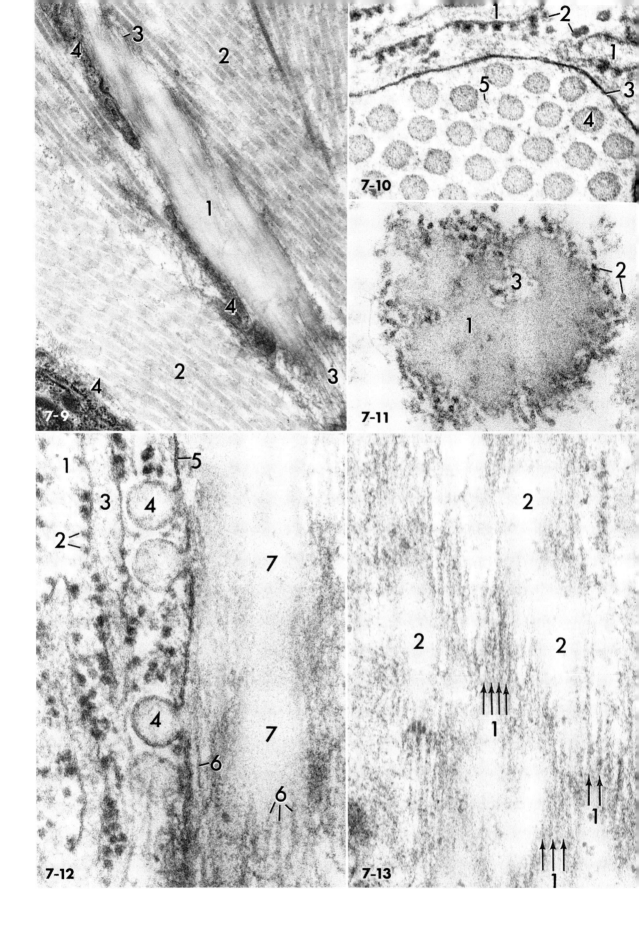

ually become less numerous with age. They average 130 Å in width and appear tubular with a light central core. (Fig. 7-11) The microfibrils may exhibit an indistinct segmentation and are usually arranged in parallel array. (Fig. 7-13) The **amorphous substance** increases in amount with increasing age, forming large structureless masses. (Fig. 7-12) The microfibrils form a peripheral envelope or mantle around the central amorphous substance. They may also occur singly or in small groups unrelated to the amorphous substance but associated with a variety of structures such as collagenous fibrils, boundary membranes, basal laminae, lymphatic channels, and subendothelial basement membranes. Biochemical analyses of elastic fibers indicate that the amino acid composition of the amorphous substance is poor in hydroxyproline and rich in valine, glycine, proline, and alanine. This corresponds roughly to the postulated characteristic protein of elastic fibers which has been termed **elastin.** The large polypeptide molecules of the elastin are not oriented to one another in a definite pattern similar to collagen. The microfibrils consist of a different connective tissue protein that is neither collagen nor elastin. It contains far less glycine and proline but -more hydroxyproline. Since the microfibrils form an aggregate structure before the appearance of the amorphous component, it is assumed that they determine the shape of the elastic fibers in various tissues.

The elastic fibers can be stretched to about 1.5 times their original length, and they return almost completely to their original length when released after stretching. The synthesis of the elastic fiber is controlled by fibroblasts and smooth muscle cells (see p. 152). The microfibrils are usually in close apposition to the cell membrane of these cells, often in niches or infoldings of the cell. With the appearance of amorphous substance, the elastic fibers move away from the fibroblasts or smooth muscle cells.

Reticular fibers. The reticular fibers form a delicate network (reticulum) in which the individual fibers vary in diameter from 1000 Å to 1.5 μ. The fibers are **argyrophilic,** that is, they can be made visible under the light microscope by special silver impregnation techniques. (Fig. 7-14) The fibers are permanent components of the fibrous framework of lymphoid and myeloid tissues. They form a fine meshwork as part of the basement membrane of surface epithelia and endothelia of capillaries and blood vessels. (Fig. 7-15) They also surround fat cells and form the connective tissue stroma of the liver, pancreas, and many other parenchymatous organs. In the lymphoid and myeloid tissues, the reticular fibers are closely related to the reticular cells (fixed macrophages) and are often embraced by sheets of reticular cell cytoplasm. In other tissues, they are closely related to fibroblasts and smooth muscle cells. Fibers reminiscent of reticular fibers are present abundantly in the mesenchyme of the fetus and the newborn.

Each reticular fiber consists of a large

Fig. 7-14. Reticular fibers in red pulp. Silver impregnation. Spleen. Rat. L.M. X 665. **1.** Lumen of blood vessel. **2.** Wall of blood vessel. **3.** Reticular fibers; width between bars 1.5μ. **4.** Individual cells of red pulp cannot be categorized at this magnification.

Fig. 7-15. Wall of venule. Medullary cord. Lymph node. Enlargement of area similar to rectangle in Fig. 7-14. Rat. E.M. X 4800. **1.** Lumen of venule. **2.** Nucleus of endothelial cell. **3.** Cytoplasmic strands of pericytes. **4.** Reticular fibrils form a loose network in the vascular wall. Bar is 1.5 μ. **5.** Nucleus of granular leukocyte. **6.** Lymphocyte.

Figs. 7-16 & 7-17. Details of reticular fibrils. Synovial membrane. Knee joint. Enlargement of area similar to rectangle in Fig. 7-15. Rat. E.M. X 156,000. **1.** Reticular fibrils: width between bars 250 Å. **2.** Arrow: axial banding with no apparent regular periodicity. **3.** Elastic microfibrils with light core: width 90 Å. **4.** Apparent axial periodicity in this reticular fibril: distance between arrows 250 Å. **5.** Thin cytoplasmic strand of fibroblast. **6.** Delicate collagenous fibril; width 400 Å.

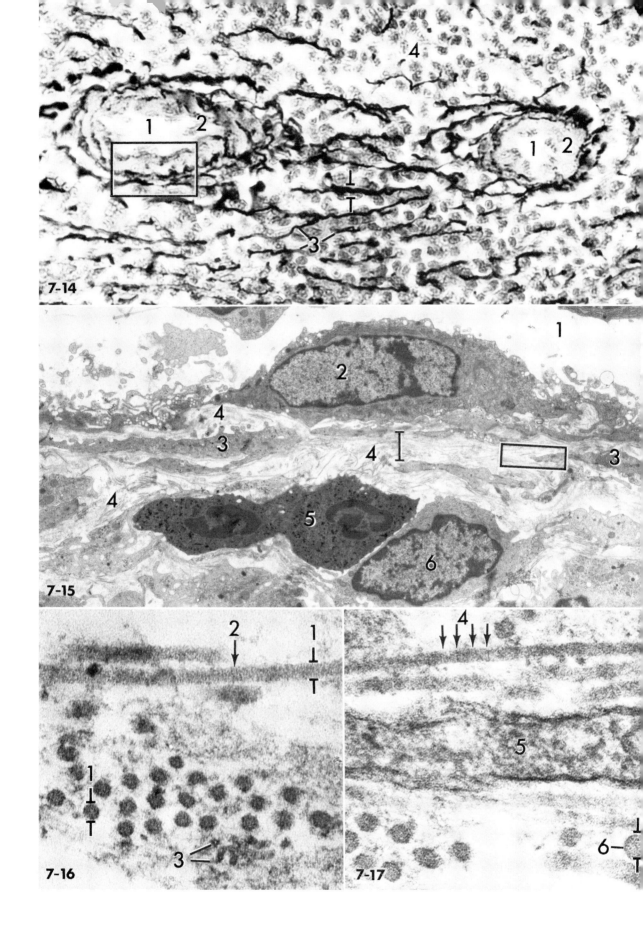

number of **reticular fibrils** averaging 300 Å in diameter and characterized by a 250 Å periodic cross-banding. (Figs. 7-16, 7-17) It is generally believed that the reticular fibrils represent delicate collagenous fibrils which can either remain small for an indefinite length of time or may enlarge to become "mature" collagenous fibrils by an increase in cross-sectional diameter.

GROUND SUBSTANCE

The ground substance of the connective tissue proper contains 1) fluid; 2) interstitial matrix; and 3) basement membranes.

Fluid. The water-rich phase of the ground substance is probably quite restricted and small under normal circumstances. After tissue injury and during inflammation, free fluid accumulates rapidly, most of it derived from leaky blood capillaries.

Interstitial matrix. The colloid-rich phase of the ground substance is a gelatinous matrix which exists at varied levels of water binding. The matrix is made up of **mucoproteins** and of two major mucopolysaccharides; hyaluronic acid (mostly in loose connective tissue) and chondroitin sulfuric acid (high concentrations in cartilage matrix). Under the electron microscope, this intercellular matrix is poorly defined and shows up as a medium dense, homogeneous or slightly flocculent substance. It has been suggested that fibroblasts and possibly smooth muscle cells, where present, participate in the synthesis of the intercellular matrix by discharging protein-polysaccharide complexes via coated vesicles.

Basement membranes. The basement membranes are interstitital condensations, continuous with the ground substance of the connective tissue proper. They underlie most epithelial membranes and enclose fat cells, muscle cells, Schwann cells of peripheral nerves, and capillaries. In light microscopy, the basement membrane is resolved as a zone of varied thickness, de-

pending on tissue and organ. With the aid of the electron microscope (Fig. 7-18), it can be seen that the basement membrane consists of essentially two parts: 1) a thin basal lamina facing the cell membrane of related cells; and 2) a network of reticular fibrils, microfibrils similar to those associated with elastic fibers, and fine collagenous fibrils blending with other adjacent connective tissue fibrils. The **basal lamina** (synonyms: boundary membrane; external lamina; lamina densa) is 300–700 Å thick. (Fig. 7-19) In exceptional cases, it can attain widths of up to 3000 Å even under normal circumstances (human glomerular filtration membrane; zona pellucida of the ovarian follicle; Descemet's membrane in the cornea).

The basal lamina is composed of a diffusely flocculent or often finely filamentous material. (Fig. 7-20) Biochemical analyses indicate that the basal lamina is rich in mucopolysaccharides and proteins with amino acid composition similar to

Fig. 7-18. Basement membrane. Epidermis. Human. E.M. X 18,000. **1.** Basal processes of basal cells. **2.** Basal lamina; width 1000 Å. **3.** Reticular fibrils. **4.** Aggregations of elastic microfibrils. **5.** Delicate collagenous fibrils. **6.** Cytoplasmic strand of fibroblast.

Fig. 7-19. Basement membrane. Intestine. Rat. E.M. X 48,000. **1.** Base of epithelial cells in crypt of Lieberkühn. **2.** Basal lamina; width 400 Å. **3.** Reticular fibrils; width 300 Å. **4.** Cytoplasmic strand of fibroblast. **5.** Delicate collagenous or reticular fibrils; width 300 Å. **6.** Elastic microfibrils, unassociated with amorphous elastic substance, form a finely filamentous network. **7.** Endothelial cell of lymph capillary. Note absence of basal lamina underneath lymphatic endothelium. **8.** Lumen of capillary. **9.** Mitochondrion. **10.** Coated vesicle.

Fig. 7-20. Comparison of two basal laminae. Kidney. Rat. E.M. X 60,000. **1.** Basal processes of proximal tubule cell. **2.** Basal lamina of proximal tubule. This is exceptionally thick in rat (width 5000 Å) and some of the basal cell processes are lodged partly in the basal lamina. **3.** Small interstitial space. **4.** Basal lamina of peritubular blood capillary; width 330 Å. **5.** Fenestrated capillary endothelium. **6.** Capillary lumen.

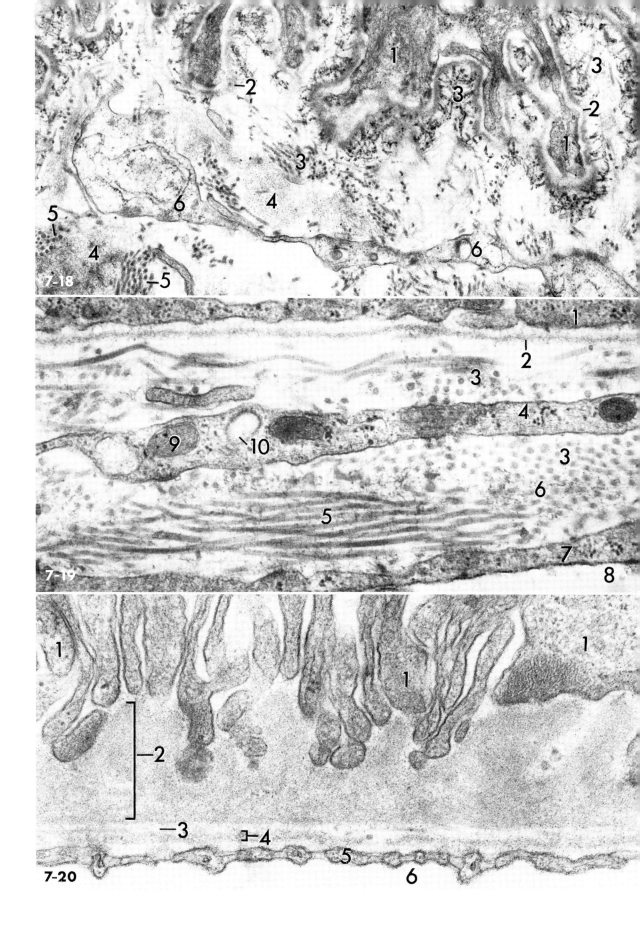

that of collagen. It is likely that the finely fibrillar content is the collagenous component and the amorphous material is the non-collagenous fraction. Recent investigations have shown convincingly that the basal lamina is synthesized by the related cells, although, in the past, one strongly believed that there was a connective tissue control of this synthesis. The basal lamina establishes a microenvironment for the related cells and acts as a diffusion barrier to rapid ion exchanges.

CELLS

Fibroblasts and reticular cells are the **specific fixed cells** of connective tissue proper. As a rule, mast cells and fat cells are also encountered regularly, whereas macrophages, granular leukocytes, lymphocytes, plasma cells, and monocytes are **wandering cells** and therefore more transient. Pigment-containing cells (melanocytes) occur in the connective tissue of the skin.

Fibroblasts. The term fibroblast is generally used for the active specific connective tissue cell that is responsible for the synthesis of most of the extracellular material, both fibers and ground substance. The term **fibrocyte** refers to the same cell in resting or less active phase with less cytoplasm and much diminished fine structure. (Fig. 7-21) The fibroblast is derived from the mesenchyme and it closely resembles the mesenchymal cell (see p. 140). The number of fibroblasts varies greatly with the type of connective tissue. There are only a few in loose connective tissue, whereas there is a relative abundance in dense connective tissue. Superficially, the loose connective tissue is rich in cells, but the majority of these cells are not fibroblasts.

The **fibroblast** is spindle-shaped or stellate with long, thin cytoplasmic processes, some of which lie parallel to, and often partly surround, collagenous fibers. The cytoplasm is relatively scarce, and does not show up well in routine light microscope preparations. The nucleus is oval and

slightly indented with a thin marginal zone of dense heterochromatin and several nucleoli. The granular endoplasmic reticulum is well developed with long interconnecting cisternae, some of which vary greatly in shape and show marked dilatations. (Fig. 7-22) The cisternae often contain a medium dense, homogeneous substance. There occur numerous free ribosomes. The Golgi zone is large and well developed with some dilated sacs, numerous vacuoles and vesicles, the latter of both the smooth and the coated (acanthosome) variety. Profiles of elongated, membrane-bound granules with apparent filamentous content may be present. Mitochondria are large but scarce, and lipid droplets occur occasionally. Filaments, 50–70 Å thick, may be present in small numbers throughout the cytoplasm and in aggregations at certain points along the cell membrane. Coated vesicles and numerous smooth, micropinocytotic vesicles are connected with the cell membrane. (Fig. 7-23) There is no external lamina (basal lamina) associated with fibroblasts.

Fig. 7-21. Fibrocytes. Enlargement of rectangle in Fig. 7-32. Submucosa. Tertiary bronchus. Cat. E.M. X 9500. **1.** Nuclei of fibrocytes. **2.** Cytoplasm is sparse and the cells spindle-shaped. There is only a small amount of granular endoplasmic reticulum, indicating that this is a resting fibrocyte rather than an active fibroblast. **3.** Collagenous fibers, each made up of numerous collagenous fibrils. **4.** Ground substance of connective tissue.

Fig. 7-22. Fibroblast (tendon cell). Enlargement of area similar to rectangle in Fig. 7-35. Tendon. Tail. Rat. E.M. X 9500. **1.** Nucleoli of fibroblast. **2.** Nuclear membrane. **3.** Golgi zone (small). **4.** Dilated cisternae of granular endoplasmic reticulum. **5.** Mitochondria. **6.** Sheet-like cytoplasmic processes. **7.** Collagenous fibers.

Fig. 7-23. Fibroblast. Synovial membrane. Knee joint. E.M. X 37,000. **1.** Nucleus of fibroblast. **2.** Mitochondria. **3.** Ribosomes. **4.** Smooth surfaced micropinocytotic invaginations. **5.** Coated invagination. **6.** Coated invagination (flattening out or starting to invaginate). **7.** Flocculent ground substance. **8.** Reticular and delicate collagenous fibrils; width 300 Å.

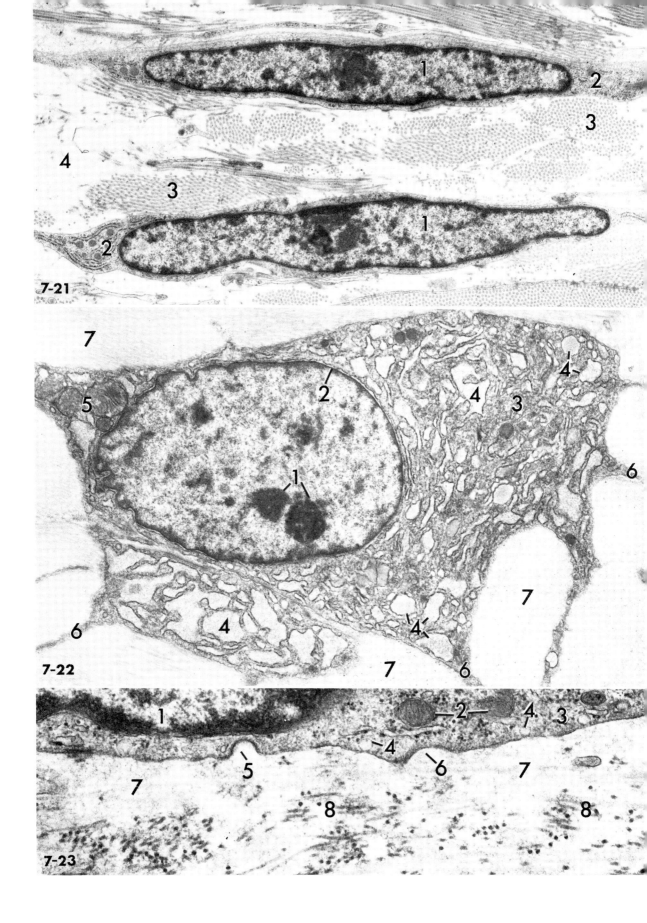

7-21

7-22

7-23

The **function** of the fibroblast relates to the synthesis of collagenous, elastic and reticular fibers and the production of mucopolysaccharides for the ground substance. The precise intracellular events that precede **collagen fiber formation** is not clear, and there are presently two theories. On the one hand, it is believed that the amino acids and polypeptides of the tropocollagen are formed and assembled on the ribosomes, shed into the cisterna of the endoplasmic reticulum, and then moved to the vesicles and sacs of the Golgi zone. Subsequently, these vesicles and dilated sacs, some of which contain condensed, and even filamentous material, move to the periphery of the cell and discharge their contents of tropocollagen, or its precursors, into the extracellular space. On the other hand, it has been shown that a major portion of the collagenous proline passes directly from the cisternae of the endoplasmic reticulum to the extracellular space without going through the Golgi zone.

In either case, the cell surface of the fibroblast is the site of accumulation of newly released **tropocollagen units** (14 Å × 2800 Å), and the cell surface provides structural substrate for the polymerization of these units into a periodic thread, the **procollagen filament** (40 Å × 7000 Å) with nodules at 640 Å intervals. When this filament is formed, it is released from the cell to join end-to-end with other procollagen filaments. The procollagen filament serves as a template for the continued polymerization of tropocollagen. Replication of another procollagen filament in register with the parent filament yields a double **beaded filament** composed of two 40 Å filaments linked in parallel with one another by means of beads at intervals of 640 Å along the length of the filament. An aggregation of double beaded filaments together with associated procollagen filaments is recognized as an **immature collagenous fibril.** Maturation occurs by progressive cross-linking between beaded filaments to form the cohesive **adult col-**lagenous fibrils, the most delicate represented by **reticular fibrils.**

In **elastic fiber formation,** it is believed that both fibroblasts and smooth muscle cells can synthesize and assemble the amino acids and polypeptides that form the peripheral microfibrils and the central amorphous substance of the elastic fiber. The microfibrils are formed first and may polymerize at the cell surface in a similar way that is postulated for the tropocollagen units. The amorphous substance of the elastic fiber which appears subsequent to the microfibrils may arise by a fusion of microfibrils, or it may be discharged from the fibroblast in a separate process, or it may be formed by a combination of both processes. The possibility has been suggested that the elastic microfibrils represent precursors of all connective tissue fibers, including reticular, collagenous, and elastic fibrils. If so, they would most closely correspond to the immature collagenous fibrils.

The **formation** of the **ground substance** of the connective tissue proper is not well understood, but it may arise from a discharge of coated vesicles of the fibroblasts.

Reticular cells. The reticular cell is a close relative of the fibroblast, since one of its primary functions is to synthesize reticular fibers and delicate collagenous fibrils. The reticular cell is also related to the macrophage, since it serves in the combined capacity of synthesizing reticular

Fig. 7-24. Mast cell. Lymph node. Rat. E.M. X 24,000. **1.** Nuclear euchromatin.
2. Heterochromatin. **3.** Golgi zone.
4. Mitochondria. **5.** Ribosomes. **6.** Short profiles of granular endoplasmic reticulum.
7. Secretory granules. **8.** Vacuoles, possibly remnants of discharged secretory granules.
9. Microvilli. **10.** Cell membrane.

Fig. 7-25. Detail of mast cell. Tracheal submucosa. Human. E.M. X 54,000. **1.** Cell membrane. **2.** Ribosomes. **3.** Mitochondria.
4. Matrix of secretory granules. **5.** "Scrolls" cross-sectioned. **6.** "Scrolls" sectioned longitudinally. **7.** Poorly preserved boundary membrane of secretory granule.

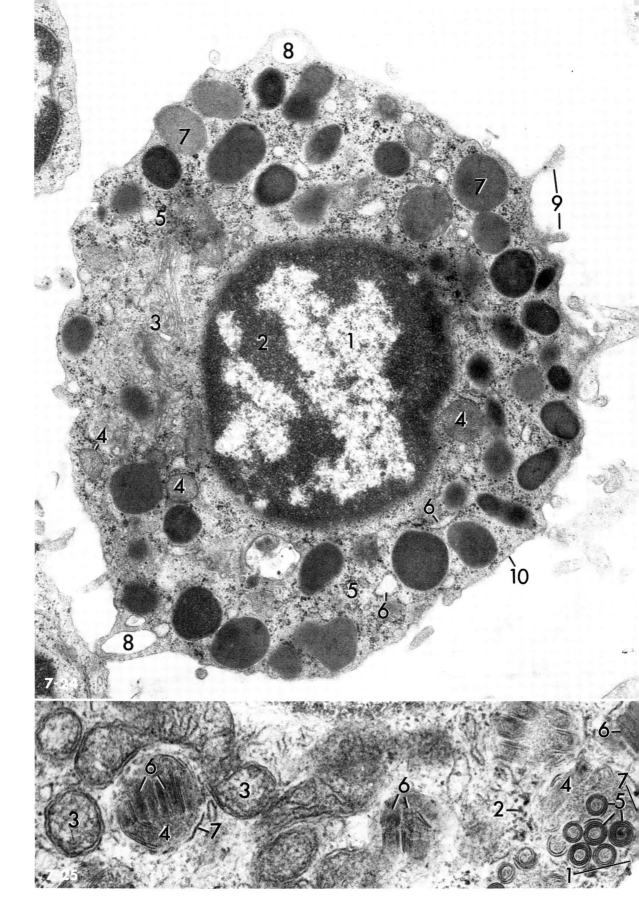

fibers and phagocytosing particles and foreign proteins. The reticular cells form a delicate network in the bone marrow. Their possible role as precursors of blood cells in myeloid tissue, has been questioned lately, and is discussed on p. 112. In the lymph nodes, the reticular cells form a relatively dense network of highly phagocytic cells. Their role in the immunological defense system of the body by digesting antigenic proteins is discussed on p. 382. In the spleen (p. 402) the reticular cells also form a wide network, but, as a rule, are less phagocytic than in lymph nodes. The parenchyma of the thymus is permeated by a wide network of cells termed epithelial reticular cells (p. 418), which represent a separate group of supporting cells with an ectodermal rather than a mesenchymal origin, and with no apparent phagocytic properties.

Mast cells. Among the more permanent cells of the connective tissue proper is the mast cell. It is prevalent in the dermis of man and rodents, in the liver of the dog, and in the lungs of the guinea pig. It is generally found in the loose connective tissue along small blood vessels and near fat cells. It originates from mesenchymal cells in the fetus, but it has not been possible to trace its precursors in adult tissue.

The mast cell is round or oval, averaging 12–15 μ in width. It has a small, round nucleus and an abundant cytoplasm filled with numerous secretion granules. (Fig. 7-24) In ordinary light microscope preparations the nucleus is obscured by the many granules. The cell surface is smooth with a varied number of short microvilli. The cytoplasm is lightly basophilic due to a small number of free ribosomes and short profiles of granular endoplasmic reticulum. The Golgi zone is well developed and the mitochondria are round and few in number. The **secretory granules** average 1 μ in width. They are bounded by a thin membrane, in human tissues difficult to preserve undisrupted. (Fig. 7-25) It surrounds a finely granular matrix which contains a heterogenous population

of membranous structures, reminiscent of scrolls. In the rodent these membranous whorls are missing. The secretory granules are basophilic, water soluble, and metachromatic. **Metachromasia** is the term used for staining reactions in which the stained material takes on a color (purplered) different from that of the applied dye (toluidine blue). The phenomenon is due to the presence of sulfated acid mucopolysaccharides. The secretory granules contain **heparin,** a complex of sulfated mucopolysaccharides and basic protein, as well as **histamine** and **serotonin,** the latter stored in an ionic linkage to the heparin-protein complex. The core of the granule is discharged at the cell surface by a process of exocytosis whereby the perigranular membrane fuses with the cell membrane. There is no external lamina (basal lamina) associated with mast cells.

The **functions** of the mast cell relate to the action by its secretory products. Heparin is an anticoagulant substance, and serotonin is a vasoconstrictor agent. The effect of histamine is on the endothelium of postcapillary venules, increasing their permeability to plasma proteins and stim-

Fig. 7-26. Free macrophage. Spleen. Rat. E.M. X 19,000. **1.** Nucleolus. **2.** Euchromatin. **3.** Heterochromatin. **4.** Golgi zone. **5.** Mitochondria. **6.** Granular endoplasmic reticulum. **7.** Small primary lysosomes. **8.** Secondary lysosomes. **9.** Microvilli. **10.** Interstitial space of red splenic pulp.

Fig. 7-27. Primary lysosomes. Kupffer cell. Liver. Rat. E.M. X 120,000. **1.** Matrix of primary lysosomes. **2.** Trilaminar lysosomal boundary membrane; width 70 Å. **3.** Matrix of this primary lysosome is denser, possibly indicating ingested material. **4.** Ribosomes. **5.** Small vesicle, possibly part of nearby Golgi zone.

Fig. 7-28. Secondary lysosome. Macrophage. Spleen. Rat. E.M. X 60,000. **1.** Interior of secondary lysosome filled with dense matrix and layered structures. **2.** Lysosomal boundary membrane. **3.** Two small primary lysosomes, one of which apparently merges (arrows) with secondary lysosome. **4.** Part of Golgi zone. **5.** Ribosomes.

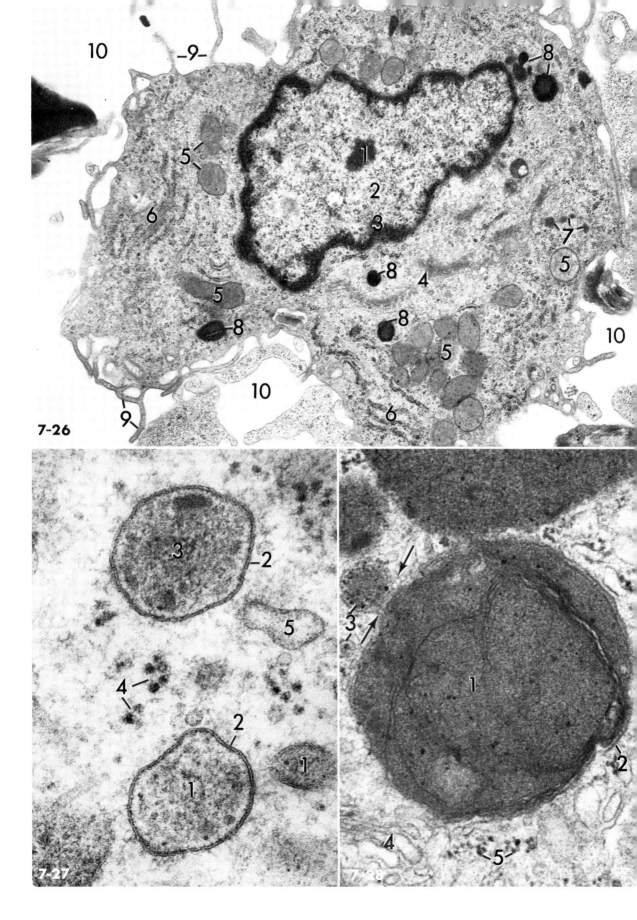

ulating diapedesis of leukocytes. In addition, the enzyme hyaluronidase may be synthesized and discharged by the mast cell. It increases connective tissue permeability by reducing the viscosity of the ground substance. The proximity of mast cells to small blood vessels seems to indicate that the mast cells participate in maintaining normal, functional relationship between blood vessels and the connective tissue compartment.

Macrophages. Macrophages (phagocytes, histiocytes) are present in virtually every organ where there is loose and richly vascularized connective tissue. The macrophages can be classified into two major categories: fixed macrophages (resting wandering cells) and free macrophages (true wandering cells). Macrophages represent an essential part of the defense system of the mammalian body against invading microorganisms, foreign proteins (antigens), and inert foreign matter. They are also functionally important since they pick up tissue debris and effete cells (erythrocytes, lymphocytes, plasma cells, thymocytes). The macrophages appear in many shapes and locations throughout the body, and they are often collectively referred to as the **reticuloendothelial system (R.E.S.).** This system consists of phagocytic cells placed at certain strategic positions where they come in contact with interstitial fluid, lymph, and the circulating blood. The reticular cells of the spleen (p. 402) and lymph nodes (p. 382) are part of this system, as are the endothelial (Kupffer) cells of the liver sinusoids (p. 584), the lining (littoral) cells of the splenic (p. 408) lymph node (p. 380) and bone marrow (p. 198) sinuses.

The macrophages originate from mesenchymal cells and subsequently arise by mitosis from existing macrophages. Blood monocytes readily become macrophages upon leaving the vascular channels, and it is possible that both lymphocytes and fibroblasts can be transformed into macrophages at times of great demand for these cells.

The fixed macrophages generally are flat, spindle-shaped, or multiangular, whereas the free macrophages are mostly round or oval. The following description pertains to all macrophages with only slight exceptions. The nucleus is oval with several indentations. It contains several nucleoli and an abundance of dense peripheral heterochromatin. The nuclear membrane is exceptionally porous. The cell surface varies tremendously, depending on the location of the cell, but microvilli and pseudopods are numerous in the actively phagocytic cells, particularly in the free macrophages which probably are highly ameboid. (Fig. 7-26) The cytoplasm is abundant and contains a moderate amount of free ribosomes and, depending on the species, either a large amount of granular endoplasmic reticulum (mouse, rat) or a small amount (man). The Golgi zone is prominent with numerous vesicles of both the smooth and the coated variety. Mitochondria are oval and few in number. The surface membrane has numerous pinocytotic invaginations, most of which are smooth but some are typically coated (acanthosomes). There is no external lamina (basal lamina) associated with macrophages. The macrophage is filled with a varied number of vesicles, vacuoles, lysosomes, and residual bodies. These structures are part of a process referred to as **phagocytosis,** which is an uptake (ingestion) of particulate matter by an invagination of the cell membrane. The invaginated cell membrane encloses the phagocytosed particle in a smooth-walled vesicle or vacuole which is referred to as

Fig. 7-29. Plasma cell. Bone marrow. Human. E.M. X 16,000. **1.** Nucleolus. **2.** Euchromatin. **3.** Heterochromatin. **4.** Golgi zone. **5.** Centrioles. **6.** Mitochondria. **7.** Granular endoplasmic reticulum. **8.** Ribosomes. **9.** Primary lysosomes. **10.** Microvillus. **11.** Cell membrane. **12.** Pseudopod. **13.** Flocculent intercellular matrix of bone marrow cavity. **14.** Part of arteriolar smooth muscle cells.

7-29

a **phagosome** once it has become detached and moved away from the cell surface. Organic material is digested by proteolytic enzymes, mainly hydrolases, derived from **primary lysosomes.** (Fig. 7-27) These are membrane-bound vesicles, or dense bodies, derived from the Golgi sacs, which fuse with the phagosomes to form **secondary** lysosomes (Fig. 7-28); and as lysis progresses they are called **residual bodies.** The latter may contain lipid droplets, bacteria, dye particles, or iron-rich degradation products depending on the ingested matter.

One of the main **functions** of the macrophage is therefore to serve as scavenger cell throughout the body and to dispose of effete cells and extraneous matter. In the dermis, macrophages pick up and retain indefinitely inert foreign matter such as dye particles (the basis for the tatoo process). In the lungs, alveolar macrophages pick up inhaled carbon and dust particles and are subsequently carried via the lymphatics to regional lymph nodes, or become lodged in the connective tissue, giving rise to the black pattern seen at the surface of the lungs. The macrophages contribute to the antibody response of the body by trapping, processing, and storing antigens, and by presenting specific information to the antibody forming lymphocytes or plasma cells in the form of fragments of antigens coupled to ribonucleic acid (p. 382). The macrophage also plays an important role in iron metabolism. Upon ingestion of erythrocytes, the hemoglobin becomes digested. The iron and the protein are retained by the macrophage and utilized in erythropoiesis, whereas some of the hemoglobin is transformed to bilirubin and eliminated via bile secretion in the liver. Under the stimulus of inflammatory conditions, macrophages become especially active in ingesting tissue and cellular debris.

Plasma cells. Plasma cells are the main source of antibody synthesis, and these cells therefore represent an important link in the immunological defense system of the mammalian body. Plasma cells are particularly numerous in the medullary cords of lymph nodes, but they are also abundant in germinal centers of lymphoid tissue. There are only a few in loose connective tissue, except in the lamina propria of the gastrointestinal tract and the respiratory passages. Plasma cells increase greatly in number under conditions of chronic inflammation such as tuberculosis.

The plasma cells are egg-shaped cells with an intensely basophilic, non-granular homogeneous cytoplasm as seen under the light microscope. The origin and precursors of plasma cells are discussed in detail on p. 390. In short, their immediate precursors are the medium or large lymphocytes, the latter often referred to as lymphoblasts. The mature plasma cell is an ameboid cell. Its nucleus is spherical or oval and eccentrically placed in the cell. There is an abundance of dense heterochromatin. (Fig. 6-29) It distribution in relation to the light euchromatin often produces a pattern reminiscent of the spokes of a wheel. The cell surface is

Fig. 7-30. Reticular connective tissue. Medullary cord. Lymph node. Rat. E.M. X 4500.
  1. Lumen of arteriole. **2.** Endothelium.
  3. Reticular fibers. **4.** Reticular cells. In this location, these cells are only phagocytic to a limited extent and resemble fibroblasts.
  5. Small lymphocytes. **6.** Large lymphocyte (lymphoblast). **7.** Monocyte. **8.** Plasma cells.
  9. Cytoplasmic strand of macrophage.
  10. Smooth muscle cells.

Fig. 7-31. Loose connective tissue. Core of villus. Small intestine. Rat. E.M. X 17,000.
  1. Venous capillary. **2.** Lumen of postcapillary venule. **3.** Endothelial cells. **4.** Pericyte.
  5. Fibroblasts. **6.** Smooth muscle cells.
  7. Macrophages. **8.** Lymphocytes. **9.** Plasma cell. **10.** Mast cells. **11.** Eosinophil polymorphonuclear leukocyte. **12.** Monocyte.
  13. Reticular and delicate collagenous fibers are scarce. **14.** Interstitial spaces (areolae) filled with tissue fluid. *Note:* The identifcation of cell types and location of fibers is based on analysis of this field of view at higher magnifications.

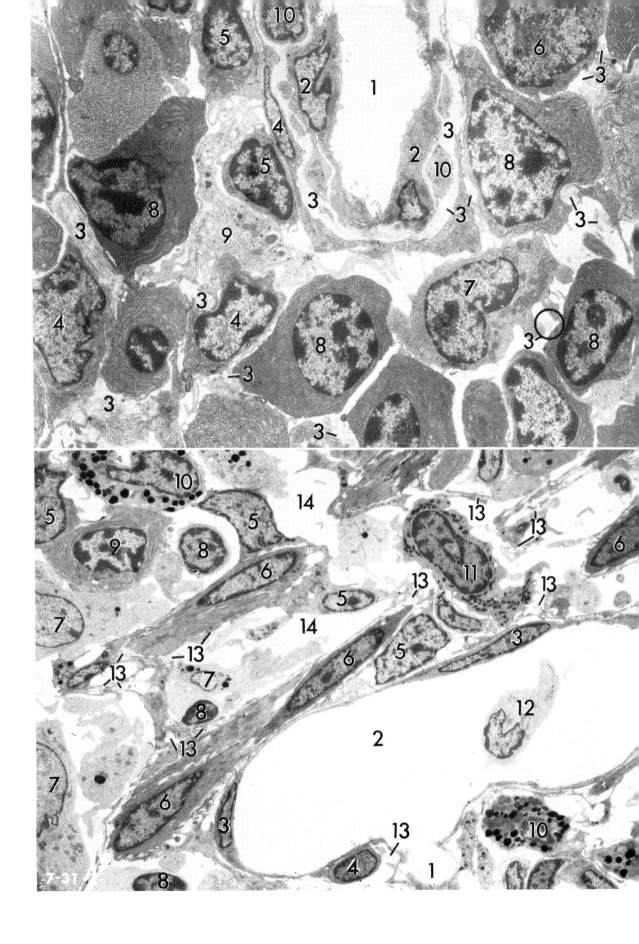

7-31

smooth, with only very few microvilli, and occasionally, pseudopods. There is only a restricted number of smooth pinocytotic invaginations of the cell membrane, and rarely does one find coated vesicles. There is no external lamina (basal lamina) associated with the plasma cell. The basophilic cytoplasm is filled with numerous free ribosomes and an extensive **granular endoplasmic reticulum,** except for the paranuclear region occupied by the Golgi zone. The cisternae of the granular endoplasmic reticulum are flat and in parallel arrangement (Fig. 7-29), but may become greatly extended and appear as a collection of ribosome-studded vacuoles, especially in plasma cells actively synthesizing antibodies. The cisternae often contain a medium dense, finely granular, substance. The Golgi zone is well developed with both membranous sacs and vesicles. Small membrane-bound granules may be present near the Golgi zone in addition to occasional primary lysosomes (dense bodies). Mitochondria are large and round, but scarce. A pair of centrioles occurs as a rule.

The **function** of the plasma cells is to produce, and temporarily store, immune gamma-globulins (antibodies) against foreign body proteins (antigens). The process of detecting the antigens involves both small lymphocytes and macrophages and is not fully understood at the moment. This problem is discussed further on p. 394 in relation to the structure and function of lymphoid tissue in general. In short, the small lymphocyte may respond directly to an antigen stimulation and develop into a plasma cell; or a macrophage may trap the foreign protein, digest it, and pass the antigen to the lymphocyte which then develops into a plasma cell. In either case, the antibodies first appear in the perinuclear space of the immature plasma cell (also referred to as lymphoblast or plasmablast). As this cell gradually develops a granular endoplasmic reticulum, the antibodies appear in the cisternae near the nucleus. In the fully developed plasma cell, the antibodies are present throughout all cisternae of the granular endoplasmic reticulum, and sometimes also overflow to fill the cytoplasm. The saccules of the Golgi zone usually contain antibodies throughout the plasma cell development, but they do not seem to participate in the same way this organelle does in some protein-secreting cells by accumulating, condensing, and packaging the secretory products as secretory granules. The mode of excretion of antibody from the plasma cell is not known. One possibility is that a transient communication is established between the cisternae of the granular endoplasmic reticulum and the cell membrane. It is also possible that a diffusion of the relatively low molecular weight gamma globulins occurs through the cell membrane. A third possibility is expressed by the hypothesis that plasma cells release their antibody content by cellular disintegration, since the plasma cell generally is considered to be a terminal cell.

Other cells. The connective tissue proper contains several other cell types. **Monocytes** enter from the blood vessels

Fig. 7-32. Comparison of loose and dense connective tissues. Lamina propria and submucosa of tertiary bronchus. Lung. Cat. E.M. X 1800. **1.** Lumen of tertiary bronchus. **2.** Ciliated respiratory epithelium. **3.** Lamina propria (loose connective tissue). **4.** Submucosa (irregular dense fibrous connective tissue). **5.** Lumen of bronchial gland. **6.** Fibroblasts and fibrocytes. Rectangle enlarged in Fig. 7-17. **7.** Loosely arranged collagenous fibers. **8.** Cross-sectioned elastic fibers. **9.** Densely arranged collagenous fibers. **10.** Plasma cells. **11.** Mast cells. **12.** Macrophages. **13.** Nerve bundle. **14.** Perineural cell nucleus. **15.** Nucleus of Schwann cell. **16.** Fat cell with two fat globules. **17.** Blood capillary. **18.** Tangentially sectioned bronchial glands. *Note:* The identification of cell types, fibers and other structures is based on analysis at higher magnifications. For description of respiratory epithelium and bronchial glands, turn to p. 618 and p. 628.

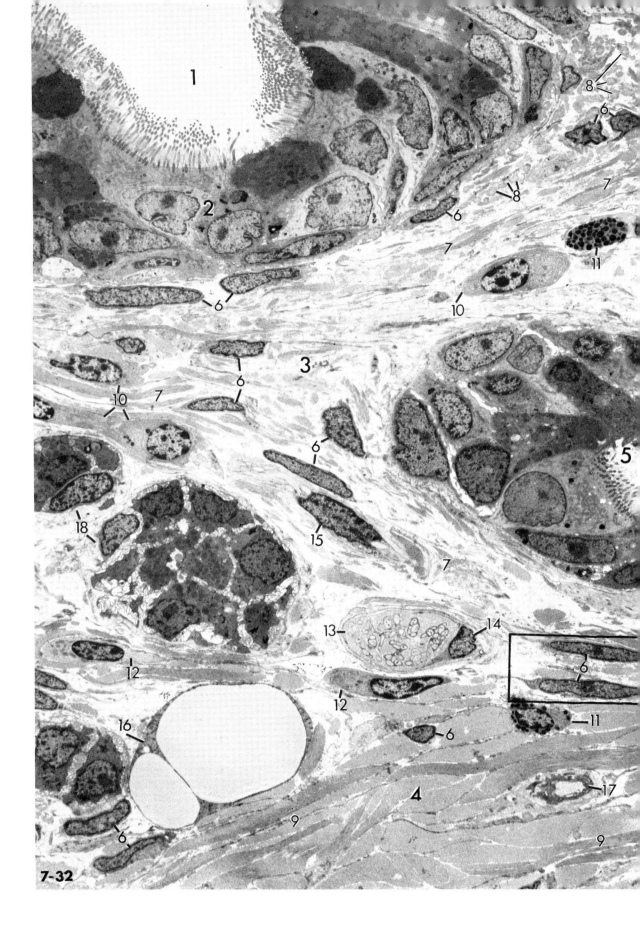

and are transformed into macrophages. Their structure is described on p. 106. **Lymphocytes** are transient but represent an essential part of the connective tissue proper. They are discussed on p. 104 and p. 388. Granular polymorphonuclear **leukocytes** leave the circulating blood to enter the connective tissue proper in response to a variety of stimuli. These cells are described on p. 98 and p. 100. **Melanocytes** are sometimes present in the connective tissue of the human skin. Their structure is described on p. 484. **Fat cells** are encountered particularly in loose connective tissue. They are discussed on p. 168 under adipose tissue.

Types of Connective Tissue Proper

There are generally four types of adult connective tissue proper: 1) reticular connective tissue; 2) loose (areolar) connective tissue; 3) dense fibrous connective tissue; and 4) adipose tissue.

RETICULAR CONNECTIVE TISSUE

This tissue occurs in lymphoid organs (lymph node, spleen) and in the bone marrow. It is an extremely loose connective tissue, which consists of a varied number of **reticular cells** and a wide, delicate meshwork of **reticular** fibers. The reticular cells serve the dual function of being macrophages and fibroblasts, and they form, collectively, the structural basis for the reticuloendothelial system (p. 156). The reticular fibers are delicate bundles of thin collagenous fibrils which are difficult to resolve under the light microscope, but can be made visible by silver impregnation (p. 146).

The reticular tissue forms an integral and delicate part of the lymphoid and myeloid organs, and only the resolving power of the electron microscope settled the question of the nature of the reticular fibers and the relationship of fibers to the reticular cells. (Fig. 7-30) The reticular

fibers are completely surrounded by sheets of the reticular cell cytoplasm in the red pulp of the spleen, and in the medullary sinuses of lymph nodes, where blood plasma percolates constantly. In the white pulp of the spleen, in the germinal centers and medullary cords of lymph nodes, the reticular fibers travel freely between cellular elements. For the purpose of keeping a simple classification, one may still refer to reticular tissue as a special kind of connective tissue. However, since it has been demonstrated that the fibers are collagenous in nature, it might be more appropriate to include reticular tissue with the loose connective tissue.

LOOSE CONNECTIVE TISSUE

The loose connective tissue acts as a support for epithelial surfaces and makes up the **stroma** of most organs, including glands and muscles. It is especially prominent in the thin connective tissue **septa** of some organs, and it forms a sleeve around blood vessels, capillaries and nerves. The **lamina propria** of the gastrointestinal tract is made up largely of loose connective tissue. (Fig. 7-31) This kind of connective tissue, rich in cells but poor in fibers, abounds in gelatinous ground substance. The fibers are collagenous, reticu-

Fig. 7-33. Subepithelial connective tissue. This is an example of a cell-rich tissue which represents an intermediate type between loose and dense connective tissue. Pars cavernosa of male urethra. Rat. E.M. X 5000.
1. Base of urethral epithelium. **2.** Lumina of postcapillary venules. **3.** Lumina of capillaries. **4.** Cross-sectioned non-myelinated nerve fibers. **5.** Axons of myelinated nerves. **6.** Nuclei of endothelial cells. **7.** Nucleus of pericyte. **8.** Nuclei of fibroblasts. **9.** Cytoplasmic strands of smooth muscle cells. Smooth muscle cells are abundant in the cavernous tissue which lies under this connective tissue. **10.** Nucleus of smooth muscle cell. **11.** Nucleus of macrophage. **12.** Part of macrophage cytoplasm. **13.** Erythrocytes. **14.** Platelets. **15.** Irregularly arranged collagenous fibers completely fill the intercellular spaces.

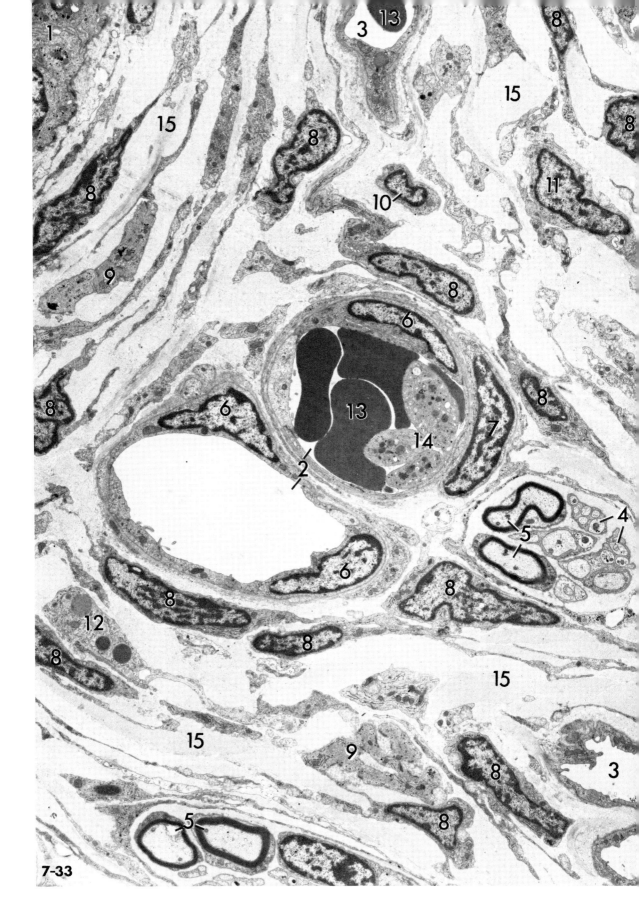

7-33

lar, and elastic, forming a spongy cobweb in which are found numerous cells, both fixed and transient. The fixed cells are fibroblasts, fat cells, and mast cells, whereas cells such as macrophages, granular leukocytes, lymphocytes, and plasma cells move about. The fibroblasts are usually in the minority among the cells of the loose connective tissue, and their relationship to the fibers is not very intimate. The fibers may touch the surface of the fibroblasts, but more often the fibers course freely through the loose connective tissue.

Loose connective tissue is sometimes referred to as **areolar tissue** (Latin, **areola,** small space) because of its apparent spaces filled by tissue fluid and viscous ground substance. Fat cells often accumulate in loose connective tissue, gradually changing it to an adipose tissue. Loose connective tissue has a rich microvascular bed, and the reticular fibers present are usually concentrated in the connective tissue sleeve around these vessels. The loose connective tissue serves as a flexible support for blood vessels and nerves.

DENSE FIBROUS CONNECTIVE TISSUE

In some instances, the distinction between loose and dense fibrous connective tissue is quite arbitrary, since gradual transition between the two can easily be observed. (Fig. 7-32, 7-33) In general, dense fibrous connective tissue is characterized by an abundance of fibers and a paucity of cells. The fibers are large and collagenous, although elastic components may also be present. The cells are mostly fibroblasts with occasional macrophages and mast cells.

The bundles of collagenous fibers are arranged according to local functional demands and the direction of the pull exerted upon them. Also, the number of collagenous fibers increases if the pulling forces are strong. Dense **irregular** connective tissue contains fiber bundles which are interwoven and criss-cross each other in many directions because of the many-

directional pull to which the tissue is subjected. Irregular dense connective tissue forms the **capsules,** large septa, and **trabeculae** of many organs, the deep fasciae of the muscles, the dermis, the periosteum, the perichondrium, and the dura mater. The fibers of dense irregular connective tissue are mostly collagenous in nature with a small admixture of reticular and elastic fibers. The collagenous fibers vary greatly in width and length. The fibroblasts are usually flat or spindle-shaped with long processes reaching out in between the fiber bundles. (Fig. 7-33) Dense **regular** connective tissue contains fiber bundles which are in parallel arrangement, arising through pulling forces from usually only two directions. Regular dense connective tissue forms aponeuroses, tendons, and ligaments. In the **aponeurosis,** which represents a flattened tendon, the parallel fiber bundles are gathered in sheets, each with the fibers arranged in a direction that crosses the fiber direction of the sheet above or below. In the ligaments and tendons the collagenous bundles are arranged in parallel bundles, forming thick bands which either connect bone to bone (ligaments) or muscle to bone (tendons). In the **tendon** (Fig.

Fig. 7-34. Tendon. Longitudinal section. Rabbit. L.M. X 185. **1.** Nuclei of fibroblasts. **2.** Collagenous fibers.
Fig. 7-35. Tendon. Cross section. Tail. Rat. E.M. X 1000. **1** Fibroblasts (tendon cells). **2.** Collagenous fibers. Rectangle enlarged in Fig. 7-22.
Fig. 7-36. Tendon. Longitudinal section. Tail. Rat. E.M. X 1600. **1.** Nuclei of fibroblasts (tendon cells). **2.** Nucleus of unidentified cell. **3.** Cytoplasmic processes of fibroblasts. **4.** Collagenous fibers.
Fig. 7-37. Detail of fibroblast (tendon cell). Tendon. Longitudinal section. Tail. Rat. E.M. X 9500. **1.** Nucleoli. **2.** Nuclear membrane. **3.** Golgi zone. **4.** Granular endoplasmic reticulum. **5.** Mitochondrion. **6.** Sheet-like cytoplasmic processes. **7.** Collagenous fibers composed of numerous collagenous fibrils. **8.** Cell membrane. **9.** Narrow cleft between two adjoining fibroblasts.

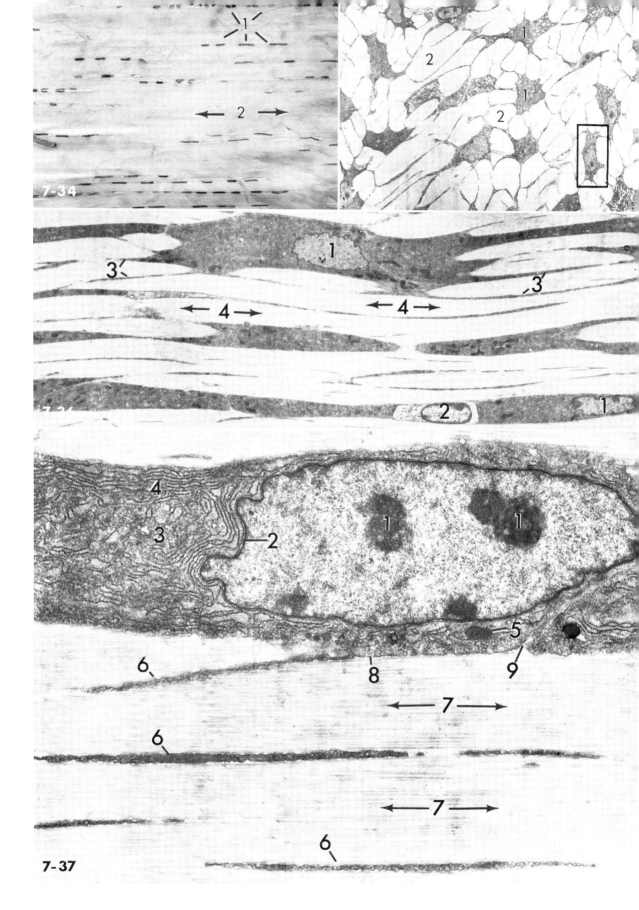

7-34), the fibroblasts, often referred to as tendon cells, are arranged in parallel rows, and their cytoplasm extends laterally in broad sheet-like processes which embrace individual fibers, or groups of them. (Fig. 7-37) The processes contact those of neighboring cells. Groups of collagenous fibers and fibroblasts form fascicles which are separated from other fascicles by loose connective tissue, sometimes called **endotendineum**. Groups of fascicles are held together by an irregular dense connective tissue, peritendineum. A fibrous sheath, vagina fibrosa, or **epitendineum** surrounds the tendon. This fibrous sheath may contain a cavity filled with fluid, facilitating the movements of the tendon.

In the **ligaments,** fibroblasts are irregularly arranged and less numerous than in tendons. The fiber bundles are extremely thick, and the fibroblasts do not have processes which surround them. In some ligaments there is a preponderance of elastic fibers. One example is the ligamenta flava, which connect the arches of the vertebrae of the spinal column.

ADIPOSE TISSUE

General considerations. Adipose tissue is a large accumulation of fat-storing cells which form lobular masses supported by connective tissue septa. (Fig. 7-38) Adipose tissue always develops in loose connective tissue, and there are clear, regional differences in its sites of predilection. The hypodermal region invariably contains fat, except in a few places such as the eyelids and the scrotum. Fat cells also accumulate around kidneys and adrenals, in the coronary sulcus of the heart, in bone marrow, mesentery, and omentum. Adipose tissue serves the functions of being a store for reserve energy, insulation against heat loss through the skin, and a protective padding of certain organs. There is a rapid turnover of stored fat, and with only a few exceptions (orbit, major joints, sole of the foot) the adipose tissue can be used up almost completely during starvation.

Components. The adipose tissue con-

sists of a varied number of large globular **fat cells** which store drops of fat, with the cytoplasm forming a thin pellicle around the fat droplets, and the nucleus displaced to a corner of the cell with a small amount of cytoplasm. (Fig. 7-39) The fat cells are surrounded by a meshwork of fine collagenous and reticular **fibers,** as well as by a rich **capillary** network.

Development. In the fetus, the newborn, and the child, the fat cells develop from fusiform or stellate mesenchymal cells by a gradual accumulation of fat droplets. It is believed that the number of fat cells that developed in the fetus and child remain fairly constant in the adult, since dividing cells are not observed; and it has been postulated that it is only the degree of storage that varies. It has also been assumed that fibroblasts, macrophages, and endothelial cells can develop into fat cells, but these hypotheses have been seriously questioned lately. The generally occurring adipose tissue is referred to as **white adipose tissue.** It has a yellow tint in man. A special kind of adipose tissue, **brown fat,** is abundant in childhood, and occurs near the kidneys in the adult. Brown fat is also present in hibernating species. It contains fat cells in which the lipid droplets do not coalesce

Fig. 7-38. Adipose tissue. Hypodermis. Lip. Human. L.M. X 121. **1.** Fat cells. Lipid dissolved. **2.** Collagenous fiber bundles.

Fig. 7-39. Adipose tissue. Hypodermis. Thigh. Rabbit. E.M. X 600. **1.** Fat cells. Lipid preserved by osmic acid fixation. **2.** Nucleus of fat cell. **3.** Loose connective tissue. **4.** Capillaries.

Fig. 7-40. Developing adipose tissue. Newborn kitten. E.M. X 1750. **1.** Nuclei of fat cells. **2.** Lipid droplets. **3.** Capillaries. **4.** Nucleus of fibroblast. **5.** Interstitial space.

Fig. 7-41. Developing fat cell. Newborn kitten. E.M. X 9000. **1.** Nucleus. **2.** Lipid droplets in various stages of development. **3.** Mitochondria. **4.** Lysosome. **5.** Parts of capillary endothelium. **6.** Narrow interstitial space with reticular and delicate collagenous fibrils. A thin external (basal) lamina invests each fat cell.

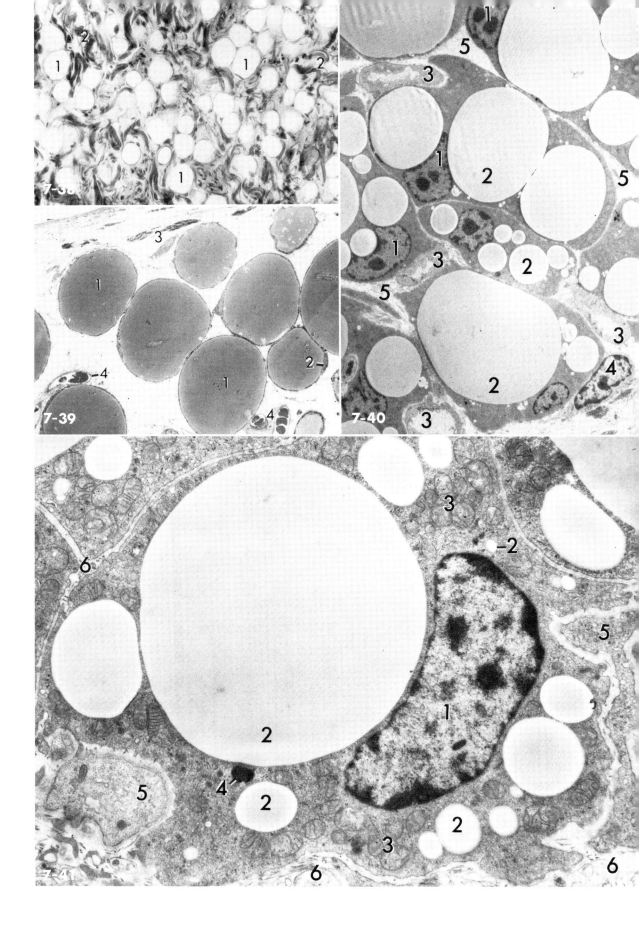

as readily as in regular white adipose tissue. The mitochondria of brown fat cells are numerous, large, and have a complex internal fine structure. The brown color is derived from a rich vascular network and abundant lysosomes (pigment-like residual bodies) in the fat cells. Some investigators believe that brown fat can be transformed into white adipose tissue.

Fat cells. The fully developed fat cell in white adipose tissue is a large, ovoid or spherical cell, averaging 50–75 μ in width. The nucleus is round or oval in young fat cells, but is cup-shaped and displaced to the periphery by a large fat droplet in the mature cell. (Fig. 7-41) The cytoplasm is stretched to form a thin sheath around the fat globule, but a relatively large volume is concentrated around the nucleus. A thin external lamina (basal lamina) surrounds the cell. The smooth cell membrane shows no microvilli but has abundant smooth micropinocytotic invaginations. These often fuse to form small vacuoles and appear as rosettes during this process. (Fig. 7-42) Mitochondria are few in number. They are spherical or oval with loosely arranged membranous cristae. The Golgi zone is small. The cytoplasm is filled with free ribosomes (Fig. 7-43), but contains only a limited number of short profiles of the granular endoplasmic reticulum. Occasional lysosomes can be found but they are not as numerous as in brown fat. In the fully developed fat cell there are one or two large fat globules which develop gradually through a coalescence of **lipid droplets.** They contain a mixture of neutral fats, triglycerides, fatty acids, phospholipids, and cholesterol. They become dissolved by alcohol and leave empty spaces which contribute to the sponge-like appearance of adipose tissue in routine preparations for light microscopy. In formaldehyde-fixed tissue stained with Sudan III, the lipid droplets appear orange to red; and in osmic acid-preserved tissue they emerge black or gray. A thin interface membrane separates the lipid droplet from the cytoplasmic matrix. Peripheral to this membrane occurs a system of parallel meridional thin filaments. (Fig. 7-44) Agranular endoplasmic reticulum occurs throughout the cytoplasm as short tubules and vesicles. These profiles also form an incomplete casing or fenestrated flattened envelope around both small and large lipid droplets.

The accumulation of lipid by the fat cell does not involve the absorption of preformed substances such as chylomicra. It is probably due to a cellular synthesis involving both the pinocytotic invaginations and the vesicles of the agranular endoplasmic reticulum. The mechanism of release is not known, but the lipid droplets decrease in size when lipid is mobilized during starvation. Under normal conditions, the fat cell undergoes cyclic changes of synthesis, storage, and release, since a rapid turnover of fat occurs under the influence of hormones from the thyroid gland and the pituitary.

Fig. 7-42. Detail of developing fat cell. Newborn kitten. E.M. X 54,000. **1.** Mitochondria. **2.** Lipid droplets. **3.** Ribosomes. **4.** Agranular endoplasmic reticulum. **5.** Micropinocytotic invaginations of cell membrane merging to form rosette-like configurations. **6.** Parallel microfilaments are seen in this tangential section of a lipid droplet.

Fig. 7-43. Part of developing fat cell. Newborn kitten. E.M. X 90,000. **1.** External (basal) lamina. **2.** Cell membrane. **3.** Micropinocytotic invaginations. **4.** Merging vesicles. **5.** Small Golgi zone. **6.** Enlarging Golgi vesicle. **7.** Ribosomes. **8.** Outer mitochondrial membrane. **9.** Membranous cristae. **10** Matrix of mitochondrion. **11.** Intramitochondrial dense granules.

Fig. 7-44. Detail of developing fat cell. Enlargement of rectangle in Fig. 7-37. Newborn kitten. E.M. X 120,000. **1.** Center of lipid droplet. **2.** Interface membrane. **3.** Arrows point to cross-sectioned, equally spaced filaments outside of the interface membrane. **4.** Agranular endoplasmic reticulum. **5.** Tangential section of lipid droplet. **6.** Peripheral filaments, longitudinally cut. **7.** Ribosomes.

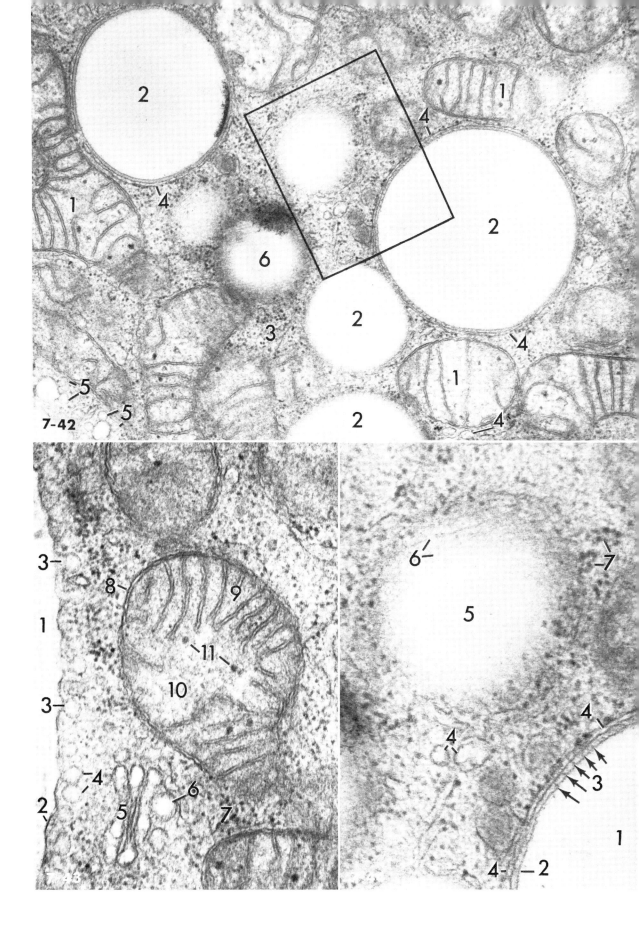

References

FIBERS

Bairati, A., Petruccioli, M. G. and Torri Tarelli, L. Studies on the ultrastructure of collagen fibrils. 1. Morphological evaluation of the periodic structure. J. Submicr. Cytol. *1*: 113–141 (1969).

Bruns, R. R. A symmetrical, extracellular fibril. J. Cell Biol. *42*: 418–430 (1969).

Fernando, N. V., von Erkel, G. A. and Movat, H. Z. The fine structure of connective tissue. IV. The intercellular elements. Exp. Molec. Path. *3*: 529–545 (1964).

Gomori, G. Silver impregnation of reticulum in paraffin sections. Am. J. Path. *13*: 993–1002 (1937).

Grant, R. A., Horne, R. W. and Cox, R. W. New model for the tropocollagen macromolecule and its mode of aggregation. Nature *207*: 822–826 (1965).

Greenlee, T. K., Jr., Ross, R. and Hartman, J. L. The fine structure of elastic fibers. J. Cell Biol. *30*: 59–71 (1966).

Gross, J. The behavior of collagen units as a model in morphogenesis. J. Biophys. Biochem. Cytol. (Suppl.) *2*: 261–274 (1956).

Hall, D. A. The fibrous components of connective tissue with special reference to the elastic fiber. Int. Rev. Cytol. *8*: 212–252 (1959).

Haust, M. D. Fine fibrils of extracellular space (microfibrils): their structure and role in connective tissue organization. Am. J. Path. *47*: 1113–1137 (1965).

Hayes, R. L. and Allen, E. R. Electron microscopic studies on a double-stranded beaded filament of embryonic collagen. J. Cell Sci. *2*: 419–434 (1967).

Low, F. N. Extracellular connective tissue fibrils in the chick embryo. Anat. Rec. *160*: 93–108 (1968).

Rhodin, J. and Dalhamn, T. Electron microscopy of collagen and elastin in lamina propria of the tracheal mucosa of rat. Exp. Cell Res. *9*: 371–375 (1955).

Ross, R. and Bornstein, P. The elastic fiber. I. The separation and partial characterization of its macromolecular components. J. Cell Biol. *40*: 366–381 (1969).

Ross, R. and Bornstein, P. Elastic fibers in the body. Sci. American *224*: 44–59 (1971).

Taylor, J. J. and Yeager, V. L. The fine structure of elastic fibers in the fibrous periosteum of the rat femur. Anat. Rec. *156*: 129–142 (1966).

Torri Tarelli, L. and Petruccioli, M. G. Studies on the ultrastructure of collagen fibrils. II. Filamentous structure with negative staining. J. Submicr. Cytol. *3*: 153–170 (1971).

Wassermann, F. Fibrillogenesis in the regenerating rat tendon with special reference to growth and composition of the collagenous fibril. Am. J. Anat. *94*: 399–438 (1954).

GROUND SUBSTANCE

Briggaman, R. A., Dalldorf, F. G. and Wheeler, C. E., Jr. Formation and origin of basal lamina and anchoring fibrils in adult human skin. J. Cell Biol. *51*: 384–395 (1971).

Gersh, I. and Catchpole, H. R. The nature of ground substance of connective tissue. Perspectives in Biology and Medicine *3*: 282–319 (1969).

Goel, S. C. and Jurand, A. Electron microscopic observations on the basal lamina of chick limb buds after trypsin and EDTA treatment. J. Cell Sci. *3*: 373–389 (1968).

Low, F. N. and Burkel, W. E. A boundary membrane concept of ultrastructural morphology. Anat. Rec. *151*: 489–490 (1965).

Meyer, K. The chemistry of the mesodermal ground substance. Harvey Lectures *51*: 88–112 (1955).

Pierce, G. B. and Nakane, P. K. Basement membranes, synthesis and deposition in response to cellular injury. Lab. Investig. *21*: 27–41 (1969).

Scalleta, L. J. and MacCallum, D. K. A fine structural study of divalent cation-mediated epithelial union with connective tissue in human oral mucosa. Am. J. Anat. *133*: 431–454 (1972).

FIBROBLASTS

Alpert, E. N. Developing elastic tissue. Am. J. Path. *69*: 89–102 (1972).

Fahrenbach, W. H., Sandberg, L. D. and Cleary, E. G. Ultrastructural studies on early elastogenesis. Anat. Rec. *155*: 563–576 (1966).

Fernando, N. V. and Movat, H. Z. Fibrillogenesis in regenerating tendon. Lab. Investig. *12*: 214–229 (1963).

Goldberg, B. and Green, H. An analysis of collagen secretion by established mouse fibroblast lines. J. Cell Biol. *22*: 227–258 (1964).

Greenlee, T. K., Jr. and Ross, R. The development of the rat flexor digital tendon, a fine structure study. J. Ultrastruct. Res. *18*: 354–376 (1967).

Haust, M. D. and More, R. H. Electron microscopy of connective tissue and elastogenesis. *In* The Connective Tissue (Eds. B. M. Wagner and B. E. Smith), pp. 352–376. Williams & Wilkins, Baltimore, 1967.

Haust, M. D., More, R. H., Bencosme, S. A. and Balis, J. V. Elastogenesis in human aorta: an electron microscopic study. Exp. Molec. Path. *4*: 508–524 (1965).

Movat, H. Z. and Fernando, N. V. The fine structure of connective tissue. I. The fibroblast. Exp. Molec. Path. *1*: 509–534 (1962).

Parry, E. W. Some electron microscope observations on the mesenchymal structures of full-term umbilical cord. J. Anat. *107*: 505–518 (1970).

Porter, K. R. and Pappas, G. C. Collagen formation by fibroblasts of the chick embryo dermis. J. Biophys. Biochem. Cytol. *5*: 153–166 (1959).

Reith, E. J. Collagen formation in developing molar teeth of rat. J. Ultrastruct. Res. *21*: 383–414 (1968).

Rhodin, J. A. G. Organization and ultrastructure of connective tissue. *In* The Connective Tissue (Eds. B. M. Wagner and D. E. Smith), pp. 1–16. Williams & Wilkins, Baltimore, 1967.

Ross, R. The connective tissue fiber forming cell. *In* Treatise on Collagan (Ed.: B. S. Gould) *2*: 1–75 (1968) Academic Press, New York.

Ross, R. and Benditt, E. P. Wound healing and collagen formation. V. Quantitative electron microscope radioautographic observations of proline-H³ utilization by fibroblasts. J. Cell Biol. *27*: 83–106 (1965).

Van Winkle, W., Jr. The fibroblast in wound healing. Surg. Gynec. Obstet. *124*: 369–386 (1967).

Weinstock, M. Collagen formation. Observations on its intracellular packaging and transport. Z. Zellforsch. *129*: 455–470 (1972).

MAST CELLS

Combs, J. W. Maturation of rat mast cells. An electron microscope study. J. Cell Biol. *31*: 563–575 (1966).

Fernando, N. V. and Movat, H. Z. The fine structure of connective tissue. III. The mast cell. Exp. Molec. Path. *2*: 450–463 (1963).

Kobayasi, T., Midtgard, K. and Asboe-Hansen, G. Ultrastructure of human mast cell granules. J. Ultrastruct. Res. *23*: 153–165 (1968).

Padawer, J. The reaction of rat mast cells to polylysine. J. Cell Biol. *47*: 352–372 (1970).

Röhlich, P., Anderson, P. and Uvnäs, B. Electron microscope observations on compound 48/80-induced degranulation in rat mast cells. Evidence for sequential exocytosis of storage granules. J. Cell Biol. *51*: 465–483 (1971).

Smith, D. E. The tissue mast cell. Int. Rev. Cytol. *14*: 327–386 (1963).

Weinstock, A. and Albright, J. T. The fine structure of mast cells in normal human gingiva. J. Ultrastruct. Res. *17*: 245–256 (1967).

MACROPHAGES

Pearsall, N. N. and Weiser, R. S. The Macrophage. Lea & Febiger, Philadelphia, 1970.

PLASMA CELLS

dePetris, S., Karlsbad, G. and Connolly, J. M. Localization of antibodies in plasma cells by electron microscopy. J. Exp. Med. *117*: 849–862 (1963).

Leduc, E. H., Avrameas, S. and Bouteille, M. Ultrastructural localization of antibody in differentiating plasma cells. J. Exp. Med. *127*: 109–118 (1968).

Movat, H. Z. and Fernando, N. V. The fine structure of connective tissue. II. The plasma cell. Exp. Molec. Path. *1*: 535–553 (1962).

FAT CELLS

Barnard, T. The ultrastructural differentiation of brown adipose tissue in the rat. J. Ultrastruct. Res. *29*: 311–332 (1969).

Cushman, S. W. Structure-function relationship in the adipose cell. I. Ultrastructure of the isolated adipose cell. J. Cell Biol. *46*: 326–341 (1970).

Dyer, R. F. Morphological features of brown adipose cell maturation in vivo and in vitro. Am. J. Anat. *123*: 255–282 (1968).

Napolitano, L. The differentiation of white adipose cells. An electron microscope study. J. Cell Biol. *18*: 663–679 (1963).

Napolitano, L. The fine structure of adipose tissue. *In* Handbook of Physiology. Section *5*: 109–124 (1965).

Sheldon, H. The fine structure of the fat cell. *In* Fat as a Tissue (Eds. K. Rodahl and B. Issekutz), pp. 41–68. McGraw-Hill, New York, 1964.

Slavin, B. G. The cytophysiology of mammalian adipose cells. Int. Rev. Cytol. *33*: 297–334 (1972).

Wood, E. M. An ordered complex of filaments surrounding the lipid droplets in developing adipose cells. Anat. Rec. *157*: 437–448 (1967).

8 Cartilage

GENERAL CONSIDERATIONS

Cartilage is an avascular dense connective tissue which consists of cells and solid intercellular matrix. Cartilage is for support and protection. In the embryo it serves as a model for many developing bones, and in childhood and adolescence it constitutes a vital part of the growing ends (epiphyses) of the long bones. It protects the articular surfaces of bones which make up the synovial joints; it connects the ribs to the sternum; it makes up the intervertebral disks; and it forms a supporting part of the nose, epiglottis, larynx, trachea, bronchi, and the external ear (pinna). There are essentially three kinds of cartilage: hyaline, elastic, and fibrocartilage. The classification is based on the prevalent fiber type occurring in the intercellular matrix.

The **matrix** of cartilage is made up of fibers and ground substance. The **fibers** are of the collagenous and. in some cases, elastic type. The **ground substance** of the matrix is rich in acid mucopolysaccharides (predominantly chondroitin sulfates) which render the cartilage a solid firmness coupled with a certain resilience and elasticity. The young and immature cells are referred to as **chondroblasts,** the mature cells as **chondrocytes.** The cells occur singly or in nests of two or three. There are no cytoplasmic connections between cells or nests of cells. (Fig. 8-2) A membranous layer of dense irregular connective tissue, the **perichondrium** surrounds the cartilage on all outer surfaces with two exceptions: the articular surfaces of joints and the fibrocartilages. The perichondrium is richly vascularized, and the cartilage receives its nutrition from its blood vessels. The metabolites reach the chondrocytes by diffusing through the cartilage matrix. Although cartilage normally is avascular, blood vessels can penetrate cartilage by forming tunnels through an erosion of the matrix as part of a process referred to as endochondral bone formation (p. 212). This process is associated with a calcification of the cartilage matrix, a phenomenon which also may occur in cartilage not undergoing endochondral bone formation, but as a result of old age or poor nutritional conditions.

Development and Growth

Cartilage develops from mesenchyme. The mesenchymal cells initially change from a stellate to a round shape, and the intercellular space is diminished through a mitotic increase of the mesenchymal cells, now referred to as **chondroblasts.** The cells become crowded into masses or centers of chondrification, known as **precartilage.** Around each chondroblast is deposited a layer of cartilage matrix which, by a gradual increase in thickness, separates chondroblasts more and more. The cells are then referred to as **chondrocytes.**

The continued growth of cartilage follows essentially two routes: interstitial growth and appositional growth. The cartilage increases in size rapidly by **interstitial** (endogenous) growth through mitosis of existing chondrocytes and a continued deposition of an increasing amount of intercellular matrix. The chondrocytes first form nests or groups of **isogenous** cells, in which all cells present have descended by mitoses from a single cell. Subsequently, matrix is deposited between isogenous cells, and the chondrocytes become separated. Interstitial growth occurs as long as the cartilage matrix is soft and yielding, continuing until the cartilage has reached its definite size and shape. During childhood and adolescence, interstitial growth of cartilage is a factor

Fig. 8-1. Hyaline cartilage. Pulmonary bronchus. Cat. L.M. X 225. **1.** Perichondrium. **2.** Matrix of hyaline cartilage. **3.** Chondrocytes.

Fig. 8-2. Hyaline cartilage. Pulmonary bronchus. Cat. Enlargement of area similar to rectangle in Fig. 8-1. E.M. X 2600. **1.** Nucleus of fibroblast in perichondrium. **2.** Collagenous fibrils of perichondrium. **3.** Fibroblasts differentiating into chondrocytes. **4.** Nuclei of young chondrocytes. **5.** Nuclei of mature chondrocytes. **6.** Matrix. **7.** Lipid droplets.

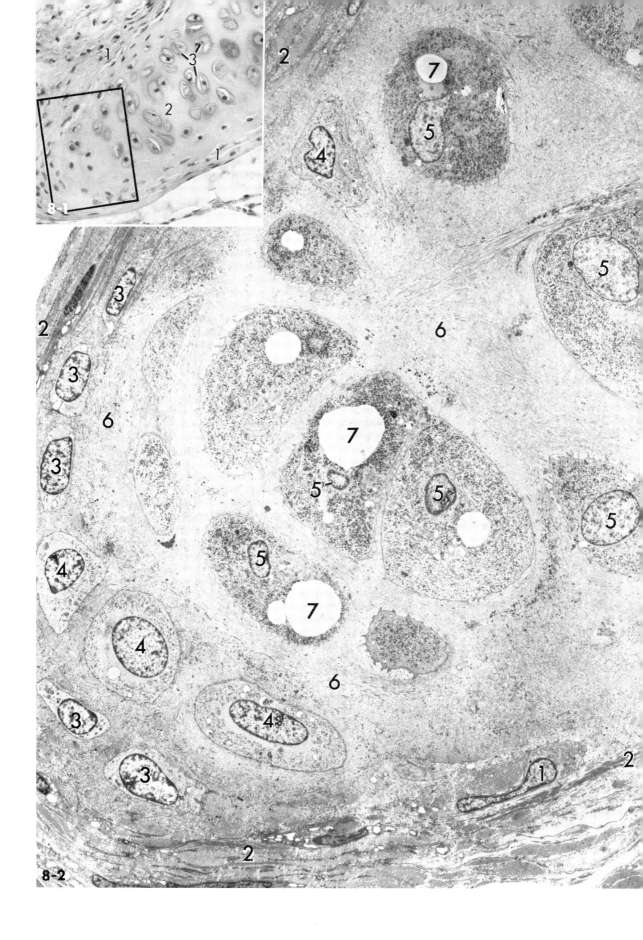

of particular importance in the lengthening of long bones by the growth of epiphyseal cartilage (p. 214).

In contrast, **appositional** (exogenous) growth of cartilage occurs from the perichondrium. Precursor cells are the fibroblasts which differentiate to chondroblasts, and by surrounding themselves with a cartilage matrix gradually turn into chondrocytes and increase the size of the cartilage by adding to the surface. Appositional growth starts somewhat later than interstitial growth but it continues throughout life. In fact, it is the only type of growth that can occur in mature cartilage since a solidified cartilage matrix makes interstitial growth impossible.

Types of Cartilage

There are three types of cartilage: 1) hyaline; 2) elastic; and 3) fibrocartilage.

HYALINE CARTILAGE

Hyaline cartilage occurs in the epiphyseal plate of growing bones, in the pieces of cartilage which connect the ribs to the sternum, and in the nose, larynx, trachea, and bronchi. Traditionally, articular cartilage has been categorized as hyaline cartilage. For reasons given below, this author finds it more appropriate to include articular cartilage with fibrocartilage. Hyaline cartilage consists of **matrix** and **chondrocytes**. The matrix is made up of fine fibrils and ground substance. (Fig. 8-3)

Fibrils. The hyaline cartilage fibrils cannot be resolved under the light microscope. Electron microscopy reveals an interlacing dense feltwork of **delicate fibrils** with diameters ranging from 60 to 250 Å. The fibrils have no apparent periodic cross-banding but it is assumed that they are collagenous in nature. (Figs. 8-5, 8-6) It has been postulated that the presence of acid mucopolysaccharides in cartilage matrix interferes with the polymerization of tropocollagen units and blocks

the formation of native collagenous fibrils with an axial banding. Under normal conditions, only occasional native collagenous fibrils with 640 Å axial periodicity course through the matrix of hyaline cartilage. The matrix of articular cartilage is composed of abundant collagenous fibrils, arranged in well-ordered bundles. A 640 Å banding is constantly present. This fact is justification for including articular cartilage with fibrocartilage (p. 200).

Ground substance. The ground substance is solid in cartilage matrix as opposed to connective tissue proper. It contains varied numbers of electron-dense, irregularly spherical **matrix granules** with diameters ranging from 100 to 400 Å. Most granules are freely dispersed among the delicate fibrils but many are closely associated with the fibrils. (Fig. 8-6) The granules most likely represent randomly disposed protein-polysaccharide macromolecular complexes. These complexes are rich in chondroitin sulfates (acid mucopolysaccharides) which are linked to a protein backbone. This in turn is bound to the delicate collagenous fibrils. The matrix of hyaline cartilage is metachromatic because of the presence of the acid mucopolysaccharides. There is a loss of normal cartilage turgor and metachromasia when chondroitin sulfates are removed from the matrix. This can be accomplished by an intravenous injection of the enzyme papain.

In epiphyseal cartilage, small electron-dense, **membrane-bound granules** (vesicles, globules) are present in varied numbers.

Fig. 8-3. Chondrocyte. Hyaline cartilage. Pulmonary bronchus. Cat. E.M. X 12,300.
1. Nucleus. 2. Golgi zone. 3. Lipid droplet. 4. Accumulations of particulate glycogen. 5. Mitochondria. 6. Profiles of granular endoplasmic reticulum. 7. Bundle of cytoplasmic filaments. 8. Vacuoles with some flocculent content. 9. Scalloped cell surface. 10. Capsular region. 11. Cartilage matrix. 12. Part of neighboring chondrocyte.

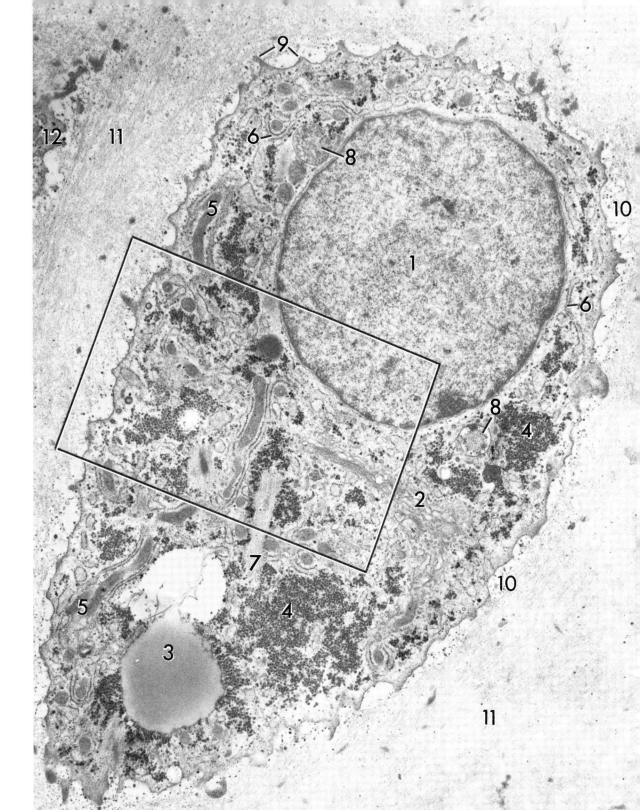

The origin of these structures is uncertain but it has been assumed that they are shed from the cytoplasm of the chondrocytes. The dense granules are rich in acid and alkaline phosphatases and probably represent sites of early calcification as this process spreads through the cartilage matrix.

Chondrocytes. Chondrocytes represent the specific cells of cartilage. They vary greatly in size and shape, depending on location. They are flat or watchglass-shaped near the surface of the cartilage, whereas they vary from round to oval and multiangular in the central parts of cartilages. The nucleus is small with evenly distributed chromatin. The cell surface is scalloped and provided with short, irregularly arranged ridges. (Fig. 8-3) These ridges protrude into the so-called **capsule,** a pericellular region in which the delicate collagenous fibrils are less closely arrayed. In light microscope preparations, this zone stains more intensely basophilic than the rest of the matrix and shows a high degree of metachromasia, presumably because of a high concentration of acid mucopolysaccharides. Since the chondrocytes are soft and the surrounding matrix is solid, it is said that the chondrocyte is located in a **lacuna.** However, there is no free space between the cell membrane and the matrix except in preparations distorted by poor fixation, or at times when the chondrocyte is disintegrating because of progressing calcification of the cartilage matrix.

The cytoplasm of the chondrocyte contains a variable amount of glycogen particles. (Fig. 8-4) Some cells have enormous quantities and other cells only a little. Mitochondria are small and scarce. Lipid droplets occur as a rule and may become as large as the nucleus. Cytoplasmic filaments are often present, either singly or in aggregations of varied extent. Free ribosomes are abundant and the granular endoplasmic reticulum is relatively well developed, often with dilated cisternae. The Golgi zone is large and consists of

saccules, vesicles, and vacuoles. Some vacuoles contain, at times, a finely fibrillar matrix. Coated vesicles are present both throughout the cytoplasm and in connection with the cell membrane.

There is general agreement that the chondrocytes synthesize and secrete both the extracellular fibrils and the ground substance of the cartilage matrix. The non-collagenous protein of the matrix is presumably synthesized by ribosomes, aggregated in the cisternae of the granular endoplasmic reticulum and transferred to the Golgi vacuoles. The synthesis of mucopolysaccharides and the addition of the carbohydrate moiety to the proteins occur in the Golgi zone. As a final step, Golgi vacuoles and/or coated vesicles, containing the protein-polysaccharide complexes, fuse with the cell membrane and discharge the complexes into the extracellular space. The synthesis and secretion of collagenous protein may follow the same route just described, or may bypass the Golgi zone as suggested for the secretion of tropocollagen by fibroblasts in connective tissue proper (p. 152).

Fig. 8-4. Detail of chondrocyte in hyaline cartilage. Enlargement of rectangle in Fig. 8-3. E.M. X 33,000. **1.** Nucleus. **2.** Golgi zone. **3.** Particulate glycogen. **4.** Mitochondria. **5.** Granular endoplasmic reticulum. **6.** Ribosomes. **7.** Cytoplasmic filaments. **8.** Coated vesicles. **9.** Cell membrane. **10.** Pericellular region (capsule).

Fig. 8-5. Detail of chondrocyte. Hyaline cartilage. Same preparation as in Fig. 8-4. E.M. X 66,000. **1.** Cisterna of granular endoplasmic reticulum. **2.** Ribosomes. **3.** Particulate glycogen; average width 400 Å. **4.** Cell membrane. **5.** Dense feltwork of delicate fibrils; average width 100 Å. **6.** Matrix granules; average width 150 Å.

Fig. 8-6. Detail of chondrocyte. Hyaline cartilage. Same preparation as in Fig. 8-4. E.M. X 66,000. **1.** Cell membrane. **2.** This region represents a coated vesicle which just fused with the cell membrane. **3.** Dense feltwork of fibrils; average width 300 Å. No axial periodicity. **4.** Large matrix granules; average width 500 Å. **5.** Small matrix granules; average width 150 Å.

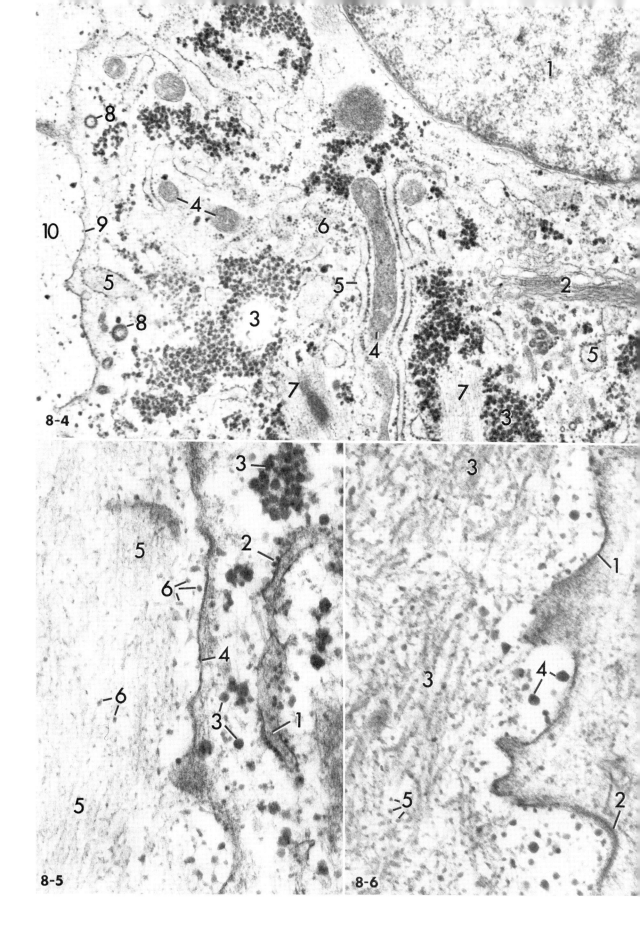

ELASTIC CARTILAGE

Elastic cartilage predominates the cartilages of the auricle of the ear (pinna); the auditory (Eustachian) tube; the epiglottis; the corniculate, cuneiform, and the vocal processes of the arytenoid cartilages of the larynx. The structure of the elastic cartilage is similar to that of hyaline cartilage except that the matrix contains elastic plates which render to the cartilage a high elasticity and flexibility and make it more susceptible to deformation than other types of cartilage. Elastic cartilage is predominantly cellular with the minor part occupied by intercellular matrix. (Figs. 8-7, 8-8)

Matrix. The matrix consists of a loose meshwork of branched fibrils, 60–250 Å thick with irregularly spaced matrix granules, averaging 200 Å in thickness. The fibrils are relatively sparse near the chondrocytes but form a dense network 1–2 μ from the cell surface. (Fig. 8-10) In this area, the fibrils are reinforced by fenestrated, 1–2 μ-thick plates of elastic substance. In the mature elastic cartilage, the elastic plates consist largely of amorphous substance, and elastic microfibrils occur only in the dense fibrous connective tissue of the perichondrium. In contrast to elastic fibers elsewhere, the development of elastic substance in the elastic cartilage is not preceded by the formation of elastic microfibrils. Native collagenous fibrils with the characteristic 640 Å axial periodicity do not occur as a rule in the matrix of elastic cartilage except near the perichondrium.

Chondrocytes. The chondrocytes, which are round or oval, vary in size and occur singly and are rarely seen to form nests of cells. It is not uncommon to find two nuclei in one cell. Distribution and appearance of cell organelles and inclusions are similar to that of the chondrocytes of hyaline cartilage (Fig. 8-9) except that the accumulations of lipid can reach such enormous proportions in elastic cartilage that the chondrocyte acquires the appearance of a fat cell. The chondrocytes synthesize and secrete both the proteinaceous matrix and the elastic component of the elastic cartilage. Therefore, the chondrocyte is the second cell type, in addition to the fibroblast, that controls the production of both collagenous and elastic fibrils. The third cell type with this dual function is the smooth muscle cell of the vascular wall (p. 342).

FIBROCARTILAGE

Fibrocartilage is intermediate in structure between hyaline cartilage and regular dense fibrous connective tissue. The presence of collagenous fibers adds to the firm, pliable cartilage ground substance a quality of durability and resistance to compression, pressure, and tension. Fibrocartilage occurs in the intervertebral disks (Fig. 8-11), in the symphysis pubis and in the articular disks of the mandibular, sternoclavicular, and knee joints. It is also present in the cartilage which borders the glenoid fossa of the shoulder joint (glenoid ligament) and in the acetabulum of the hip joint (cotyloid ligament). Fibrocartilage also blends in with tendons and ligaments, particularly at their junction

Fig. 8-7. Elastic cartilage. External ear (pinna). Mouse. L.M. X 200. **1.** Perichondrium. **2.** Matrix of elastic cartilage. **3.** Chondrocytes.

Fig. 8-8. Elastic cartilage. Pinna. Mouse. Enlargement of area similar to rectangle in Fig. 8-7. E.M. X 1100. **1.** Fibroblasts of perichondrium. **2.** Elastic fibers in cartilage matrix. **3.** Nuclei of chondrocytes. **4.** Lipid droplets in cytoplasm of chondrocytes.

Fig. 8-9. Chondrocyte. Elastic cartilage. Same preparations as in Fig. 8-8. E.M. X 9600. **1.** Nucleus. **2.** Mitochondria. **3.** Large accumulation of cytoplasmic filaments. **4.** Scalloped cell surface with microvilli. **5.** Fibrillar cartilage matrix. **6.** Elastic fibers.

Fig. 8-10. Detail of elastic cartilage. Enlargement of area similar to rectangle in Fig. 8-9. E.M. X 68,000. **1.** Part of chondrocyte cytoplasm. **2.** Feltwork of delicate fibrils; average width 200 Å. **3.** Elastic fibrils. **4.** Small matrix granules; average width 200 Å. **5.** Large matrix granule; width 500 Å.

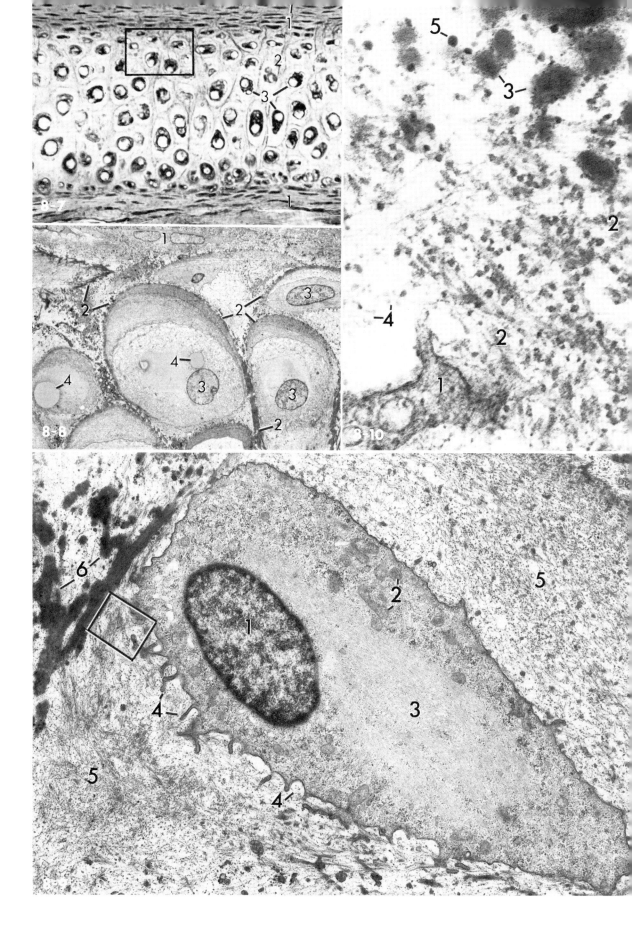

8-7

8-8

8-10

with bones. A delicate type of fibrocartilage occurs in the articular cartilage of synovial joints. Fibrocartilage is dominated by fibers, whereas the chondrocytes are relatively scarce.

Chondrocytes. The chondrocytes occur singly and are often arranged in rows reminiscent of tendon cells. The chondrocytes vary in shape from round to oval or even spindle-shaped (Fig. 8-12), and it is sometimes difficult to tell them from fibroblasts under the light microscope. From an ultrastructural point of view the chondrocytes are characterized by a well-developed granular endoplasmic reticulum, with a finely stippled material filling most of those cisternae which are dilated. (Fig. 8-13) There are numerous free ribosomes, a compact Golgi zone with flattened sacs and small vesicles. Mitochondria are elongated but scarce, and glycogen particles occur in small accumulations throughout the cell. A fair number of lysosomes occurs but accumulations of cytoplasmic filaments and lipid droplets, so prevalent in the chondrocytes of hyaline and elastic cartilage, are not found. The cell surface is provided with short and narrow microvilli, whereas the system of surface ridges seen in chondrocytes of hyaline and elastic cartilage is missing.

Extracellular material. Each chondrocyte or row of chondrocytes is surrounded by an electron-lucent zone 1–2 μ wide, occupied by a system of 60–250 Å-thick **fibrils,** arranged haphazardly to form a dense network. (Fig. 8-14) Some dense granules, 100–200 Å in diameter occur among the filaments. This pericellular zone represents an area of solid hyaline cartilage matrix in which native collagenous fibrils with 640 Å-axial periodicity are not demonstrable. The rest of the extracellular space of the fibrocartilage is dominated by an extensive system of interwoven thick bundles of collagenous **fibers,** each fiber being composed of numerous, 400–800 Å-thick collagenous fibrils with the characteristic 640 Å-axial pattern.

The collagenous fibers do not intermingle as a rule but are demarcated by either a thin strip of ground substance or a wider zone containing a few disoriented strands of collagen. Areas with chondrocytes and collagenous bundles of fibers can border on and mix with areas of fibroblasts and regular dense fibrous connective tissue, but a **perichondrium** in the true sense of the word **does not exist** in fibrocartilage.

References

Anderson, D. R. Ultrastructure of hyaline and elastic cartilage of the rat. Am. J. Anat. *114*: 403–434 (1964).

Anderson, H. C. Electron microscopic studies on induced cartilage development and calcification. J. Cell Biol. *35*: 81–101 (1967).

Anderson, H. C. Vesicles associated with calcification in the matrix of epiphyseal cartilage. J. Cell Biol. *41*: 59–72 (1969).

Anderson, H. C. and Matsuzawa, T. Membranous particles in calcifying cartilage matrix. Trans. N.Y. Acad. Sci. Series II, *22*: 619–630 (1970).

Bonucci, E. Fine structure of early cartilage calcification. J. Ultrastruct. Res. *20*: 33–50 (1967).

Fig. 8-11. Fibrous cartilage. Annulus fibrosus. Intervertebral disk. Human. L.M. × 250. **1.** Rows of chondrocytes. **2.** Layers of collagenous fibers.

Fig. 8-12. Fibrous cartilage. Annulus fibrosus. Intervertebral disk. Mouse. Enlargement of area similar to rectangle in Fig. 8-11. E.M. × 2000. **1.** Nuclei of chondrocytes. **2.** Collagenous fibers.

Fig. 8-13. Chondrocyte. Fibrous cartilage. Enlargement of rectangle in Fig. 8-12. E.M. × 11,100. **1.** Nucleus. **2.** Granular endoplasmic reticulum. **3.** Golgi zone. **4.** Centrioles. **5.** Pericellular capsule of cartilage matrix. **6.** Longitudinally sectioned collagenous fibrils. **7.** Cross-sectioned collagenous fibrils.

Fig. 8-14. Detail of fibrous cartilage. Annulus fibrosus. Intervertebral disk. Mouse. Enlargement of area similar to rectangle in Fig. 8-13. E.M. × 68,000. **1.** Part of chondrocyte cytoplasm. **2.** Cell membrane. **3.** Feltwork of delicate fibrils make up the pericellular capsule of cartilage matrix. Width of fibrils averages 80 Å. **4.** Cross-sectioned collagenous fibrils: A) width 800 Å; B) width 300 Å.

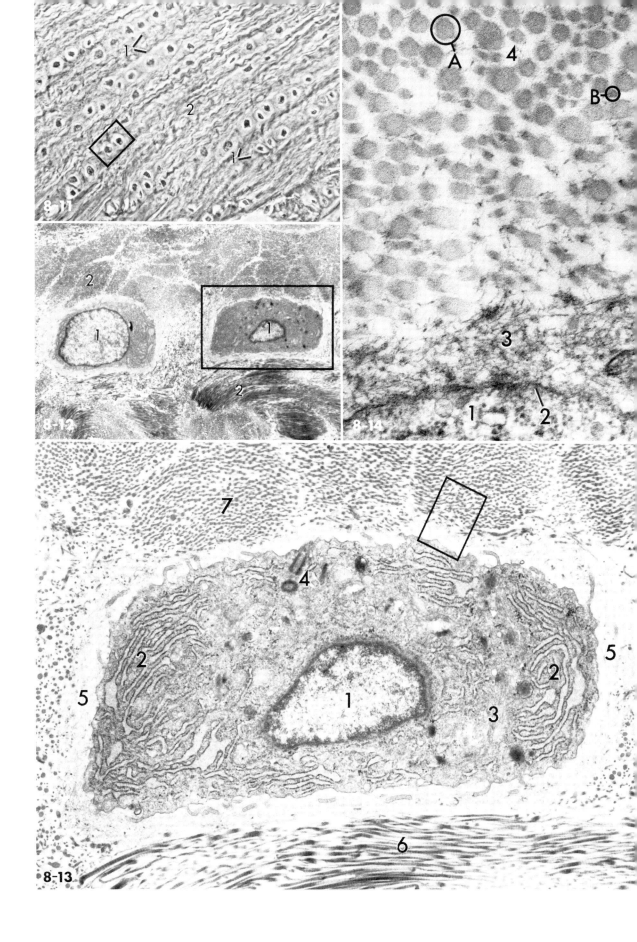

Cooper, G. W. and Prockop, D. J. Intracellular accumulation of protocollagen and extrusion of collagen by embryonic cartilage cells. J. Cell Biol. *38*: 523–537 (1968).

Godman, G. C. and Lane, N. On the site of sulfation in the chondrocyte. J. Cell Biol. *21*: 353–366 (1964).

Godman, G. C. and Porter, K. R. Chondrogenesis, studied with the electron microscope. J. Biophys. Biochem. Cytol. *8*: 719–760 (1960).

Goel, S. C. Electron microscopic studies on developing cartilage. I. The membrane system related to the synthesis and secretion of extracellular materials. J. Embryol. Exp. Morph. *23*: 169–184 (1970).

Horwitz, A. L. and Dorfman, A. Subcellular sites for synthesis of chondromucoprotein of cartilage. J. Cell Biol. *38*: 358–368 (1968).

Matukas, V. J., Panner, B. J. and Orbison, J. L. Studies on ultrastructural identification and distribution of protein polysaccharide in cartilage matrix. J. Cell Biol. *32*: 365–378 (1964).

Minor, R. R. Somite chondrogenesis. A structural study. J. Cell Biol. *56*: 27–50 (1973).

Palfrey, A. J. and Davies, D. V. The fine structure of chondrocytes. J. Anat. *100*: 213–226 (1966).

Revel, J. P. and Hay, E. D. An autoradiographic and electron microscopic study of collagen synthesis in differentiating cartilage. Z. Zellforsch. *61*: 110–144 (1963).

Seegmiller, R., Ferguson, C. C. and Sheldon, H. Studies on cartilage. IV. A genetically determined defect in tracheal cartilage. J. Ultrastruct. Res. *38*: 288–301 (1972).

Sheldon, H. Cartilage. *In* Electron Microscopic Anatomy (Ed. S. M. Kurtz), pp. 295–313. Academic Press, New York, 1964.

Sheldon, H. and Kimball, F. B. Studies on cartilage. III. The occurence of collagen within vacuoles of the Golgi apparatus. J. Cell Biol. *12*: 599–613 (1962).

Sheldon, H. and Robinson, R. A. Studies on cartilage: electron microscope observations on normal rabbit ear cartilage. J. Biophys. Biochem. Cytol. *4*: 401–406 (1958).

Silberberg, R. Ultrastructure of articular cartilage in health and disease. Clin. Orthop. *57*: 233–257 (1968).

Silva, D. G. and Hart, J. A. L. Ultrastructural observations on the mandibular condyle of the guinea pig. J. Ultrastruct. Res. *20*: 227–243 (1967).

Silva, D. G. Further ultrastructural studies on the temporo-mandibular joint in the guinea pig. J. Ultrastruct. Res. *26*: 148–162 (1969).

Smith, J. W. and Serafini-Fracassini, A. The distribution of the protein-polysaccharide complex in the nucleus pulposus matrix in young rabbits. J. Cell Sci. *3*: 33–40 (1968).

Smith, J. W., Peters, T. J. and Serafini-Fracassini, A. Observations on the distribution of the protein-polysaccharide complex and collagen in bovine articular cartilage. J. Cell Sci. *2*: 129–136 (1967).

Thyberg, J. Ultrastructural localization of aryl sulfatase activity in epiphyseal plate. J. Ultrastruct. Res. *38*: 332–342 (1972).

Thyberg, J. and Friberg, U. Ultrastructure and acid phosphatase activity of matrix vesicles and cytoplasmic dense bodies in the epiphyseal plate. J. Ultrastruct. Res. *33*: 554–573 (1970).

9 Bone

GENERAL CONSIDERATIONS

Bone is a hard, rigid connective tissue composed of an extensive vascular network, specific bone cells (osteocytes, osteoclasts, osteoblasts), and a matrix consisting of collagenous fibrils and inorganic salts. Bone tissue forms the **skeleton** which provides attachment for skeletal muscles and thereby represents an essential part of the locomotion system. Bone also has a protective function, since it forms the bony cages of the skull, chest, and pelvis. Bones serve as a hemopoietic organ by harboring marrow within their cavities, and bones play an important role in the mineral homeostasis of the body by storing well over 90% of the amount of calcium salts in the body.

There are in the human body, long bones, flat bones, and short irregular bones. The **long bones** consist of a central shaft (diaphysis) and two articular ends (epiphysis); typical examples are the humerus and the femur. The flat bones and the short irregular bones vary greatly in shape, with the parietal bone a good example of a **flat bone**; the carpal bones and the vertebrae are examples of **short irregular bones.** Two types of bone tissue make up the bones, regardless of their shape: compact bone and spongy bone. The **compact bone** tissue forms the exterior part of all bones. (Fig. 9-4) It is particularly thick in the shaft (diaphysis) of long bones, and very thin in the epiphyses. In the flat bones, compact bone tissue forms two exterior plates, whereas in the short irregular bones it is found as an exterior thin layer. **Spongy bone** makes up the epiphyses of long bones and the interior of all other bones. (Fig. 9-3) In flat bones, the interior, spongy part is extremely thin and referred to as diploë.

Compact and spongy bone tissues are continuous with each other. Both are made up of bone cells and extracellular matrix, but the main difference relates to the degree of vascularization and the arrangement of the bone cells in reference to the vascular ramifications. The compact bone is permeated by numerous blood vessels which travel in small channels (Haversian canals). Bone cells are arranged concentrically around these channels. Spongy bone, on the other hand, is composed of delicate bony trabeculae and spicules with irregularly dispersed bone cells. The blood vessels are largely confined to the hemopoietic tissue which fills the cavernous spaces between the trabeculae.

Hemopoietic, **myeloid tissue** occupies in adults all areas of the skeleton where spongy bone is present. This is the red bone marrow. The central cavity of the diaphysis of long bones contains largely adipose tissue (yellow bone marrow), which can be reverted to red, myeloid tissue in case of a great demand for new blood formation, as for instance, after extensive blood loss through hemorrhage.

A thin layer of dense fibrous connective tissue, the **periosteum,** surrounds the bones on all sides (Fig. 9-4), except where they meet in a synovial joint. The interior surfaces of the bone, including the larger Haversian canals, are lined by a thin single layer of osteoprogenitor cells, the **endosteum.**

Fig. 9-1. Section of upper end of dry femur. Adult. Human. L.M. X 1.0. **1.** Spongy bone of epiphysis. **2.** Compact bone of distal part of diaphysis. **3.** Marrow cavity. **4.** Trabeculae follow major lines of stress. Note absence of epiphyseal cartilage plate.

Fig. 9-2. Sagittal section of femoral condyle. Young rabbit. L.M. X 4.2. **1.** Articular cartilage. **2.** Spongy bone of epiphysis. **3.** Marrow cavity. **4.** Narrow epiphyseal cartilage plate. **5.** Compact bone of diaphysis. **6.** Bone marrow.

Fig. 9-3. Survey of spongy bone. Enlargement of area similar to rectangle (A) in Fig. 9-2. Epiphysis. Femur. Young cat. L.M. X 72. **1.** Spicules. **2.** Bone marrow. **3.** Trabeculae. **4.** Marrow spaces simulating Haversian canals.

Fig. 9-4. Compact cortical bone. Enlargement of rectangle (B) in Fig. 9-2. L.M. X 88. **1.** Periosteum. **2.** Compact bone. **3.** Haversian canals. **4.** Trabeculae. **5.** Bone marrow. **6.** Nutrient foramen and canal.

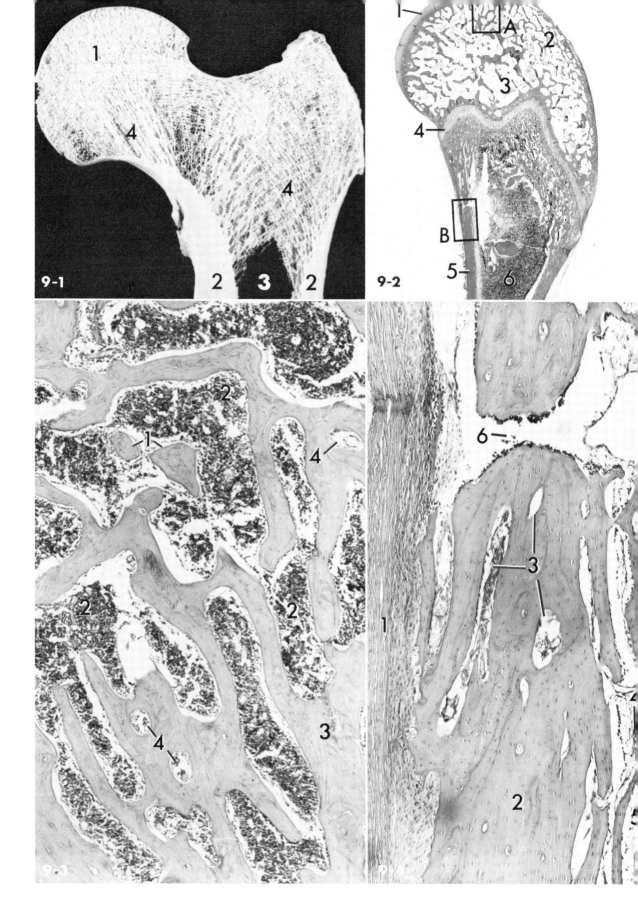

The epiphyseal surfaces of the bones, forming **synovial joints** are covered by a thin layer of fibrous or hyaline cartilage. A dense fibrous connective tissue capsule surrounds the joint and holds the bones together. Ligaments reinforce the capsule. The inner surface of the capsule is differentiated into a synovial membrane which secretes a viscous synovial fluid into the narrow space of the joint cavity.

ARCHITECTURE OF BONE

The architectural organization of mature adult bone tissue is primarily the result of physical forces on a particular bone or part of the bone during development and growth. Secondarily, it depends on the pattern of vascularization which develops as a result of these forces. The tubular structure of long bones is the best construction for resisting bending forces in any direction, whereas the pattern of the spongy bone is superior in withstanding and resisting forces of compression and disruption.

Compact bone. Compact (cortical) bone forms the shafts of long bones and surrounds all bones as a layer of varied thickness. The central part of thick compact bone is referred to as **Haversian bone.** It consists of a system of numerous small channels (Fig. 9-6), **Haversian canals,** which serve as tunnels for small blood vessels, usually arterioles, venules, and capillaries. The channels are parallel to each other and to the long axis of the bone. The blood vessels reach the Haversian canals either from the periosteum or from the marrow cavity through **Volkmann's canals,** which are less abundant than the Haversian canals and run perpendicular to the long axis of the bone. The Haversian canal, with its blood vessels, forms the center of a functional unit, the **osteon.** (Fig. 9-7) In addition to the blood vessels the osteon consists of scattered, concentrically arranged **osteocytes** (Fig. 9-8), and 10–15 bony **circular lamellae** averaging 5 μ in thickness. The osteocytes are lodged in small **lacunae** and communicate with

each other through long cell processes which travel in a vast system of narrow **canaliculi** (Fig. 9-9) in the bony lamellae. The circular (concentric) lamellae make up the extracellular matrix and consist of numerous collagenous fibrils, a small amount of ground substance, and inorganic calcium salts which are present both in soluble and crystalline form. The crystals are deposited upon and within the framework of collagenous fibrils. There is great variation in the degree of mineralization of the different osteons. As a rule newly formed osteons are less mineralized than old ones. The Haversian canals vary considerably in size. A large canal is usually an indication that an active resorption of bone matrix is taking place (or has taken place) and that it will be followed by new bone formation. This is discussed further on p. 218.

The osteon has the same length as its central blood vessel, and because of the dependence on the blood vessels, osteons are also branching structures. The periph-

Fig. 9-5. Cross section through diaphysis of dry femur. Human. L.M. X 0.8. **1.** Compact bone. **2.** Trabeculae. **3.** Marrow cavity.

Fig. 9-6. Cross section of tibia. Enlargement of area similar to rectangle in Fig. 9-5. Human. L.M. X 70. **1.** Periosteum (removed). **2.** External circumferential lamellae. **3.** Haversian canals. **4.** Circle: osteon. **5.** Traces of interstitial lamellae. **6.** Erosion tunnel. **7.** Volkmann's canals. **8.** Internal circumferential lamellae. Each small dot represents an osteocyte in a lacuna. **9.** Bone marrow.

Fig. 9-7. Osteon (Haversian system). Ground cross section through compact bone of diaphysis. Femur. Human. L.M. X 1000. **1.** Cementing line. **2.** Lacunae. **3.** Haversian canal.

Fig. 9-8. Central part of osteon. Decalcified preparation to demonstrate bony lamellae. Rib. Human. L.M. X 360. **1.** Haversian canal. **2.** Osteocytes in lacunae. **3.** Bony circular lamellae.

Fig. 9-9. Central part of osteon. Ground section. Same preparation as in Fig. 9-7. L.M. X 1300. **1.** Haversian canal. **2.** Canaliculi; some reach the Haversian canal. **3.** Lacunae.

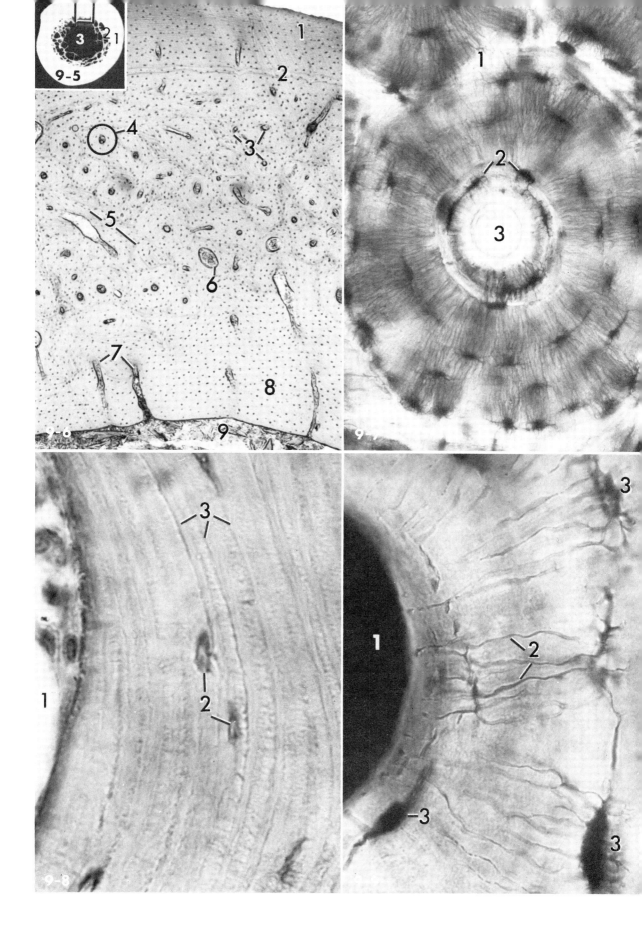

eral boundary of an osteon, the **cementing line,** stands out as a refractive border because of the difference in orientation of collagenous fibrils within the osteon, as compared to adjoining bony lamellae of other osteons or interstitial bony lamellae.

The lamellar arrangement of the matrix in the osteon reflects a very fundamental way in which bone is formed, since bands of matrix, interspersed with osteocytes, are laid down in regular layers (see p. 206). The most superficial parts of compact bone similarly contain bony lamellae which are parallel with the periosteal and endosteal surfaces forming the **external** or the **internal circumferential lamellae.** This part of the compact bone is often referred to as **lamellar bone** (as opposed to Haversian bone) because of its pronounced lamellation without Haversian canals. (Fig. 9-6) Between concentric lamellae of the osteons are the **interstitial lamellae,** areas of highly mineralized matrix left by a remodeling process of old Haversian osteons or peripheral lamellar bone.

Spongy bone. Spongy (cancellous, trabecular) bone forms the interior of short bones and the ends of long bones. There is a small amount present in the flat bones. The spongy bone tissue receives its name from the numerous, delicate **trabeculae** and **spicules** which form a spongy meshwork. The arrangement of the trabeculae of the spongy bone follows, generally, the major lines of stress to which a bone or its epiphysis are subjected. The intertrabecular spaces vary greatly in size and shape. They are occupied by hemopoietic, myeloid tissue and some fat cells.

The trabeculae consists of osteocytes, lodged in lacunae (Fig. 9-10), and irregularly arranged bony lamellae. There are only a few osteons with the typical arrangement of a blood vessel in a Haversian canal surrounded by concentric bony lamellae. The osteocytes of the narrow trabeculae, as a rule, do not seem to require a blood vessel of a Haversian canal for their survival, probably because no osteocyte is very far way from the rich

capillary network of the bone marrow in the intertrabecular spaces. The surfaces of the trabeculae are covered by a thin layer of osteoprogenitor cells and occasional osteoclasts.

Bone matrix. The intercellular substance of bone contains an organic matrix with collagenous fibrils (Fig. 9-12), an amorphous ground substance and inorganic salts of high concentrations. The **collagenous fibrils** make up the lamellae of the bone matrix. The fibrils are arranged parallel within each lamella, often with a helical course around the central axis of an osteon. The direction of the fibrils is different in adjoining lamellae, often making a $90°$ angle with the fibrils of

Fig. 9-10. Osteocyte in lacuna. Mandible. Decalcified preparation. Newborn rat. E.M. X 7000. **1.** Nucleus of osteocyte. **2.** Mitochondria. **3.** Granular endoplasmic reticulum. **4.** Coated vesicle. **5.** Pericellular zone of lacuna. **6.** Cytoplasmic processes. **7.** Bone matrix.

Fig. 9-11. Detail of osteocyte. Enlargement of area similar to rectangle (A) in Fig. 9-10. Diaphysis of radius. Partly decalcified preparation. Two-day-old rat. E.M. X 34,000. **1.** Nucleus of osteocyte. **2.** Ribosomes. **3.** Granular endoplasmic reticulum. **4.** Cytoplasmic process without ribosomes, entering canaliculus. **5.** Collagenous fibrils in pericellular zone of lacuna. **6.** Bone matrix: apatite crystals removed in white areas, remaining in black areas.

Fig. 9-12. Detail of osteocyte lacuna and bone matrix. Enlargement of area similar to rectangle (B) in Fig. 9-10. Diaphysis of radius. Partly decalcified preparation. Two-day-old rat. E.M. X 72,000. **1.** Bone matrix dominated by hydroxyapatite crystals which obscure the collagenous fibrils. **2.** Cross-sectioned collagenous fibrils immediately before mineralization. **3.** Periosteocytic space of the lacuna with collagenous fibrils.

Fig. 9-13. Detail of bone matrix. Enlargement of area similar to rectangle in Fig. 9-12. Head of humerus. Two-day-old rat. E.M. X 200,000. Hydroxyapatite crystals (15 Å X 300 Å) dominate in the matrix, completely obscuring the collagenous fibrils.

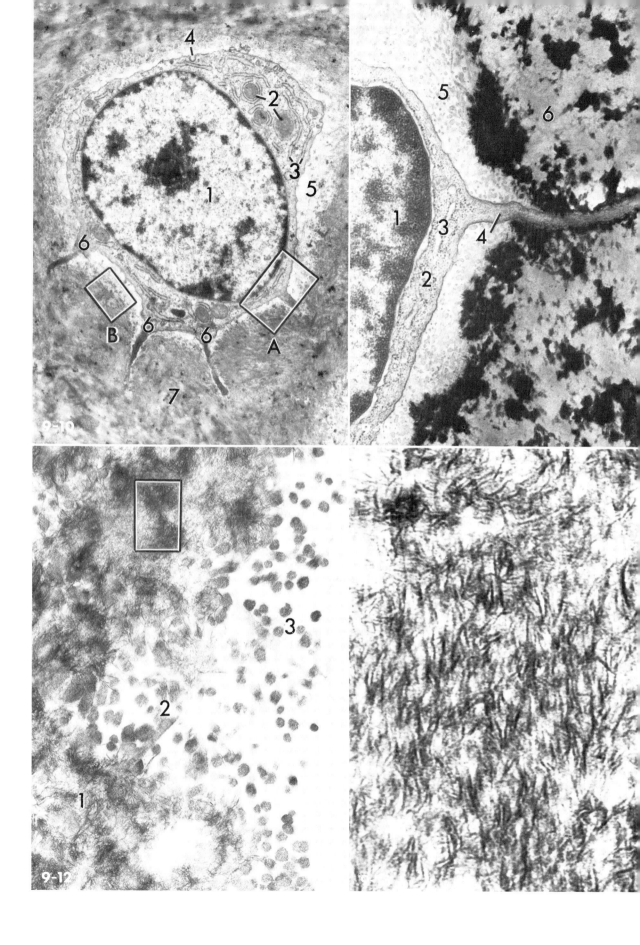

9-10

9-12

these lamellae. The difference in fibril direction constitutes the basis for the obvious lamellation of bone matrix which can be observed also in ordinary light microscope preparations. The collagenous fibrils vary in diameter but they are all characterized by the typical 640 Å-axial periodicity. (Fig. 9-16) In preparations for electron microscopy which have not been decalcified the large amount of inorganic salt crystals may obscure this periodicity, but it becomes apparent after decalcification of the tissue.

The non-collagenous, amorphous **ground substance** consists of protein-polysaccharides and glycoproteins. In the protein-polysaccharides, long polysaccharide chains are attached to a protein core, whereas the carbohydrate chains are short in a glycoprotein such as sialoprotein, the only one isolated so far from bone. The amount of sulfated polysaccharides (chondroitin sulfates) is low as opposed to the high content in cartilage. As a result bone matrix is acidophilic, whereas cartilage matrix is basophilic and metachromatic (p. 176).

The **inorganic salts** make up 65% of the bone weight. They consist mostly of calcium phosphate, calcium carbonate, and sodium. In addition there are small amounts of calcium fluoride, magnesium chloride, citrate, and potassium. Calcium is present mainly in the form of hydroxyapatite crystals, and some of the other inorganic components are adsorbed on the surface of the crystals or go into the hydration shell. The hydroxyapatite crystals are needle-shaped, averaging $15 Å \times 300 Å$. (Fig. 9-13) The crystals are bound mainly to the collagenous fibrils both at the surface and within the fibrils. The crystals are arranged in parallel with the long axis of the fibrils. (Fig. 9-17) Some crystals may also be present in the ground substance between the collagenous fibrils. (Fig. 9-16) The precise interrelationship of the hydroxyapatite crystal to the tropocollagen molecules is not known. It has been suggested that the polypeptide chains of the collagen are folded or wrapped around the hydroxyapatite crystal.

Bone cells. The matrix of bone is synthesized, laid down, maintained, and remodeled by four kinds of bone cells: 1) osteocytes; 2) osteoblasts; 3) preosteoblasts; and 4) osteoclasts. These cells are essential for the processes of bone formation and bone resorption which are discussed in detail in Chapter 10 (p. 206). However, the structures and functions of these cells will be described here.

The **osteocytes** are small, often almond-shaped cells which are lodged in a **lacuna**, completely surrounded by fully mineralized bone matrix with the exception of a $1-2$ μ-wide zone near the osteocyte cell membrane. This zone is occupied generally by native collagenous fibrils without

Fig. 9-14. Osteoblast. Diaphysis of radius. Two-day-old rat. E.M. X 9000. **1.** Nucleus of osteoblast. **2.** Golgi zone. **3.** Mitochondria. **4.** Granular endoplasmic reticulum. **5.** Lysosomes. **6.** Short microvillus. **7.** Long microvillus. **8.** Osteoid.

Fig. 9-15. Detail of osteoblast. Same preparation as in Fig. 9-14. E.M. X 46,000. **1.** Components of Golgi zone. **2.** Granular endoplasmic reticulum. **3.** Lysosome. **4.** Coated vesicles, the uppermost just fusing with the cell membrane. **5.** Coated vesicle completing its fusion with the cell membrane. **6.** Periosteoblastic space with some collagenous fibrils. **7.** Bone matrix.

Fig. 9-16. Detail of osteoid. Enlargement of area similar to rectangle in Fig. 9-14. Head of humerus. Two-day-old rat. E.M. X 99,000. **1.** Osteoblast cell membrane. **2.** Collagenous fibrils with 610 Å axial periodicity (between each bar). **3.** Initial calcification loci. **4.** Hydroxyapatite crystal, parallel to long axis of collagenous fibril. **5.** Crystals perpendicular to long axis of collagenous fibril.

Fig. 9-17. Detail of mineralized collagenous fibril. Same preparation as in Fig. 9-16. E.M. X 111,000. **1.** Arrows indicate sites where the hydroxyapatite crystals are oriented parallel to the long axis of the collagenous fibril. They seem to be both at the surface and within the fibril. **2.** The lower part of the fibril shows clear axial periodicity without crystals.

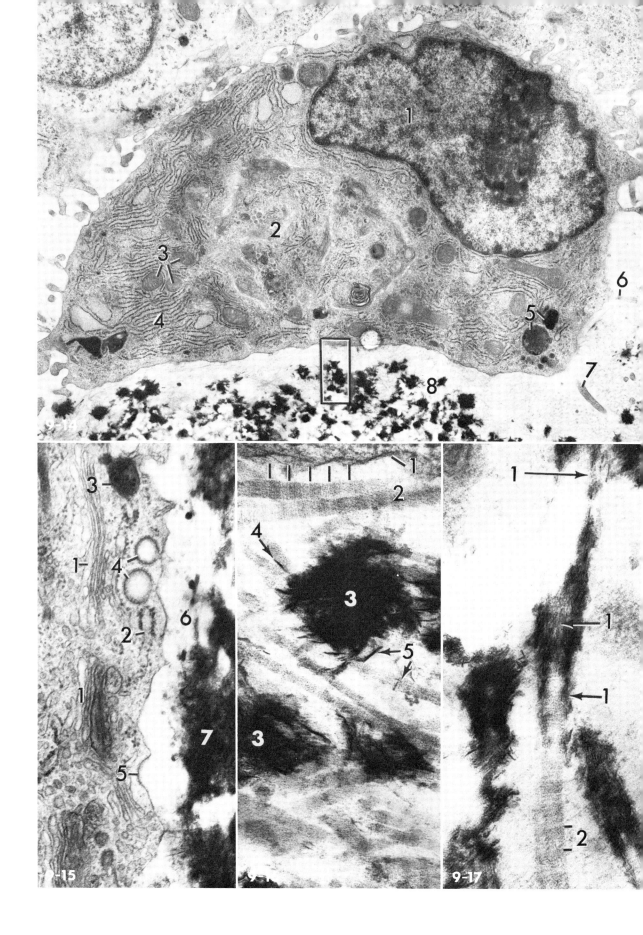

apatite crystals. The osteocyte has several narrow and extremely long cytoplasmic processes which pierce the bone matrix in small tunnels of their own called **canaliculi.** (Fig. 9-11) There is a narrow space around the cell processes, approximately 0.1 μ-wide which is not occupied by collagenous fibrils. It is assumed that interstitial fluid and metabolites circulate in this narrow space. The osteocyte has a small nucleus and a relatively sparse cytoplasm. The Golgi apparatus is small and mitochondria are few. Some lysosomes are present. The granular endoplasmic reticulum varies greatly depending on the age and state of activity of the osteocyte. A young osteocyte near the periosteal bone surface, which is in the process of actively synthesizing collagenous fibrils, contains a large amount of granular endoplasmic reticulum, whereas an old osteocyte, lodged deeply in the bony matrix of an osteon, is poor in granular endoplasmic reticulum. Therefore, it is presumably less actively manufacturing collagen. In fact, it has been suggested that old osteocytes may enter a resorptive phase.

The **osteoblasts** are small round, ovoid, or flat cells, forming a single layer on the surface of young bone. They form the active periosteal layer of the diaphysis of long bones. They also line all inner surfaces of spongy and compact bones. However, here they may not form a complete layer since they are often interspersed with osteoclasts and early hemopoietic cells. In general, the ultrastructure of the osteoblast is very similar to that of a plasma cell (compare Figs. 9-14 and 7-25). The osteoblast has a large ovoid nucleus, often placed eccentrically. (Fig. 9-14) The Golgi zone is relatively large; mitochondria are numerous; and the granular endoplasmic reticulum is extensive. Lysosomes and coated vesicles are present. The coated vesicles are frequently fusing with the cell membrane. Accumulations of particulate glycogen often occur. The cell surface is provided with a small num-

ber of short microvilli. These microvilli become increasingly longer and coarser as the osteoblast is transformed into an osteocyte by a mineralization of the surrounding matrix. There is no doubt that the osteoblast participates actively in the synthesis and formation of the collagenous fibrils and ground substance of the bone matrix. The mechanism is very likely similar to that described for the fibroblast (p. 152). It has been suggested that the osteoblasts are also instrumental in the movement and binding of apatite crystals to the collagenous fibrils, giving rise to a preosseus tissue, **osteoid,** but the precise mechanism is not known. (Fig. 9-14) The formation of osteoid is discussed further on p. 208.

The **preosteoblasts** or osteoprogenitor cells are spindle-shaped or slightly flattened cells which occur in the loose connective tissue of the bone marrow, especially around capillaries and small blood vessels. They also occur in great abundance in the preosteoblastic layer of the periosteum of the midshaft of long bones between the fibroblasts and the fully differentiated osteoblasts (see Fig. 10-5). The

Fig. 9-18. Remodeling of spongy bone. Rib. Human. L.M. X 350. **1.** Bone marrow. **2.** Trabeculum. **3.** Bone matrix. **4.** Osteocytes. **5.** Osteoblasts. **6.** Osteoclasts.

Fig. 9-19. Osteoclast. Enlargement of area simiar to rectangle in Fig. 9-18. Head of humerus. Two-day-old rat. E.M. X 2300. **1.** Nucleus of osteoclast. **2.** Extensive cytoplasm. **3.** Bone matrix. **4.** Nucleus of neighboring osteoblast.

Fig. 9-20. Part of osteoclast. Enlargement of area similar to rectangle in Fig. 9-19. Same preparation as in Fig. 9-19. E.M. X 9000. **1.** Nuclei of osteoclast. **2.** Golgi zone. **3.** Mitochondria. **4.** Ruffled border. **5.** Bone matrix.

Fig. 9-21. Detail of osteoclast ruffled border. Enlargement of lower half of Fig. 9-20. E.M. X 17,000. **1.** Mitochondria. **2.** Phagocytic vacuoles containing small, needle-shaped crystals. **3.** Microvilli of ruffled border. **4.** Delicate mineralized collagenous fibrils of bone matrix.

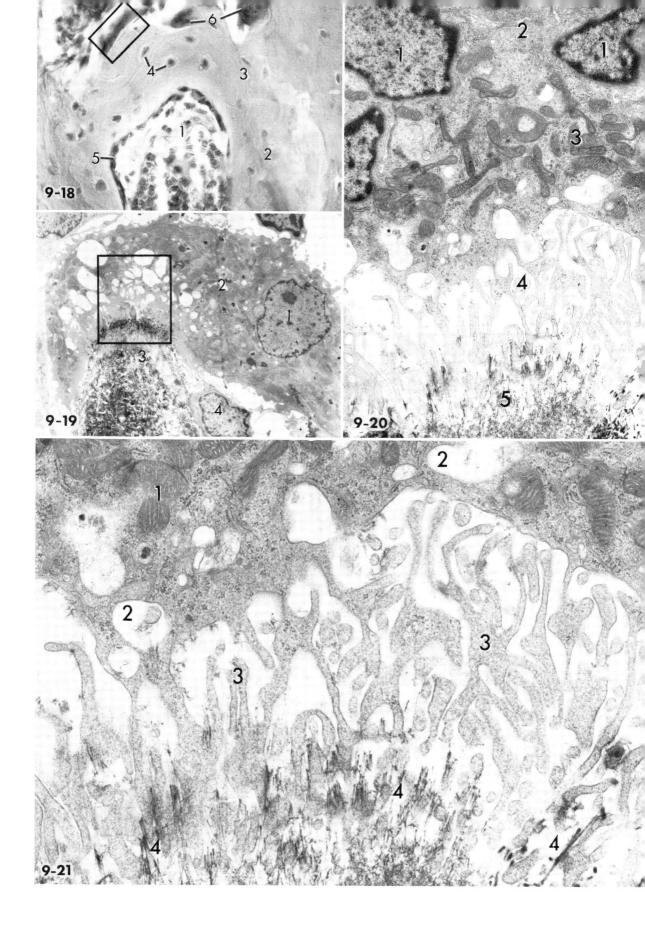

9-18

9-19

9-20

9-21

fine structure of the cytoplasm of the preosteoblast resembles that of a primitive mesenchymal cell with the exception that the preosteoblasts often contain large accumulations of particulate glycogen. The preosteoblasts are engaged mainly in cell proliferation to provide for a population of cells which differentiate into osteoblasts as the bone formation progresses, or to osteoclasts under an appropriate stimulus.

The **osteoclasts** are large, multinucleated cells, occurring singly on the inner surfaces of spongy and compact bones. (Fig. 9-18) Their cytoplasm contains numerous mitochondria, moderate amounts of loosely organized granular endoplasmic reticulum, and several well-developed perinuclear Golgi zones. Vacuoles of varied sizes are abundantly present, together with primary and secondary lysosomes. The surface of the osteoclast, which lies adjacent to the bone matrix, is differentiated into two areas: 1) the clear zone and 2) the ruffled border. The clear zone is devoid of organelles and is characterized by a moderately dense granular cytoplasm. The ruffled border is an area with deep invaginations of the cell membrane and numerous cytoplasmic microvilli. (Fig. 9-21) The cytoplasm deep to the ruffled border contains many smooth and coated vesicles as well as phagosomes and residual bodies. The clear zone surrounds the zone with the ruffled border. It is generally accepted that the ruffled border serves as an active site of resorption, and that the clear zone seals off the zone of resorption from the extracellular space lateral to the osteoclast. Thus, the main function of the osteoclast is bone resorption. This conclusion is based on the observations that the immediately adjacent bone usually appears demineralized, and that hydroxyapatite crystals are present between microvilli of the ruffled border, and within phagocytic vacuoles and secondary lysosomes. There is no information on the mechanism that promotes the differentiation of an osteoprogenitor cell

into an osteoclast, although it has been suggested that the parathyroid hormone may be instrumental in initiating this differentiation.

Periosteum. The outer surface of bone is covered by periosteum, a dense fibrous, irregular connective tissue membrane. The periosteum contains numerous bundles of collagenous and elastic fibers. Some of the collagenous bundles enter the compact bone at right angles, particularly where tendons are attached to bone, and penetrate the outer bony lamellae to become anchored deep inside the bone. These fibers are referred to as **Sharpey's perforating fibers.** The periosteum consists of superficial, flattened fibroblasts, a middle layer of indifferent, osteoprogenitor cells (preosteoblasts), and of an innermost layer of osteoblasts (see Fig. 10-5). The periosteal membrane is richly vascularized and contains many sensory nerves. During development and growth, the periosteum is a source of new, subperiosteal bone which is laid down through appositional growth. This is described in more detail on p. 210. In the adult, the periosteum lacks the layer of osteoblasts, but the bone-forming ability is retained by the fibroblasts and the osteoprogenitor cells which become very active bone-forming cells during the healing and knitting of fractured bones.

Endosteum. The inner surfaces of the marrow cavities and the larger Haversian

Fig. 9-22. Cross section of a 23 μ-wide Haversian canal in frontal bone of a four-week-old kitten. Specimen fixed by vascular perfusion with subsequent decalcification. E.M. X 6000. **1.** Lumen of venous capillary. **2.** Endothelial nucleus. **3.** Continuous thin endothelium; basal lamina incomplete. **4.** Collagenous fibrils. **5.** Nuclei of osteoprogenitor cells and resting, flat osteoblasts. These cells form an endosteal lining of the Haversian canal. Distance between asterisks is 23 μ. **6.** Nucleus of macrophage. **7.** Cross section of small capillary, probably in a state of sprouting growth, judging from the narrow, slit-like lumen. **8.** Osteoid. **9.** Calcified bone matrix.

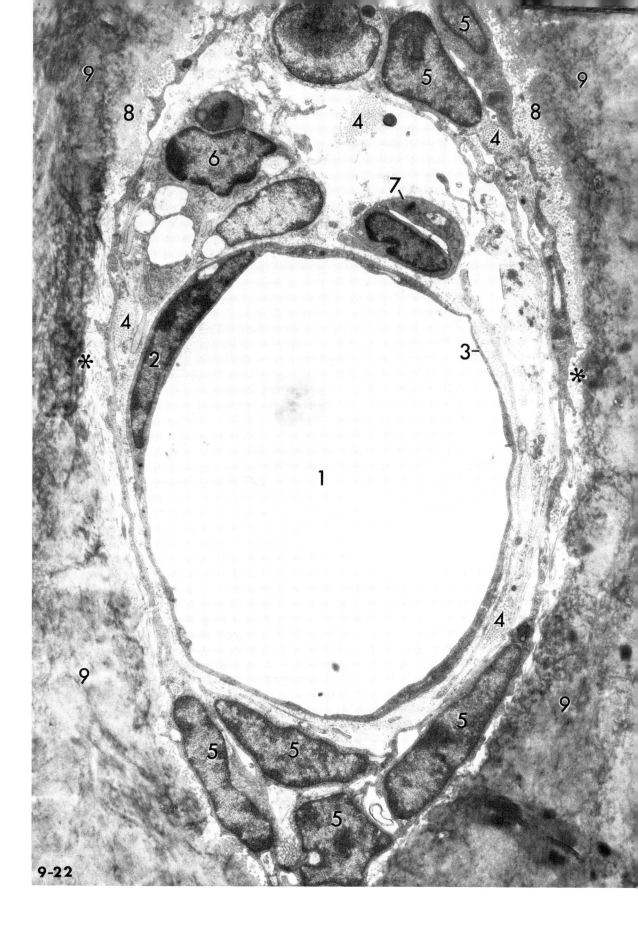

canals in bone are lined by endosteum, a thin layer of osteoprogenitor cells or osteoblasts. (Fig. 9-22) During the development and growth, the osteoblasts often form a layer of cuboidal cells, simulating an epithelial layer. Among the osteoblasts occur also osteoclasts (p. 196). In the adult, the endosteum consists of flat squamous, inactive cells which retain the potential to become osteoblasts upon stimulation.

BLOOD VESSELS IN BONE AND MARROW

The vascular systems of the cortical compact bone, the epiphyseal spongy bone, and the bone marrow anastomose relatively freely and make bone an extremely vascular tissue. The **compact bone** receives its blood supply from the bone marrow and from the periosteum. The nutrient (medullary) arteries reach the marrow cavity through the nutrient foramina. Most long bones have only one such foramen, except the femur and the clavicle which have two. In the marrow the artery gives off ascending and descending branches which, on the one hand, supply the bone marrow with capillaries and sinusoids; on the other hand, many branches turn radially, go through the endosteum, enter Volkmann's canals, and from there branch into the Haversian canals. The vascular network of the periosteum also sends many small arteries and arterioles via Volkmann's canals into the Haversian canals of the compact cortical bone. The blood vessels in the Haversian canals are generally both arterial and venous capillaries, but many canals contain only one vessel. (Fig. 9-22) The endothelium of these vessels is mostly continuous, but in some instances, fenestrated endothelium occurs. A basal lamina is present in some species. The pericapillary cells are pericytes, fibroblasts, and undifferentiated cells. By the nature of their location, the latter can properly be called osteoprogenitor cells. These cells also form an incomplete lining of the canal, in which case they should be re-

ferred to as endosteum. Schwann cells accompanying non-myelinated axons are also present in the perivascular space of the Haversian canals. The **spongy bone** in the epiphyses of long bones is supplied by periarticular arterial branches which usually enter the bone through the capsule of the joint, or via a ligament. When the epiphyseal growth plate is closed in the adult bone, some branches of the medullary artery reach the epiphysis and establish anastomoses with the epiphyseal blood vessels. The **bone marrow** itself receives its blood supply almost exclusively from the nutrient artery. Short arterioles and arterial capillaries feed into a multitude of sinusoids of greatly varied diameters. (Fig. 9-23) The bone marrow sinusoids are extremely thin-walled. The endothelium is greatly attenuated (Fig. 9-24), but as a rule not fenestrated, although large gaps may be present here

Fig. 9-23. Survey of bone marrow. Diaphysis. Two-day-old rat. E.M. X 600. **1.** Wide sinusoids. **2.** Narrow blood capillaries. **3.** Remnants of bone trabeculae with core of calcified cartilage. **4.** Layer of osteoblasts (endosteum). **5.** Reticular cells (fixed macrophages). **6.** Megakaryoblasts. **7.** Osteoclasts. **8.** Circles: cells in mitosis. *Note:* Identification of cells is based on analysis of this field at higher magnifications. No attempt has been made to identify the varied stages of cells in hemopoietic development.

Fig. 9-24. Detail of bone marrow sinusoid. Enlargement of area similar to rectangle in Fig. 9-23. Same preparation. E.M. X 15,000. **1.** Lumen of sinusoid. **2.** Nucleus of endothelial (lining) cell. **3.** Coated vesicles. **4.** Phagocytic vacuole. **5.** Thin attenuated continuous endothelial cytoplasm.

Fig. 9-25. Detail of endothelial cell in bone marrow sinusoid. E.M. X 49,000. **1.** Lumen of sinusoid. **2.** Endothelial cells. **3.** Cell junction. **4.** Perisinusoidal space. Note absence of basal lamina.

Fig. 9-26. Detail of endothelial cell in bone marrow sinusoid. Same preparation as in Fig. 9-24. E.M. X 72,000. **1.** Lumen of sinusoid. **2.** Nucleus of endothelial (lining) cell. **3.** Phagocytic vacuole. **4.** Small Golgi zone. **5.** Mitochondria. **6.** Perisinusoidal space.

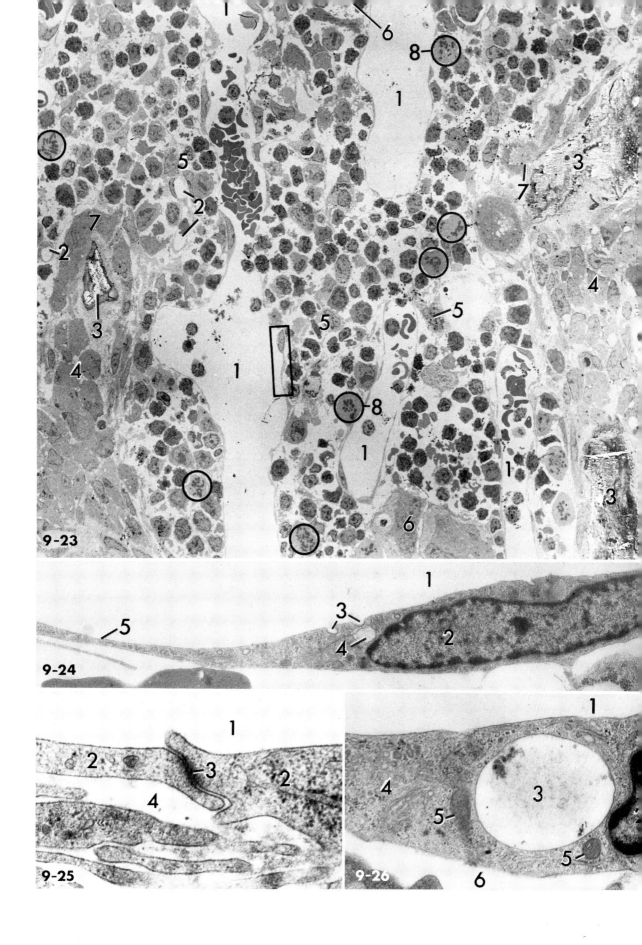

and there. The endothelial cells are highly phagocytic as witnessed by the many phagocytic vacuoles and lysosomes. (Fig. 9-26). Micropinocytotic invaginations and vesicles abound. Maturing blood cells enter the lumen of the sinusoids through diapedesis, crossing mostly at endothelial cell junctions, but also utilizing the endothelial gaps when available. In most species, there is no basal lamina present beneath the endothelium. The perisinusoidal cells are undifferentiated reticular cells which can develop into osteoprogenitor cells upon proper stimulation. These cells are not pericytes since they lack an external (basal) lamina. The possible role of the reticular cells in hemopoiesis is discussed on p. 112.

The **venous drainage** of the marrow and the bone tissue itself follows essentially the routes of the arterial supply. Most of the blood flows toward a large central longitudinal vein in the marrow. The central vein connects with the nutrient vein. The walls of the veins are usually quite thin.

Lymphatic vessels have been convincingly demonstrated in the periosteum and in some Haversian canals. There is still no clear evidence that lymphatic capillaries exist in the bone marrow. The sinusoids probably serve as lymphatic capillaries since they have a similar endothelium and generally lack a basal lamina.

SYNOVIAL JOINTS

Synovial or **diarthrodial** joints are categorized as joints where the two apposed surfaces of bone, covered by articular cartilage, are separated by a small cavity filled with synovial fluid, and held together by an articular capsule.

The **articular cartilage** covers the two apposed surfaces of bone. (Fig. 9-27) It is mostly made up of fibrous cartilage (p. 180), but, in some instances, it consists of hyaline cartilage. Perichondrium and periosteum are not present in synovial joints. The two apposed bones are held together by an **articular capsule** which

often is supported and reinforced by ligaments. (Fig. 9-28) The capsule consists of: 1) an outer layer of strong, dense fibroelastic connective tissue which is continuous with the periosteum of the diaphysis of the bone; 2) a middle layer of subsynovial loose fibrous connective tissue rich in blood vessels, lymphatics, and adipose tissue; and 3) a synovial membrane forming the innermost layer of the capsule. Parts of the capsule project into the joint cavity in the shape of coarse **folds** and club-shaped villi. The synovial membrane and parts of the capsule evaginate between adjoining tendons, muscles, and bones as **bursae.** The **synovial membrane** lines the inside of the capsule, villi, folds, and bursae. (Fig. 9-29) The membrane consists of an incomplete layer of flattened fibroblasts (synovial cells), and an underlying layer of reticular fibrils intermingled with a medium dense, diffusely distributed basement membrane-like material or connective tissue matrix. (Fig. 9-30) A distinct, true thin basal lamina is missing. The joint cavity forms from the mesenchyme, but it is not lined by meso-

Fig. 9-27. Survey of synovial joint. Finger. Monkey. Four months old. L.M. X 10.5. **1.** Epiphyseal growth plate. **2.** Spongy bone of epiphysis. **3.** Epiphyseal and articular cartilages. **4.** Joint cavity. **5.** Articular capsule.

Fig. 9-28. Detail of joint. Enlargement of rectangle in Fig. 9-27. L.M. X 163. **1.** Epiphyseal cartilage. **2.** Articular cartilage. **3.** Joint cavity. **4.** Synovial membrane. **5.** Articular capsule.

Fig. 9-29. Articular capsule. Knee joint. Enlargement of area similar to rectangle in Fig. 9-28. Rat. E.M. X 1800. **1.** Joint cavity. **2.** Synovial membrane. **3.** Nucleus of fibroblast. **4.** Collagenous fiber bundles in articular capsule. **5.** Lymph vessel. **6.** Blood capillary. **7.** Nerve.

Fig. 9-30. Synovial membrane. Enlargement of rectangle in Fig. 9-29. E.M. X 18,000. **1.** Nuclei of synovial cells. **2.** Basement membrane-like material. **3.** Reticular fibrils. **4.** Collagenous fibrils. **5.** Golgi zone. **6.** Granular endoplasmic reticulum. **7.** Mitochondria. **8.** Coated vesicles.

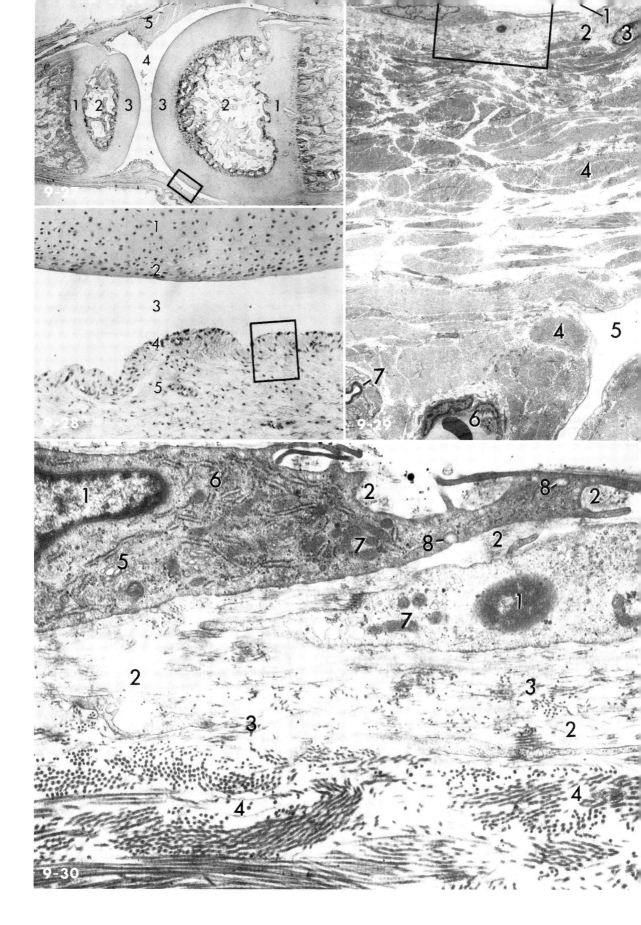

thelial cells. The lining cells are definitely flattened fibroblasts with a large amount of granular endoplasmic reticulum, an extensive Golgi zone, and numerous micropinocytotic vesicles and coated vesicles. A certain variation in number and distribution of these organelles has led some investigators to categorize the synovial cells (fibroblasts) into types A and B. The fibroblasts are not held together by junctional complexes. Areas exist where the flattened fibroblasts do not overlap but leave connective tissue fibers exposed to the joint cavity.

The function of the synovial membrane is to secrete the **synovial fluid,** a viscous substance which contains about 95% water, the rest being made up of proteins, mucopolysaccharides, and salts. It is not known how the synovial fluid is formed, but its composition seems to indicate that it is a protein-containing dialysate of blood with added mucin. It is likely that the proximity of capillaries and lymphatics in the subsynovial connective tissue facilitates the formation of the synovial fluid. The mucopolysaccharide components of the synovial fluid, composed mainly of hyaluronic acid, may be synthesized by the flattened fibroblasts (synovial cells). The many coated vesicles could be the ultrastructural indication of this activity. The synovial fluid lubricates the articular surfaces of the joint and helps to maintain nutrition of the articular cartilage.

References

Barland, P., Novikoff, A. B. and Hamerman, D. Electron microscopy of the human synovial membrane. J. Cell Biol. *14*: 207–220 (1962).

Baud, C. G. Submicroscopic structure and functional aspects of the osteocyte. Clin. Orthop. *56*: 227–236 (1968).

Brookes, M. The vascular architecture of tubular bone in the rat. Anat. Rec. *132*: 25–41 (1958).

Cabrini, R. L. Histochemistry of ossification. Int. Rev. Cytol. *11*: 283–306 (1961).

Cameron, D. A. The fine structure of osteoblasts in the metaphysis of the tibia of young rat. J. Biophys. Biochem. Cytol. *9*: 583–595 (1961).

Cameron, D. A. The fine structure of bone and calcified cartilage. Clin. Orthop. *26*: 199–228 (1963).

Cohen, J. and Harris, W. H. The three-dimensional anatomy of Haversian systems. J. Bone and Joint Surg. *40-A*: 419–434 (1958).

Cooper, R. R., Milgram, J. W. and Robinson, R. A. Morphology of the osteon. An electron microscopic study. J. Bone and Joint Surg. *48-A*: 1239–1271 (1966).

Drinker, C. K., Drinker, K. R. and Lund, C. C. The circulation in the mammalian bone marrow. Am. J. Physiol. *62*: 1–92 (1922).

Dudley, H. R. and Spiro, D. The fine structure of bone cells J. Biophys. Biochem. Cytol. *11*: 627–649 (1961).

Engström, A. Structure of bone from the anatomical to the molecular level. Ciba Foundation Symposium on Bone Structure and Metabolism. (Eds. G. E. W. Wolstenholme and C. M. O'Connor), pp. 3–10. Churchill, London, 1956.

Ghadially, F. N. and Roy, S. Ultrastructure of Synovial Joints in Health and Disease. Butterworths, London, 1969.

Glimcher, M. J. Molecular biology of mineralized tissues with particular reference to bone. Rev. Mod. Phys. *31*: 359–393 (1959).

Glimcher, M. J. and Krane, S. M. The organization and structure of bone, and the mechanism of calcification. *In* Treatise on Collagen (Ed. B. S. Gould), Vol. 2, part B. Academic Press, New York, 1968.

Herring, G. M. A review of recent advances in the chemistry of calcifying cartilage and bone matrix. Calc. Tiss. Res. *4*, Suppl. 17 (1970).

Hohling, H. J., Kreilos, R., Neubauer, G. and Boyde, A. Electron microscopy and electron microscopical measurements of collagen mineralization in hard tissue. Z. Zellforsch. *122*: 36–52 (1971).

Jande, S. S. Fine structural study of osteocytes and their surrounding bone matrix with respect to their age in young chicks. J. Ultrastruct. Res. *37*: 279–300 (1971).

Jande, S. S. and Belanger, L. F. Electron microscopy of osteocytes and the pericellular matrix in rat trabecular bone. Calc. Tiss. Res. *6*: 280–289 (1971).

Kallio, D. M., Garant, P. R. and Minkin, C. Evidence of coated membranes in the ruffled border of the osteoclast. J. Ultrastruct. Res. *37*: 169–177 (1971).

Lacroix, P. Bone and cartilage. *In* The Cell (Eds. J. Brachet and A. E. Mirsky) Vol. 5: 219–266. Academic Press, New York, 1961.

Mjör, I. A. The bone matrix adjacent to lacunae and canaliculi. Anat. Rec. *144*: 327–339 (1962).

Robinson, R. A. and Cameron, D. A. Bone. *In*: Electron Microscopic Anatomy (Ed. S. M. Kurtz), pp. 315–340. Academic Press, New York, 1964.

Rohr, H. Die Kollagensynthese in ihrer Beziehung zur submikroskopischen Struktur des Osteoblasten. Virchows Arch. Path. Anat. *338*: 342–354 (1965).

Roy, S. and Ghadially, F. N. Ultrastructure of normal rat synovial membrane. Ann. Rheum. Dis. *26*: 26–38 (1967).

Scherft, J. P. The lamina limitans of the organic matrix of calcified cartilage and bone. J. Ultrastruct. Res. *38*: 318–331 (1972).

Scott, B. L. The occurrence of specific cytoplasmic granules in the osteoclast. J. Ultrastruct. Res. *19*: 417–431 (1967).

Scott, B. L. and Glimcher, M. J. Distribution of glycogen in osteoblasts of the fetal rat. J. Ultrastruct. Res. *36*: 565–586 (1971).

Talmage, R. V. Morphological and physiological considerations in a new concept of calcium transport in bone. Am. J. Anat. *129*: 467–476 (1970).

Vaughan, J. M. The Physiology of Bone. Oxford University Press, London, 1970.

Wassermann, F. and Yaeger, J. A. Fine structure of the osteocyte capsule and the wall of the lacunae in bone. Z. Zellforsch. *67*: 636–652 (1965).

Yoffey, J. M. Structural peculiarities of the blood vessels of the bone marrow. Bibl. Anat. (Basel) 7: 298–303 (1965).

Zamboni, L. and Pease, D. C. The vascular bed of red bone marrow. J. Ultrastruct. Res. *5*: 65–85 (1961).

10 Bone development

GENERAL CONSIDERATIONS

Bone tissue develops from mesenchymal connective tissue. This development requires osteoprogenitor cells and a proper milieu for the formation of extracellular organic matrix and its subsequent mineralization. Under normal conditions, bone tissue does not develop unless blood capillaries supply the area richly with nutrients, salts, and oxygen. Therefore, the presence of blood vessels is another requirement for bone tissue to form. The osteoprogenitor cells may be present as undifferentiated mesenchymal cells, or they may be brought in by the blood vessels. In any case, these cells are induced to form the collagenous fibrils and the ground substance upon and within which the hydroxyapatite crystals are formed during the mineralization of the bone matrix.

Traditionally, one considers that bone is formed in two ways: 1) intramembranous, direct bone formation; 2) endochondral (intracartilaginous), indirect bone formation. The **intramembranous** bone formation is direct in the sense that the osteoprogenitor cells aggregate and form bone tissue locally without a preformed cartilage model. Most flat bones are formed by intramembranous bone formation. The **endochondral** bone formation is said to be indirect because it occurs within and upon a framework of a previously formed model consisting of cartilage cells and cartilage matrix. The cartilage model is gradually removed by absorption and replaced by bone. Most bones, including long bones, are formed through endochondral bone formation. The great advantage of this kind of bone formation is that these bones continue to grow as long as they retain plates of cartilage in their growth zones. However, there is no difference in the basic processes of intramembranous and endochondral bone formation since each involves appositional growth and mineralization of a matrix of collagenous fibrils

by agency of the same cell, the osteoblast. This will be discussed further.

One of the most important reasons for discussing and studying bone formation in detail is that one must be aware of the fact that there is a long and continuous process of bone formation and bone absorption throughout life. This remodeling is required since each developmental stage puts a different demand on the strength of the bone and the ability of that bone to resist bending forces as well as compression and disruption.

The first (**primary**) bone that is formed either in intramembranous or intracartilaginous bone formation is spongy bone. In this, the collagenous fibers are intertwined, giving rise to a **woven bone** in which one rarely can identify Haversian systems. Remodeling in later development changes the primary spongy bone to secondary compact bone where such bone is required. In the compact bone, the collagenous fibers are laid down in an orderly fashion and in alternate directions, giving rise to the lamellated bone with the typical Haversian systems and osteons. Where

Fig. 10-1. Intramembranous bone formation. Calvaria. Rat fetus. L.M. X 560. **1.** Fusiform mesenchymal cells of future periosteum. **2.** Mesenchymal cells, proliferating, aggregating, and becoming spherical. **3.** Osteoblasts. **4.** Osteocytes. **5.** Spicules of osteoid and bone matrix forming primitive trabeculae and primary spongy bone. **6.** Capillaries. **7.** Mesenchymal cells aggregating to form future dura mater (endosteum).

Fig. 10-2. Intramembranous bone formation. Enlargement of area similar to rectangle in Fig. 10-1. Mandible. Newborn rat. Decalcified preparation. E.M. X 1900. **1.** Nuclei of osteocytes. **2.** Osteoid. **3.** Bone matrix, partly mineralized.

Fig. 10-3. Osteocyte. Same preparation as in Fig. 10-2. E.M. X 9000. **1.** Nucleus. **2.** Golgi zone. **3.** Granular endoplasmic reticulum. **4.** Mitochondria. **5.** Lysosomes. **6.** Coated vesicles. **7.** Cell processes. **8.** Pericellular space with non-mineralized osteoid. **9.** Fully mineralized bone matrix.

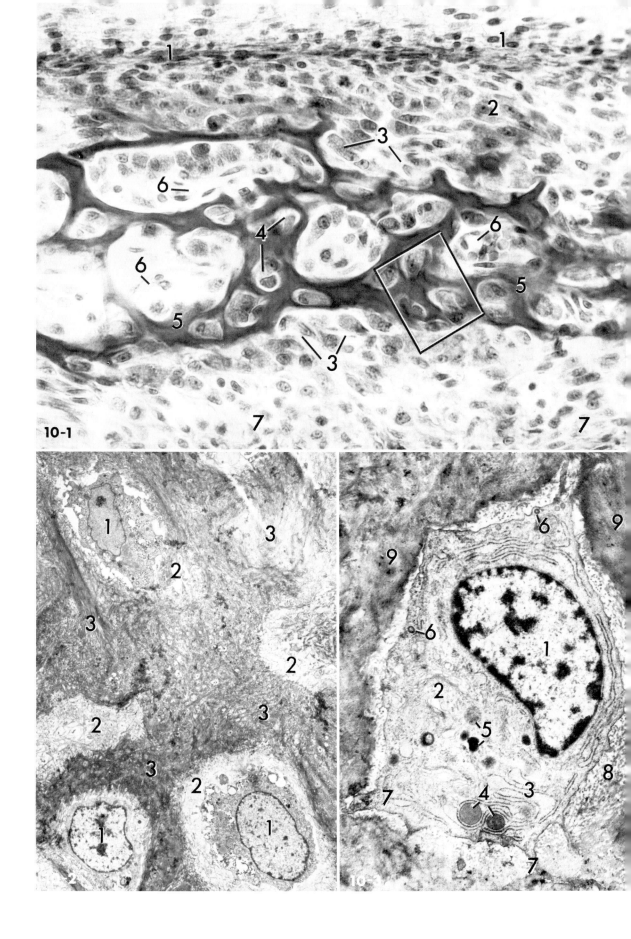

spongy bone is ultimately required, the primary spongy bone is replaced by secondary spongy bone.

INTRAMEMBRANOUS BONE FORMATION

The vault of the cranium and the flat bones of the face are formed by an intramembranous bone formation. (Fig. 10-1) This includes the nasal bones, frontal bone, interparietal bones, squama and tympanic part of temporal bone, medial pterygoid plate of the sphenoid bone, nasal bones, vomer, maxilla, and part of the mandible. In addition, the shaft of long bones and parts of several other bones are formed by an intramembranous process which originates from the periosteum. However, the ultimate remodeling of the diaphysis during growth and development occurs by a combination of intramembranous (subperiosteal) and endochondral ossification, which is further discussed on p. 216.

Flat bones of fetus. The first indication of an intramembranous bone formation in the flat bones of the face is a spotty proliferation of mesenchymal connective tissue cells. (Fig. 10-1) The cells become round, enlarge, and form small groups over large areas, which together associate in the form of an irregular connective tissue membrane. The cells are now recognized as **osteoblasts** with an abundance of granular endoplasmic reticulum, a large Golgi zone, and numerous coated vesicles. (Fig. 10-3) These osteoblasts synthesize and surround themselves with irregular bundles of collagenous fibrils. Increasing numbers of capillaries appear around and within the groups of osteoblasts. At some point in time, the large irregular bundles of collagenous fibrils are difficult to resolve by light microscopy since they become obscured by a hyaline, eosinophilic ground substance. These areas are said to contain **osteoid**, defined as collagenous fibers masked by a hyaline ground substance just before mineralization (calcification) sets in. Ultrastructurally, osteoid consists of coarse collagenous fibrils mixed

in with a few loci of initial calcification with hydroxyapatite crystals. (Fig. 10-5) The collagenous fibrils of the osteoid tend to fuse laterally with each other in a process that is poorly understood, but which may form the basis for the hyaline substance observed by light microscopy. Gradually, the osteoid becomes fully mineralized, and small irregularly shaped islands of bone, called **spicules** appear, surrounded by a single layer of osteoblasts. Adjoining spicules merge to form trabeculae of the primary spongy bone. Soon osteoblasts become surrounded and trapped by calcified matrix and turn into **osteocytes.** Osteocytes maintain contact with each other and with the vascularized mesenchymal tissue by means of their long cytoplasmic processes which also become surrounded by mineralized bone matrix and are lodged in the tunnel-shaped canaliculi.

The center part of the membranous flat bone takes shape by the appearance of an increasing number of trabeculae which arise in the manner described for the initial spicules. The spicules and the trabeculae unite into a bony sponge-like structure, the meshes of which contain a rich vascular mesenchyme and primary bone marrow. The peripheral limits of the definite bone are formed by fusiform mesenchymal cells which aggregate in a

Fig. 10-4. Cross section at the level of the diaphysis of the radius. Two-day-old rat. E.M. X 660. **1.** Periosteum. **2.** Primary spongy bone. **3.** Single layer of osteoblasts forming endosteum. **4.** Osteocytes. **5.** Venule, part of periosteal sprout. **6.** Capillaries. **7.** Primary bone marrow cells.

Fig. 10-5. Periosteum. Diaphysis of radius. Enlargement of area similar to rectangle in Fig. 10-4. Two-day-old rat. E.M. X 5600. **1.** Nuclei of fibroblasts. **2.** Collagenous fibers. **3.** Nuclei of osteoprogenitor cells. **4.** Nuclei of osteoblasts. **5.** Osteoid. **6.** Mineralized bone matrix (some minerals partly removed during preparation process). **7.** Osteoblast in the process of being completely surrounded by mineralized bone matrix. **8.** Osteocyte in bone lacuna.

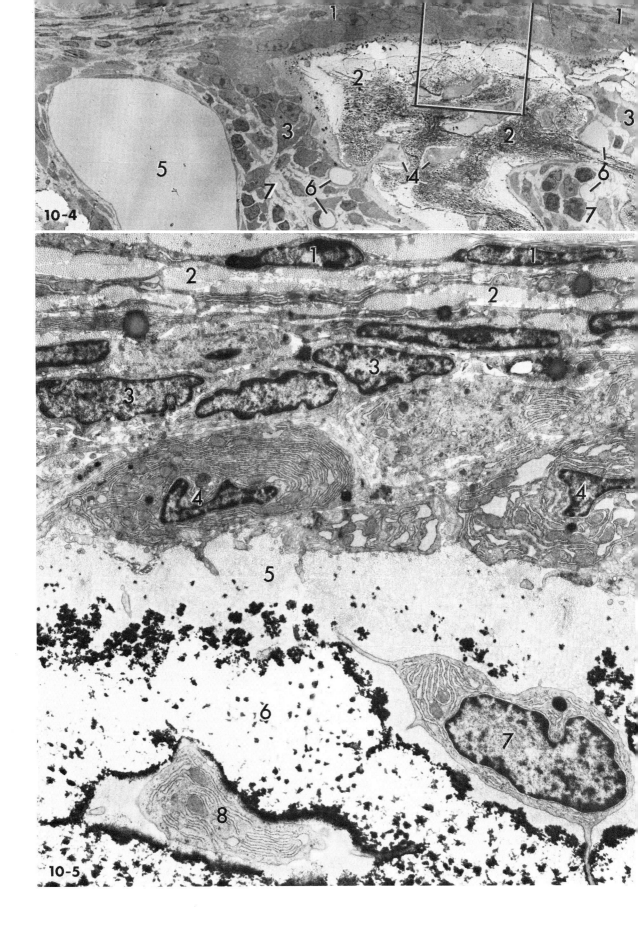

primitive periosteum. The more external plates of the flat membranous bones are formed by the osteoblastic inner layer of this primitive periosteum. The initial spongy bone is later replaced by compact bone by filling the spaces of the spongy bone with concentric lamellar bone, creating an inner and an outer plate or table. Between the plates, the spongy bone remains as a largely unchanged, narrow zone, the diploë.

Periosteum of long bones. The perichondrium (future periosteum) which surrounds the shaft of the cartilage model of long bones in the fetus is also the site of an intramembranous bone formation. In contrast to the somewhat disorderly bone formation in the flat bones of the skull which starts in many areas, the perichondrial (periosteal) intramembranous bone formation is orderly and highly polarized. The perichondrium consists of several peripheral layers of flattened fibroblasts, one or two middle layers of osteoprogenitor cells, and an inner single layer of osteoblasts. (Figs. 10-4, 10-5, 10-6) At some point in time of the development of the cartilage model, the osteoblasts of the perichondrium start to lay down a thin cylindrical sleeve of osteoid on the outer surface of the cartilage model. Subsequently, the osteoid is transformed to bone by a mineralization process, and osteoblasts become trapped in the bone matrix as the cylindrical sleeve increases in thickness. The perichondrium is now more properly referred to as periosteum. The layering of the periosteum and the precise apportionment of synthetic work among cells in the various layers make the periosteum an ideal place to study bone formation. The peripheral layers of **fibroblasts** manufacture the many bundles of collagenous and elastic fibrils present in these layers. The collagenous fibrils are relatively coarse. (Fig. 10-7) Cells and fibrils together establish a strong membrane which protects and holds together the cartilage model and the newly formed bone collar. The middle layers consist of

osteoprogenitor cells and a fine capillary network. The osteoprogenitor cells have a more rounded shape than the fibroblasts. These cells are considered to be stem cells. By frequent mitoses they give rise to osteoblasts as well as other osteoprogenitor stem cells. They have a scant cytoplasm with numerous free ribosomes and a limited amount of granular endoplasmic reticulum. They frequently hold large accumulations of particulate glycogen and contain many coated vesicles. In the narrow space between osteoprogenitor cells appear bundles of delicate collagenous fibrils. Their average width is about 200 Å (Fig. 10-8), which puts them in the category of reticular fibrils (p. 148). The homogeneous ground substance is prominent around these delicate fibrils. The ap-

Fig. 10-6. Periosteum. Diaphysis of radius. Two-day-old rat. E.M. X 12,000. **1.** Nuclei of fibroblasts in superficial layers of periosteum. **2.** Bundles of collagenous fibrils. **3.** Cytoplasmic strands of fibroblasts. **4.** Nuclei of osteoprogenitor cells in middle part of periosteum. **5.** Cytoplasm of osteoblasts. **6.** Osteoid. **7.** Fully calcified bone matrix (some mineral salts removed during preparation of specimen).

Fig. 10-7. Detail of fibroblast layer of periosteum. Enlargement of area similar to rectangle (A) in Fig. 10-6. Same preparation. E.M. X 50,000. **1.** Cytoplasm of fibroblast. **2.** Cross-sectioned collagenous fibrils; average width 400 Å. **3.** Elastic fibrils.

Fig. 10-8. Details of osteoprogenitor layers of periosteum. Enlargement of area similar to rectangle (B) in Fig. 10-6. Same preparation. E.M. X 48,000. **1.** Granular endoplasmic reticulum of osteoprogenitor cells. **2.** Mitochondrion. **3.** Accumulation of particulate glycogen. **4.** Cross-sectioned delicate collagenous (reticular) fibrils; average width 200 Å. **5.** Cross-sectioned cell processes.

Fig. 10-9. Detail of osteoid. Enlargement of area similar to rectangle (C) in Fig. 10-6. Same preparation. E.M. X 48,000. **1.** Cross-sectioned cell processes. **2.** Collagenous fibrils near surface of osteoblast are delicate, newly formed. **3.** Collagenous fibrils further away from osteoblast cell surface increase in size. **4.** Collagenous fibrils still further away are coarse and tend to fuse laterally. **5.** Loci of initial calcification.

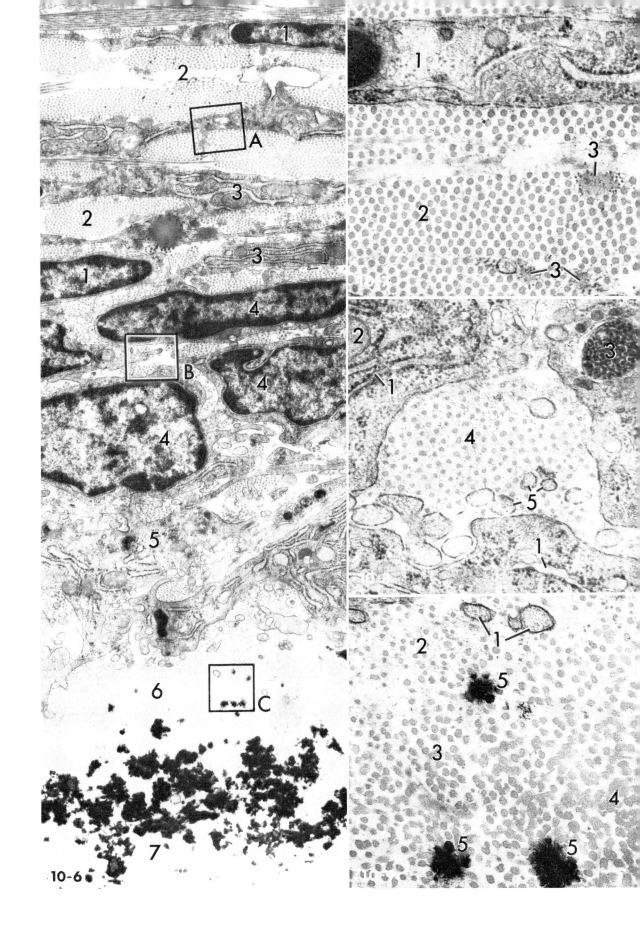

10-6

pearance of the fibrils and the ground substance is the first sign of an osteoid being synthesized by the osteoprogenitor cells. The innermost layer of cells of the periosteum consists of osteoblasts. They have a large Golgi zone and a vast amount of granular endoplasmic reticulum. They are engaged in a heavy synthesis of collagenous fibrils. The fibrils increase in cross-sectional diameter as they become further removed from the osteoblasts. (Fig. 10-9) Gradually, each osteoblast develops long slender cytoplasmic processes, surrounds itself with collagenous fibrils on all sides, and finally turns into an **osteocyte** at the moment when it is completely enclosed in fully mineralized bone matrix.

ENDOCHONDRAL BONE FORMATION

Most bones are formed by an endochondral (intracartilaginous) ossification. Miniature hyaline cartilaginous models of the bones (Fig. 10-10) are formed from mesenchymal cells in the manner described on p. 174. These cartilage models continue to grow by both interstitial and appositional growth. In a long bone, such as the humerus, the first sign of an imminent endochondral bone formation appears in the center of the diaphysis at the beginning of the eighth week in the human embryo, giving rise to a primary center of ossification. Other bones start their ossification at other time points of the gestation, and one cartilage model may have more than one primary ossification center.

Formation of primary ossification centers. First, the chondrocytes in the center of the diaphysis become large and vacuolated, and they arrange themselves in long rows parallel to the long axis of the cartilage model. Subsequently, the lacunar spaces hypertrophy and the cartilage matrix becomes calcified and impregnated with an amorphous form of calcium salts. The calcification of the cartilage matrix is a deposition of lime salts in a haphazard manner with no orderly arrangement in relation to the fine collagenous

fibrils of the hyaline cartilage matrix. These fibrils, it is recalled, do not have the typical axial periodicity of regular native collagenous fibrils (p. 176). The calcification inhibits or hampers the transport of nutrients across the cartilage matrix, and most of the chondrocytes degenerate and die. Simultaneously, a subperiosteal sleeve of intramembranous bone (Fig. 10-11) has formed around the diaphysis as described on p. 210. Originating from the periosteum, sprouts of tissue erode the sleeve of periosteal bone

Fig. 10-10. Cartilage model. Longitudinal section. Os coxae. Mouse embryo. L.M. X 55. **1.** Hyaline cartilage of epiphysis. **2.** Diaphysis. **3.** Perichondrium: enlarging chondrocytes signify onset of endochondral ossification.

Fig. 10-11. Cartilage model. Longitudinal section. Humerus. Mouse embryo. L.M. X 43. **1.** Epiphysis. **2.** Enlarging chondrocytes in center of diaphysis. **3.** Subperichondrial (periosteal) sleeve of bone starting to form by intramembranous ossification.

Fig. 10-12. Endochondral ossification. Longitudinal section. Metatarsal bone. newborn rat. L.M. X 36. **1.** Epiphysis. **2.** Primitive bone marrow of primary ossification center. **3.** Enlarging subperiosteal bone sleeve. **4.** Endochondral ossification progresses in opposite directions (arrows) towards the epiphyses.

Fig. 10-13. Progressing endochondral ossification. Longitudinal section. Femur. Newborn mouse. L.M. X 20. **1.** Epiphysis with future head and major trochanter of femur clearly outlined. **2.** Primary ossification of entire diaphysis. **3.** Epiphysis with future condyles of femur.

Fig. 10-14. Early stages of endochondral ossification. Sphenoid bone. Rat fetus. L.M. X 168. **1.** Periosteum. **2.** Subperiosteal bone collar. **3.** Bone eroded by periosteal sprouts. **4.** Hypertrophied chondrocytes. **5.** Periosteal sprouts invading cartilage lacunae.

Fig. 10-15. Endochondral ossification. Enlargement of rectangle in Fig. 10-14. L.M. X 290. **1.** Periosteum. **2.** Subperiosteal bone collar. **3.** Periosteal sprout growing into cartilage. **4.** Hypertrophied cartilage lacunae. **5.** Capillaries and osteoprogenitor cells in enlarged cartilage lacunae. **6.** Calcified cartilage matrix.

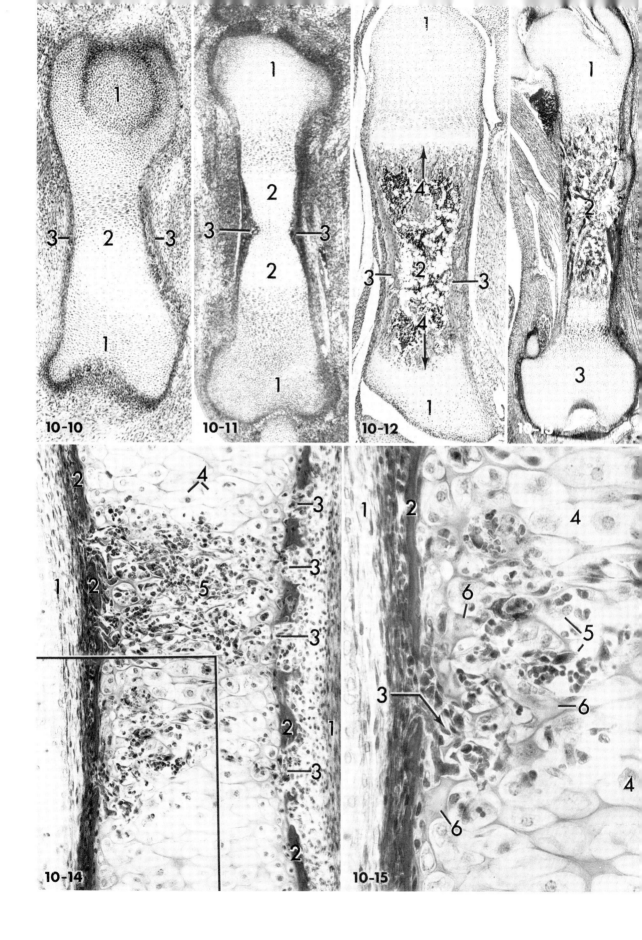

and grow into the enlarged cartilaginous lacunae. The sprouts consist of blood capillaries, osteoprogenitor cells, and osteoblasts derived from the periosteum. (Figs. 10-14, 10-15) The periosteal sprouts further erode the remnants of the calcified cartilage matrix and remove some of the matrix by absorption. The osteoprogenitor cells now proliferate and form numerous osteoblasts which start to lay down osteoid and subsequently mineralized **primary bone,** using the remnants of the calcified cartilage matrix as a temporary scaffolding. At the ultrastructural level this process of bone formation is similar to that described for intramembranous ossification (p. 208).

Through this process arises a system of interconnected bone spicules and trabeculae with a central core of calcified cartilage matrix. Most hypertrophied chondrocytes degenerate, die, and become absorbed as the vascular sprouts enter the lacunae of the cartilage. However, there is some evidence that a certain number of liberated chondrocytes may survive and change into osteogenic cells or cells engaged specifically in resorption (osteoclasts, chondroclasts). The primary bone formed on the surface of the calcified cartilaginous spicules is gradually broken down by osteoclasts and absorbed. By this process, the trabeculae and partitions of the primary spongy bone are removed and a primitive bone marrow cavity formed. (Fig. 10-12) The osteogenic buds from the periosteum also bring in or induce the formation of hemopoietic stem cells, resulting in the establishment of a primary bone marrow and a vascularization of the primitive bone marrow cavity.

Extension of primary ossification centers. The calcification of cartilage matrix and the ossification which originated in the center of the diaphysis now extends in two directions toward the epiphyses (ends of cartilage model). This expanding process takes place by a regular sequence of changes in the cartilage, and is present not only in the fetal long bones, but also in the growth zones (epiphyseal plates) of the child and adolescent. (Fig. 10-16) The **epiphyseal plate** can be divided into zones, each of which exhibits a different and special activity. (Fig. 10-17)

The **zone of resting cartilage** (reserve cartilage) is the most distal, consisting of small chondrocytes which are distributed at random. Next, toward the diaphysis, is the **zone of chondrocyte multiplication.** The chondrocytes here are engaged in a heavy mitotic activity, dividing transversely and becoming arranged in rows parallel to the long axis of the cartilage model. There is also an intense deposition of additional cartilage matrix between the newly formed chondrocytes. This activity results in a lengthening of the bone, justifying the term "growth zone" for this part of the bone. Further toward the diaphysis is the **zone of chondrocyte hypertrophy** and lacunar enlargement. The enlargement of the chondrocytes entails accumulation of particulate glycogen and lipid droplets in the cytoplasm. The nuclei enlarge and gradually become either vacuo-

Fig. 10-16. Endochondral ossification extending toward epiphysis. Longitudinal section. Metatarsal bone. Newborn rat. L.M. X 116.
1. Epiphyseal cartilage. **2.** Periosteum.
3. Subperiosteal bone collar of diaphysis.
4. Primary bone marrow.

Fig. 10-17. Endochondral ossification. Enlargement of area similar to rectangle in Fig. 10-16. Femur. Rabbit. L.M. X 127.
1. Zone of chondrocyte multiplication with parallel rows of cells. **2.** Zone of chondrocyte hypertrophy. **3.** Zone of cartilage matrix calcification. **4.** Capillaries invade lacunar spaces. **5.** Spicules and trabeculae of calcified cartilage covered with bone. **6.** Primary bone marrow.

Fig. 10-18. Endochondral ossification. Enlargement of area similar to rectangle in Fig. 10-17. Epiphyseal growth plate. Humerus. Two-day-old rat. E.M. X 1800.
1. Chondrocytes proliferating. **2.** Matrix of hyaline cartilage. **3.** Hypertrophying chondrocytes. **4.** Degenerating and dying chondrocytes. **5.** Nodules of calcified cartilage matrix. **6.** Erythrocytes in lumina of capillaries invading cartilage lacunae.

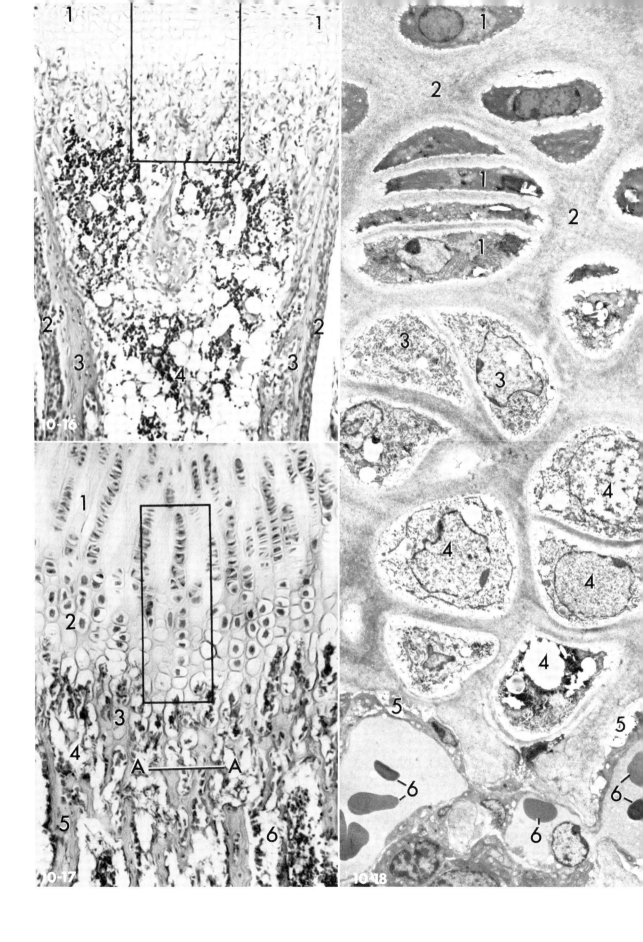

lated or pyknotic, indicating degeneration and approaching cell death. Next, is the **zone of cartilage calcification.** The thin lamellae of cartilage matrix become impregnated with small spherical calcification nodules in a relatively narrow zone. The transverse walls of the lacunae become dissolved, leaving longitudinal walls of ragged spicules of calcified cartilage matrix. The calcified zone is now gradually transformed into a **zone of cartilage removal and bone deposition.** Capillary sprouts from the approaching primary bone marrow grow into the lacunae (Fig. 10-18) and supply osteoprogenitor cells and osteoblasts to the area; they in turn start to lay down osteoid and bone on the surface of the calcified cartilage spicules and trabeculae. The increased vascularization of this zone facilitates also the resorption of calcified cartilage matrix (Fig. 10-19), and the subsequent resorption of the bony spicules and trabeculae of the primary spongy bone, creating more space for the steadily increasing volume of the bone marrow.

Formation of secondary ossification centers. At the time of birth, and several years after birth, centers of secondary ossification are formed in the epiphyses of the long bones. (Fig. 10-20) The process is similar to that which occurs initially when the primary ossification center is formed in the diaphysis. The chondrocytes in the center of the epiphysis hypertrophy, the lacunae enlarge, and a slight calcification of the cartilage matrix occurs. From the perichondrium of the epiphysis, a bud of osteogenic tissue and blood capillaries enters the enlarged lacunae (Fig. 10-22), and the invading osteoblasts lay down osteoid and bone, giving rise to the typical spongy bone of the epiphysis. The ossification extends radially within the epiphysis, and a small bone marrow cavity is formed. Between the epiphysis and the diaphysis remains a layer of cartilage, the **epiphyseal plate.** This plate allows further growth in length until the 18th to 20th years.

REMODELING AND GROWTH

As indicated in the general considerations of bone formation on p. 206, bone remodeling and growth occurs throughout life. To facilitate the understanding of the many processes involved, one can simplify the matter by dividing the processes into several principal events: 1) early bone resorption; 2) growth in length and width; 3) conversion of spongy bone to compact bone; 4) remodeling of compact bone.

Early bone resorption. From the very first bone spicule formed by osteoblasts, a resorption of bone matrix occurs through the action of osteoclasts and the presence of blood capillaries. As indicated, the main reason for this resorption is to remove unnecessary trabeculae and to create space for bone marrow. This process continues until the growth process of the bone is completed.

Growth in length and width. Bones grow in length through a continuous multiplication of chondrocytes within the epiphyseal plates of long bones. The closure of the epiphyseal plate terminates

Fig. 10-19. Endochondral ossification. Zone of cartilage calcification and early bone deposition. This survey demonstrates the invading capillary sprouts as they bring in osteoprogenitor cells and osteoblasts to the cartilage lacunae. Cross section of bone at the level indicated by the line A—A in Fig. 10-17. Specimen fixed by vascular perfusion with subsequent decalcification. Upper epiphysis of humerus. Two-day-old rat. E.M. X 1800. **1.** Lumina of invading capillaries. **2.** Ragged spicules of calcified cartilage matrix. The decalcification process of specimen preparation has removed the calcium crystals, causing the white unstained background. **3.** Thin layer of osteoid deposited on the surface of the calcified cartilage matrix. **4.** Nuclei of osteoblasts. **5.** Nuclei of osteoprogenitor cells. **6.** Osteoprogenitor cell in mitosis. **7.** Nuclei of endothelial cells. **8.** Erythrocytes. **9.** Lymphocyte. *Note:* Identification of cells and other structures in this survey is based on analysis of this field at higher magnification.

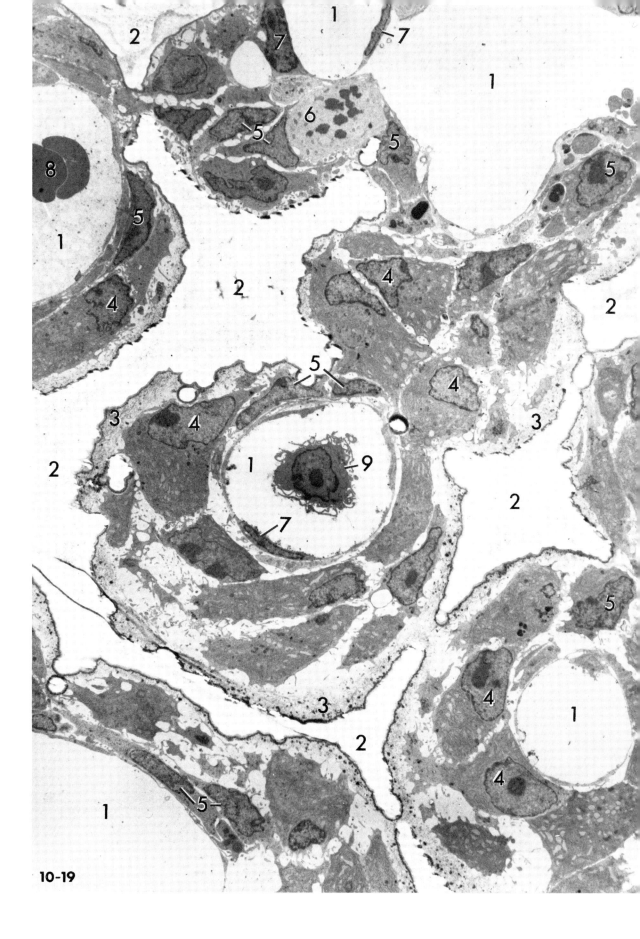

the lengthening process. Bones grow in width by appositional deposition of subperiosteal bone in a process of intramembranous ossification described on p. 208. Simultaneously, bone is resorbed from the endosteal side in order to maintain the appropriate thickness of the tubular shaft of the bone and to enlarge the marrow cavity.

Conversion of spongy bone to compact bone. All primary bone is spongy. The spongy bone of the diaphysis and the cortical regions of epiphyses is gradually converted into compact bone in order to make these parts of the bone stronger. This is accomplished by a deposition of collagenous lamellae and mineralized bone matrix progressively inward on the surface of the cavities of the spongy bone until these cavities are reduced to narrow canals with a central blood vessel. Since this kind of bone is similar to the adult compact bone, the narrow canals with surrounding bone are referred to as **primitive Haversian systems.**

Starting at the age of one year in man, this bone is in turn replaced by the final type of bone present in the adult compact bone. Vascular sprouts grow into the compact bone from either the periosteum or the marrow cavity. By intense osteoclastic activity, these sprouts make tunnels and cavities in the bone. Once an **erosion tunnel** has reached a certain diameter, osteoprogenitor cells of the vascular sprouts differentiate into osteoblasts and start to line the walls of the erosion tunnel, laying down concentric layers of osteoid and bone. Gradually, osteoblasts become enclosed by bone matrix, turning into osteocytes. The end result is an osteon with a central Haversian canal containing the original blood vessels of the eroding vascular sprout, surrounded by layers of mineralized collagenous fibers and osteocytes contained in their lacunae. Through these processes the primary spongy bone is converted to the compact cortical type of adult bone.

Remodeling of compact bone. Stress and strain on cortical compact bone throughout life make it necessary to remodel repeatedly existing osteons and Haversian systems. This occurs through a process similar to the one just described. Vascular sprouts erode the compact bone and destroy, partly or entirely, old Haversian systems. Subsequently, new osteons are laid down as indicated above. The interstitial lamellae present in compact bone are an indication of older, eroded Haversian systems. The external and internal circumferential lamellae of cortical compact bone are laid down from the periosteum and endosteum, respectively, in a final process of establishing the bony architecture of the diaphysis.

Fig. 10-20. Longitudinal section of tibia. Newborn rat. L.M. X 41. **1.** Rectangle: epiphyseal ingrowth of perichondrial sprout, indicating beginning of a secondary ossification center. **2.** Zone of chondrocyte multiplication. **3.** Zone of chondrocyte hypertrophy. **4.** Primary ossification center extending toward the epiphysis. **5.** Bone marrow of diaphysis.

Fig. 10-21. Perichondrial sprout. Enlargement of rectangle in Fig. 10-20. L.M. X 218. **1.** Ordinary chondrocytes. **2.** Capillaries. **3.** Osteoprogenitor cells. **4.** Slightly calcified cartilage matrix. **5.** Hypertrophied cartilage lacunae with degenerating chondrocytes.

Fig. 10-22. Longitudinal section of phalanx. Monkey. Four months old. L.M. X 17. **1.** Articular capsule. **2.** Joint cavity. **3.** Articular and epiphyseal cartilage. **4.** Secondary ossification center with spongy bone. **5.** Epiphyseal growth plate. **6.** Primary ossification center extending toward the epiphysis. **7.** Bone marrow cavity of diaphysis. **8.** Compact cortical bone. **9.** Nutrient blood vessels.

Fig. 10-23. Epiphyseal growth plate. Enlargement of rectangle in Fig. 10-22. L.M. X 120. **1.** Marrow cavity. **2.** Bone and calcified cartilage matrix. **3.** Zone of resting cartilage cells. **4.** Vascular sprout establishing connection between primary and secondary ossification centers. **5.** Zone of chondrocyte proliferation. **6.** Zone of chondrocyte hypertrophy. **7.** Trabeculae of endochondral bone with center of calcified cartilage matrix.

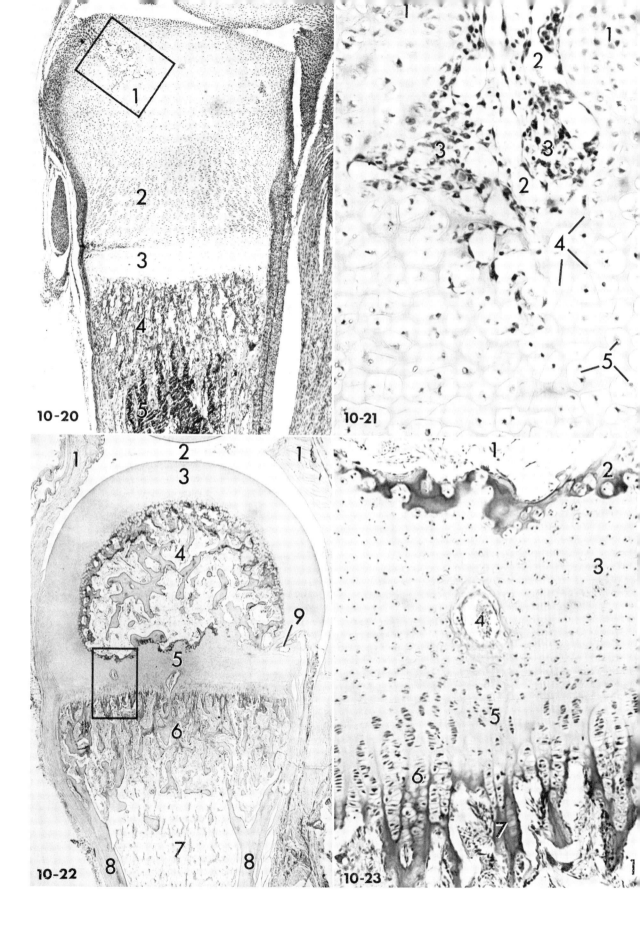

10-20

10-21

10-22

10-23

References

Amprino, R. On the growth of cortical bone and the mechanism of osteon formation. Acta. Anat. *52*: 177–187 (1963).

Anderson, C. E. and Parker, J. Invasion and resorption in endochondrial ossification. An electron microscopic study. J. Bone and Joint Surg. *48-A*: 899–914 (1966).

Ascenzi, A. and Bendetti, E. L. An electron microscopic study of the foetal membranous ossification. Acta Anat. *37*: 370–385 (1959).

Ascenzi, A., Bonucci, E. and Bocciarelli, D. S. An electron microscope study on the primary periosteal bone. J. Ultrastruct. Res. *18*: 605–618 (1967).

Bernard, G. W. and Pease, D. C. An electron microscopic study of initial intramembranous osteogenesis. Am. J. Anat. *125*: 271–290 (1969).

Bonucci, E. Further investigations on the organic/inorganic relationships in calcifying cartilage. Calc. Tiss. Res. *3*: 38–64 (1968).

Decker, J. D. An electron microscopic investigation of osteogenesis in the embryonic chick. Am. J. Anat. *118*: 591–641 (1966).

Engfeldt, B. Studies on the epiphysial growth zone. III. Electronmicroscopic studies on the normal epiphysial growth zone. Acta Path. Microbiol. Scand. *75*: 201–219 (1969).

Fitton-Jackson, S. The fine structure of the developing bone in the embryonic fowl. Proc. Roy. Soc. Lond. *146B*: 270–280 (1957).

Gonzales, F. and Karnovsky, M. J. Electron microscopy of osteoclasts in healing fractures of rat bone. J. Biophys. Biochem. Cytol. *9*: 299–316 (1961).

Knese, K. H. and Knoop, A. M. Elektronenoptische Untersuchungen über die periostale Osteogenese. Z. Zellforsch. *48*: 455–478 (1958).

Knese, K.-H. Osteoklasten, Chondroklasten, Mineraloklasten, Kollagenoklasten. Acta Anat. *83*: 275–288 (1972).

Owen, M. Uptake of (^{3}H) uridine into precursor pools and RNA in osteogenic cells. J. Cell Sci. *2*: 39–56 (1967).

Owen, M. The origin of bone cells. Int. Rev. Cytol. *28*: 213–238 (1970).

Schenk, R. K., Spiro, D. and Wiener, J. Cartilage resorption in the tibial epiphyseal plate of growing rats. J. Cell Biol. *34*: 275–291 (1967).

Schenk, R. K., Wiener, J. and Spiro, D. Fine structural aspects of vascular invasion of the tibial epiphyseal plate of growing rats. Acta Anat. *69*: 1–17 (1968).

Scott, B. L. Thymidine-^{3}H electron microscope radioautography of osteogenic cells in the fetal rat. J. Cell Biol. *35*: 115–126 (1967).

Scott, B. L. and Pease, D. C. Electron microscopy of the epiphyseal apparatus. Anat. Rec. *126*: 465–495 (1956).

Smith, J. W. The disposition of proteinpolysaccharide in the epiphysial plate cartilage of the young rabbit. J. Cell Sci. *6*: 843–864 (1970).

Thyberg, J. and Friberg, U. Ultrastructure and acid phosphatase activity of matrix vesicles and cytoplasmic dense bodies in the epiphyseal plate. J. Ultrastruct. Res. *33*: 554–573 (1970).

Young, R. W. Cell proliferation and specialization during endochondral osteogenesis in young rats. J. Cell Biol. *14*: 357–370 (1962).

Urist, M. R. Origins of current ideas about calcification. Clin. Orthop. Rel. Res. *44*: 13–39 (1966).

11 Muscular tissue

GENERAL CONSIDERATIONS

Muscular tissue is the primary tissue of motion. Together with the bones of the skeleton, it moves and limits the movements of the many parts of the body as well as the entire individual. The muscle tissue consists of: 1) **muscle cells,** often referred to as muscle fibers; 2) **connective tissue elements** such as fibroblasts and collagenous fibers which hold the muscle cells together to form a muscle as recognized by the unaided eye; 3) a rich network of **capillaries** to secure the great demand for nutrients and rapid exchange of oxygen and carbon dioxide between the muscle and the vascular system; and 4) **nerves** and nerve endings. (Fig. 11-4) Adult muscular tissue can be divided into two classes based on their structure: a) striated muscle; b) nonstriated smooth muscle. On a functional basis, three classes can be identified: A) skeletal, voluntary muscle; B) cardiac involuntary muscle; and C) smooth involuntary muscle. **Skeletal,** somatic muscle is striated and concentrated to the skeleton. **Cardiac** muscle is also striated and is located mainly in the heart. **Smooth** muscle is generally limited to the viscera.

Muscle cells are usually elongated and spindle-shaped. (Fig. 11-3) They function by shortening their length, approximating the two opposite points which are attached to connective tissue structures such as septa, trabeculae, fasciae, tendons, periosteum, or bone. The skeletal muscles as a rule act across joints, moving one bone in relation to another bone. The cardiac muscle cells, by their arrangement in the wall of the heart, upon shortening reduce the size of the heart chambers. The smooth muscle cells of the gut upon shortening narrow the lumen of the intestine in a wave-like movement, propelling the content of the lumen forward.

The shortening of the muscle cell is called **contraction.** The contractile property of muscle cells is determined by the presence of the filamentous contractile proteins, **actin** and **myosin.** In the striated muscles, actin and myosin filaments are arranged in an orderly, registered manner, giving rise to the typical cross-banding or transverse striations. In the smooth muscle, a less orderly arrangement of actin and myosin filaments is recorded. The striated muscle cells have a rapid contraction and become easily fatigued, whereas the smooth muscle cells have a relatively slow contraction and are capable of a sustained contraction. The **voluntary** muscles (skeletal) are innervated by the cerebrospinal system of nerves and are under the control of the highest functional levels of the cerebral cortex. The **involuntary** muscles (cardiac, smooth) are innervated by the autonomic nervous system and are not under the direct control of the cerebral cortex.

Skeletal Muscle

The shape and size of skeletal muscles are greatly variable, and textbooks of Gross Anatomy should be consulted for a

Fig. 11-1. Skeletal muscle. Longitudinal section. Human. L.M. X 290. **1.** Arrow: longitudinal axis of a skeletal muscle fiber (cell). **2.** Width of muscle fiber between bars: 25 μ. **3.** Muscle cell nuclei. **4.** Intercellular space. **5.** Transverse striations.

Fig. 11-2. Skeletal muscle. Cross section. Tongue. Monkey. L.M. X 460. **1.** Width of muscle fiber between bars: 20 μ. **2.** Muscle cell nuclei. **3.** Capillaries. **4.** Intercellular space with endomysium. **5.** Perimysium around muscle fascicle.

Fig. 11-3. Skeletal muscle. Longitudinal section. Rat. E.M. X 600. **1.** Arrow: longitudinal axis of muscle fiber. **2.** Width of muscle fiber: 38 μ. **3.** Muscle cell nuclei. **4.** Intercellular space and endomysium. **5.** Capillaries. **6.** Transverse striations.

Fig. 11-4. Skeletal muscle, fixed by intravascular perfusion. Cross section of nerve-vascular bundle and muscle cells. Rat. E.M. X 600. **1.** Myelinated nerves. **2.** Small artery; width of lumen 55 μ; wall thickness 2 μ. **3.** Small veins. **4.** Periaxial space of neuromuscular spindle with intrafusal muscle fibers. **5.** Small lymphatic vessel. **6.** Arteriole. **7.** Venule. **8.** Blood capillaries. **9.** Muscle fibers. **10.** Width of muscle fiber 37 μ. **11.** Loose connective tissue.

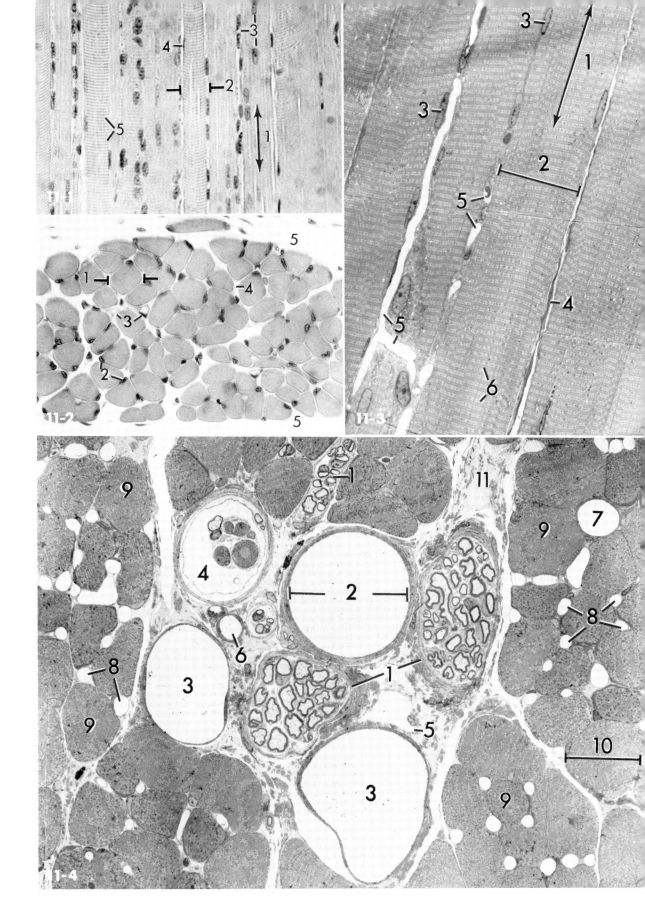

review of this topic. Each individual skeletal muscle is invested by a layer of dense connective tissue, the **epimysium.** The muscle is composed of **fasciculi,** which are bundles of skeletal muscle cells, each fascicle being surrounded by its own connective tissue sheet, the **perimysium.** (Fig. 11-2) The fascicle is composed of many muscle fibers (the word "fiber" is synonymous with cell). Each muscle fiber is invested by a delicate connective tissue sheet, the **endomysium.** (Fig. 11-6) This arrangement of compartmentalized connective tissue investment greatly facilitates the process of muscle contraction, since groups of muscle fibers or fasciculi can contract independently of neighboring fibers and fasciculi. As a general principle, there is more connective tissue present in muscles capable of finely graded movements as compared with muscles that do not have this capability.

MUSCLE FIBERS

General organization. The skeletal muscle fibers are long and cylindrical, multinuclear cells with transverse striations and tapering ends. Their dimensions vary from 1 to 40 mm in length and 10 to 100 μ in width. (Fig. 11-1) Most skeletal muscles are longer than their component muscle fibers, with the tapered ends of the fibers attached to connective tissue septa within the muscle. In cross section, the muscle cells are rounded or polygonal. (Fig. 11-2) Each fiber is bordered by a cell membrane, **sarcolemma,** and contains over a hundred oval and flattened **nuclei** scattered throughout the cell in peripheral positions just under the sarcolemma. The cytoplasm of the muscle cell, the **sarcoplasm,** is largely made up of longitudinally arranged columns of **myofibrils.** The extrafibrillar sarcoplasm consists of mitochondria, lipid droplets, glycogen, and an extensive system of agranular endoplasmic reticulum. (Fig. 11-9)

Sarcolemma. Originally, the term "sarcolemma" referred to a tough elastic membrane surrounding muscle cells. Electron microscopy revealed this membrane to be a compound structure consisting of the cell membrane, an external (basal) lamina, and a thin network of reticular and delicate collagenous fibrils. Presently, the external lamina and the reticular fibrils are collectively called endomysium, and the term "sarcolemma" is reserved for the cell membrane of the muscle cell.

The sarcolemma is a 90 Å trilaminar membrane which tightly encloses the sarcoplasm. (Fig. 11-8) Some micropinocytotic invaginations occur. In addition, the sarcolemma extends to the interior of the muscle fibers in the shape of narrow tubular invaginations, **transverse tubules.** The lumen of each tubule is continuous with the extracellular space. In the mammalian skeletal muscle cells, the transverse tubules surround the myofibrils at the levels of the junctions between the light and the dark transverse striations (A-I junctions), establishing the so-called **T-system** which participates in spreading the excitation impulse of muscle contraction (p. 232), acting as a conduction pathway from the outer sarcolemma to the interior of the cell. (Fig. 11-10)

Myofibrils. The fibrils are densely packed, lengthwise oriented, and arranged in parallel. (Fig. 11-5) In the light microscope they appear as 1–2 μ-wide cylindrical columns, and in cross section their cut ends look like small dots. Electron microscopy of well-preserved specimens has demonstrated that adjacent myofibrils

Fig. 11-5. Skeletal muscle. Longitudinal section. Rat. E.M. X 2100. **1.** Lumina of capillaries. **2.** Nuclei of muscle cells. **3.** Nucleus of endothelial cell. **4.** Intercellular space and endomysium. **5.** A-bands of transverse striations. **6.** I-bands with bisecting Z-line. **7.** Arrow: longitudinal axis of muscle cell.

Fig. 11-6. Skeletal muscle. Cross section. Rat. E.M. X 2100. **1.** Lumina of blood capillaries. **2.** Nuclei of muscle cells. **3.** Myofibrils. **4.** Extrafibrillar sarcoplasm. **5.** Mitochondria. **6.** Intercellular space with endomysium. **7.** Nucleus of fibroblast. **8.** Cytoplasm of fibroblast. **9.** Small myelinated nerve.

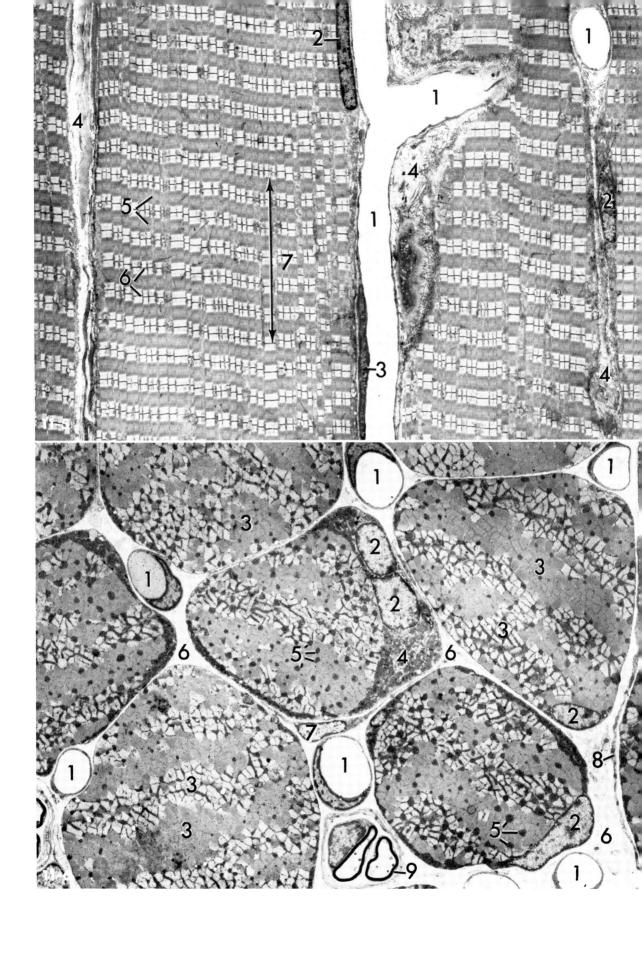

often are continuous, forming irregularly shaped columns. Fixation and preparation procedures for ordinary light microscopy separate artificially these irregularly shaped columns, in cross section making them appear as large, distinct areas, referred to earlier as **fields of Cohnheim**. These fields are absent in well-preserved specimens. (Fig. 11-7) The number of myofibrils varies greatly and can be used to subdivide muscle cells into white and red fibers. In man, red and white fibers are always intermingled in any single muscle, but in other species the fibers may be separated. **White fibers** are large cells, rich in myofibrils and poor in mitochondria. These fibers are numerous, for instance, in the biceps muscle. They have a rapid rate of contraction over long periods and do not fatigue easily. **Red fibers** are small cells with relatively few myofibrils, numerous small mitochondria, and a rich supply of myoglobin, the muscle cell pigment which contributes to their predominent red color. These fibers are present abundantly in the muscles of respiration, mastication, and the eyeball. They have a slow and powerful contraction but fatigue more easily than white fibers.

In sections stained with hematoxylin and eosin for ordinary light microscopy, as well as in specimens preserved for electron microscopy, myofibrils have alternating dark (**A-band**) and light (**I-band**) portions which are arranged in register with those of adjoining myofibrils, resulting in transverse striations. (Fig. 11-10) The light portion is bisected by a thin dense area, the **Z-line**, whereas the center of the dark portion is occupied by a less dense zone, the **H-band**. The part between two Z-lines is called **sarcomere**. When observed in the darkfield of a polarizing microscope, the dark A-band appears light and is doubly refractive (anisotropic or birefringent), reflecting a regular molecular arrangement of submicroscopic **myofilaments**. The light I-band is invisible and singly refractive in

the darkfield of the polarizing microscope (isotropic or non-birefringent), reflecting a less regular molecular arrangement. The essential protein of the muscle is **actomyosin**. This is a combination of myosin and actin, proteins making up the submicroscopic myofilaments of the myofibril.

Myofilaments. Each myofibril consists of 1000–2000 regularly arranged filaments of two categories: thick myofilaments and thin myofilaments. There are approximately twice as many thin filaments as there are thick. The **thick myofilaments** are concentrated to the dense A-band and made up of **myosin**. (Fig. 11-10) They are about 1.5 μ long, 100 Å thick, and consist of **heavy meromyosin**, which are short, rod-like structures each with a globular head; and **light meromyosin**, which are long rods arranged longitudinally in, and

Fig. 11-7. Skeletal muscle. Cross section demonstrating the close relationship between muscle cells and blood capillaries. Rat. E.M. × 4800. 1 mm=0.2 μ. **1.** Lumina of blood capillaries. Width indicated by bars: 5.5 μ. **2.** Nuclei of endothelial cells. **3.** Nuclei of muscle cells. **4.** Width of muscle fiber: 19 μ. **5.** Narrow intercellular space.

Fig. 11-8. Detail of edges of two skeletal muscle cells in cross section. Rat. E.M. × 19,000. **1.** Nucleus of muscle cell. **2.** Nucleolus. **3.** Mitochondria in paranuclear sarcoplasm. **4.** Sarcolemma. **5.** Intercellular space with reticular and delicate collagenous fibrils of endomysium. **6.** Cytoplasmic process of fibroblast. **7.** Nucleus of satellite cell. **8.** Cytoplasm of satellite cell. **9.** Cell membrane of satellite cell borders on the sarcolemma of the host muscle cell. **10.** Myofilaments of host cell. **11.** External (basal) lamina encloses host cell and satellite cell.

Fig. 11-9. Detail of cross-sectioned skeletal muscle cell. Enlargement of rectangle in Fig. 11-7. Rat. E.M. X 27,000. **1.** Narrow intercellular space with apposing external (basal) laminae alone forming the endomysium. **2.** Sarcolemma. **3.** Mitochondria (sarcosomes). **4.** Myofibrils sectioned at level of I-band. **5.** Myofibril sectioned at level of A-band. **6.** Sarcoplasmic reticulum. **7.** Lipid droplet. After studying this enlargement, go back to Fig. 11-7 and try to identify details of other parts of that field of view.

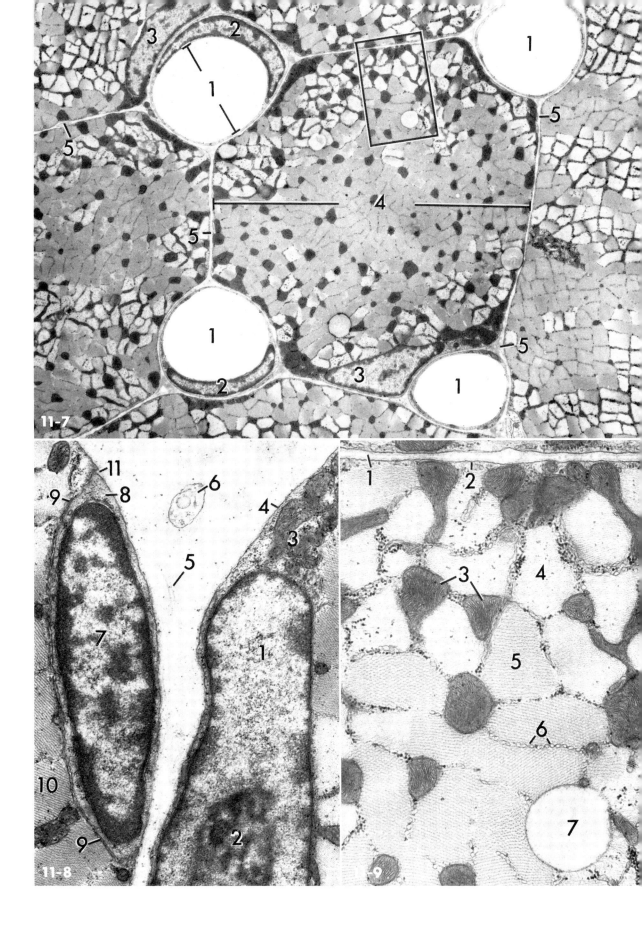

forming, the core of the thick myosin filament. Each thick filament has six longitudinal rows of minute, short lateral projections arranged helically around the filament in a staggered fashion. These lateral projections (spines; cross-bridges) probably correspond to the globular heads of the heavy meromyosin. In the middle of each thick filament appears a local swelling. Thin strands, 40 Å thick, extend in this region between thick filaments. The local swelling, a light zone on either side, and the cross links are collectively referred to as the **M-band.**

The **thin myofilaments** are made up of **actin** and average 1 μ in length and 50 Å in width. They are composed of two coiled strands of **F-actin** (fibrous actin), each of which is a polymere of **G-actin,** a monomeric globular unit. The thin filaments originate with delicate strands from both sides of the Z-line, actually forming this zone by an intermeshing of their thin strands of origin in a zigzag, square pattern. From the Z-line, the thin myofilaments extend in opposite directions, forming the I-band and passing between the ends of the thick myofilaments within the A-band. The degree of interdigitation of thin and thick filaments depends on the state of muscle contraction and relaxation. (Figs. 11-13, 11-14) The zone between the ends of the thin myofilaments, in which only thick myofilaments are present, is the **H-band.** This zone disappears in fully contracted myofibrils. According to present understanding of the contraction process, the thin myofilaments of the I-band slide in between the thick myofilaments of the A-band. This is discussed under muscle contraction on p. 232.

The arrangement of interdigitating thin and thick filaments becomes more obvious in cross sections through this area of the myofibril. (Fig. 11-12) The thick myosin filaments are arranged in a hexagonal pattern, about 450 Å apart, with six thin actin filaments grouped around each thick filament. Each thin filament is shared by three thick filaments. It appears that the lateral projections of the thick filaments (globular heads of the heavy meromyosin) reach the thin filaments, bridging the interfilamentous gap, which measures about 150 Å.

Extrafibrillar sarcoplasm. A very small part of the muscle cell is occupied by structures in the extrafibrillar sarcoplasm. **Mitochondria** (also called sarcosomes) are disposed in longitudinal rows between myofibrils, often opposite the I-bands or Z-lines. They are numerous near the nucleus and in a narrow zone beneath the sarcolemma. They are elongated or round with numerous, closely packed membra-

Fig. 11-10. Detail of myofibrils and myofilaments. Relaxed skeletal muscle. Longitudinal section. Rat. E.M. X 62,000. 1 mm = 161 Å. See legend Fig. 11-12.

Fig. 11-11. Relaxed skeletal muscle. Cross section. Rat. E.M. × 62,000. See legend Fig. 11-12.

Fig. 11-12. A, B, C, D and E are enlargements of areas similar to rectangle A–E in Fig. 11-11. Relaxed skeletal muscle. Cross section. Rat. E.M. × 120,000. 1 mm = 83 Å. **1.** Z-line. Distance between two Z-lines equals one sarcomere. **2.** I-band with only thin filaments. **3.** Ends of thick myofilaments; also border between I-band and A-band. **4.** Zone of interdigitating thin and thick myofilaments. **5.** Ends of thin filaments. **6.** H-band with only thick myofilaments. **7.** M-band: local swelling of thick myofilaments with cross-linking filaments. **8.** Extent of two thin myofilaments, indicated by lines (1 μ). **9.** Extent of one thick myofilament, indicated by line, marks extent of A-band (1.5 μ). **10.** Profiles of sarcoplasmic reticulum. **11.** Terminal cisterna of sarcoplasmic reticulum. **12.** Glycogen particles. **13.** Transverse tubule of T-system. **14.** Triad. **15.** Mitochondria. **16.** Thin myofilaments. **17.** Thick myofilaments. **A.** Cross section of interdigitating thin and thick filaments (level 4 in Fig. 11-10). Six thin filaments surround one thick filament; one thin filament shared by three thick filaments. **B.** Cross section of M-band. (level 7 in Fig. 11-10). **C.** Cross section of H-band (level 6 in Fig. 11-10). **D.** Cross section of I-band (level 2 in Fig. 11-10). **E.** Cross section of Z-line with square pattern of thin filaments (level 1 in Fig. 11-10).

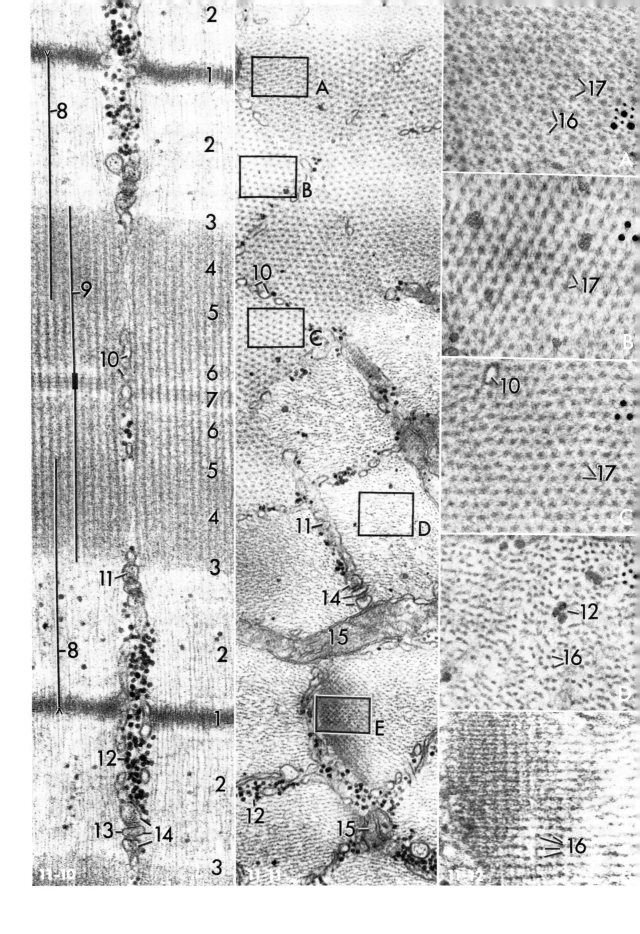

nous cristae. The **Golgi zones** are small, located near the poles of the nuclei. **Lipid droplets,** which are relatively frequent and usually near mitochondria, are normal components of the cell but increase in number with age. **Glycogen particles** are present throughout with larger accumulations between myofibrils at the level of I-bands. The **sarcoplasmic reticulum** is a modified or special type of agranular endoplasmic reticulum, consisting of tubules and cisternae arranged longitudinally and transversely around each myofibril in a loose basketweave pattern. The transverse tubules are the largest and form **terminal cisternae** at the level of the A-I junctions (Fig. 11-16), where two terminal cisternae are interposed by a small invagination of the sarcolemma, the transverse tubule (p. 224) giving rise to the so-called **triad.** (Fig. 11-15) Each sarcomere, therefore, has two triads which, in mammals, are located at the A-I junctions, and in amphibians at the level of the Z-line. Ribosomes and profiles of the granular endoplasmic reticulum are normally absent in mature muscle cells.

CONNECTIVE TISSUE

The **endomysium** is a thin connective tissue sheet around each muscle fiber, consisting of an external (basal) lamina close to the sarcolemma, and a thin layer of loosely arranged reticular and delicate collagenous fibrils. Occasional fibroblasts are present. So-called **satellite cells** are rare in adult muscle tissue. (Fig. 11-8) If present, they are located underneath the endomysium with direct contact between the satellite cell membrane and the sarcolemma. These cells are undifferentiated cells, probably myoblasts, but definitely do not represent fibroblasts. The narrow intercellular connective tissue space of the endomysium conveys small nerves and a vast network of blood capillaries. The **perimysium** surrounds a group of muscle cells referred to as fascicle. It is thicker than the endomysium and contains bun-

dles of collagenous fibrils, some elastic fibers and several fibroblasts. Arterioles and venules are present in the perimysium and carry with them mast cells and macrophages. The perimysium also contains larger nerves and neuromuscular spindles. The **epimysium** is a dense regular connective tissue with coarse bundles of collagenous fibers. It connects the muscle to the tendon at the **myotendinal junction.** A thin layer of reticular fibrils and elastic microfibrils is interposed between the sarcolemma and the coarse collagenous fibers of the tendon.

BLOOD AND LYMPHATIC VESSELS

The muscle cells are extremely well supplied with blood capillaries which are closely apposed to the sarcolemma. The capillaries run longitudinally between the muscle fibers with frequent short transverse anastomoses, resulting in a capillary

Fig. 11-13. *Relaxed* skeletal muscle. Longitudinal section. Rat. E.M. X 24,000. 1 mm = 0.0417 μ. **1.** M-band 0.13 μ. **2.** Z-line 0.08 μ. **3.** I-band 1.3 μ. **4.** A-band 1.5 μ. **5.** Sarcomere (Z-Z) 2.7 μ. **6.** H-band 0.63 μ.

Fig. 11-14. *Contracted* skeletal muscle. Longitudinal section. Mouse. E.M. X 24,000. Comparison of lengths of bands in contracted myofibrils with those of relaxed myofibrils. **1.** M-band 0.13 μ. **2.** Z-line 0.08 μ. **3.** I-band 0.63 μ. **4.** A-band 1.5 μ. **5.** Sarcomere (Z-Z) 2.1 μ. *Note:* H-band obliterated at maximum contraction.

Fig. 11-15. Topography of I-band and related structures. Skeletal muscle. Longitudinal section. Rat. E.M. X 90,000. **1.** Ends of thick filaments. **2.** I-band with thin filaments. **3.** Terminal cisternae of sarcoplasmic reticulum. **4.** T-tubule. **5.** Triads. **6.** Z-line. **7.** Particulate glycogen.

Fig. 11-16. Detail of I-band and related structures. Skeletal muscle. Cross section. E.M. X 126,000. **1.** Myofilaments of four adjacent myofibrils. **2.** Mitochondrion. **3.** Particulate glycogen. **4.** Tubular elements of sarcoplasmic reticulum. **5.** Terminal cisterna of sarcoplasmic reticulum.

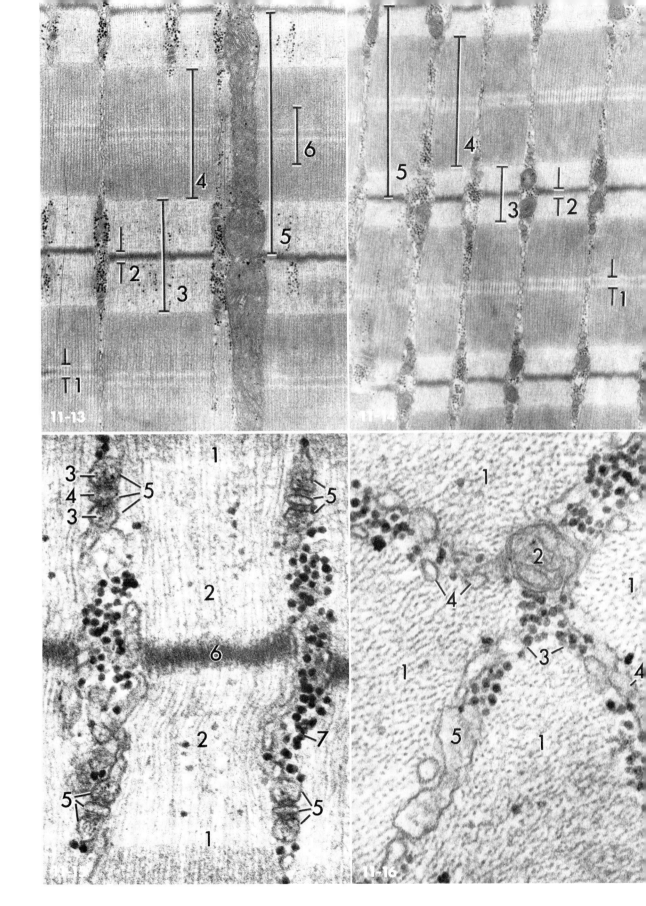

network with narrow oblong meshes. (Fig. 11-5) The capillary endothelium is of the thick, continuous type, provided with numerous micropinocytotic vesicles (p. 352). Lymphatic capillaries and vessels are not present in the endomysium but occur in the epimysium and perimysium.

NERVE ENDINGS

Contraction of skeletal muscles and coordination of muscle activity is controlled by two kinds of nerve endings: **motor nerve endings** represented by the motor end-plates, and **sensory nerve endings,** represented by the neuromuscular spindles and the neurotendinous endings. Each skeletal muscle cell is provided with one **motor end plate,** consisting of a branching axon terminal lodged in trench-like recesses of the muscle cell surface. (Figs. 11-17, 11-18) Efferent nerve impulses reach the sarcolemma in the motor end-plate, initiating muscle contraction. From a functional point of view, a muscle is composed of **motor units,** each unit consisting of a motor nerve cell, its axon, and the group of muscle cells contacted by this axon. If many muscle cells are innervated by the same nerve cell, contraction results in gross movements; whereas fine movements are accomplished by muscles where a motor neuron innervates only one or very few muscle cells. **Neuromuscular spindles** consist of groups of delicate muscle cells enclosed in a capsule. Afferent sensory nerves contact the muscle cells of the spindle, and contraction of these muscle cells stimulates the nerve terminals. The main function of the neuromuscular spindle is to control muscle contraction subconsciously via a monosynaptic reflex arc. **Neurotendinous endings** are located in tendons near the myotendinal junction. Axons terminate freely as leaf-like expansions among the collagenous fiber bundles. The nerve endings are stimulated by stretching or pulling the tendon. The afferent nerve impulse inhibits extreme tension in contracting muscles via a disynaptic reflex arc. These nerve endings are discussed further on p. 296.

SKELETAL MUSCLE CONTRACTION

There is a long chain of events related to skeletal muscle contraction. This is a brief summary of some of the major steps, based on present ultrastructural and biochemical information, as well as on current functional hypotheses. Textbooks of physiology and biochemistry should be consulted for a comprehensive discussion of muscle contraction.

1. As the efferent nerve impulse reaches the axon terminal of the motor end plate, acetylcholine is released and reaches the sarcolemma, depolarizing this membrane and its invaginations, the tranverse tubules.

2. By the depolarization of the sarcolemma and the proximity of the T-system to the sarcoplasmic reticulum at the tri-

Fig. 11-17. Topography of motor end plate. Skeletal muscle. Cross section. Rat. E.M. X 9000. **1.** Nucleus of fibroblast. **2.** Nucleus of Schwann cell (teloglial cell). **3.** Nucleus of muscle cell. **4.** Terminal nerve branches. **5.** Muscle cell mitochondria (sarcosomes). **6.** Myofibrils. **7.** Sarcolemma.

Fig. 11-18. Motor end plate. Slight enlargement of area similar to rectangle in Fig. 11-17. Skeletal muscle. Rat. E.M. X 22,000. **1.** Nerve axon terminal in synaptic trough. **2.** Mitochondria. **3.** Synaptic vesicles. **4.** Subneural clefts filled with external (basal) lamina. **5.** Sarcolemma. **6.** Nucleus of muscle cell. **7.** Golgi zone. **8.** Myofilaments.

Fig. 11-19. Myotendinal junction. Papillary muscle. Heart. Rat. E.M. X 6900. **1.** Bundles of collagenous fibrils. **2.** Network of delicate collagenous fibrils, reticular fibrils, and elastic microfibrils. **3.** Invaginations of sarcolemma. **4.** Myofibrils.

Fig. 11-20. Detail of myotendinal junction. Enlargement of area similar to rectangle in Fig. 11-19. Skeletal muscle. Mouse. E.M. X 30,000. **1.** Delicate collagenous fibrils. **2.** Myofilaments. **3.** Sarcolemma with attached dense cytoplasm. Myofilaments seem to anchor in this region. **4.** External (basal) lamina.

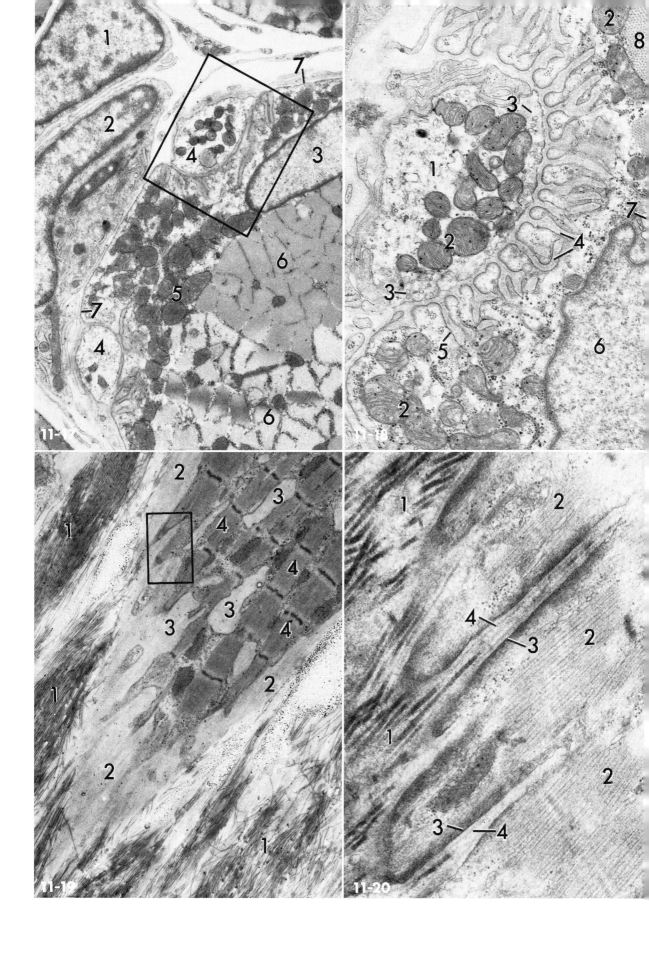

ads, calcium ions, stored in the sarco-plasmic reticulum are released into the sarcoplasm and reach the thin actin fila-ments. Calcium ions become bound to the G-actin, activating these sites.

3. ATP-ase is located in the globular heads of the heavy meromyosin of the thick filaments. The ATP (adenosine triphosphate) of the mitochondria is made available and splits to ADP (adenosinedi-phosphate) by the action of ATP-ase, re-leasing free phosphate ions and delivering the energy for contraction.

4. At this point, the latent chemical energy of the carbohydrates is transformed into mechanical energy. It is postulated that the energy set free by the splitting of the terminal phosphate bonds of the ATP makes the heavy meromyosin mole-cules swing to join the G-actin sites of the thin filaments which were activated by the calcium ions set free from the sarco-plasmic reticulum and attached to the G-actin sites.

5. Each globular head of the heavy meromyosin molecule (also referred to as spines or cross-bridges) is attracted by a succession of G-actin sites on the thin filament to form the contractile mole-cule, actomyosin, in a ratchet-like action, resulting in a pulling or sliding of the thin filaments into the spaces between the thick filaments.

6. As a result, the H-band (zone be-tween ends of thin filaments) is narrowed, the I-band diminished, the distance be-tween the Z-lines (sarcomere) reduced, and the entire myofibril shortened. All myo-fibrils in a cell contract simultaneously and instantly.

7. At the end of the contraction, cal-cium ions return to the sarcoplasmic re-ticulum and muscle relaxation sets in.

8. A skeletal muscle cell cannot con-tract at different degrees of intensity. It follows the "all-or-none" law, which means that if the muscle cell contracts it does so to maximum capacity or not at all. To increase the contraction power more motor units are made to contract.

Cardiac Muscle

The cardiac muscle consists of striated muscle cells but, in contrast to the skele-tal muscle, the cardiac muscle contraction is not normally subject to voluntary con-trol. Although innervated by the auto-nomic nervous system, the inherent prop-erties of cardiac muscle cells to contract spontaneously and rhythmically are only moderated by this nervous system. The muscular tissue of the heart (myocardium) contains two types of muscle fibers (cells): 1) **cardiac muscle fibers** and 2) **specialized cells of conducting system.** The cells of both types have structural and functional

Fig. 11-21. Cardiac muscle. Longitudinal section. Interventricular septum of steer heart. L.M. × 115. 1. Myocardium. 2. Part of right branch of common bundle of impulse conducting system. Width between bars: 97 μ. 3. Endocardial connective tissue. 4. Lumen of ventricle.

Fig. 11-22. Enlargement of rectangle in Fig. 11-21. L.M. X 350. 1. Nuclei of cardiac muscle cells. 2. Erythrocytes in capillary. 3. Width of cardiac muscle cell: 12 μ. 4. Connective tissue. 5. Myofibrils of Purkinje fibers. 6. Nuclei.

Fig. 11-23. Cross section of a branch of the common bundle. Interventricular septum of steer heart. L.M. X 350. 1. Sheath of connective tissue. 2. Nuclei of Purkinje fibers (cells). 3. Cell borders of Purkinje fibers enhanced by accumulations of peripheral myofibrils. 4. Nuclei of fibroblasts.

Fig. 11-24. Cardiac muscle cells. Cross section. Left ventricle of steer heart. L.M. X 350. 1. Nuclei of cardiac muscle cells. 2. Cardiac muscle cell; width 14 μ. 3. Endomysium. 4. Perimysium enclosing muscle fascicle. 5. Fine stippling of sarcoplasm represents cross-sectioned myofibrils. 6. Rectangle enlarged in Fig. 11-28.

Fig. 11-25. Cardiac muscle cells. Longitudinal section. Enlargement of area similar to rectangle in Fig. 11-22. Heart. Rat. E.M. X 1900. 1. Erythrocytes in lumina of blood capillaries. 2. Nuclei of endothelial cells. 3. Nucleus of fibroblast. 4. Nuclei of cardiac muscle cells. 5. Width of cardiac muscle cell: 19 μ. 6. Myofibrils. 7. Rows of mitochondria. 8. Intercalated disks.

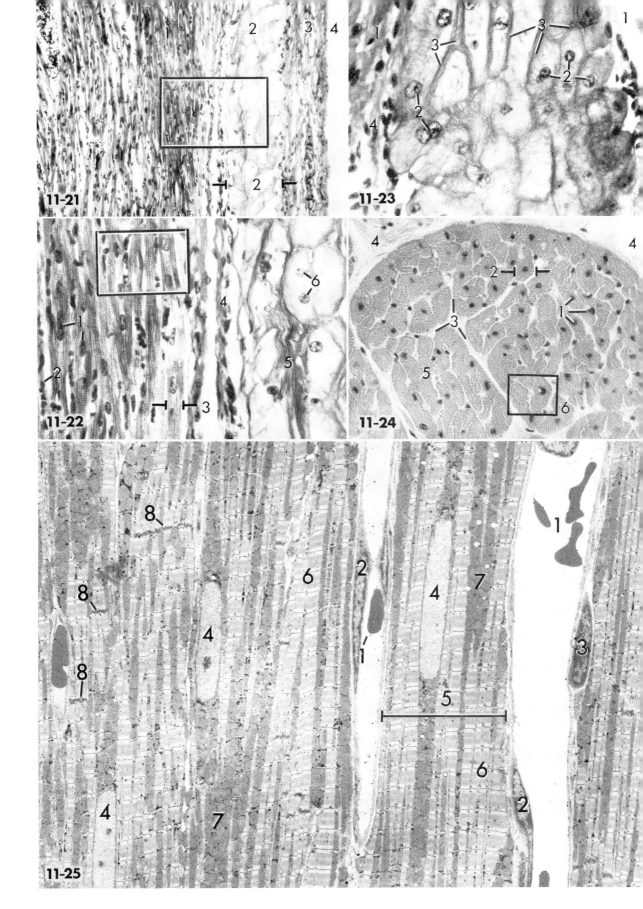

similarities as well as dissimilarities. (Fig. 11-22) The cardiac muscle fibers dominate the myocardium and reduce the size of the heart chambers upon contraction, whereas the cells of the conducting system are concentrated to knots and strands of tissue, serving as a special impulse conducting system within the myocardium. By contractions, this system initiates and disseminates to the cardiac muscle fibers an impulse to contract, and it coordinates the contraction of the four heart chambers.

CARDIAC MUSCLE FIBERS

General organization. The cardiac muscle is composed of cylindrical cells which average 100–150 μ in length and 10–20 μ in width. (Fig. 11-25) They branch, bifurcate, and anastomose rather freely. The cells, as well as their branches, meet end-to-end in junctional complexes called intercalated disks. A thin endomysium surrounds each cell but is not interposed at the intercalated disks. The endomysium consists of an external (basal) lamina and a thin network of reticular and delicate collagenous fibrils. The cardiac muscle fibers are arranged in thin layers, parallel to each other within each layer but at an angle to fibers of adjacent layers. To form the myocardium, the muscle layers are arranged in a wide spiral which stretches from the base to the apex of the heart. The **nucleus** of the cardiac cell is elongated, cigar-shaped. There is usually one, sometimes two, nuclei per cell in a central position. The cells are bordered by the sarcolemma. The **sarcoplasm** contains fewer myofibrils, and the extrafibrillar components are more numerous than in skeletal muscle fibers.

Sarcolemma. The sarcolemma is a 90 Å trilaminar cell membrane provided with a moderate number of **micropinocytotic** invaginations and surface vesicles. In the cells of the ventricles there are long, intracellular tubular invaginations, forming a **T-system** at the level of the Z-lines of the myofibrils. The tubules are larger than in skeletal muscle cells, and the external (basal) lamina of the cell is carried along as a thin intratubular coating. (Figs. 11-31, 11-32, 11-33) The T-system is absent in the cells of the atria in most mammalian species.

The sarcolemma is highly specialized in relation to the **intercalated disks,** where it is differentiated into zones of desmosome (macula adhaerens), intermediate junction (fascia adhaerens), and gap-junction (nexus). (Fig. 11-29) The intercalated disks are transverse structures, occurring at the level of the Z-lines representing areas where the cardiac muscle cells and their branches meet end-to-end. Often these junctions are not in register laterally but arranged as steps in a staircase. This can be observed in iron-hematoxylin stained preparations with the light microscope. At the ultrastructural level, short, blunt cell processes are seen to protrude from apposing cell surfaces in an interdigitating manner. It is these processes which are provided with the three categories of junctional specializations men-

Fig. 11-26. Cardiac muscle cells. Longitudinal section. Heart. Rat. E.M. X 7500.
1. Erythrocyte. **2.** Lumen of longitudinally sectioned capillary. **3.** Endothelium.
4. Extracellular space with endomysium.
5. Nucleus of cardiac muscle cell.
6. Nucleolus. **7.** Extrafibrillar sarcoplasm in central conical space. **8.** Small Golgi zones. **9.** Mitochondria. **10.** Z-lines of myofibrils. **11.** Part of intercalated disk.

Fig. 11-27. Cardiac muscle cell. Longitudinal section. Heart. Rat. E.M. X 19,000.
1. Transverse part of intercalated disk.
2. Longitudinal part of intercalated disk.
3. Mitochondria. **4.** Z-lines of myofibrils.
5. Particulate glycogen.

Fig. 11-28. Cardiac muscle cells. Cross section. Enlargement of area similar to rectangle in Fig. 11-24. Heart. Rat. E.M. × 9000.
1. Nucleus of cardiac muscle cell. **2.** Small Golgi zone. **3.** Myofibrils. **4.** Mitochondria.
5. Endomysium of extracellular space.
6. Intercalated disk; lateral junction of two cells. **7.** Lumen of blood capillary with erythrocytes. **8.** Nucleus of endothelial cell.

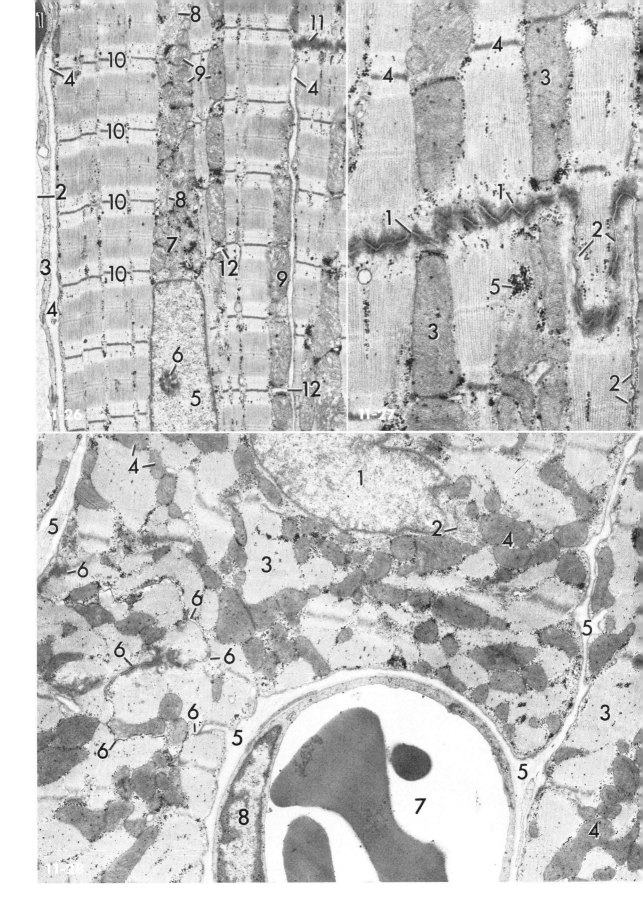

tioned. In addition, longer stretches of nexuses or gap-junctions occur in areas where the surface of the apposing cell membranes is parallel to the long axis of the cell (vertical part of the "steps in the staircase"). Myofilaments connect with a web of fine cytoplasmic filaments that adheres to the cytoplasmic aspect of the sarcolemma, particularly in relation to the desmosomes and the fasciae adhaerentes of the intercalated disk. These disks aid in cell cohesion, as well as in transmitting tension and contraction impulses from cell to cell. They become more complex and numerous with age.

Myofibrils. The myofibrils are less numerous than in skeletal muscle fibers. They usually form a continuum of irregularly shaped, longitudinally arranged columns throughout the cell. The pattern of transverse bands described for the skeletal myofibril (p. 226) also characterizes the cardiac myofibril. (Fig. 11-31) The same two sets of filaments, thick myosin filaments and thin actin filaments, are present and they interdigitate.

Extrafibrillar sarcoplasm. A relatively large part of the cardiac muscle cell is occupied by structures in the extrafibrillar sarcoplasm. **Mitochondria** occur abundantly in rows between myofibrils as well as in subsarcolemmal aggregations and in cone-shaped, elongated zones extending from either pole of the nucleus. The mitochondria are round or elongated and provided with numerous, closely arranged membranous cristae. The Golgi zone is small and located at one pole of the nucleus. **Lipid droplets** are spherical and occur both near the sarcolemma and between myofibrils, often in contact with mitochondria. Brown to yellow **lipofuscin** pigment granules occur sparingly in the central cone-shaped zones and become increasingly more numerous with age. They represent accumulations of secondary lysosomes, and are particularly common in the so-called brown myocardial atrophy. **Glycogen** particles are more numerous

than in skeletal muscle fibers, occurring everywhere. In atrial muscle cells occur **dense granules** (also referred to as atrial granules) which average 0.3μ in diameter. They are numerous in the perinuclear and central conical areas, often associated with the Golgi zone. They were initially thought to represent a storage form of catecholamines, but this has not been confirmed. The **sarcoplasmic reticulum** is abundantly present as richly interconnected, smooth tubules with less regular arrangement compared with the situation in the skeletal muscle. The longitudinal arrangement is not as prominent, and there are no clear-cut transverse terminal cisternae, but only short terminal expansions in ventricular muscle cells which aggregate around the transverse tubules of the T-system to form one small **triad** at the level of each Z-line.

Fig. 11-29. Detail of intercalated disk. Heart. Rat. E.M. X 99,000. **1.** Desmosomes (maculae adhaerentes). **2.** Intermediate junctions (fasciae adhaerentes). **3.** Rectangle: gap-junction (nexus). **4.** Web of fine cytoplasmic filaments. **5.** Myofilaments. **6.** Z-line. **7.** Glycogen particles. **8.** Outer mitochondrial membrane.

Fig. 11-30. Nexus (gap-junction). Enlargement of area similar to rectangle in Fig. 11-29. Intercalated disk. Heart. Rat. E.M. X 250,000. **1.** Apposing sarcolemmae. **2.** Intermembranous gap, about 20 Å wide. **3.** Glycogen particles.

Fig. 11-31. Periphery of cardiac muscle cell. Rat. E.M. X 64,000. **1.** Delicate collagenous fibrils. **2.** External (basal) lamina. **3.** Sarcolemma. **4.** Invagination of sarcolemma (T-tubule) with external lamina. **5.** Myofilaments. **6.** Mitochondria. **7.** Profiles of tubular sarcoplasmic reticulum. **8.** Glycogen particles.

Fig. 11-32. Longitudinal section of cardiac muscle cell. Rat. E.M. X 32,000. **1.** Z-lines. **2.** Mitochondria. **3.** Transverse tubule of T-system. **4.** Glycogen particles.

Fig. 11-33. Topography of Z-line in cardiac muscle cell. Rat. E.M. X 96,000. **1.** Z-lines. **2.** Thin filaments. **3.** Terminal portions of sarcoplasmic reticulum. **4.** Transverse tubule of T-system. **5.** Triad. **6.** Glycogen particles.

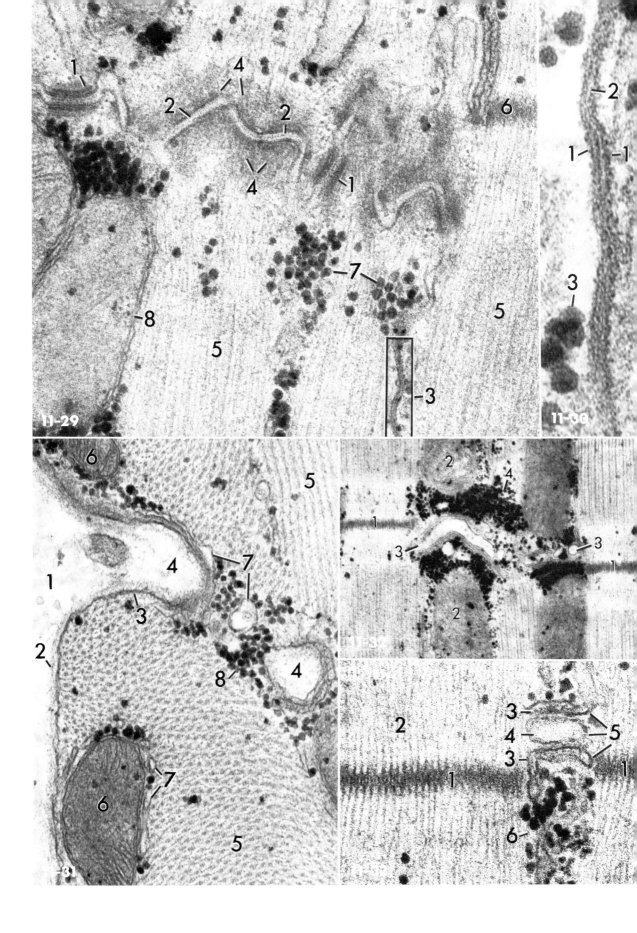

SPECIALIZED CELLS
OF CONDUCTING SYSTEM

The specialized cells are modified cardiac muscle cells with a structure slightly different from the ordinary cardiac muscle cells. The specialized cells can only be detected in areas where they are aggregated into small nodes and strands, and separated from the rest of the myocardium by a connective tissue sheath of varied thickness. The aggregations of specialized cells are generously supplied with sympathetic and parasympathetic nerve fibers, and they have a rich capillary bed. By their location in the heart, as well as distribution and ultrastructural characteristics, the specialized cardiac muscle cells serve as pacemakers for the heart beat, distributors of the contraction impulse throughout the heart, and coordinators of the contraction of the four heart chambers.

The conducting system of the mammalian heart consists of: 1) sinuatrial (SA) node of Keith and Flack; 2) atrioventricular (AV) node of Tawara; 3) atrioventricular (common) bundle of His; 4) right and left branches on either side of the interventricular septum; and 5) terminal ramifications of the right and left branches, leading to papillary muscle and the walls of the ventricles. Textbooks of anatomy should be consulted for topographic details of this system.

Cells of nodes. The SA-node and AV-node consist of small specialized fusiform cells, forming a compact, branching network. The cells are smaller than ordinary cardiac muscle cells, averaging 10μ in width and 25μ in length, but they are ultrastructurally quite similar with reference to myofibrils and extrafibrillar sarcolemma, except for the transverse tubules of the T-system, which are missing. They differ through their arrangement, since they often form cord-like clusters of cells in which the cells are mutually interconnected, mostly side to side because of their fusiform shape. Intercalated disks do not occur, but all three categories of junctional specializations of the

sarcolemma, present in the intercalated disks, occur here also, distributed along the surfaces making the contact. (Fig. 11-37) Undifferentiated regions of cell junction are large in the specialized nodal muscle tissue. A thin external (basal) lamina and a thin layer of connective tissue fibrils invest the cord-like clusters of specialized cells. The specialized muscle cells of the nodal tissue make contact with the atrial muscle cells.

Cells of AV-bundle and branches. The major part of the AV-bundle is made up of specialized cells similar to those found in the nodes. In the distal parts of the bundle, and throughout the interventricular branches, the specialized cells in many mammals are large and change from fusiform to elongated cylindrical, meeting end to end, as well as side to side, within the strands of the conducting system. These cells are referred to as **Purkinje**

Fig. 11-34. Comparison between Purkinje fibers and ordinary cardiac muscle fibers. Interventricular septum. Steer heart. E.M. X 1800. **1.** Nuclei of ordinary cardiac muscle fibers. **2.** Width of fiber 10 μ. **3.** Bundles of collagenous fibrils. **4.** Nuclei of Purkinje fibers; width indicated 20 μ. **5.** Cell borders (sarcolemmae) of adjacent Purkinje fibers in close contact. Their course is easily seen because of differences in sarcoplasmic density of the Purkinje fibers. **6.** Cross-sectioned myofibrils. **7.** Blood capillaries.

Fig. 11-35. Longitudinal section of Purkinje fibers (cells). Steer heart. E.M. X 1800. **1.** Cells with dense sarcoplasm. **2.** Cell border. **3.** Cell with light sarcoplasm. **4.** Myofibrils. **5.** Mitochondria.

Fig. 11-36. Enlargement of area similar to rectangle in Fig. 11-35. Steer heart. E.M. X 9000. **1.** Density of sarcoplasm caused by large accumulations of particulate glycogen. **2.** Cell border. **3.** Glycogen particles present to limited extent in the sarcoplasm of this cell. **4.** Z-lines of myofibril.

Fig. 11-37. Detail of sarcolemmal specializations. Purkinje fibers. Steer heart. E.M. × 86,000. **1.** Gap-junction (nexus). **2.** Intermediate junction (fascia adhaerens). **3.** Desmosome (macula adhaerens). **4.** Myofilaments. **5.** Sarcoplasmic reticulum. **6.** Glycogen particles.

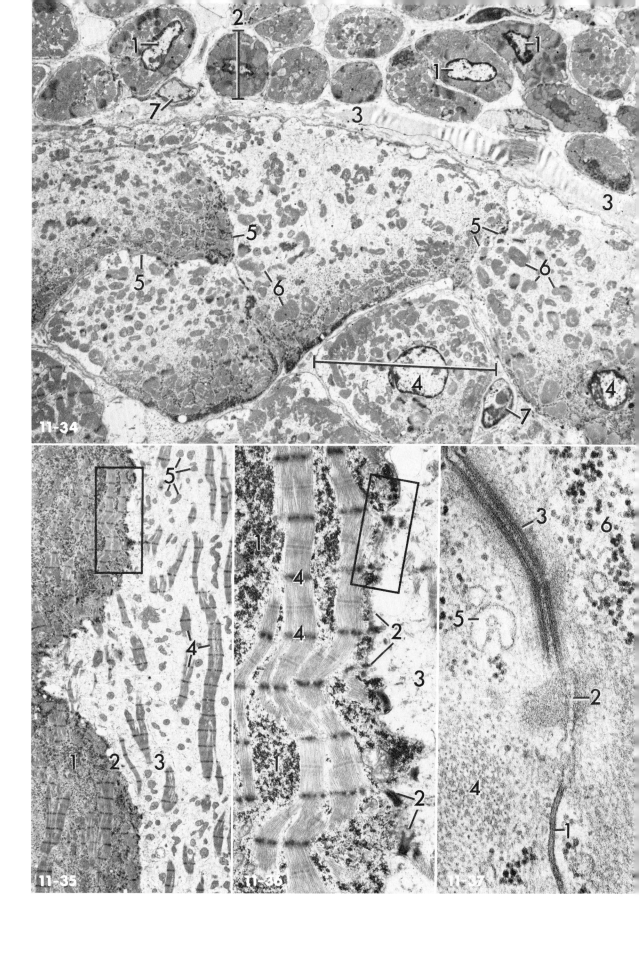

fibers, and average 50μ in width and 100μ in length. (Fig. 11-34) In the human heart, the typical large Purkinje fibers are first present in the branches of the conducting system halfway down the interventricular system.

CONNECTIVE TISSUE

The myocardium contains a small amount of connective tissue, mostly of the loose variety, which is associated with blood capillaries in the spaces between cardiac cells. In adition, a thin sheath of endomysium surrounds the cardiac cells. It is made up of a thin external (basal) lamina and some reticular and delicate collagenous fibrils. Sheaths of perimysial connective tissue surround groups of cardiac muscle cells to form fascicles. The amount of myocardial connective tissue increases in older hearts. The connective tissue skeleton of the heart itself is described on p. 336. The conducting system of the heart is separated from the regular cardiac muscle cells by sheaths of connective tissue.

BLOOD AND LYMPHATIC VESSELS

The capillary bed of the myocardium is very dense, and the **blood capillaries** form an intricate network throughout the slit-like spaces between cardiac muscle cells. In contrast to skeletal muscle, the myocardium has a fair number of **lymphatic capillaries.** The endocardial system of lymphatics courses through the myocardium via transverse branches to the epicardial collecting lymphatic vessels.

NERVES

The myocardium and the impulse conducting system of the heart are richly innervated by nerves from the autonomic nervous system. The nerve endings make contact with, or are closely apposed to, the muscle cells, but motor end-plates do not exist.

Preganglionic **parasympathetic** efferent nerve fibers from the cardiac branches of the vagus synapse with ganglion cells in the myocardium. Postganglionic nerves reach cardiac muscle cells and specialized cells of the SA-node and AV-node. Postganglionic **sympathetic** nerve fibers from cervical sympathetic and upper thoracic ganglia reach cardiac muscle cells, as well as nodal tissue and branches of the conducting system.

CARDIAC MUSCLE CONTRACTION

In summary, there is a chain of events leading to and encompassing myocardial contractions. Spontaneous, myogenic contractions occur in cardiac cells from early embryonic life. The contraction mechanism of the myofibrils at the molecular level is similar to that described for skeletal muscle (p. 232).

The specialized muscle cells of the SA-node serve as pacemaker cells, controlling the contraction rate of the cardiac muscle fibers. The parasympathetic nerve endings within the nodal tissue have an inhibitory effect on this rate, whereas the sympathetic nerve endings have an excitatory effect, increasing the rate of contraction. The spread of excitation impulse from the specialized muscle cells of the SA-node to the atrial muscle cells and further across the atrium is facilitated by

Fig. 11-38. Smooth muscle cells of myometrium. Uterus. Human. L.M. X 315.
1. Cross-sectioned smooth muscle cells.
2. Obliquely sectioned smooth muscle cells.
3. Longitudinally sectioned smooth muscle cells.

Fig. 11-39. Smooth muscle cells. Ductus deferens. Rat. E.M. X 13,000. 1. Nuclei of longitudinally sectioned smooth muscle cells. 2. Nuclei of cross-sectioned smooth muscle cells. 3. Narrow intercellular space with reticular and delicate collagenous fibrils. 4. Denuded axon of nerve terminal. 5. Narrow cell processes establishing intercellular contact. 6. Golgi zones. 7. Centriole. 8. Mitochondria. 9. Granular endoplasmic reticulum. 10. Surface (micropinocytotic) vesicles. 11. Fusiform densities. 12. Longitudinal axis of myofilaments in sarcoplasm.

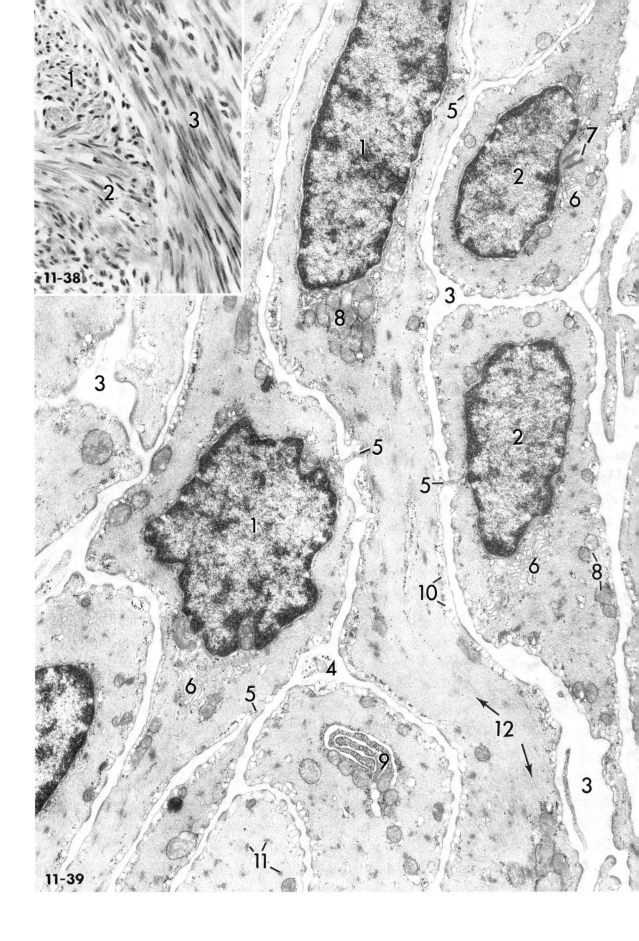

11-38

11-39

the presence of nexuses at the cell junctions. The nexus (gap-junction) represents a low resistance electrical pathway for the propagation of impulses.

The excitation impulse is picked up by the specialized muscle cells of the AV-node. Then the atrioventricular (common) bundle of His carries the impulse across the connective tissue septum separating the atrial myocardium from the ventricular myocardium. Via the Purkinje fibers of the right and left branches of the conducting system on either side of the interventricular system, the impulse reaches the papillary muscles and ventricular myocardium with a speed ten times faster than the rate of conduction across the myocardium itself. This has been attributed to the large ratio of nexus area to total junctional area within the strands of Purkinje fibers.

Smooth Muscle

Smooth muscle tissue consists of elongated, narrow, spindle-shaped cells, devoid of transverse striations. They are arranged with their tapered ends overlapping to form cords, bundles, and sheets. Smooth muscle cells are not under voluntary control. Their activity is regulated by the autonomic nervous system and they have an ability to perform work for long periods of time since their contraction is slow and sustained. Smooth muscle tissue is often referred to as a **visceral muscle** since it regulates the internal environment of a great many systems and organs. Smooth muscle of **mesodermal** origin is present in the wall of almost the entire gastrointestinal tract, in the gall bladder and in some ducts of the liver and the pancreas. It is an essential part of the cardiovascular system, notably the endocardium, the walls of arteries, veins, larger lymphatic vessels, and in minute quantities in the spleen. It is found in the respiratory system as part of the tracheal and bronchial walls. In the urinary tract it is present in the ureter, urinary bladder, and urethra. In the male reproductive system it is found in the duct system (Fig. 11-39), the prostate, and the cavernous tissue of the penis. In the female reproductive system it is particularly abundant in the uterus (Fig. 11-38), and to a lesser extent in the oviducts and the vagina. Smooth muscle of **ectodermal** origin is located in the iris and the ciliary body of the eye, and in the dermis of the skin. In mammary, salivary, sweat, and lacrimal glands, smooth muscle cells are present among epithelial cells and are referred to as **myoepithelial** cells.

Fig. 11-40. Smooth muscle cell. Longitudinally sectioned. Prostate. E.M. × 32,000. **1.** Nucleus. **2.** Golgi zone. **3.** Mitochondria. **4.** Cisternae of granular endoplasmic reticulum. **5.** Myofilamentous part of sarcoplasm. **6.** Fusiform density (indistinct). **7.** Sarcolemma. **8.** Intercellular space. **9.** Membranous contact between two smooth muscle cells. Similar area enlarged in Fig. 11-49. **10.** Glycogen particles. **11.** Adjacent smooth muscle cell.

Fig. 11-41. Detail of sarcolemmae of two apposing smooth muscle cells. Enlargement of area similar to rectangle (A) in Fig. 11-40. Ductus deferens. Mouse. E.M. X 90,000. **1.** Sarcoplasm. **2.** Dense body (attachment plaque). **3.** Sarcolemma. **4.** Narrow intercellular space, about 900 Å wide, occupied only by thin external (basal) laminae. **5.** Surface (micropinocytotic) vesicles. **6.** Element of sarcoplasmic reticulum, in close proximity ("coupling") to sarcolemma. **7.** Glycogen particles.

Fig. 11-42. Myofilaments of smooth muscle cell, sectioned longitudinally. Enlargement of area similar to rectangle (B) in Fig. 11-40. Prostate. Rat. E.M. × 90,000. **1.** Only one kind of filaments present in this preparation, averaging 60 Å in width. **2.** Fusiform density (dense oval body).

Fig. 11-43. Subsarcolemmal topography of smooth muscle cell. Prostate. Rat. E.M. × 90,000. **1.** Myofilaments. **2.** Fusiform density. **3.** Mitochondrion. **4.** Tubules of sarcoplasmic reticulum near sarcolemma ("coupling"). **5.** Surface vesicles. **6.** Sarcolemma. **7.** External (basal) lamina. **8.** Particulate glycogen.

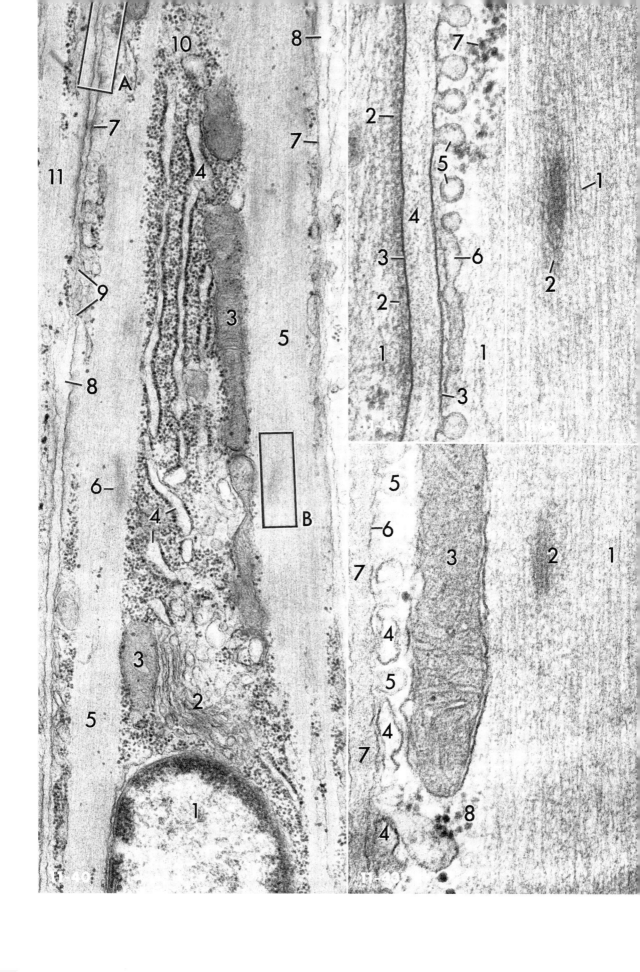

SMOOTH MUSCLE FIBERS

General organization. The smooth muscle fiber is a slender, fusiform, cylindrical, slightly flattened cell, occasionally branching. Its length varies from 500 μ in the pregnant uterus, 100 μ–50 μ in the intestines, to 20 μ in small arteries. The width averages 5–10 μ in most cases. Each smooth muscle cell is invested by a thin external (basal) lamina and a thin layer of reticular fibrils. In an overlapping, staggered fashion, the cells form layers, sheets, or bundles in which the fibers are parallel to one another. The sheets and bundles are surrounded by loose connective tissue sheaths, and the fiber direction of one set of smooth muscle fibers is usually different from adjacent ones. Each smooth muscle fiber has a single, eliptical, or rod-shaped **nucleus** which becomes twisted spirally in contracted cells. Several nucleoli are present. The smooth muscle cell is bordered by a sarcolemma and is almost completely filled with myofilaments. The extrafibrillar sarcoplasm is largely restricted to a conical space at the poles of the nucleus. (Fig. 11-40)

Sarcolemma. The sarcolemma is a 70 Å trilaminar cell membrane provided with a large number of micropinocytotic invaginations or smooth **surface vesicles.** (Fig. 11-41) The cell sends out a varied number of blunt, or short, narrow finger-like projections which make contact with, and often are connected to adjacent cells in a peg-and-socket arrangement. These areas of membrane contact may be differentiated into **nexuses** (gap-junctions) in which the outer leaflets of the apposing trilaminar cell membranes are either fused or separated by a narrow, 20 Å, space. Gap-junctions are discussed on p. 14. Attached to the cytoplasmic aspect of the sarcolemma at varied intervals are areas of high electron density referred to as **dense bodies** or attachment plaques (Fig. 11-41), structurally resembling half-desmosomes (p. 14). These are long (3–5 μ) and numerous in vascular smooth muscle, but short (0.5 μ–1 μ) and scarce in intestinal

smooth muscle. Tubular invaginations of the sarcolemma, similar to the transverse tubules of the T-system of skeletal muscle, are not present in smooth muscle cells.

Myofilaments. Myofibrils do not appear in smooth muscle cells of well-preserved specimens. Faint longitudinal striations may be seen in light microscope preparations and can be enhanced by macer-

Fig. 11-44. Cross-sectioned smooth muscle cells. Ureter. Rat. E.M. X 62,000.
1. Mitochondrion. **2.** Nucleus.
3. Myofilaments. **4.** Microtubules. **5.** Glycogen particles. **6.** Surface (micropinocytotic) vesicles. **7.** Dense bodies (attachment plaques). **8.** Narrow intercellular space with external (basal) laminae. **9.** Points of sarcolemmal contact.

Fig. 11-45. Cross-sectioned myofilaments. Smooth muscle. Ductus deferens. Mouse. E.M. X 32,000. See legend Fig. 11-47.

Fig. 11-46. Cross-sectioned myofilaments in lattice-like bundles. Smooth muscle. Muscularis externa. Large intestine. Rat. E.M. X 64,000. See legend Fig. 11-47.

Fig. 11-47 Cross-sectioned myofilaments. Smooth muscle. Ductus deferens. Mouse. E.M. X 96,000. **1.** Fusiform densities (dense oval bodies). **2.** Thick myofilaments (about 150 Å). **3.** Intermediate size myofilaments (about 100 Å). **4.** Thin myofilaments (about 50 Å). **5.** Mitochondria. **6.** Tubules of sarcoplasmic reticulum.

Fig. 11-48. Myoneural junctions. Smooth muscle. Ductus deferens. Rat. E.M. X 9000.
1. Nucleus of smooth muscle cell.
2. Intercellular space. **3.** Sarcolemmal contacts between adjacent smooth muscle cells.
4. Fusiform densities. **5.** Denuded axons of autonomic nerve endings.

Fig. 11-49. Sarcolemmal point of contact. Enlargement of area similar to rectangle (A) in Fig. 11-48. E.M. X 90,000.
1. Sarcolemma. **2.** Gap-junction. **3.** Surface vesicles. **4.** Glycogen particles. **5.** Ribosomes.

Fig. 11-50. Myoneural junction. Smooth muscle. Enlargement of area similar to rectangle (B) in Fig. 11-48. E.M. X 63,000.
1. Sarcolemma. **2.** Intercellular space.
3. Axolemma of autonomic nerve ending.
4. Subneural sarcolemma. **5.** Granulated synaptic vesicles of nerve ending.
6. Sarcoplasmic reticulum. **7.** Glycogen particles. **8.** Mitochondrion.

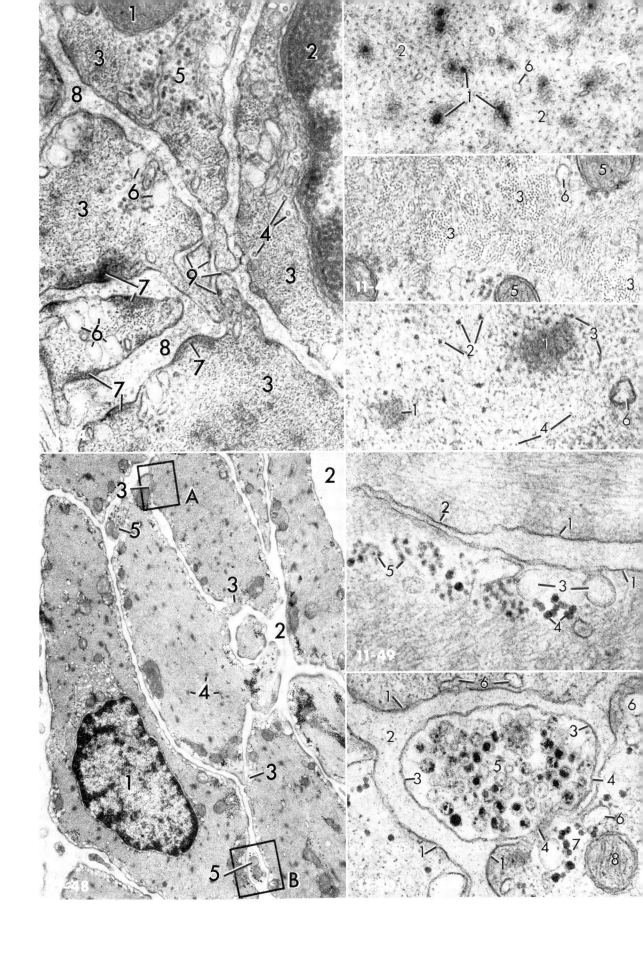

ation, but are strictly artificial. The contractile sarcoplasm of the smooth muscle fiber is made up of three sets of myofilaments: thick, intermediate-size, and thin. They are oriented parallel to the long axis of the smooth muscle fiber. (Fig. 11-43) Some of the filaments, especially the thick ones, are difficult to preserve properly, since they become dispersed in response to changes in extracellular calcium-ion concentration, and are readily disturbed during fixation. The **thick** filaments average 150 Å in width and about 0.6 μ in length. (Fig. 11-45) They are straight filaments with irregular outlines, often surrounded by a narrow zone of amorphous ground substance. The thick filaments probably contain myosin. This assumption is based on X-ray diffraction data and quantitative biochemical analyses. The **intermediate-size** filaments average 100 Å in width. Their length is not known. They may form lattice-like bundles between the thick filaments. (Fig. 11-46) These filaments are few in number but less labile than the thick filaments; their protein composition is not known. The **thin** filaments average 50 Å in width. (Fig. 11-47) Their length has not been measured since they have a wavy course and are difficult to resolve in longitudinal sections. Two or three rows of thin filaments may surround a thick filament to form rosette-like configurations. They are generally considered to contain actin. In vertebrate smooth muscle, the thin-to-thick filament ratio is high. The thin filaments are held closely together as they course through **fusiform densities,** dense oval bodies, 0.5 μ long and 0.1 μ wide, which are distributed widely among the filamentous part of the sarcoplasm. (Figs. 11-42, 11-48) They are similar but not identical to the Z-lines of skeletal and cardiac muscles. The thin filaments attach to the dense bodies along the sarcolemma. Possible mechanisms related to smooth muscle contraction are discussed on p. 232.

Extrafibrillar sarcoplasm. A small part of the smooth muscle fiber is occupied by structures in the extrafibrillar sarcoplasm. **Mitochondria** are relatively scarce, spherical or rod-shaped, with a few membranous cristae. They are present in the conical central space at the nuclear poles, in a subsarcolemmal position, or distributed singly among the myofilaments. The Golgi zone is relatively large and situated near the nuclear pole together with a few **lipid droplets,** profiles of the **granular sarcoplasmic reticulum** of varied lengths, and many free **ribosomes.** Coursing through, and parallel to the myofilamentous sarcoplasm occur several **microtubules,** averaging 250 Å in width. **Glycogen** particles are abundant between

Fig. 11-51. Myoepithelial cells associated with sweat glands. Axilla. Human. E.M. X 600.
1. Lumina of odoriferous sweat glands.
2. Lumen of ordinary sweat gland.
3. Connective tissue. **4.** Blood capillaries.
5. Longitudinally sectioned myoepithelial cell. The gland is also sectioned longitudinally. **6.** Cross-sectioned myoepithelial cells.

Fig. 11-52. Myoepithelial cells. associated with odoriferous sweat gland, sectioned in the plane indicated by the bar A-A in Fig. 11-51. Axilla. Human. E.M. X 3600.
1. Nucleus of myoepithelial cell.
2. Cytoplasm of myoepithelial cells contains numerous fusiform densities. The myoepithelial cells of the odoriferous gland are all arranged quite regularly and in parallel with the long axis of the tubular gland. **3.** Secretory epithelial cells alternate with myoepithelial cells. **4.** Collagenous fibrils.

Fig. 11-53. Part of ordinary sweat gland. Axilla. Human. E.M. X 4000. **1.** Lumen of gland.
2. Nuclei of dark (mucoid) cells. **3.** Nucleus of clear cell. **4.** Intercellular canaliculi.
5. Nucleus of longitudinally sectioned myoepithelial cell. **6.** Filamentous part of sarcoplasm. **7.** Cell processes. **8.** Basal lamina (unusually thick). **9.** Connective tissue.

Fig. 11-54. Detail of myoepithelial cell of ordinary sweat gland. Enlargement of area similar to rectangle (B) in Fig. 11-51. Axilla. Human. E.M. X 9000. **1.** Nucleus
2. Small perinuclear non-fibrillar part of sarcoplasm. **3.** Filamentous part of sarcoplasm.
4. Cell processes. **5.** Basal lamina.

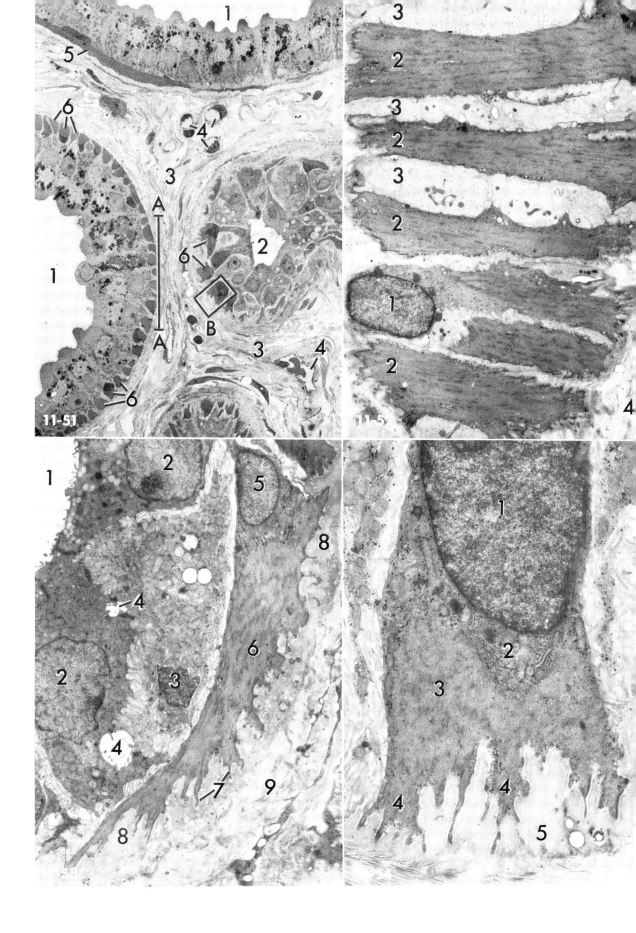

myofilaments, near the sarcoplasm, and in the conical zones at the nuclear poles. The **sarcoplasmic reticulum** (agranular) consists of smooth tubular elements. They are not in continuity with the sarcolemma, although they occur mostly near the periphery of the cell adjacent to the surface vesicles, and often surround the vesicles in a lace-like network. Some tubules are located among the myofilaments, parallel to their long axis, and in the conical areas near the nuclear poles, where they are often mixed with components of the Golgi zone. Peripheral tubules and sac-like dilatations of the sarcoplasmic reticulum form couplings with the sarcolemma and close contacts with the surface vesicles, the apposed membranes separated by gaps of about 100 Å. Regions of the sarcolemma occupied by dense bodies are devoid of sarcoplasmic reticulum.

CONNECTIVE TISSUE

Each smooth muscle fiber (cell) is surrounded by an external (basal) lamina and a thin meshwork of reticular fibrils, delicate collagenous fibrils, and elastic fibrils, forming an endomysium throughout the muscle tissue, except in regions occupied by the nexuses. Coarser connective tissue fibers separate layers and bundles of smooth muscle cells. Tendons do not occur in smooth muscle tissue.

BLOOD AND LYMPHATIC VESSELS

Both blood capillaries and lymphatic capillaries are present, but smooth muscle tissue is not as vascular as either skeletal or cardiac muscle. The blood capillaries are of the continuous, thick endothelial type with abundant micropinocytotic vesicles.

NERVES AND NERVE ENDINGS

Smooth muscle cells receive a double **motor innervation** from the autonomic nervous system: a **sympathetic** innervation from the thoracic autonomic nerves and a **parasympathetic** innervation from the cranial and pelvic autonomic nerves.

Although one set of nerves produces contraction and the other set of nerves relaxation, there are great differences in the effect of sympathetic and parasympathetic innervation on the varied sites of smooth muscle tissue. Textbooks of physiology should be consulted for a comprehensive discussion of this subject. Nerve fibers exerting an influence on the smooth muscle cells are all postganglionic and nonmyelinated. The axons form delicate branches or various terminals. The application of the nerve endings to the smooth muscle cells varies somewhat. In the ductus deferens, practically every cell receives one or several nerve endings which make membranous contact, and may even be lodged in shallow impressions of the cell surface. (Fig. 11-50) In the intestine, only very few cells receive nerve endings that make membranous contacts. The majority of smooth muscle cells in the intestine are surrounded by nerve endings, located in the endomysium at a distance from the cell that varies from 0.5 μ to several microns. In vascular smooth muscle, as a rule, no cells receive nerve endings that make membranous contacts. The nerves and their endings form a large plexus that accompanies the blood vessels at a distance of several microns from the cells of the smooth muscle media of the vessel, and only occasional nerve endings get to within a distance of 0.5 μ or less of the smooth muscle sarcolemma.

Sensory nerve endings may be present; if so, they probably serve as stretch receptors as in the tendinous organ of skeletal muscle.

MYOEPITHELIAL CELLS

Myoepithelial cells are smooth muscle cells which lie between the glandular epithelial cells and the basal lamina of the secretory alveoli (acini) of salivary glands, sweat glands, lacrimal glands, and mammary glands. They develop with the epithelial cells from the embryonic ectoderm. Because of their branching, stellate shape, and their position near the base of the alveolus they are also referred to as basket (basal) cells. They contain a single nucleus. The sarcoplasm is occupied largely by contractile filaments with dimensions and distribution similar to those of other smooth muscle cells. (Fig. 11-54) The myoepithelial cells expel the secretion from the acini to the ducts of the glands by contraction.

SMOOTH MUSCLE CONTRACTION

Smooth muscle tissue is characterized by rhythmic contraction and relaxation, processes which are spontaneous and automatic without the necessity of a neural stimulus. However, the activity of smooth muscle cells is moderated and controlled by the autonomic nervous system. Excitation-contraction impulses are conveyed by chemical transmission of neurotransmitter substances which are released from the nerve endings and reach the sarcolemma of the smooth muscle, in most cases after diffusion through the connective tissue barrier of the endomysium. The agent that ultimately controls the mechanical activity of smooth muscle fibers at the cellular level is the calcium ion. The sarcoplasmic reticulum may function as a calcium store in the process of excitation-contraction and inhibition-relaxation coupling. Calcium ions are released to the myofilaments during excitation-contraction. The release is triggered by the action potential initiated by the neurotransmitters acting at the α-receptor or β-receptor sites, but the mechanism of signal transmission between the sarcolemma and the sarcoplasmic reticulum is not known at the moment. The precise mode of interaction of thick, thin, and intermediate-size filaments is still unclear, but a process of interdigitation and sliding of thin actin filaments in relation to thick myosin filaments has been postulated. The role of the intermediate-size filaments in this process is not known. For the development of maximum tension, smooth muscle requires large percentage changes in length, and it is

believed that the sliding-interaction zone between actin and myosin is at least ten times the length of this zone in skeletal muscle.

Smooth muscle tissue has a united and integrated multicellular activity which does not depend on contact between nerve endings and muscle cells in most types of smooth muscle tissue, but rather the mode of intercellular attachment, notably the nexus. By means of this junctional specialization, excitation-contraction impulses are propagated from cell to cell in much the same way they are in cardiac muscle.

References

SKELETAL MUSCLE

Ashley, C. C. Calcium and the activation of skeletal muscle. Endeavour 30: 18–25 (1971).
Bourne, G. H. (Ed.). The Structure and Function of Muscle Vol. I: Structure. Academic Press, New York, 1960.
Franzini-Armstrong, C. Studies on the triad. I. Structure of the junction in frog twitch fibers. J. Cell Biol. 47: 488–499 (1970).
Franzini-Armstrong, C. Studies on the triad. II. Penetration of tracers into the junctional gap. J. Cell Biol. 49: 196–203 (1971).
Franzini-Armstrong, C. and Porter, K. R. The Z disc of skeletal muscle fibrils. Z. Zellforsch. 61: 661–672 (1964).
Hess, A. and Rosner, S. The satellite cell bud and myoblast in denervated mammalian muscle fibers. Am. J. Anat. 129: 21–40 (1970).
Huxley, H. E. The mechanism of muscular contraction. Sci. Amer. 213: 18–27 (1965).
Huxley, H. E. The mechanism of muscular contraction. Science 164: 1356–1366 (1969).
Huxley, H. E. and Hanson, J. Molecular basis of contraction in cross-striated muscle. In Structure and Function of Muscle (Ed. G. H. Bourne), Vol. I, pp. 183–227. Academic Press, New York, 1960.
Kelly, D. E. Models of muscle Z-band fine structure based on a looping filament configuration. J. Cell Biol. 34: 827–840 (1967).
Kelly, D. E. The fine structure of skeletal muscle triad junctions. J. Ultrastruct. Res. 29: 37–49 (1969).
Kelly, D. E. and Cahill, M. A. Filamentous and matrix components of skeletal muscle Z-disks. Anat. Rec. 172: 623–642 (1972).
Knappeis, G. G. and Carlsen, F. The ultrastructure of the Z-disc in skeletal muscle. J. Cell Biol. 13: 323–331 (1962).
Mauro, A. Satellite cell of skeletal muscle fibers. J. Biophys. Biochem. Cytol. 9: 493–495 (1961).
Porter, K. R. The sarcoplasmic reticulum. Its recent history and present status. J. Biophys. Biochem. Cytol. 10: (Suppl.) 219–226 (1961).

Rowe, R. W. Ultrastructure of the Z line of skeletal muscle fibers. J. Cell Biol. *51*: 674–685 (1971).

Schiaffino, S., Hanzlikova, V. and Pierobon, S. Relations between structure and function in rat skeletal muscle fibers. J. Cell Biol. *47*: 107–119 (1970).

Shafiq, S. A. Gorycki, M. Goldstone, L. and Milhorat, A. T. The fine structure of fiber types in normal human muscle. Anat. Rec. *156*: 283–302 (1966).

CARDIAC MUSCLE

Barr, L., Dewey, M. M. and Berger, W. Propagation of action potentials and the structure of the nexus in cardiac muscle. J. Gen. Physiol. *48*: 797–824 (1965).

Challice, C. E. Microstructure of specialized tissues in the mammalian heart. Ann. N.Y. Acad. Sci. *156*: 14–33 (1969).

DeFelice, L. J. and Challice, C. E. Anatomical and ultrastructural study of the electrophysiological atrioventricular node of the rabbit. Circulation Res. *24*: 457–474 (1969).

Fawcett, D. W. and McNutt, N. S. The ultrastructure of the cat myocardium. I. Ventricular papillary muscle. J. Cell Biol. *42*: 1–45 (1969).

Fishman, A. P. (Ed.) The Myocardium—Its Biochemistry and Biophysics. Circulation *24*: 323–548 (1961).

Hibbs, R. G. and Ferrans, V. J. An ultrastructural and histochemical study of rat atrial myocardium. Am. J. Anat. *124*: 251–280 (1969).

Jamieson, J. D. and Palade, G. E. Specific granules in atrial muscle cells. J. Cell Biol. *23*: 151–172 (1964).

Kawamura, K. and James, T. N. Comparative ultrastructure of cellular junctions in working myocardium and the conduction system under normal and pathological conditions. J. Molec. Cell Cardiol. *3*: 31–60 (1971).

Kim, S. and Baba, N. Atrioventricular node and Purkinje fibers in the guinea pig heart. Am. J. Anat. *132*: 339–354 (1971).

Leak, L. V. The ultrastructure of myofibers in a reptilian heart: the boa constrictor. Am. J. Anat. *120*: 553–582 (1967).

McNutt, N. S. and Fawcett, D. W. A comparison of the T system and sarcoplasmic reticulum in atrial and ventricular heart muscle. J. Cell Biol. *35*: 90A (1967).

McNutt, N. S. and Fawcett, D. W. The ultrastructure of the cat myocardium. II. Atrial muscle. J. Cell Biol. *42*: 46–67 (1969).

McNutt, N. S. and Weinstein, R. S. The ultrastructure of the nexus. A correlated thin-section and freeze-cleavage study. J. Cell Biol. *47*: 666–688 (1970).

Simpson, F. O. and Rayns, D. G. The relationship between the transverse tubular system and other tubules at the Z disc levels of myocardial cells in the ferret. Am. J. Anat. *122*: 193–208 (1968).

Simpson, F. O. and Oertelis, S. J. The fine structure of sheep myocardial cells: sarcolemmal invaginations and the transverse tubular system. J. Cell Biol. *12*: 91–100 (1962).

Sjöstrand, F. S., Andersson-Cedergren, E. and Dewey, M. M. The ultrastructure of the intercalated discs of frog, mouse and guinea pig cardiac muscle. J. Ultrastruct. Res. *1*: 271–287 (1958).

Sommer, J. R. and Johnson, E. A. A comparative study of Purkinje fibers and ventricular fibers. J. Cell Biol. *36*: 497–526 (1968).

Sonnenblick, E. H. Correlation of myocardial structure and function. Circulation *38*: 29–44 (1968).

Sperelakis, N., Rubio, R. and Radnick, J. Sharp discontinuity in sarcomere lengths across intercalated disks of fibrillating cat hearts. J. Ultrastruct. Res. *30*: 503–532 (1970).

Stenger, R. J. and Spiro, D. The ultrastructure of mammalian cardiac muscle. J. Biophys. Biochem. Cytol. *9*: 325–353 (1961).

Thaemert, J. C. Atrioventricular node innervation in ultrastructural three dimensions. Am. J. Anat. *128*: 239–264 (1970).

Thaemert, J. C. Fine structure of the atrioventricular node as viewed in serial sections. Am. J. Anat. *136*: 43–66 (1973).

SMOOTH MUSCLE

Bo, W. J., Odor, D. L. and Rothrock, M. L. Ultrastructure of uterine smooth muscle following progesterone or progesterone-estrogen treatment. Anat. Rec. *163*: 121–132 (1969).

Cobb, J. L. S. and Bennett, T. A study of nexuses in visceral smooth muscle. J. Cell Biol. *41*: 287–297 (1969).

Cooke, P. H. and Fay, F. S. Correlation between fiber length, ultrastructure, and the length-tension relationship of mammalian smooth muscle. J. Cell Biol. *52*: 105–116 (1971).

Dewey, M. M. and Barr, L. A study of the structure and distribution of the nexus. J. Cell Biol. *23*: 553–585 (1964).

Devine, C. E. and Somlyo, A. P. Thick filaments in vascular smooth muscle. J. Cell Biol. *49*: 636–649 (1971).

Devine, C. E., Somlyo, A. V. and Somlyo, A. P. Sarcoplasmic reticulum and excitation-contraction in mammalian smooth muscles. J. Cell Biol. *52*: 690–718 (1972).

Fay, F. S. and Cooke, P. H. Reversible disaggregation of myofilaments in vertebrate smooth muscle. J. Cell Biol. *56*: 399–411 (1973).

Goldstein, D. J. On the origin and morphology of myoepithelial cells of apocrine sweat glands. J. Investig. Dermatol. *37*: 301–309 (1961).

Kelly, R. E. and Arnold, J. W. Myofilaments of the pupillary muscles of the iris fixed in situ. J. Ultrastruct. Res. *40*: 532–545 (1972).

Kelly, R. E. and Rice, R. V. Localization of myosin filaments in smooth muscle. J. Cell Biol. *37*: 105–116 (1968).

Kelly, R. E. and Rice, R. V. Ultrastructural studies on the contractile mechanism of smooth muscle. J. Cell Biol. *42*: 683–694 (1969).

Leeson, C. R. The electron microscopy of the myoepithelium in the rat exorbital lacrimal gland. Anat. Rec. *137*: 45–56 (1960).

Merrillees, N. C. R. The nervous environment of individual smooth muscle cells of the guinea pig vas deferens. J. Cell Biol. *37*: 794–317 (1968).

Nonomura, Y. Myofilaments in smooth muscle of guinea pig taenia coli. J. Cell Biol. *39*: 741–745 (1968).

Panner, B. J. and Honig, C. R. Filament ultrastructure and organization in vertebrate smooth muscle. Contraction hypothesis based on localization of actin and myosin. J. Cell Biol. *35*: 303–321 (1967).

Panner, B. J. and Honig, C. R. Locus and state of aggregation of myosin in tissue sections of vertebrate smooth muscle. J. Cell Biol. *44*: 52–61 (1970).

Rice, R. V., Moses, J. A., McManus, G. M., Brady, A. C. and Blasik, L. M. The organization of contractile filaments in mammalian smooth muscle. J. Cell Biol. *47*: 183–196 (1970).

Richardson, K. C. The fine structure of autonomic nerve endings in smooth muscle of the rat vas deferens. J. Anat. Lond. *96*: 427–442 (1962).

Rhodin, J. A. G. Fine structure of vascular walls in mammals with special reference to smooth muscle component. Physiol. Rev. *42* (Suppl.): 48–81 (1962).

Somlyo, A. P. and Somlyo, A. V. Vascular smooth muscle. I. Normal structure, pathology, biochemistry and biophysics. Pharmacol. Rev. *20*: 197–272 (1968).

Somlyo, A. P., Devine, C. E., Somlyo, A. V. and North, S. R. Sarcoplasmic reticulum and the temperature-dependent contraction of smooth muscle in calcium-free solutions. J. Cell Biol. *51*: 722–741 (1971).

Tandler, B. Ultrastructure of the human submaxillary gland. III. Myoepithelium. Z. Zellforsch. *68*: 852–863 (1965).

Uehara, Y. and Burnstock, G. Postsynaptic specialization of smooth muscle at close neuromuscular junctions in the guinea pig sphincter pupillae. J. Cell Biol. *53*: 849–853 (1972).

Uehara, Y., Campbell, G. R. and Burnstock, G. Cytoplasmic filaments in developing and adult vertebrate smooth muscle. J. Cell Biol. *50*: 484–497 (1971).

12 Nervous system—organization

GENERAL CONSIDERATIONS

The nervous system consists of many **nerve cells** provided with a number of cell processes of varied lengths and diameters, the **axons** and the **dendrites.** The axons conduct signals over considerable distances, whereas the dendrites are ramified elaborate extensions of the cell body and assist the latter in collecting impulses. Each nerve cell has a **nucleus** surrounded by a cytoplasmic mass, the **perikaryon.** The nerve cell and its processes form the **neuron,** which constitutes the functional and anatomical unit of the nervous system. Neurons are connected by **synapses,** membranous contacts where axons of one neuron touch the cell membrane of other neurons. The synapses establish a multitude of pathways in the nervous system and connect all parts of the body with the nervous system.

In addition to neurons the nervous system contains specialized **neuroglial cells** which are intimately related to and surround the perikarya and cell processes in a very special way. **Blood vessels** form an integral part of the nervous system. The vascular channels are accompanied by connective tissue, but otherwise extensive accumulations of connective tissue fibers and fibroblasts or other connective tissue cell types are lacking within the nervous system.

The different parts of the nervous system may be classified according to their function. **Anatomically,** the nervous system is made up of the central nervous system (CNS) and the peripheral nervous system (PNS).

The **CNS** consists of the **brain** and the **spinal cord,** whereas the **PNS** is formed by the **cranial** and the **spinal nerves,** as well as by the **spinal** and **autonomic ganglia.**

Functionally, the nervous system is divided into a somatic (cerebrospinal, largely voluntary) system and a visceral (autonomic, largely involuntary) system. The **somatic system** comprises appropriate parts of the CNS, the cranial and

spinal ganglia, and the nerves to the skin and skeletal muscles. The **visceral system** consists of certain parts of the CNS, the autonomic ganglia, and the nerves to smooth muscle cells, cardiac muscle cells, and glands.

DISTRIBUTION OF NEURAL ELEMENTS

Nerve cells are aggregated in certain parts of the nervous system and the nerve processes in others, but a mixture of the two components occurs in many locations. The **nerve cells** (nucleus and perikaryon) are extremely numerous in the gray matter of the brain and spinal cord and in the spinal and sympathetic ganglia. They also occur in small groups as parasympathetic ganglia in locations such as the intestinal wall, the myocardium, and the conducting portion of the respiratory tract. The **nerve fibers** (axons) dominate the white

Fig. 12-1. Principal disposition of neurons in the central and peripheral nervous system. Arrows indicate direction of nerve impulses. **1.** Rectangle: central nervous system (brain and spinal cord). **2.** Peripheral nervous system (outside rectangle). **3.** Sense organ. **4.** Pseudo-unipolar nerve cell in sensory ganglion. **5.** Nerve cells in spinal cord and brain. **6.** Motor nerve cells. **7.** Skeletal muscle. **8.** Multipolar nerve cells in autonomic ganglion. **9.** Viscera (non-skeletal muscle and glands). **10.** Synapses.

Fig. 12-2. Purkinje nerve cell, made visible by gold impregnation technique. Cerebellum. Cat. L.M. X 450. **1.** Axon. **2.** Perikaryon (nucleus obliterated by impregnation technique). **3.** Dendrites. **4.** Dendritic arborization.

Fig. 12-3. Motor neuron. Anterior horn. Spinal cord. Gold chloride. Cat. L.M. X 800. **1.** Nucleus. **2.** Perikaryon with neurofilamentous network. **3.** Axon hillock. **4.** Axon. **5.** Dendrites. **6.** Artificial perineuronal shrinkage space. **1.** Neuropil with network of axons and dendrites.

Fig. 12-4. Pseudo-unipolar nerve cells. Spinal (sensory) ganglion. Cat. E.M. X 880. **1.** Nucleus of large nerve cell. **2.** Nucleus of small nerve cell. **3.** Perikaryon. **4.** Nuclei of satellite cells. **5.** Nucleus of Schwann cell. **6.** Myelinated nerve processes. **7.** Capsule cells.

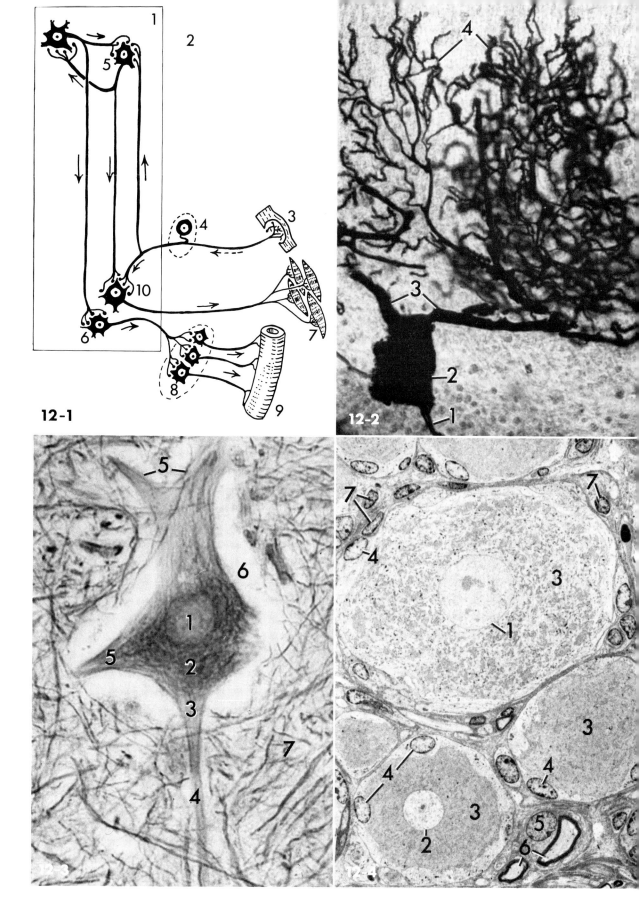

12-1

12-2

12-3

12-4

matter of the brain and spinal cord as fiber tracts and they alone make up the peripheral nerves.

At the level of sense organs and **afferent nerve endings** a stimulus is transformed into a nervous impulse which travels in the peripheral process of a spinal ganglion cell (in a **peripheral spinal nerve**) indicated by the broken arrow in Fig. 12-1. The impulse continues via the central process of the cell and enters (as the dorsal root of the spinal nerve) the spinal cord. The impulse undergoes dispersal by numerous collateral branches within the CNS and reaches many levels of cord and brain. A fantastic number of synaptic links form highly complex circuits which initiate and govern **integration** of reflexes, sensation, volition, memory storage, regulation of fundamental vital activities, and emotive functions. Finally, certain **motor cells** are singled out for carrying out responses. A **somatic efferent** neuron does it via the **ventral root** by means of its axon which contacts a number of muscle cells with its collaterals. A **visceral efferent** neuron sends its axon, also via the **ventral root,** to an **autonomic ganglion.** Here the axon branches and contacts synaptically several autonomic ganglion cells which send their axons to visceral target areas.

STAINING CHARACTERISTICS

The structural and ultrastructural details of nerve cells, nerve processes, and non-neural structures can be visualized simultaneously only with the electron microscope. They are described in Chapters 13 (p. 272), 14 (p. 294), and 15 (p. 314). However, before studying these details, it is necessary to be familiar with the different histological stains and their selectivity with reference to the nervous tissue. Most important is the realization that there exists no histological stain which will bring out simultaneously nerve cells, nerve processes, and neuroglial cells. Electron microscopical techniques bring out all these details (Fig. 12-4), but the depth of the observed field is limited by the short

focal depth of the electron beam and the extreme thinness of the section.

Nerve processes. A large number of nerve cell processes in both the central and peripheral nervous systems are surrounded by **myelin sheaths,** a phospho-lipid material (p. 286) which appears **white** in the living tissue. The white myelin therefore contributes to the color of the white matter of the central nervous system and the white glistening appearance of the peripheral nerves. The myelin sheaths stain **black** with osmic acid impregnation, **deep blue** with Klüver-Barrera staining method, and **blue-black** with Weigert's stain. In these preparations, the white matter appears dark, and the gray matter appears light. In sections impregnated with heavy metals, usually silver and gold (Figs. 12-2 and 12-3) according to methods described by Golgi, Cajal, Bodian, and others, nerve cell processes and terminals appear dark, nuclei and perikarya in less intense shades of rose or gold; but myelin sheaths do not accept the impregnation.

Figs. 12-5 & 12-6. *Frontal section through the cerebral hemispheres, thalami, and ventral pons.*

Fig. 12-5 is stained with cresyl-violet, showing nerve cells dark, and nerve processes light.

Fig. 12-6 is stained with the Weigert method, showing nerve cells light and myelinated nerve processes black. Human. X 1.4. **1.** Parietal lobe. **2.** Lateral fissure. **3.** Temporal lobe. **4.** Insula. **5.** Pons. **6.** Cerebral peduncle. **7.** Thalamus. **8.** Internal capsule. **9.** Lateral ventricle. **10.** Corpus callosum. **11.** Longitudinal cerebral fissure.

Fig. 12-7. Cerebral (temporal) cortex. Enlargement of area similar to rectangle in Fig. 12-5. Human. L.M. X 40. **1.** Surface of brain. **2.** Molecular layer of cortex (layer I). **3.** Cortex (nerve cell layers II–VI). **4.** Medulla (white matter).

Fig. 12-8. Detail of cerebral cortex (gray matter). Enlargement of area similar to rectangle in Fig. 12-7, corresponding to approximately nerve cell layers III–IV. Human. L.M. X 385. **1.** Pyramidal nerve cells of layer III. **2.** Stellate-shaped (granule) cells of layer IV. **3.** Neuroglial cells.

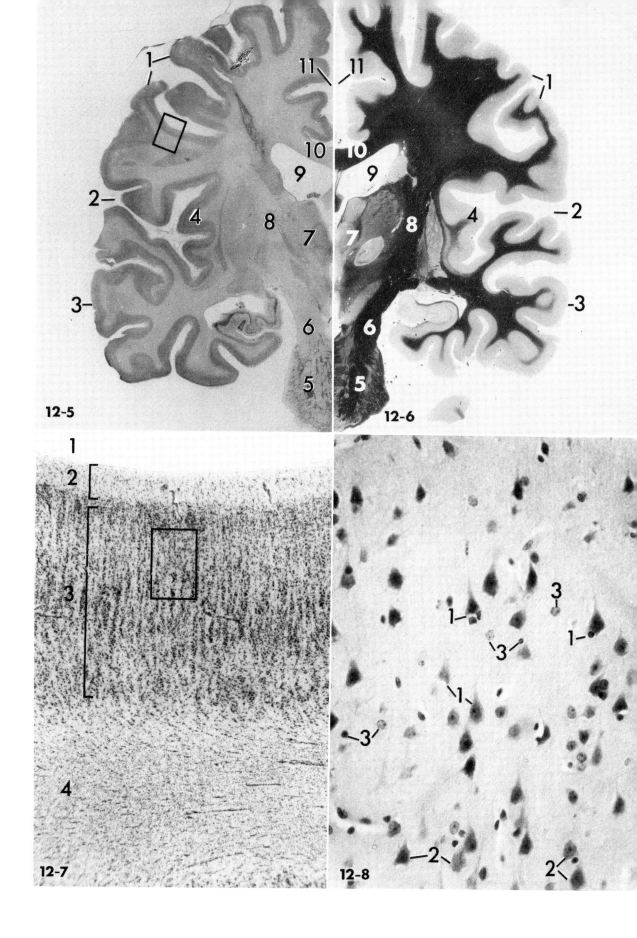

12-5

12-6

12-7

12-8

Nerve cells. Common histological staining methods such as hematoxylin and eosin, or basic dyes such as toluidine blue, cresyl-violet, or thionine, bring out the granular endoplasmic reticulum (Nissl substance), chromatin, and other cell components, but not the cell bodies of neuroglia. Therefore, the gray matter of the brain and spinal cord appears blue or violet, the white matter very pale. (Fig. 12-5)

Neuroglial cells. Neuroglial cells and their varied types of cell processes are visible in sections impregnated with silver and gold (methods according to Golgi and Rio Hortega), but the techniques are difficult and the results quite variable.

Arrangement of Nervous Tissue

For the purpose of orientation, here follows a short survey of the basic patterns of organization in the major parts of the nervous system. For a comprehensive coverage, the student is referred to textbooks of neuroanatomy.

BRAIN

The brain consists of telencephalon (2 cerebral hemispheres, the cerebellum, and the brain stem), diencephalon, midbrain, pons, and medulla oblongata. The most superficial part of the telencephalon and cerebellum, the **cortex**, is occupied by gray matter (Figs. 12-5, 12-6), whereas the central region of these areas of the brain, the **medulla**, contains white matter, made up of numerous fiber tracts, in which are lodged clusters of nerve cells (nuclei) such as the basal ganglia (telencephalon) and the internal nuclei (cerebellum). The diencephalon, midbrain, pons, and medulla oblongata lack a cortex but have numerous fiber tracts and many nuclei such as thalamus (diencephalon) and nuclei of the cranial nerves: midbrain (nerves III and IV); pons (nerves V, VI, and VII); medulla oblongata (nerves VIII, IX, X, XI, and XII).

Cerebral cortex. The nerve cells which form the gray matter of the cerebral cortex are arranged in six more or less distinctive, ill-defined layers, parallel to the surface of the cortical convolutions. (Fig. 12-7) Only the phylogenetically oldest areas have fewer layers, whilst subdivision into more than six layers has been recognized in certain other cortical fields. The nerve cells vary greatly in size. The largest are referred to as **pyramidal cells** (Fig. 12-8) and are especially numerous in the fifth layer (counted from the surface) of the motor area. Smaller pyramidal nerve cells form the third layer, whereas small polymorphous (stellate, fusiform, granule) cells dominate the second and the sixth layers. The most superficial, plexiform or molecular, layer is formed by a network of fine dendrites (neuropil) and few if any nerve cells.

Cerebellar cortex. The cerebellar cortex (Figs. 12-9, 12-10) is divisible into two layers, both of considerable depth: an inner granular (nuclear) and an outer molecular (plexiform) layer. Between these two layers is a single layer of thinly spaced, large conspicuous nerve cells, the **Purkinje cells.** The

Fig. 12-9. Horizontal section of the cerebellum. Section stained with the Weigert method; myelinated nerve processes black. Human. L.M. X 1.1. **1.** Vermis of cerebellum. **2.** Cerebellar hemispheres.

Fig. 12-10. Cerebellar folia. Enlargement of area similar to rectangle in Fig. 12-9. Weigert staining method. Human. L.M. X 7.3. **1.** Folia. **2.** Sulci. **3.** Cerebellar cortex (gray matter). **4.** Cerebellar medulla (white matter).

Fig. 12-11. Cerebellar folium. Enlargement of area similar to rectangle in Fig. 12-10. Weigert staining method. Human. L.M. X 69. **1.** Interfoliary sulcus. **2.** Molecular layer of cerebellar cortex. **3.** Purkinje cell layer. **4.** Granule cell layer. **5.** White matter of folium (myelinated nerve processes).

Fig. 12-12. Detail of cerebellar cortex. Enlargement of area similar to rectangle in Fig. 12-11. Human. L.M. X 770. **1.** Nerve cells (basket cells). **2.** Purkinje nerve cells. **3.** Nuclei of granule cells. **4.** Golgi type II nerve cell. **5.** Nuclei of neuroglial cell.

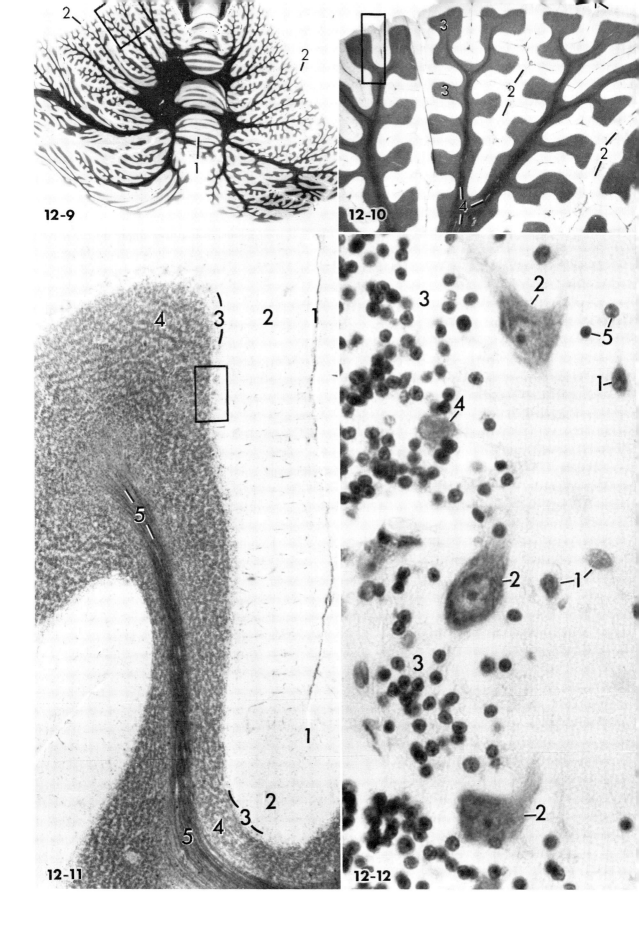

12-9

12-10

12-11

12-12

outer molecular layer consists of small cortical nerve cells, large cortical (basket) nerve cells, and a network of dendrites (neuropil). The inner granular layer is formed by a multitude of densely packed granule cells and some stellate nerve cells. (Figs. 12-11, 12-12)

MEDULLA OF TELENCEPHALON
AND CEREBELLUM

The white matter (or the medulla) is composed of bands and bundles of nerve fibers which radiate to and from the cortex or curve from one cortical area to another. These fibers are either myelinated or nonmyelinated and display great variations in caliber. They are grouped to form major pathways of ascending and descending fiber tracts. The nerve cells of the basal ganglia, the internal nuclei of the cerebellum, and the nuclei of the brain stem are small, medium, or large size polymorphic cells. They often contain pigments and iron granules, as in the substantia nigra of the midbrain. Both the cortex and medulla of the brain contain abundant neuroglial cells.

SPINAL CORD

The spinal cord consists of a central mass of gray matter surrounded by a layer of myelinated and non-myelinated nerve fibers, the white matter. In cross section the gray matter resembles the letter H: two lateral columns, each with a broad **anterior horn** (column) and a narrow **posterior horn** (column) united by the **central** (gray) commissure. (Figs. 12-13, 12-14) In addition, **lateral horns** (columns) are present in the thoracic and the two first lumbar segments of the spinal cord. The cross-sectional diameter of the cord, the profile of the central gray matter, and the thickness of the peripheral layer of white matter vary according to the segmental level of the cord.

The **anterior horns** contain (Fig. 12-15) large nerve cells (motor neurons) which send axons via the ventral spinal roots to skeletal muscles of corresponding somatic

segments, terminating in motor end plates. The **posterior horns** contain small nerve cells which receive afferent impulses from the sensory nerve cells of the spinal ganglion cells via the dorsal spinal roots. The cells of the posterior horns relay the impulses to upper or lower segments of the spinal cord either on the same side (ipsilaterally) or on the opposite side (contralaterally); in the latter case they cross over in the central commissure. The **lateral horns** have intermediate size nerve cells which send their axons to autonomic ganglia.

The peripheral white matter of the

Fig. 12-13. Cross section through the spinal cord. Lumbar segment (L5). Weigert staining method; myelinated nerve processes black. Human. L.M. X 8.8. **1.** Dorsal root. **2.** Dorsal median septum. **3.** Dorsal funiculus (white matter). **4.** Posterior horn (gray matter). **5.** Lateral funiculus. **6.** Anterior horn. **7.** Gray commissure. **8.** Ventral median fissure. **9.** Anterior funiculus. **10.** Ventral roots.

Fig. 12-14. Enlargement of rectangle in Fig. 12-13. L.M. X 26. **1.** Columns of white matter (myelinated nerve processes). **2.** Motor neurons in anterior horn of gray matter. **3.** Myelinated and non-myelinated nerve processes form an irregular loose network in the gray matter of the spinal cord.

Fig. 12-15. Motor neuron. Anterior horn. Spinal cord. Thoracic segment. Enlargement of area similar to rectangle (A) in Fig. 12-14. Rat. E.M. X 780. **1.** Nucleus of motor neuron. **2.** Perikaryon. **3.** Dendrites. **4.** Axon. **5.** Network of myelinated and non-myelinated nerve processes. **6.** Lumen of capillary. This neuron is enlarged further in Fig. 13-1.

Fig. 12-16. Cross section of anterior funiculus. Spinal cord. Thoracic segment. Enlargement of area similar to rectangle (B) in Fig. 12-14. Rat. E.M. X 640. **1.** Motor neuron in anterior horn of gray matter. **2.** Myelinated nerve processes of varied diameters; arranged in parallel, make up the columns of white matter of the spinal cord. **3.** Lumen of capillary. **4.** Myelinated nerve processes (axons) traversing the white column on their way to the ventral root of the spinal nerve. **5.** Nuclei of neuroglial cells. Further enlargements of this area are seen in Figs. 13-9 and 13-10.

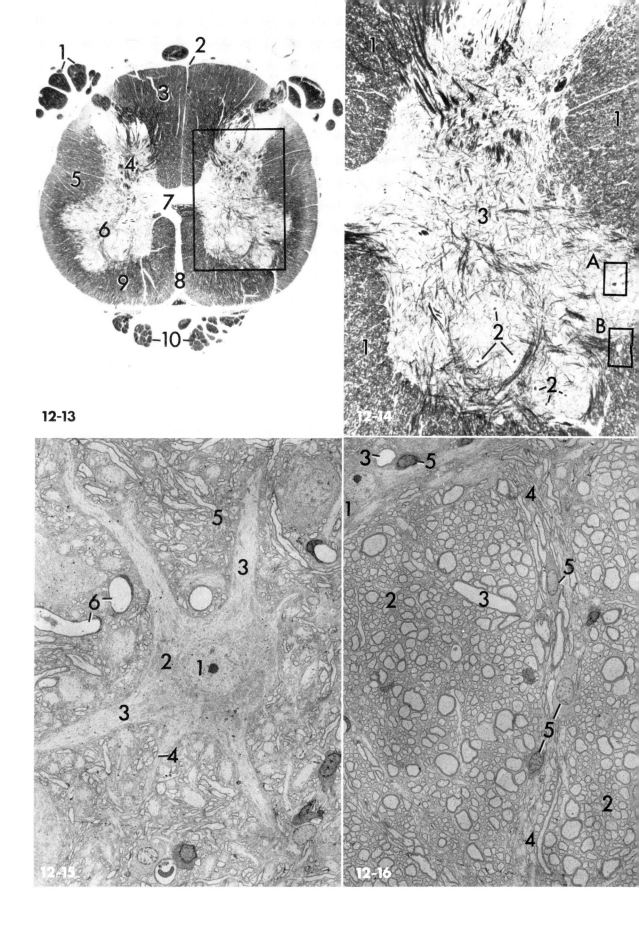

12-13

12-14

12-15

12-16

spinal cord is divided into several longitudinal columns containing ascending and descending fiber tracts. (Fig. 12-16)

PERIPHERAL NERVES

Peripheral nerves are formed by bundles of nerve fibers (Figs. 12-17, 12-20) which originate from nerve cells in the anterior horns of the gray matter of the spinal cord, and in the spinal ganglia. The term **nerve fiber** applies to long nerve cell processes. The peripheral nerve contains myelinated and non-myelinated nerve fibers of varied cross-sectional diameters. (Figs. 12-18, 12-19). Furthermore, in all peripheral nerves, afferent (sensory) and efferent (motor) nerve fibers are intermingled and structurally indistinguishable. The spinal roots are exceptions to this rule, since the dorsal roots contain only afferent nerve fibers, and the ventral roots only efferent nerve fibers. The dorsal and ventral roots unite in the intervertebral foramen to form a **mixed spinal nerve.** The spinal nerves supply segmentally the body wall with mixed (sensory and motor) peripheral nerves. The twelve cranial nerves arise from the brain stem and show a rather rudimentary segmentation. Four of them are mixed nerves.

The peripheral nerves do not contain perikarya of nerve cells. The majority of cell nuclei present in the peripheral nerves belong to Schwann cells (p. 284) which cover the nerve processes, arranged side by side along the processes. The adjoining ends of Schwann cells are slightly constricted. These areas are called **nodes of Ranvier.** (Figs. 12-21 and 12-22) The Schwann cell cytoplasm forms the multilayered **myelin sheath.** The peripheral part of the Schwann cell is traditionally referred to as **neurolemma.** The Schwann cell is surrounded by a small quantity of loose connective tissue, the **endoneurium.** The fibroblast nuclei of this sheath make up a minority of nuclei seen in the peripheral nerves. Individual nerve fibers are grouped to form **nerve fascicles,** surrounded by a sheath of dense connective

tissue, the **perineurium.** The entire peripheral nerve (trunk) is covered by loose connective tissue, the **epineurium.**

NERVE GANGLIA

Groups of nerve cells are located outside of the CNS, forming ganglia. There are two kinds: sensory ganglia and autonomic ganglia.

Sensory ganglia. To this group belong the spinal (dorsal root) ganglia (Figs. 12-23, 12-24) and the ganglia associated with afferent nerve fibers of the cranial nerves. The **spinal ganglia** are located in the intervertebral foramina. The sensory **ganglion cells** which make up these dorsal

Fig. 12-17. Peripheral nerve. Cross section. Sciatic nerve. Human. L.M. X 27. **1.** Bundles of nerve fibers (nerve fascicles). **2.** Loose connective tissue (epineurium). **3.** Perineurium. **4.** Blood vessels.

Fig. 12-18. Bundle of nerve fibers. Cross section. Enlargement of area similar to rectangle in Fig. 12-17. Specimen fixed by osmium tetroxide. Monkey. L.M. X 220. **1.** Perineurium. **2.** Myelin sheaths show up as black rings. **3.** Nerve processes, largely unstained.

Fig. 12-19. Bundle of nerve fibers. Cross section. Enlargement of area similar to rectangle in Fig. 12-18. Rat. E.M. X 640. **1.** Perineurium. **2.** Myelin sheaths. **3.** Nerve processes. **4.** Schwann cells (neurolemma). **5.** Lumen of blood vessels. **6.** Endoneurium. Further enlargement of this area is seen in Fig. 13-18.

Fig. 12-20. Peripheral nerves. Longitudinal section. Sciatic nerve. Human. L.M. X 28. **1.** Bundles of nerve fibers. There is a great resemblance to tendons at this magnification. **2.** Epineurium. **3.** Perineurium.

Fig. 12-21. Bundle of nerve fibers. Longitudinal section. Specimen fixed by osmium tetroxide. Enlargement of area similar to rectangle in Fig. 12-20. Monkey. L.M. X 400. **1.** Myelin sheaths. **2.** Nodes of Ranvier. **3.** Schmidt-Lanterman's incisure.

Fig. 12-22. Bundle of nerve fibers. Longitudinal section. Enlargement of area similar to rectangle in Fig. 12-21. Rat. E.M. X 580. **1.** Myelin sheaths. **2.** Nerve processes. **3.** Node of Ranvier. **4.** Schmidt-Lanterman's incisure. **5.** Schwann cell (neurolemma). **6.** Blood vessel. Further enlargements of this area are seen in Figs. 13-20 to 13-24.

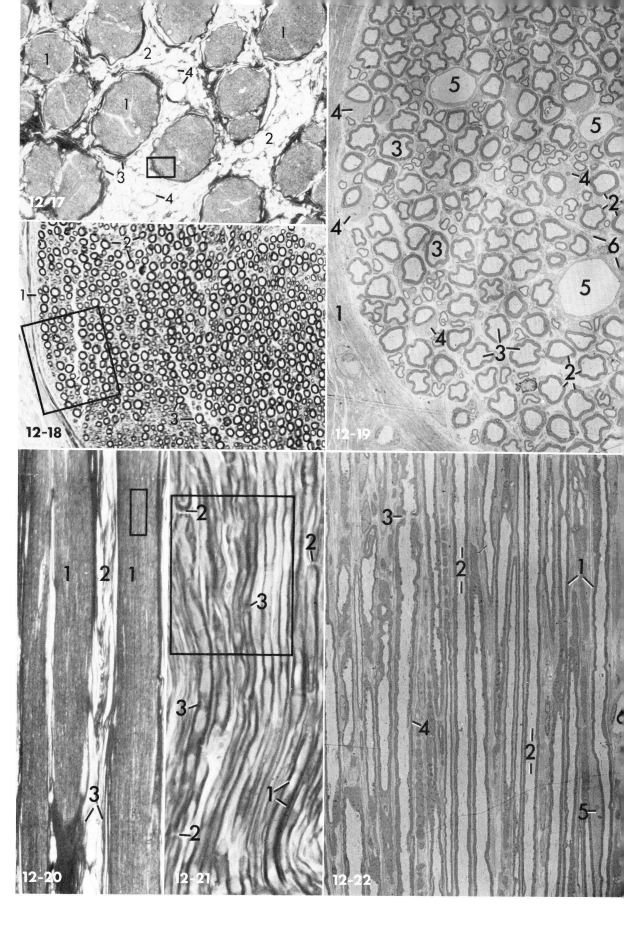

root ganglia receive afferent impulses through very long peripheral nerve fibers which conduct toward the cell as "peripheral processes." These fibers have the physiological and histological features of axons but have often been classified among dendrites because of the cellulopetal direction of the impulses they conduct. Having passed the cell, the impulses travel in "central processes" via the dorsal root of the spinal nerve to neurons in the CNS. The **ganglia** of the **cranial nerves** include the **trigeminal** (Gasserian) **ganglion,** which has a large sensory root and a minor motor root for the trigeminal nerve (V); the **geniculate ganglion** which is the sensory ganglion of the facial nerve (VII); the **spiral ganglion** of the cochlea and the **vestibular ganglion,** both part of the acoustic nerve (VIII); the **superior** and **inferior ganglia** of the glossopharyngeal nerve (IX); and the superior and inferior ganglia of the vagus (X) (formerly jugular and nodose ganglia).

Autonomic ganglia. To this group belong sympathetic and parasympathetic ganglia. The **sympathetic ganglia** occur as sympathetic chain ganglia and as collateral ganglia. (Figs. 12-27, 12-28) They both represent **peripheral motor ganglia** and contain cell bodies of nerve cells, the processes of which convey impulses to smooth muscle cells, myocardium, and various glands throughout the body. Preganglionic nerve fibers arise in the lateral horns of the spinal cord (Th1—L2) and make synaptic contacts with the ganglion cells in the sympathetic ganglia. Postganglionic nerve fibers emerge from the ganglia seeking out smooth muscle cells, myocardium, and glands. The **sympathetic chain ganglia** form a bilateral, segmental series which extends from the skull to the coccyx along the lateral aspect of the vertebral column. The **collateral ganglia** consist of the celiac ganglia, aorticorenal ganglia, superior and inferior mesenteric ganglia. These ganglia are non-segmental and located in the midline in front of the spine.

The **parasympathetic ganglia** are scat-

tered throughout the body, and are always located in or near the organs they innervate. They are known by their anatomical names, such as ciliary ganglion, otic ganglion, pterygopalatine ganglion, submandibular ganglion, and the small peripheral ganglia in all viscera of the neck, thorax, and abdomen. (Fig. 29-41) The parasympathetic ganglia contain cell bodies of nerve cells, the postganglionic nerve processes of which convey impulses to smooth muscle cells, myocardium, and glands. Their influence on these structures opposes that exerted by the sympathetic nerve fibers. Preganglionic nerve fibers arise with the cranial nerves oculomotor (III), facial (VII), glossopharyngeal (IX), and vagus (X), and with the spinal nerves S2, S3, and S4.

Autonomic Nervous System

The autonomic or visceral nervous system consists of: 1) appropriate parts of the central nervous system; 2) autonomic gan-

Fig. 12-23. Spinal (dorsal) root ganglion. Human. L.M. X 17. **1.** Spinal (sensory) ganglion.
2. Dorsal nerve root. **3.** Ventral nerve root.
4. Connective tissue capsule.
Fig. 12-24. Spinal root ganglion. Enlargement of area similar to rectangle in Fig. 12-23. Cat. L.M. X 110. **1.** Connective tissue capsule.
2. Nerve cells. **3.** Myelinated nerve processes.
Fig. 12-25. Pseudo-unipolar nerve cells. Spinal ganglion. Enlargement of area similar to rectangle in Fig. 12-24. Cat. E.M. X 600.
1. Large spinal ganglion cell. **2.** Small spinal ganglion cell. **3.** Myelinated nerve processes.
4. Connective tissue elements.
Fig. 12-26. Pseudo-unipolar (sensory) ganglion cell. Spinal root ganglion. Cat. E.M. X 2400.
1. Nucleus of ganglion cell. **2.** Nucleolus.
3. Perikaryon. Note: origin of single nerve process of this pseudo-unipolar cell is not in the plane of section. **4.** Nucleus of satellite cell. **5.** Cytoplasm of satellite cells.
6. Nucleus of Schwann cell. **7.** Nerve processes surrounded by cytoplasm of Schwann cell. **8.** Myelinated nerve processes.
9. Nuclei of capsule cells. **10.** Lumen of capillary with erythrocytes.

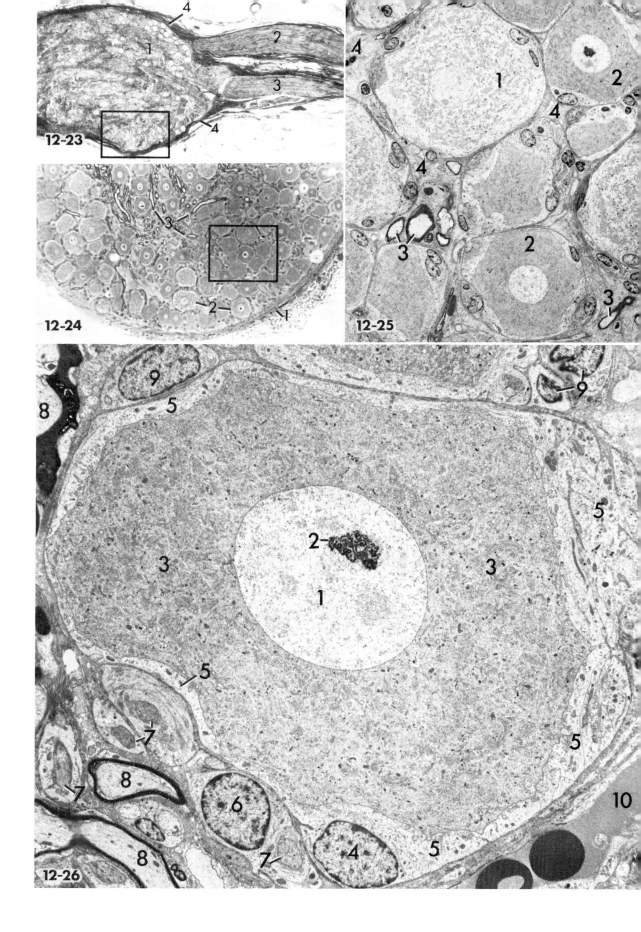

12-23

12-24

12-25

12-26

glia (sympathetic and parasympathetic); 3) preganglionic nerve fibers (which connect the CNS with the autonomic ganglia); and 4) postganglionic nerve fibers (which connect the autonomic ganglia with the effector organs).

Almost all organs receive both sympathetic and parasympathetic innervation. The two systems are usually antagonistic. For a review of the specific actions of the sympathetic and the parasympathetic nervous systems on each organ, consult textbooks of neuroanatomy and physiology.

SYMPATHETIC NERVOUS SYSTEM

The **preganglionic** nerve fibers arise from nerve cells in the lateral horns of the spinal cord (Th 1–L 2). They leave the cord via the anterior roots and white rami communicantes. Preganglionic fibers, which innervate vascular smooth muscle, glands of body walls, and viscera of head and neck, synapse in the sympathetic chain ganglia. Preganglionic fibers, which innervate the viscera of the abdomen, pass through the chain ganglia and reach as splanchnic nerves the sympathetic collateral ganglia, where they synapse.

The **postganglionic** nerve fibers from the sympathetic chain ganglia leave as gray rami communicantes and rejoin the spinal nerves to reach the periphery. In the head they follow a less regular course and partly accompany arteries. The postganglionic nerve fibers from the sympathetic collateral ganglia reach the viscera directly by their association with arteries.

PARASYMPATHETIC NERVOUS SYSTEM

The **preganglionic** nerve fibers arise from neurons in the visceral nuclei of the following cranial nerves: oculomotor (III; Edinger-Westphal's nucleus); facial (VII; superior salivatory nucleus); glossopharyngeal (IX; inferior salivatory nucleus); and vagus (X; dorsal motor nucleus). Fibers also arise with the spinal nerves S 2, S 3, and S 4. In both instances, these fibers first accompany their parent nerves. Subsequently they may accompany perivascular sympathetic nerves, or they proceed as bundles of their own to seek out the parasympathetic ganglia in or near the wall of the organs where they synapse.

The **postganglionic** nerve fibers are short and travel only a few millimeters to reach the effector organs.

References

Babel, J. Ultrastructure of the Peripheral Nervous System. C. V. Mosby, St. Louis, 1970.

Barr, M. L. The Human Nervous System. Harper & Row, New York, 1972.

Bourne, G. H. (Ed.). The Structure and Function of Nervous Tissue. Vol. 1: Structure I. Academic Press, New York, 1968.

Everett, N. B. Functional Neuroanatomy. Lea & Febiger, Philadelphia, 1971.

Ford, D. H. and Schade, J. P. Atlas of Human Brain. Elsevier, Amsterdam, 1966.

Klüver, H. and Barrera, E. A method for the combined staining of cells and fibers in the nervous system. J. Neuropath. & Exper. Neurol. *12*: 400–403 (1953).

Noback, C. The Human Nervous System. McGraw-Hill, New York, 1967.

Rexed, B. A cytoarchitectonic atlas of the spinal cord in the cat. J. Comp. Neurol. *100*: 297–380 (1954).

Rodahl, K. and Issekutz, D. (Eds.). Nerve as a Tissue. Harper & Row, New York, 1966.

Truex, R. C. and Carpenter, M. B. Strong and Elwyn's Human Neuroanatomy. Williams & Wilkins, Baltimore, 1969.

Willis, W. D., Jr. and Grossman, R. G. Medical Neurobiology. Neuroanatomical and neurophysiological principles basic to clinical neuroscience. C. V. Mosby, St. Louis, 1973.

Fig. 12-27. Sympathetic ganglion. Thorax. Human. L.M. X 15.5. **1.** Sympathetic (motor) ganglion. **2.** Bundle of visceral nerve fibers. **3.** Connective tissue capsule.

Fig. 12-28. Sympathetic ganglion. Human. L.M. X 290. **1.** Nerve cells. **2.** Satellite cells. **3.** Non-myelinated nerve fibers. **4.** Loose connective tissue.

Fig. 12-29. Multipolar nerve cells. Sympathetic ganglion. Abdomen. Cat. E.M. X 600. **1.** Ganglion cells. **2.** Binucleate ganglion cell. **3.** Non-myelinated nerve fibers. **4.** Connective tissue elements.

Fig. 12-30. Multipolar sympathetic (motor) ganglion cell. Sympathetic ganglion. Abdomen. Cat. E.M. X 4600. **1.** Nucleus of ganglion cell. **2.** Nucleolus. **3.** Perikaryon. **4.** Cell process, presumably axon. **5.** Nucleus of satellite cells. **6.** Non-myelinated nerve fibers. **7.** Connective tissue fibers. **8.** Nuclei of endothelial cells. **9.** Lumen of capillary.

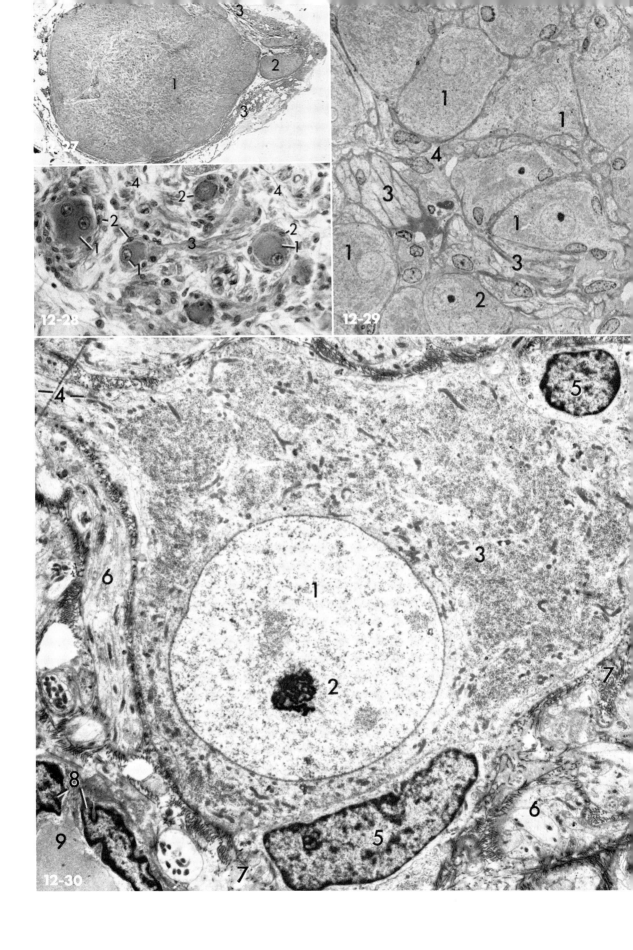

13 Nervous tissue— the neuron

GENERAL CONSIDERATIONS

The nerve cell (neuron) is unique compared with other cells of the mammalian body, since enormously long processes emerge from the cell body, reaching areas located at distances of up to 3 feet away. Furthermore, a chain of nerve cells is established through membranous contacts between the termination of cell processes and the cell body or short cell processes of other nerve cells. The nerve processes may also contact other cells such as epithelial cells and muscle cells. In addition to these anatomical peculiarities, nerve cells have fundamental physiological and biochemical properties that make them different from other cells. The cell membrane of nerve cells is characterized by its high degree of excitability, by its ability to initiate electrochemical activities—called nerve impulses—and by its highly developed capacity to propagate these impulses (conductivity). In addition, the terminations of the nerve processes can transmit these impulses via membranous contacts to other neurons as well as to muscle cells, glands, and surface epithelial cells. By these contacts, the nerve cells either receive stimuli from surface or other outlying cells (receptors) or transmit nervous impulses to muscle cells or glands (effectors).

Neuron

The neuron (nerve cell) consists of the cell body, **perikaryon,** and the cell processes, the **axon** and the **dendrites.** (Fig. 13-1) Nerve cells vary somewhat in size and shape, and there are particularly great variations in the morphology of the nerve processes. This is used as basis for the classification of neurons and is discussed on p. 280. However, it is appropriate to give a general description of the structure and ultrastructure of certain features common to all neurons before discussing differences.

PERIKARYON

The mass of cytoplasm which surrounds the nucleus is called cell body or perikaryon. This cytoplasm contains organelles and inclusions, typically encountered in most mammalian cells.

Nucleus. Most nerve cells have only one nucleus, but two or more nuclei may be present in autonomic ganglion cells. The nucleus is spherical, and varies in size between 3μ and 18μ. It is located centrally in most nerve cells. The nuclear membrane is provided with numerous pores. The dense heterochromatin is widely dispersed and rarely shows margination. The **nucleolus** is prominent and markedly basophilic. (Fig. 13-2) It contains large amounts of RNA and a diffuse coating of DNA. Several nucleoli may be present in the nuclei of nerve cells.

Cell membrane. The cell membrane of nerve cells is a trilaminar structure, averaging 70–80 Å in width. Localized modifications occur in the synaptic regions and adhesive junctions, characterized by focal aggregations of dense material in the cytoplasm on one or the other sides of the junctions. **Micropinocytotic (surface) vesicles** are rarely seen in connection with the cell membrane. The membrane regulates the interchange of materials and ions between the nerve cell and its environment, as do other cell membranes. It also participates in the reception and transmission of electric potentials (nerve impulses) from one nerve cell to another. However, in spite of these properties, the fine structure of the cell membrane of nerve cells does not differ from that of other mammalian cells.

Fig. 13-1. Multipolar motor neuron. Anterior horn. Spinal cord. Thoracic segment. Rat. E.M. X 1920. **1.** Nucleus. **2.** Nucleolus. **3.** Nissl substance (granular endoplasmic reticulum). **4.** Axon hillock. **5.** Axon. **6.** Dendrites. **7.** Cross-sectioned dendrites. **8.** Myelinated nerve processes of the spinal cord gray matter. **9.** Lumen of capillary. **10.** Part of neighboring motor neuron.

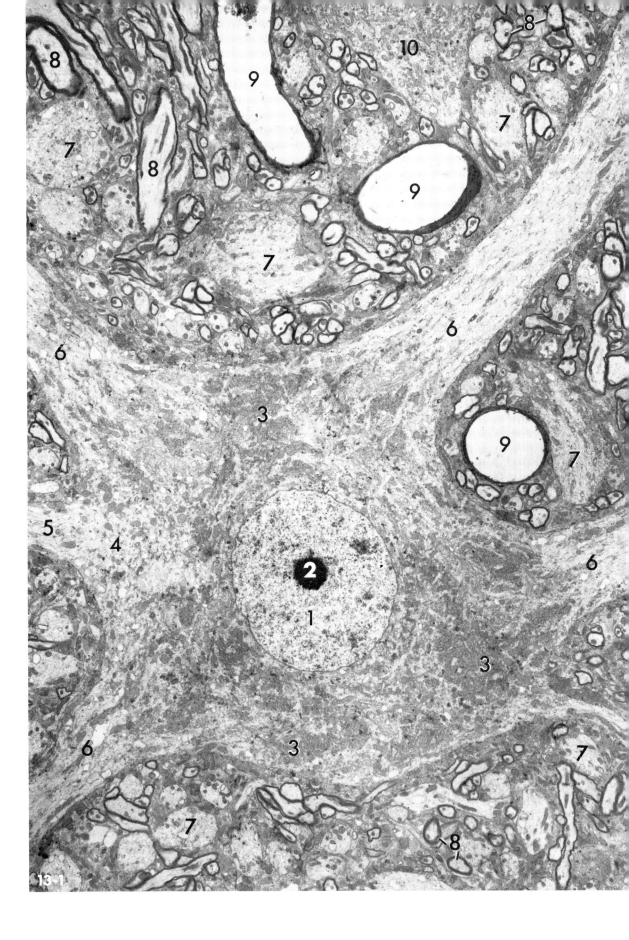

Cell organelles. The perikaryon contains a relatively large number of spherical and elongated **mitochondria** (Fig. 13-3) with diameters averaging 0.1 μ. The mitochondrial cristae are of both the lamellar and the tubular variety. There are only a few dense matrix granules in the mitochondria. The **Golgi zone** is well developed in most neurons. It forms a perinuclear network of flattened membranous sacs and cisternae with associated small vesicles, many of which are of the coated variety. The function of the Golgi zone in nerve cells is obscure. **Multivesicular bodies** are often associated with the Golgi zone. Their function is not known, but it has been suggested that they represent secondary lysosomes.

The **Nissl substance** (synonyms: Nissl bodies; tigroid substance; chromophil substance) represents the **granular endoplasmic reticulum** of nerve cells. It is widely distributed and abundant in large motor neurons (Fig. 13-3), and less abundant in sensory neurons. It is present in dendrites but absent in axons. It consists of stacks of flat, short cisternae of varied size, in addition to tubular and vesicular components. The membranes are studded with ribosomes. Clusters of free monoribosomes and polysomes occur abundantly between the cisternae. The Nissl substance is the principal protein-synthesizing organelle of the nerve cell. Proteins are continuously consumed during the normal physiological activity of neurons, and there seems to be a continuous flow of proteins from the perikaryon to axons and nerve endings as part of a replacement mechanism. **Agranular endoplasmic reticulum** is almost entirely absent from the perikaryon, but is present in both dendrites and axons as tubules (Fig. 13-27), cisternae, and irregular vesicles. **Neurofibrils** abound in perikarya, dendrites, and axons. They are aggregates of submicroscopic microtubules and neurofilaments, made visible in light microscope preparations by staining techniques involving silver and gold impregnation. (Fig. 12-3) **Microtubules** aver-

age 200-300 Å in diameter. (Figs. 13-10, 13-26) They are similar to microtubules in other cells and have an outer smooth membrane and a light central core. A thin central filament is present in many microtubules of neurons but absent in microtubules elsewhere. The **neurofilaments** average 70–100 Å. (Figs. 13-10, 13-27) They also have a light core and closely resemble cytoplasmic filaments of other cells. The functions of microtubules and neurofilaments are not known. It has been suggested that they are involved in intracellular transport of ions and metabolites, and that they support the cytoplasm of the neuron.

Many neurons have a single **cilium** which originates from a **basal body** and projects above the cell surface. A neuronal cilium may also have an associated **centriole** suspended in the cytoplasm at right angles below the basal body. Paired centrioles are present in neuroblasts, but usually do not occur in adult neurons except in association with the basal body of a cilium. The neuronal cilia are non-motile, and most likely have a sensory function. This is certainly the case in the bipolar neurons of the olfactory epithelium, as well as in the retina, where a cilium, albeit highly modified, forms an essential part of the bipolar neurons of the rods and cones. Cilia of neurons in the CNS are probably vestigial in nature without apparent function. The absence of cen-

Fig. 13-2. Purkinje nerve cell. Cerebellar cortex. Rat. E.M. X 9000. **1.** Nucleus. **2.** Nucleolus. **3.** Nuclear membrane. **4.** Golgi zone. **5.** Mitochondria. **6.** Lysosomes. **7.** Granular endoplasmic reticulum (Nissl substance). **8.** Multivesicular bodies. **9.** Axon terminals. **10** Axo-somatic synapses.

Fig. 13-3. Detail of motor neuron. Anterior horn. Spinal cord. Thoracic segment. Rat. E.M. X 37,000. **1.** Nucleus. **2.** Nuclear membrane. **3.** Golgi zone. **4.** Mitochondria. **5.** Lysosome. **6.** Granular endoplasmic reticulum (Nissl substance). **7.** Cisternae of granular endoplasmic reticulum. **8.** Polyribosomes. **9.** Axon terminal (bouton terminal). **10.** Axo-somatic synapse.

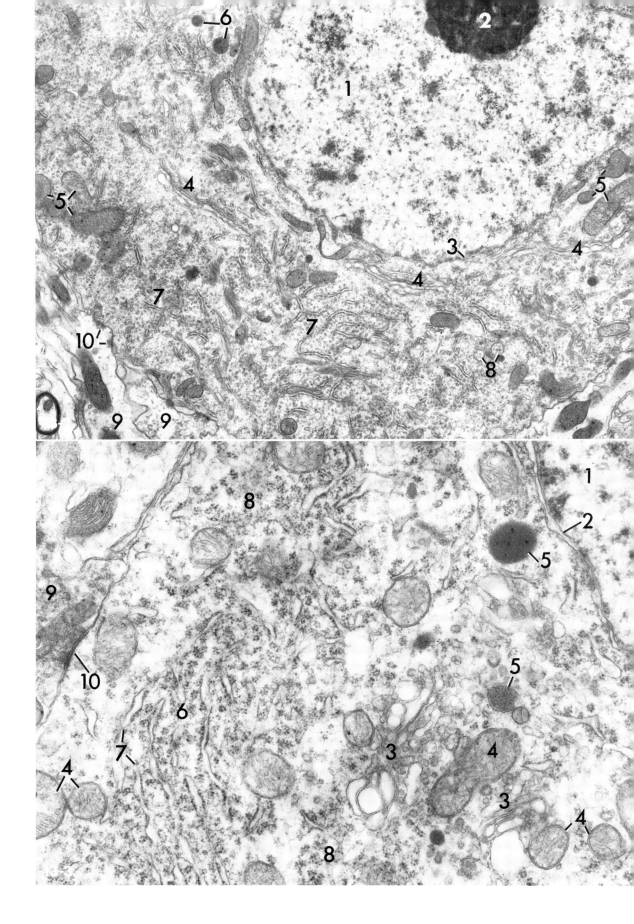

trioles in most neurons may correlate with the fact that mature nerve cells do not undergo mitosis.

Nerve cells contain many **primary lysosomes,** often in close proximity to the Golgi zone. (Fig. 13-3) Lysosomes of neurons are probably engaged in the degradation of unsaturated lipids and the detoxification of end products of neuronal cellular activity. As a result, the number of **secondary lysosomes** (residual bodies) increases with age. It is now generally accepted that the yellow-brown pigment granules, also referred to as **lipofuscin granules,** and which can be identified in light microscope preparations, represent secondary lysosomes. Dark brown pigment granules also occur in some nerve cells, especially the substantia nigra and locus ceruleus of the brain stem. These are true **melanin granules** and must not be confused with the lipofuscin granules. Peculiar laminar and fibrillary **inclusions** are present in some neurons, but their origin and significance are not known.

DENDRITES

Dendrites are generally short, abundant, and widely branching cell processes which protrude from the perikaryon. (Fig. 13-1) They lack myelin sheaths. (Figs. 13-4 and 13-5)

The dendrites are bordered by the cell membrane. The surface is irregular and provided with projecting **dendritic spines** (thorns). The spines vary considerably in size and shape. In most instances, their length averages 0.2μ. They consist of a narrow neck and an ovoid terminal bulb. Most of the axo-dendritic synapses occur on these spines. The dendrites contain several microtubules but only few neurofilaments. (Fig. 13-6) Both structures are arranged parallel to the long axis of the dendrite. These structures do not enter the dendritic spines, which are dominated by a finely filamentous material and sometimes by several flat, membranous cisternae alternating with thin laminae of dense material, the spine apparatus. Large

dendrites contain Nissl substance, but small dendrites are devoid of this organelle, which makes it difficult to differentiate between small dendrites and small axons. Elongated mitochondria occur in the dendrites together with a limited number of tubular profiles of the agranular endoplasmic reticulum. The terminal portion of the dendrites are often enlarged to form a knob-like swelling. The peripheral processes of sensory ganglion cells are afferent nerve fibers and have all the characteristics of axons of the peripheral nervous system, as described next.

AXONS

Axons are defined as nerve processes which carry nerve impulses over considerable distances. They are, with few exceptions, long processes, each with a relatively constant diameter. There are great variations in diameter between individual axons, varying from about 1μ to 20μ. It has been established that axons with the larger diameters conduct nerve impulses faster than the small diameter axons. Most axons have a myelin sheath, the structure of which is described on p. 284.

Each axon originates from the **axon hillock,** a cone-shaped elevation of the perikaryon. (Fig. 13-7) The axon gives off **collaterals** (side-branches) a short distance

Fig. 13-4. Irregularly arranged dendrites. Molecular layer. Cerebral cortex. Rat. E.M. X 4800. **1.** Large dendrite: longitudinal section. **2.** Cross-sectioned large dendrites. **3.** Myelinated nerve process. **4.** Part of neuroglial cell. **5.** Neuropil: a mixture of abundant, delicate branching axon terminals (telodendria); small dendrites; and neuroglial cell processes.

Fig. 13-5. Cross-sectioned dendrites, arranged in parallel. Gray matter. Spinal cord. Rat. E.M. X 9000. **1.** Dendrites. **2.** Myelinated nerve processes. **3.** Axon terminals.

Fig. 13-6. Enlargement of cross-sectioned dendrite. Gray matter. Spinal cord. E.M. X 60,000. **1.** Dendritic cytoplasm. **2.** Microtubules. **3.** Profiles of tubular, agranular endoplasmic reticulum. **4.** Mitochondria. **5.** Axo-dendritic synapses. **6.** Axon terminals. **7.** Synaptic vesicles.

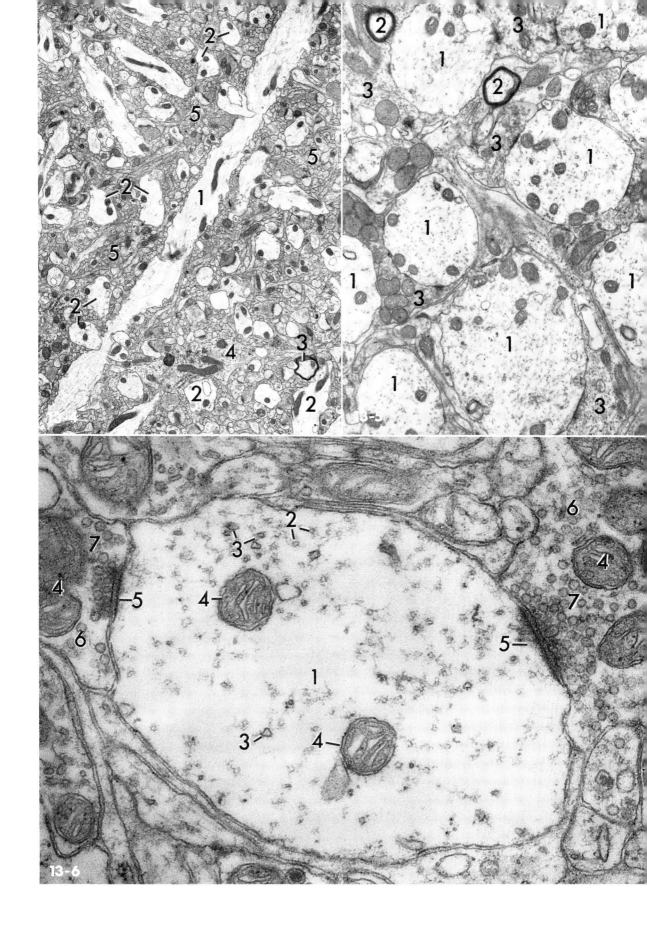

from the hillock. The axon ends as **telodendria,** an arborization of delicate branching nerve terminations. These nerve endings make contact with other neurons, **synapses,** which are described below. The nerve endings also have characteristic associations with effector organs such as muscles. These are described on p. 294.

The surface of the axon is smooth. It is covered by the cell membrane, often referred to as **axolemma.** The initial segment of the axons from neurons in the central nervous system, and the axon segment at the nodes of Ranvier (p. 286), have an "undercoating" of dense cytoplasmic material beneath the axolemma. The cytoplasm of the axon contains thin, long mitochondria, abundant microtubules, and neurofilaments (Fig. 13-10), as well as vesicular and tubular profiles of the agranular endoplasmic reticulum (Fig. 13-9), and occasional multivesicular bodies. Ribosomes and profiles of the granular endoplasmic reticulum (Nissl substance) do not occur in the axoplasm but may be present in the axon hillock. The initial segment of the axon has an abundance of microtubules (Fig. 13-8) often arranged in fascicles, whereas neurofilaments are relatively sparse here. Ribosomes may also be present in this segment. Neurofilaments predominate in large axons, but the ratio of neurofilaments to microtubules decreases in smaller axons.

SYNAPSES

A synapse is a specialized membranous contact between the axon ending of one neuron and the dendrite (axo-dendritic synapse) or perikaryon (axo-somatic synapse) of another neuron. The preterminal part of an axon is expanded to form a **bouton terminal** (end-bulb). In addition, bead-like swellings, **boutons en passant,** occur along the axon, each of which can make synaptic contacts with another neuron. End-bulbs occur at the terminations of both myelinated and non-myelinated axons. Bead-like swellings are most often

present in non-myelinated axons, but may be present at the nodes of Ranvier of myelinated axons.

The end-bulbs and the bead-like swellings contain a varied number of small mitochondria and small vesicles, the majority of which have an electron-lucent center. (Figs. 13-11, 13-12) These are collectively called **synaptic vesicles** and are assumed to contain neurotransmitter substances. The specialized regions of the membranous contacts consist of the **presynaptic membrane** of the axon, the **postsynaptic membrane** of the dendrite or perikaryon, and an intermembranous **synaptic cleft,** averaging 200–300 Å and containing some medium dense amorphous material. Dense filamentous material is accumulated at the cytoplasmic aspect of the postsynaptic membrane, the **subsynaptic web.** This gives the synaptic region a polarized, asymmetric appearance. (Figs. 13-13, 13-14)

Fig. 13-7. Pseudo-unipolar neuron. Spinal root ganglion. Cat. E.M. X 4800. **1.** Nissl substance (granular endoplasmic reticulum) of spinal ganglion cell. **2.** Hillock. **3.** Initial segment of single nerve process of pseudo-unipolar neuron. **4.** Cell processes of satellite cells ensheath the nerve process. Axon terminals and synapses are not present in association with spinal (sensory) ganglion cells.

Fig. 13-8. Initial segment of single nerve process of pseudo-unipolar ganglion cell. Enlargement of rectangle in Fig. 13-7. Spinal root ganglion. Cat. E.M. X 18,000. **1.** Mitochondria. **2.** Lysosomes. **3.** Microtubules and neurofilaments. **4.** Cell processes of satellite cells with numerous glial filaments.

Fig. 13-9. Myelinated nerve processes of varied diameters. White matter. Spinal cord. Cross section. Rat. E.M. X 9000. **1.** Axon cytoplasm. **2.** Mitochondria. **3.** Profiles of agranular endoplasmic reticulum. **4.** Myelin sheaths. **5.** Cytoplasm of neuroglial cells.

Fig. 13-10. Detail of myelinated nerve process. White matter. Spinal cord. Rat. E.M. X 124,000. **1.** Axon cytoplasm. **2.** Neurofilaments. **3.** Microtubules. **4.** Axolemma. **5.** Myelin sheath. **6.** Ad-axonal oligodendroglial cytoplasm.

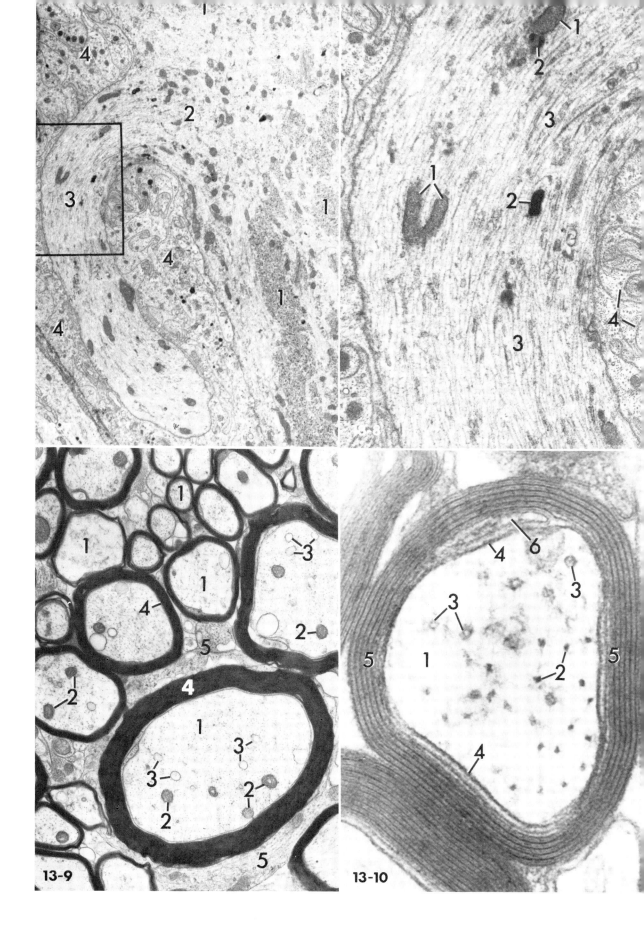

13-9

13-10

This kind of synapse is the most common in mammals and is referred to as **chemical synapse,** since the chemical transmitters of the synaptic vesicles are assumed to become extruded into the synaptic cleft for action on the postsynaptic membrane. This involves an alteration of the permeability of the postsynaptic membrane, thereby producing a small change in the membrane potential, resulting in a transmission of the nerve impulse across the synaptic cleft. From a functional point of view, both **excitatory** and **inhibitory** synapses are known to exist. Some structural differences have been identified, and it is believed that excitatory endings have a predominance of round synaptic vesicles, whereas inhibitory nerve terminals have many oval or flat synaptic vesicles.

In lower vertebrates and invertebrates, **electrical synapses** have been described. In these synapses the apposed membranes are separated by a synaptic cleft of about 20–40 Å. They resemble gap-junctions or nexuses of mammalian cardiac and smooth muscle cells. The electrical resistance between the cells is low at these junctions, and ions diffuse freely through these points. Therefore, no chemical transmitters are required for passing nerve impulses from one cell to the next.

Classification of Neurons

Based on the shape of the cell bodies and the number of cell processes, neurons may be classified as: 1) bipolar neurons; 2) pseudo-unipolar neurons; and 3) multipolar neurons.

Bipolar neurons. These neurons have two processes, one peripheral and one central, emerging opposite each other from the cell body. All processes may branch. Bipolar neurons are present in the vestibular and spiral ganglia of the VIII cranial (acoustic) nerve, and in the middle layer of neurons in the retina.

Pseudo-unipolar neurons. During development, the two processes of these neu-

rons come together and fuse at their bases to form a single short stem. In the fully developed neuron, a single nerve process emerges from the perikaryon. (Fig. 13-7) This process bifurcates and gives rise to a peripheral and a central fiber, both of which are myelinated. The round cell bodies of these neurons are located in the spinal and cranial sensory ganglia. The peripheral fiber takes its origin in a sense organ, and the central process synapses with other neurons in the central nervous system.

Multipolar neurons. These neurons are characterized by their many dendrites and their irregularly shaped cell body. The multipolarity is difficult, if not impossible, to observe in ordinary hematoxylin and eosin preparations, but is clearly evident in sections impregnated with silver. These neurons can be subdivided into two types: Golgi I and II. **Golgi type I** neurons have a long axon and many dendrites. To this

Fig. 13-11. Axo-somatic synapses. Motor neuron. Anterior horn. Spinal cord. Rat. E.M. X 37,000. **1.** Cytoplasm of motor neuron. **2.** Polysomes. **3.** Mitochondria. **4.** Cytoplasm and part of nucleus of perineuronal neuroglial cell (oligodendrocyte). **5.** Axon terminals with axo-somatic synapses.

Fig. 13-12. Axo-somatic synapses. Enlargement of area similar to rectangle in Fig. 13-11. Motor neuron. Anterior horn. Spinal cord. Rat. E.M. X 93,000. **1.** Cytoplasm of motor neuron. **2.** Ribosomes. **3.** Cell membrane of motor neuron. **4.** Axoplasm of bouton terminal (axon terminal). **5.** Mitochondria. **6.** Oval or flat synaptic vesicles. **7.** Synaptic region. **8.** Axolemma. **9.** Enlarged intercellular space.

Fig. 13-13. Axo-dendritic synapse. Molecular layer. Cerebellar cortex. Rat. E.M. X 172,000. **1.** Axon terminal. **2.** Dendrite. **3.** Mitochondrion. **4.** Round synaptic vesicles. **5.** Presynaptic membrane. **6.** Synaptic cleft. **7.** Postsynaptic membrane. **8.** Subsynaptic web.

Fig. 13-14. Detail of synaptic region. Axo-dendritic synapse. Gray matter. Spinal cord. Rat. E.M. X 172,000. **1.** Cytoplasm of axon terminal. **2.** Synaptic vesicles. **3.** Presynaptic membrane. **4.** Synaptic cleft. **5.** Postsynaptic membrane. **6.** Subsynaptic web. **7.** Cytoplasm of dendrite.

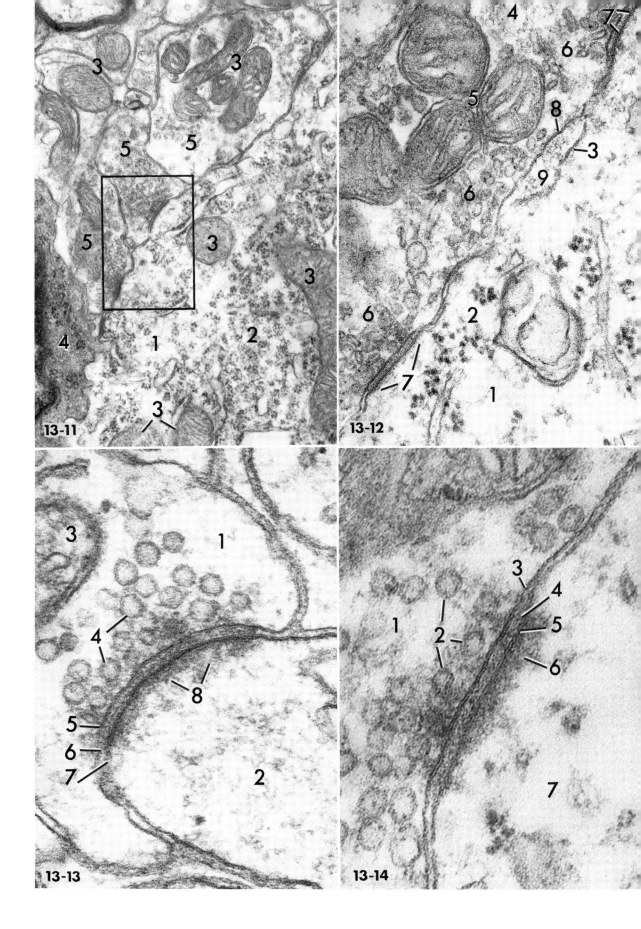

group belong, among others, the sympathetic (Fig. 12-30) and parasympathetic ganglion cells, the pyramidal cells of the cerebral cortex, the Purkinje cells of the cerebellar cortex (Fig. 12-2), and the motor neurons of the spinal cord. These neurons relay nerve impulses over long distances. **Golgi type II** neurons have a short axon and an abundance of widely branching dendrites. To this group belong many cells in the central nervous system. Examples are the stellate, basket, and granule cells of the cerebellar cortex, the Martinotti and granule cells of the cerebral cortex, as well as the internuncial neurons of the spinal cord. These neurons disseminate nerve impulses to a large number of neurons.

Modifications of Neurons

Some neurons do not fit into the scheme above. For instance, **rods** and **cones** of the **retina** are modified bipolar neurons, in which the dendritic process is differentiated into a specialized photoreceptor sense organ, responsible for the light absorption and initiation of the visual stimulus. The axon is short, synapsing with the true bipolar cells of the retina (p. 764). In the nasal cavity the **olfactory cells** represent modified bipolar neurons, each with the cell body and its peripheral process located in the olfactory surface epithelium (p. 610). This outlying process is provided with special cilia which respond to various odors and initiate nerve impulses. The axon is long, leaving the epithelium and synapsing with a second neuron in the olfactory bulb. The **cells of the adrenal medulla** are highly modified autonomic ganglion cells without dendrites and axons (p. 462). These cells receive preganglionic sympathetic nerve fibers provided with synaptic nerve endings. The cytoplasm of the cells is filled with numerous secretory granules containing catecholamines, which are re-

leased into the bloodstream upon the arrival of nerve impulses.

Yet another kind of modification is found in the nerve cells which are located in the paraventricular and supraoptic nuclei of the hypothalamus. Their axons terminate at various levels in the neurohypophysis (p. 436) and contain and transport neurosecretory granules. These cells are modified neurons, **neurosecretory cells,** which synthesize and release hormones in a fashion similar to the adrenal medullary cells. However, the neurosecretory cells of the hypothalamus release their secretions along the axons rather than from the perikaryon.

Sheaths of Neurons

The nerve cell bodies and their processes are surrounded by special cells and their sheet-like cytoplasmic processes. In the peripheral nervous system these cells are called **Schwann cells** and **satellite cells,** whereas in the central nervous system they are referred to as **oligodendrocytes,** a spe-

Fig. 13-15. Sheath surrounding spinal root ganglion cell. Cat. E.M. X 2500. **1.** Nucleus of pseudo-unipolar neuron. **2.** Perikaryon. **3.** Nucleus of satellite cell. **4.** Nucleus of capsule cell or Schwann cell. **5.** Nerve cell processes surrounded by cytoplasmic sheath of satellite or Schwann cells.

Fig. 13-16. Satellite cell. Enlargement of rectangle in Fig. 13-15. Spinal root ganglion. Cat. E.M. X 9000. **1.** Cytoplasm of spinal ganglion cell. **2.** Nissl substance (granular endoplasmic reticulum). **3.** Nucleus of satellite cell. **4.** Nucleolus. **5.** Cell membrane of satellite cell borders directly on cell membrane of ganglion cell. **6.** Cytoplasmic processes ensheathing the ganglion cell. **7.** Pericellular connective tissue fibrils.

Fig. 13-17. Detail of ganglion cell and satellite cell. Trigeminal (sensory) ganglion (Gasserian). Cat. E.M. X 28,000. **1.** Nucleus of satellite cell. **2.** Electron-dense cytoplasm of satellite cell. **3.** Electron-lucent cytoplasm of ganglion cell. **4.** Profiles of granular endoplasmic reticulum. **5.** Mitochondria. **6.** Lysosomes. **7.** Golgi zone. **8.** External (basal) lamina.

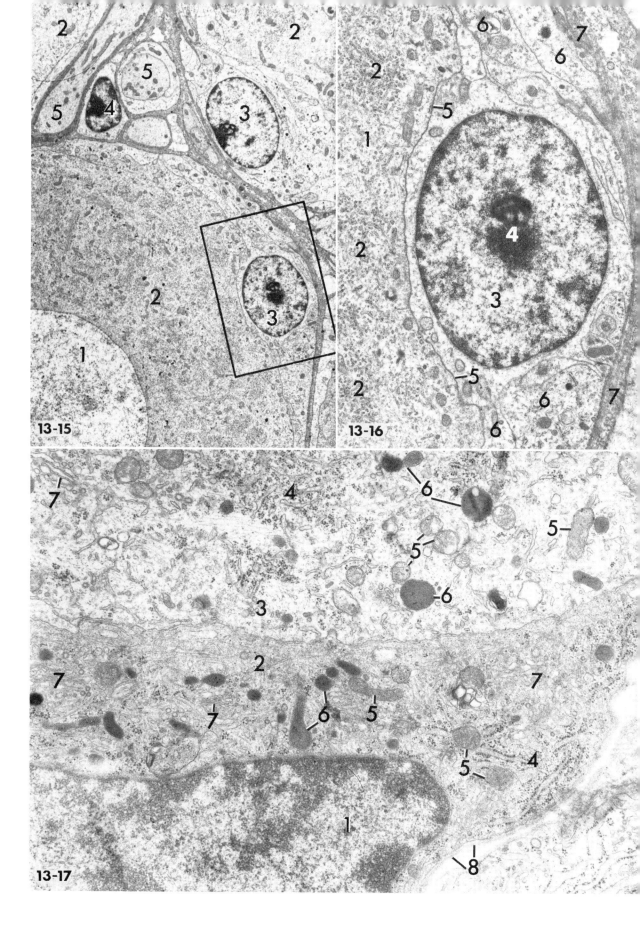

13-15

13-16

13-17

cific type of neuroglial cell. The basic function of all these cells is to protect and support the neuron, and to aid in the metabolic exchange processes of the nerve cell membrane and cytoplasm, functions fundamental to the initiation and propagation of nerve impulses.

SHEATHS OF PERIKARYA AND DENDRITES

In the **peripheral nervous system,** the perikarya of the spinal, cranial, and large autonomic ganglia are surrounded by a single layer of saucer-shaped **satellite cells.** (Figs. 13-15, 13-16) Their nucleus is round, smaller than that of the ganglion cell, and provided with more dense heterochromatin. The perinuclear cytoplasm is rich in ribosomes, granular endoplasmic reticulum, and mitochondria. (Fig. 13-17) Lysosomes also occur, mostly in the proximity of the Golgi zone, which is rather prominent. There is a 150-200 Å intercellular gap between the neuronal cell membrane and the satellite cell membrane. Junctional complexes and other specializations are not associated with these cell membranes. The satellite cell surface is irregular and is provided with small microvillous projections. Dendrites often pierce the satellite cytoplasm. The peripheral surface of the satellite cell is covered by a thin **external** (basal) **lamina.** In many instances, the layer of satellite cells is surrounded peripherally by an incomplete layer of flat fibroblasts, **capsule cells** with elongated nuclei. They form part of the connective tissue network of fibers and cells that exists in peripheral ganglia and nerves. The satellite cells which surround the ganglion cells of the VIII cranial (acoustic) nerve often form myelin sheaths around the perikarya and the dendrites of these bipolar cells. The myelin formation is similar to that of axons, described on p. 286. Nowhere else in mammals are myelin sheaths known to occur around perikarya.

In the **central nervous system** the perikarya of nerve cells are surrounded by an incomplete layer of neuroglial cells.

Among these, the oligodendrocytes are more frequent than the astrocytes. The structure of these cells is described on p. 314. Dendrites in the central nervous system are surrounded by processes from neuroglial cells as well as by other dendritic and axonal processes in an entanglement, collectively referred to as the neuropil. (Fig. 13-4)

SHEATHS OF AXONS

Axons in the peripheral and the central nervous systems are surrounded by sheetlike processes, extending from the Schwann cells (PNS) and the oligodendrocytes (CNS). The cytoplasmic encasement of the axons can be simple, in which case one refers to the axon as **non-myelinated.** It can also involve a complicated, multilayered enclosure; then the axon is said to be **myelinated.**

In the **peripheral nervous system,** Schwann cells are associated with axons in the following fashion. In **myelinated** nerves, Schwann cells are arranged side by side along the axons. (Fig. 13-21) Each

Fig. 13-18. Myelinated peripheral nerve processes with associated myelin sheaths and Schwann cell cytoplasm. Sciatic nerve. Rat. E.M. X 25,000. **1.** Nucleus of Schwann cell. **2.** Nuclear membrane. **3.** Cytoplasm (neurolemma). **4.** Golgi zone. **5.** Profiles of granular endoplasmic reticulum. **6.** External (basal) lamina. **7.** Myelin sheath. **8.** Nerve cell process (could be either peripheral process of sensory neuron or axon of motor neuron). **9.** Mitochondria. **10.** Outer mesaxon (point where membrane spiral of myelin sheath ends). **11.** Collagenous fibrils of endoneurium.

Fig. 13-19. Myelinated nerve process in the central nervous system. White matter of spinal cord. Rat. E.M. X 168,000. **1.** Nerve cell process (could be either central process of sensory neuron or axon of neuron located within the central nervous system). **2.** Microtubules. **3.** Neurofilaments. **4.** Axolemma. **5.** Internal mesaxon (point where membrane spiral of myelin sheath begins). **6.** Interperiod membrane of myelin sheath. **7.** Major period membrane. **8.** External tongue process of oligodendrocyte. **9.** Internal tongue process of oligodendrocyte (ad-axonal cytoplasm).

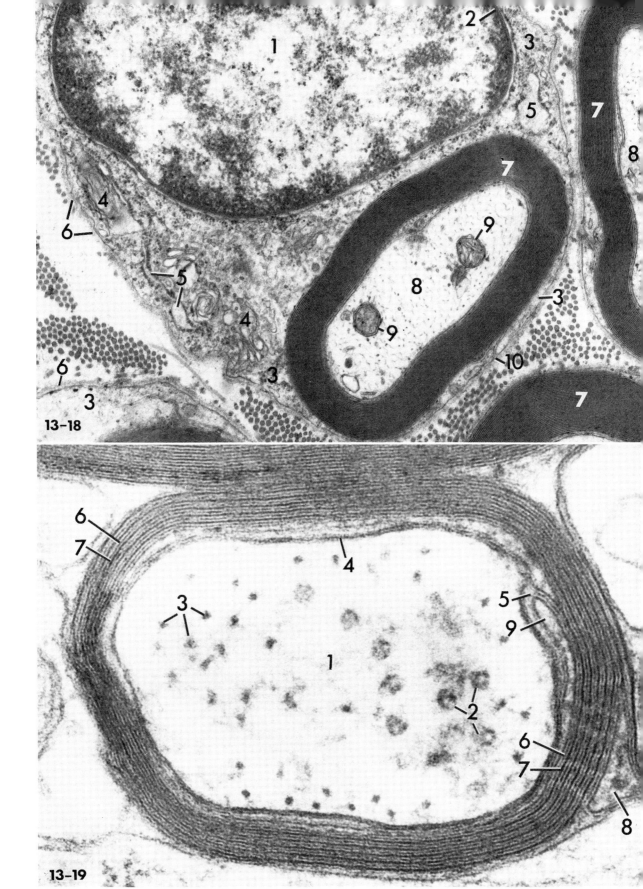

13-18

13-19

Schwann cell covers an axon segment (internode; internodal segment) ranging in length from 25 μ to 1000 μ. The thicker the nerve fibers the longer the segments. The region where adjoining Schwann cells are juxtaposed, the **node of Ranvier,** is slightly constricted. (Fig. 13-22) The outermost part of the Schwann cell is called **neurolemma.** (Fig. 13-18) It contains most of the cytoplasm with mitochondria, Golgi zone, ribosomes, and the nucleus, the last located at the midpoint of the extent of each cell. The outer surface of the Schwann cell is surrounded by a thin **external lamina.** (Fig. 13-25) The innermost portion of the Schwann cell cytoplasm is concentrically wrapped around the axon, forming the **myelin sheath.** (Fig. 13-19) The number of cytoplasmic layers in the "jelly-roll" configuration of myelin sheaths varies from very few to about fifty. From a developmental point of view, a gradual myelinization occurs in the fetus and the newborn and continues for many years at a decreasing rate. During the wrapping process the cytoplasm of the sheet-like process is flattened out and disappears. As a result the inner leaflets of the trilaminar cell membranes fuse to form a 30 Å thick membrane, giving rise to the typical pattern observed in sections of myelin sheaths: concentric layers of lipoprotein membranes. The average distance between inner fused leaflets is about 150 Å, referred to as **major period.** The juxtaposed outer leaflets of apposed cell membranes form a 20 Å thick membrane bisecting the major period as an **interperiod membrane.**

In the myelin sheaths occur at regular intervals, funnel-shaped, oblique clefts, termed **incisures of Schmidt-Lantermann.** (Fig. 13-20) These are shearing defects in the lamellae, and were initially thought of as fixation artifacts. (Fig. 13-23) The possibility exists that they serve as channels for exchange of nutrients and gases between the axon and the neurolemma. At the **nodes of Ranvier,** the condensed cytoplasmic laminae of the myelin sheath open up along the major 30 Å thick membranes to enclose pockets of paranodal cytoplasm. (Figs. 13-22, 13-24)

In the **non-myelinated** peripheral nerves (Fig. 13-28), Schwann cells are similarly arranged in a series side by side. In this case, however, several axons invaginate the cytoplasm of one Schwann cell. The cytoplasm thereby encloses each axon by a simple folding and overlapping of the cytoplasmic sheet. (Figs. 13-29, 13-30) Adjoining regions of juxtaposed Schwann cells interdigitate, and nodes of Ranvier do not exist. Non-myelinated nerves represent mostly postganglionic nerve fibers of the autonomic nervous system, and some pain-conducting fibers.

Fig. 13-20 & 13-21. Peripheral myelinated nerve process. Longitudinal section. Sciatic nerve. Rat. E.M. X 4500. **1.** Nerve process ("axon"). **2.** Myelin sheath. **3.** Nucleus of Schwann cell. **4.** Cytoplasm of Schwann cell (neurolemma). **5.** Collagenous fibrils of endoneurium. **6.** Incisure of Schmidt-Lantermann. **7.** Nuclear region of cytoplasm indents locally the myelin sheath.

Fig. 13-22. Node of Ranvier. Peripheral myelinated nerve process. Longitudinal section. Sciatic nerve. Rat. E.M. X 9000. **1.** Nerve process ("axon"). **2.** Myelin sheath. **3.** Nodal area of nerve process. **4.** Schwann cell processes. **5.** Outer collar of Schwann cell processes. **6.** Schwann cell cytoplasm (neurolemma). **7.** Collagenous fibrils of endoneurium.

Fig. 13-23. Detail of incisure of Schmidt-Lantermann. Enlargement of area similar to rectangle in Fig. 13-20. Sciatic nerve. E.M. X 18,000. **1.** Axoplasm with microtubules and neurofilaments. **2.** Myelin sheath. **3.** Schwann cell cytoplasm is retained in the region of the incisure, since the fusion of the inner leaflets of the cell membrane is locally opened up at these points. **4.** Schwann cell cytoplasm (neurolemma). **5.** External lamina.

Fig. 13-24. Detail of node of Ranvier. Enlargement of rectangle in Fig. 13-22. E.M. X 39,000. **1.** Nodal axoplasm with microtubules and neurofilaments. **2.** Myelin sheath. **3.** Successive laminae of the myelin sheath terminate as paranodal cytoplasmic swellings. **4.** Outer collar of Schwann cell processes. **5.** External (basal) lamina. **6.** Collagenous fibrils of endoneurium.

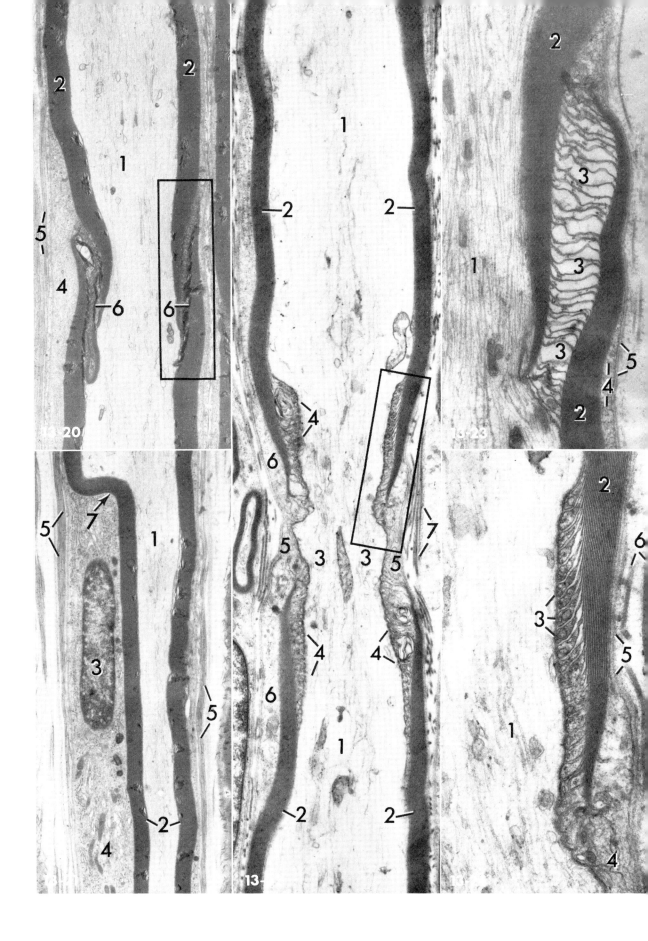

In the **central nervous system,** axons become **myelinated** by the cytoplasm of the oligodendrocytes. (Figs. 13-9, 13-10) These neuroglial cells are arranged along the axons, sending out trunk-like processes in several directions. Each process spreads out as a sheet-like envelope, which encircles an axon and forms a myelin sheath, the fine structure of which is similar to that of peripheral nerves. (Fig. 13-10) One oligodendrocyte forms the myelin sheath of several axons, whereas the Schwann cell of the peripheral nervous system participates in the myelinization of only one axon. Junctional complexes, reminiscent of synaptic junctions, may be present between the cell membrane of the oligodendrocytes and the axolemma. Oligodendrocytes do not always border on each other, but leave the axon without sheath for a short distance. There is a multitude of **non-myelinated** axons in the central nervous system. They are not covered by oligodendrocytes but meander through a matrix of neuroglial cells, dendrites, and other axons, the **neuropil.** (Fig. 13-4)

Functional Considerations

There is a long chain of events related to initiation, propagation, and transmission of nerve impulses. This is a brief summary of some of the major steps based on present ultrastructural, biochemical, and physiological information and current functional hypotheses. Textbooks of physiology should be consulted for a comprehensive discussion of this subject.

Sensory nerve endings are stimulated mechanically, chemically, and thermally through specially designed **sensory receptors** (p. 294) which act as **transducers,** structures that transform one kind of energy into another. At rest an electrical potential exists across the cell membrane of the sensory nerve endings (or any neuron) and is referred to as **resting potential.** This potential is present since the resting cell membrane is slightly permeable to sodium ions, and highly permeable to potassium ions. The concentration of sodium ions is high on the outside surface (positive charge) and low on the inside surface (negative charge).

The stimulation of the sensory nerve endings makes the cell membrane of the nerve ending temporarily permeable to sodium ions, which then flow freely into the cytoplasm of the nerve process, causing decreased electronegativity on the inside. The influx of ions sets up an electrotonic current which depolarizes adjacent parts of the cell membrane, giving rise to what is known as a **generator potential,** which in turn elicits an **action potential.** The action potential is self-propagating, advancing as a wave of depolarization along the nerve process. The **nerve impulse** is therefore the migration of the change in potential from the resting to the active state in consecutive regions of the cell membrane.

When the action potential reaches a presynaptic terminal, the membrane de-

Fig. 13-25. Detail of myelin sheath. Longitudinal section. Sciatic nerve. E.M. X 130,000.
1. Collagenous fibrils of endoneurium.
2. External (basal) lamina. **3.** Cell membrane of Schwann cell. **4.** Thin rim of Schwann cell cytoplasm (neurolemma). **5.** Myelin sheath: major period membranes are clearly resolved; interperiod membranes indistinct. **6.** Thin rim of ad-axonal Schwann cell cytoplasm.
7. Axolemma. **8.** Cytoplasm of nerve cell process (axon).

Figs. 13-26 & 13-27. Detail of myelinated peripheral nerve process. Longitudinal section. Sciatic nerve. Rat. E.M. Fig. 13-26: X 102,000. Fig. 13-27: X 96,000.
1. Microtubules; average width 225 Å.
2. Neurofilaments; average width 85 Å.
3. Tubular profile of agranular endoplasmic reticulum; average width 400 Å.

Fig. 13-28. Autonomic nerve, consisting largely of non-myelinated nerve fibers. Cross section. Kidney. Rat. E.M. X 1700. **1.** Epineurium (in this case also perineurium). **2.** Nuclei of Schwann cells. **3.** Small circular profiles are non-myelinated nerve processes. **4.** Myelinated nerve processes. **5.** Lumen of capillary.
6. Area similar to rectangle is enlarged in Fig. 13-29.

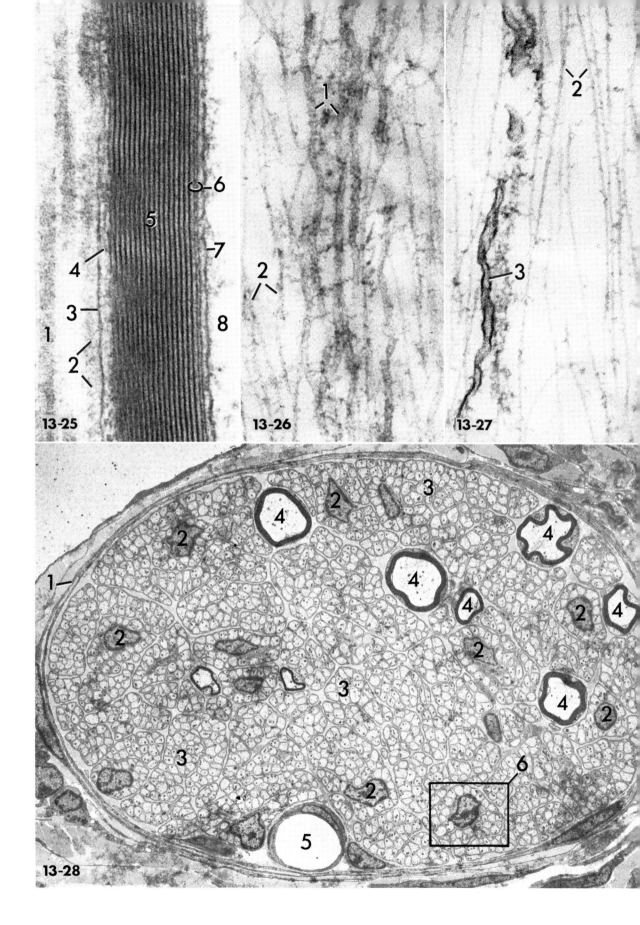

13-25

13-26

13-27

13-28

polarization brings about a discharge of neurotransmitter substances from the synaptic vesicles. The transmitters diffuse across the synaptic cleft and act as chemical stimuli on the postsynaptic membrane of a dendrite or perikaryon which becomes depolarized. Generally, several synaptic inputs are required to cause a depolarization strong enough to reach and excite the initial axon segment. Through this process a **synaptic transmission** of the nerve impulse is accomplished from the nerve terminal of one neuron to the nerve cell body of a second neuron. (Fig. 13-11)

A wave of depolarization now originates at the initial axon segment of the second neuron and is propagated along the axolemma. In the **myelinated** axons, the electrotonic current flow is greatly speeded up by the presence of nodes of Ranvier. According to one hypothesis the current remains confined to, and flows forward in, the axon because of the insulating myelin sheath of the internodal segment. A regeneration of the action potential cannot occur until the next node is reached, where the myelin is interrupted. The electrotonic current "leaps" from one node to the next, a phenomenon referred to as **saltatory conduction.** Another theory suggests that the action potential reaches the extracellular fluid at the node and is propagated via the interstitial space to the next node. The electrotonic current flow is slower in the **non-myelinated** axons, which has been attributed to the absence of nodes of Ranvier.

Finally, transmission of efferent nerve impulses occurs at the axon terminals by the discharge of neurotransmitter substances (p. 278). The substances diffuse across the synaptic cleft or interstitial connective tissue to reach neurons, muscle cells, or glands, the cell membranes of which become depolarized, resulting in a stimulation of and action by these effector cells. The special topographic relationships between nerve endings and receptor or effector cells is discussed in the chapter on nerve endings, p. 294.

References

Bischoff, A. and Moor, H. Ultrastructural differences between the myelin sheaths of peripheral nerve fibers and CNS white matter. Z. Zellforsch. *81*: 303–310 (1967).

Bodian, D. The generalized vertebrate neuron. Science *137*: 323–326 (1962).

Brunk, U. and Ericsson, J. L. E. Electron microscopical studies on rat brain neurons. Localization of acid phosphatase and mode of formation of lipofuscin bodies. J. Ultrastruct. Res. *38*: 1–15 (1972).

Burkel, W. E. The histological fine structure of perineurium. Anat. Rec. *158*: 177–190 (1967).

de Robertis, E. Submicroscopic morphology of the synapse. Int. Rev. Cytol. *8*: 61–96 (1959).

de Robertis, E. Ultrastructure and cytochemistry of the synaptic region. Science *156*: 907–914 (1967).

Eccles, J. C. The Physiology of Synapses. Academic Press, New York, 1964.

Elfvin, L. G. The ultrastructure of the superior cervical sympathetic ganglion of the cat. 1. The structure of the ganglion processes as studied by serial sections. J. Ultrastruct. Res. *8*: 403–440 (1963).

Friede, R. L. and Samorajski, T. The clefts of Schmidt-Lanterman: a quantative electron microscopic study of their structure in developing and adult sciatic nerves of the rat. Anat. Rec. *165*: 89–102 (1969).

Geren, B. B. The formation from the Schwann cell surface of myelin in the peripheral nerves of chick embryos. Exper. Cell Res. *7*: 558–562 (1954).

Gobel, S. Electron microscopical studies of the cerebellar molecular layer. J. Ultrastruct. Res. *21*: 430–458 (1968).

Fig. 13-29. Non-myelinated nerve processes. Cross section. Enlargement of area similar to rectangle in Fig. 13-28. Sciatic nerve. Rat. E.M. X 21,000. **1.** Nucleus of Schwann cell. **2.** Schwann cell cytoplasm. **3.** Cytoplasm of adjoining Schwann cell, interdigitating with neighboring cell. **4.** Golgi zone. **5.** Nerve cell processes partly or completely surrounded by Schwann cell cytoplasm. **6.** External (basal) lamina. **7.** Collagenous fibrils of endoneurium.

Fig. 13-30. Small non-myelinated nerve processes. Cross section. Smooth muscle layer. Ureter. Rat. E.M. X 90,000. **1.** Schwann cell cytoplasm. **2.** Delicate nerve processes. **3.** Bead-like swellings of nerve processes (boutons en passant). One is seen in longitudinal section in Fig. 16-58. **4.** Mitochondria. **5.** Clear synaptic vesicles. **6.** Granulated (dense-core) synaptic vesicles. **7.** Large granulated vesicles. **8.** Microtubules. **9.** Neurofilaments. **10.** Extremely delicate external (basal) lamina. **11.** Cross-sectioned collagenous fibrils.

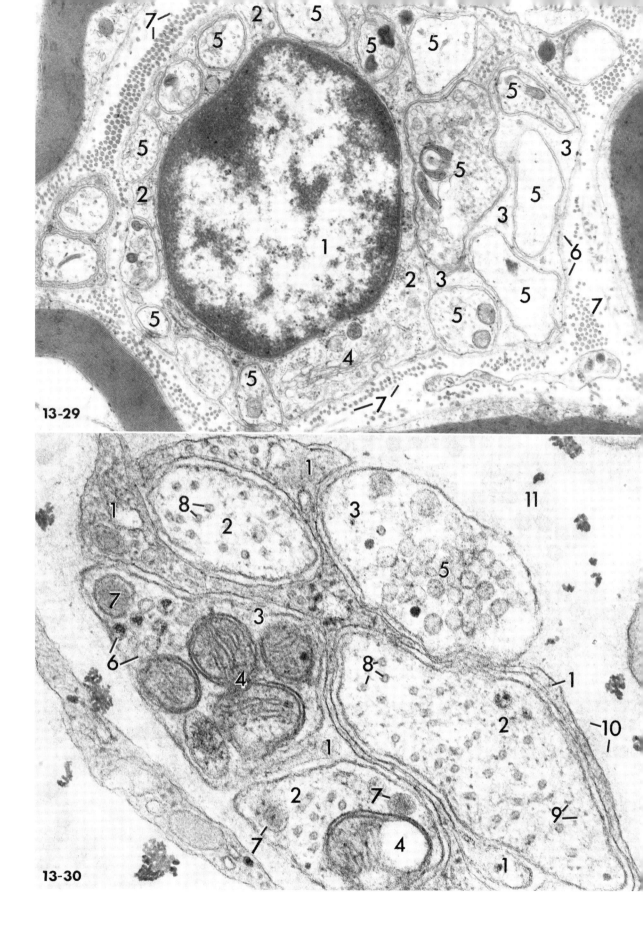

13-29

13-30

Gray, E. G. and Guillery, R. W. Synaptic morphology in the normal and degenerating nervous system. Int. Rev. Cytol. *19*: 111–182 (1966).

Herndon, R. M. The fine structure of the Purkinje cell. J. Cell Biol. *18*: 167–180 (1963).

Hirano, A. and Dembitzer, H. M. A structural analysis of the myelin sheath in the central nervous system. J. Cell Biol. *34*: 555–567 (1967).

Hydén, H. (Ed.). The Neuron. Elsevier, Amsterdam, 1967.

Karlsson, U. Three-dimensional studies of neurons in the lateral geniculate nucleus of the rat. II. Environment of perikarya and proximal part of their branches. J. Ultrastruct. Res. *16*: 482–504 (1966).

Metuzals, J. Ultrastructure of the nodes of Ranvier and their surrounding structures in the central nervous system. Z. Zellforsch. *65*: 719–759 (1965).

Palay, S. L. The morphology of synapses in the central nervous system. Exper. Cell Res. Suppl. *5*, 275–293 (1958).

Palay, S. L. and Palade, G. E. The fine structure of neurons. J. Biophys. Biochem. Cytol. *1*: 69–88 (1955).

Peters, A. and Kaiserman-Abramof, I. T. The small pyramidal neuron of the rat cerebral cortex. The perikaryon, dendrites and spines. Am. J. Anat. *127*: 321–356 (1970).

Peters, A. Stellate cells of the rat parietal cortex. J. Comp. Neurol. *141*: 345–373 (1971).

Peters, A., Palay, S. L. and Webster, H. de F. The Fine Structure of the Nervous System. The cells and their processes. Harper & Row, New York, 1970.

Pick, J., de Lemos, C. and Gerdin, C. The fine structure of sympathetic neurons in man. J. Comp. Neurol. *122*: 19–67 (1964).

Revel, J.-P. and Hamilton, D. W. The double nature of the intermediate dense line in peripheral nerve myelin. Anat. Rec. *163*: 7–16 (1969).

Siegesmund, K. A. The fine structure of subsurface cisterns. Anat. Rec. *162*: 187–196 (1968).

Sjöstrand, F. S. The lamellated structure of the nerve myelin sheath as revealed by high resolution electron microscopy. Experientia *9*: 68–69 (1953).

Sotelo, C. The fine structural localization of norepinephrine-^{3}H in the substantia nigra and area postrema of the rat. An autoradiographic study. J. Ultrastruct. Res. *36*: 824–841 (1971).

Steer, J. M. Some observations on the fine structure of rat dorsal spinal nerve roots. J. Anat. *109*: 467–485 (1971).

Uga, S. and Ikui, H. Membrane modification occurring between neurons and Schwann cells. J. Electron Micr. *17*: 155 (1968).

Uzman, B. G. The spiral configuration of myelin lamellae. J. Ultrastruct. Res. *2*: 208–212 (1964).

van der Loos, H. Fine structure of synapses in the cerebral cortex. Z. Zellforsch. *60*: 815–825 (1963).

Wuerker, R. B. and Kirkpatrick, J. B. Neuronal microtubules, neurofilaments, and microtubules. Int. Rev. Cytol. *33*: 45–75 (1972).

14 Nervous tissue—nerve endings

GENERAL CONSIDERATIONS

Peripheral nerve endings are terminations of nerve fibers outside of the central nervous system. Nerve endings of peripheral processes of sensory ganglion cells initiate nerve impulses which are propagated toward the central nervous system by **afferent** nerve fibers. Nerve endings of axons in the peripheral nervous system relate to effector organs such as muscles and glands and are **efferent** in nature. The majority are associated with the initiation of muscular contraction, and are therefore referred to as **motor** nerve endings.

The majority of the afferent nerve endings are associated with special **sensory receptors** which serve as **transducers,** converting one kind of energy to another. The sensory receptors are divided into: 1) local sensory receptors; 2) baroreceptors; 3) chemoreceptors; and 4) receptors of special sense organs.

From a **functional point of view,** the sensory receptors are divided into: 1) **exteroceptive,** responding to stimuli from outside the body (touch, light pressure, cutaneous pain, temperature, olfaction, taste, vision, hearing); 2) **interoceptive,** responding to stimuli from within the viscera (visceral pain, chemoreceptors of the aortic and carotid bodies, baroreceptors of carotid sinuses); and 3) **proprioceptive,** responding to stimuli from within skeletal muscles, tendons, and joints (tension, deep pressure, orientation, awareness of position and movement).

The efferent nerve endings are divided into: 1) somatic efferent, terminating as motor end-plates on skeletal muscle cells; 2) visceral efferent, associated with smooth muscle cells, cardiac muscle, and glands.

From a **structural point of view,** nerve endings can be subdivided according to the following scheme:

I. **Afferent** nerve endings (sensory)
  1. **Free** (naked; non-encapsulated; denuded)
    a) simple: skin, connective tissue, cornea: pain/touch
    b) elaborate: Golgi tendon organ: stretch (proprioceptive sense)
    c) more elaborate: neuromuscular spindle: muscle proprioceptive sense
  2. **Encapsulated**
    a) Pacini's corpuscles: pressure; touch
    b) Meissner's corpuscles: touch
    c) Ruffini's corpuscles: possibly heat receptors; touch
    d) Krause's end-bulbs: possibly cold receptors; touch
  3. **Baroreceptors:** in the wall of carotid sinuses
  4. **Chemoreceptors:** carotid and aortic bodies; olfaction, taste
  5. **Special sense organs:** vision, hearing
II. **Efferent** nerve endings (motor)
  1. Somatic: motor end plates
  2. Visceral:
    a) smooth muscle
    b) cardiac muscle
    c) glands

No attempt will be made to describe in detail the varied structural appearance of all the nerve endings above.

Fig. 14-1. Free nerve endings (sensory). Silver impregnation method. Cornea. Flat mount. Mouse (4 days old). L.M. X 225. **1.** Irregularly patterned background represents corneal epithelial cells and their nuclei. **2.** Myelinated nerves located in corneal connective tissue stroma. **3.** Points where myelin sheath is shed. **4.** Denuded nerve endings among corneal epithelial cells.

Fig. 14-2. Free nerve endings (sensory). Skin. Rat. E.M. X 31,000. **1.** Base of epidermis. **2.** Basal lamina. **3.** Nerve process within epithelium. **4.** Nerve processes in subepithelial connective tissue. **5.** Schwann cell cytoplasm. **6.** Network of reticulum and delicate collagenous fibrils.

Fig. 14-3. Termination of myelinated nerve process. Papillary layer of dermis. Rat. E.M. X 31,000. **1.** Peripheral nerve process of sensory neuron. **2.** Microtubules. **3.** Mitochondria. **4.** Myelin sheath. **5.** Successive laminae of the myelin sheath terminate as cytoplasmic swellings. **6.** Schwann cell cytoplasm (neurolemma). **7.** Level at which the nerve process becomes denuded. **8.** External (basal) lamina. **9.** A limited number of delicate cytoplasmic processes of the Schwann cell surround loosely the denuded nerve process. **10.** Connective tissue fibrils.

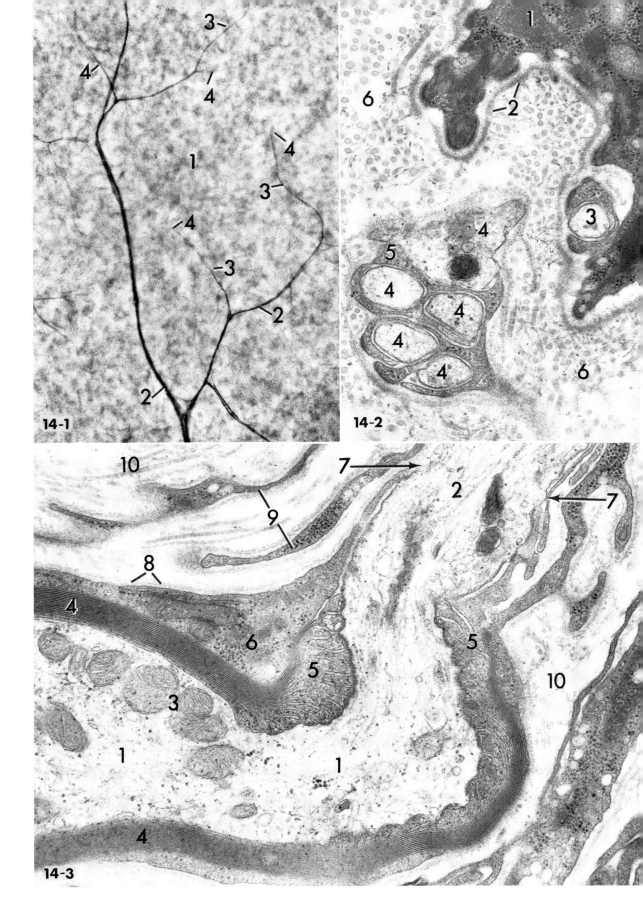

14-1

14-2

14-3

FREE NERVE ENDINGS

Sensory afferent nerve fibers, unassociated with special receptors are located between the cells of the germinative layer of the epidermis, in dermal connective tissue, periosteum, joint surfaces, intestinal and vascular connective tissue, and in the stratified epithelia of the oral cavity and the cornea. (Fig. 14-1) The nerve fibers lose their Schwann cell encasements some distance from their terminations (Fig. 14-3), making them free (denuded; naked; non-encapsulated). The terminal ramifications are abundant and may be as small as 0.2μ in diameter (Fig. 14-2), terminating in little knob-like swellings. Many of these nerve endings are derived from non-myelinated nerves.

The free nerve endings, described here, are sensory receptors for pain, touch, and perhaps heat and cold. The mechanism by which they are stimulated is not known. It is assumed that some chemical substances, perhaps proteolytic enzymes and/or bradykinin, are released from damaged cells, exciting the nerve endings. However, free nerve endings respond also to mechanical, chemical, and thermal stimuli provided they are of considerable intensity.

GOLGI TENDON ORGAN

The Golgi tendon organs are also referred to as tendon (neurotendinous) spindles. These sensory organs are located in tendons near the junctions with muscle. They are small, spindle-shaped bodies, consisting of several collagenous fiber bundles and surrounded by a thin capsule. The arborizations of the free nerve endings terminate around and upon the collagenous bundles. (Figs. 14-11, 14-12) The nerve terminations are completely denuded of Schwann cell cytoplasm, and their club-shaped endings are filled with numerous mitochondria.

A varied or constant tension on the tendon is transmitted to the nerve endings of the Golgi tendon organ (mechanical stimulation). The nerve endings become stimulated by stretching or by contraction of the related muscle. Therefore, these nerve endings record any tension which occurs in the muscle. The nerve impulse is transmitted to local areas of the spinal cord and through the spinocerebellar tracts to the cerebellum. In the cord, the nerve impulse is transmitted to ventral horn motor cells via internuncial neurons. Upon muscle contraction, the Golgi tendon organ becomes activated, inhibits the motor neurons, and therefore prevents the muscle from contracting too much or from being overextended.

NEUROMUSCULAR SPINDLES

The neuromuscular spindle is a small sense organ located in the belly or near the tendon of skeletal muscle. It consists of modified (intrafusal) muscle cells, sensory and motor nerves, and is enclosed by a capsule. (Figs. 14-4, 14-5) The neuromuscular spindle is oriented in parallel with the main (extrafusal) muscle cells and registers mechanical distortion of the extrafusal muscle fibers.

The spindle is fusiform with a wide equatorial region and two narrow polar regions. It averages 2 mm in length and 0.1 mm in width. It contains 3–10 delicate fusiform striated intrafusal muscle fibers of two different types. (Fig. 14-6) The **nuclear bag fiber** contains numerous nu-

Fig. 14-4. Neuromuscular spindle. Cross section. Equatorial region. Triceps surae muscle. Rat. Embryo, 2 days before birth. E.M. $\times$ 1200. (From: Jacqueline H. Levy, 1972). **1.** Extrafusal skeletal muscle fibers. **2.** Lumen of blood capillary. **3.** Outer capsule. **4.** Periaxial space. **5.** Inner capsule. **6.** Myelinated nerve fibers. **7.** Intrafusal nuclear chain muscle fibers. **8.** Nuclear bag muscle fibers. **9.** Fibroblasts. **10.** Loose connective tissue.

Fig. 14-5. Neuromuscular spindle. Cross section. Juxta-equatorial region. Front leg muscle. Newborn rat. E.M. X 1900. **1.** Extrafusal skeletal muscle fibers. **2.** Lumen of capillary. **3.** Outer capsule. **4.** Periaxial space. **5.** Inner capsule. **6.** Myelinated nerve fibers. **7.** Nuclear chain muscle fibers. **8.** Nuclear bag muscle fibers. Rectangle enlarged in Fig. 14-6.

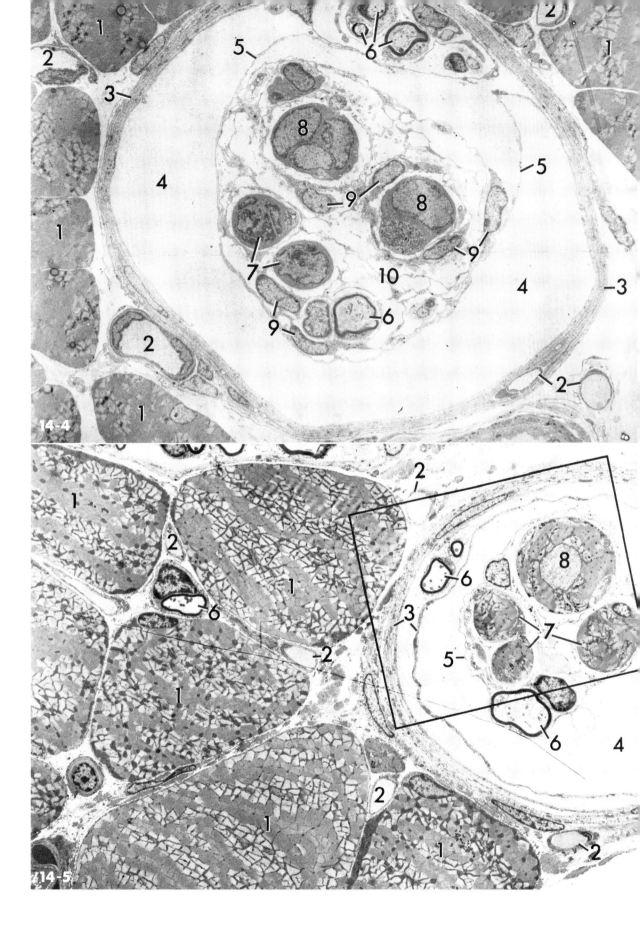

clei in the middle of the cell, and only a limited number of striated myofibrils. The **nuclear chain fiber** contains a single row of nuclei and a relative abundance of delicate myofibrils. The intrafusal muscle fibers are enclosed by a **capsule,** consisting of concentrically arranged flat cells with an external (basal) lamina on either side of each layer. The nature of these cells is uncertain, but the presence of an external lamina indicates their possible relationship to Schwann cells rather than fibroblasts. The capsule is continuous with the perimysium of the extrafusal fibers and with the Schwann cells of entering nerves. There is a **periaxial space** between the intrafusal muscle cells and the capsule. It varies in size and contains nerve fibers, small blood vessels, fibroblasts, and tissue fluid.

The spindle is supplied with two sets of sensory nerve fibers and one set of motor nerve fibers. The sensory nerve fibers have two types of endings. The **annulospiral endings** are denuded nerve terminals which are wrapped spirally around the equatorial region of the intrafusal nuclear bag fibers. The axolemma and the sarcolemma are separated by a 200 Å intercellular space. An occasional zonula adhaerens may be present. The external (basal) lamina of the intrafusal muscle cell encloses the nerve terminal. The nerve terminal is filled with small spherical mitochondria, clear vesicles, and neurofilaments. The second type of sensory nerve terminations, the **flower-spray** (or **secondary) endings,** is grouped around the juxta-equatorial region of the intrafusal nuclear chain fiber. Ultrastructurally, both types of sensory nerve endings are similar. (Fig. 14-7)

The **efferent gamma fibers** from the small gamma motor neurons of the spinal cord terminate on the intrafusal fibers with modified motor end plates.

From a **functional** point of view, the annulospiral and flower-spray nerve endings represent stretch receptors, which are stimulated mechanically when the extra-fusal muscle fibers are stretched and thus increase in length. The nerve impulse thus generated exerts, in the spinal cord, an excitatory influence on the motor neurons to the same muscle via a direct reflex connection. The efferent gamma nerve fibers shorten the intrafusal muscle fibers, thereby increasing the sensitivity of the muscle spindle to stretch. Consult textbooks of neurophysiology for functional differences between annulospiral and flower-spray endings.

PACINI'S CORPUSCLES

The lamellated corpuscle of Pacini is a sense organ which is stimulated by pressure. The Pacinian corpuscles are located in the deep layers of the skin, particularly in the finger pads (Fig. 14-8), around viscera and walls of large vessels, in the peritoneum, and on tendons and ligaments.

The corpuscle has the shape of an onion, averaging 2 mm in width and 4 mm in length. The **outer part** consists of some 50 lamellae, arranged loosely and concentrically. The lamellae are made up of thin flat endothelial-like cells, connective tissue fibers and interstitial fluid. The central core consists of compactly and concentrically arranged flat cells. (Fig. 14-9) A large myelinated nerve pierces the cor-

Fig. 14-6. Neuromuscular spindle. Cross section. Juxta-equatorial region. Enlargement of rectangle in Fig. 14-5. E.M. X 4500. **1.** Part of extrafusal muscle fiber. **2.** Lumen of capillary. **3.** Sheet-like cells of outer capsule. **4.** Myelinated nerve fibers. **5.** Periaxial space. **6.** Inner capsule. **7.** Nucleus of fibroblast. **8.** Nucleus of Schwann cell. **9.** Nucleus of nuclear bag fiber. **10.** Polar ends of nuclear chain fibers. **11.** Satellite muscle cell. **12.** Sensory nerve endings.

Fig. 14-7. Sensory nerve ending. Neuromuscular spindle. Enlargement of rectangle in Fig. 14-6. E.M. X 60,000. **1.** Myofilaments of intrafusal nuclear chain muscle fiber. **2.** Sensory nerve ending. **3.** Mitochondria. **4.** Membranous contact between sarcolemma and cell membrane of nerve ending. **5.** Zonula adhaerens junction. **6.** External (basal) lamina.

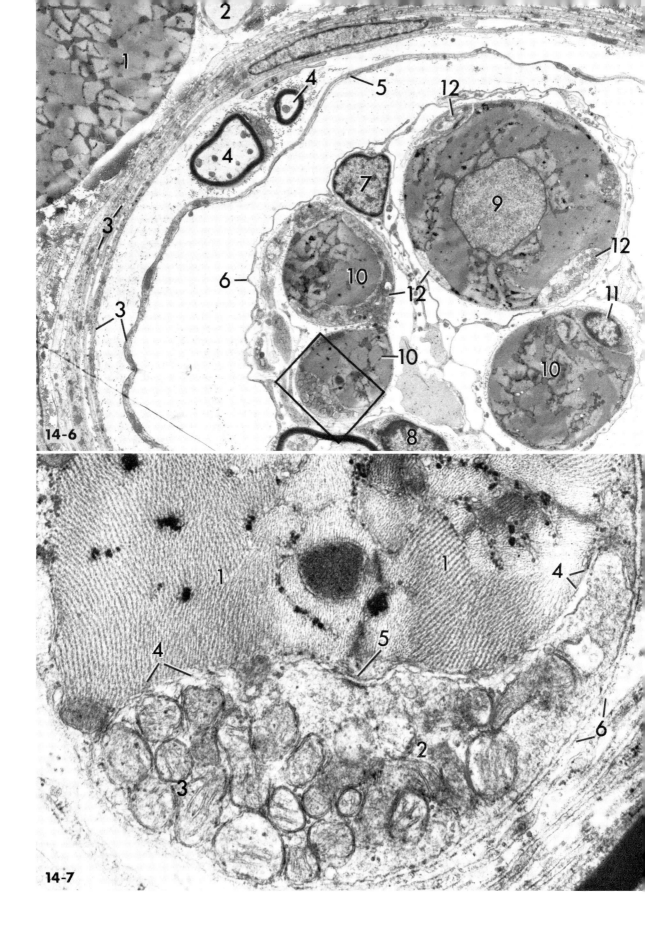

14-6

14-7

puscle at one pole and continues as a long straight, non-branching non-meylinated nerve fiber through the middle of the central core. (Fig. 14-10) The nerve ending is filled with small spherical mitochondria and clear synaptic vesicles.

The Pacinian corpuscle is a transducer which responds to mechanical vibrations, pressure, and tension. In the skin it responds to tactile pressure, whereas it registers movements and positions in joint capsules and tendons, providing a mechanism for proprioception. A compression or distortion of the corpuscle is probably amplified by the lamellae and the interlamellar fluid, deforming the central core, whereby the axolemma of the nerve ending is stretched and deformed. This deformation changes the permeability of the axolemma, giving rise to a generator potential, which in turn initiates action potentials in the nerve fiber.

MEISSNER'S CORPUSCLES

Meissner's corpuscles are small, ovoid or cylindrical touch receptors, especially numerous in the dermal papillae of the finger pads. (Fig. 14-13) They also occur in the lips, edges of the eyelids, and genital skin. Each corpuscle consists of a series of elongated, flat, or slightly conical connective tissue cells of mesodermal origin, which are stacked transversely to form the corpuscle. (Fig. 14-14) A thin connective tissue capsule surrounds some corpuscles. Non-myelinated nerve endings form a ramified plexus around and between the stacked, conical cells. They join to form a large, myelinated nerve fiber outside the capsule of the corpuscle.

Meissner's corpuscle is a mechanoreceptor, sensitive to touch. The arrangement of the nerve terminals in relation to the transversely stacked mesodermal cells facilitates and enhances the deformation of the nerve endings, initiating the nerve impulses.

RUFFINI'S CORPUSCLES

These receptors are also referred to as **spray endings** and are structurally similar to the Golgi tendon organ. The corpuscles of Ruffini occur in the dermis of fingers, and the soles of the foot, in the capsules of joints and in the walls of blood vessels. The spindle-shaped corpuscles may be surrounded by a thin connective tissue capsule. As the myelinated nerve approaches the corpuscle, it branches to form a terminal arborization of delicate, denuded nerve fibers, each provided with a small knob-like ending. The endings are intimately associated with collagenous fibers and fibroblasts of the connective tissue in which they occur.

It has been suggested that the corpuscles of Ruffini represent receptors of heat and warmth. In addition, they probably also act as transducers which respond to touch, vibrations, and mechanical distortion, registering changes in position as well as motion and therefore participating in proprioception.

KRAUSE'S END-BULBS

These receptors are present in the outer zone of the dermis, in the conjunctiva, lips, and oral cavity. The spherical corpuscle is surrounded by a thick capsule of fibroblasts and collagenous fibrils. The afferent nerve fiber loses its myelin sheath as it penetrates the capsule of the endbulb. The denuded nerve fiber branches

Fig. **14-8.** Hypodermal region. Skin of palm of hand. Human. L.M. X 56. **1.** Pacinian corpuscles. **2.** Outer part. **3.** Central core. **4.** Bundle of nerve fibers. **5.** Artery. **6.** Veins. **7.** Adipose tissue.

Fig. **14-9.** Pacini's corpuscle. Cross section. Central core. Enlargement of area similar to rectangle in Fig. 14-8. Pancreas. Cat. E.M. X 1800. **1.** Nuclei of flattened fibroblasts in outer part of corpuscle. **2.** Cytoplasmic lamellae of central core. **3.** Nerve fiber.

Fig. **14-10.** Pacini's corpuscle. Cross section. Central core and nerve ending. Enlargement of area similar to rectangle in Fig. 14-9. Pancreas. Cat. E.M. X 16,000. **1.** Interdigitating lamellar cell processes of inner core. **2.** Mitochondria. **3.** Nerve ending. **4.** Cell membrane of nerve process. **5.** Neurofilaments.

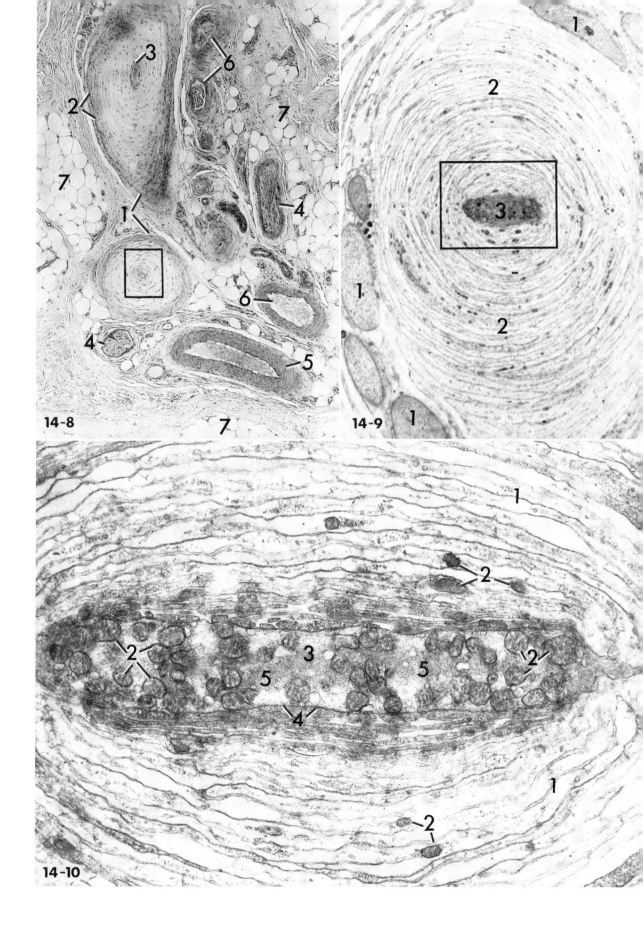

14-8

14-9

14-10

repeatedly within the center of the bulb, giving rise to a rich terminal arborization.

In the subepithelial connective tissue of the glans penis and clitoris occur **genital corpuscles,** which are structurally similar to but larger than Krause's end-bulbs.

Krause's end-bulbs are thought to represent receptors of cold. However, one should be aware of the fact that the free nerve endings of the skin can be stimulated thermally, responding to gradations of cold and heat. Therefore, it is quite possible that Krause's end-bulbs, as well as Ruffini's corpuscles, function solely as mechanoreceptors.

The tactile stimulation of the genital corpuscles activates the axolemma of the nerve endings and initiate afferent nerve impulses. As a response, this leads to vasodilation and engorgement of the corpora cavernosa of the penis and clitoris, secretion of mucus from the glands of Bartholin in the vagina, and the sexual sensations and motor phenomena that form the orgasm and precede or accompany ejaculation.

BARORECEPTORS

Baroreceptors (or pressoreceptors) are mechanoreceptors present in the walls of large arteries. They respond to pressure or tension as the vascular walls become distended during an elevation of blood pressure.

The receptors consist of free, spray-type nerve endings in the adventitia of all large arteries in the neck and thorax. They are particularly abundant in the aortic wall and the carotid sinus, the dilatation of the common carotid artery near its bifurcation into the internal and external arteries. The nerve endings represent the terminal arborization of the carotid sinus (Hering's) nerve, a branch of the glossopharyngeal nerve which originates from the medulla oblongata. The afferent nerve endings in the arch of the aorta are derived from the vagus nerve.

The baroreceptors are transducers in a negative feedback system, regulating the arterial blood pressure. An elevation in blood pressure stretches the nerve endings and elicits a carotid sinus reflex. The afferent nerve impulses inhibit the vasomotor centers of the medulla and excite the vagal center. The arterial blood pressure is then lowered as a result of a general vasodilatation and a decreased cardiac rate via the autonomic nervous system.

CHEMORECEPTORS

Chemoreceptors are transducers, sensitive to chemical substances, converting chemical stimuli into nerve impulses. The **olfactory epithelium** of the nose and the **taste buds** of the tongue are examples of chemoreceptors. They are discussed on p. 610 and p. 512.

Another chemoreceptor which is sensitive to changes in concentrations of blood oxygen, carbon dioxide, and hydrogen ion is represented by the **aortic** and **carotid bodies** and **glomus pulmonale.** The carotid bodies are located at the bifurcation of the common carotid artery. The aortic body lies between the arch of the aorta

Fig. 14-11. Golgi tendon organ. Teased skeletal muscle. Impregnation method. Rat. L.M. X 154. **1.** Striated skeletal muscle fibers (cells). **2.** Muscle-tendon junction. **3.** Peripheral (sensory) nerve fiber. **4.** Arborization of nerve termination (tendon organ).

Fig. 14-12. Golgi tendon organ. Enlargement of rectangle in Fig. 14-11. L.M. X 418. **1.** Tendon. **2.** Peripheral (sensory) nerve fiber. **3.** Branching of nerve fiber. **4.** Terminal arborization of nerve fiber with club-shaped endings.

Fig. 14-13. Meissner's corpuscle. Skin. Human. L.M. X 385. **1.** Stratum granulosum of epidermis. **2.** Stratum spinosum. **3.** Stratum basale of epidermis. **4.** Papillary layer of dermis. **5.** Meissner's corpuscle. **6.** Dermal capillaries and venules.

Fig. 14-14. Meissner's corpuscle. Enlargement of rectangle in Fig. 14-13. L.M. X 600. **1.** Stratum basale of epidermis. **2.** Level of basal lamina. **3.** Connective tissue of dermal papillary layer. **4.** Nuclei of flat, transversely stacked fibroblasts. **5.** Distribution of terminal arborization of nerve fiber indicated by solid and dotted lines. **6.** Capillary.

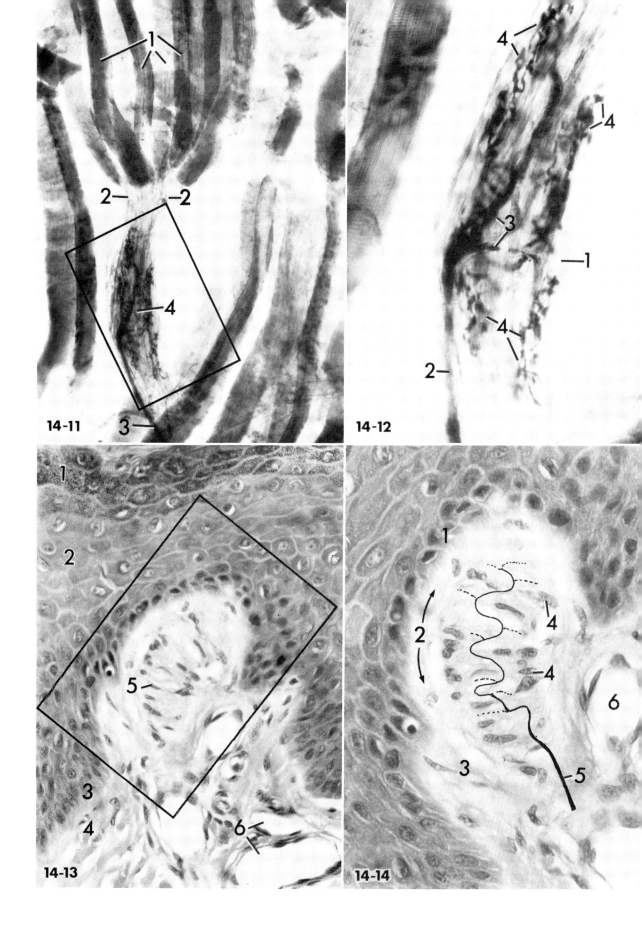

14-11

14-12

14-13

14-14

and the pulmonary artery. The glomus pulmonale is situated in the wall of the pulmonary arteries near the root of the lungs. They are round or oval bodies, averaging 2–3 mm in diameter, consisting of densely arranged glomus cells, some autonomic ganglion cells, and denuded nerve fibers. Each body is perforated by a rich capillary network (Fig. 14-15), which receives its blood supply directly from the adjacent arterial trunk via a small artery.

Several types of glomus cells have been described. It is presently agreed that the most common cell, **type I glomus cell** (chief cell), is large and rounded and has a round nucleus with abundant light euchromatin and a cytoplasm filled with numerous small, membrane-bound dense-core granules. **Type II glomus cell** (supporting cell) is less common. It is flat, branching, and has an oval nucleus rich in dense heterochromatin. The cytoplasm contains some dense-core granules. (Fig. 14-16) Other glomus cells have been described, but it is presently not known if they represent functional variations of glomus cells I and II. The dense-core granules of the glomus cells have been demonstrated to contain catecholamines (noradrenalin, dopamine, and perhaps 5-hydroxytryptamine). It is therefore conceivable that these cells are unrelated to the chemoreceptor function of the aortic and carotid bodies. Efferent nerve fibers in the sinus nerve and the postganglionic branches of the sympathetic superior cervical ganglia contact the glomus cells synaptically with nerve endings containing clear and dense-core vesicles. It has been suggested that the glomus cells, upon arrival of efferent nerve impulses, liberate catecholamines into the bloodstream, similar to the cells of the adrenal medulla (p. 462).

Several delicate, sensory type, denuded nerve fibers occur in the aortic and carotid bodies. (Fig. 14-17) Many of them are closely applied to the walls of blood capillaries. They are believed to represent true chemoreceptor nerve endings of the sinus

and vagus nerves. When the oxygen concentration in the arterial blood falls below a certain level, these chemoreceptors become stimulated, and excitatory nerve impulses are transmitted to the vasomotor center of the medulla oblongata. As a result, arterial blood pressure is elevated and the quantity of oxygen offered to the tissues increased. Increased blood concentrations of carbon dioxide as well as hydrogen ion also stimulate the chemoreceptors of the aortic and carotid bodies, resulting in an increased respiratory activity.

The participation of the aortic and carotid bodies and the glomus pulmonale in chemoreception has been clearly established. However, the structural complexity seems to indicate that these bodies also have endocrine functions that could be, but may not necessarily be, related to chemoreception.

SPECIAL SENSE ORGANS

The receptors and sensory nerve endings for the special senses of vision and hearing are described elsewhere: vision (p. 749); hearing (p. 773).

MOTOR END PLATES

The motor end plates (synonyms: neuromuscular junctions; myoneural junctions)

Fig. 14-15. Carotid body. Rat. E.M. X 640.
  1. Lumen of small arteriole. **2.** Lumen of capillary. **3.** Glomus cells.
Fig. 14-16. Carotid body. Glomus cells. Enlargement of area similar to rectangle in Fig. 14-15. Rat. E.M. X 9000. **1.** Nucleus of type I glomus cell (chief cell). **2.** Nucleus of type II glomus cell (supporting cell.) **3.** Lumen of capillary. **4.** Nucleus of endothelial cell. **5.** Dense-core granules. **6.** Mitochondria. **7.** Effector type (motor) nerve processes with dense-core vesicles. **8.** Sensory type nerve process.
Fig. 14-17. Detail of glomus cells. Carotid body. Enlargement of area similar to rectangle in Fig. 14-16. Rat. E.M. X 58,000. **1.** Sensory type nerve fiber with microtubules. **2.** Cytoplasmic processes of type II glomus cell, encircling nerve fiber. **3.** Dense-core granules of type I glomus cell.

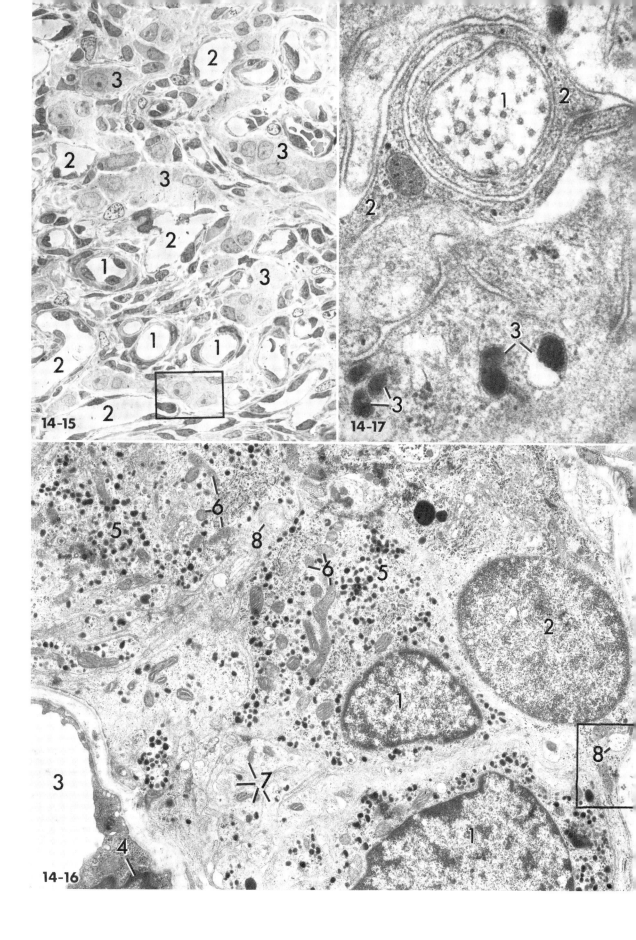

14-15

14-17

14-16

represent somatic efferent nerve endings of ventral horn motor neurons which establish contact with every striated skeletal muscle fiber (cell) and mediate the nerve impulses which result in muscle contraction. (Fig. 14-18)

The motor end plate is a flat, oval structure, averaging 40–60 μ in diameter. (Fig. 14-19) It is slightly recessed at the muscle cell surface and located midway along the length of each muscle cell. The efferent nerve abruptly loses its myelin sheath as it approaches the motor end plate (Fig. 14-20), and is subsequently protected by the neurolemmal sheath of several Schwann (teloglial) cells. Peripherally is a thin sheath of endoneurial connective tissue which is continuous with the endomysium of the muscle fiber.

The denuded axon divides into several processes, each terminating as a small bulbous expansion above the external (basal) lamina of the muscle cell. The terminal arborization is reminiscent of a flat cluster of grapes. The end knobs contain many small mitochondria, and numerous clear **synaptic vesicles** of both the round (excitatory?) and flat (inhibitory?) variety. (Figs. 14-22, 14-23) Synaptic vesicles often fuse with the presynaptic membrane. (Fig. 14-21) Since they are believed to contain the cholinergic neurotransmitter substance acetylcholine, this fusion is interpreted as a process of discharging (exocytosis) the neurotransmitter into the synaptic cleft. Neurofilaments are present in the preterminal part of the axon, but do not continue into the nerve end expansion.

The bulbous nerve expansions occupy a recess (trough) of the muscle surface. The subneural, postsynaptic sarcolemma is thrown into **junctional folds,** establishing a complex system of parallel primary and secondary clefts, which bifurcate and communicate. (Fig. 14-21) These folds increase greatly the postsynaptic surface. Acetylcholinesterase is associated with the postsynaptic membrane of the folds. The **synaptic cleft** ranges from 200 Å to 500 Å

in width, and contains a glycoprotein material which is similar to and continuous with the external (basal) lamina of the muscle cell. The subneural sarcoplasm, the **sole plate,** is devoid of myofibrils but rich in small mitochondria, particulate glycogen, microtubules, and nuclei.

By the action of the efferent nerve impulses, acetylcholine is discharged from the synaptic vesicles into the synaptic cleft. It reaches and depolarizes the postsynaptic muscle cell membrane (sarcolemma). This results in an action potential which spreads over the entire sarcolemma, and also reaches the interior of the muscle cell via the transverse tubular system (T-system), resulting in muscle contraction (see p. 232). Subsequently, the acetylcholinesterase hydrolyses the acetylcholine and stops its action. The resting potential of the postsynaptic membrane is thereby restored, and the sarcolemma can react to a new discharge of acetylcholine.

VISCERAL EFFERENT NERVE ENDINGS

Efferent non-myelinated, autonomic nerve fibers and their terminals contain and release neurotransmitter substances which depolarize the cell membranes of smooth

Fig. 14-18. Motor nerve endings. Skeletal muscle. Gold chloride method. Human. L.M. X 200. **1.** Striated muscle fibers. **2.** Bundle of myelinated nerve fibers. **3.** Motor end plates.

Fig. 14-19. Motor end plates. Gold chloride method. Skeletal muscle. Human. L.M. X 600. **1.** Efferent nerve fibers. **2.** Motor end plate in surface view. **3.** Motor end plate in side view. **4.** Striated skeletal muscle fibers.

Fig. 14-20. Motor end plate. Skeletal muscle. Enlargement of area approximately similar to rectangle in Fig. 14-19. Rat. E.M. X 30,000. **1.** Efferent nerve process (axon). **2.** Myelin sheath. **3.** Successive laminae of the myelin sheath terminate as cytoplasmic swellings. **4.** Cytoplasm of Schwann cell (neurolemma). **5.** Endoneurial connective tissue. **6.** Cytoplasm of teloglial cell (Schwann cell). **7.** Axon terminal (end knob). **8.** Synaptic trough (recess). **9.** Mitochondria. **10.** Subneural, synaptic clefts. **11.** Nucleus of skeletal muscle cell. **12.** Myofibrils. **13.** External (basal) lamina.

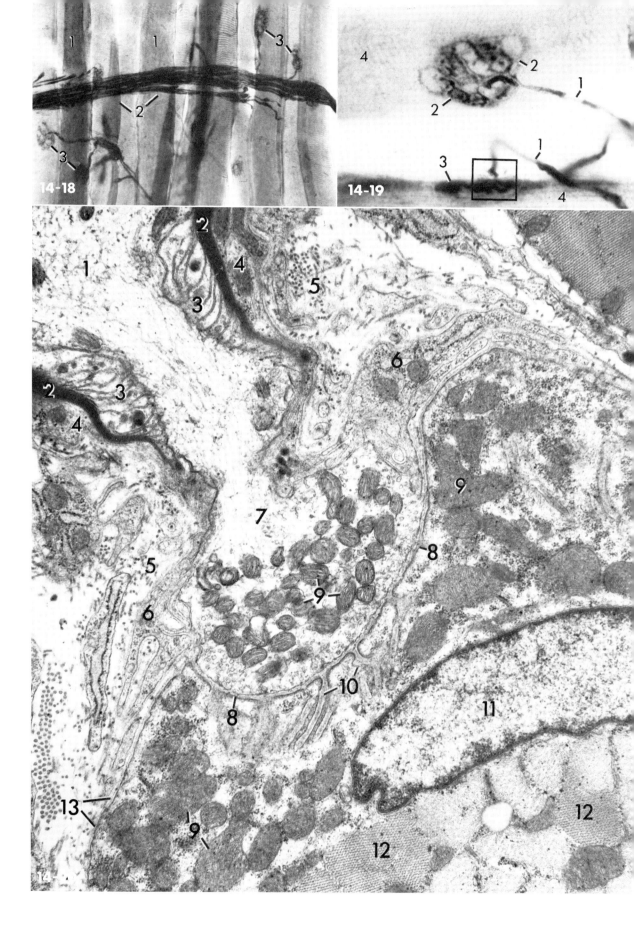

muscle cells, cardiac muscle cells, and glandular cells. The nerve fibers are highly branched, forming both dense and loose plexuses. The non-myelinated axons are provided with bead-like swellings (varicosities) along their length, and have nodular thickenings at their terminals. (Fig. 16-58) These swellings contain adrenergic neurotransmitters in the sympathetic nervous system, and cholinergic neurotransmitters in the parasympathetic nervous system.

The relationship of these nerve fibers to the various effector organs differs considerably. In most cases, the nerves of the plexus stay near the surface of the organ or tissue, but in some cases the nerve fibers permeate and surround individual cells. Structures similar to the somatic efferent motor end plates do not exist. In **vascular** smooth muscle, membranous contacts are not established between axolemma and sarcolemma, and the intervening extracellular space averages $0.1\ \mu$. (Figs. 14-24, 14-25, 16-59). In **intestinal, respiratory,** and **female reproductive** tracts, as well as in the **urinary bladder** smooth muscle, an occasional membranous contact is established between nerve fiber and smooth muscle cell, but the majority of nerve axons remain at a distance of $0.1\ \mu$ from the effector cell. In the **cardiac** muscle, **urinary** (ureter) and **male reproductive** (ductus deferens) tract smooth muscle (Fig. 14-26), as well as endocrine and exocrine glandular cells, a membranous contact is established in the majority of cases, the intervening space averaging 200 Å or less.

An area of the varicosities of the nonmyelinated visceral efferent nerves is often exposed to the interstitial space, denuded of the accompanying Schwann cell cytoplasm. The terminals are almost exclusively denuded nerve endings.

The varicosities and the terminations contain an accumulation of vesicular structures which can be subdivided into three categories: 1) small granulated vesicles; 2) large granulated vesicles; and 3) clear vesicles. (Figs. 14-25, 14-26) The **small granulated vesicles** average 300–500 Å in diameter. They have a dense core which is assumed to contain norepinephrine. The **large granulated vesicles** average 800–1000 Å in diameter. Their internal content varies in density. These granules are probably synthesized in the perikaryon and transported along the axon. They are assumed to represent storage sites of monoamines (norepinephrine and 5-hydroxytryptamine) and precursor structures of the small granulated vesicles, although undisputed evidence for these hypotheses is still missing. The **clear vesicles** of parasympathetic nerves are assumed to contain acetylcholine as do similar vesicles in the synaptic terminations of motor end plates. It is presently not known if the clear vesicles of adrenergic nerve endings represent acetyl-containing structures, or if they are membranous ghosts, representing the final stage of a continuous transition from large to small granulated vesicles.

The neurotransmitter substances are probably discharged by exocytosis. They subsequently diffuse across the extracellular space and interact with membrane-bound receptors on or near the cell membrane of the effector cell.

Fig. 14-21. Detail of motor end plate. Skeletal muscle. Rat. E.M. X 60,000. **1.** Axon terminal. **2.** Cytoplasm of muscle cell (sole plate). **3.** Mitochondria. **4.** Flat synaptic vesicles. **5.** Round synaptic vesicles. **6.** Presynaptic membrane. **7.** Synaptic cleft with glycoprotein material. **8.** Postsynaptic, junctional folds. **9.** Subneural primary and secondary clefts. **10.** Postsynaptic sarcolemma. **11.** Synaptic vesicles fusing with presynaptic membrane. **12.** Microtubules. **13.** Ribosomes.

Figs. 14-22 & 14-23. Detail of synaptic junctions of motor end plate. Skeletal muscle. Rat. E.M. X 124,000. **1.** Presynaptic cell membrane of axon terminal. **2.** Synaptic cleft. **3.** Postsynaptic sarcolemma. **4.** Round (excitatory?) electron-lucent, synaptic vesicles, bounded by a delicate, trilaminar membrane. **5.** Flat (inhibitory?) synaptic vesicles.

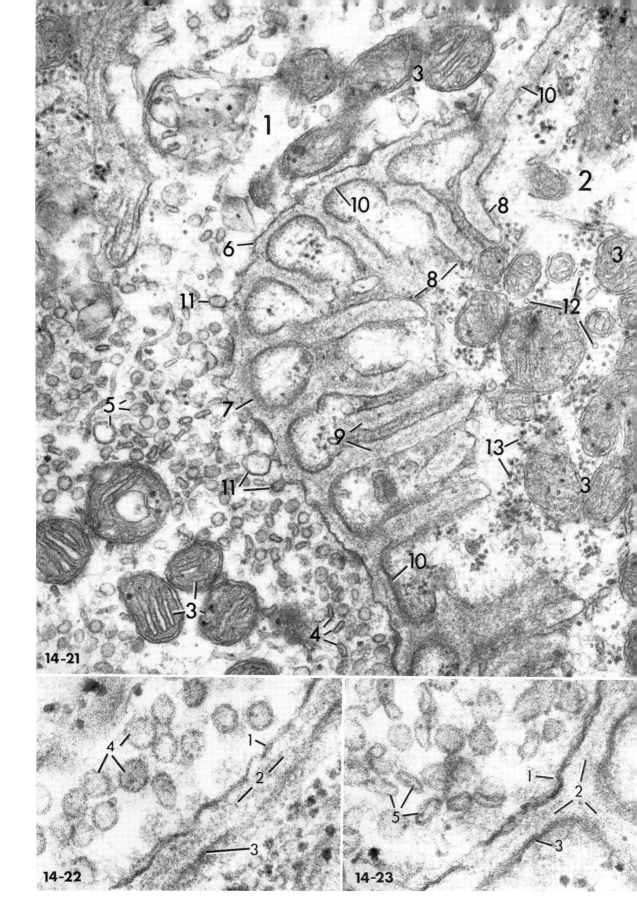

14-21

14-22

14-23

References

Adal, M. N. The fine structure of the sensory region of cat muscle spindles. J. Ultrastruct. Res. 26: 332–354 (1969).

Abbott, C. P. and Howe, A. Ultrastructure of aortic body tissue in the cat. Acta Anat. 81: 609–619 (1972).

Andersson-Cedergren, E. Ultrastructure of motor end-plate and sarcoplasmic components of mouse skeletal muscle fiber. J. Ultrastruct. Res. Suppl. 1, 1959.

Banker, B. Q. and Girvin, J. P. The ultrastructural features of the mammalian muscle spindle. J. Neuropath. Exp. Neurol. 30: 155–195 (1971).

Biscoe, T. J. and Stehbens, W. E. Ultrastructure of the carotid body. J. Cell Biol. 30: 563–578 (1966).

Böck, P., Stockinger, L. and Vyslonzil, E. Die Feinstruktur des Glomus caroticum beim Menschen. Z. Zellforsch. 105: 543–568 (1970).

Bridgman, C. F. The structure of tendon organs in the cat: a proposed mechanism for responding to muscle tension. Anat. Rec. 162: 209–220 (1968).

Cauna, N. and Ross, L. L. The fine structure of Meissner's touch corpuscles of human fingers. J. Biophys. Biochem. Cytol. 8: 467–482 (1960).

Cauna, N. Structure of digital touch corpuscles. Acta Anat. 32: 1–23 (1958).

Cauna, N. The mode of termination of the sensory nerves and its significance. J. Comp. Neurol. 113: 169–210 (1959).

Chiba, T. and Yamauchi, A. On the fine structure of the nerve terminals in the human myocardium. Z. Zellforsch. 108: 324–338 (1970).

Coërs, C. Structure and organization of the myoneural junction. Int. Rev. Cytol. 22: 239–268 (1967).

Coleridge, H. M., Coleridge, J. C. G. and Howe, A. Thoracic chemoreceptors in the dog. A histological and electrophysiological study of the location, innervation and blood supply of the aortic bodies. Circ. Res. 26: 235–247 (1970).

Devine, C. E. and Simpson, F. O. The fine structure of vascular sympathetic neuromuscular contacts in the rat. Am. J. Anat. 121: 153–174 (1967).

Edwards, C., Heath, D. and Harris, P. Ultrastructure of the carotid body in high-altitude guinea-pigs. J. Path. 107: 131–136 (1971).

Geffin, L. B., Livett, B. G. and Rush, R. A. Transmitter economy of sympathetic neurons. Circ. Res. 26: Suppl. II, 33–39 (1970).

Hökfelt, T. Distribution of noradrenaline storing particles in peripheral adrenergic neurons as revealed by electron microscopy. Acta Physiol. Scand. 76: 427–440 (1969).

Iggo, A. and Muir, A. R. The structure and function of a slowly adapting touch corpuscle in hairy skin. J. Physiol. 200: 763–796 (1969).

Levy, J. H. Development of the neuromuscular spindle in the rat: light and electron microscopy. Ph.D. Thesis 1972. Graduate School of Basic Medical Science. New York Medical College, Valhalla, N.Y. 10595.

Morita, E., Chiocchio, S. R. and Tramezzani, J. H. Four types of main cells in the carotid body of the cat. J. Ultrastruct. Res. 28: 399–410 (1969).

Niedorf, H. R., Rode, J. and Blümcke, S. Feinstruktur und Catecholamingehalt des Glomus caroticum der Ratte nach einmaliger Reserpin-injektion. Virchows Arch., Part B, Zellpath. 5: 113–123 (1970).

Ovalle, W. K., Jr. Fine structure of rat intrafusal muscle fibers. The polar region. J. Cell Biol. 51: 83–103 (1971).

Ovalle, W. K., Jr. Motor nerve terminals on rat intrafusal muscle fibers, a correlated light and electron microscopic study. J. Anat. 111: 239–252 (1972).

Ovalle, W. K., Jr. Fine structure of rat intrafusal muscle fibers. The equatorial region. J. Cell Biol. 52: 382–396 (1972).

Padykula, H. A. and Gauthier, G. F. The ultrastructure of the neuromuscular junctions of mammalian red, white and intermediate skeletal muscle fibers. J. Cell Biol. 46: 27–41 (1970).

Pick, J. Fine structure of nerve terminals in the human gut. Anat. Rec. 159: 131–145 (1967).

Quilliam, T. A. and Armstrong, J. Mechanoreceptors. Endeavour, 22: 55–60 (1963).

Rees, P. M. The distribution of biogenic amines in the carotid bifurcation region. J. Physiol. 193: 245–253 (1967).

Rees, P. M. Observations on the fine structure and distribution of presumptive baroreceptor nerves at the carotid sinus. J. Comp. Neurol. 131: 517–548 (1967).

Richardson, K. C. The fine structure of autonomic nerve endings in smooth muscle of the rat vas deferens. J. Anat. 96: 427–442 (1962).

Fig. 14-24. Vasomotor nerve endings. Large helicine arteriole. Corpus cavernosum penis. Rat. E.M. X 31,000. 1. Nucleus of Schwann cell. 2. Centriole. 3. Microtubules. 4. Schwann cell cytoplasm. 5. Sympathetic (adrenergic) nerve endings. 6. Denuded adrenergic nerve endings. 7. Cytoplasm of vascular smooth muscle cells. 8. Collagenous fibrils. 9. External (basal) lamina.

Fig. 14-25. Sympathetic (adrenergic) vasomotor nerve ending. Helicine arteriole. Corpus cavernosum penis. Rat. E.M. X 60,000. 1. Vascular smooth muscle cell. 2. External lamina. 3. Perivascular connective tissue space. 4. Adrenergic axon terminal with numerous small, granulated (dense-core) vesicles and some large granulated (dense-core) vesicles. 5. Mitochondria. 6. Schwann cell cytoplasm with microtubules. 7. Minimum diffusion gap between axolemma and sarcolemma (indicated by T-bars) is 0.27 μ in this section.

Fig. 14-26. Myoneural junction. Smooth muscle. Ductus deferens. Rat. E.M. X 90,000. 1. Sarcolemma of smooth muscle cells. 2. Axolemma of sympathetic nerve ending. 3. Intercellular space. 4. Myoneural junction; intercellular space 175 Å. 5. Clear vesicles. 6. Small granulated vesicles. 7. Large granulated vesicles.

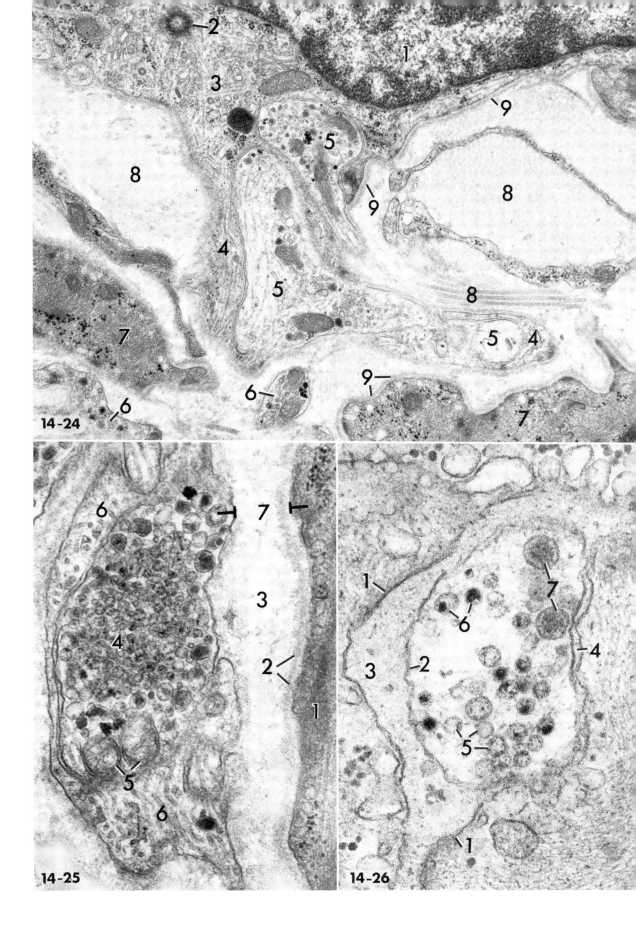

14-24

14-25

14-26

Rumpelt, H.-J. and Schmalbruch, H. Zur Morphologie der Bauelements von Muskelspindeln bei Mensch und Ratte. Z. Zellforsch. *102*: 601–630 (1969).

Scalzi, H. A. and Price, H. M. The arrangement and sensory innervation of the intrafusal fibers in the feline muscle spindle. J. Ultrastruct. Res. *36*: 375–390 (1971).

Shuangshoti, S. and Netsky, M. G. Human choroid plexus: morphologic and histochemical alterations with age. Am. J. Anat. *128*: 73–96 (1970).

Yates, R. D., Chen, I. and Duncan, D. Effects of sinus nerve stimulation on carotid body glomus cells. J. Cell Biol. *46*: 544–552 (1970).

15 Nervous tissue— non-neural structures

The nervous tissue contains, and is surrounded by, cells which do not represent nerve cells, although embryologically some of them may have developed from the same dermal layer as the neurons. Among the non-neural structures discussed in this chapter are: 1) neuroglia; 2) ependyma; 3) choroid plexus; 5) meninges; and 6) blood vessels.

Neuroglia

The neuroglia of the central nervous system consists of cells with a highly branched cytoplasm, filling in the spaces between the nerve cells, and forming the sheaths of the myelinated nerve fibers. These cells make up about 40 percent of the total volume of the CNS with a glia:neuron ratio of about 2:1. The glial cells assist in the regulation of the neuronal microenvironment through supportive, protective, and nutritive processes. Hypothetically, the glial cells may also have properties which are related to the storage of inherited and acquired behavioral patterns.

The neuroglial cells are smaller than the nerve cells, and their processes shorter. The visualization of the neuroglial cells is difficult. The classical histology relied mostly on nuclear size and shape, and on gold and silver impregnation techniques of cell body and processes (Golgi, Cajal), but these methods are technically difficult and the results erratic. (Fig. 15-1) Early electron microscope analyses did not help to clarify the problem of cell identification, but rather confused the issue further. Only during the last few years, improved fixation and embedding techniques for electron microscopy have contributed to a better, albeit preliminary, understanding of the several types of neuroglial cells. It is anticipated that research during the next decade will further our knowledge considerably concerning the relationship and functions of the neuroglial cells. According to present knowledge, the neu-roglial cells are divided into: 1) oligodendroglia; 2) astroglia; and 3) microglia. Ependymal cells are usually also considered glial elements, but are described separately on p. 318.

Oligodendroglia. Oligodendroglia or oligodendrocytes are small, angular cells of neural ectodermal origin which occur in both the white and gray matter of the CNS. In the white matter, oligodendrocytes are **interfascicular** (Fig. 15-3), providing the myelin sheath for the nerve fibers. In the gray matter, oligodendrocytes are often **perineuronal,** closely associated with nerve cell perikarya in a satellite position. (Fig. 15-2) Oligodendrocytes average 6–8 μ in diameter. The nucleus is round or oval and rich in dense heterochromatin. (Fig. 15-4) The cytoplasm occupies a thin perinuclear rim which has an electron-dense appearance because of the presence of numerous free ribosomes and profiles of the granular endoplasmic reticulum. (Fig. 15-5) The Golgi zone is small, and the irregularly shaped mito-

Fig. 15-1. Neuroglial cells. Cerebellar cortex. Impregnation method. Cat. L.M. X 242.
1. Molecular layer. 2. Purkinje nerve cells.
3. Granule cell layer. 4. Neuroglial cells.
Fig. 15-2. Oligodendrocytes. Gray matter. Spinal cord. Rat. E.M. X 1800. 1. Nucleus of neuron in anterior horn. 2. Nuclei of perineuronal (satellite) oligodendrocytes. 3. Myelinated nerves.
Fig. 15-3. Oligodendroycytes. White matter. Spinal cord. Cross section. Rat. E.M. X 1800.
1. Nuclei of interfascicular oligodendrocytes.
2. Myelinated nerve processes of varied diameters.
Fig. 15-4. Oligodendrocyte. White matter. Spinal cord. Cross section. Rat. E.M. X 9000.
1. Nucleus of oligodendrocyte. 2. Golgi zone.
3. Centriole. 4. Mitochondria. 5. Myelinated nerve processes. Sheet-like processes of the oligodendrocytes form the myelin sheaths of the central nervous system.
Fig. 15-5. Detail of oligodendrocyte. Gray matter. Spinal cord. Rat. E.M. X 62,000.
1. Golgi zone. 2. Mitochondria. 3. Lysosome.
4. Cisternae of granular endoplasmic reticulum. 5. Polyribosomes and monoribosomes in electron-dense cytoplasm.

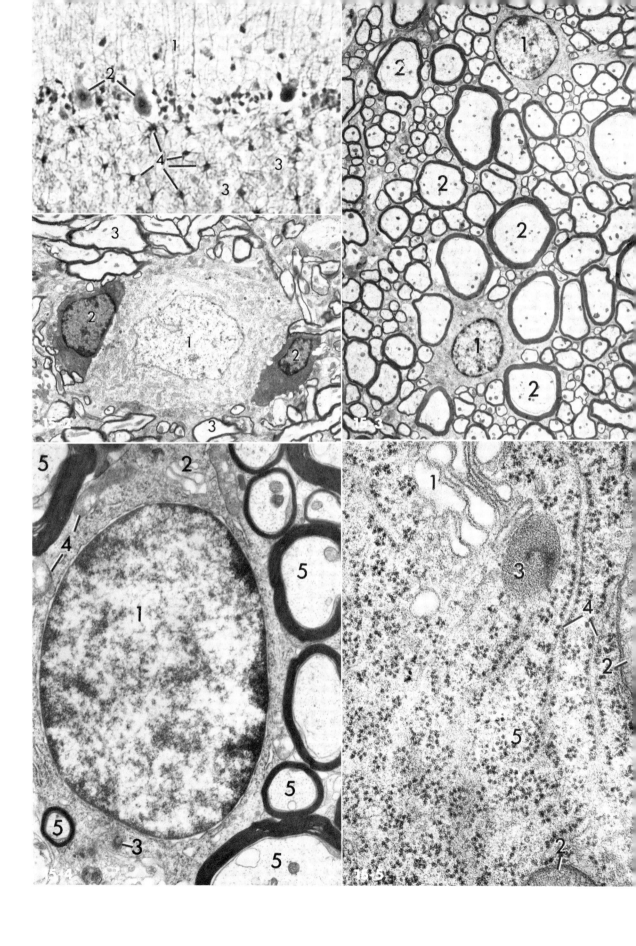

chondria are provided with tubular cristae. Some microtubules are present in the cytoplasm, but filaments are rare. Particulate glycogen is not present.

The cytoplasm extends into a limited number of trunk-like processes which spread out and become sheet-like as they form the myelin sheaths of several nerve processes of the CNS. (Fig. 13-19) The primary function of the oligodendrocytes is the formation of the myelin sheath, and indirectly, they therefore play a certain role in nerve impulse transmission within the CNS. The function of the perineuronal (satellite) oligodendrocyte is not clear, although it has been suggested that some kind of symbiotic relationship exists, possibly consisting of a transfer of RNA between glia and neurons.

Astroglia. Astroglia or astrocytes are stellate cells of neuronal ectoderm origin which occur in the gray matter as **protoplasmic astrocytes,** and in the white matter of the brain and spinal cord chiefly as **fibrous astrocytes.** (Fig. 15-6) It is generally accepted that the two types of astrocytes are varieties of the same kind of cell. The cells average 8–10 μ in diameter, thus being slightly larger than the oligodendrocytes. The nucleus is irregularly ovoid and is pale because of an abundance of light euchromatin.

The cytoplasm, which occupies a relatively broad perinuclear area, is electron lucent because of a scarcity of free ribosomes and profiles of granular endoplasmic reticulum. (Fig. 15-7) Particulate glycogen is relatively abundant. Mitochondria are few in number and large, the Golgi zone often elaborate, and lysosomes are always present. The cytoplasm is drawn out into many, either broad or slender, highly branching processes which fill in most of the interneuronal spaces of the CNS. Some processes have terminal expansions which are applied to the walls of capillaries and other blood vessels, forming an incomplete layer of hydrated plate-like **perivascular feet.** Similar processes also form a complete layer of **subpial**

feet beneath the pia mater, covering the surface of the CNS.

The cytoplasmic processes, as well as the perinuclear cytoplasm contains a varied amount of fibrils. These are sheets and bundles of filaments, the individual filament averaging 60–100 Å. (Figs. 15-8, 15-9) Depending on the amount of these fibrils, one may subdivide the astroglia into fibrous and protoplasmic astrocytes.

The astrocytes serve as support for tracts of nerve fibers. They cover the non-synaptic surfaces of neurons, probably in order to establish a microenvironment for the neuron. It is also believed that the cytoplasmic processes which contact blood vessels (Fig. 15-26) and pia mater (Fig. 15-21) participate in an exchange of fluid, gases and metabolites between the nervous tissue and the blood and cerebrospinal fluid. Fibrous astrocytes participate in

Fig. 15-6. Astrocyte. White matter. Spinal cord. Rat. E.M. X 15,000. **1.** Nucleus of fibrous astrocyte. **2.** Bundles of filaments in electron-lucent cytoplasm. **3.** Myelinated nerve processes. **4.** Non-myelinated nerve processes. **5.** Subpial feet of astrocyte. **6.** Nucleus of pia mater fibroblast. **7.** Cytoplasm of fibroblast. Rectangle (A) is enlarged further in Fig. 15-21.

Fig. 15-7. Astrocyte. Enlargement of rectangle (B) in Fig. 15-6. E.M. X 32,000. **1.** Nucleus. **2.** Mitochondria. **3.** Profiles of granular endoplasmic reticulum. **4.** Longitudinally sectioned glial filaments. **5.** Cross-sectioned glial filaments. **6.** Myelin sheaths. **7.** Axoplasm with microtubules.

Fig. 15-8. Detail of astrocyte. White matter. Spinal cord. Rat. E.M. X 47,000. **1.** Mitochondria. **2.** Cross-sectioned bundles of glial filaments. **3.** Profiles of granular endoplasmic reticulum. **4.** Electron-lucent astrocyte cytoplasm. **5.** Astrocyte cell membranes.

Fig. 15-9. Detail of astrocyte. White matter. Spinal cord. Rat. E.M. X 62,000. **1.** Nucleus. **2.** Granular endoplasmic reticulum. **3.** Lysosome. **4.** Glial filaments, longitudinally sectioned. **5.** External tongue process of oligodendrocyte. **6.** Myelin sheath, formed by oligodendrocyte. **7.** Nerve process with microtubules.

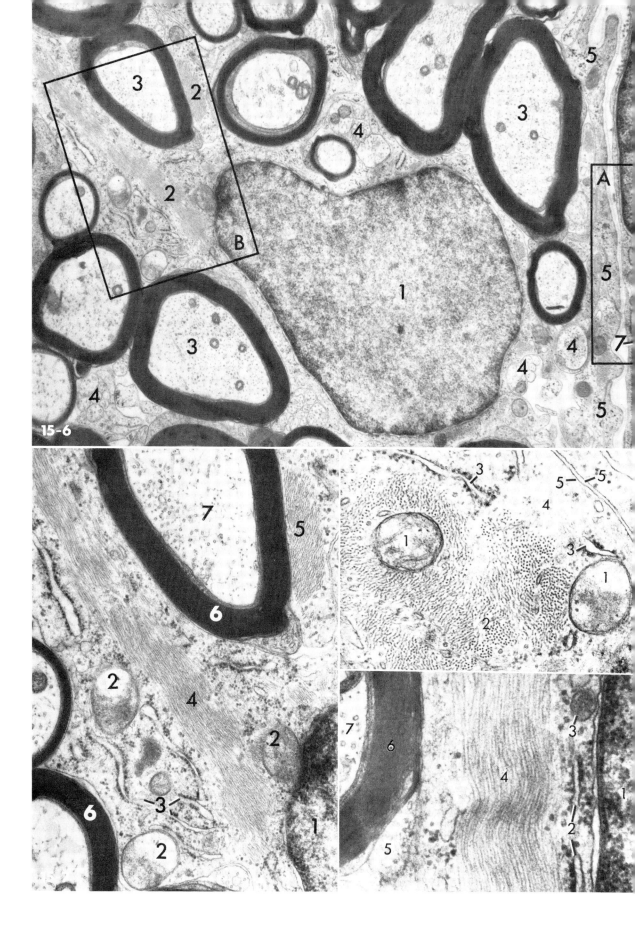

forming glial scar tissue (gliosis) after trauma and injury to the CNS.

Microglia. A limited number of multipolar cells which are smaller than the oligodendrocytes have been identified near blood vessels by impregnation methods in the gray and white matter of the CNS. They are collectively referred to as **microglial cells** (synonym: mesoglia). However, electron microscope analyses have not yet been able to positively identify specific microglial cells. The following is a summary of the present knowledge of the so-called microglia and cells of similar appearance.

Associated with blood vessels of the CNS are perivascular cells of mesodermal origin which are identical to pericytes (p. 354) in other tissues and organs. These pericytes are surrounded by an external (basal) lamina and have an ultrastructure which makes them appear as a combination of fibroblasts and macrophages. Other cells in close proximity to the blood vessels of the CNS, structurally reminiscent of these pericytes but without external (basal) lamina, have been referred to as **perivascular microglial cells.** Other small cells with dense, lobulated nucleus and a minimum quantity of cytoplasm may, under normal circumstances, occasionally be present at some distance from the vascular channels. These cells have been referred to as **interstitial microglial cells.** Some investigators claim that the presence of granular inclusions, probably lysosomes, in the cytoplasm of these cells, positively identifies them as microglial cells. Other investigators insist that the interstitial microglial cells can not be differentiated structurally from small oligodendrocytes, since they both may contain lysosomes, and also have other structural features in common.

It has long been claimed that microglial cells can become ameboid, and that their migration away from the vascular channels through the interstices of the nervous tissue is prompted by their ability to serve as macrophages within the CNS. The origin of the many phagocytic cells that appear as a result of degenerative and injurious processes in the CNS is still uncertain. Some investigators have concluded that they arise from pre-existing microglial cells, oligodendrocytes, or astrocytes. Others claim that the phagocytic cells form from pericytes, monocytes, or leukocytes. Further research in this area is required before a more definite account can be given of the origin, structure, and function of cells which now are collectively referred to as microglial cells.

Ependyma

The ependyma lines the ventricles and the central canal of the spinal cord. (Figs. 15-10, 15-11) The ventricular system of the brain consists of the two lateral ventricles, the 3rd and 4th ventricles, the latter two united via the cerebral aqueduct. For a detailed review of the system of ventricles, consult textbooks of gross anatomy and neuroanatomy. The ependyma is a true epithelium, derived from the superficial

Fig. 15-10. Diencephalon. Frontal section. Rat. L.M. × 134. 1. Thalamus. 2. Hypothalamus. 3. Third ventricle. 4. Choroid plexus. 5. Roof of third ventricle (tela choroidea: pia mater + ependyma). 6. Venous sinus. 7. Arachnoid.

Fig. 15-11. Choroid plexus. Enlargement of area indicated by rectangle in Fig. 15-10. E.M. × 640. 1. Capillaries of choroid plexus with erythrocytes. 2. Single layer of modified, non-ciliated ependymal cells. 3. Third ventricle. 4. Single layer of ciliated ependymal cells lining the third ventricle. 5. Neurons of thalamus.

Fig. 15-12. Ependyma. Third ventricle. Enlargement of area similar to rectangle in Fig. 15-11. Rat. E.M. × 2100. 1. Nuclei of ependymal cells. 2. Cilia. 3. Microvilli. 4. Mitochondria. 5. Lumen of capillary. 6. Nuclei of neurons in thalamus. 7. Nuclei of neuroglial cells. 8. Myelinated and non-myelinated nerve processes border directly on the basal cell membrane of the ependymal cells. No basal lamina present. 9. Neuropil of the thalamus.

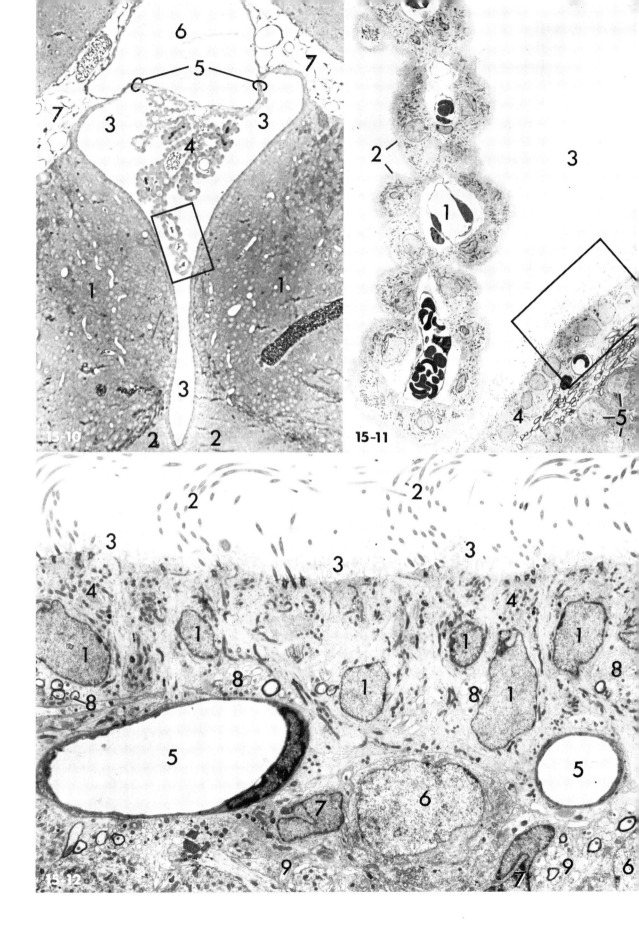

15-10

15-11

15-12

layer of the neural ectoderm. It consists of a single layer of closely packed columnar cells. (Fig. 15-12) A basal lamina does not separate the ependymal layer from the underlying neuropil. From the tapered base of the ependymal cell, a long, slender, and branching process descends into the neuropil.

A varied number of cilia project from the free surface of the cell in addition to a large number of short and slender microvilli. (Fig. 15-12) Occasional micropinocytotic invaginations of the coated variety occur at the ventricular surface. The lateral surfaces are irregular, and short, broad cytoplasmic processes link adjacent cells. The junctional arrangement of adjacent cell membranes includes zonulae occludentes, adhaerentes, and gap-junctions. The nucleus is round or oval, occupying a large part of the cell. Spherical and slightly elongated mitochondria abound. The Golgi zone is small, and the number of granular endoplasmic reticulum profiles and free ribosomes are limited. Particulate glycogen is abundantly present. Occasional microtubules and some filaments are present.

The ependymal cells form a selective barrier between the nervous tissue and the cerebrospinal fluid of the ventricular system. They may help to form and/or modify this fluid by secretory or absorptive processes. The junctional complexes of adjacent cell membranes probably determine to a large degree what is transferred across the epithelium. Since the cilia are not present in the adult individual as abundantly as during embryonic life, these structures are probably rudimentary, and the ciliary beat may have little influence on the circulation of the cerebrospinal fluid.

Choroid Plexus

The choroid plexus consists of tufts of capillaries, protruding into the two lateral ventricles, as well as the 3rd and 4th ventricles. (Fig. 15-10) It is directly involved in the production of cerebrospinal fluid.

The roof of the 3rd and 4th ventricles consists of connective tissue elements of the arachnoid, a thin layer of pia mater, and an inner layer of ependymal cells. From this roof extensive intrusions of the highly vascularized pia mater project into the ventricular cavity and the cerebrospinal fluid. (Fig. 15-11) The intrusions are covered by a single, continuous layer of **modified ependymal cells.** These ependymal cells are cuboidal with a large, round central nucleus. The cells rest on a **basal lamina,** which is derived from the pia-arachnoid connective tissue of the choroid plexus.

The free surface of the modified ependymal cells is provided with numerous, irregularly shaped, bulbous microvilli. (Fig. 15-13) Cilia do not occur as a rule. The lateral and basal surfaces are highly folded and interdigitations of adjacent cells are common. The cells are rich in mitochondria, free ribosomes, profiles of granular endoplasmic reticulum, and lysosomes. The Golgi zone is rather prominent.

The blood vessels and capillaries of the choroid plexus are highly tortuous and generally thin-walled. The capillary endothelium is of the fenestrated variety. (Fig. 15-13)

It is generally accepted that the **cerebrospinal fluid** is formed through an excre-

Fig. 15-13. Details of choroid plexus. Ependymal cells of the modified type that covers the vascular tufts of the choroid plexus. Diencephalon. Third ventricle. Rat. E.M. X 13,000. **1.** Third ventricle. **2.** Bulbous microvilli. **3.** Junctional specialization of apposing cell membranes. **4.** Profiles of granular endoplasmic reticulum. **5.** Mitochondria. **6.** Golgi zone. **7.** Nuclei. **8.** Lysosomes. **9.** Infolded and interdigitated basal cell membranes. **10.** Basal lamina. **11.** Pial connective tissue fibrils. **12.** Pericyte. **13.** Fenestrated thin endothelium. **14.** Nucleus of endothelial cell. **15.** Lumen of capillary. **16.** Erythrocyte.

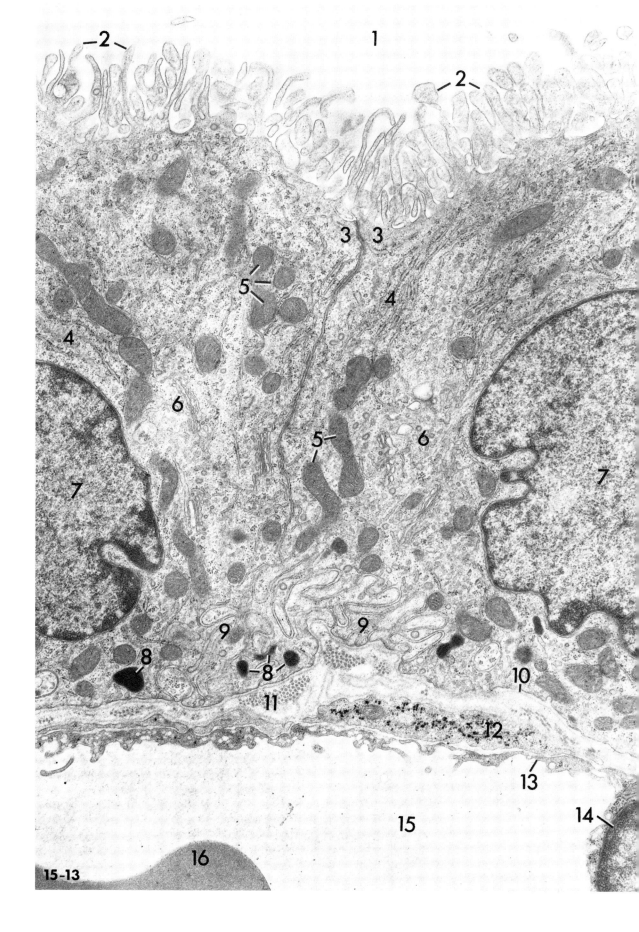

15-13

tory process across the modified ependymal cells of the choroid plexus. This occurs through active transport of sodium and chloride across the cells, and a passive transport of water. Small amounts of protein and glucose are also transported across this epithelium and appear in the cerebrospinal fluid.

The cerebrospinal fluid leaves the ventricular system of the brain and the central canal of the spinal cord via the median aperture of Magendie and the two lateral apertures of Luschka in the 4th ventricle. Through these openings it reaches the subarachnoidal space, which is also filled with cerebrospinal fluid. The fluid of the subarachnoidal space in turn drains into venous channels of the skull via arachnoid granulations (villi) which protrude into veins, and similarly along the vertebral column near the roots of the spinal nerves.

Meninges

The central nervous system is primarily protected by the bony structures of the cranium and vertebral column, and by the cerebrospinal fluid. A third kind of mechanical protection and support is provided by the meninges, which are delicate sheets of connective tissue, consisting of flattened fibroblasts and bundles of collagenous fibrils. There are three meninges: 1) dura mater; 2) arachnoid; and 3) pia mater. (Figs. 15-14, 15-15) Dura mater is the most superficial, and also the toughest. It is often referred to as **pachymeninx**. Arachnoid and pia mater are quite delicate membranes, structurally indistinguishable, but topographically identifiable under the light microscope, except where the cerebrospinal fluid intervenes. They are referred to as the pia-arachnoid membrane or **leptomeninx**. Of the two, pia mater is the innermost sheet.

Dura mater. The dura mater is attached to the inner periosteum of the cranium and does not follow closely the contours of the brain. In the spinal column the dura mater is separated from the periosteum of the vertebrae by a narrow **epidural space** which does not exist in the skull.

The dura mater of the skull consists of an outer layer and an inner layer. (Fig. 15-14) The **outer layer** corresponds to the internal periosteum and is made up of densely packed bundles of collagenous fibrils mixed in with fibroblasts. It is a typical dense fibrous connective tissue, as illustrated at higher magnifications in Figs. 10-6 and 10-7 (p. 211). The outer layer contains blood vessels for its own nutrition and for the bone. Enclosed in this layer are also large, non-muscular veins, the **venous sinuses** of the skull. Sensory nerve fibers and autonomic nerve fibers for the blood vessels are also present in the dura mater.

The **inner layer** of the dura mater is a relatively thin sheet of dense connective

Figs. 15-14 & 15-15. Architecture of meninges. Survey. Parietal region. Frontal section. Kitten. E.M. X 640. **1.** Matrix of parietal bone. **2.** Osteocytes in bone lacunae. **3.** Outer layer of dura mater (= inner periosteum). **4.** Blood vessels. **5.** Inner layer of dura mater. **6.** Subdural space filled with lymph. **7.** Cellular membrane of arachnoid. **8.** Arachnoid trabeculae. **9.** Arachnoid space filled with cerebrospinal fluid. **10.** Small artery ("pial" blood vessel). **11.** Pia mater. **12.** Cortical nervous tissue of cerebral hemisphere.

Fig. 15-16. Arachnoid. Enlargement of area similar to rectangle (A) in Fig. 15-15. Parietal region. Kitten. E.M. X 9000. **1.** Subdural space. **2.** Nuclei of fibroblasts. **3.** Flat processes of cells forming the arachnoid cellular membrane. **4.** Bundles of collagenous fibrils. **5.** Arachnoid trabeculae. **6.** Arachnoid space. **7.** Nucleus of trabecular fibroblast.

Fig. 15-17. Pia-arachnoid membrane. Enlargement of area similar to rectangle (B) in Fig. 15-15. Parietal region. Kitten. E.M. X 9000. **1.** Arachnoid trabeculae. **2.** Nucleus of macrophage. **3.** Arachnoid space. **4.** Collagenous fibrils. **5.** Fibroblast of pial membrane. **6.** Nucleus. **7.** Subpial astroglial feet.

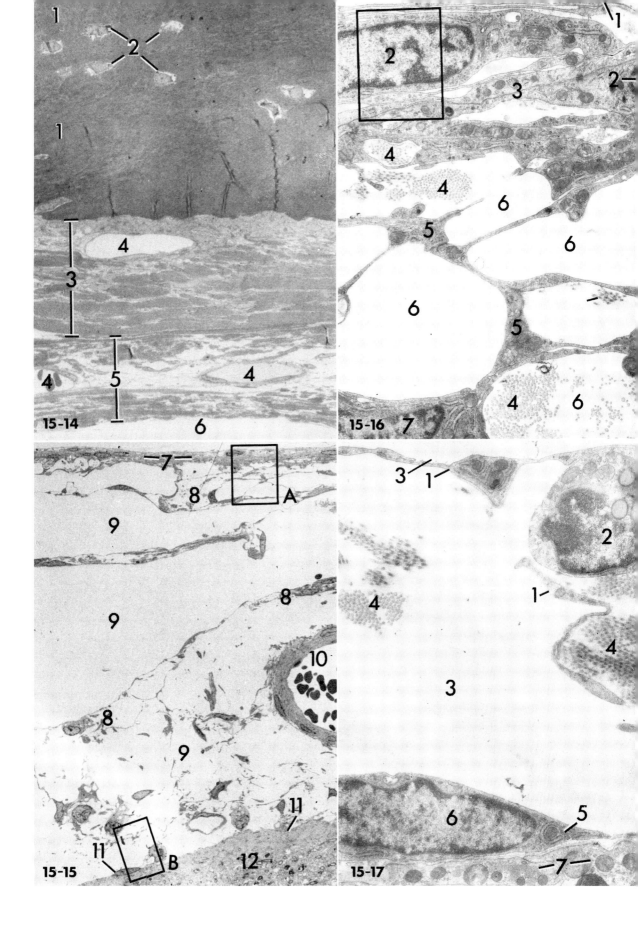

15-14

15-16

15-15

15-17

tissue, which represents the proper dura mater in the spinal canal. A very narrow **subdural space** has been described in some locations in the brain and spinal cord. It is filled with lymph or interstitial fluid, but definitely not cerebrospinal fluid.

It is presently uncertain whether flattened fibroblasts (synonyms: mesothelium; neurothelium; intermediate cellular layer) form a complete lining of the subdural surface of the inner connective tissue sheet of the dura. In the dura mater of the kitten, prepared by the author for the illustrations of this chapter (Fig. 15-14), an incomplete layer of flattened fibroblasts is present. Since the dura mater is of mesodermal origin it is conceivable that connective tissue spaces may arise, and flattening of fibroblasts occur as a result of functional demands, as in the development of joint cavities (see p. 200).

Arachnoid. The arachnoid membrane follows the brain contours more closely than the dura mater but does not go into all crevices of the brain surface. It consists of a cellular membrane and trabeculae.

The **membrane** is outermost, bordering on the narrow subdural space. (Fig. 15-15) It consists of 5–8 layers of flattened, densely packed fibroblasts. These cells are highly reminiscent of primitive mesenchymal cells without emphasis on a particular cell organelle. (Fig. 15-18) The cells are held together by frequent and extensive nexuses (gap-junctions). These junctional specializations may explain the alleged inability of the cerebrospinal fluid to reach the subdural space from the arachnoidal space. Underneath the cellular membrane, the **trabeculae** are present as delicate thin pillars, forming a three-dimensional spider-web pattern between the pia mater and the cellular membrane of the arachnoid. (Fig. 15-16) The trabeculae consist of narrow, thin cytoplasmic processes of fibroblasts, and bundles of collagenous fibrils. The fibroblasts have a fair amount of mitochondria, free ribosomes, and granular endoplasmic reticu-

lum. (Fig. 15-20) The fibroblasts of the trabeculae are frequently held together by desmosomes. (Fig. 15-19)

Between the cellular membrane of the arachnoid and the pia mater is the **arachnoidal space,** which is traversed by the trabeculae and is filled with cerebrospinal fluid. There are also blood vessels which traverse the arachnoidal space on their way to the pia mater and the nervous tissue of the brain and spinal cord. Occasional macrophages, lymphocytes, and perivascular mast cells occur in the arachnoidal space.

Pia mater. Pia mater is the most internal membrane, adhering to the nervous tissue of the brain, spinal cord, and roots of the nerves. It invests all surfaces, including indentations, sulci, and fissures.

According to recent investigations, the pia mater consists of one or several layers of flattened fibroblasts, which are closely applied to the surface of the brain tissue. (Fig. 15-17) Occasional thin collagenous fibrils may be scattered between the flat fibroblasts, or be present between the innermost layer of fibroblasts and the nervous tissue. Astrocytic cell processes form a layer of **subpial feet,** and a thin **basal**

Fig. 15-18. Detail of arachnoid cellular membrane. Enlargement of area similar to ▸ rectangle in Fig. 15-16. Parietal region. Kitten. E.M. X 31,000. **1.** Nucleus of fibroblast. **2.** Many closely apposed, delicate, squamous fibroblasts make up the arachnoid membrane. **3.** Gap-junctions.

Fig. 15-19 & 15-20. Arachnoid trabecular fibroblasts. Parietal region. Kitten. E.M. X 31,000. **1.** Arachnoid space. **2.** Slender cell processes. **3.** Mitochondria. **4.** Cisternae of granular endoplasmic reticulum. **5.** Desmosome.

Fig. 15-21. Pia-glial membrane. Enlargement of rectangle (A) in Fig. 15-6. Spinal cord. Rat. E.M. X 62,000. **1.** Arachnoid space. **2.** Nucleus of pial fibroblast. **3.** Mitochondria. **4.** Cisternae of granular endoplasmic reticulum. **5.** Lysosomes. **6.** External (basal) lamina of the brain tissue of the central nervous system. **7.** Astrocytic cytoplasm of subpial feet. **8.** Gap-junction. **9.** Astrocytic filaments.

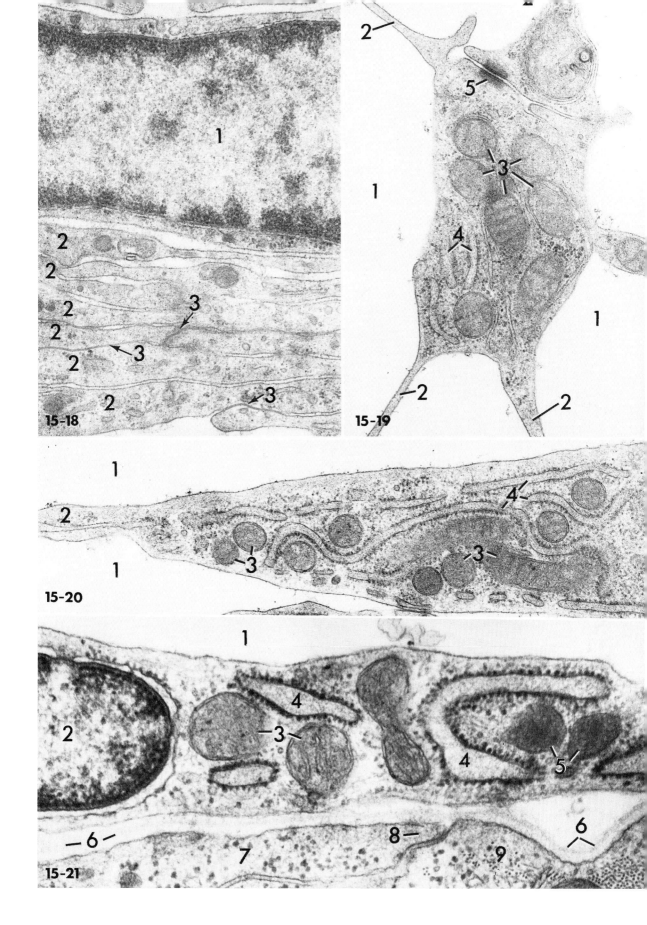

15-18

15-19

15-20

15-21

(external) **lamina** adheres closely to the pial surface of these feet, interposed between the innermost layer of pial fibroblasts and the glial feet. (Fig. 15-21) Occasionally, gaps or discontinuities in the cytoplasm of the flattened pial fibroblasts may expose the subpial (astrocytic) basal lamina to the cerebrospinal fluid of the subarachnoidal space.

Earlier accounts of the pia mater included a superficial (epipial) layer of collagenous fibrils and fibroblasts. In the present description, these structures are included as part of the trabecular network in the arachnoidal space. The recent observations on the ultrastructural architecture of the arachnoid and the pia mater confirm the opinions of some early investigators who considered the arachnoid and pial membranes as one (pia-arachnoid membrane; leptomeninx), mainly because the two meninges were structurally indistinguishable at the light microscope level.

There is no subpial space comparable to the subdural and arachnoidal space. However, instead of pial fibroblasts, macrophages may be present adjacent to the subpial basal lamina, particularly in the perivascular areas.

Blood Vessels

The arteries of the brain are derived from the internal carotid arteries, the basilar artery and the circle of Willis. The spinal cord is supplied by anterior and posterior spinal arteries, as well as branches of segmental arteries. Branches from these arteries travel and anastomose freely within the pia-arachnoid membrane. From the pia-arachnoid vessels, branches are given off at right angles to the surface of the brain and spinal cord, reaching deeper parts of the nervous tissue, where they give rise to capillaries. The number of capillaries is larger in the gray matter than in the white, and capillaries are especially numerous in the cerebral cortex. The blood vessels of the brain and spinal

cord are considered to be **end-arteries,** which implies that there are essentially no anastomoses, resulting in a highly inadequate collateral circulation. The venous system of the nervous tissue of the brain and spinal cord does not follow closely the arterial system. Lymphatic vessels and lymphatic capillaries are not present in the central nervous system.

Arteries and arterioles. The small arteries and arterioles of the central nervous system have a thin media, consisting of 2–3 layers of smooth muscle cells; a distinct inner elastic membrane; and squamous endothelial cells. (Figs. 15-22, 15-23) Myoendothelial junctions (p. 348) have not been identified. A thin cuff of pial fibroblasts and some collagenous fibrils surround the initial part of the arteries and arterioles as they descend into the neuropil. No perivascular space can be seen in relation to well-preserved arteries and arterioles in the brain and spinal cord. (Fig. 15-24) The arterial vessels of the central nervous system are accompa-

Fig. 15-22. Pia-arachnoid blood vessels. Cerebral cortex. Rat. E.M. X 600.
1. Arachnoid space. 2. Pial membrane.
3. Small pial artery; lumen 70 μ. 4. Arteriole entering the molecular layer of the cerebral cortex; lumen 25 μ. 5. Small pial venule; lumen 40 μ. 6. Brain capillary; lumen 5 μ.
7. Molecular layer of cerebral cortex.

Fig. 15-23. Pia-arachnoid blood vessels. Enlargement of rectangle in Fig. 15-22. E.M. X 1500. 1. Arachnoid space. 2. Arachnoid macrophage. 3. Nuclei of pial fibroblasts.
4. Wall of arteriole; thickness 5 μ. 5. Smooth muscle cell. 6. Elastic membrane.
7. Endothelium. 8. Nucleus of astrocyte.
9. Molecular layer of cerebral cortex.
10. Small arteriole; lumen 25 μ.

Fig. 15-24. Topography of perivascular space in the brain tissue. Enlargement of area similar to rectangle in Fig. 15-23. Cerebral cortex. Rat. E.M. X 60,000. 1. Lumen of arteriole; 25 μ. 2. Endothelial cytoplasm. 3. Tight junction. 4. Basal lamina. 5. Smooth muscle cells. 6. External lamina of smooth muscle cells. 7. Pial fibroblast. 8. Subpial collagenous fibrils. 9. Subpial astrocytic feet. 10. Junctional specializations of apposed cell membranes of the glial feet.

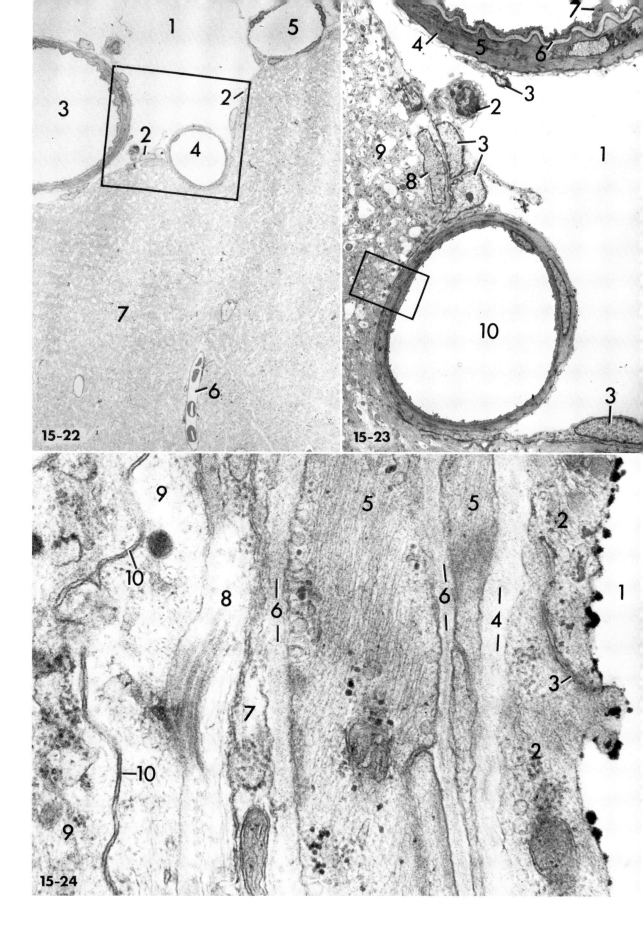

15-22

15-23

15-24

nied by a loose plexus of autonomic nerves. However, these vessels are relatively unresponsive to the stimulation of vasomotor nerves and to vasoactive drugs.

Capillaries. The capillaries of the nervous tissue have an endothelium which has been classified as continuous, thin and non-fenestrated (p. 354), containing few vesicles. (Fig. 15-25) Exceptions are found in the capillaries of the choroid plexus, area postrema, and median eminens where the endothelium is fenestrated. (Fig. 15-13) The junctions of endothelial cells of the brain capillaries are closed by a fusion of the outer leaflets of the apposing cell membranes (tight junctions). The endothelium is surrounded by a thin basal lamina. Occasional pericytes are present, and they are always enclosed by the same basal lamina. The perivascular cuff of pial cells does not exist in relation to the capillaries of the central nervous system. A relatively complete layer of plate-like astrocytic foot-processes invests the periphery of these capillaries. (Fig. 15-26) Extracellular, perivascular space is extremely narrow, measuring 200–300 Å.

Blood-brain barrier. The non-fenestrated capillaries of the CNS are less permeable than similarly structured capillaries in other locations. This selective physiological barrier, often referred to as blood-brain barrier, determines the size of the molecules which will be allowed to leave or enter the capillary lumen. It is probably the result of the tight junctions of the capillary endothelial cells. (Fig. 15-27) The perivascular glial end-feet seem to play a less important role in this physiological barrier.

References

Baron, M. and Gallego, A. The relation of the microglia with the pericytes in the cat cerebral cortex. Z. Zellforsch. *128*: 42–57 (1972).

Blakemore, W. F. The ultrastructure of the subependymal plate in the rat. J. Anat. *104*: 423–433 (1969).

Bondareff, W. and McLone, D. G. The external glial limiting membrane in Macaca: ultrastructure of a laminated glioepithelium. Am. J. Anat. *136*: 277–296 (1973).

Brightman, M. W. and Paley, S. L. The fine structure of ependyma in the brain of the rat. J. Cell Biol. *19*: 415–439 (1963).

Brightman, M. W. and Reese, T. S. Junctions between intimately apposed cell membranes in the vertebrate brain. J. Cell Biol. *40*: 648–677 (1969).

Bunge, R. Glial cells and the central myelin sheath. Physiol. Rev. *48*: 197–251 (1968).

Cammermeyer, J. Morphologic distinctions between oligodendrocytes and microglia cells in the rabbit cerebral cortex. Am. J. Anat. *118*: 227–248 (1966).

Cancilla, P. A., Baker, R. N., Pollock, P. S. and Frommes, S. P. The reaction of pericytes of the central nervous system to exogenous protein. Lab. Investig. *26*: 376–383 (1972).

Cserr, H. F. Physiology of the choroid plexus. Physiol. Rev. *51*: 273–311 (1971).

Davson, H. Physiology of the Cerebrospinal Fluid. Little, Brown, Boston, 1967.

Frederickson, R. G. and Low, F. N. Blood vessels and tissue space associated with the brain of the rat. Am. J. Anat. *125*: 123–146 (1969).

Himango, W. A. and Low, F. N. The fine structure of a lateral recess of the subarachnoid space in rat. Anat. Rec. *171*: 1–20 (1971).

Hirano, A. and Zimmerman, H. M. Some new cytological observations of the normal rat ependymal cell. Anat. Rec. *158*: 293–302 (1967).

Hydén, H. and Pigon, A. A cytophysiological study of the functional relationship between oligodendroglial cells of Deiters' nucleus. J. Neurochem. *6*: 57–72 (1960).

Jones, E. G. On the mode of entry of blood vessels into the cerebral cortex. J. Anat. *106*: 507–520 (1970).

Fig. 15-25. Brain capillary. Molecular layer. Cerebral cortex. Rat. E.M. × 21,500.
1. Lumen; 5 μ. **2.** Nucleus of endothelial cell. **3.** Non-fenestrated, continuous endothelium. **4.** Pericytic process. **5.** Perivascular feet of astrocytes. **6.** Neuropil.

Fig. 15-26. Brain capillary. Molecular layer. Cerebral cortex. Rat. E.M. X 8400.
1. Erythrocyte. **2.** Capillary lumen; 8 μ. **3.** Endothelium. **4.** Cytoplasm of pericyte. **5.** Nucleus. **6.** Endothelial-pericytic junction. **7.** Basal lamina. **8.** Glial perivascular feet of astrocytes. **9.** Mitochondria. **10.** Neuropil of molecular layer of cerebral cortex.

Fig. 15-27. Blood-brain barrier. Brain capillary. Enlargement of area similar to rectangle in Fig. 15-25. Molecular layer. Cerebral cortex. Rat. E.M. X 120,000.
1. Capillary lumen. **2.** Overlapping endothelial processes. **3.** Trilaminar endothelial cell membrane. **4.** Tight junction (= fusion of outer leaflets of apposing cell membranes). **5.** Cell membranes sectioned obliquely between arrows. **6.** Basal lamina. **7.** Perivascular astroglial end-feet. **8.** Junctional specialization: gap-junctions.

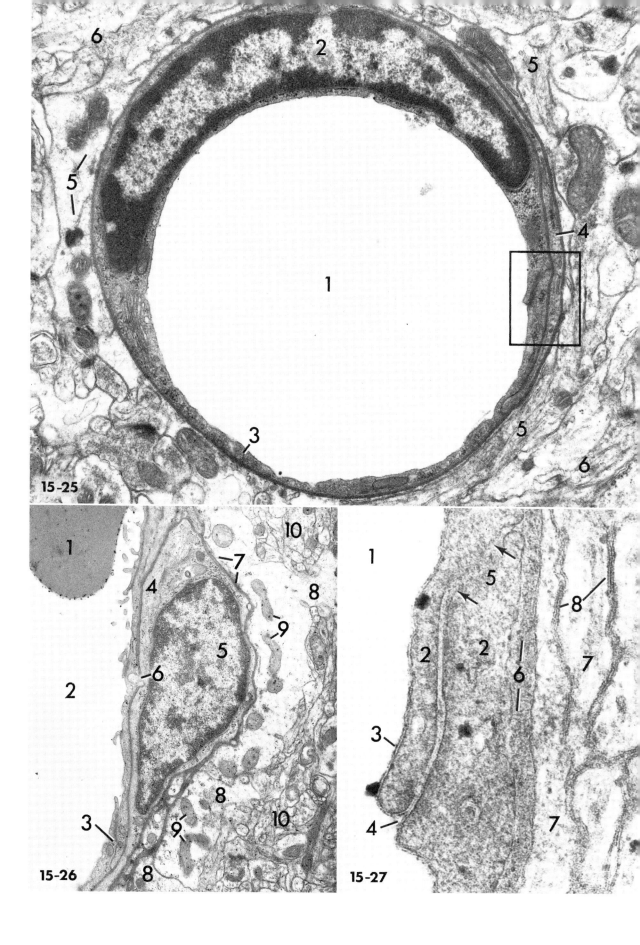

15-25

15-26

15-27

Kruger, L. and Maxwell, D. S. Electron microscopy of oligodendrocytes in normal rat cerebrum. Am. J. Anat. *118*: 411–436 (1966).

Kuffler, S. W. and Nicholls, J. G. The physiology of neuroglial cells. Ergebn. Physiol. *57*: 1–90 (1966).

McCabe, J. S. and Low, F. N. The subarachnoid angle: an area of transition in peripheral nerve. Anat. Rec. *164*: 15–34 (1969).

Morse, D. E. and Low, F. N. The fine structure of the pia mater of the rat. Am. J. Anat. *133*: 349–368 (1972).

Millhouse, O. E. Light and electron microscopic studies of the ventricular wall. Z. Zellforsch. *127*: 149–174 (1972).

Nakai, J. Morphology of Neuroglia. C. C. Thomas, Springfield, Ill., 1963.

Peters, A. Anatomical considerations of the site of the blood-brain barrier. J. Anat. *95* (suppl): 20–22 (1961).

Pease, D. C. and Schultz, R. L. Electron microscopy of rat cranial meninges. Am. J. Anat. *102*: 301–313 (1958).

Vaughn, J. E. and Peters, A. Electron microscopy of the early postnatal development of fibrous astrocytes. Am. J. Anat. *121*: 131–152 (1967).

16 Cardiovascular system

The cardiovascular system consists of 1) heart; 2) arteries; 3) microvascular bed; 4) veins; and 5) lymphatic vessels. The **heart** serves as a pump, forcing the blood via the **arteries** to the microvascular beds of various organs and parts of the body. In the **microvascular bed,** which consists of a rich **capillary network** supplied by **arterioles** and drained by **venules,** an exchange takes place between the vascular channels and their environment. It is an exchange of mainly oxygen, carbon dioxide, metabolites, salts, water, and metabolic waste products. The **veins** conduct the blood back to the heart. Some of the extravasated blood plasma, now referred to as lymph, is returned to the venous system via the lymphatic vessels which connect with the larger veins at a few limited points. Extravascular substances such as lipids and large molecular proteins are also returned to the blood via the lymphatic vessels.

Heart

The heart is a propulsive, muscular pump composed of four chambers, two **atria** and two **ventricles.** The right atrium receives the deoxygenated venous blood from the venae cavae and passes it on to the right ventricle through the right atrioventricular orifice. The right ventricle propels the blood via the pulmonary artery to the lungs. Freshly oxygenated blood is returned from the lungs to the left atrium by the pulmonary veins, and from here reaches the left ventricle through the left atrioventricular orifice. By forceful contraction, the left ventricle drives the blood via the aorta and its many branches to all parts of the body. Valves are positioned at the pulmonary and aortic orifices, as well as at the right and left atrioventricular orifices to prevent backflow of blood. Together with the impulse-conducting system of the heart, these valves make it possible for the left atrium and ventricle to function in synchrony with the right side of the heart. (Fig. 16-1)

The heart wall consists mainly of three layers: endocardium, myocardium, and epicardium. Here the blood supply is very rich, especially that to the myocardium, which consists of cardiac muscle fibers, contracting rhythmically, and continuously moderated by the autonomic nervous system.

ENDOCARDIUM

The endocardium is a membrane which covers all inner surfaces of the heart. It is very thin and transparent in the ventri-

Fig. 16-1. Schematic drawing of human heart. For simplicity, aorta and arteria pulmonalis are not shown. **1.** Right atrium. **2.** Left atrium. **3.** Right ventricle. **4.** Left ventricle. **5.** Venae cavae. **6.** Pulmonary veins. **7.** Right artioventricular valve (tricuspid). **8.** Left atrioventricular valve (bicuspid). **9.** Interatrial septum. **10.** Interventricular septum. **11.** SA-node. **12.** AV-node. **13.** AV-bundle. **14.** Right and left branches of impulse-conducting system. **15.** Terminal ramifications.

Fig. 16-2. Part of atrial and ventricular wall. Corresponds to area indicated by rectangle (A) in Fig. 16-1. Heart. Monkey. L.M. X 7. **1.** Wall of atrium, 1 mm thick. **2.** Wall of ventricle, 10 mm thick. **3.** Cusp of atrioventricular valve. **4.** Papillary muscles. **5.** Chordae tendineae (indicated by dashed lines). **6.** Delicate trabeculae carneae. **7.** Adipose tissue in coronary sulcus. **8.** Coronary artery.

Fig. 16-3. Ventricular wall. Human heart. Enlargement of area similar to rectangle (B) in Fig. 16-1. L.M. X 11. **1.** Ventricle. **2.** Cross-sectioned papillary muscles. **3.** Myocardium: bundles and layers of cardiac muscle cells with markedly alternating fiber directions. **4.** Connective tissue septa (perimysium). **5.** Blood vessel. **6.** Surface of heart (thin epicardium).

Fig. 16-4. Atrial wall. Monkey heart. Enlargement of rectangle (A) in Fig. 16-2. L.M. X 128. **1.** Endocardium, several times thicker than in ventricle. **2.** Myocardium: bundles and layers of cardiac muscle fibers. **3.** Coronary sulcus.

Fig. 16-5. Juncture of atrium and ventricle. Monkey heart. Enlargement of rectangle (B) in Fig. 16-2. L.M. X 30. **1.** Atrial wall. **2.** Annulus fibrosus. **3.** Ventricular wall. **4.** Base of cusp in atrioventricular valve. **5.** Adipose tissue in coronary sulcus.

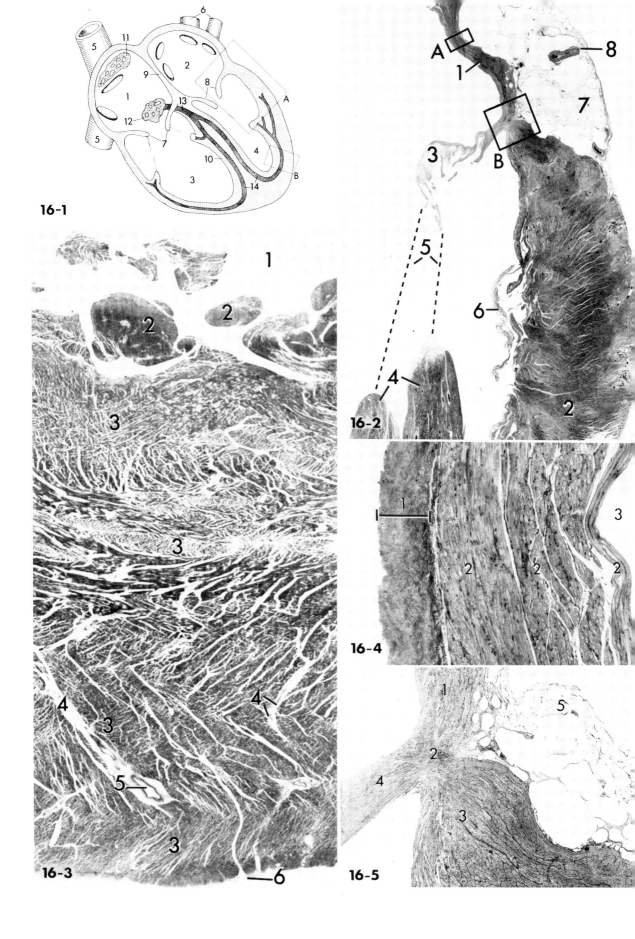

16-1

16-2

16-3

16-4

16-5

cles, but thick, milky, and less transparent in the atria. (Fig. 16-4) It consists of a single layer of flat, polygonal **endothelial cells** which rest on a thin **basement membrane,** consisting of a thin basal lamina and a layer of reticular fibrils. (Fig. 16-6) The endothelial cytoplasm contains numerous delicate filaments, averaging 100 Å in diameter, in addition to a small number of mitochondria and a small Golgi zone. (Fig. 16-7) Numerous surface (micropinocytotic) vesicles are attached to the cell membrane. The endothelial cells are held together by junctional specializations among which the gap-junction is closest to the heart chamber.

Peripheral to the basement membrane is a dense **fibroelastic layer** which accounts for the variation in thickness between atrial and ventricular endocardium. Smooth muscle cells may be present in this layer. A **subendocardial layer** consists of loose connective tissue with some adipose tissue mixed in. Small blood vessels, nerves, and branches of the impulse conducting system of the heart are present in this layer, which also connects the endocardium to the perimysium of the myocardium.

MYOCARDIUM

The myocardium consists of cardiac muscle fibers, grouped to form bundles and layers, separated by connective tissue septa (perimysium). The myocardium is quite thin in the atria (Fig. 16-2), but it is of medium thickness in the right ventricle and very thick in the left ventricle. A superficial layer of cardiac fibers surrounds both **atria,** whereas a longitudinal deep layer surrounds each atrium individually. Ridges of myocardium (pectinate muscles) project into the atrial cavity in the auricles. In the **ventricles,** both the superficial and the deep muscular layers originate from the dense rings of connective tissue around the atrioventricular orifices. The muscle fibers terminate in the papillary muscles on the side opposite their origin. (Fig. 16-3) The **papillary muscles** emerge

from the myocardium, traverse the ventricular cavity, and become attached to the atrioventricular valves via delicate tendons (chordae tendineae). The superficial muscle layer surrounds both ventricles, whereas the deep layer goes through the interventricular septum and encircles each individual ventricle. Ridges and bars of myocardium (trabeculae carneae) project into and traverse the ventricular cavity. The structure and ultrastructure of the cardiac muscle fibers are described on p. 234.

EPICARDIUM

Epicardium, the visceral layer of the pericardium, is a thin, transparent serous membrane covering the outer surface of the heart. It consists of a single layer of mesothelial cells resting on a basal lamina, and a thin layer of loose connective tissue. (Fig. 16-8) The main characteristic of the **mesothelial cells** are the numerous microvilli and the many surface (micropinocy-

Fig. 16-6. Endocardium. Left atrium. Rat. E.M. X 1800. **1.** Atrial cavity. **2.** Endothelial cells. **3.** Basement membrane. **4.** Fibroelastic layer. **5.** Subendocardial layer. **6.** Smooth muscle cell. **7.** Fibroblasts.

Fig. 16-7. Detail of endocardium. Left ventricle. Rat. E.M. X 29,000. **1.** Nucleus of endothelial cell. **2.** Cytoplasmic filaments. **3.** Delicate and incomplete basal lamina. **4.** Reticular and elastic microfibrils. **5.** Nucleus of smooth muscle cell. **6.** Cytoplasmic processes of smooth muscle cells containing delicate bundles of myofilaments. **7.** Mitochondria. **8.** Collagenous fibrils.

Fig. 16-8. Epicardium. Right atrium. Rat. E.M. X 1800. **1.** Cavity of pericardial sac. **2.** Mesothelial cells. **3.** Loose connective tissue with bundles of collagenous fibrils. **4.** Pericardial lymphatic vessel. **5.** Cardiac muscle fibers of atrial myocardium. **6.** Blood capillaries. **7.** Connective tissue septum.

Fig. 16-9. Detail of epicardial mesothelial cells. Right atrium. Rat. E.M. X 62,000. **1.** Pericardial cavity. **2.** Microvilli. **3.** Surface (micropinocytotic) vesicles. **4.** Desmosome. **5.** Gap-junction. **6.** Thin basal lamina. **7.** Delicate collagenous (or reticular) fibrils 350 Å thick.

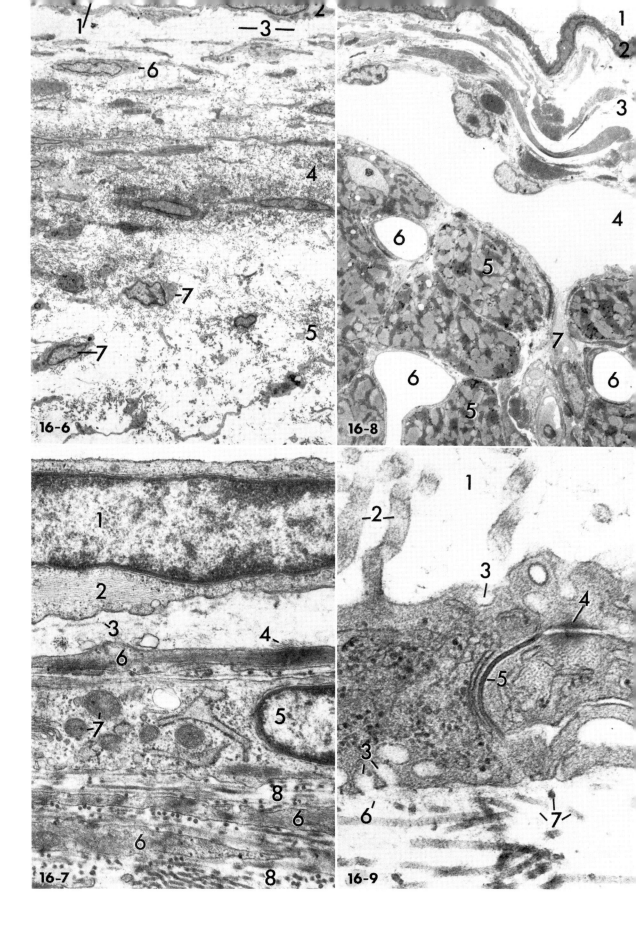

totic) vesicles. (Fig. 16-9) The ultrastructure of the mesothelial cell is quite similar to that of mesothelial cells in the peritoneum (Fig. 29-47) and in the pleura (Fig. 31-71). The connective tissue contains many large blood vessels, lymphatic vessels, nerves, and adipose tissue. The last is particularly abundant around the larger blood vessels.

CONNECTIVE TISSUE

In addition to connective tissue elements of the endocardium, myocardium, and epicardium, the heart contains small areas of very dense connective tissue. These areas are: 1) cardiac valves; 2) annuli fibrosi; 3) trigona fibrosa; 4) septum membranosum; and 5) chordae tendineae.

Cardiac valves. The aortic and pulmonary orifices each have three crescentic semilunar folds (cusps). The right atrioventricular orifice has three folds (tricuspid valve) and the left atrioventricular orifice has two folds (bicuspid or mitral valve). Each cusp is an endocardial fold with a central plate of dense fibroelastic tissue. (Fig. 16-10) The elastic components are concentrated near the ventricular surface of the cusp. Cardiac and smooth muscle cells may occur near the base of the cusps of the AV-orifices but are absent in the aortic and pulmonary valves. Normally, blood capillaries are not present in the cusps beyond the muscle cells.

Annuli fibrosi. The valves are surrounded by a ring of dense fibrous connective tissue which serves as attachment for the cusps. (Fig. 16-5)

Trigona fibrosa. These are small, central triangular areas of dense connective tissue, located between and connecting the annuli fibrosi. The connective tissue matrix of the trigona and the annuli may become chondroid and even calcified in certain large mammals such as the ox, giving rise to either fibrous cartilage or bone tissue. The annuli and the trigona together form a fibrous separation of the atrial and ventricular myocardia, penetrated only by a narrow muscular trunk,

the atrioventricular (common) bundle of His — a part of the impulse-conducting system of the heart.

Septum membranosum forms part of the interventricular septum. It also consists of dense connective tissue.

Chordae tendineae. These are delicate tendons which unite the apex of each papillary muscle to the ventricular surfaces of the cusps of the mitral and tricuspid valves. (Fig. 16-2) The chordae contain parallel, dense bundles of collagenous fibrils mixed with some elastic elements. They are covered by a thin endocardium. (Figs. 16-11, 16-12)

IMPULSE-CONDUCTING SYSTEM

The impulse-conducting system of the heart serves as a pace maker for the heartbeat, distributes the contraction impulse throughout the heart, and coordinates the contraction of the four heart chambers. It consists of: 1) sinuatrial (SA) node of Keith and Flack; 2) atrioventricular (AV) node of Tawara; 3) atrioventricular (common) bundle of His; 4) right and left branches on either side of the interventricular septum; and 5) terminal ramifications of the right and left branches, leading to papillary muscles and the walls of the ventricles. Textbooks of anatomy should be consulted for topographic de-

Fig. 16-10. Cusp of left atrioventricular valve. Rat. E.M. X 1900. **1.** Left atrium. **2.** Left ventricle. **3.** Nuclei of endothelial cells. **4.** Nuclei of fibroblasts. **5.** Loose connective tissue. **6.** Dense connective tissue. **7.** Erythrocytes.

Fig. 16-11. Chorda tendinea. Longitudinal section. Left ventricle. Heart. Rat. E.M. X 1100. **1.** Ventricular cavity. **2.** Nuclei of endothelial cells of thin endocardium. **3.** Collagenous fiber bundles. **4.** Nuclei of fibroblasts.

Fig. 16-12. Chorda tendinea. Cross section. Left ventricle. Heart. Rat. E.M. X 1500. **1.** Ventricular cavity. **2.** Nuclei of endothelial cells. **3.** Subendothelial loose connective tissue. **4.** Elastic fibers (dark dots). **5.** Circle: enlargement of this area is found in Fig. 7-7 (p. 143). **6.** Collagenous fibers. **7.** Fibroblasts.

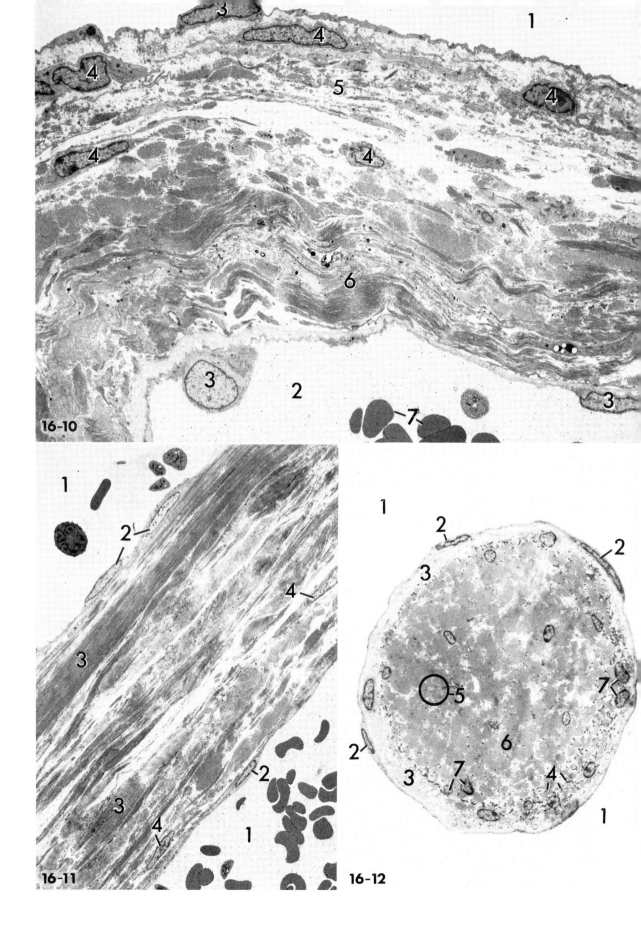

tails of this system. The structure and function of the impulse-conducting system of the heart is described on p. 240.

BLOOD AND LYMPHATIC VESSELS

The myocardium receives a rich blood supply through the **coronary arteries,** which are the first branches of the aorta. They are vessels of the muscular artery type, often with longitudinally arranged smooth muscle cells in the intima. The major branches of the coronary arteries are located in the deeper parts of the epicardium before they turn into the myocardium and give rise to an extensive, richly anastomosing **capillary network** around the cardiac muscle cells. The impulse-conducting system is also highly vascularized. The AV-node, the common bundle, and the larger branches receive their blood supply from the right coronary artery, mainly from its posterior interventricular branch. **Veins** return the blood from the capillary plexus and pursue a course similar to that of the arteries, draining into the large venous coronary sinus. In some instances, small veins open up directly to the heart chambers. These are particularly prevalent in the right atrium. **Lymphatic capillaries** are present in the myocardium and also form a subendocardial as well as a subepicardial plexus. (Fig. 16-8)

NERVES

The cardiac muscle cells and the specialized cells of the impulse-conducting system are innervated by the so-called **cardiac plexus,** which consists of postganglionic nerve fibers from the parasympathetic as well as the sympathetic nervous systems. The nerve endings of the cardiac plexus make contacts (myoneural junctions) with both cardiac and conducting system muscle fibers. The nerve endings do not form special motor end plates of the type found in skeletal muscle. They are simply denuded axons containing agranular and granular vesicles, located near the mus-

cle fiber or recessed in grooves of the muscle cell surface. Preganglionic **parasympathetic** nerve fibers from the cardiac branches of the vagus nerve synapse with ganglionic cells in the myocardium. Postganglionic fibers form one of the two components of the cardiac plexus. The parasympathetic outflow restrains the action of the heart by decreasing the rate and force of contraction, and by decreasing myocardial excitability and conductivity. Postganglionic **sympathetic** nerve fibers from the cervical sympathetic and upper thoracic ganglia form the second component of the cardiac plexus. The sympathetic outflow accelerates the action of the heart by increasing the rate and force of contraction, and by increasing myocardial excitability and conductivity.

Fig. 16-13. Aorta. Cross section. Human. L.M. X 5. **1.** Wall thickness averages 1.5 mm. **2.** Diameter of lumen: max. distance 14 mm; min. distance 7 mm. **3.** Small artery in tunica adventitia.

Fig. 16-14. Aorta. Cross section. Human. Elastic stain. Enlargement of area similar to rectangle in Fig. 16-13. L.M. X 65. **1.** Intima (108 μ). **2.** Media. (820 μ). Elastic membranes of media stained black. No distinct inner or outer elastic membrane. **3.** Adventitia (215 μ) with peripheral adipose tissue.

Fig. 16-15. Aorta. Cross. section. Human. Hematoxylin and eosin stain. Area similar to Fig. 16-14. L.M. X 89. **1.** Intima. **2.** Media. Nuclei of smooth muscle cells appear as dark dots. **3.** Elastic membranes appear as faintly stained, slightly refractive, wavy lines.

Fig. 16-16. Aorta. Cross section. Squirrel monkey. E.M. X 380. **1.** Intima. **2.** Media.

Fig. 16-17. Aorta. Cross section. Enlargements of areas similar to rectangles in Fig. 16-16. **A** (intima), **B** (media), **C** (media-adventitia). Squirrel monkey. E.M. X 1800. **1.** Nuclei of endothelial cells. **2.** Longitudinally arranged smooth muscle cells. **3.** Circularly arranged smooth-muscle cells. **4.** Nuclei of smooth muscle cells. **5.** Irregularly arranged collagenous and elastic fibers. **6.** Elastic membranes. **7.** Nucleus of fibroblast in adventitia. **8.** Coarse bundles of collagenous fibrils in adventitia.

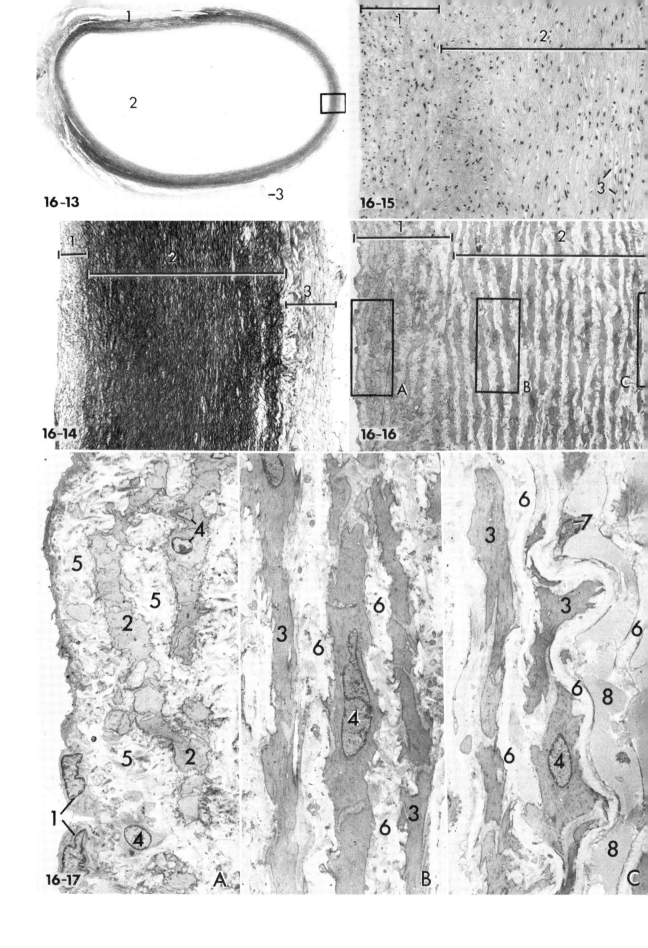

16-13

16-15

16-14

16-16

16-17

Arteries

Arteries have a thick muscular wall with a varied amount of elastic components. They can be recognized in a section because their wall is thick and prevents a collapse of the vascular lumen. Veins are thin-walled and often appear with a collapsed lumen. Large arteries, such as the aorta (Fig. 16-13) and pulmonary arteries, are called **elastic arteries** because of their high content of elastic membranes and fibrils. As the large arteries branch and give rise to successively smaller arteries, the thickness of the wall decreases, the elastic components gradually become scarcer, and the smooth muscle cells prevail. These vessels are the most numerous. They are referred to as **muscular arteries** and are generally of medium and small caliber. (Fig. 16-22) The last ramifications of the arterial blood vessels, the **arterioles** form an essential part of the microvascular bed.

The walls of the arteries consist of three coats (tunics): 1) intima; 2) media; 3) adventitia. **Tunica intima** is composed of an innermost lining of endothelial cells, a thin layer of subendothelial connective tissue, and an internal elastic membrane. **Tunica media** is composed of alternating layers of concentric elastic membranes (sheets) and smooth muscle cells. **Tunica adventitia** consists of fibrous connective tissue with an external elastic membrane establishing the border between media and adventitia. The adventitia also contains small blood vessels, **vasa vasorum,** which supply the vascular wall, lymphatic vessels, and nerves.

ELASTIC ARTERIES

Elastic arteries have a large diameter and do not vary greatly in size. To this category belong the aorta, pulmonary arteries, innominate artery (brachiocephalic trunk), as well as the subclavian, common carotid, and common iliac arteries. They are often referred to as **conducting** arteries because of their obvious function in the cardiovascular system.

Tunica intima. This coat averages 100 μ in thickness. (Fig. 16-14) The **endothelial cells** are polygonal, rounded, or flat, with the nucleus causing a local luminal protrusion of the cell. (Fig. 16-17A) Several processes project from the luminal surface. Some of these resemble microvilli; others are leaf-like. The base of the cell has many small, branching, foot-like processes, descending into the subendothelial connective tissue. (Fig. 16-18) The cells are held together by junctional complexes, usually with a gap-junction near the lumen. (Fig. 16-19) There are numerous surface (micropinocytotic) vesicles attached to all parts of the cell membrane. The cytoplasm contains a small Golgi zone, a limited number of small mitochondria, and a varied number of **specific granules,** 0.1–0.2 μ in diameter. They are bounded by a trilaminar membrane and have a finely granular, dense matrix in

Fig. 16-18. Endothelium. Aorta. Cross section. Squirrel monkey. E.M. X 24,000. **1.** Lumen of aorta. **2.** Nucleus of endothelial cell. **3.** Junction of endothelial cells. **4.** Specific endothelial granules. **5.** Basal lamina. **6.** Elastic fibers with both amorphous substance and elastic microfibrils. **7.** Collagenous fibrils.

Fig. 16-19. Detail of aortic endothelial cells. Squirrel monkey. E.M. X 87,000. **1.** Lumen of aorta. **2.** Surface (micropinocytotic) vesicles. **3.** Specific endothelial granules without apparent inner microtubules. **4.** Mitochondrion. **5.** Cytoplasmic filaments. **6.** Gap-junction. **7.** Non-specialized junction of cell membranes. **8.** Indistinct basal lamina.

Fig. 16-20. Detail of aortic media. Squirrel monkey. E.M. X 24,000. **1.** Part of smooth muscle cell. **2.** Elastic membrane, consisting mostly of amorphous substance. **3.** Delicate bundles of collagenous fibrils.

Fig. 16-21. Detail of media-adventitia transitional zone. Squirrel monkey. E.M. X 24,000. **1.** Part of smooth muscle cell. **2.** Elastic membrane, consisting almost entirely of amorphous substance. **3.** Large accumulation of collagenous fibrils. **4.** Non-myelinated nerve fibers.

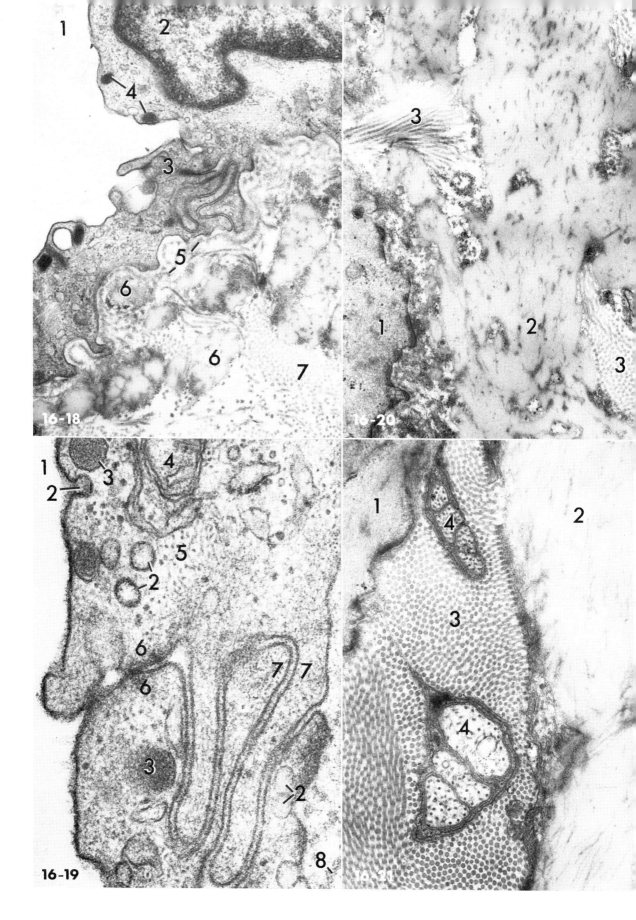

which varied numbers of microtubules about 150 Å thick are often embedded. The function of this specific endothelial organelle has not been determined, although it has been suggested that the granules may contain a procoagulative substance which becomes discharged into the vascular lumen in response to high plasma concentrations of epinephrine. The cells also contain a varied number of cytoplasmic filaments, often arranged in bundles. A thin **basal lamina** separates the endothelial cells from the underlying thin **intermediate layer** of connective tissue which often contains small bundles of longitudinally arranged smooth muscle cells (Fig. 16-17) in addition to branched, fibroblast-like cells and a network of fine collagenous and elastic microfibrils. There is no distinct internal elastic membrane present in elastic arteries.

Tunica media. This coat averages 500 μ in thickness and consists of 50–75 fenestrated **elastic membranes** or sheets, arranged concentrically, each with a thickness of 2–3 μ. (Fig. 16-16) The elastic membranes are composed of a central amorphous substance, and peripherally arranged elastic microfibrils. (Fig. 16-20) The space between the elastic membranes is occupied by relatively short, spindle-shaped **smooth muscle cells** provided with numerous short cytoplasmic branches, attached to and embedded in the elastic membranes. (Fig. 16-17B) The smooth muscle cells are arranged spirally around the lumen, their ends making membranous contacts. The number of smooth muscle cells per square unit is smaller in elastic arteries than in muscular arteries. Near the heart, the media of the aorta and the pulmonary arteries may contain cardiac muscle fibers. Fibroblasts do not occur in the media. Scattered delicate elastic fibrils and small collagenous fibers occur in between and surrounding the smooth muscle cells, in addition to an amorphous, basophilic (metachromatic) ground substance rich in mucopolysaccharides.

Tunica adventitia. The adventitia of elastic arteries is extremely thin. (Fig. 16-14) It consists of bundles of collagenous and elastic fibrils pursuing a spiral or longitudinal course. (Fig. 16-17C) A distinct external elastic membrane is missing. The adventitia merges with adjacent connective tissue. It contains small blood vessels and lymphatic vessels (vasa vasorum) as well as myelinated and non-myelinated nerves.

Functional aspects. The elastic arteries are looked upon as shock absorbers which must withstand the rapid and great changes of the pulse pressure. These vessels dilate passively with each systole (heart contraction). Through their distensibility, the elastic membranes pick up the force of the heart contraction, and by

Fig. 16-22. Muscular artery. Finger. Human. L.M. $\times$ 27. **1.** Lumen; max. width 3 mm (3000 μ). **2.** Intima and media; width 250 μ. **3.** Adventitia; width 80 μ. **4.** Perivascular connective tissue. **5.** Tear (preparation artifact).

Fig. 16-23. Small muscular artery. Mesentery. Rabbit. L.M. $\times$ 135. **1.** Lumen; max. width 0.5 mm (500 μ). **2.** Intima and media; width 75 μ. **3.** Adventitia; width 22 μ. **4.** Internal elastic membrane (scalloped line). **5.** Perivascular adipose tissue. **6.** Lumen of small vein (entire vein seen in Fig. 16-48). **7.** Wall of vein; width 20 μ.

Fig. 16-24. Renal artery and vein. Cross section. Fixed by intra-arterial perfusion. Rat. E.M. $\times$ 660. **1.** Lumen of artery preserved in non-collapsed condition; width 650 μ. **2.** Lumen of vein; width 2600 μ. **3.** Endothelium and internal elastic membrane. **4.** Media; width 25 μ. **5.** Adventitia blending with perivascular connective tissue; width approx. 20 μ. **6.** Intima and media of vein; width averages 5 μ. **7.** Tear (preparation artifact). **8.** Adventitia. **9.** Fibroblasts.

Fig. 16-25. Wall of small muscular artery. Enlargement of area similar to rectangle in Fig. 16-24. Renal artery. Cross section. Rat. E.M. $\times$ 5000. **1.** Lumen. **2.** Nucleus of endothelial cell. **3.** Internal elastic lamina. **4.** Nuclei of smooth muscle cells. **5.** Circularly arranged smooth muscle cells. **6.** Elastic fibers. **7.** Collagenous fibrils. **8.** Profiles of incomplete external elastic membrane. **9.** Non-myelinated nerve axons.

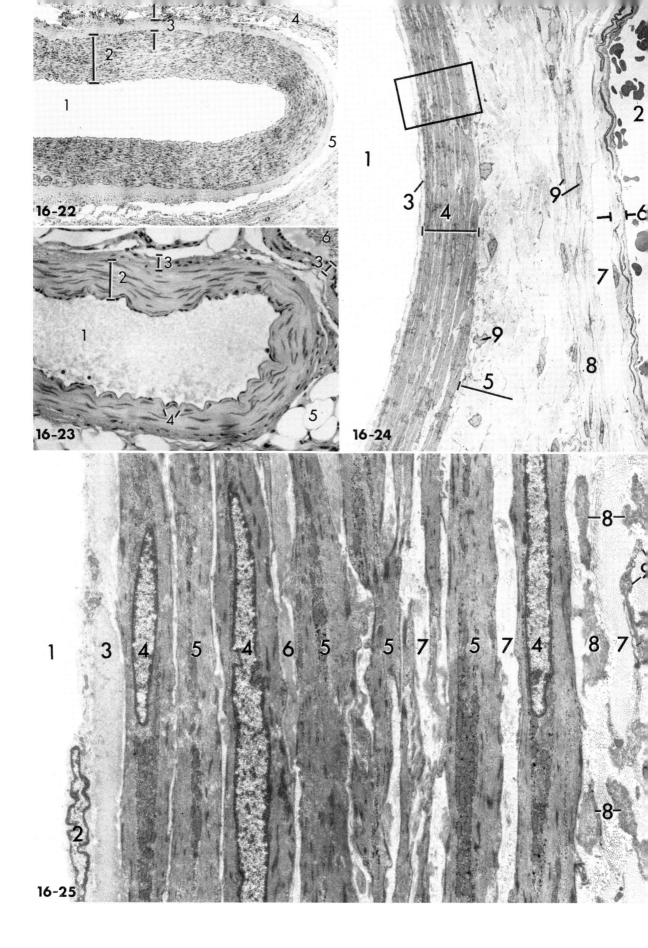

16-22

16-23

16-24

16-25

a recoil propel the blood onward during diastole (heart relaxation). The smooth muscle cells greatly facilitate this recoil by contracting. However, the smooth muscle cells are poorly innervated and do not contract actively. They are therefore unable to close down the lumen of the elastic artery. The activities and properties of the components of the wall of elastic arteries result in a relatively smooth flow of blood instead of a pronounced pulsatile flow.

MUSCULAR ARTERIES

Muscular arteries vary considerably in size, their cross-sectional diameter ranging from about 10 mm to about 0.3 mm (300 μ). To this category belong most arteries of the mammalian body (Figs. 16-22, 16-23), except those included with the elastic arteries on p. 340. They are often referred to as **distributing** arteries, since they control the flow to the various organs of the body by an active vascular constriction.

Tunica intima. In the **small** muscular arteries, the intima consists of a single layer of squamous endothelial cells, resting on a thin inner elastic membrane. (Figs. 16-23, 16-24) In all **large** muscular arteries, there is a relatively thick layer of collagenous and reticular fibrils interposed between the elastica and the endothelial lining. In addition, longitudinally oriented smooth muscle cells may be present in this connective tissue layer in a number of arteries such as the coronary, splenic, and renal arteries, the dorsal penile artery, the helicine arteries of the cavernous tissue of the penis (Fig. 16-28), as well as the ovarian and coiled uterine arteries. These smooth muscle aggregations can reach large proportions and take the shape of **intima cushions,** serving as valves. (Fig. 16-29)

The **endothelial cells** are similar to those present in the elastic arteries with the exception that specific endothelial granules are less common. A thin **basal lamina** is always present in the larger ves-

sels, but is often substituted for the internal elastic membrane in the smaller vessels. (Fig. 16-26) The **internal elastic membrane** is prominent in all muscular arteries except in the umbilical artery where it is missing. It is a fenestrated sheet, which appears as a refractive narrow zone with a wavy outline when collapsed muscular arteries are viewed in histological sections.

Tunica media. In the large muscular arteries, this coat is thick in proportion to the size of the vascular lumen. It consists of 10–40 layers of spindle-shaped, closely packed, interdigitating smooth muscle cells which encircle the lumen in a helical manner. In small arteries, only 3–4 smooth muscle layers are present. The media of the umbilical artery has an inner layer of longitudinally arranged smooth muscle cells (Fig. 34-52) and an outer layer of circularly arranged smooth muscle cells. Fenestrated elastic membranes occur in muscular arteries near their origin from the elastic arteries, but they are not prominent in muscular arteries of small caliber.

Fig. 16-26. Detail of tunica intima of cross-sectioned muscular artery. Renal artery. Rat. E.M. X 17,000. **1.** Lumen. **2.** Nuclei of endothelial cells. **3.** Junctional area of adjacent endothelial cells. **4.** Internal elastic membrane, 1.6 μ thick. Note absence of subendothelial basal lamina. **5.** Mitochondria of smooth muscle cell. **6.** Slender cytoplasmic processes of smooth muscle cell reach toward the endothelial cell across an interruption (fenestra) of the elastic membrane.
7. External lamina of smooth muscle cell. **8.** Small bundles of delicate collagenous fibrils.

Fig. 16-27. Detail of border zone between tunica media and tunica adventitia of cross-sectioned muscular artery. Renal artery. Rat. E.M. X 17,000. **1.** Fusiform densities of smooth muscle cell myofilaments.
2. Delicate cytoplasmic processes, some of which establish membranous contacts with neighboring cell. **3.** External lamina of smooth muscle cell. **4.** Collagenous fibrils.
5. Elastic fibers forming an incomplete external elastic membrane. **6.** Attachment plaque (dense body).

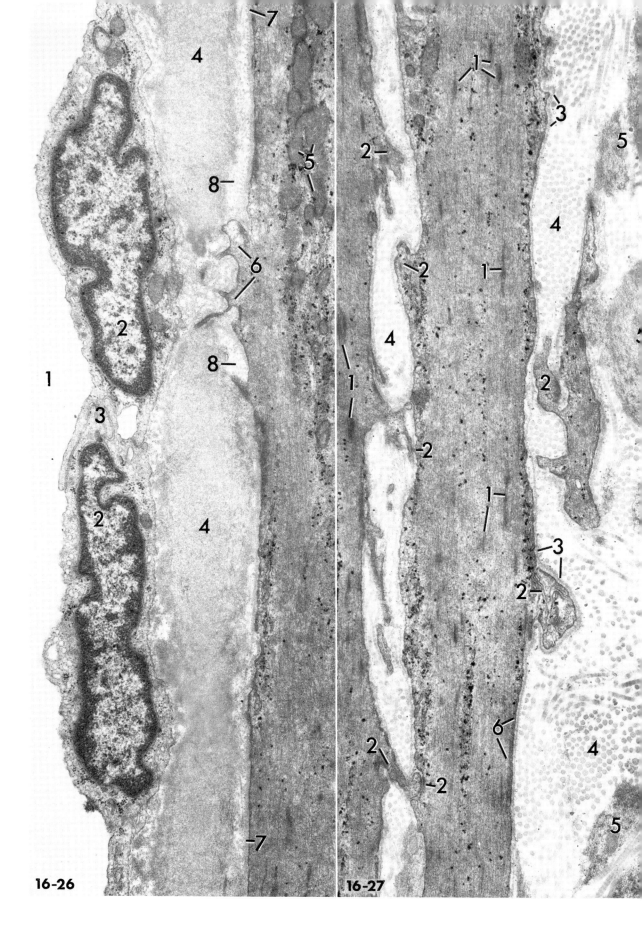

16-26

16-27

The renal arteries have well-developed elastic membranes in the media, whereas they are inconspicuous in meningeal and cerebral arteries, as well as in branches of the pulmonary arteries. Arteries in the latter three locations also have a relatively thin media. As a rule, the smooth muscle cells in muscular arteries are surrounded individually by an external lamina and delicate strands of collagenous fibrils. (Fig. 16-27) Fibroblasts do not occur in the media.

Tunica adventitia. The adventitia of muscular arteries is relatively thick, and consists of an inner layer of dense fibrous connective tissue, and an outer layer of loose connective tissue. The collagenous and elastic fibrils are arranged mostly longitudinally. (Fig. 16-25) The **external elastic membrane** forms a distinct border between media and adventitia in the larger muscular arteries, but is indistinct or absent in the small muscular arteries. Longitudinally arranged smooth muscle cells sometimes occur in the adventitia of coronary and splenic arteries. The adventitia also contains many nerves, vasa vasorum, and fat cells. The nerves penetrate only as far as the most superficial layer of the media.

Functional aspects. The muscular arteries control the amount of blood distributed to a specific region of the body, or to a particular organ. This is accomplished by reducing the lumen through contraction, although the lumen cannot be completely obliterated. The smooth muscle cells of the media are under nervous control, but very few if any myoneural junctions exist. The nervous influence on the vascular smooth muscle is indirect in that the chemical transmitters from the terminal axons are released into the interstitial space of the adventitia and the most superficial layer of the media. The transmitters diffuse via the tissue fluid, reaching and influencing many smooth muscle cells. The innervation of blood vessels is discussed further on p. 366.

Microvascular Bed

The microvascular bed is that part of the cardiovascular system which is concerned with exchange of gases, nutrients, and metabolic waste products. The major part of these processes takes place in the **capillaries** which form the most essential part of the microcirculatory bed. The smallest components of the arterial system, the **arterioles** and the **precapillary sphincter** area, monitor blood flow into the capillary network, and are often referred to as peripheral resistance vessels because of their influence on the blood pressure. The capillary bed is drained by a system of channels with increasingly larger diameters as they leave the capillary bed. In the direction of the blood flow, these are the **postcapillary venules,** the **collecting venules,** and the **muscular venules.** The venous part of the microcirculatory bed is involved largely in recapturing tissue fluid, small molecular proteins, water, and metabolites.

ARTERIOLES

An exact point cannot be indicated at which a small artery changes to an arteriole since this transition is gradual. However, it is generally agreed that arterioles are microvessels with a diameter of

Fig. 16-28. Small helicine artery. Cross section. Fixed by intra-arterial perfusion. Cavernous tissue. Penis. Rat. E.M. X 800. **1.** Lumen; width between arrows 110 μ. **2.** Endothelium. **3.** Longitudinally arranged smooth muscle cells of intima. Aggregations of these cells form intima cushions. **4.** Circularly arranged smooth muscle cells of media. **5.** Adventitia.

Fig. 16-29. Wall of small helicine artery. Enlargement of rectangle in Fig. 16-28. E.M. X 4500. **1.** Lumen. **2.** Nuclei of endothelial cells. **3.** Nuclei of longitudinally arranged smooth muscle cells. **4.** Elastic fibers and scattered collagenous fibrils. **5.** Nuclei of circularly arranged smooth muscle cells. **6.** Nucleus of fibroblast. **7.** Bundles of collagenous fibrils.

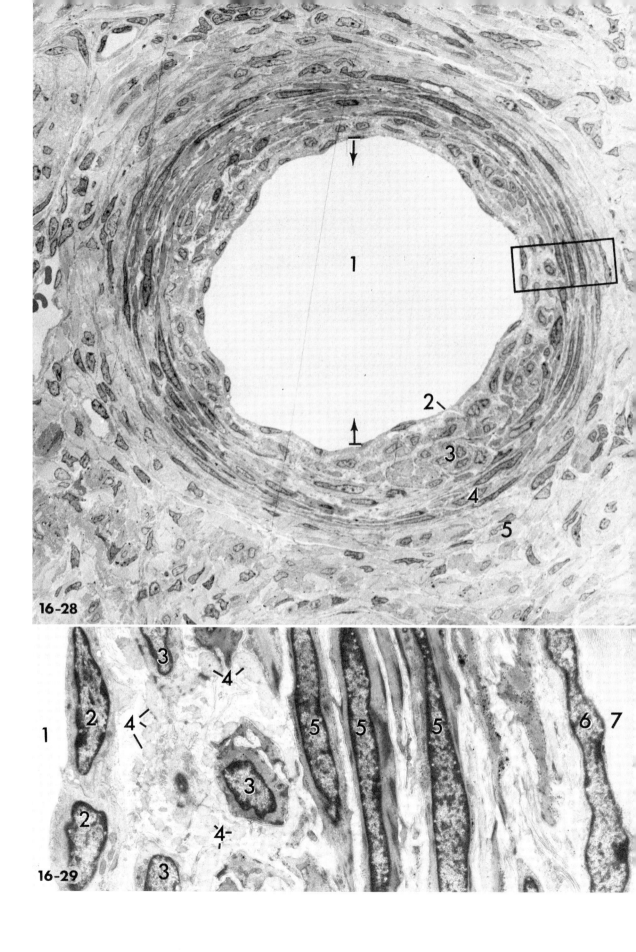

16-28

16-29

less than 300 μ and a wall which contains no more than 1 or 2 circularly arranged, layers of smooth muscle cells. The wall of the arteriole also contains an endothelial lining, an indistinct internal elastic lamina, and a thin connective tissue sleeve. (Fig. 16-30)

Endothelium. The endothelial cells are elongated, squamous, and arranged longitudinally. They are connected laterally via junctional specializations. In the central nervous system, one of these specializations is a tight junction where the outer laminae of apposing cell membranes have fused. (Fig. 16-40) In all other organs and tissues, gap-junctions and desmosomes establish junctions between endothelial cells. (Fig. 16-39) The nucleus is flattened out and makes the cell surface bulge, only slightly, into the lumen. A small number of short microvilli project from the luminal surface. In most tissues and organs, cytoplasmic filaments are numerous in the endothelial cells of the arterioles. Their function is probably supportive, but the possibility that they also are contractile cannot be excluded. Other organelles are present in limited number, with the exception of surface (micropinocytotic) vesicles. They are the structural evidence for a metabolic exchange between the cell and its environment, and they may also represent a type of transport vehicle across the endothelial cell.

In the larger arterioles, a thin **internal elastic membrane** separates the endothelial cells from the smooth muscle cells. In small arterioles with a luminal diameter of 50 μ and less, this elastic membrane is replaced by a basal lamina. Exception to this rule is found in the afferent glomerular arterioles of the kidney, where a thin elastic, often fenestrated, membrane is present in arterioles which have a luminal diameter of 10–15 μ. (Fig. 16-30)

An occasional foot-like process emerges from the base of the endothelial cells in the larger arterioles, and in the smaller arterioles a relatively large number of similar projections occur. They penetrate the thin elastic membrane as well as the basal lamina, and establish membranous contacts (gap-junctions) with the smooth muscle cells in an arrangement referred to as **myoendothelial junctions.** (Fig. 16-31)

One or two layers of **smooth muscle cells** are arranged circularly, sometimes spirally, around the long axis of the arterioles. These are spindle-shaped cells with their polar ends divided into several long processes. Each muscle cell is invested by an external (basal) lamina (Fig. 16-31) except for areas where adjacent muscle cells, their processes, and endothelial projections make membranous contacts (gap-junctions). Delicate collagenous and reticular fibrils are present between smooth muscle cells of the larger arterioles, but fibroblasts do not exist here.

Peripherally to the smooth muscle cells is a thin sleeve of loose connective tissue consisting of a few fibroblasts, collagenous and elastic fibrils, occasional macrophages, mast cells, non-myelinated nerve fibers, and denuded terminal axons with agranular and granular vesicles.

Precapillary sphincter area. This is the terminal part of an arteriole, also referred to as metarteriole. Classically, a precapillary sphincter was thought of as one or two smooth muscle cells surrounding the

Fig. 16-30. Afferent arteriole. Cross section. Kidney. Rat. E.M. X 7000. **1.** Lumen; width 18 μ. **2.** Nuclei of endothelial cells. **3.** Nucleus of spirally arranged smooth muscle cell. **4.** Nuclei of perivascular connective tissue cells. **5.** Non-myelinated nerve axons. **6.** Collagenous fibrils. **7.** Profiles of incomplete internal elastic membrane. **8.** Mitochondria. **9.** Centriole.

Fig. 16-31. Afferent arteriole. Longitudinal section. Kidney. Rat. E.M. X 31,000. **1.** Lumen. **2.** Endothelial cytoplasm. **3.** Basal lamina. **4.** Nucleus of smooth muscle cell. **5.** Mitochondria. **6.** Glycogen particles. **7.** Myofilaments. **8.** Myoendothelial junction. **9.** Junctional area of smooth muscle cells. **10.** Attachment plaques (dense bodies). **11.** External (basal) lamina.

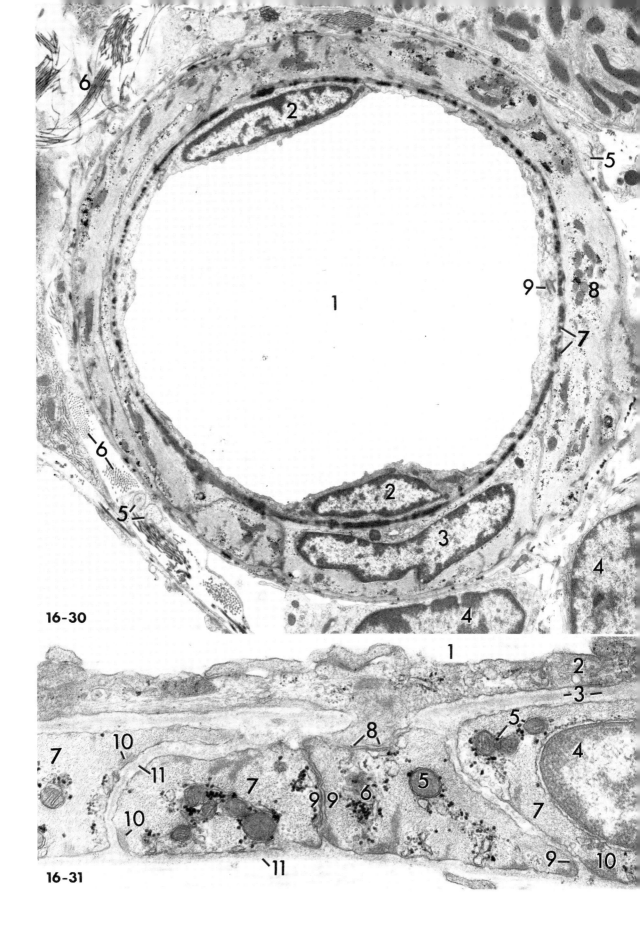

16-30

16-31

capillary at the point where it branches off from the arteriole. Contemporary evaluations of the functional significance of a precapillary sphincter tend to look upon the terminal part of the arteriolar system as a region of varied lengths which controls the blood flow to the capillary bed by an increase or reduction of luminal diameter, or by a complete obliteration of the lumen, shunting the blood to other parts of the microvascular bed or bypassing it completely.

The precapillary sphincter area, then, is variable in length, ranging from 5 μ to 100 μ or more, and with a luminal diameter which ranges between 30 μ and 5 μ. (Fig. 16-32) The **endothelial cells** of these small arterioles are structurally similar to those of the larger arterioles. The cells rest on a thin basal lamina. Within the precapillary sphincter area, the number of basal endothelial processes which establish **myoendothelial junctions** increases gradually toward the periphery and reaches a maximum at the last smooth muscle cells before the capillary branches off from the arteriole. (Fig. 16-34) Exceptions to this are found in the arterioles of the central nervous system which are largely devoid of myoendothelial junctions.

The **smooth muscle cells** are small and few in number. They disappear gradually as the arteriole is transformed into an arterial capillary. In the afferent glomerular arteriole of the kidney, and in the cavernous tissue of the penis, the termination of smooth muscle cells is very abrupt, whereas in organs such as the lung, intestine, and skeletal muscle, there is a gradual decrease in number of smooth muscle cells.

There is a sparse perivascular **connective tissue** which forms a narrow sleeve around the precapillary sphincter area, and which merges imperceptibly with the connective tissue of the organ through which the microvessels pursue their course. Non-myelinated nerves and denuded terminal axons with agranular and granular

vesicles are present near the smooth muscle cells of the precapillary sphincter area. (Fig. 16-33)

From a **functional** point of view, arterioles and precapillary sphincter areas are collectively called peripheral resistance vessels, since it is the state of tonic contraction or relaxation of the arteriolar smooth muscle that determines the peripheral resistance and the diastolic blood pressure. The fundamental hemodynamic change of diastolic hypertension involves sustained contraction and increased resistance in the arterioles. The arterioles are under the control of the autonomic nervous system,

Fig. 16-32. Precapillary sphincter area. Longitudinal section. Dermis. Rabbit. E.M. $\times$ 1600. Arrows indicate direction of blood flow. **1.** Lumen of 30 μ arteriole. **2.** Lumen of 12 μ terminal arteriole. **3.** Beginning of arterial capillary; lumen 7.5 μ wide. **4.** Nuclei of smooth muscle cells. **5.** Nuclei of endothelial cells. **6.** Nuclei of fibroblasts. **7.** Nuclei of smooth muscle cells. In this position around the origin of an arterial capillary, these smooth muscle cells form a true precapillary sphincter. **8.** Bundles of collagenous fibrils. **9.** Lymphatic capillary (After Rhodin: J. Ultrastr. Res. *18*, 181, 1967).

Fig. 16-33. Precapillary sphincter area. Cross section in the plane indicated by line A-A in Fig. 16-32. Enlarged detail of Fig. 11-4 (p. 223). Skeletal muscle. Rat. E.M. $\times$ 9000. **1.** Lumen of terminal arteriole; width 10 μ. **2.** Lumen of beginning of arterial capillary; width 5 μ. **3.** Nuclei of endothelial cells. **4.** Cytoplasm of smooth muscle cells. **5.** Fibroblast cytoplasm. **6.** Non-myelinated nerve axons. **7.** Lamellated capsular cells of neuromuscular spindle.

Fig. 16-34. Myoendothelial junction in arteriole. Enlargement of area indicated by rectangle in Fig. 16-33, several sections deeper. Skeletal muscle. Rat. E.M. $\times$ 47,000. **1.** Lumen. **2.** Junctional area of endothelial cells. **3.** Foot-like process from base of endothelial cell. **4.** Basal lamina. **5.** Cytoplasm of smooth muscle cell. **6.** Junctional area of smooth muscle cell and endothelial cell (myoendothelial junction). **7.** External lamina. **8.** Mitochondrion. **9.** Profiles of granular endoplasmic reticulum. **10.** Microtubules. **11.** Ribosomes.

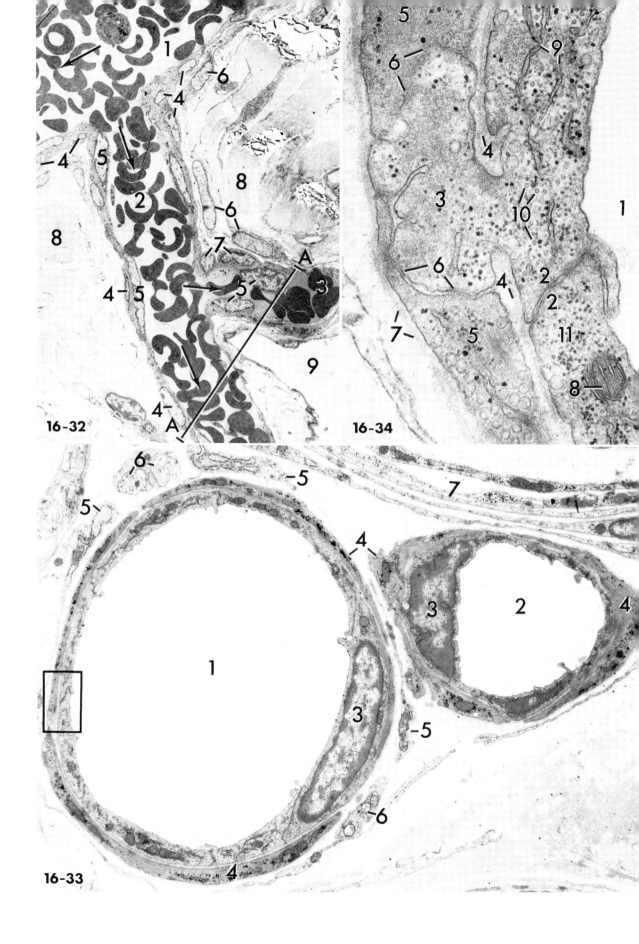

16-32

16-34

16-33

but they also respond to blood-borne neurotransmitter substances, and chemical mediators, as well as to local metabolic processes. The last-mentioned phenomenon is referred to as **autoregulation,** since it is believed that the arterioles of the precapillary sphincter area may dilate in response to a build-up of metabolic waste products and low oxygen tension. The arterioles, on the other hand, reduce the blood flow to a certain region when adequate oxygen tension of that region is reached. The alternating contractions and dilatations of the arterioles of the precapillary sphincter area are called **vasomotion.** It has been suggested that the myoendothelial junctions may facilitate an ionic exchange between endothelial and smooth muscle cells. They may, therefore, help to initiate contraction of the smooth muscle cells, either by a mechanical stretch of the smooth muscle membrane (Bayliss' effect), or by initiating a change in membrane potential through the action of neurotransmitter substances.

CAPILLARIES

Capillaries are the most delicate branches of the blood vessels. The luminal diameter of true capillaries ranges from $3\ \mu$ to $10\ \mu$. The upper limit is indicated and restricted by the ultrastructure of the capillary wall which consists of a single layer of **endothelial cells,** a **basal lamina,** and an occasional **pericyte** (pericapillary cell). In earlier literature, the somewhat larger postcapillary venules were often included among the capillaries, but recent investigations have demonstrated that they differ structurally and functionally from true capillaries. Until recently it was also believed that all capillaries had the same general structure, but it is now recognized that there are several types of capillaries and that different organs and different tissues have their own type of capillary. In addition, there are indications that some structural differences exist between arterial and venous capillaries in some organs. The pattern of the capillary ramifications

of the vascular tree varies greatly with the tissue and the organ, but capillaries generally form an interconnected network, the **capillary bed** (Fig. 16-35), in which the length of the component capillaries varies from about $25\ \mu$ to several thousand microns.

Types of capillaries. Capillaries can be subdivided into several types, based mainly on certain variations in the fine structure of the endothelial cells, although the basal lamina and the pericapillary cells (pericytes) are also subject to variation.

Continuous thick endothelium (Fig. 16-36) is present in the true capillaries of skeletal, cardiac, and smooth muscle tissue and, to some extent, in the testis and ovary. The endothelial cells, which have

Fig. 16-35. Capillary network. Longitudinal section. Connective tissue core of intestinal villus. Rat. E.M. X 1900. Arrows indicate assumed direction of blood flow. **1.** True capillaries. Lumen averages $4\ \mu$ in width. **2.** Postcapillary venule; lumen $9\ \mu$ wide. **3.** Erythrocyte. **4.** Nuclei of endothelial cells. **5.** Pericyte. **6.** Fibroblast. **7.** Schwann cell nucleus. **8.** Non-myelinated nerve axons. **9.** Plasma cell. **10.** Macrophage. **11.** Leukocytes. **12.** Loose network of collagenous fibrils. **13.** Stretches of fenestrated endothelium near the venous end of the capillary network. (After Rhodin: Topics in the Study of Life; The Bio Source Book. Harper & Row, 1971.)

Fig. 16-36. True capillary. Cross section. Cardiac muscle. Rat. E.M. X 19,000. **1.** Lumen; width $3.5\ \mu$. **2.** Nucleus of endothelial cell. **3.** Junction of cytoplasmic arms of same endothelial cell. **4.** Cytoplasm rich in micropinocytotic vesicles. **5.** Basal lamina. **6.** Cytoplasmic process of pericyte. **7.** Pericapillary connective tissue space. **8.** Part of cardiac muscle cells.

Fig. 16-37. Peritubular capillary. Kidney. Rat. E.M. X 16,000. **1.** Lumen; width $5\ \mu$. **2.** Nucleus of endothelial cell. **3.** Junction of endothelial cytoplasmic arms. **4.** Highly fenestrated cytoplasm. Each fenestra closed by a thin membrane (diaphragm). **5.** Basal lamina. **6.** Part of pericyte. **7.** Pericapillary connective tissue space. **8.** Base of kidney tubule cell. **9.** Nucleus of fibroblast. **10.** Golgi zone. **11.** Centrioles.

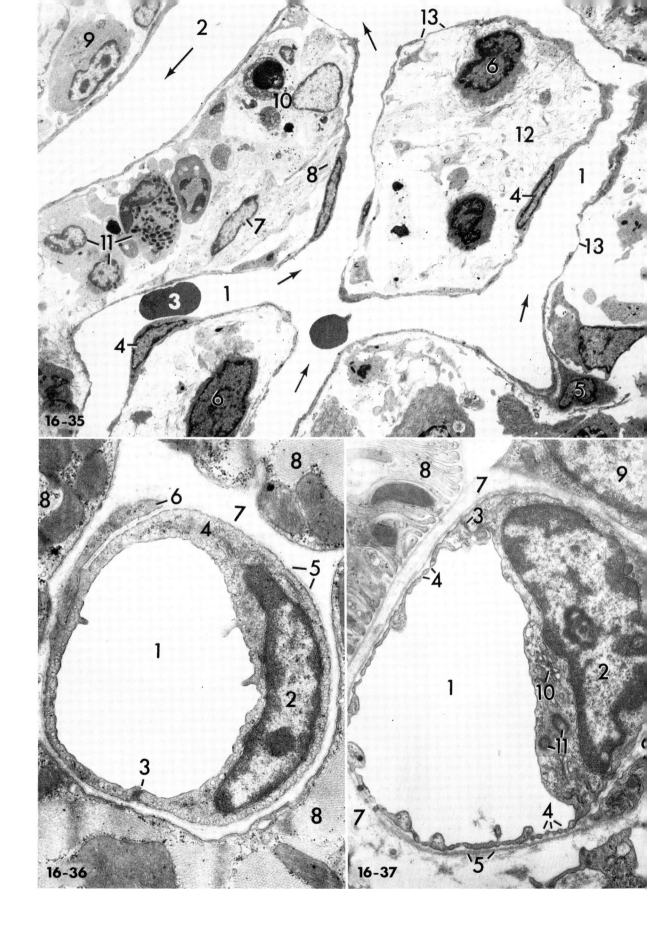

16-35

16-36

16-37

an average thickness of 0.2 μ, are provided with many micropinocytotic vesicles, both at the luminal and basal surfaces as well as within the cytoplasm. (Fig. 16-38A) Cytoplasmic filaments and microtubules occur in varied numbers. The endothelial cells are held together by gap-junctions (nexuses), and occasional desmosomes (maculae adhaerentes). There is always a thin basal lamina which envelops the endothelium. Spread out along this type of true capillary are occasional **pericytes**. These are elongated, slender pericapillary cells with a highly branched cytoplasm embracing the capillary endothelium. Each cell is invested by an external (basal) lamina, which is absent in the regions where the cell membranes of the endothelial cells and the pericytes make contact. The pericyte contains a large nucleus, and the ultrastructure of the cytoplasm and its organelles is very similar to that of a fibroblast, except that the pericyte contains a larger number of cytoplasmic filaments, some dense bodies attached to the cytoplasmic aspect of the cell membrane, and is invested by its own external lamina. (Fig. 16-44)

Continuous thin endothelium is present in the true capillaries of the central nervous system, the lung (Fig. 16-38B), arterial capillaries of the dermis, vasa recta of the kidney, and the spleen, as well as in capillaries of the thymus, lymph nodes, bone marrow, and Haversian systems of the bone. The endothelial cells have an average thickness of 0.1 μ. Their cytoplasm contains a small number of micropinocytotic vesicles and cytoplasmic filaments. The cells are held together by gap-junctions and occasional desmosomes, except in the central nervous system, where true tight junctions exist. A basal lamina is present in the lung, dermis, and nervous tissue, but is many times incomplete and even missing in bone and in myeloid and lymphoid tissues. In all locations pericytes are scarce in this type of capillary.

Fenestrated thin endothelium (Fig. 16-37) is present in the true capillaries of the urinary system (kidney, bladder), endocrine glands, choroid plexus of the brain, ciliary body of the eye, and the venous capillaries of the dermis and intestinal connective tissue, and the venous part of the vasa recta of the kidney. The endothelium averages 0.08 μ (800 Å) in thick-

Fig. 16-38. A comparison of capillary walls in rat tissue. E.M. $\times$ 60,000. (A–E). **A.** Continuous thick endothelium. Cardiac muscle. **B.** Continuous thin endothelium. Lung. **C.** Fenestrated thin endothelium. Kidney. Peritubular capillary. **D.** Fenestrated thin endothelium. Kidney. Glomerular capillary. **E.** Discontinuous endothelium. Liver. Sinusoid. **1.** Lumen of capillary. **2.** Endothelial cytoplasm. **3.** Basal lamina. **4.** Pericapillary space. **5.** Surface (micropinocytotic) vesicles. **6.** Cytoplasm of alveolar epithelial cell. **7.** Cytoplasm of visceral epithelial cell of Bowman's capsule. **8.** Pulmonary alveolus (air sac). **9.** Urinary space. **10.** Fenestration bridged by a thin membrane (diaphragm). **11.** Open fenestrations. **12.** Cytoplasmic holes (gaps). **13.** Microvilli of hepatic parenchymal cell. **14.** Pericapillary space of Disse. (After Rhodin: Topics in the Study of Life: The Bio Source Book. Harper & Row, 1971.)

Fig. 16-39. Junctional area. Capillary. Skeletal muscle. Rat. E.M. $\times$ 120,000. **1.** Lumen. **2.** Trilaminar cell membrane. **3.** Gap-junction. **4.** Basal lamina.

Fig. 16-40. Junctional area. Capillary. Cerebral cortex. Rat. E.M. $\times$ 120,000. **1.** Lumen. **2.** Trilaminar cell membrane. **3.** True tight junction (fusion of outer leaflets of apposing trilaminar cell membranes).

Fig. 16-41. Routes of transport across capillary endothelial cells are schematized in this composite drawing. The transport may occur in either direction across the cell. F1, F2, and F3 are adjoining segments of endothelial cells. The cell membrane is composed of a superficial glycoprotein layer (illustrated as pegs) and three laminae (leaflets). **A.** Capillary lumen. **B.** Basal lamina. **C.** Pericapillary space. **D.** True tight junction. **E.** Gap-junction. *Transport routes:* **1.** Through plasma membrane. **2.** Surface (micropinocytotic) vesicles. **3.** True tight junction (impenetrable). **4.** Gap-junction (penetrable). **5.** Fenestrations (with closing membrane). **6.** Fenestrations (open). **7.** Holes (gaps). (After Rhodin: Topics in the Study of Life: The Bio Source Book. Harper & Row 1971.)

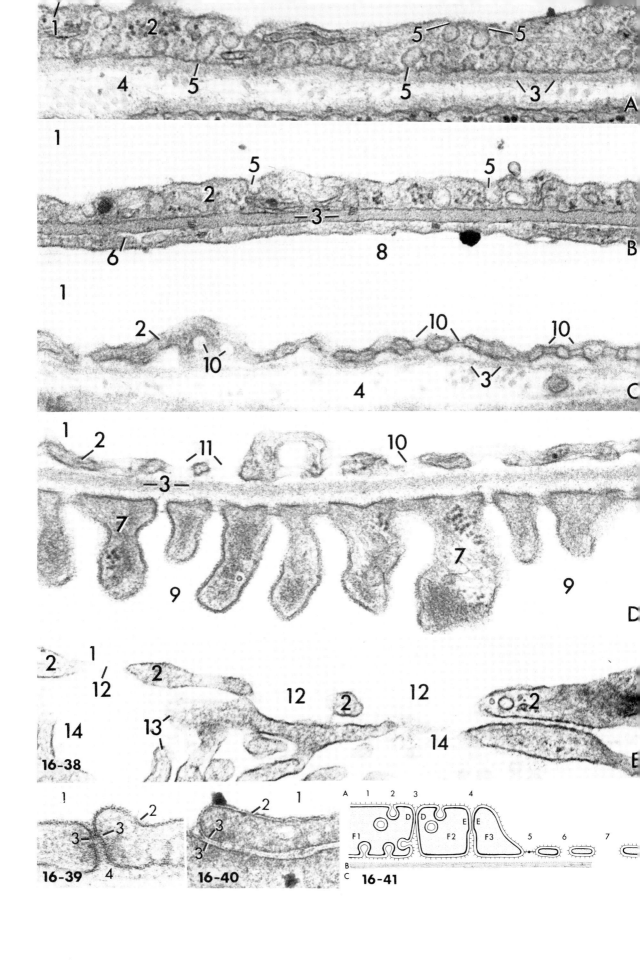

16-38

16-39

16-40

16-41

ness. (Fig. 16-38C) The fenestrations are round with a diameter of about 700 Å and spaced regularly, averaging 30 per square micron. The fenestrations are closed by a thin single-layered membrane with a central knob-like swelling. An exception to this is found in the glomerular capillaries of the kidney where the majority of fenestrations are open and not bridged by a thin membrane. (Fig. 16-38D) The cells are joined by gap-junctions. The cytoplasm contains occasional micropinocytotic vesicles, but other organelles are sparse. A basal lamina is always present, but pericytes are rare.

Discontinuous endothelium is found only in the large capillaries (sinusoids; sinuses) of the liver parenchyma. (Fig. 16-38E) The endothelial cells contain cytoplasmic holes, the diameter of which ranges between 0.5 μ to 2 μ. On rare occasions, a thin membrane closes off the smaller holes. These endothelial cells, also referred to as Kupffer cells, are highly phagocytic, and the cytoplasm contains a varied number of primary and secondary lysosomes in addition to many coated vesicles, some of which are connected to the cell membrane. Cytoplasmic filaments are rare, but microtubules are relatively abundant. The cells are held together by gap-junctions in most instances, but sometimes the edges of adjacent endothelial cells simply overlap without junctional specialization, similar to the arrangement in lymphatic capillaries (p. 372). A basal lamina is absent in most species. Occasional pericytes occur.

Arterial and venous capillaries. In some organs and tissues the endothelial cells at the venous end of capillaries are structurally different from those at the arterial end. The endothelial cells of venous capillaries have fenestrations, bridged by a thin membrane in the dermis (Fig. 16-42), intestinal connective tissue (Fig. 16-35), and the venous capillary part of the vasa recta of the kidney, whereas the arterial end of capillaries in these locations is of the continuous thick or thin endothelial variety.

Sinusoids (sinuses). In some organs, the luminal diameter of capillaries is very much larger than indicated above for true capillaries. Traditionally, these large capillaries are referred to as sinusoids or sinuses. They are found in the liver, bone marrow, spleen, adrenal glands, and hypophysis. Since the endothelial cells of sinusoids vary greatly in their fine structure, it is necessary to regard sinusoids as specialized capillaries adapted to the functional demands of each particular organ. The endothelial cells of the sinusoids in the liver and bone marrow, as well as in the lymphatic sinuses of lymph nodes, are highly phagocytic and belong to the reticuloendothelial system (p. 156). The endothelial cells of the splenic sinuses are less phagocytic, and those of the adrenal glands and the hypophysis hardly ever phagocytose.

Pericapillary space. The extent of the pericapillary space varies greatly with the organ. It is rather wide in loose connec-

Fig. 16-42. Connection between venous capillary and postcapillary venule. Longitudinal section. Dermis. Rabbit. E.M. X 2300. Arrows indicate direction of blood flow. **1.** Lumen of venous capillary; width averages 8 μ. **2.** Lumen of postcapillary venule; lumen averages 12 μ. **3.** Nuclei of endothelial cells. **4.** Nuclei of pericytes. **5.** Fibroblast. **6.** Collagenous fibrils. **7.** Stretch of fenestrated endothelium. **8.** Erythrocytes. **9.** Processes of pericytic cytoplasm surround junction of capillary and postcapillary venule. Smooth muscle cells do not occur here.

Fig. 16-43. Cross section of postcapillary venule, corresponding approximately to level indicated by line A-A in Fig. 16-42. Interstitial tissue. Testis. Rat. E.M. X 7000. **1.** Lumen; width 10 μ. **2.** Nucleus of endothelial cell. **3.** Nucleus of pericyte. **4.** Junctions of endothelial cells. **5.** Strands of pericytic cytoplasm. **6.** Junctions of pericytes and endothelial cells. **7.** Basal lamina.

Fig. 16-44. Postcapillary venule. Longitudinal section. Dermis. Rat. E.M. X 20,000. **1.** Lumen. **2.** Erythrocyte. **3.** Junction of endothelial cells. **4.** Mitochondria. **5.** Nucleus of pericyte. **6.** Golgi zone. **7.** Lysosomes. **8.** Profiles of granular endoplasmic reticulum. **9.** Basal (external) lamina.

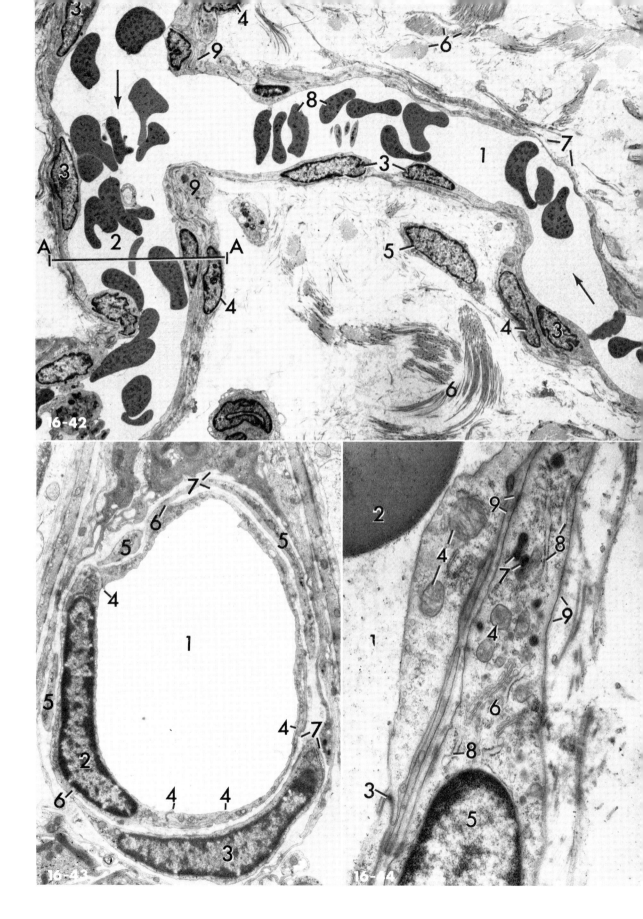

tive tissue, narrow in the liver and lung, and minimal in muscle and nervous tissue. It contains a loosely woven network of reticular and delicate collagenous fibrils, together with occasional fibroblasts, some of which have thin, extensive cytoplasm, and therefore are sometimes referred to as veil cells.

Capillary functions. Gases, nutrients, and metabolic waste products are exchanged across the capillary wall. It is generally accepted that the micropinocytotic (surface) vesicles of the capillary endothelial cells participate in carrying metabolites, large molecular proteins, and perhaps fluids across the capillary wall— a two-directional transport. (Fig. 16-41) The fenestrations and the intercellular narrow space (20–50 Å) of the gap-junctions probably represent sites for easy diffusion of low molecular substances and water. In the brain capillaries, the junctions are closed by a fusion of the outer leaflets of the apposing cell membranes (tight junctions), possibly creating the so-called blood-brain barrier. The basal lamina represents only a crude barrier to large molecular substances, and to the formed elements of the blood. The large holes of the liver sinusoids clearly offer preferential channels for exchange. Experimental evidence is not yet available to suggest the formulation of hypotheses of whether the capillary fenestrations are stationary or transient, whether they are more abundant during increased capillary permeability, and whether they occur permanently more often near the venous end of capillaries of certain organs. The cytoplasmic filaments of the endothelial cytoplasm may indicate a potential contractility of the capillary. If so, this is probably a very slow contraction, more in the nature of ameboid movements than the relatively fast contraction of smooth muscle cells. The pericytes were thought of earlier as contractile cells and were referred to as **Rouget cells.** Recent experimental investigations have failed to demonstrate contractile properties in the pericyte.

VENULES

The capillary bed is drained by increasingly larger vessels, the venules. Immediately connected to the capillaries are the **postcapillary venules.** These channels range in diameter from 10 μ to 30 μ, and in length from 50 μ to 500 μ. The wall consists of an endothelial lining, a basal lamina, an incomplete layer of pericytes, and occasional peripheral fibroblasts. (Fig. 16-43) The endothelium is thin, continuous, averaging 0.4 μ in thickness. The lymph nodes, in which cuboidal endothelial cells line the postcapillary venules, are an exception. (Fig. 17-33) Micropinocytotic (surface) vesicles, ribosomes, and filaments are generally abundant, in addition to profiles of the granular endoplasmic reticulum. The edges of adjacent endothelial cells often overlap. Gap-junctions sometimes occur in these regions, but often junctional specializations are missing. Long and narrow basal projections of the endothelial cytoplasm penetrate the basal lamina and make membranous contacts with the peripheral

Fig. 16-45. Connection between collecting venule and muscular venule. Longitudinal section. Dermis. Rabbit. E.M. X 1800. Arrows indicate direction of blood flow. **1.** Lumen of collecting venule; width averages 50 μ. **2.** Lumen of muscular venule; width averages 90 μ. **3.** Nuclei of endothelial cells. **4.** Nuclei of pericytes. **5.** Smooth muscle cells. **6.** Erythrocytes.

Fig. 16-46. Muscular venule. Cross section. Submucosa. Small intestine. Rat. E.M. X 1200. **1.** Lumen; width 70 μ. **2.** Nuclei of endothelial cells. **3.** Nuclei of smooth muscle cells. **4.** Base of crypt of Lieberkühn. **5.** Lumen of capillary; width 7 μ. **6.** Loosely arranged collagenous fibrils.

Fig. 16-47. Wall of cross-sectioned muscular venule. Enlargement of area similar to rectangle in Fig. 16-46. Skeletal muscle. Rat. E.M. X 47,000. **1.** Lumen of venule; width 80 μ. **2.** Junction of endothelial cells. **3.** Mitochondrion. **4.** Specific endothelial granules. **5.** Basal lamina. **6.** Delicate elastic fibers. **7.** Smooth muscle cell. **8.** External lamina. **9.** Collagenous fibrils. **10.** Cytoplasm of fibroblast.

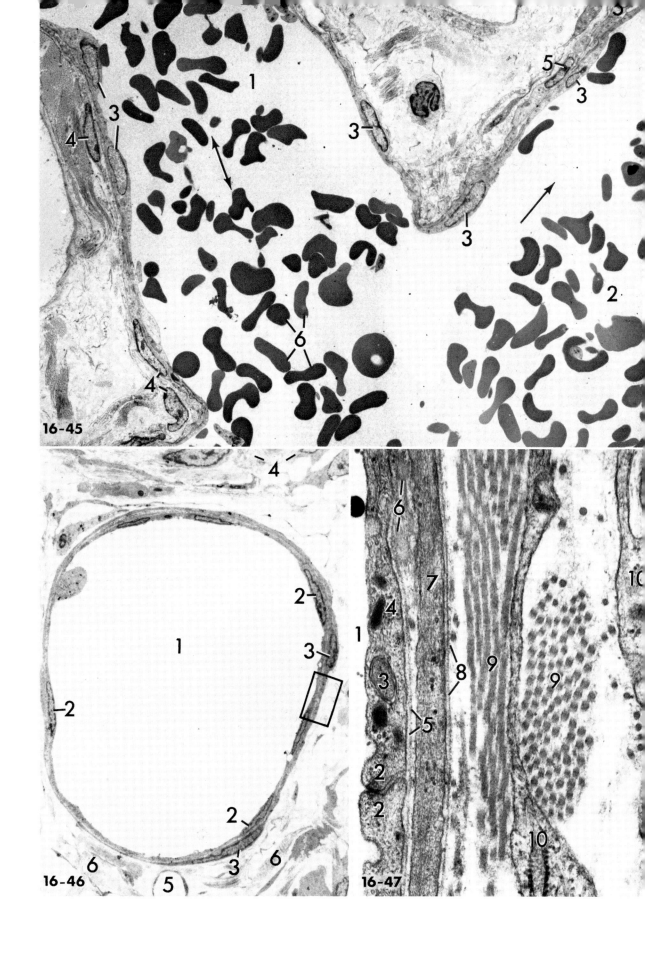

16-45

16-46

16-47

layer of flat pericytes. The pericytes are more numerous, but are structurally similar to those associated with the true capillaries. (Fig. 16-44)

Collecting venules are vessels which connect postcapillary venules to muscular venules. They range in diameter from 30μ to about 50μ. (Fig. 16-45) The endothelial cells are structurally similar to those of postcapillary venules. The pericytes form a complete layer of highly branched cells, each invested by an external lamina. The cytoplasm of these pericytes contains more filaments and dense bodies attached to the cell membrane than do pericytes of other locations. The cells, therefore, resemble smooth muscle cells. One important structural difference is the glycogen particles which are numerous in smooth muscle cells but apparently absent in pericytes of collecting venules.

Muscular venules range in diameter from 50μ to about 1000μ (1 mm). These are the small blood vessels (Fig. 16-46) which traditionally are referred to as simply "venules." They are recognized in light microscope preparations as microvessels with thin walls accompanying an arteriole with slightly thicker walls. In routine histological preparations, the lumen of the arteriole is often round or oval, whereas the lumen of the muscular venule is irregularly oval or collapsed. (Fig. 16-48) The endothelium of the muscular venules is squamous but relatively thick, often containing specific endothelial granules (p. 340), cytoplasmic filaments, microtubules, and profiles of the granular endoplasmic reticulum. (Fig. 16-47) There are generally one or two layers of elongated, flat, smooth muscle cells in most muscular venules, but in organs such as the kidney and the spleen, venules with a diameter of over 300μ may contain only an incomplete layer of smooth muscle cells. A basal lamina separates the endothelial cells from the smooth muscle cells, except in areas of myoendothelial junctions. Collagenous and elastic fibrils occur in varied numbers between the endothelium and the smooth

muscle cells, but an elastic membrane is never present. The perivascular connective tissue contains a few fibroblasts (Fig. 16-47) which are sometimes called **veil cells** because of their peculiar shape and extremely attenuated thin cytoplasm. Nonmyelinated nerves occur sparingly in this perivascular connective tissue.

Functions of venules. Venules generally collect the blood from the capillary beds and return it to the heart via the veins. The function of the **postcapillary venules** is closely related to that of the true capillaries, since this segment normally aids in the transcapillary exchange of metabolites, ion and fluid. In contrast to true capillaries, postcapillary venules are easily affected by inflammation, allergic reactions, and extreme temperatures, reacting to these factors by opening up the junc-

Fig. 16-48. Small vein. Mesentery. Rabbit. L.M. X 190. **1.** Lumen (max. width 570 μ) with coagulated blood. **2.** Intima and media; width 20 μ. **3.** Adventitia blending with perivascular connective tissue. **4.** Adipose tissue **5.** Wall of small artery (width 90 μ).

Fig. 16-49. Wall of cross-sectioned renal vein. Same preparation as in Fig. 16-24. Rat. E.M. X 4500. **1.** Lumen; width 2600 μ. **2.** Erythrocytes. **3.** Nuclei of endothelial cells. **4.** Elastic fibers, unevenly distributed immediately adjacent to the endothelial cells in the subendothelial connective tissue. **5.** Smooth muscle cells. **6.** Collagenous fibrils between smooth muscle cells. **7.** Bundles of collagenous fibrils in adventitia. **8.** Non-myelinated nerve axons.

Fig. 16-50. Junctional area of endothelial cells. Renal vein. Enlargement of rectangle in Fig. 16-49. Rat. E.M. X 64,000. **1.** Lumen. **2.** Nucleus. **3.** Mitochondria. **4.** Gap-junction. **5.** Intermediate-type junction with adjacent accumulation of cytoplasmic filaments. **6.** Microtubules. **7.** Surface (micropinocytotic) vesicles. **8.** Specific endothelial granules. **9.** Longitudinally sectioned specific endothelial granule. **10.** Indistinct basal lamina. **11.** Cross-sectioned microfibrils of elastic fiber. **12.** Amorphous substance of elastic fiber. **13.** Inset: Enlargement (X 128,000) of specific endothelial granule, showing its boundary membrane and component small tubules which are not present in all specific endothelial granules.

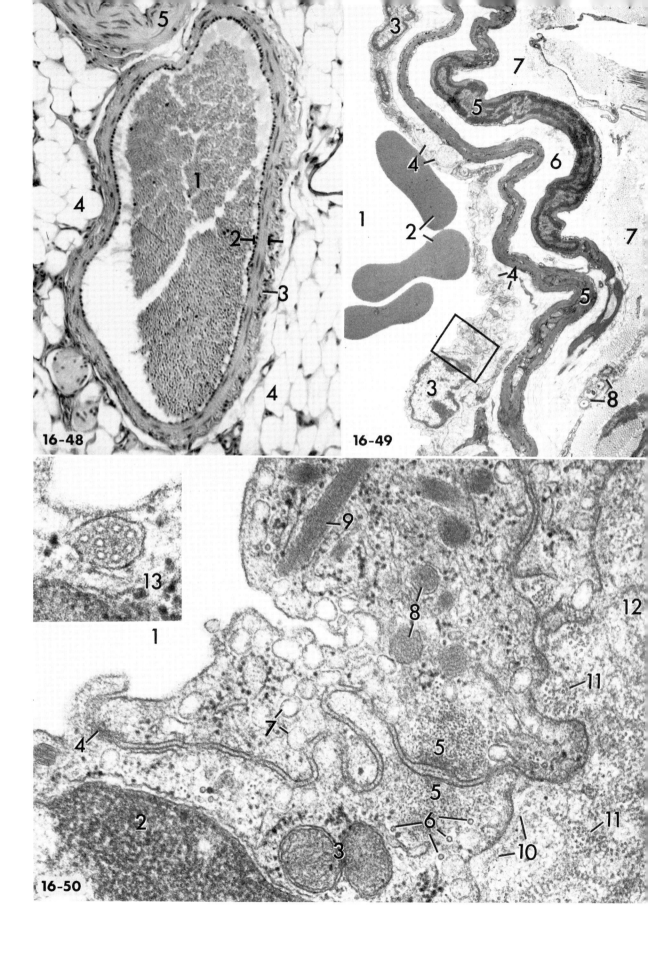

16-48

16-49

16-50

tional specializations. This results in an increase in outward diffusion of plasma (edema) and an extravasation of formed elements of the blood, especially the granular leukocytes.

The **collecting venules** are far less sensitive to pathogens and other abnormal factors. Here the presence of a larger number of pericytes may be of some protective importance. The increase in cytoplasmic filaments and dense bodies in the pericytes of this segment is probably an indication that pericytes represent incompletely differentiated smooth muscle cells. Upon the proper stimulus, they may develop into smooth muscle cells, but the possibility also exists that they are precursors of fat cells, fibroblasts, chondroblasts, and osteoblasts.

The **muscular venules** are under the control of the autonomic nervous system, but their contractile ability is weak. They do not serve as very effective postcapillary sphincters, and reduce only slightly the lumen of the venule when they contract.

Veins

Veins have a larger diameter than the arterial vessel they accompany, and their lumen is often slightly collapsed in routine preparations for the light microscope. Veins have thinner walls than their arterial companion, and the venous wall contains an abundance of fibrous connective tissue, whereas elastic components and smooth muscle cells occur in small numbers.

The wall of the veins consists of three indistinct coats: 1) tunica intima; 2) tunica media; 3) tunica adventitia. However, there are great variations in the composition of these coats in various locations of the body, and it is not possible to categorize veins into elastic and muscular types as it is with arteries. It is customary to group the veins into two categories according to size: 1) small and medium-sized veins; 2) large veins.

SMALL AND MEDIUM-SIZED VEINS

The diameter of these veins ranges from about 1 mm to 10 mm. The **small veins** are very similar to the largest muscular venules (p. 360). With an increase in vascular diameter, there occur, as a rule, at least two complete layers of smooth muscle cells, arranged largely in a circular manner. (Fig. 16-49)

To the group of **medium-sized veins** belong most of the superficial veins, as well as the veins of the viscera. The **tunica intima** consists of a single layer of flat, round, or polygonal endothelial cells, held

Fig. 16-51. Vena cava. Cross section. Human. L.M. $\times$ 5. **1.** Lumen, highly collapsed; width 21 mm. **2.** Wall thickness approximately 700 μ (0.7 mm).

Fig. 16-52. Wall of cross-sectioned vena cava. Enlargement of area similar to rectangle in Fig. 16-51. Human. L.M. X 100. **1.** Lumen **2.** Intima and media (100 μ) with circularly arranged smooth muscle cells. **3.** Adventitia (600 μ) with longitudinally arranged smooth muscle cells.

Fig. 16-53. Intima and media of cross-sectioned vena cava. Enlargement of area similar to rectangle (A) in Fig. 16-52. Squirrel monkey. E.M. X 5100. **1.** Lumen. **2.** Nucleus of endothelial cell. **3.** Subendothelial elastic fibers, forming an incomplete internal elastic membrane. **4.** Nucleus of circularly arranged smooth muscle cell. **5.** Nucleus of longitudinally arranged smooth muscle cell. **6.** Bundles of collagenous fibrils. **7.** Elastic fibers.

Fig. 16-54. Adventitia of cross-sectioned vena cava. Enlargement of area similar to rectangle (B) in Fig. 16-52. Squirrel monkey. E.M. X 5100. **1.** Coarse bundles of collagenous fibrils. **2.** Scattered elastic fibers. **3.** Nuclei of longitudinally arranged smooth muscle cells. **4.** Circle: non-myelinated nerve axons. **5.** Scattered collagenous fibrils.

Fig. 16-55. Detail of vena cava. Enlargement of area similar to rectangle in Fig. 16-53. Squirrel monkey. E.M. $\times$ 27,000. **1.** Lumen. **2.** Specific granules of endothelial cell. **3.** Mitochondria. **4.** Elastic fibers. **5.** Collagenous fibrils. **6.** Nucleus of circularly arranged smooth muscle cell. **7.** Slender cytoplasmic processes of smooth muscle cell establish contacts with endothelial cell. **8.** Myoendothelial junctions. **9.** Non-myelinated nerve axons.

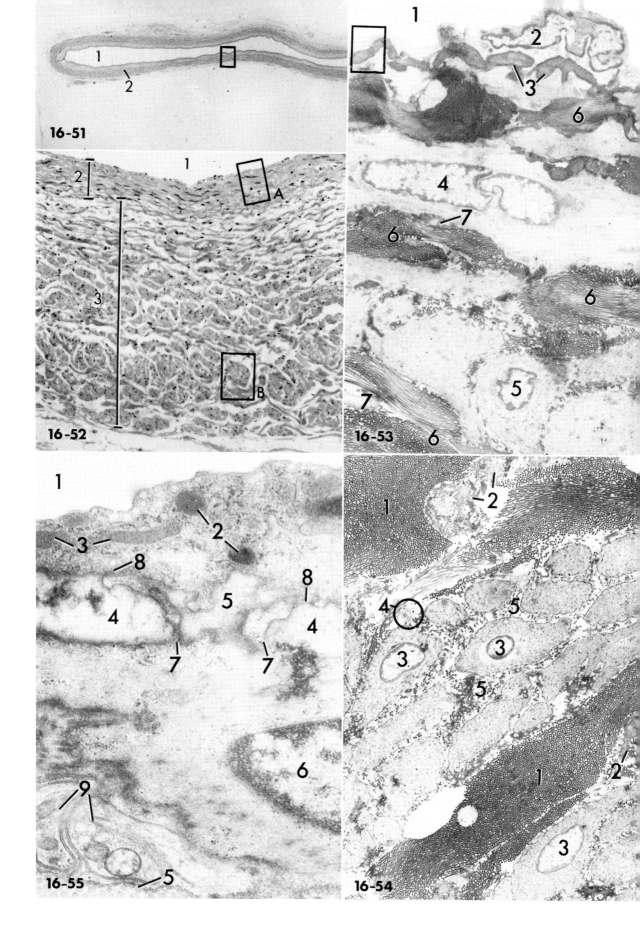

16-51

16-52

16-53

16-55

16-54

together by gap-junctions. Specific endothelial granules occur in relative abundance. (Fig. 16-50) A thin but distinct basal lamina separates the endothelial cells from a very thin layer of subendothelial connective tissue, which consists of delicate collagenous and reticular fibrils. Scattered elastic fibers occur here, but they do not form a distinct internal elastic membrane. In veins larger than 2 mm in diameter, **valves** consisting of pairs of semilunar folds of the endothelium with a central core of connective tissue occur at regular intervals. Valves of larger medium-sized veins may contain an occasional smooth muscle cell. Valves are present only in certain veins, notably those which conduct blood against gravity, preventing a backflow of blood. They are missing in cerebral veins and in veins of viscera and bone marrow.

The **tunica media** is thin and indistinct, consisting mostly of 2–3 layers of circularly arranged, flat and slender smooth muscle cells. The layers are far apart, separated by bundles of collagenous and elastic fibers. (Fig. 16-49) Veins of the legs generally have a thicker media than veins in other locations. The smooth muscle cells are invested by a prominent external (basal) lamina, except for areas where they contact adjacent smooth muscle cells or endothelial basal projections (myoendothelial junctions).

The **tunica adventitia** is the thickest part of the wall, blending with the media. It consists mostly of thick collagenous fibers arranged longitudinally. Some elastic fibers and smooth muscle cells may also be present, together with non-myelinated nerves, lymphatic vessels, and small vasa vasorum.

LARGE VEINS

These vessels all have a diameter larger than 10 mm. To this group belong the venae cavae (Fig. 16-51), pulmonary veins, portal vein, innominates, azygos, as well as the renal, adrenal, splenic, and superior mesenteric veins. The **tunica intima** con-

sists of a single layer of squamous or polygonal endothelial cells joined by gap-junctions. (Figs. 16-53, 16-55) The cytoplasm is richly provided with micropinocytotic (surface) vesicles and specific endothelial granules. In the large veins of most species, there is no distinct basal lamina underneath the endothelium. Instead, a network of delicate fibrils, mixed with elastic fibers, forms, in some large veins, a fragmented or widely fenestrated internal elastic membrane. Valves do not exist in large veins. The **tunica media** is poorly developed and very thin in most large veins, and contains a limited number of circularly arranged smooth muscle cells. Some of these smooth muscle cells make extensive membranous contact with the endothelial cells (myoendothelial junctions). In the venae cavae and the pulmonary veins, the media may contain cardiac muscle fibers near the heart.

The **tunica adventitia** is extremely thick, consisting of longitudinally arranged bundles of collagenous and elastic fibers as well as smooth muscle cells. (Fig.

Fig. 16-56. Helicine arteriole. Cavernous tissue. Penis. Rat. E.M. X 9000. **1.** Lumen; width 15 μ. **2.** Nuclei of endothelial cells. **3.** Smooth muscle cells. **4.** Nucleus of Schwann cell. **5.** Non-myelinated nerve axons. **6.** Fibroblast. **7.** Collagenous fibrils.

Fig. 16-57. Helicine arteriole. Enlargement of rectangle in Fig. 16-56. Cavernous tissue. Penis. Rat. E.M. X 36,000. **1.** Lumen. **2.** Nucleus of endothelial cell. **3.** Mitochondria. **4.** Smooth muscle cells. **5.** External lamina. **6.** Non-myelinated nerve axons with synaptic vesicles and mitochondria. **7.** Nucleus of Schwann cell. **8.** External lamina.

Fig. 16-58. Sympathetic nerve axon terminal. Afferent arteriole at the level of the juxtaglomerular (JG) cells. Kidney. Rat. E.M. X 31,000. **1.** Denuded nerve axon terminal, cut longitudinally. **2.** Local swelling (widening) of terminal axon. **3.** Granulated (dense-core) vesicles. **4.** Mitochondria. **5.** Secondary lysosome. **6.** External lamina. **7.** Secretory granule of juxtaglomerular (JG) cells. **8.** Minimum diffusion gap between axolemma and sarcolemma is 670 Å. **9.** Schwann cell cytoplasm.

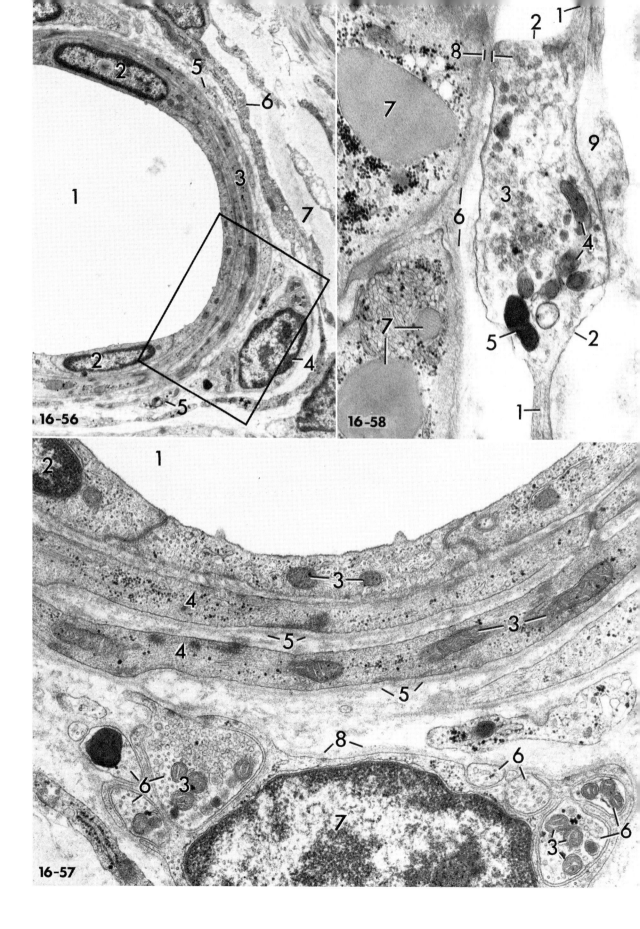

16-56

16-58

16-57

16-54) Non-myelinated nerves form a rich plexus in this adventitia, and the superficial part contains many vasa vasorum and lymphatic vessels.

FUNCTIONAL ASPECTS

The main function of the veins is to return the blood from the capillary beds to the heart. Since the blood pressure in the venous blood vessels is extremely low, the return of blood to the heart is accomplished either by gravity or by the pressure from contracting skeletal muscles exerted on the walls of the veins. To a limited extent, a small intravenous pressure is achieved at the beginning of the venous system near the capillary bed by the diffusion of tissue fluid into the venules.

ARTERIOVENOUS ANASTOMOSES

Blood can bypass the capillary bed by being shunted via a specialized vascular channel connecting a small artery or arteriole directly with a small vein or venule. These **true** arteriovenous anastomoses are present mostly in the skin of the fingertips and toes, in the nail beds, lips, and nose. They also form an essential part of the carotide and aortic bodies (p. 302) as well as the coccygeal body. The anastomoses are short, coiled, and twisted vessels with a pronounced accumulation of special smooth muscle cells in the wall. These cells, often referred to as **epithelioid cells,** have lost many of the characteristic features of smooth muscle cells, being short and thick with few myofilaments, and sometimes accumulations of secretory granules. The adventitia of these anastomoses is rich in both myelinated and non-myelinated nerve fibers.

The true arteriovenous anastomoses regulate the loss of heat from the areas of the skin where they are present. In the aortic and carotid bodies, they are related to sensory chemoreceptors. The function of the coccygeal body is not known.

The precapillary sphincter area of many microvascular beds can serve as a func-tional arteriovenous anastomosis, since so-called thoroughfare channels are often present. These are small arterioles which connect directly with venules. In the erectile tissue, helicine arterioles, in a sense, also represent arteriovenous anastomoses. These arterioles open directly into the cavernous spaces without an intervening capillary bed.

Vascular Nerves

VASOMOTOR NERVES

Innervation of vascular smooth muscle is derived from the autonomic nervous system. The vascular nerves are **mainly sympathetic** and adrenergic, causing contraction of vascular smooth muscle. They are usually referred to as vasomotor nerves because they constantly keep the blood vessels in a state of partial contraction (steady tone). The nerve impulses may also give rise to vasodilation, but it is presently not known if there are separate sets of sympathetic vasodilator and vasoconstrictor nerves, or whether it is a variation in neurotransmitter release and influence on the smooth muscle cells which determines the effect. As a general rule, the release of norepinephrine brings about a vasoconstriction, and the release of acetylcholine a vasodilatation. However, there are regional exceptions to this rule, and

Fig. 16-59. Detail of vascular smooth muscle innervation. Afferent arteriole. Kidney. Rat. E.M. X 68,000. **1.** Myofilaments of smooth muscle cell. **2.** Mitochondria. **3.** Fusiform density. **4.** Attachment plaque (dense body). **5.** Cell membrane of smooth muscle cell. **6.** Junctional area of smooth muscle cell membranes. **7.** External laminae. **8.** Delicate elastic fibers. **9.** Microtubules of non-myelinated nerve axons. **10.** Axolemma. **11.** Mixture of granulated (dense-core) and non-granulated vesicles of non-myelinated nerve axon swellings. **12.** Minimum diffusion gap between axolemma and sarcolemma (for neurotransmitter substances) is $0.1\ \mu$ (indicated by T-bars). **13.** Nuclear membrane of Schwann cell nucleus. **14.** Dense heterochromatin. **15.** Light euchromatin.

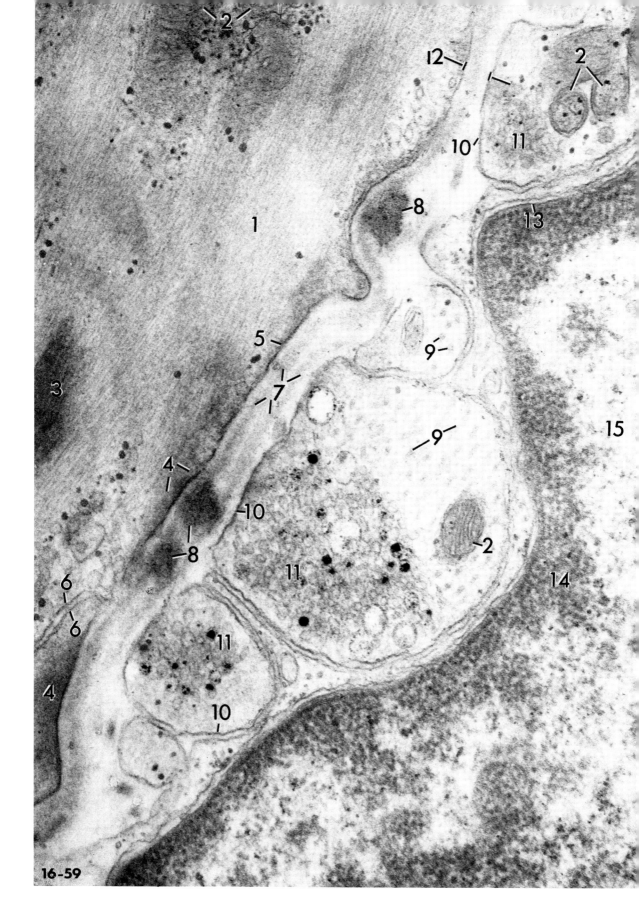

16-59

textbooks of physiology should be consulted for a comprehensive discussion of this topic.

Nerve cells in the intermediolateral column (lateral horn) of the thoracic and upper lumbar levels of the spinal cord send preganglionic myelinated nerve fibers via the ventral roots and white communicating rami to the vertebral ganglia of the sympathetic trunk where they synapse. Postganglionic sympathetic vasomotor nerve fibers, which innervate blood vessels in the **wall of the body** and the **extremities,** originate from visceral motor neurons of vertebral sympathetic ganglia and travel via the gray communicating rami and spinal nerves to the blood vessels. Postganglionic sympathetic vasomotor nerve fibers for the blood vessels of the **heart** and **viscera** travel via the sympathetic cardiac and splanchnic nerves.

Coronary and thoracic blood vessels receive postganglionic **parasympathetic** (cholinergic) nerve fibers from the ganglia of the cardiac and pulmonary plexuses. The preganglionic fibers are derived from the vagus nerve. Other vessels in the body probably also have a parasympathetic innervation, but its pathway has not been conclusively established.

It can be demonstrated with silver staining and fluorescent techniques that arteries, arterioles, venules, and veins are accompanied mostly by non-myelinated nerves which form a plexus in the adventitia of the vessels. Elastic arteries and small veins have a loose nerve plexus, whereas it is dense in muscular arteries and large veins. Arterioles and venules have a very delicate plexus, and capillaries are accompanied only by an occasional delicate nerve fiber.

The exact termination of the vascular nerves has not been fully explored in all mammalian organs and tissue. A combination of fluorescence and electron microscope techniques indicates that nerve terminals lie near the most peripheral layer of smooth muscle cells (Figs. 16-56, 16-58), and that they sometimes penetrate this layer to surround individual smooth muscle cells. The infiltration of nerve terminals among vascular smooth muscle cells is more pronounced in veins than in arteries.

Most of the **nerve terminals** are denuded axons with a beaded appearance and provided with small, irregularly spaced, widened areas. These swellings contain a mixture of agranular vesicles and dense-core vesicles, presumably representing precursors of the chemical mediators (neurotransmitters) acetylcholine and norepinephrine, respectively. As a rule, the nerve terminals do not make membranous contacts with vascular smooth muscle cells, as discussed on p. 250. The distance between axolemma and sarcolemma can be as short as 0.1 μ and as wide as several microns. (Fig. 16-59) The neurotransmitters, upon release, rapidly diffuse across the interstitial space to reach and activate receptor sites assumed to be associated with the cell membrane (sarcolemma), or some other part of the smooth muscle cells, as discussed on p. 250. The **alpha-receptors,** upon stimulation, initiate a smooth muscle contraction, whereas stimulation of a second type, the **beta-receptors,** results in smooth muscle relaxation. Obviously, many details remain to be worked out regarding vascular motor innervation.

SENSORY NERVES

Sensory nerves are also present in the wall of blood vessels. They are myelinated, and register a sensation of pain caused by a penetrating object, or a sudden distension of the vessel. In the carotid and aortic bodies, the sensory nerve endings register changes in blood pressure and carbon dioxide tension (see p. 304). Impulses from these sensory nerve endings affect the autonomic centers of the brain stem.

Lymphatic Vessels

These are described with the lymphatic system (Chapter 17), on p. 374.

References

HEART

Chiba, T. and Yamauchi, A. On the fine structure of the nerve terminals in the human myocardium. Z. Zellforsch. *108*: 324–338 (1970).

Forssmann, W. G. and Girardier, L. A study of the T-system in rat heart. J. Cell Biol. *44*: 1–19 (1970).

Hirano, H. and Ogawa, K. Ultrastructural localization of cholinesterase activity in the guinea pig heart. J. Electron Micr. *16*: 313–321 (1967).

Kolb, R., Pischinger, A. and Stockinger, L. Ultrastruktur der Pulmonalisklappe des Meerschweinchens. Zeitschr. mikr. anat. Forsch. *76*: 184–211 (1967).

Lannigan, R. A. and Zaki, S. A. Ultrastructure of the normal atrial endocardium. Brit. Heart J. *28*: 785–795 (1966).

Luisada, A. A. (Ed.). Development and Structure of the Cardiovascular System. McGraw-Hill, New York, 1961.

Mitomo, Y., Nakao, K. and Angrist, A. The fine structure of the heart valves in the chicken. I. Mitral valve. Am. J. Anat. *125*: 147–167 (1969).

Novi, A. M. An electron microscopic study of the innervation of papillary muscles in the rat. Anat. Rec. *160*: 123–142 (1968).

Rhodin, J. A. G., Del Missier, P. and Reid, L. C. The structure of the specialized impulse-conducting system of the steer heart. Circulation *24*: 349–367 (1969).

Stotler, W. A. and McMahon, R. A. The innervation and structure of the conductive system of the human heart. J. Comp. Neurol. *87*: 57–83 (1947).

Thaemert, J. C. Fine structure of neuromuscular relationships in mouse heart. Anat. Rec. *163*: 575–586 (1969).

ARTERIES AND VEINS

Abramson, D. I. (Ed.). Blood Vessels and Lymphatics. Academic Press, New York, 1962.

Albert, E. N. and Pease, D. C. An electron microscopic study of uterine arteries during pregnancy. Am. J. Anat. *123*: 165–194 (1968).

Bucciante, L. Microscopie optique de la paroi veineuse. Angiologica *2*: part II, 211–308 (1966).

Bunce, D. F. M. Structural differences between distended and collapsed arteries. Angiology *16*: 53–56 (1965).

Burri, P. H. and Weibel, E. R. Beeinflussung einer spezifischen cytoplasmatischen Organelle von Endothelzellen durch Adrenalin. Z. Zellforsch. *88*: 426–440 (1968).

Devine, C. E. and Simpson, F. O. The fine structure of vascular sympathetic neuromuscular contacts in the rat. Am. J. Anat. *121*: 153–173 (1967).

Fillenz, M. Innervation of pulmonary and bronchial blood vessels of the dog. J. Anat. *106*: 449–461 (1970).

Lang, J. Mikroskopische Anatomie der Arterien. Angiologica *2*: part I, 225–284 (1965).

Pease, D. C. and Paule, W. J. Electron microscopy of elastic arteries; the thoracic aorta of the rat. J. Ultrastruct. Res. *3*: 469–483 (1960).

Pease, D. C. and Molinari, S. Electron microscopy of muscular arteries: pial vessels of the cat and monkey. J. Ultrastruct. Res. *3*: 447–468 (1960).

Peters, T. J., Müller, M. and de Duve, C. Lysosomes of the arterial wall. I. Isolation and subcellular fractionation of cells from normal rabbit aorta. J. Exp. Med. *136*: 1117–1139 (1972).

Piezzi, R. S., Santolaya, R. S. and Bertini, F. The fine structure of endothelial cells of toad arteries. Anat. Rec. *165*: 229–236 (1969).

Ratschow, M. (Ed.). Angiologie. George Thieme, Stuttgart, 1959.

Reale, E. and Ruska, H. Die Feinstruktur der Gefässwände. Angiologica *2*: part I, 314–366 (1965).

Rhodin, J. A. G. Fine structure of vascular walls in mammals with special reference to smooth muscle component. Physiol. Rev. *42*: 48–87 (1962).

Sato, S. An electron microscopic study on the innervation of the intracranial artery of the rat. Am. J. Anat. *118*: 873–890 (1966).

Schwartz, S. M. and Benditt, E. P. Studies on aortic intima. I. Structure and permeability of rat thoracic aortic intima. Am. J. Path. *66*: 241–264 (1972).

Sengel, A. and Stoebner, P. Golgi origin of tubular inclusions in endothelial cells. J. Cell Biol. *44*: 223–226 (1970).

Silva, D. G. and Ikeda, M. Ultrastructural and acetylcholinesterase studies on the innervation of the ductus arteriosus, pulmonary trunk and aorta of the fetal lamb. J. Ultrastruct. Res. *34*: 358–374 (1971).

Takayanagi, T., Rennels, M. L. and Nelson, E. An electron microscopic study of intimal cushions in intracranial arteries of the cat. Am. J. Anat. *133*: 415–430 (1972).

Ts'ao, C., Glagov, S. and Kelsey, B. F. Structure of mammalian portal vein: postnatal establishment of two mutually perpendicular medial muscle zones in the rat. Anat. Rec. *171*: 457–470 (1971).

Weibel, E. R. and Palade, G. E. New cytoplasmic components in arterial endothelia. J. Cell Biol. *23*: 101–112 (1964).

Wissler, R. W. The arterial medial cell, smooth muscle or multifunctional mesenchyme? J. Atherosclerosis Res. *8*: 201–213 (1968).

Wood, E. The venous system. Sci. American *218*: 86–96 (1968).

MICROVASCULAR BED

Bennett, H. S., Luft, J. H. and Hampton, J. C. Morphological classification of vertebrate blood capillaries. Am. J. Physiol. *196*: 381–390 (1959).

Bensley, R. R. and Vintrup, B. On the nature of the Rouget cells of capillaries. Anat. Rec. *39*: 37–55 (1929).

Brightman, M. W. and Reese, T. S. Junctions between intimately apposed cell membranes in the vertebrate brain. J. Cell Biol. *40*: 648–677 (1969).

Bruns, R. R. and Palade, G. E. Studies on blood capillaries. I. General organization of blood capillaries in muscle. J. Cell Biol. *37*: 244–276 (1968).

Bruns, R. R. and Palade, G. E. Studies on blood capillaries. II. Transport of ferritin molecules across the wall of muscle capillaries. J. Cell Biol. *37*: 277–299 (1968).

Cecio, A. Ultrastructural features of cytofilaments within mammalian endothelial cells. Z. Zellforsch. *83*: 40–48 (1967).

Clementi, F. and Palade, G. E. Intestinal capillaries. I. Permeability to peroxidase and ferritin. J. Cell Biol. *41*: 33–58 (1969).

Clementi, F. and Palade, G. E. Intestinal capillaries. II. Structural effects of EDTA and histamine. J. Cell Biol. *42*: 706–714 (1969).

Crone, C. and Lassen, N. A. (Eds.). Capillary Permeability. Academic Press, New York, 1970.

Fernando, N. V. P. and Movat, H. Z. The fine structure of the terminal vascular bed. II. The smallest arterial vessels: terminal arterioles and metarterioles. Exp. Molec. Path. *3*: 1–9 (1964).

Fernando, N. V. P. and Movat, H. Z. Fine structure of the terminal vascular bed. III. Capillaries. Exp. Molec. Path. *3*: 87–97 (1964).

Karnovsky, M. J. The ultrastructural basis of capillary permeability studied with peroxidase as a tracer. J. Cell Biol. *35*: 213–236 (1967).

Lever, J. D., Spriggs, T. L. B. and Graham, J. D. P. A formol-fluorescence, fine-structural and autoradiographic study of the adrenergic innervation of the vascular tree in the intact and sympathectomized pancreas of the cat. J. Anat. *103*: 15–34 (1968).

Majno, G. Ultrastructure of the vascular membrane. *In* Handbook of Physiology, Section 2, Vol. III, Circulation, 1965, pp. 2293–2375.

Majno, G., Shea, S. M. and Leventhal, M. Endothelial contraction induced by histamine-type mediators. An electron microscopic study. J. Cell Biol. *42*: 647–672 (1969).

Marchesi, V. T. The role of pinocytic vesicles in the transport of material across the walls of small blood vessels. Investig. Ophthalmol. *4*: 1111–1121 (1965).

Maul, G. G. Structure and formation of pores in fenestrated capillaries. J. Ultrastruct. Res. *36*: 768–782 (1971).

Movat, H. Z. and Fernando, N. V. P. The fine structure of the terminal vascular bed. II. Small arteries with an internal elastic lamina. Exp. Molec. Path. *2*: 549–563 (1963).

Movat, H. Z. and Fernando, N. V. P. The fine structure of the terminal vascular bed. IV. The venules and their perivascular cells. Exp. Molec. Path. *3*: 98–114 (1963).

Pappenheimer, J. R. Passage of molecules through capillary walls. Physiol. Rev. *33*: 386–423 (1953).

Phelps, P. C. and Luft, J. H. Electron microscopical study of relaxation and constriction in frog arterioles. Am. J. Anat. *125*: 399–428 (1969).

Reese, T. S. and Karnovsky, M. J. Fine structural localization of a blood brain barrier to exogenous peroxidase. J. Cell Biol. *34*: 207–217 (1962).

Rhodin, J. A. G. The diaphragm of capillary endothelial fenestrations. J. Ultrastruct. Res. *6*: 171–185 (1962).

Rhodin, J. A. G. The ultrastructure of mammalian arterioles and precapillary sphincters. J. Ultrastruct. Res. *18*: 181–223 (1967).

Rhodin, J. A. G. Ultrastructure of mammalian venous capillaries, venules, and small collecting veins. J. Ultrastruct. Res. *25*: 452–500 (1968).

Rhodin, J. A. G. Fine structure of capillaries. *In* Topics in the Study of Life. The Bio Source Book (Ed. H. Ris), pp. 215–224. Harper & Row, New York, 1971.

Simon, G. Ultrastructure des capillaires. Angiologica *2*: part I, 370–434 (1965).

Venkatachalam, M. A. and Karnovsky, M. J. Extravascular protein in the kidney. An ultrastructural study of its relation to renal peritubular capillary permeability using protein tracers. Lab. Investig. *27*: 435–444 (1972).

Wolff, J. and Merker, H. J. Ultrastruktur und Bildung von Poren im Endothel von porösen und geschlossenen Kapillaren. Z. Zellforsch. *73*: 174–191 (1966).

17 Lymphatic system

GENERAL

The lymphatic system consists of: 1) a system of widely interconnected capillaries; 2) lymphatic vessels and ducts; 3) an infiltration by lymphocytes in epithelia and subepithelial connective tissue, either diffusely or densely forming nodules; 4) aggregated nodules; 5) tonsils; and 6) lymph nodes. In addition, the spleen and the thymus represent organs in which an unusually large accumulation of lymphoid cells has taken place.

The **lymph** is composed of a fluid, and formed elements, the lymphocytes. Lymph fluid circulates within the lymphatic capillaries and vessels. Lymphocytes occur both within these vessels and in the interstitial spaces. There is also fluid in the extracellular spaces, but it is referred to there as tissue fluid, its composition of proteins being almost identical to that of lymph fluid. The lymphatic capillaries and vessels drain the tissues and organs of extravasated materials except for erythrocytes and polymorphonuclear leukocytes. The function of the lymphocytes is largely to serve as precursor cells for plasma cells, a transformation that occurs in response to foreign-body proteins collectively called antigens. The plasma cells synthesize antibodies against these antigens. The nodules and nodes serve as filters for the lymph, and also as centers for lymphocyte production.

LYMPHATIC CAPILLARIES

Lymphatic capillaries are present in most mammalian tissues and organs with the exception of the central nervous system and the intralobular portion of the liver. They form a widely interconnected system of thin-walled channels, and they vary greatly in cross-sectional diameter, ranging from $10\,\mu$ to $50\,\mu$. (Fig. 17-1) The beginnings of the lymphatic capillaries are not easily identified. There is good evidence, however, that they originate as blind terminal endings, often with a bulb-like dilatation, particularly in the core of the intestinal villi. However, since the lymphatic capillaries form such a vast system of interconnected channels, the question of how this system originates is mostly academic.

The wall of the lymphatic capillaries consists of endothelial cells only. The **endothelium** forms a thin, continuous sheath with an average thickness of about $0.3\,\mu$. (Fig. 17-2) As a rule, there is **no** basal lamina to support the endothelium. Fine collagenous and **reticular fibrils** form a thin layer around most lymphatic capillaries. In some instances, there seems to be specific areas at the abluminal surface of the endothelium where bundles of collagenous fibrils (anchoring filaments) attach more closely than elsewhere. Adventitial cells or pericytes are not present.

Adjoining endothelial cells overlap each other to some extent. (Fig. 17-4) There are no special junctional complexes present with the exception of an occasional tight junction in some tissues. Interdigitations and foldings of abutting surfaces occur often. The luminal surface is smooth and generally without microvilli. The nucleus is elongated, and makes the endothelial cell protrude locally into the capillary lumen. The cytoplasm contains a small number of round mitochondria, a small Golgi complex, some ribosomes, and pro-

Fig. 17-1. Longitudinal section of lymphatic capillaries and venules in the dermal connective tissue. Skin. Rabbit. E.M. X 600. **1.** Lymphatic capillaries of varied cross-sectional diameters. These vessels drain the skin and are largely devoid of lymphocytes before reaching the first lymph node. **2.** Venules. **3.** Small vein (diameter about $90\,\mu$). Arrows indicate direction of blood flow. **4.** Marginated granulocytes. **5.** Fat cells. **6.** Collagenous fibers.

Fig. 17-2. Microvascular dimensions. Cross section of vascular bundle. Mesentery. Rat. E.M. X 870. **1.** Lymphatic capillary: lumen $30\,\mu$; wall $0.1\,\mu$. **2.** Arteriole: lumen $85\,\mu$; wall $5\,\mu$. **3.** Arteriole: lumen $45\,\mu$; wall $2.5\,\mu$. **4.** Precapillary arteriole; lumen $14\,\mu$; wall $2\,\mu$. **5.** Capillary: lumen $5\,\mu$; wall $0.2\,\mu$. **6.** Venule: lumen $40\,\mu$; wall $1\,\mu$. **7.** Non-myelinated nerves. **8.** Fat cell. **9.** Loose connective tissue.

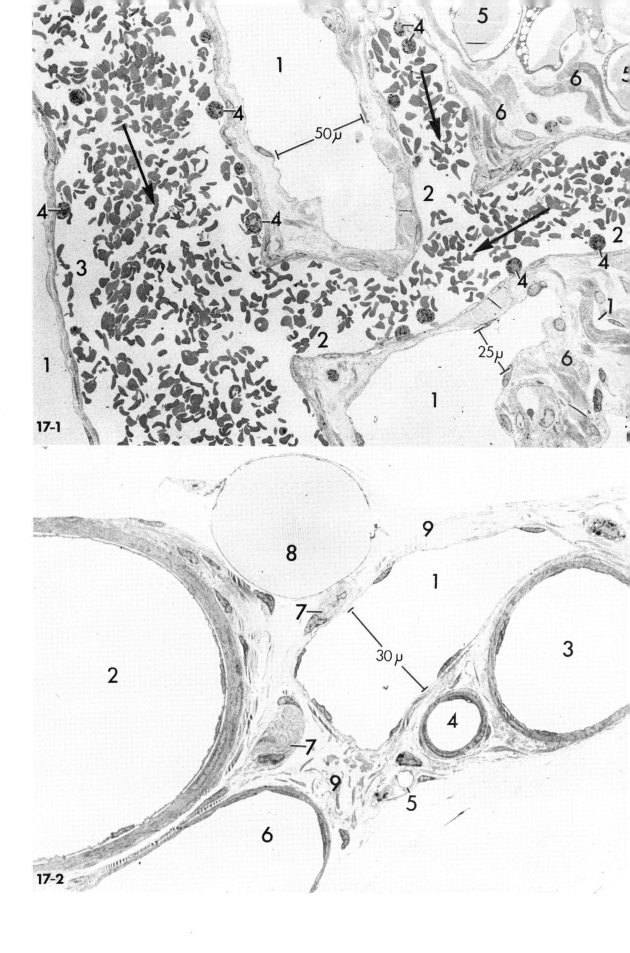

files of tubular endoplasmic reticulum of the granular variety. Bundles of fine filaments may be present, in addition to a limited number of micropinocytotic vesicles arising from both the luminal and abluminal surfaces of the endothelial cell membrane. A moderate number of smooth surfaced vesicles occur in the cytoplasm.

The **functions** of the lymphatic capillaries relate to the reabsorption of part of the water and electrolytes and most of the proteins that continually leave the blood capillaries and form the tissue fluid. The endothelium of the lymphatic capillaries is highly permeable. It is believed that the absence of junctional complexes and a basal lamina, in combination with a thin endothelium provided with micropinocytotic vesicles, are factors that contribute to the high permeability. The lymph fluid is moved from the most peripheral capillaries and their blind terminations to the lymphatic vessels by an elevation of interstitial pressure brought about either by contraction of skeletal muscles or by increased filtration from blood capillaries. In some instances, such as the subcutaneous lymphatic capillaries of the bat wing, contractions of the endothelium itself have been observed. These contractions are most likely brought about by the filaments of the endothelial cells.

LYMPHATIC VESSELS AND DUCTS

From the lymphatic capillaries, the lymph is picked up by collecting lymphatic vessels which conduct the lymph to and through a sequence of regional lymph nodes. After filtration through the nodes, the lymph is delivered to the venous system by either the thoracic duct or the right lymphatic duct.

The walls of the **collecting lymphatic vessels** consist of a thin endothelial lining, a thin sheath of reticular fibrils, an incomplete layer of smooth muscle cells (Fig. 17-6), and an adventitial layer of connective tissue. In addition, there are many **valves** in these vessels, often placed closely together along the vessel. (Fig. 17-5) The valves are usually formed of two cusps which are simply two layers of endothelium separated by a narrow plate of fine collagenous and reticular fibrils. The cusps project into the lumen of the vessel in the direction of the lymph flow. The collecting lymphatic vessels contract rhythmically and thereby aid considerably in forwarding the lymph.

The **lymphatic ducts** are larger in diameter than the collecting lymphatic vessels. Their luminal diameter rarely exceeds 5 mm. The three layers of the vascular wall are more clearly defined, particularly the tunica media which may contain bundles of smooth muscle cells oriented both longitudinally and circularly.

SUBEPITHELIAL LYMPHATIC TISSUE

Lymphocytes occur freely in loose connective tissue among collagenous fibrils and fibroblasts that form the framework of this tissue. A **diffuse infiltration** of lymphocytes is always present in the subepithelial connective tissue of the intestinal tract (Fig. 17-7), in specific areas of the genitourinary tracts such as the vagina, and often also in the air-conducting

Fig. 17-3. Cross section of intestinal lymphatic capillary (lacteal). Small intestine. Rat. E.M. × 1400. **1.** Lumen (50 μ). **2.** Nucleus of endothelial cell. **3.** Endothelial cytoplasm. **4.** Bundles of collagenous fibrils. **5.** Smooth muscle cells of lamina muscularis mucosae (not part of the wall of the lacteal).

Fig. 17-4. Enlargement of area similar to rectangle in Fig. 17-3. Wall of lymphatic capillary. Mouse. E.M. × 64,000. **1.** Lumen. **2.** Overlapping edges of the endothelial cells. No special junctional arrangements. **3.** Pinocytotic vesicles. *No basal lamina.*

Fig. 17-5. Longitudinal section of collecting lymphatic vessel. Ovary. Rat. E.M. × 2800. **1.** Lumen. **2.** Endothelium. **3.** Valves. **4.** Nuclei of endothelial cells in the cusps. Arrow indicates direction of lymph flow.

Fig. 17-6. Cross section of part of afferent lymphatic vessel near entrance to lymph node. Rat. E.M. × 4000. **1.** Lumen. **2.** Nucleus of endothelial cell. **3.** Nucleus of smooth muscle cell. **4.** Nuclei of fibroblasts. **5.** Collagenous fibrils.

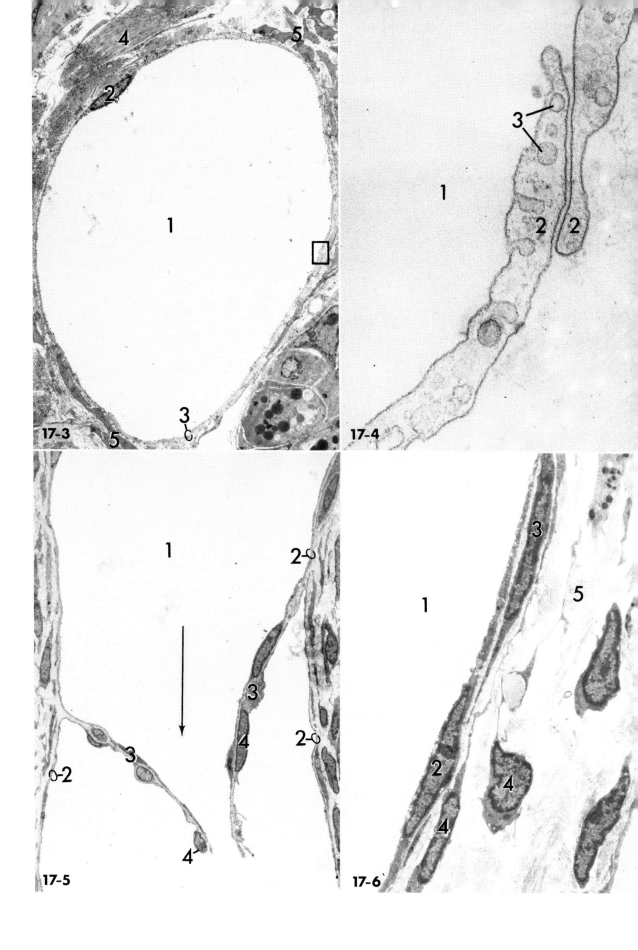

17-3

17-4

17-5

17-6

system of the respiratory tract. An invasion of the epithelium itself by lymphocytes is particularly common in relation to the tonsils of the oropharyngeal region (Fig. 17-8), but occurs also to a limited degree in the intestine.

The subepithelial infiltration may become pronounced in certain areas referred to as **lymphatic nodules** which are small, spherical, or oval aggregations of densely packed lymphocytes. The nodules are not encapsulated by connective tissue but there is often a concentration of small lymphocytes at the peripheral zone of the nodule. (Fig. 17-9) This is particularly evident at the time of active lymphocyte production which occurs in the inner part of the nodule, the **germinal center** (also referred to as secondary nodule). At this point, lymphocytopoietic cells with large nuclei and abundant cytoplasm arise, causing the center of the nodule to appear less densely populated than the periphery. The mechanism of lymphocytopoiesis and the cells involved is discussed in detail on p. 384. It is important to remember that lymphatic nodules without germinal centers reflect an inactive or a resting phase of that particular lymphatic tissue. The lymphatic nodules may be **solitary** or they may occur in small or large groups. In the case of large groups, they are referred to as **aggregated** nodules. Examples of these large accumulations of nodules are the Peyer's patches (Fig. 17-11), which characterize one part of the small intestine, the ileum.

TONSILS

The several types of tonsils, forming a ring around the oropharynx, represent a special form of subepithelial lymphatic tissue. They are called: 1) lingual tonsils; 2) pharyngeal tonsils; and 3) palatine tonsils. The **lingual tonsils** generally occur either as a diffuse infiltration of lymphocytes or as multiple small nodules below the epithelium of the posterior third of the tongue in similarity with the general description above. The overlying stratified

squamous epithelium is usually invaded by lymphocytes to a varying degree. The **pharyngeal tonsils** are situated in the posterior wall of the nasopharynx and contain large aggregations of lymphatic nodules. The pharyngeal tonsils are often greatly enlarged in some individuals during childhood and adolescence, in which case they are called **adenoids.** The largest accumulations of lymphatic tissue in the oropharynx are the **palatine tonsils** lying between the glossopalatine and pharyngopalatine arches. (Fig. 17-10) The base and sides of these tonsils are separated from the nearby muscles and glands by a dense connective tissue capsule. From this capsule arise delicate connective tissue septa which divide incompletely the lymphatic tissue. The palatine tonsils typically contain **crypts** which are deep, pit-like invaginations of the surface epithelium. As a rule, this epithelium is heavily invaded by lymphocytes on their way to the

Fig. 17-7. Lingual tonsil. Monkey. L.M. X 100. **1.** Stratified squamous, non-keratinized epithelium of upper surface of base of tongue. **2.** Aggregation of lymphocytes, forming a lymphatic nodule without germinal center. **3.** Ducts of salivary gland.

Fig. 17-8. Lingual tonsil. Detail. Monkey. L.M. X 260. **1.** Surface epithelium **2.** Subepithelial aggregation of lymphocytes. **3.** Extensive infiltration of surface epithelium by invading lymphocytes. **4.** Level of basement membrane. **5.** The most superficial layers of the squamous epithelium are not invaded by lymphocytes.

Fig. 17-9. Solitary lymphatic nodule. Appendix. Human. L.M. X 185. **1.** Germinal center of solitary lymphatic nodule. **2.** Peripheral aggregation of small lymphocytes. **3.** Diffuse infiltration of lamina propria by lymphocytes. **4.** Lumen of appendix. **5.** Crypts of Lieberkühn.

Fig. 17-10. Palatine tonsil. Human. L.M. X 14. **1.** Oropharyngeal cavity. **2.** Surface epithelium. **3.** Longitudinally sectioned crypt. **4.** Cross-sectioned crypt. **5.** Multiple lymphatic nodules with germinal centers. **6.** Capsule.

Fig. 17-11. Peyer's patch. Ileum. Monkey. L.M. X 39. **1.** Lumen of gut. **2.** Intestinal villi. **3.** Crypts of Lieberkühn. **4.** Multiple lymphatic nodules without germinal centers. **5.** Muscularis externa.

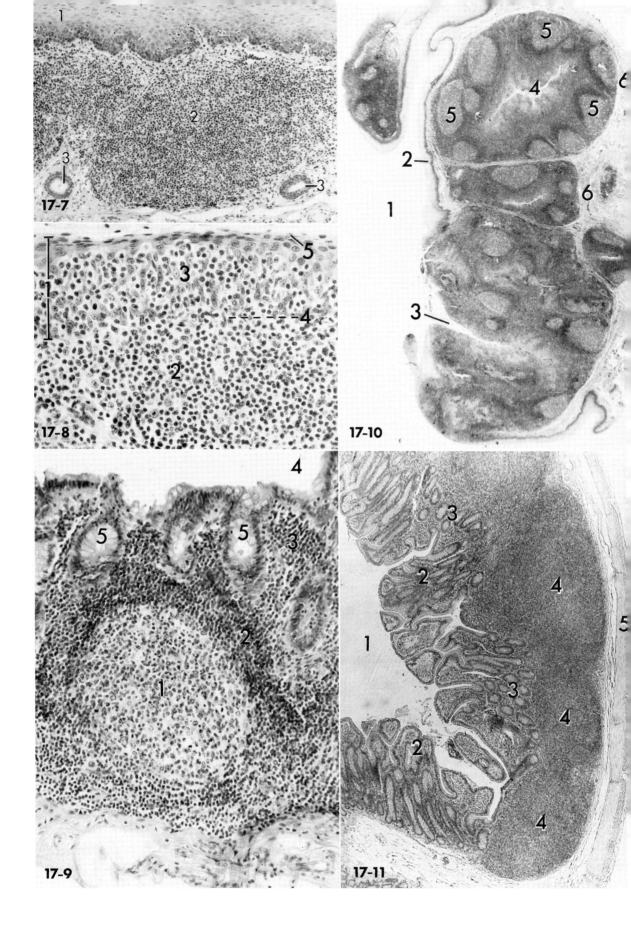

17-7

17-8

17-9

17-10

17-11

free surface. The crypts become filled by a mixture of these lymphocytes, desquamated epithelial cells, and bacteria even under normal circumstances. The lymphocytes that are encountered in the saliva are referred to as **salivary corpuscles.** The bulk of the palatine tonsil is made up of many lymphatic nodules in which germinal centers are present at the time of lymphocyte regeneration. There are lymphatic capillaries and efferent lymphatic vessels around and near the base of the palatine tonsils as opposed to other types of tonsils.

Functions. The subepithelial lymphatic tissue and tonsils are situated in areas where the lymphoid elements can readily defend the body against invading bacteria, viruses, and other foreign proteins by an early chemical or physical contact with the invaders. The foreign antigens stimulate the production of antibodies in plasma cells. The plasma cells are derived from lymphocytes which in turn are generated in the germinal centers of the lymphatic nodules.

LYMPH NODES

Lymph nodes are accumulations of dense lymphatic tissue, surrounded by a capsule of dense connective tissue. Collecting lymphatic vessels, termed afferent lymphatic vessels, discharge the lymph beneath this capsule, and efferent lymphatic vessels drain the node. Foreign materials are removed from the lymph during this filtration process and lymphocytes, produced in the germinal centers of the many lymph nodules within the node, are added to the lymph. The lymphatic tissue of the node is permeated by arteries, blood capillaries, venules, and veins in contradistinction to subepithelial lymphatic tissue and tonsils which are poor in blood vessels.

General. There are a great number of lymph nodes in the mammalian body, and the position of each group is relatively constant, receiving lymph from specific regions of the body. Lymph nodes are round, oval, or kidney-shaped, averaging

about 15 mm in longitudinal diameter. (Fig. 17-12) Many afferent lymphatic vessels go through the capsule on the convex side of the node, and blood vessels enter and leave the node together with a single efferent lymphatic vessel on the concave side, the **hilus.** There is a connective tissue framework or **stroma** composed of a dense connective tissue **capsule** and **trabeculae,** extending from the capsule and converging on the hilus. There is also a dense meshwork of reticular cells and fine **collagenous** and **reticular fibrils** that permeates the entire lymph node. There is a dense accumulation of lymphocytes that forms the **cortex** of the node. (Fig. 17-14) The dense accumulation of lymphocytes continues and extends toward the hilus as **medullary cords** to make up the major part of the **medulla** of the node. The lymph percolates through the node via wide intercellular spaces, collectively called **sinuses.** A **subcapsular** sinus receives the lymph from the afferent lymphatic vessels and passes it on toward the medulla via **penetrating** and **medullary** sinuses. Therefore, the cortex of the node is made up mostly of lymph nodules, whereas the medulla contains a large number of sinuses. The larger blood vessels

Fig. 17-12. Section of entire lymph node. Monkey. L.M. X 9. **1.** Capsule. **2.** Cortex. **3.** Medulla. **4.** Hilus. **5.** Blood vessels and efferent lymphatic vessel.

Fig. 17-13. Enlargement of area similar to rectangle (A) in Fig. 17-12. Lymph node. L.M. X 91. **1.** Capsule. **2.** Part of trabecula. **3.** Subcapsular sinus. **4.** Germinal center of lymphatic nodule. **5.** Penetrating sinus. **6.** Medullary sinuses. **7.** Medullary cords.

Fig. 17-14. Enlargement of area similar to square in Fig. 17-13. Lymph node. Rat. E.M. X 620. **1.** Capsule. **2.** Subcapsular sinus. **3.** Penetrating sinus. Arrows indicate direction of lymph flow. **4.** Germinal center of lymphatic nodule. Dominated by lymphoblasts and medium-sized lymphocytes. **5.** Peripheral aggregation of small lymphocytes (corona). **6.** Blood capillaries, fixed by intravascular perfusion. Rectangle (A) enlarged in Fig. 17-15; rectangle (B) in Fig. 17-16.

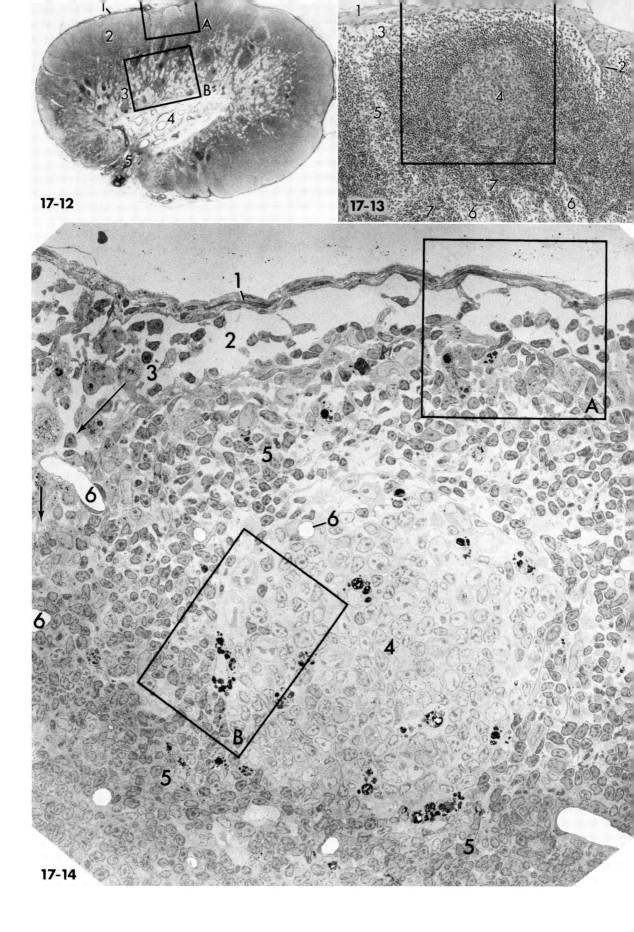

17-12

17-13

17-14

mostly follow the connective tissue trabeculae, whereas the capillary network and the postcapillary venules permeate the dense lymphatic tissue. In some lymphatic nodes of certain mammals, there is a mixture of lymph and erythrocytes in the sinuses, giving rise to **hemal nodes.** The mixture is established by some arterial capillaries opening up directly to the intercellular sinuses of these nodes. This is identical to the situation in the spleen where, similarly, an "open" circulation exists. As a rule, hemal nodes are rare in man but common in ruminants. The hemal nodes function as sites of antibody formation in response to both blood-borne and lymph-borne antigens.

Sinuses of the node. The sinuses form a system of continuous, interconnected irregular spaces throughout the node. Depending on location, there are subcapsular, penetrating (or trabecular), and medullary sinuses. The **subcapsular** sinus is a narrow space (Fig. 17-14) which does not show up in all histological preparations due to its tendency to collapse upon removal of the lymph node. The **penetrating** (trabecular) sinuses originate from the subcapsular sinus. They represent narrow clefts which subdivide the dense lymphatic tissue. They vary greatly in size and shape depending upon the reactive state of the lymphatic tissue, i.e. whether germinal centers are present or not. The **medullary** sinuses dominate the medulla and the area around the hilus of the node by forming a wide meshwork in which only narrow strands of lymphoid tissue, the medullary cords, are present. (Fig. 17-17) The lymphatic sinuses of nodes do not represent endothelial tubes, as in the liver or the adrenal cortex, since their shape is highly irregular. The sinuses are separated from the capsule, the trabeculae, and the accumulations of dense lymphoid tissue by **littoral cells.** (Fig. 17-15) These are squamous lining cells of endothelial nature which form a layer that can readily be traversed by lymphocytes, as these cells emerge from the nodules and medullary

cords to enter the sinuses. The littoral cell is provided with a few primary lysosomes, but is generally not engaged in phagocytic work unless stimulated by an excess amount of foreign materials. A thin **basal lamina** separates the littoral cells from the connective tissue of the capsule and the trabeculae. It is virtually absent between the littoral cells and the dense lymphoid tissue. The sinuses are bridged by numerous **reticular cells,** interconnected by thin strands of cytoplasmic processes to form a three-dimensional network, particularly prominent in the wide medullary sinuses. The reticular cell has a peculiar mixture of structural properties, usually found in endothelial cells, fibroblasts, and macrophages. It is considered to be an essential part of the stroma of the lymph node.

Stroma of the lymph node. The capsule, the trabeculae, and the reticular cells form the stroma of the lymph nodes. The stroma is composed of connective tissue fibers and cells. In the **capsule,** the predominant cell is a fibroblast. However, many of the fibroblasts show cytoplasmic differentiations such as filamentous bundles, glycogen accumulations, local den-

Fig. 17-15. Survey of subcapsular lymph sinus. Enlargement of rectangle (A) in Fig. 17-14. Lymph node. Rat. E.M. × 1800. **1.** Collagenous fibers of capsule. **2.** Lumen of subcapsular sinus. **3.** Littoral (lining) cell, endothelial in nature. **4.** Narrow bundles of collagenous fibrils, covered by thin cytoplasm of littoral cells, crossing sinus. **5.** Reticular cells. **6.** Macrophages. **7.** Monocytes (or macrophages). **8.** Small lymphocytes. **9.** Medium-sized lymphocytes. **10.** Small lymphocyte going through wall of lymph sinus.

Fig. 17-16. Survey of area between germinal center and peripheral corona of lymph nodule. Enlargement of rectangle (B) in Fig. 17-14. Lymph node. Rat. E.M. X 1800. **1.** Small lymphocytes of corona. **2.** Medium-sized lymphocytes. **3.** Macrophage at border between germinal center of corona. **4.** Large lymphocytes (lymphoblasts). Rectangle enlarged in Fig. 17-27. **5.** Small lymphocytes of germinal center. **6.** Lymphoid cell in mitosis.

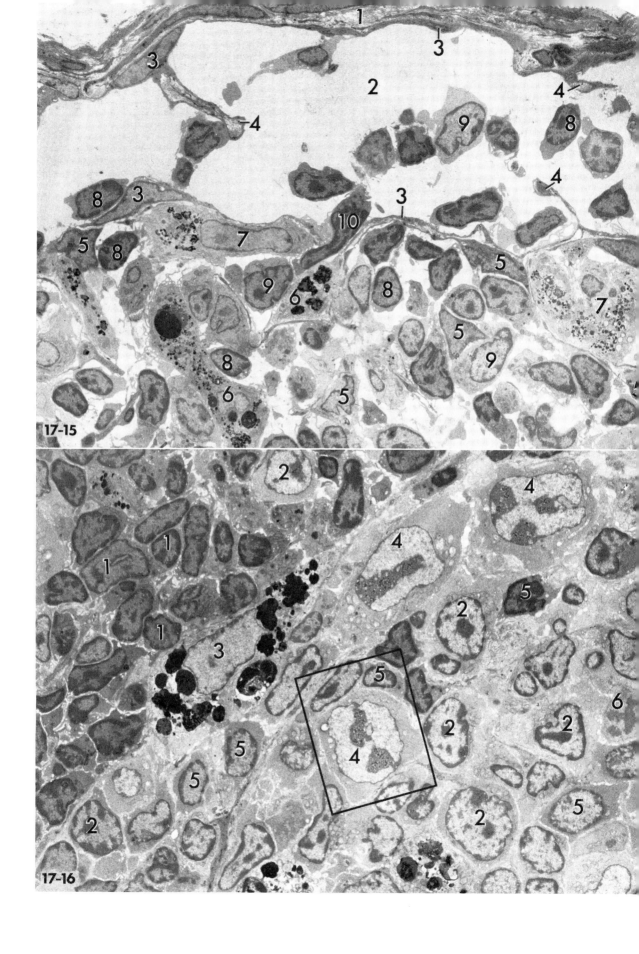

17-15

17-16

sities along the cell membrane, and stretches of basal lamina which make it difficult to separate these cells from smooth muscle cells. Yet, other cells in the capsule clearly represent true smooth muscle cells. The connective tissue fibers are largely of collagenous nature with some elastic fibers mixed in. In the **trabeculae,** most of the cells are regular fibroblasts. (Fig. 17-20) Since the trabeculae also contain nerves and blood vessels, cells such as pericytes, Schwann cells, and ordinary macrophages may also be present. Smooth muscle cells are absent. Collagenous fibrils predominate in the intercellular space of the trabeculae, although many fibrils are extremely fine and therefore could be classified as either young collagenous or reticular in nature. The remainder of the stroma of the lymph nodes is made up of **reticular cells** and the extracellular fibers that invariably are associated with these cells: reticular fibrils and delicate collagenous fibrils. The reticular stroma is particularly prominent as it forms a three-dimensional network throughout the sinuses. However, it is also present in the cortical nodules as well as in the medullary cords but to a lesser extent in these locations. The reticular cell is structurally similar to a macrophage, and by virtue of its close association with extracellular connective tissue fibers, is a **fixed macrophage.** (Fig. 17-21) There is a great abundance of primary and secondary lysosomes, a large Golgi complex, some mitochondria, a few profiles of granular endoplasmic reticulum, and free ribosomes. The entire cytoplasm is pervaded by small vesicles of both the coated and uncoated variety. Depending on its reactive stage, the cells contain a varying number of phagosomes. The surface of the reticular cell is extremely irregular with long cytoplasmic processes extending for long distances. Because of this appearance, the reticular cell is sometimes referred to as dendritic macrophage. The **reticular fibrils** consist largely of delicate collagenous fibrils. (Fig. 17-21) Whether they represent only young

collagenous fibrils or a special category of delicate collagenous fibrils which do not attain the diameter of large collagenous fibrils is not known. Originally they were classified as a special kind of fibril, based on the fact that they could be impregnated with silver (argyrophil fibers). The reticular fibrils deeply indent the long cytoplasmic processes of the reticular cells as they stretch across the lymphatic sinuses. This is not always the case as they traverse the lymphatic nodules and the medullary cords. In the sinuses, the collagenous and reticular fibrils are always completely separated from the circulating lymph fluid by the cytoplasm of the reticular cells, whereas in the dense lymphoid tissue, the fibrils make their way in between cells and touch the surface of a great variety of cell types.

From a **functional** point of view, the reticular cell is primarily engaged in **phagocytosis.** Its presence in the midst of the circulating lymph makes it come in contact with particles and foreign material that must be removed from the lymph and made harmless through lyso-

Fig. 17-17. Medulla of lymph node.
Enlargement of rectangle (B) in Fig. 17-12. Lymph node. Monkey. L.M. X 40.
1. Medullary cords. **2.** Medullary sinuses.

Fig. 17-18. Survey of medullary cord and sinus. Enlargement of area similar to rectangle (A) in Fig. 17-17. Lymph node. Cat. E.M. X 640.
1. Medullary cord of densely packed plasma cells and lymphocytes. **2.** Medullary lymph sinus with a variety of circulating lymphoid cells. **3.** Trabeculae of dense connective tissue. Area similar to rectangle (A) is enlarged in Fig. 17-20 and area similar to rectangle (B) is enlarged in Fig. 17-30.

Fig. 17-19. Survey of medullary sinus near hilus. Enlargement of area similar to rectangle (B) in Fig. 17-17. Lymph node. Rat. E.M. X 570.
1. Lumen of sinus with circulating lymphoid cells. **2.** Cells forming a reticular network across sinus represent fixed macrophages.
3. Small artery. **4.** Small veins. **5.** Capillaries.
6. Dotted lines indicate trabeculae of loose connective tissue. Blood vessels of lymph nodes travel within the trabecular connective tissue compartment.

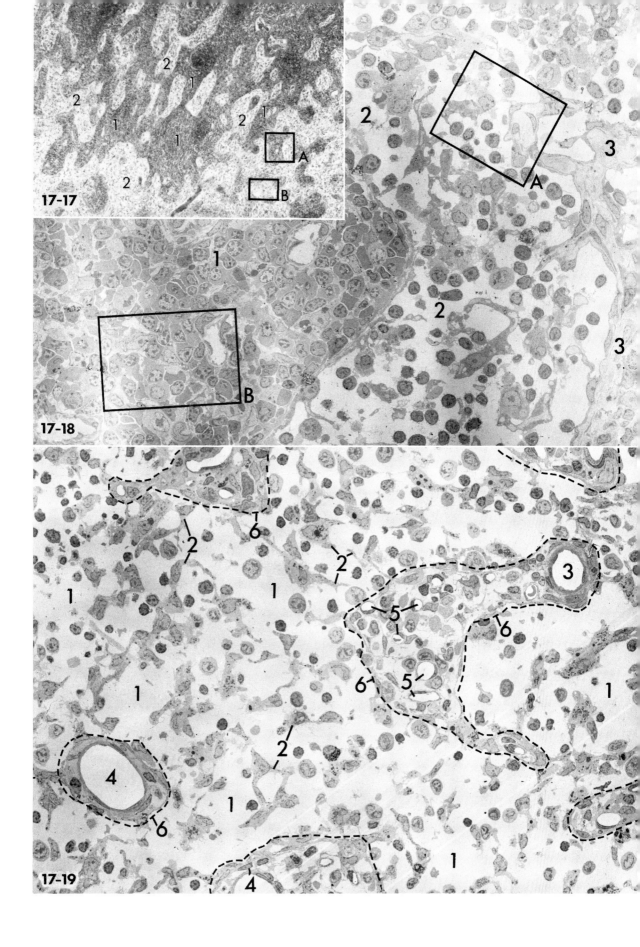

17-17

17-18

17-19

somal action. Soluble and particulate antigenic proteins are undoubtedly also taken up by the reticular cells. If so, they must be brought into association with immunologically competent lymphocytes for antigen identification or initiation of antibody formation. It is possible that the matrix in which the reticular fibrils are embedded, may act as diffusion channels to carry the antigens from the reticular cells to the perimeter of the lymphatic nodule. According to one theory, the reticular cell also represents a **stem cell** in lymphatic and myeloid tissues, with the potentialities of developing into either a hemocytoblast (lymphoblast in lymphoid tissue), monocyte, or fixed macrophage. It is possible that the reticular cells of the dense lymphoid tissue serve as such stem cells for lymphoblasts (large lymphocytes) more often than the reticular cells that bridge the lymphatic sinuses, the latter more likely giving rise to monocytes and macrophages. There is no doubt that the reticular cells, particularly those bridging the lymphatic sinuses, actively synthesize and lay down collagenous and reticular fibrils in view of the fact that this cell embraces the collagenous fibrils during its passage across the sinuses. By this cytoplasmic embrace, the extracellular milieu necessary for the collagenous fibrils to exist is created and maintained.

LYMPHATIC NODULES

The lymphatic nodules, whether located in lymph nodes, spleens, or subepithelial lymphatic tissue, are composed of densely packed lymphocytes. As indicated above, a fine **stroma of reticular** cells and reticular fibrils permeate the nodule. The nodules contain **germinal centers** at the time of active lymphocytopoiesis and a peripheral **corona** of small and densely packed lymphocytes. (Fig. 17-14) There are several sizes of lymphoid cells making up the nodule and its germinal center: small lymphocytes, medium-sized lymphocytes, and large lymphocytes, the latter also referred to as lymphoblasts. (Fig. 17-25)

Plasma cells occur but are far more numerous in the medullary cords. Only the small and medium-sized lymphocytes reach the cardiovascular system. Under normal conditions, large lymphocytes and plasma cells do not circulate.

PRODUCTION OF LYMPHOCYTES

Before a description of lymphocytes is given, it may be useful to summarize the present concepts of how lymphocytes are formed and their roles in the immunological defense system of the body.

The central part of the lymphatic nodules contains, at times, a large number of dividing cells, most of which are relatively large, each containing a large, pale nucleus and prominent nucleoli prior to mitosis. (Fig. 17-16) These cells are mostly large lymphocytes but some may repre-

Fig. 17-20. Survey of medullary sinus. Enlargement of area similar to rectangle (A) in Fig. 17-18. Lymph node. Cat. E.M. X 1800. **1.** Lumen of sinus. **2.** Densely packed collagenous fibrils in trabeculae. **3.** Fibroblasts. **4.** Littoral cells cover the large dense connective tissue trabeculae. **5.** Fixed macrophages cover the narrow bundles of collagenous fibrils (asterisks). **6.** Small lymphocytes. **7.** Medium-sized lymphocytes. **8.** Unclassified lymphoid cells, similar to the cell enlarged in Fig. 17-29. These cells are probably intermediate between medium-sized and larger lymphocytes and/or plasma cells. **9.** Erythrocytes occasionally in the lymph sinus.

Fig. 17-21. Fixed macrophage in medullary lymph sinus. Lymph node. Cat. E.M. X 3300. **1.** Lumen of sinus. **2.** Nucleus of fixed macrophage. **3.** Golgi zone. **4.** Mitochondria. **5.** Lysosomes. **6.** Small numerous profiles most of which represent pinocytotic vesicles. **7.** Narrow bundles of fine and densely packed collagenous fibrils, surrounded by cytoplasmic processes of the macrophage.

Fig. 17-22. Enlargement of square in Fig. 17-21. Lymph node. Cat. E.M. X 25,000. **1.** Cross-sectioned narrow bundle of fine collagenous fibrils. **2.** Cytoplasmic arms of macrophage surround extracellular bundle of collagenous fibrils. **3.** Nucleus **4.** Filamentous layer of cell membrane (glycocalyx).

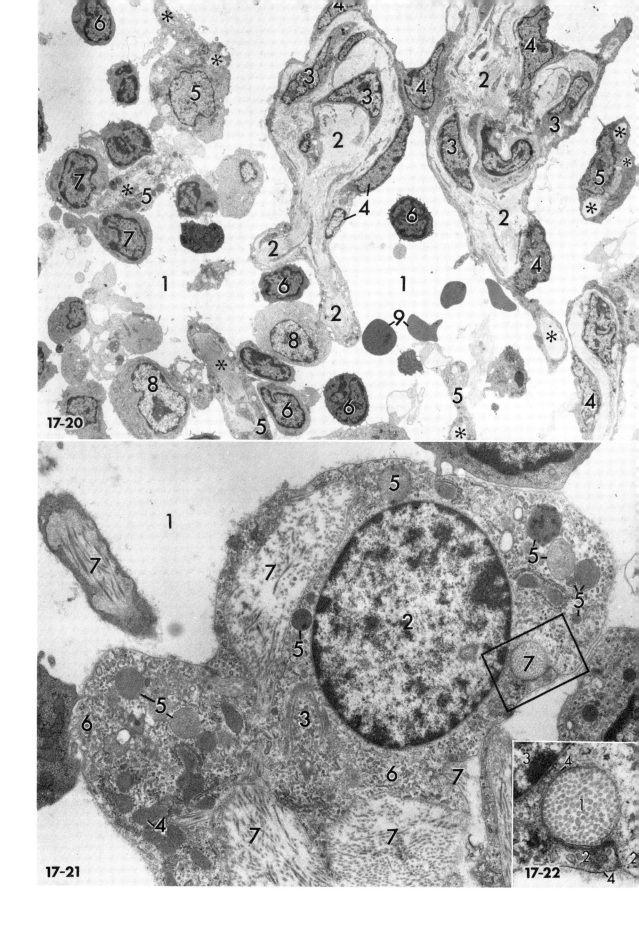

sent reticular cells. In the opinion of most investigators, the name **large lymphocyte** should be considered synonymous with the term **lymphoblast** since ultrastructurally, and probably also functionally, they are indistinguishable. Upon division, the large lymphocytes give rise to **medium-sized lymphocytes**. These, in turn, divide and give rise to **small lymphocytes**. The stimulus to divide comes through the invasion of proteins foreign to the body, collectively referred to as **antigens**. However, a second reaction to the invasion of foreign-body proteins is the formation of a large number of **plasma cells**, usually in the medullary cords of the lymph nodes or in the germinal centers of the lymphatic nodules. The plasma cells are the key cells responsible for the synthesis of antigen specific **antibodies**, a gamma globulin. The details of the formation of plasma cells are not fully understood. It is fairly well established that the large lymphocytes, upon division, give rise to not only medium-sized lymphocytes but also to cells which are called plasmablasts which, in turn, divide and differentiate into plasma cells. However, it is also believed that an antigen can influence a small lymphocyte to proliferate and/or differentiate into a plasma cell. During this process, the small lymphocyte goes through stages during which it is structurally indistinguishable from medium-sized and large lymphocytes. The development of a small lymphocyte into a plasma cell via intermediate stages can occur only if the small lymphocyte is **immunologically competent**. This term refers to the fact that lymphocytes, which were formed as a result of an earlier invasion of a certain antigen, retain at their surface, or somewhere in their cytoplasm, the memory of that particular antigen. They have acquired the ability to form antibodies against this antigen if they were to encounter it at a later time. It has been established that the majority of small lymphocytes have a life span of 6–12 months, whereas the rest disappear in 1–2 weeks.

It is the long-lived small lymphocytes that are referred to as **memory cells**. They are responsible for a delayed hypersensitivity reaction to foreign-body proteins. The short-lived small lymphocytes probably serve to counter an acute invasion of antigens, some having been produced specifically in response to the invasion. However, both long- and short-lived lymphocytes are ultrastructurally similar and little is known about the mechanisms which determine the life span of a small lymphocyte.

STRUCTURE OF LYMPHOCYTES

With the knowledge that lymphocytes, most of the time, are in a state of differentiation, proliferation, or division, it becomes clear that the classical description and subdivision of lymphocytes into small, medium-sized, and large must be rather arbitrary. Recent electron microscope investigations have made this obvious, since there are any number of intermediate stages and variations in ultrastructural architecture of lymphocytes. The following description summarizes some of the major ultrastructural features, but a more complete account will have to await the numerous structural and functional studies presently under way to explore these

Fig. 17-23. Small lymphocyte (5 μ in diameter) in medullary sinus of lymph node. Cat. E.M. X 32,000. **1.** Heterochromatin of nucleus. **2.** Euchromatin of nucleus. **3.** Nuclear pore areas. **4.** Nuclear membrane. **5.** Free ribosomes in narrow zone of cytoplasm. **6.** Small granule. **7.** Microvilli. **8.** Surface membrane.

Fig. 17-24. Medium-sized lymphocyte (7 μ in diameter) in medullary sinus of lymph node. Cat. E.M. X 33,000. **1.** Heterochromatin of nucleus. **2.** Euchromatin of nucleus. **3.** Nuclear pore areas. **4.** Nuclear membrane. **5.** Numerous free ribosomes. Cytoplasmic zone is wider than in a small lymphocyte. **6.** Some free polysomes. **7.** Short profiles of granular endoplasmic reticulum. **8.** Mitochondria. **9.** Small granules. **10.** Microvilli. **11.** Surface membrane.

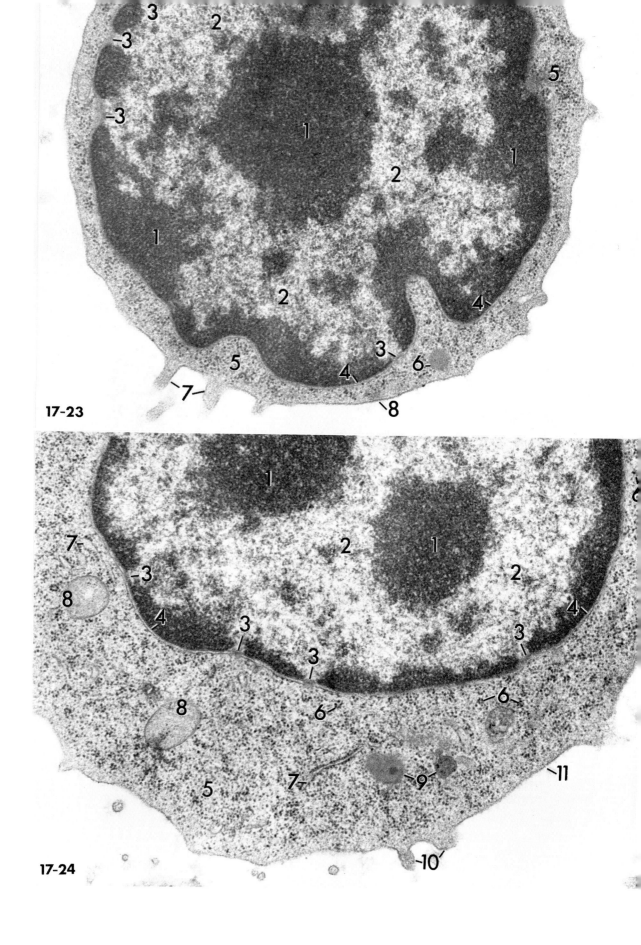

17-23

17-24

cells which are of such vital importance in the immunological defense mechanism of the body.

Small lymphocytes. The description given here applies to both circulating small lymphocytes and those lodged in the coronal zone of a lymphatic nodule. The size of the small lymphocytes in sectioned material is about 6 μ. In smear preparations of peripheral blood, the diameter may be larger, since cells become flattened and enlarged through the smearing process. The **nucleus** is usually round with minor shallow indentations. In sectioned material, it has an average diameter of about 5 μ which results in a high nuclear-cytoplasmic ratio. (Fig. 17-23) The heterochromatin is highly condensed into masses near the nuclear membrane, but also fills the major part of the interior of the nucleus. In routine histological preparations the **cytoplasm** is pale staining and visible as a small peripheral rim around the nucleus. The cell surface is provided with occasional short and narrow microvilli. At the ultrastructural level, the cytoplasm is dominated by monoribosomes. A small portion of the small lymphocyte population has an intensely basophilic cytoplasm because of a high number of monoribosomes and some polyribosomes. These cells are believed to be immunologically committed. Profiles of granular endoplasmic reticulum are scarce and the Golgi complex small. There is a small number of spherical mitochondria and occasionally an inclusion body, the structure of which is reminiscent of a primary or secondary lysosome. By light microscopical investigation, it has been established that 10% of the small lymphocytes contain a small number of granules. The granules have an affinity for the methylene azure of blood stains. They are referred to as azurophilic granules but their function is not known.

Large lymphocytes. The description of large lymphocytes refers to cells in germinal centers of lymphatic nodules in Peyer's patches (Fig. 17-27), lymph nodes and spleens. (Fig. 17-26) As indicated above, the account given of lymphocytopoiesis in this book is based on the assumption that large lymphocytes and lymphoblasts are identical cells. Some investigators believe that the reticular cell of lymphoid tissue is the precursor of the lymphoblast. However, this has not been convincingly demonstrated, and one must await further proof for this theory before it can be generally accepted. According to the outline of lymphocyte production on p. 384, we assume that the precursor of the large lymphocyte (lymphoblast) is the small lymphocyte. It is also assumed here, that the large lymphocytes (lymphoblasts) do not reach the cardiovascular system and therefore cannot be found among circulating blood cells under normal conditions.

The large lymphocytes (**lymphoblasts**) are round or slightly oval cells, averaging about 13 μ in diameter. (Fig. 17-27) The **nucleus** is usually round but may have surface indentations which are deeper than those present in small lymphocytes. The heterochromatin is concentrated to a thin rim near the nuclear membrane. Large and coarsely granular nucleoli are very characteristic for the nucleus of the large lymphocyte. One part of the nucleoli is generally connected to the chromatin near the nuclear membrane. The **cytoplasm** occupies a zone of about 2 μ around the nucleus. The cell surface is slightly irregular with an occasional short microvillus. The cytoplasm is occupied by a

Fig. 17-25. Survey of germinal center in nodule of white pulp of spleen. Same preparation and area as seen in Fig. 18-6. Rat. E.M. × 2500.
1. Small lymphocytes (average 5 μ in width).
2. Medium-sized lymphocytes (average 8 μ in width). **3.** Large lymphocytes or lymphoblasts (average 12 μ in width).
4. Large lymphocyte in prophase of mitotic division. Further enlarged in Fig. 17-26.
5. Reticular cells. **6.** *Asterisks* indicate bundles of collagenous fibrils. Note that some of the lymphoid cells in this field of view cannot be categorized with certainty unless they are studied at higher magnifications.

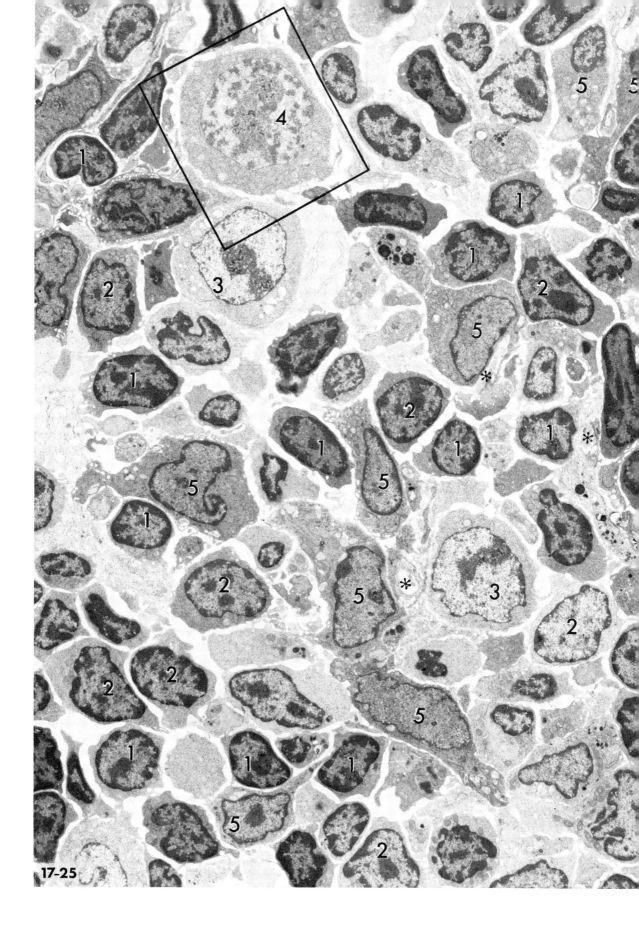

multitude of free polyribosomes which render the cytoplasm of large lymphocytes deeply basophilic under the light microscope. Spherical mitochondria and short profiles of granular endoplasmic reticulum occur in limited number. As a rule, a Golgi apparatus is not seen. In lymph nodules with large germinal centers, the number of large lymphocytes is high. Occasionally, large lymphocytes can be observed in a medullary sinus of a lymph node, but most cells in these sinuses are small and medium-sized lymphocytes.

The ultrastructure of the large lymphocytes (lymphoblasts) resembles closely that of the primitive cells of bone marrow (see p. 118) which are referred to as **hemocytoblasts,** serving as stem cells for myeloid and erythroid blood cells. Therefore, it has been suggested by several investigators that there may exist pluripotential stem cells whose progeny are capable of differentiating not only into myeloid, erythroid, and megakaryocytic elements, but also into lymphocytes as well.

Medium-sized lymphocytes. The description here applies to medium-sized lymphocytes in the circulating blood as well as in lymph nodes. It should be kept in mind that there is a great heterogeneity in structure and function among cells which collectively and somewhat arbitrarily are referred to as "medium-sized lymphocytes."

As a **general description,** these cells are round or slightly oval, varying in size from about 6 μ to 10 μ. The **nucleus** may be slightly indented. There is a dense chromatin network and mostly one or two prominent nucleoli. The **cytoplasm** occupies a zone of about 1 μ around the nucleus. As a rule, there are more free ribosomes than in the small lymphocyte but fewer polyribosomes than in the large lymphocyte. A small Golgi region is present. There is a great variation in the amount of granular endoplasmic reticulum and mitochondria, probably depending on the direction of differentiation in which the medium-sized lymphocyte exists

at a given time. The **specific description** must be largely conjectural, based on assumptions that have not yet been verified experimentally. If **differentiation to plasma cells** is under way, the term "plasmablast" can be used for a medium-sized lymphocyte. (Fig. 17-29) As such, they would probably accumulate an increasingly large amount of granular endoplasmic reticulum. The Golgi zones would also enlarge. The nucleus would remain spherical and shift to one side of the cell, leaving one part of the cell occupied by a large portion of cytoplasm. If **differentiation to large lymphocytes** occurs, the cytoplasm of the medium-sized lymphocyte would become filled with increasingly large numbers of polyribosomes. If preparations are under way for **mitosis resulting in small lymphocytes,** it may be assumed that the cytoplasm of such medium-sized lymphocytes will contain a limited number of polysomes, a relatively large number of free ribosomes and only few mitochondria. There still remains great uncertainty in this area, particu-

Fig. 17-26. Large lymphocyte (lymphoblast) in germinal center of splenic nodule. Cell width 14 μ. Nucleus in prophase of mitotic division. Enlargement of rectangle in Fig. 17-25. Spleen. Rat. E.M. X 12,000. **1.** Nucleoli. **2.** Chromosomes. **3.** Nuclear membrane. **4.** Cytoplasm filled with polyribosomes. **5.** Mitochondria. **6.** Small Golgi zone. **7.** Small granules. **8.** Short profiles of granular endoplasmic reticulum.

Fig. 17-27. Large lymphocyte (lymphoblast) in germinal center of lymphatic nodule. Cell width 12 μ. Nucleus in interphase. Enlargement of rectangle in Fig. 17-16. Lymph node. Rat. E.M. X 12,000. **1.** Nucleoli. **2.** Narrow zone of heterochromatin. **3.** Euchromatin. **4.** Nuclear membrane. **5.** Finger-like cytoplasmic indentation of nuclear surface cut across. **6.** Cytoplasm overcrowded with polyribosomes. **7.** Mitochondria. **8.** Short profiles of granular endoplasmic reticulum. Note the great similarity in cytoplasmic ultrastructure of lymphoblasts from spleen and lymph node. **9.** Nuclei of small lymphocytes. **10.** Nucleus of reticular cell.

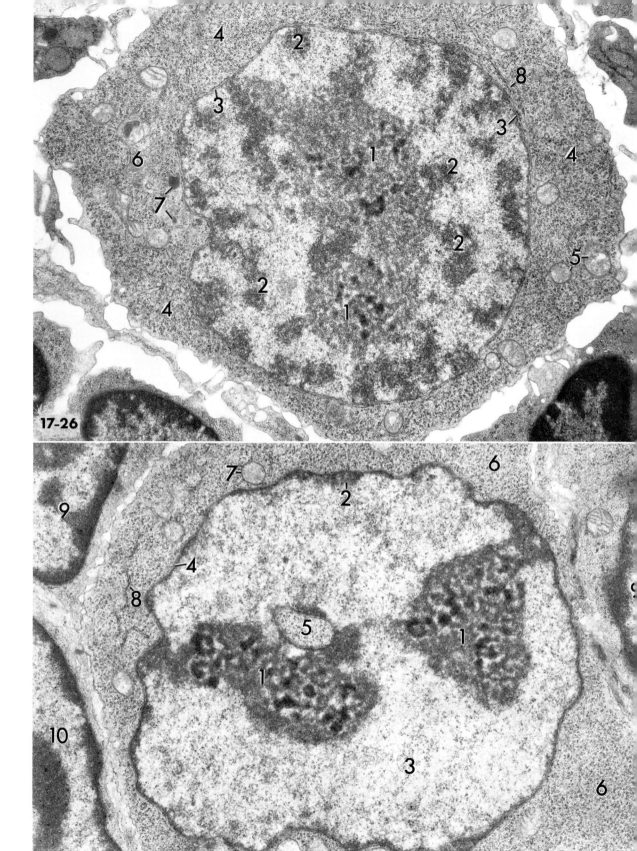

17-26

17-27

larly with reference to the direction of differentiation, and which cell represents a stem cell, and for what progeny. It must be stressed that the above description of structure and function is tentative and must await experimental confirmation.

MOVEMENTS OF LYMPHOCYTES

In areas of diffuse lymphoid infiltration and in subepithelial lymph nodules, small lymphocytes move about freely in the loose connective tissue. They also invade the epithelium itself, probably in response to an antigen stimulation, although other unknown factors may also be influential. Once a lymphocyte has invaded an epithelial lining such as the intestinal columnar epithelium, it probably does not return to the connective tissue again but becomes expelled to the intestinal lumen.

Within the lymphatic nodules, there is also a movement of lymphoid elements. This relates primarily to newly formed lymphocytes which arise in the center of the lymph nodule (germinal center) and gradually move out to the coronal zone of the nodule from where they may migrate to the surrounding connective tissue or enter nearby lymph capillaries.

Within lymph nodes, there is a constant movement of lymphoid elements from the coronal zone of the cortical nodules into subcapsular and penetrating sinuses. Most of these lymphocytes leave the lymph node via the efferent lymph vessels which drain the medullary sinuses. However, some cortical lymphocytes are transported to the medullary cords either via the lymph node sinuses or by a migration within the cords. Since the medullary cords contain a large number of plasma cells (Fig. 17-30), it is believed that the relocation of lymphocytes from cortex to medulla occurs in response to an increased demand for antibody formation.

RECIRCULATION OF LYMPHOCYTES

There is a large pool of lymphoid elements, essentially small lymphocytes which leaves the lymph node via the efferent lymph vessels, enters the cardiovascular system and then returns to the interstitial spaces of **lymph nodes** and **Peyer's patches** by going across the wall of the postcapillary venules of these areas. Although some investigators have claimed that the lymphocytes penetrate the cytoplasm of the endothelial cells of the postcapillary venules during this crossing, there is recent evidence pointing to a passage across the wall between the endothelial cells. In the **spleen,** the situation is somewhat different (see p. 408). Briefly, in this organ the circulating lymphocytes do not have to cross the walls of the blood vessels, since the majority of the arterial capillaries in the spleen have funnel-shaped terminations which open up to the interstitial spaces of

Fig. 17-28. Lymphocytes in medullary sinus. Lymph node. Cat. E.M. × 5500. This demonstrates the difficulty one encounters in trying to categorize lymphocytes solely on morphological grounds. **1.** Small lymphocytes, width indicated by line is 4.4 μ. **2.** Medium-sized lymphocyte, width indicated by line is 7.8 μ. **3.** Large lymphocyte. Width indicated by solid line is 11 μ; by dotted line 7.8 μ.

Fig. 17-29. Intermediate lymphoid cell from medullary sinus of lymph node. Cell width 10–11 μ. This is an example of the great heterogeneity among lymphoid cells. This cell could represent: a lymphoblast, a plasmablast, a monoblast, or the stem cell of the unitarian hemopoietic theory—a hemocytoblast. Lymph node. Cat. E.M. × 17,000. **1.** Nucleolus. **2.** Marginated heterochromatin. **3.** Euchromatin. **4.** Nuclear membrane. **5.** Polyribosomes. **6.** Short profiles of granular endoplasmic reticulum. **7.** Golgi zone. **8.** Mitochondria. **9.** Inclusion body (secondary lysosome). **10.** Small granules. Conclusion. If this cell is encountered in the circulating blood, it would be classified as a monocyte and not a lymphoblast, since the latter normally does not enter the peripheral circulation. Since this cell is found in a medullary lymph sinus, it probably represents a large lymphocyte (lymphoblast), possibly undergoing differentiation toward a plasma cell, particularly considering the abundant cytoplasm, the eccentric nucleus, and the relatively large number of profiles of granular endoplasmic reticulum.

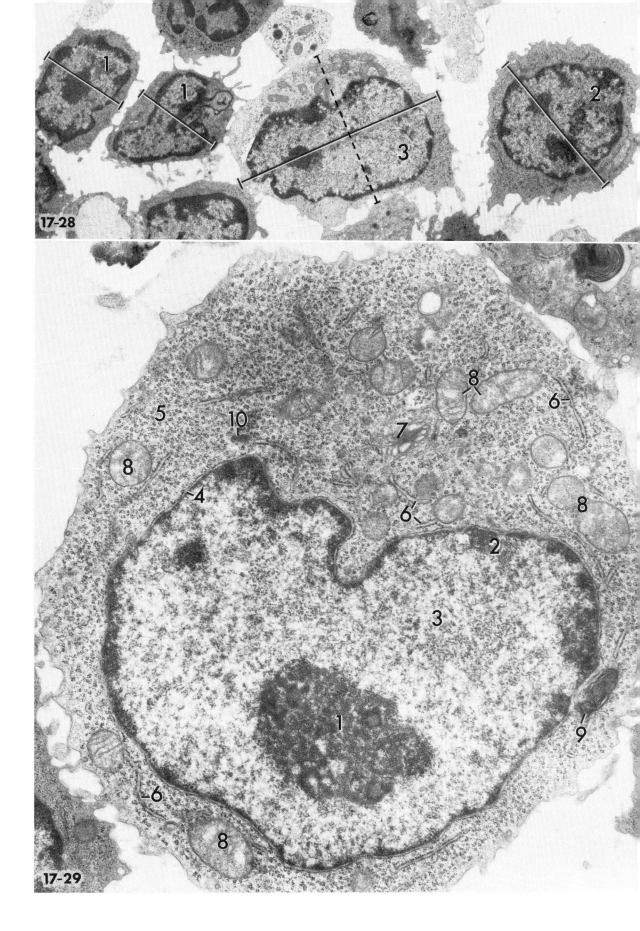

17-28

17-29

the red pulp. Furthermore, most of these terminations open up to the marginal zone between the white and the red pulp in close proximity to macrophages and lymphoid elements of the white pulp. In the **bone marrow** and **thymus,** immunologically competent lymphocytes do not leave the blood vessels under normal conditions.

The **purpose** of the recirculation of small lymphocytes is two-fold. By circulating through the cardiovascular system, the lymphocytes are constantly exposed to foreign-body proteins, wherever these antigens may enter. In addition, lymph nodes throughout the body and the spleen are kept "up to date" by the passage of immunocompetent lymphocytes, some of which settle down to divide and give rise to new cells.

BONE MARROW STEM CELLS (B CELLS)

Bone marrow is the major site for the formation of erythrocytes, granulocytes, monocytes, and megakaryocytes (see p. 112). In addition, lymphocytes are also formed in the bone marrow. How these lymphocytes arise is not clear, but their precursors probably do not represent recirculating lymphocytes. The bone marrow lymphocytes represent a distinct population which serves as stem cells for other lymphocytes. These lymphocytes are referred to as **B cells** (bone marrow lymphocytes). The lymphoid stem cells of the bone marrow (B cells) structurally are believed to be similar to small lymphocytes. These B cells enter the cardiovascular system as immunologically incompetent cells. During fetal and postnatal periods, as well as adolescence, the B cells settle down temporarily in the thymus where an induction occurs after which they and their progeny are referred to as **T cells** (thymic lymphocytes). Subsequently, they migrate to lymph nodes, Peyer's patches and spleen to become progenitors of immunologically competent cells. Recent evidence seems to indicate that the thymus may serve as an inducer to B cells not only through adolescence but also later in life in spite of the fact that the thymic parenchyma becomes greatly reduced in volume (see p. 422).

FUNCTION OF LYMPHOCYTES

To summarize some of the points already made, the lymphocytes have a key role in the initiation of the immune response. Antigen-sensitive small lymphocytes recognize a foreign protein and they store this information. At the appropriate time, they initiate an immunological response by producing immunoglobulin (antibodies) after being transformed into plasma cells. The role of the reticular cell (macrophage) in the immunological defense system is to attack, destroy, and sequester foreign materials. In the process, as a result of lysosomal activity by the macrophages, antigens are presented to the lymphocytes in molecular form.

BLOOD VESSELS OF LYMPH NODES

The blood vessels of most lymph nodes form a closed system which does not communicate with the lymph sinuses or the interstitial spaces. An exception to this is found in the hemal nodes where some arteries discharge blood into the interstitial spaces in similarity with the circulation of the spleen. However, hemal nodes are rare in the human body. An

Fig. 17-30. Survey of medullary cord. Enlargement of area similar to rectangle (B) in Fig. 17-18. Lymph node. Cat. E.M. X 1900. **1.** Lumen of blood capillary. **2.** Lumen of venule. **3.** Macrophages. **4.** Small lymphocytes. **5.** Medium-sized lymphocytes. **6.** Reticular cells. **7.** Plasma cells. **8.** Dividing plasma cells.

Fig. 17-31. Detail of medullary cord. Enlargement of rectangle in Fig. 17-30. Lymph node. Cat. E.M. X 6900. **1.** Nucleus of macrophage. **2.** Nucleus of reticular cell. **3.** Nucleus of small lymphocyte. **4.** Nuclei of plasma cells. **5.** Dividing plasma cell. **6.** Chromosomes. **7.** Granular endoplasmic reticulum. **8.** Bundles of extracellular fine collagenous and reticular fibrils. Note that they are not only associated with reticular cells but occur freely in between the plasma cells.

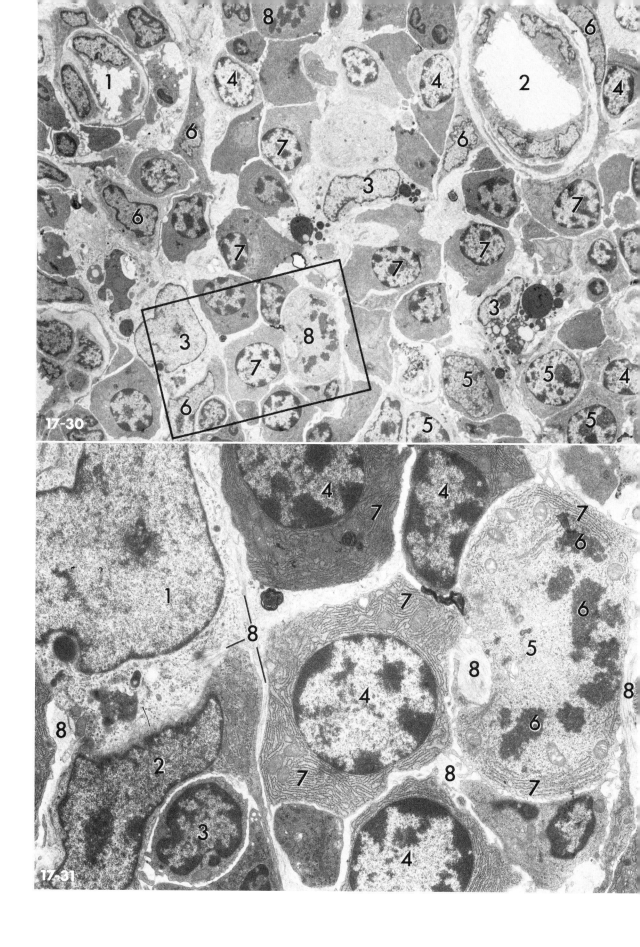

artery enters at the hilus and divides into branches which go to the connective tissue trabeculae, the medullary cords, and the dense cortical lymphatic tissue. There is a rich network of terminal **arterioles** and **capillaries** around the lymph nodules and in the medullary cords. The capillaries are lined by a continuous thin endothelium. The capillary bed is drained by a system of **postcapillary venules** which are lined by a unique endothelium. (Fig. 17-33) It consists of cuboidal and thick squamous cells. Even if the venules are preserved by intravascular perfusion, the characteristic high endothelium is present. In collapsed postcapillary venules, the height of the endothelium is accentuated. The endothelial cells are provided with large Golgi zones, a rich network of granular endoplasmic reticulum, and numerous cytoplasmic filaments. Recirculating lymphocytes leave the cardiovascular system across this endothelium to reach the dense lymphatic tissue of the nodules. The route for this passage is between endothelial cells (Fig. 17-34), although it is also maintained that lymphocytes can penetrate the endothelial cells at any point. The postcapillary venules are drained by **muscular venules** and **small veins** which accompany the arteries, leaving the node together with the efferent lymphatic vessels at the hilus.

References

Ackerman, G. A. The lymphocyte: its morphology and embryological origin. *In* The Lymphocyte in Immunology and Haematopoiesis. (Ed. J. M. Yoffey), pp. 11–30. Edward Arnold, London, 1967.

Ackerman, G. A. Structural studies of the lymphocyte and lymphocyte development. *In* Regulation of Hematopoiesis. (Ed. A. S. Gordon), Vol. 2: 1297–1338. Appleton-Century-Crofts, New York, 1970.

Bernhard, W. and Leplus, R. Fine Structure of the Normal and Malignant Human Lymph Node. Macmillan, New York, 1964.

Brooks, R. E. and Siegel, B. V. Normal human lymph node cells: an electron microscopic study. Blood 27: 687–705 (1966).

Casley-Smith, J. R. and Clark, E. L. The structure of normal small lymphatics. Q. J. Exp. Physiol. *46*: 101–106 (1961).

Cliff, W. J. and Nicoll, P. A. Structure and function of lymphatic vessels of the bat's wing. Q. J. Exp. Physiol. *55*: 112–121 (1970).

de Petris, S., Karslbad, G. and Pernis, B. Localization of antibodies in plasma cells by electron microscopy. J. Exp. Med. *117*: 849–862 (1963).

Everett, N. B. and Tyler, R. W. Lymphopoiesis in the thymus and other tissues: functional implications. Int. Rev. Cytol. 21: 205–237 (1967).

Feldman, J. D. and Nordquist, R. E. Immunologic competence of thoracic duct cells. II. Ultrastructure. Lab. Investig. *16*: 564–579 (1967).

Gowans, J. L. Life-span, recirculation and transformation of lymphocytes. Int. Rev. Exp. Path. *5*: 1–24 (1966).

Hostetler, J. R. and Ackerman, G. A. Lymphopoiesis and lymph node histogenesis in the embryonic and neonatal rabbit. Am. J. Anat. *124*: 57–76 (1969).

Leak, L. V. Studies on the permeability of lymphatic capillaries. J. Cell Biol. *50*: 300–323 (1971).

Leak, L. V. and Burke, J. F. Fine structure of the lymphatic capillary and the adjoining connective tissue area. Am. J. Anat. *118*: 785–810 (1966).

Marchesi, V. T. and Gowans, J. L. Migration of lymphocytes through the endothelium of venules in lymph nodes. An electron microscopic study. Proc. R. Soc. B. *159*: 283–290 (1964).

Mayerson, H. S. The Lymphatic System. Sci. American *208*: 80–90 (1963).

Mikata, A. and Niki, R. Permeability of postcapillary venules of the lymph node. An electron microscopic study. Exp. & Molec. Pathol. *14*: 289–305 (1971).

Fig. 17-32. Blood vessels of lymph node. Rat. E.M. × 1700. **1.** Venous capillary. Width of lumen 5 μ. Arrow indicates direction of blood flow. **2.** Postcapillary venule. Width of lumen 22 μ. **3.** Nuclei of endothelial cells.

Fig. 17-33. Cross section of lymph node postcapillary venule. Width of lumen approximately 30 μ. High endothelial cells characterize this kind of venule. Rat. E.M. × 960. **1.** Nuclei of endothelial cells. **2.** Nuclei of pericytes. **3.** Perivascular lymphocytes. **4.** Lymphocyte leaving lumen of venule (enlarged in Fig. 17-34). **5.** Lymphocyte partly surrounded by endothelial cell cytoplasm (enlarged in Fig. 17-35). **6.** Lymphocyte located between endothelium and pericytic sheath of venule (enlarged in Fig. 17-36).

Figs. 17-34, 17-35 & 17-36. Mechanism of lymphocyte recirculation. Enlargements of parts of venule in Fig. 17-33. Rat. E.M. × 4500. **1.** Nuclei of endothelial cells. **2.** Lysosomes. **3.** Basal lamina. **4.** This lymphocyte is leaving the venule by route between endothelial cells. **5.** This lymphocyte is engulfed by endothelial cell. **6.** This lymphocyte is temporarily lodged outside of endothelium.

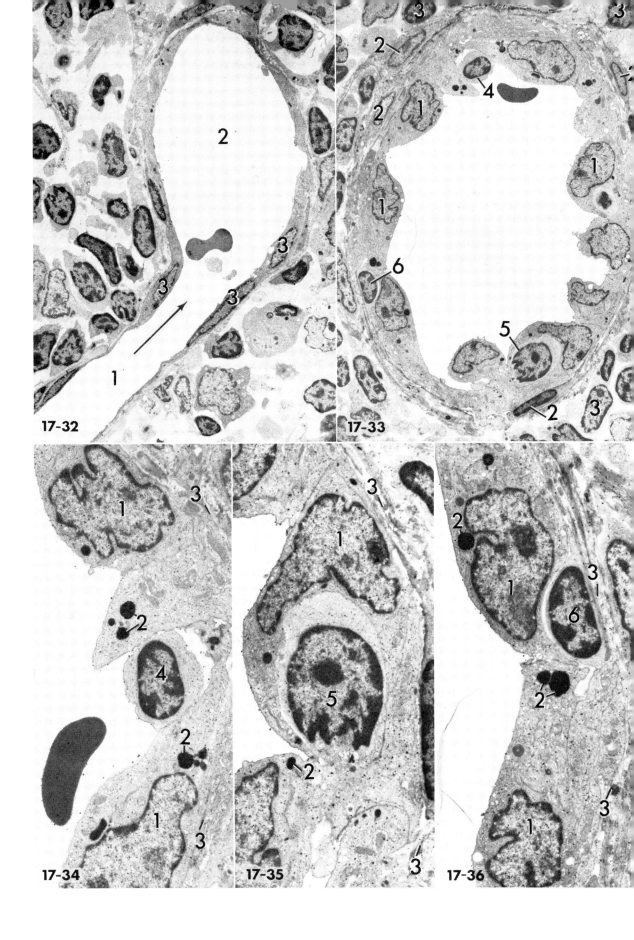

17-32

17-33

17-34

17-35

17-36

Miller, J. A. F. P., Basten, A., Sprent, J. and Cheers, C. Interaction between lymphocytes in immune responses. (Review). Cellular Immunology 2: 469–495 (1971).

Movat, H. Z. and Fernando, N. V. P. The fine structure of lymphoid tissue. Exp. & Molec. Pathol. 3: 546–568 (1964).

Movat, H. Z. and Fernando, N. V. P. The fine structure of lymphoid tissue during antibody formation. Exp. & Molec. Pathol. 4: 155–188 (1965).

Nopajaroonsri, C., Luk, S. and Simon, G. T. Ultrastructure of the normal lymph node. Am. J. Path. 65: 1–24 (1971).

Nossal, G. J. V. How cells make antibodies. Sci. American 211: 106–115 (1964).

Nossal, G. J. V. The cellular basis of immunity. Harvey Lect. Series 63: 179–211 (1968).

Nowell, P. C. and Wilson, D. B. Lymphocytes and hemic stem cells. Am. J. Path. 65: 641–652 (1971).

Sainte-Marie, G. and Sin, Y. M. Structures of the lymph node and their possible function during the immune response. Rev. Can. Biol. 27: 191–207 (1968).

Schipp, R. Der Feinstruktur filamentärer Strukturen im Endothel peripherer Lymphgefässe. Acta Anat 71: 341–351 (1968).

Schwarz, M. R. Transformation of rat small lymphocytes with allogeneic lymphoid cells. Am. J. Anat. 121: 559–570 (1967).

Smith, J. B., McIntosh, G. H. and Morris, B. The traffic of cells through tissues: a study of peripheral lymph in sheep. J. Anat. 107: 87–100 (1970).

Takada, M. The ultrastructure of lymphatic valves in rabbits and mice. Am. J. Anat. 132: 207–217 (1971).

Turner, D. R. The vascular tree of the haemal node in the rat. J. Anat. 104: 481–493 (1969).

Wenk, E. J., Orlic, D., Reith, E. J. and Rhodin, J. A. G. The ultrastructure of mouse lymph node venules and the passage of lymphocytes across their walls. J. Ultrastruct. Res. 47 (1974).

Willingham, M. C., Spicer, S. S. and Graber, C. D. Immunological labeling of calf and human lymphocyte surface antigens. Lab. Investig. 25: 211–219 (1971).

Zucker-Franklin, D. The ultrastructure of lymphocytes. Seminars in Hematology 6: 4–27 (1969).

18 Spleen

The spleen is the largest accumulation of lymphoid tissue in the body. It serves as one source of lymphocyte and antibody formation. The lymphocytes are delivered directly to the blood channels since the spleen does not have a prominent system of internal lymph vessels. Another major function of the spleen stems from its ability to break down erythrocytes toward the end of their life span. The histological architecture of the spleen reflects these two major functions, and there is a unique mixture of lymphoid tissue with that of the formed elements of the blood. The several functions of the spleen are supplemented by the activities of lymph nodes, bone marrow, and liver sinusoids. Therefore, man is not entirely dependent upon the spleen, and can live without this organ.

GENERAL

The spleen is located in the upper left region of the abdomen. Its size varies according to the state of nutrition of the body. It is usually larger after digestion and smaller after starvation. The average weight is about 200 grams. The spleen is surrounded by a fibroelastic **capsule** and contains a trabecular network and the splenic parenchyma. (Fig. 18-1) The **trabecular network** is made up of connective tissue and smooth muscle cells. The **splenic parenchyma** is divided into the **white pulp**, consisting of lymphoid tissue, and the **red pulp** which is a mixture of blood vessels, a three-dimensional network of so-called reticular cells and extravasated erythrocytes. The blood vessels and their ramifications are closely related to the functions of the spleen. At the hilus of the concave surface of the spleen, the large **splenic artery** enters the parenchyma and the **splenic vein** leaves. The arteries and the veins accompany each other initially in the connective tissue trabeculae as **trabecular arteries** and **trabecular veins**. The veins remain associated with the trabeculae whereas the arteries soon enter the splenic pulp. Once in the pulp they

are referred to as central arteries. These are surrounded by a sleeve of lymphoid tissue which represents the white pulp. The arteries gradually give rise to smaller and smaller branches. The most distal ramifications of the central arteries break up into a brush-like arrangement of vessels, the **penicilli** (Fig. 18-4), each of which has three structurally different parts: 1) arteriole of the pulp; 2) sheathed arteriole; and 3) arterial capillary. The topography and structure of these branches varies greatly with the species. The venous system starts as a widely interconnected system of **venous sinuses,** drained by **pulp veins** which, in turn, empty into the trabecular veins. The structural features of the **splenic microcirculation,** that is, the relationship between the arterial capillaries and the venous sinuses, has been a matter of controversy for well over 75 years. Recent electron microscope studies are in support of an **open** as well as a **closed** microcirculation. In rat, the majority of arterial capillaries open up into the extravascular network of reticular cells (open circulation). The extravasated

Fig. 18-1. Spleen. Human. L.M. X 10.
1. Capsule. **2.** Trabeculae. **3.** Trabeculae with vein. **4.** Red pulp. **5.** White pulp with splenic nodules.

Fig. 18-2. Spleen fixed by intra-arterial perfusion. Rat. L.M. X 50. **1.** Capsule (thin). **2.** Red pulp. **3.** White pulp. **4.** Splenic nodule. **5.** Central artery. **6.** Trabecula.

Fig. 18-3. Enlargement of rectangle (A) in Fig. 18-2. Spleen. Rat. L.M. X 240. **1.** Red pulp. **2.** Venous sinuses. **3.** Germinal center of splenic nodule. **4.** Central artery. **5.** Marginal zone. **6.** Dilated funnel-shaped terminations of arterial capillaries. **7.** Trabecula.

Fig. 18-4. Spleen. Same preparation as in Fig. 18-2. Rat. L.M. X 230. **1.** Red pulp. **2.** Trabecula. **3.** Penicilli with sleeves of lymphoid tissue (sheathed arterioles). **4.** Cross-sectioned arterial capillary, luminal diameter about 5 μ. **5.** Venous sinus.

Fig. 18-5. Enlargement of rectangle (B) in Fig. 18-2. Spleen. Rat. L.M. X 230. **1.** Pulp arteriole (first segment of penicillus). **2.** Sheathed arteriole (second segment of penicillus). **3.** Venous sinuses. **4.** Red pulp.

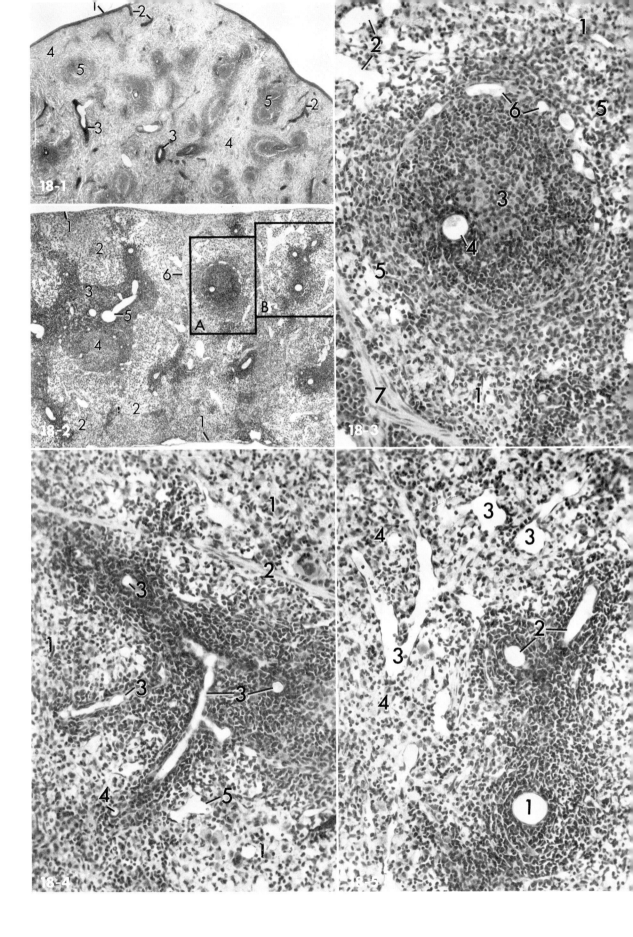

18-1

18-2

18-3

18-4

18-5

erythrocytes again enter the vascular system through numerous, slit-like openings in the walls of the venous sinuses. Some arterial capillaries, particularly those near the surface of the spleen, are directly continuous with the venous sinuses (closed circulation). This provides for two kinds of circulatory pattern: a slow extravascular, and a rapid vascular circulation.

CAPSULE, TRABECULAE, AND RETICULAR TISSUE

The capsule, the trabeculae, and the reticular tissue form the framework for the splenic pulp.

The **capsule** of the spleen in man is composed of fibroblasts, smooth muscle cells, and extracellular material such as collagen, reticular fibrils, and elastic fibers. The outer surface of the capsule is covered by the **peritoneal mesothelium.**

The **trabeculae** penetrate the parenchyma of the spleen, emerging from the inside surface of the capsule. (Fig. 18-3) The trabeculae do not acquire the shape of septa, and the formerly suggested pattern of lobulation of the spleen is not appropriate. The trabeculae consist mainly of smooth muscle cells (Fig. 18-13), fibroblasts, and bundles of collagenous fibrils. However, the number of smooth muscle cells in the capsule and trabeculae varies greatly with the species. Dogs have a large number of smooth muscle cells whereas man has few. To some extent the smooth muscle cells of the capsule and the trabeculae help in reducing the size of the spleen by contraction.

The **reticular tissue** forms a three-dimensional web of reticular cells and reticular fibrils throughout the white and red pulp. The **reticular cell** is structurally similar to the fibroblast (Fig. 18-14), but, in addition, has a few marginal bundles of cytoplasmic filaments. In the spleen, as well as in lymph nodes, this kind of cell readily ingests foreign materials including erythrocytes and thereby structurally can be identified as a **fixed macrophage.** There is good evidence that the fixed macro-phages become detached from the reticular fibrils and are then recognized as **free macrophages.** (Fig. 18-16) However, there is a strong possibility that reticular cells may also give rise to some of the many **monocytes** that occur throughout the splenic pulp. In turn, these may then give rise to free macrophages. The reticular cell may also be a precursor of the lymphocytes, and therefore in structure and function is similar to the multipotential mesenchymal cell of the embryo.

Bundles of **reticular fibrils** traverse the splenic pulp, connected to and in association with cytoplasmic processes of the reticular cells and the fixed macrophages. The reticular fibrils fall into the category of delicate, presumably young, narrow collagenous fibrils. (Fig. 18-15) Mature, wide collagenous fibrils are encountered only in association with the splenic capsule and the trabeculae.

WHITE PULP

The white pulp is represented by a sleeve of compact lymphoid tissue around the ramifications of the arterial system. (Fig. 18-6) The lymphoid tissue has a cellular composition similar to that of this tissue elsewhere in the body. Depending on the state of responsiveness of the tissue, lymphocytes aggregate to form **splenic nodules** (Malpighian corpuscles) and germinal centers. Thus, the splenic white pulp contains an assortment of small, medium, and large lymphocytes in addition to many

Fig. 18-6. Survey of white and red pulp of spleen. Fixation by intra-arterial perfusion. Rat. E.M. X 800. **1.** Central artery (lumen 30 μ) with branch (arrow) surrounded by a thick sleeve of white pulp. Details of the lymphoid tissue of the white pulp is seen in Fig. 17-25. **2.** Arteriole (lumen 11 μ) in white pulp. This is a branch of the central artery. **3.** Funnel-shaped open terminations of arterial capillaries. **4.** Marginal zone with large interstitial spaces. **5.** Venous sinuses. **6.** Red pulp. **7.** Large lymphocytes (lymphoblasts). **8.** Small lymphocytes. **9.** Reticular cells. **10.** Erythrocytes.

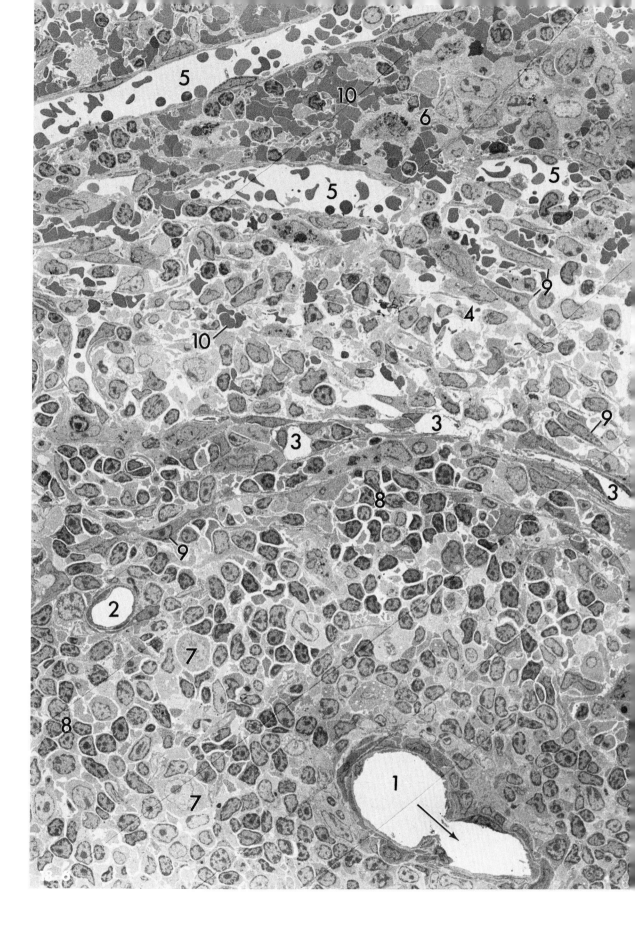

monocytes and plasma cells. Reticular cells and free macrophages also occur. The eccentrically placed arteries of the white pulp, the central arteries, give off a rich network of arterial capillaries which take care of the blood supply of the white pulp. Erythrocytes do not leave the lumina of these capillaries within the white pulp, but at the point where the capillaries terminate with funnel-shaped open ends (Fig. 18-9) in a narrow zone around the white pulp, the **marginal zone.** There is therefore no contact between erythrocytes and lymphocytes in the inner part of the white pulp. However, foreign blood-borne antigens probably reach the lymphocytes of the white pulp by diffusing from the blood through the endothelium of the capillaries of the white pulp. In addition, antigens delivered to the marginal zone can easily diffuse into the white pulp.

RED PULP

The red pulp occupies a major part of the splenic parenchyma. It consists of pulp spaces, extravasated formed elements of the blood, some lymphocytes, a spongy framework of reticular cells, the terminal part of arterial capillaries, a vast system of interconnecting venous sinuses of varying sizes, and the marginal zones bordering on the white pulp. (Fig. 18-6)

The **pulp spaces,** also referred to as the cords of Billroth, are formed by the three-dimensional web of reticular cells. The interstitial spaces are filled by free macrophages, monocytes, and all the formed elements of the blood among which the erythrocytes are the most prominent. Since many lymphocytes are also present, one may look upon the red pulp as a diffuse lymphoid tissue with an admixture of extravasated erythrocytes. From a functional point of view, the interstices of the red pulp are the spaces where reticular cells and macrophages come in contact with and phagocytose foreign materials in the blood as well as act on the older erythrocytes to destroy them and to salvage the iron of the hemoglobin. In addi-

tion, the red pulp is the location of erythropoiesis in the human fetus and in the young of rats and mice. In many species, megakaryocytes are also present, but they are rare in man under normal conditions.

The **venous sinuses** are a prominent part of the red pulp. These are thin-walled vessels of varying sizes, draining the red pulp of both the intra-arterial and extravascular blood. Their structure is described on p. 408.

The **marginal zone** is that part of the red pulp which borders on the white pulp. (Fig. 18-9) It is approximately 20–30 μ wide and characterized by a wider network of reticular cells than elsewhere in the red pulp. Most of the arterial capillaries of the white pulp terminate with funnel-shaped, open endings (ampullae) within or near the marginal zone. Contrary to earlier beliefs, the unusually wide spaces of this zone do not represent venous sinuses but widely expanded interstitial spaces. Lymphocytes derived from and formed in the white pulp are shed into the marginal zone. They subsequently traverse the zone to enter the nearest venous sinuses of the red pulp.

Fig. 18-7. Cross-sectioned central artery (arteriole) of white pulp. Spleen. Rat. E.M. X 1900. **1.** Lumen, 30 μ wide. **2.** Squamous endothelium. **3.** Media consists of 2–3 layers of smooth muscle cells. **4.** Periarteriolar sheath of lymphoid cells. Note that adventitial connective tissue cells are missing.

Fig. 18-8. Wall of central arteriole (artery) of spleen. Enlargement of rectangle in Fig. 18-7. Rat. E.M. X 14,000. **1.** Lumen. **2.** Endothelium. **3.** Basal lamina (elastica interna is missing). **4.** Smooth muscle cells. **5.** Small bundles of reticular and collagenous fibrils. **6.** Lymphocytes.

Fig. 18-9. Marginal zone of white pulp. Spleen. Rat. E.M. X 960. **1.** Edge of white pulp. **2.** Funnel-shaped open termination of arterial capillary. Arrow indicates direction of blood flow. **3.** Erythrocytes. **4.** Interstitial space, communicating with lumen of arterial capillary. **5.** Lymphocytes (mostly medium-sized). **6.** Macrophages. **7.** Reticular cells.

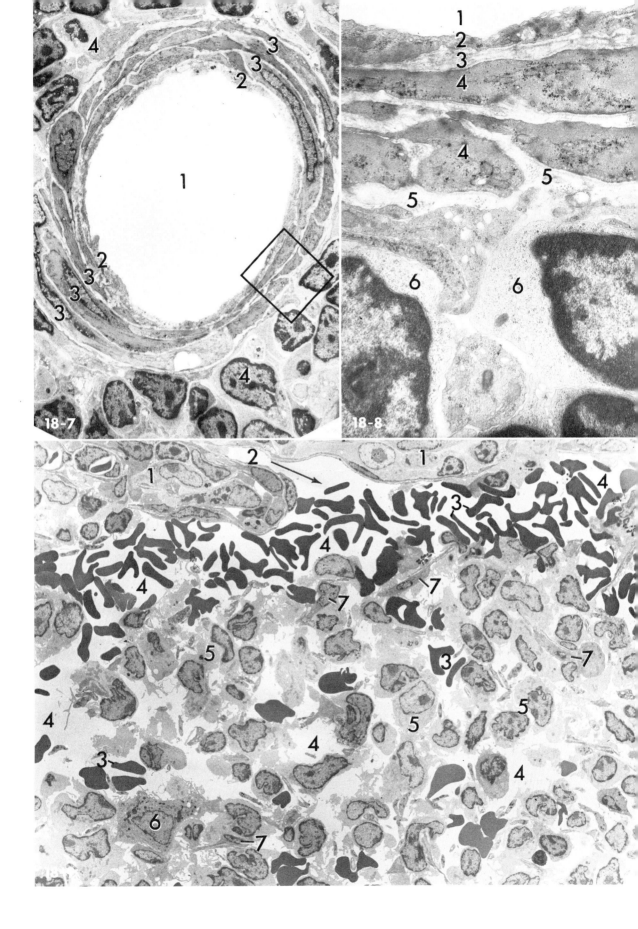

ARTERIAL BLOOD VESSELS

After the splenic artery enters the paren-chyma, it gives rise to trabecular arteries, central arteries, and penicilli.

The **trabecular arteries** are medium-sized vessels of the muscular type with a thin inner elastic membrane and a media with several layers of smooth muscle cells. Non-myelinated nerve bundles closely accompany the artery.

The **central arteries** come off from the trabecular arteries as the luminal diameter of the latter have decreased to about 0.2 mm. They traverse and subdivide in the splenic pulp surrounded by their sleeve of dense lymphoid tissue, the white pulp. The larger central arteries have a thin inner elastic membrane and a few layers of smooth muscle cells in their media. As the branching continues distally, the central arteries gradually decrease in diameter down to about 50μ (Fig. 18-7), thereby changing to **arterioles.** The inner elastic membrane disappears and there remains only one or two layers of thin, sheath-like smooth muscle cells which have a highly modified ultrastructure, reminiscent of that characterizing a pericyte. Non-myelinated nerve fibers, some without the protective Schwann cells, closely accompany all arteriolar branches of the central artery. The endothelium is relatively thin, and provided with numerous small cytoplasmic vesicles. The endothelium makes frequent contacts with the smooth muscle cells via myo-endothelial junctions. A distinct, continuous basal lamina separates endothelium from the surrounding layers of smooth muscle cells. Typical splenic reticular cells form an incomplete adventitial lining of the arterial wall establishing a connection with other reticular cells of the white pulp. The central arteries and arterioles give off **arterial capillaries** to the white pulp. The majority of these capillaries terminate in the marginal zone with open-end **ampullae,** discharging the blood to the interstices of the red pulp.

The **penicilli** represent long, brushlike terminal ramifications of the central arteries and arterioles. They are recognized as the part of the arterial blood vessel which leaves the white pulp to break up in the red pulp. The architecture and structure of the penicilli vary greatly with the species. Generally, one recognizes three subdivisions: pulp arteriole, sheathed arteriole, and arterial capillary. The **pulp arteriole** has a luminal diameter of less than 50μ. In man, mice, rabbits and guinea pigs, a thin sleeve of dense lymphoid tissue surrounds the arteriole, whereas it is missing in cats and dogs. In the **sheathed arteriole** the luminal diameter is less than 10μ. (Fig. 18-11) There is a spindle-shaped accumulation of cells (ellipsoid or sheath of Schweigger-Seidel) around these branches of the penicilli. It is prominent in cats and dogs, poorly developed in man, and absent in rats, mice, and rabbits. The wall of the sheathed arteriole has a few primitive smooth muscle cells, and the ellipsoid is composed of lymphocytes, plasma cells and reticular cells. The function of the ellipsoid is not clear. It was believed earlier to serve as a special sphincter and/or sieve, but recent investigations indicate that it merely represents another accumulation of lymphoid tissue around a specific segment of an

Fig. 18-10. Survey of spleen. Rat. E.M. X 580. **1.** Central artery (arteriole). Width of lumen 30 μ. **2.** White pulp. **3.** Sheathed arteriole (lumen 10 μ) originating from the central artery. **4.** Thin sleeve of lymphoid tissue. **5.** Funnel-shaped open terminations of arterial capillaries. **6.** Red pulp. **7.** Marginal zone.

Fig. 18-11. Sheathed arteriole. Enlargement of rectangle in Fig. 18-10. Rat. E.M. X 3700. **1.** Lumen. **2.** Erythrocytes. **3.** Endothelium. **4.** Nuclei of smooth muscle cells. **5.** Lymphocytes. **6.** Reticular cells. **7.** Bundles of collagenous fibrils.

Fig. 18-12. Wall of sheathed arteriole. Enlargement of rectangle in Fig. 18-11. Spleen. Rat. E.M. X 29,000. **1.** Lumen. **2.** Platelet. **3.** Endothelium. **4.** Smooth muscle cells. **5.** Myoendothelial junctions. **6.** Basal lamina. **7.** Thin cytoplasmic strands of reticular cells.

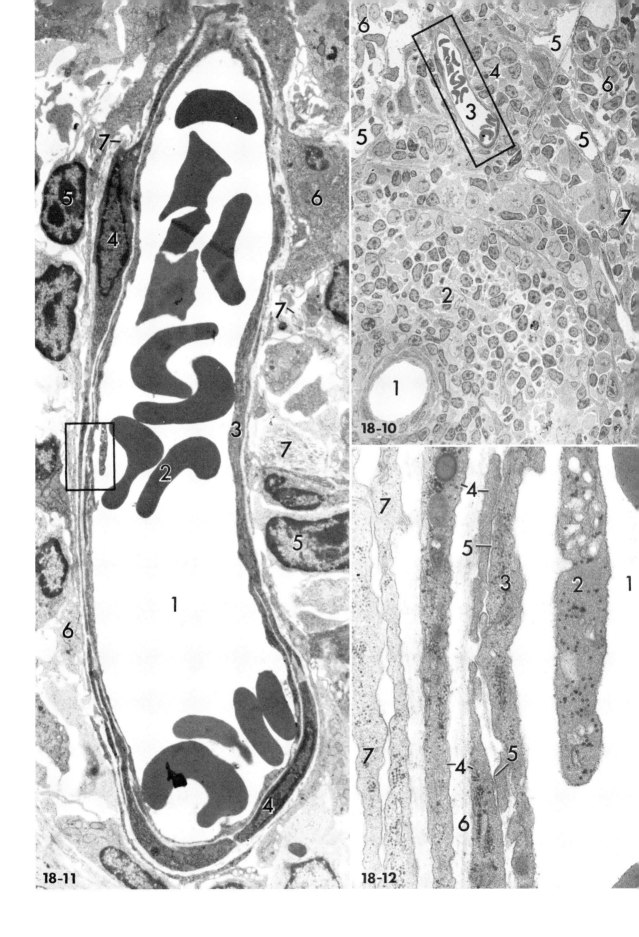

18-10

18-11

18-12

arterial blood vessel. The **arterial capillaries** form the final ramification of the penicilli. They are extremely delicate with a luminal diameter of 4–6 μ. They have a thin, continuous and vesiculated endothelium, a complete basal lamina and some reticular cells on the pulp side.

SPLENIC MICROCIRCULATION

In all other mammalian tissues and organs, an arterial capillary connects directly with a venous capillary or sinus. There is no general agreement on how the splenic arterial capillaries terminate. One school of thought maintains that they all connect with and empty into venous sinuses. This is referred to as a **closed circulation.** Other investigators hold that the arterial capillaries communicate directly with the pulp interstices. This is the **open circulation.** Recent electron microscope investigations of the rat spleen strongly indicate that the majority of arterial capillaries terminate with an open, funnel-shaped ampulla which allows the formed elements of the blood to enter the extracellular interstices of the splenic red pulp. (Fig. 18-13) From here, the blood reaches the venous sinuses through narrow slits in the sinusoidal wall. The ampullae of some arterial capillaries are gradually transformed into venous sinuses, and do not open up to the trabecular meshwork of the pulp. In rats, these connections are located mostly near the surface of the spleen. This arrangement has been demonstrated by a long series of thin sections for electron microscopy and is believed to be the most logical solution to the longstanding controversy over the splenic microcirculation. It would allow for a **rapid circulation** (closed) to assure the maintenance of a proper oxygen tension of the tissue. The **slow circulation** (open) would make it possible to test and destroy erythrocytes as these meander through the splenic interstices, being in frequent contact with the macrophages and reticular cells of the red pulp. Furthermore, through the open circulation, blood-borne antigens are generously brought into contact with macrophages of the marginal zone and lymphoid elements of the white pulp.

VENOUS BLOOD VESSELS

The venous blood vessels of the spleen consist of venous sinuses, pulp veins, and trabecular veins, all of which are drained by the splenic veins. There are no true, narrow venous capillaries.

The **venous sinuses** form a plexus of richly anastomosing channels which occupy a major portion of the red pulp in most mammals, including man, rats, dogs, and rabbits. Venous sinuses are not prominent in cats and mice. *In vivo* observations indicate that the shape and diameter of the sinuses change constantly. Some sinuses are as wide as 50 μ, and others are smaller than 15 μ. Frequently, long narrow sinuses interconnect wide ones. (Figs. 18-17, 18-18) The venous sinuses do not have open termini, and this system therefore resembles that of the lymphatic capillaries which also originates as channels with blind endings. The sinus wall is composed of elongated, spindle-shaped cells, **littoral**

Fig. 18-13. Survey of red pulp preserved by intra-arterial perfusion and serial-sectioned. This is section No. 328 in a series of 500 sections. Spleen. Rat. E.M. X 2500. **1.** Smooth muscle cells of trabecula. **2.** Elastic fibers. **3.** Bundles of collagenous fibrils. **4.** Longitudinal section of open termination of arterial capillary (end of penicillus). Arrow indicates direction of blood flow. **5.** Endothelial cells. **6.** Reticular cells. **7.** Interstitial space. **8.** Cross-sectioned venous sinuses. **9.** Littoral cells (lining cells). **10.** Macrophages. **11.** Erythrocytes. **12.** Small lymphocytes. **13.** Proerythroblasts in mitotic prophase. This is a clonal formation of erythrocytes near phagocytes. Erythropoiesis is common in the spleen of young rats. **14.** Medium-sized lymphocyte. This could possibly also represent a hemocytoblast, a precursor of the proerythroblasts. **15.** Erythrocytes passing through stomata between littoral cells. **16.** Thrombocytes (platelets).

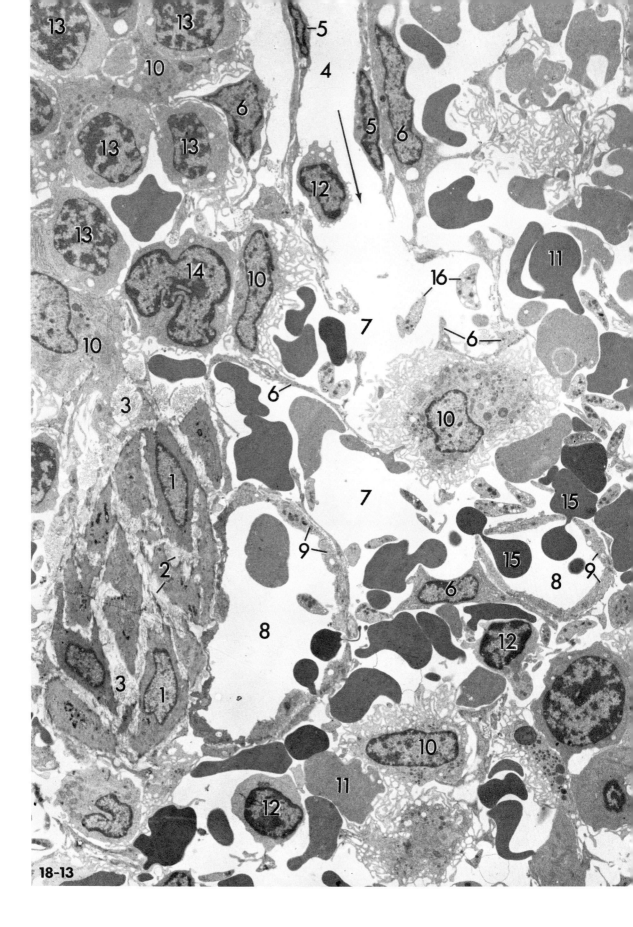

cells, which are arranged in a fence-like pattern. The cells are attached to each other at certain points via simple membranous contacts. At other points, they are separated by longitudinal oval clefts, stomata, some large enough to allow the formed elements of the blood to pass through. (Figs. 18-19, 18-20, 18-21) Reticular fibrils and irregular short strands of basal lamina establish a loose and wide-meshed framework around the littoral cells. Reticular cells form an incomplete lining of the littoral cells toward the red pulp. The littoral cell is of the same origin as the reticular cells of the stroma, but is less actively phagocytic under normal conditions. Bundles of marginated fine cytoplasmic filaments occur at the base of the littoral cells. There is some evidence that these filaments participate in changing the shape of the sinuses through a slow contraction. There is no structural evidence that the filaments are more numerous at any particular part of the sinusoidal system as indicated by some *in vivo* observations of sphincter-like contractions.

The **pulp veins** are formed by the confluence of several venous sinuses. The wall of the vein is composed of squamous endothelial cells and a complete lining of reticular cells.

The **trabecular veins** are lined by squamous endothelial cells and embedded in the trabecular fibroblasts and smooth muscle cells.

LYMPHATICS

Lymphatic capillaries are not present in the spleen. From a functional point of view, the venous sinuses serve the purpose of collecting tissue fluid and lymphocytes, since the walls of the sinuses are provided with large openings (stomata) which permit free communication between the extravascular interstitial space and the sinusoidal lumen. Lymph from the capsule and the larger trabeculae is collected by efferent lymph vessels which leave the spleen at the hilus.

NERVES

The splenic blood vessels, especially the arteries and arterioles, are accompanied by non-myelinated axons of sympathetic neurons. The nerves terminate in relation to vascular smooth muscle as well as to trabeculae and capsule in species which have smooth muscle cells in these areas. Under the influence of sympathetic stimulation, a contraction occurs which expels large amounts of stored blood from the spleen. A sympathetic inhibition brings about an expansion of the spleen which results in an accumulation of blood, particularly in the vast system of sinuses.

FUNCTIONS

Among the many functions attributed to the spleen are its ability to serve as a blood reservoir, its blood cleansing activity, and its participation in the immunological defense system of the body. During fetal life, it also serves as an erythropoietic tissue.

The spleen serves as a **blood reservoir** because of its ability to contract and expand. The venous sinuses are the primary areas for blood storage, but also the extra-

Fig. 18-14. Detail of reticular cell in red pulp of spleen. Rat. E.M. X 9500. **1.** Nucleus of reticular cell. **2.** Erythrocytes. **3.** Interstitial space of red pulp. **4.** Free ribosomes. **5.** Profiles of granular endoplasmic reticulum. **6.** Golgi zone. **7.** Mitochondria. **8.** Bundles of filaments. **9.** Reticular (extracellular) fibrils.

Fig. 18-15. Enlargement of areas similar to circles in Fig. 18-14. Spleen. Rat. E.M. X 74,000. **1.** Cytoplasmic processes of reticular cells containing densely packed filaments. **2.** Bundle of reticular fibrils with some elastic microfibrils.

Fig. 18-16. Detail of macrophage in the red pulp of spleen. Rat. E.M. X 18,000. **1.** Nucleus of macrophage. **2.** Erythrocyte. **3.** Interstitial space of red pulp. **4.** Microvilli. **5.** Micropinocytotic vesicles and vacuoles. **6.** Golgi zone. **7.** Dilated Golgi cisterna. **8.** Mitochondria. **9.** Primary lysosomes. **10.** Secondary lysosomes. **11.** Free polysomes. **12.** Profiles of granular endoplasmic reticulum.

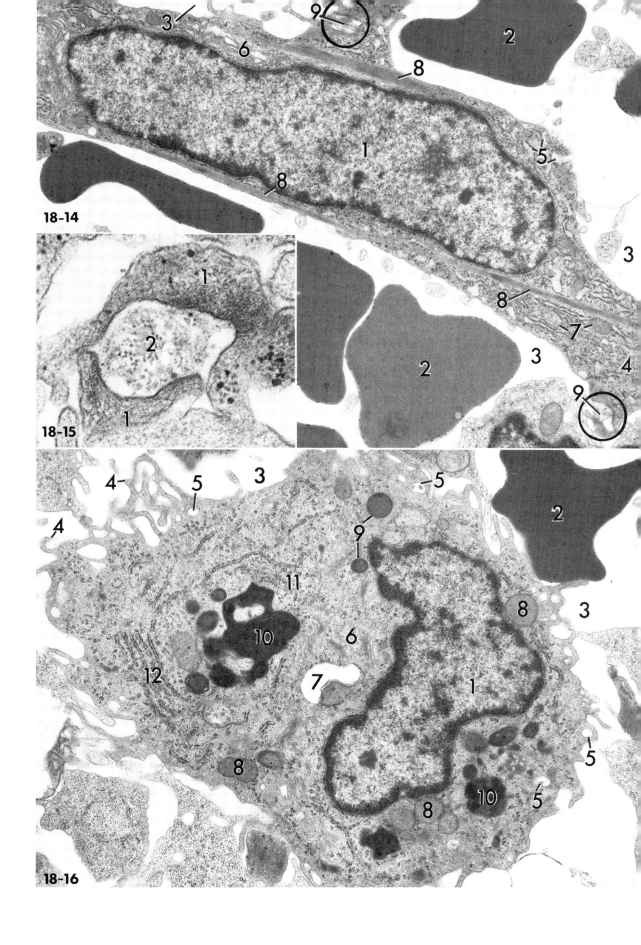

18-14

18-15

18-16

vascular spaces of the red pulp are used in highly expanded spleens. Normally, the blood moves slowly through most of the sinuses, and it is possible that large systems of sinuses, engorged with blood are temporarily shut off at some point by a sphincter action of a pulp vein. In this situation, it is obviously of great functional importance that other parts of the vascular system stay open to allow for a rapid circulation through the spleen for the purpose of oxygenation of the tissue. The direct connection between arterial capillaries and venous sinuses (the so-called closed circulation) serves this purpose.

The **blood cleansing** function involves the removal of debris, bacteria, and parasites by the reticular cells, as well as by the fixed and free macrophages. It also relates to the removal of old erythrocytes from the circulating blood as they meander through the pulp spaces. This increases the physical pressure on the red blood cells, and the pliability of the cell membrane is tested by distortion. The macrophages readily take up those erythrocytes which are near the end of their life span, and the iron-containing component of the hemoglobin is stored temporarily in the macrophage. The presence of foreign materials and old red cells in the pulp represents a constant stimulus on the reticular cells and the splenic monocytes to differentiate into macrophages, both fixed and free.

The spleen also is part of the **immunological defense system** of the body. In direct response to blood-borne and lymphogenic antigens, the plasma cells of the white pulp produce antibodies. In addition, lymphocytes are stimulated to develop into plasma cells or to give rise to other lymphocytes as part of a delayed hypersensitivity reaction. This in turn leads to an accumulation of lymphocytes and plasma cells, and germinal centers appear in the white pulp.

During fetal life, the spleen is the site for erythropoiesis. It can revert back to this function later in life, particularly if the bone marrow fails to produce an adequate amount of erythrocytes.

References

Björkman, S. E. The splenic circulation. With special reference to the function of the spleen sinus wall. Acta Med. Scand. *128*, Suppl. 191, 1–89 (1947).

Burke, J. S. and Simon, G. T. Electron microscopy of the spleen. I. Anatomy and microcirculation. Am. J. Path. *58*: 127–155 (1970).

Burke, J. S. and Simon, G. T. Electron microscopy of the spleen. II. Phagocytosis of colloid carbon. Am. J. Path. *58*: 157–181 (1970).

Edwards, V. D. and Simon, G. T. Ultrastructural aspects of red cell destruction in the normal rat spleen. J. Ultrastruct. Res. *33*: 187–201 (1970).

Hirasawa, Y. and Tokuhiro, H. Electron microscopic studies on the normal human spleen: especially on the red pulp and the reticulo-endothelial cells. Blood *35*: 201–212 (1970).

Knisely, M. H. Spleen studies. I. Microscopic observations of the circulatory system of living unstimulated mammalian spleen. Anat. Rec. *65*: 23–50 (1936).

Lewis, O. J. The blood vessels of the adult mammalian spleen. J. Anat. *91*: 245–250 (1957).

MacKenzie, D., Whipple, W. A. O. and Wintersteiner, M. P. Studies on the microscopic anatomy and physiology of living and transilluminated mammalian spleens. Am. J. Anat. *68*: 397–456 (1941).

MacNeal, W. J. The circulation of blood through the spleen pulp. Arch. Path. 7: 215–227 (1929).

Moore, R. D., Mumaw, V. R. and Schoenberg, M. D. The structure of the spleen and its functional implications. Exp. & Molec. Pathol. *3*: 31–50 (1964).

Parpart, A. K., Whipple, A. O. and Chang, J. J. The microcirculation of the spleen of the mouse. Angiology *6*: 350–362 (1955).

Peck, H. M. and Hoerr, N. L. The intermediary circulation in the red pulp of the mouse spleen. Anat. Rec. *109*: 447–477 (1951).

Pictet, R., Orci, L., Forssmann, W. G. and Girardier, L.

Fig. 18-17 & 18-18. Survey of venous sinuses traversing the red pulp. Spleen. Rat. E.M. X 1600. **1.** Cross section of venous sinus (lumen 22 μ). **2.** Longitudinally sectioned venous sinuses. **3.** Nuclei of littoral (lining) cells. **4.** Nuclei of reticular cells. **5.** Erythrocytes. **6.** Thrombocytes. **7.** Macrophages. **8.** Small lymphocytes. **9.** Medium-sized lymphocytes. **10.** Monocyte. **11.** Erythrocytes passing through stomata in wall of venous sinus. **12.** Point of confluence of two venous sinuses. **13.** Interstitial space of red pulp. **14.** Tangential section through microvillous excrescences of macrophage. **15.** Plasma cell.

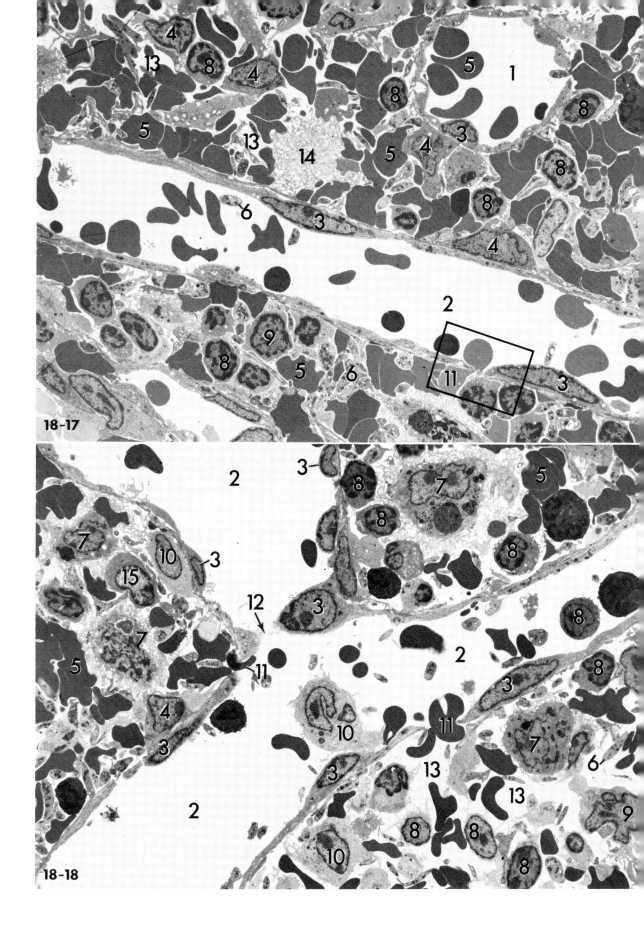

18-17

18-18

An electron microscope study of the perfusion-fixed spleen. I. The splenic circulation and the RES concept. Z. Zellforsch. *96*: 372–399 (1969).

Pictet, R., Orci, L., Forssmann, W. G. and Girardier, L. An electron microscope study of the perfusion-fixed spleen. II. Nurse cells and erythrophagocytosis. Z. Zellforsch. *96*: 400–417 (1969).

Roberts, D. K. and Latta, J. S. Electron microscopic studies on the red pulp of the rabbit spleen. Anat. Rec. *148*: 81–101 (1964).

Robinson, W. L. The vascular mechanism of the spleen. Am. J. Path. *2*: 341–355 (1926).

Simon, G. T. and Burke, J. S. Electron microscopy of the spleen. III. Erythro-leukophagocytosis. Am. J. Path. *58*: 451–469 (1970).

Simon, G. and Pictet, R. Étude au microscope électronique des sinus spléniques et des cordons de Billroth chez le rat. Acta Anat. *57*: 163–171 (1964).

Snook, T. A comparative study of the vascular arrangements in mammalian spleens. Am. J. Anat. *87*: 31–77 (1950).

Snook, T. The histology of the vascular terminations in the rabbit spleen. Anat. Rec. *130*: 711–729 (1958).

Snook, T. Studies of the perifollicular region of the rat's spleen. Anat. Rec. *148*: 149–160 (1964).

Stutte, H. J. Nature of human spleen red pulp cells with special reference to sinus lining cells. Z. Zellforsch. *91*: 300–314 (1968).

Thomas, C. E. An electron- and light-microscope study of sinus structure in perfused rabbit and dog spleens. Am. J. Anat. *120*: 527–552 (1967).

Weiss, L. The structure of the intermediate vascular pathways in the spleen of rabbits. Am. J. Anat. *113*: 51–92 (1963).

Weiss, L. The white pulp of the spleen. Bull. Johns Hopkins Hosp. *115*: 99–173 (1964).

Zwillenberg, L. O. and Zwillenberg, H. H. Zur Struktur und Funktion der Hülsenkapillaren in der Milz. Z. Zellforsch. *59*: 908–921 (1963).

Fig. 18-19. Detail of venous sinus. Longitudinal section of wall. Enlargement of rectangle in Fig. 18-17. Spleen. Rat. E.M. X 15,000. **1.** Lumen of venous sinus. **2.** Nucleus of littoral (lining) cell. **3.** Erythrocyte. **4.** Young erythrocyte (reticulocyte) passing through a stoma in the wall of the venous sinus from the interstitial space of the red pulp to the lumen of the sinus. **5.** Bundles of delicate reticular fibrils. **6.** Mitochondria. **7.** Bundles of cytoplasmic filaments. **8.** Nuclei of small lymphocytes. **9.** Golgi zone.

Fig. 18-20. Detail of wall of cross-sectioned venous sinus. Spleen. Rat. E.M. X 15,000. **1.** Lumen of sinus. **2.** Littoral cells. **3.** Stoma (opening) between two littoral (lining) cells. **4.** Erythrocyte passing through stoma. **5.** Narrow strand of basal lamina. **6.** Parts of reticular cell. **7.** Interstitial space of red pulp. **8.** Cross-sectioned cytoplasmic filaments. **9.** Junction of two littoral cells. **10.** Plane of section in Fig. 18-21.

Fig. 18-21. Stoma in the wall of venous sinus. Tangential section of littoral cells through plane indicated by dotted line between 10 and 10 in Fig. 18-20. Section No. 139 in a series of 500 sections. Spleen. Rat. E.M. X 29,000. **1.** Erythrocyte. **2.** Cytoplasm of littoral cells. **3.** Cell membranes of adjoining littoral cells. **4.** Stoma represents a true, probably permanent slit-like opening between two littoral cells. **5.** Pinocytotic vesicles. **6.** Lysosomes. **7.** Mitochondrion. **8.** Free ribosomes. **9.** Cytoplasmic filaments.

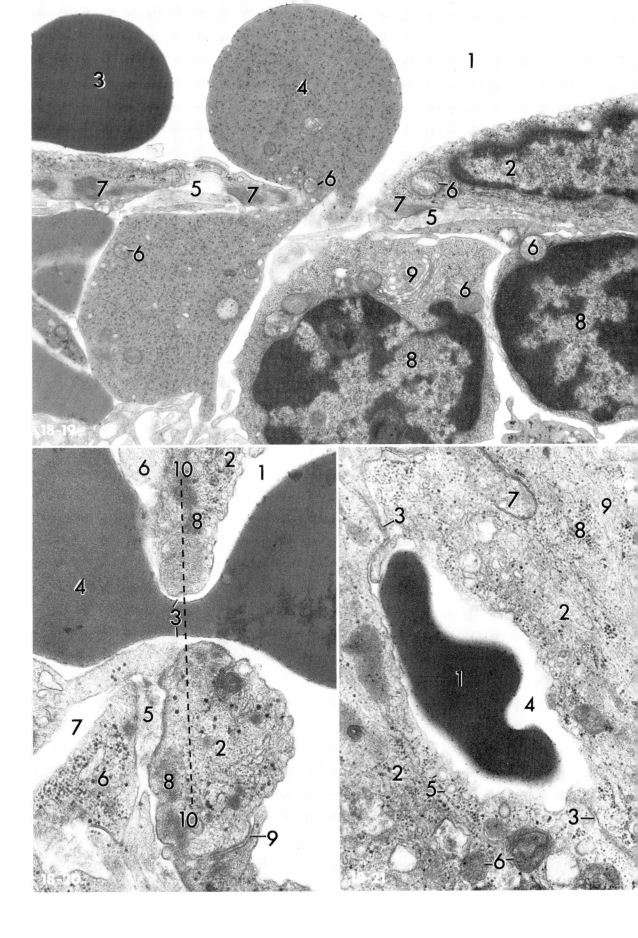

19 Thymus

The thymus gland is an accumulation of lymphoid tissue located in the superior mediastinum immediately behind the sternum. The function of the thymus has only recently been elucidated. It serves as a source of lymphocytes during the late fetal and early postnatal periods when the the thymic lymphocytes populate other lymphoid organs such as lymph nodes and spleen. Thymus is relatively large in the fetus, and reaches its maximum size during adolescence. An involution (atrophy or regression) starts after puberty and continues for several decades. By the fifth decade the thymus is largely replaced by adipose tissue.

GENERAL

The thymus has two elongated **lobes,** each surrounded by a thin connective tissue capsule. The capsule sends narrow connective tissue septa into the lymphoid tissue, dividing each lobe into numerous **lobules.** (Fig. 19-1) Each lobule consists of an outer **cortex** and an inner **medulla.** (Fig. 19-2) The medullary regions of the many lobules are in communication with each other. There is a **stroma** of epithelial reticular cells associated with delicate bundles of reticular and fine collagenous fibrils. The stroma is sparse in the cortex and rich in the medulla. In the meshwork of the reticular cells are located the thymic lymphocytes which form the lymphatic **parenchyma** of the thymus. The cortex contains numerous lymphocytes, and the medulla few. In contrast to other lymphoid organs, there are no germinal centers in the thymus under normal conditions, nor are there any afferent lymphatic vessels or lymphatic sinuses. The thymus receives its **blood supply** from branches of the internal thoracic arteries which enter at the hilus of the thymus. They are distributed throughout the gland via the connective tissue septa, and from there penetrate the medulla and the cortex, breaking up into a capillary bed in these regions. Postcapillary venules are prominent in the medulla, emptying into

veins which leave the thymus through the hilus.

DEVELOPMENT

The thymus develops as an outgrowth of the epithelium of the third branchial pouches. The accumulation of epithelial cells becomes surrounded by a thin sheath of mesodermal connective tissue. It is generally believed that mesenchymal cells from this sheath, or hemocytoblast-like cells from the blood islets of the yolk sac, enter the thymus anlage to mix with the epithelial reticular cells. In this microenvironment, the migrating cells proliferate and differentiate to form thymic lymphocytes. Yet another possibility is that the earliest thymic lymphocytes are derived by transformation from thymic epithelial reticular cells, although present evidence for this hypothesis is less convincing.

EPITHELIAL RETICULAR CELLS

The epithelial reticular cells form an interconnected meshwork by the junction of long and branching cytoplasmic processes. (Fig. 19-7) The nucleus of these cells is large and pale staining. The cytoplasm is abundant. It contains a small number of tonofibrillar bundles near the nucleus and at the periphery of the cell where they tend to insert into desmosomes connecting adjacent epithelial reticular cells. There is an average number of mitochondria, numerous ribosomes, and clusters of particulate glycogen; and in

Fig. 19-1. Thymus. Kitten. L.M. X 22.
　1. Capsule at surface of gland. **2.** Connective tissue septa. **3.** Blood vessels. **4.** Lobules.
Fig. 19-2. Part of thymic lobule. Enlargement of area similar to rectangle in Fig. 19-1. Thymus. Kitten. L.M. X 215. **1.** Capsule at surface of lobule. **2.** Cortex. **3.** Medulla. **4.** Hassall's (thymic) corpuscles.
Fig. 19-3. Survey of thymic lobule. Enlargement of area similar to rectangle in Fig. 19-2. Thymus. Kitten. E.M. X 630. **1.** Capsule. **2.** Cortex. **3.** Medulla. **4.** Hassall's corpuscles. **5.** Blood capillaries.

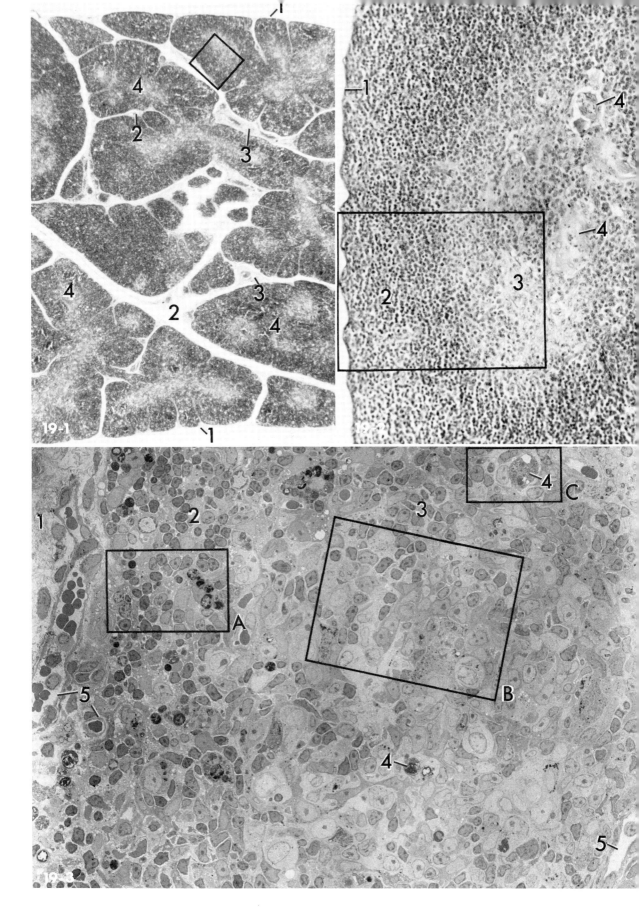

19-1

19-2

19-3

some areas, a well-developed granular endoplasmic reticulum. Several kinds of cytoplasmic inclusions are present in these cells: 1) large, dense granules, reminiscent of secondary lysosomes; 2) small, dense spherical granules, suggestive of secretory granules of the adenohypophysis; and 3) nests of spherical vacuoles, uniform in size, indented by microvillous projections of the surrounding membrane, and enclosing an amorphous material of moderate density similar to droplets of mucus in a goblet cell. The function of the epithelial reticular cells is primarily that of support or inductive instruction for the lymphoid cells. However, it cannot be excluded that they may also be responsible for the synthesis and secretion of a lymphocytic stimulating hormone, as will be discussed below. There is a slight possibility that the epithelial reticular cells may develop into macrophages and/or constitute the precursors of the thymic lymphocytes. The epithelial nature of the reticular cells is clearly expressed by the phenomenon of their forming spheres of concentrically arranged cells, the **thymic (Hassall's) corpuscles.** These are bodies which vary in size from 20 μ to 200 μ, the center cells of which may become keratinized, calcified, or cystic. (Fig. 19-10)

MACROPHAGES

The macrophages of the thymus vary in number but are generally most common in the cortical region. (Fig. 19-4) Their structure is similar to that of fixed macrophages in the spleen. Their function is to eliminate and digest thymic lymphocytes; macrophages are therefore extremely numerous during an acute involution accompanying certain diseases. Small lymphocytes in varying stages of decomposition are usually seen in the cytoplasm of the macrophage. The detecting mechanism in selecting lymphocytes for this elimination process is not known.

THYMIC LYMPHOCYTES (T CELLS)

The most common thymic lymphocyte, T cell (or thymocyte), is a small round cell

which is indistinguishable in structure from small lymphocytes elsewhere. (Fig. 19-6) The round nucleus has a dense chromatin network. The cytoplasm, limited to a thin coat around the nucleus, contains numerous ribosomes but is otherwise devoid of organelles, except for a few small mitochondria. By their concentration in the outer zone of the thymus, the thymocytes contribute to the formation of the cortex. In the medulla are located thymic lymphocytes of medium and large size. Also these cells are structurally similar to medium and large lymphocytes in other lymphoid organs. The thymic lymphocytes multiply freely, but move about in the process. This explains partly why true germinal centers do not arise in the thymus. Plasma cells are generally not present in the cortex or the medulla, but are occasionally encountered in the connective tissue septa.

CAPILLARIES AND VENULES

The capillaries and venules of the thymus have a non-fenestrated, continuous endothelium. Peripherally, there is a thin basal lamina and a pericapillary connective tissue space with fine collagenous and reticu-

Fig. 19-4. Survey of thymic cortex. Enlargement of area similar to rectangle (A) in Fig. 19-3. Thymus. Kitten. E.M. X 1800. **1.** Small thymic lymphocytes. **2.** Medium-sized thymic lymphocytes. **3.** Nuclei of epithelial reticular cells. **4.** Macrophage. **5.** Thymic lymphocytes with dense marginated nuclear chromatin. **6.** Lumen of blood capillary.

Fig. 19-5. Detail of thymic cortex. Kitten. E.M. X 4500. **1.** Nuclei of small thymic lymphocytes. **2.** Nuclei of medium-sized thymic lymphocytes. **3.** Nucleus of epithelial reticular cell. **4.** Thymic lymphocyte in mitosis. **5.** Nucleus of small thymic lymphocyte with marginated nucleoplasm, indicating imminent cell death. **6.** Digestive vacuole or secondary lysosome in cytoplasm of macrophage.

Fig. 19-6. Small thymic lymphocyte (T cell) from cortex of thymus. Cell width 5 μ. Thymus. Kitten. E.M. X 18,000.
1. Heterochromatin. **2.** Euchromatin.
3. Nuclear pores. **4.** Nuclear membrane.
5. Ribosomes. **6.** Golgi zone. **7.** Mitochondria.
8. Surface (cell) membrane.

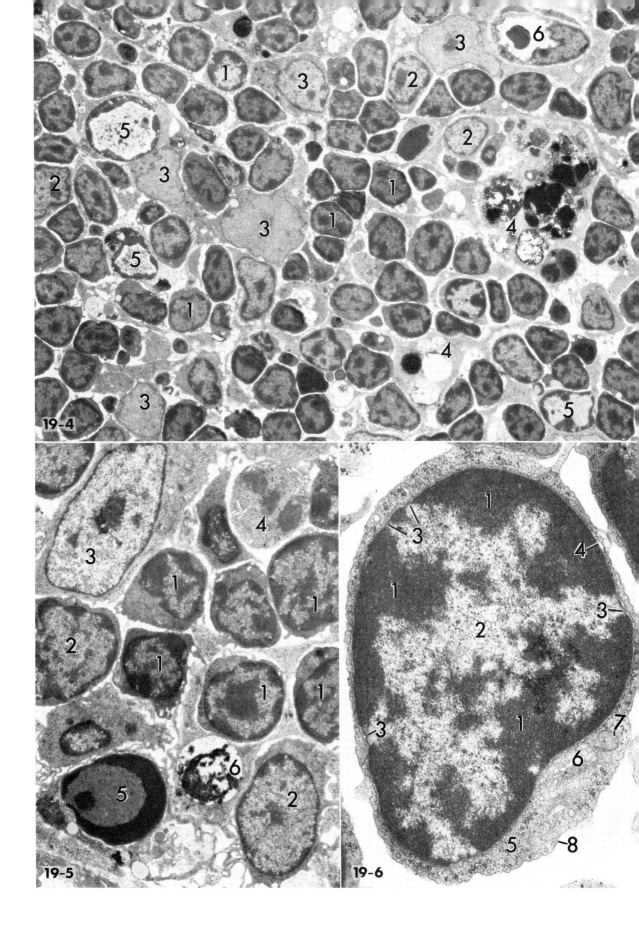

lar fibrils. (Fig. 19-12) As a rule, pericytes or epithelial reticular cells form a sleeve around the capillaries and venules. Thymic lymphocytes are seen to penetrate the vascular wall, particularly in relation to the postcapillary venules. The direction of this penetration has not been established, but it is assumed that the majority of the thymic lymphocytes leave the thymic parenchyma across the wall of the postcapillary venules during late fetal and early postnatal life. In adolescence, circulating lymphocytes, so-called B cells which are immunologically incompetent, may enter the thymic parenchyma in a process similar to what happens in lymph nodes. A structural blood-thymic barrier therefore does not seem to exist. From a functional point of view, there exists in early life a blood-thymic barrier which relates to the alleged inability of antigens to reach the thymic parenchyma in concentrations high enough to stimulate an antibody formation within the thymic parenchyma.

FUNCTIONS

The primary function of the thymus during late fetal life and early infancy is to produce thymic lymphocytes and to populate other lymphoid organs, forming stem cells for all lymphocytes. It is postulated that the thymic lymphocytes become coded to the individual's own classes of proteins or according to certain groups of antigens. Once the thymic lymphocyte encounters a foreign protein outside of the thymus it reacts by producing antibodies after being converted to plasma cells. As indicated, plasma cells do not occur in the thymic parenchyma. Therefore, antibodies are probably not produced within the thymus. The capacity of lymphocytes to respond to antigens may be induced throughout life by the thymus. It is thought that lymphocytes referred to as B cells, which are not antigen-reactive, are derived from the stem cell pool in the bone marrow. Once in circulation, these cells, which structurally resemble small lymphocytes, reach the thymus where they remain temporarily for induction. They then migrate to lymph nodes and spleen as T cells to become progenitors of immunologically competent cells. There is some indication that a humoral factor is produced in the thymus which is capable of stimulating lymphocytopoiesis in other lymphoid organs. The origin and nature of this humoral factor is not understood. It may be derived from the breakdown of lymphocytes by thymic macrophages, or it could be synthesized by the epithelial reticular cells. Further studies are required to explore this problem.

References

Ackerman, G. A. and Hostetler, J. R. Morphological studies of the embryonic rabbit thymus: the in situ epithelial versus the extrathymic derivation of the initial population of lymphocytes in the embryonic thymus. Anat. Rec. *166*: 27–46 (1970).

Burnet, M. The thymus gland. Sci. American *207*: 50–57 (1962).

Chapman, W. L. and Allen, J. R. The fine structure of the thymus of the fetal and neonatal monkey (Macaca mulatta). Z. Zellforsch. *114*: 220–233 (1971).

Fig. 19-7. Survey of thymic medulla. Enlargement of area similar to rectangle (B) in Fig. 19-3. Thymus. Kitten. E.M. X 1800. **1.** Small thymic lymphocytes. **2.** Medium-sized thymic lymphocytes. **3.** Large thymic lymphocyte. **4.** Epithelial reticular cells. **5.** Macrophages. Note that the identification of these cells is based on an analysis of each cell at higher magnifications.

Fig. 19-8. Epithelial reticular cell. Enlargement of rectangle in Fig. 19-7. Thymus. Kitten. E.M. X 13,000. **1.** Nucleus of epithelial reticular cell. **2.** Nucleolus. **3.** Desmosomes. **4.** Mitochondria. **5.** Cytoplasmic filaments. **6.** Ribosomes. **7.** Particulate glycogen. **8.** Small granules, most of which represent primary lysosomes. **9.** Adjacent epithelial reticular cell. Note that the reticular cell of the thymus is not necessarily in contact with reticular and collagenous fibrils in contrast to the reticular cells in lymph nodes and spleen.

Fig. 19-9. Small dense spherical granules in epithelial reticular cell. Enlargement of area similar to rectangle in Fig. 19-8. Thymus. Kitten. E.M. X 96,000. **1.** Core of granule. **2.** Trilaminar boundary membrane.

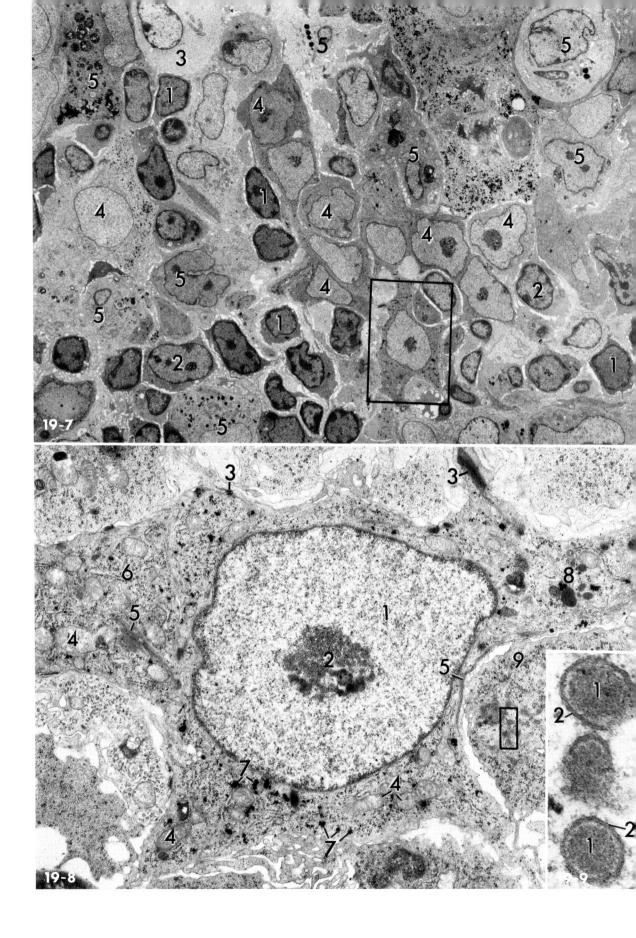

Clark, S. L., Jr. The thymus in mice of strain 129/J, studied with the electron microscope. Am. J. Anat. *112*: 1–34 (1963).

Everett, N. B. and Tyler (Caffrey), R. W. Lymphopoiesis in the thymus and other tissues: functional implications. Int. Rev. Cytol. *22*: 205–286 (1967).

Gad, P. and Clark, S. L., Jr. Involution and regeneration of the thymus in mice, induced by bacterial endotoxin and studied by quantitative histology and electron microscopy. Am. J. Anat. *122*: 573–606 (1968).

Goldstein, G. and Mackay, I. R. The Thymus, pp. 1–352. Warren H. Green, St. Louis, 1969.

Haelst, U. G. J. van. Light and electron microscopic study of the normal and pathological thymus of the rat. I. The normal thymus. Z. Zellforsch. *77*: 534–553 (1967).

Haelst, U. G. J. van. Light and electron microscopic study of the normal and pathological thymus of the rat. III. A mesenchymal histiocytic type of cell. Z. Zellforsch. *99*: 198–209 (1969).

Hoshino, T. Electron microscopic studies of the epithelial reticular cells of the mouse thymus. Z. Zellforsch. *59*: 513–529 (1963).

Ito, T. and Hoshino, T. Fine structure of the epithelial reticular cells of the medulla of the thymus in the golden hamster. Z. Zellforsch. *69*: 311–318 (1966).

Izard, J. Ultrastructure of the thymic reticulum in guinea pig. Cytological aspects of the problem of the thymic secretion. Anat. Rec. *155*: 117–132 (1966).

Kohnen, P. and Weiss, L. An electron microscopic study of thymic corpuscles in the guinea pig and the mouse. Anat. Rec. *148*: 29–57 (1964).

Fig. 19-10. Survey of Hassall's corpuscle. Enlargement of area similar to rectangle (C) in Fig. 19-3. Thymus. Kitten. E.M. X 4500. **1.** Nuclei of concentrically arranged epithelial reticular cells. **2.** Keratohyalin granules. **3.** Bundles of cytoplasmic filaments (tonofilaments). **4.** Lipid droplets. **5.** Fully keratinized epithelial reticular cell. **6.** Slightly cystic center of Hassall's corpuscle.

Fig. 19-11. Enlargement of rectangle in Fig. 19-10. Thymus. Kitten. E.M. X 18,000. **1.** Keratohyalin granule. **2.** Cross-sectioned bundles of tonofilaments. **3.** Intercellular space. **4.** Desmosomes. **5.** Membrane-coating granules. **6.** Cholesterol crystal space. **7.** Keratinized cell.

Fig. 19-12. Cross section of capillary in the medulla of the thymus. Kitten. E.M. X 4800. **1.** Lumen. **2.** Nucleus of endothelial cell. **3.** Pericytes. **4.** Basement membrane consisting of fine collagenous fibrils. **5.** Nuclei of thymic lymphocytes. **6.** Epithelial reticular cells.

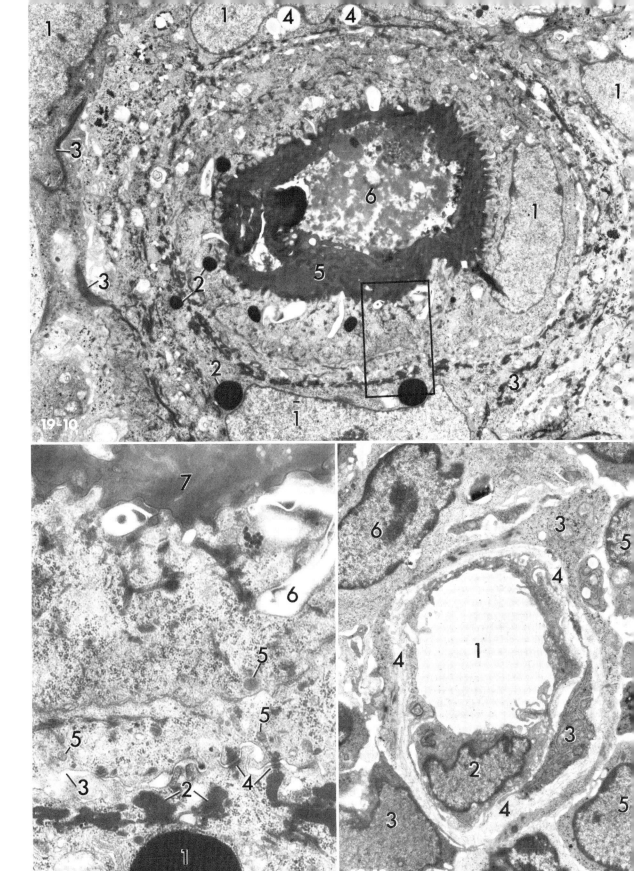

20 Hypophysis

The hypophysis (pituitary gland) is an endocrine organ, suspended from the ventral surface of the forebrain. It develops from ectoderm of two different sources. Structurally and functionally there are therefore two completely different parts, the large adenohypophysis and the small neurohypophysis. The **adenohypophysis** (glandular part) secretes several hormones, most of which are trophic, influencing the activity of the adrenal cortex, thyroid, testis, ovary, mammary glands, and general cell growth. The hormones secreted by some of these organs in turn influence the adenohypophysis in a reciprocal endocrine regulation. Some of the secretory activity of the adenohypophysis is in response to stimulation from the hypothalamus via the portal vascular system.

The **neurohypophysis** (nervous part) secretes one hormone which stimulates uterine contraction. It influences the amount of urine through another, the antidiuretic hormone, acting on the distal tubules and the collecting tubules. The hormones are elaborated by nerve cells in the supraoptic and paraventricular nuclei, transported through nerve fibers to club-like swellings and nerve terminals near capillaries in various regions of the posterior lobe where the secretion is stored or discharged. This process is called **neurosecretion.** Therefore, the pituitary is an important organ in the integration of nervous and endocrine functions.

GENERAL

The pituitary is a round organ, as large as a fresh garden pea. It is surrounded by a fibrous capsule which is an extension of the dura mater of the brain; and the diaphragm stretching across the sella turcica of the sphenoid bone in which the pituitary is lodged. A stalk connects the gland with the hypothalamus. The large anterior lobe is attached to the smaller posterior lobe by the pars intermedia, and by the pars tuberalis which surrounds the infundibulum. (Fig. 20-2) The anterior lobe stretches out laterally, whereas the posterior lobe forms a rounded structure in the sagittal plane. There is very little connective tissue in the parenchyma, and the lobes are not divided by septa. The general architecture of the pituitary is seen in Fig. 20-1, and a summary of parts and terms follows:

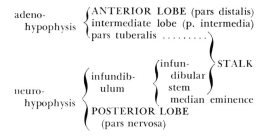

DEVELOPMENT

The **adenohypophysis** develops from evagination of the oral ectoderm (Rathke's pouch). The pouch loses its contact with the oral cavity and first forms a vesicle

Fig. 20-1. Schematic drawing of the pituitary and the hypothalamo-hypophysial tract. **1.** Anterior commissure and lamina terminalis. **2.** Optic chiasm. **3.** Tuber cinereum. **4.** Median eminence. **5.** Infundibular stalk. **6.** Mamillary body. **7.** Third ventricle. **8.** Pars tuberalis. **9.** Anterior lobe. **10.** Posterior lobe. **11.** Pars intermedia. **12.** Cleft. **13.** Superior hypophysial arteries. **14.** Portal vessels. **15.** Sinusoids of adenohypophysis. **16.** Veins to cavernous sinuses. **17.** Inferior hypophysial arteries. **18.** Veins to cavernous sinuses. **19.** Nerve cells in supraoptic nuclei. **20.** Nerve cells in paraventricular nuclei. **21.** Nerve cells in median eminence.

Fig. 20-2. Midsagittal section of pituitary. Human. L.M. X 4. **1.** Anterior lobe. **2.** Pars intermedia. **3.** Posterior lobe. **4.** Infundibular stalk.

Fig. 20-3. Survey of adenohypophysis. Human. L.M. X 340. **1.** Sinusoids (capillaries). **2.** Cords of endocrine secretory cells. **3.** Intercordal spaces. **4.** Follicle.

Fig. 20-4. Enlargement of area similar to rectangle in Fig. 20-3. Rat. E.M. X 1700. **1.** Capillaries (sinusoids). **2.** Intercellular space. **3.** Intercordal space with some collagenous fibrils. **4.** Somatotroph. **5.** Mammotroph. **6.** Gonadotroph. **7.** Thyrotroph. **8.** Adrenocorticotroph. **9.** Precursor (chromophobe) cell. The identification of these cells cannot be made accurately at this magnification. It is based on the study of these cells at higher magnifications.

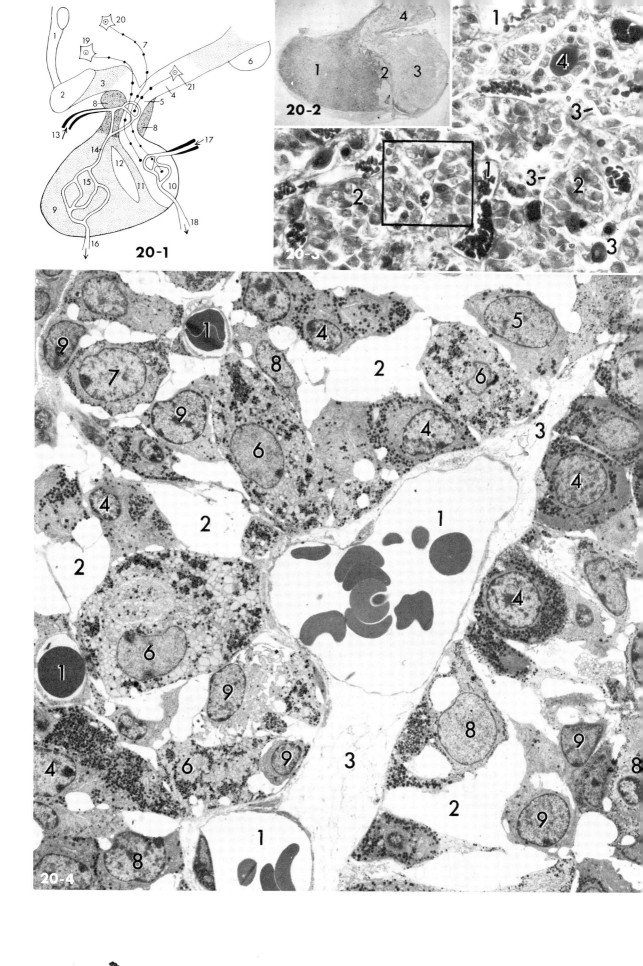

20-1

20-2

20-3

20-4

which later becomes a solid cell mass. The cavity of the vesicle at times remains as a narrow transverse slit in front of the thin posterior wall of the vesicle. This wall becomes the pars intermedia. The **neurohypophysis** develops from an infundibular, hypothalamic down-growth of the floor of the diencephalon (3rd ventricle). The down-growth, originally hollow, loses its cavity by the thickening of its walls. As a final stage in the development of the pituitary, two processes of the adenohypophysis wrap around the infundibular stalk to form the pars tuberalis.

BLOOD SUPPLY

From the internal carotid artery and the circle of Willis, the pituitary receives **inferior hypophysial arteries** which supply the posterior lobe, and **superior hypophysial arteries** which form a capillary network in the stalk. From the stalk, the blood is conducted via venous capillaries to the anterior lobe, the so-called **hypophysial portal system** of the pituitary. In the adenohypophysis these venous capillaries give rise to a widely interconnected network of thin-walled large capillaries, usually referred to as **sinusoids.** (Fig. 20-4) The endothelium of arterial and venous capillaries, as well as the sinusoids, are of the fenestrated, closed type with a thin enveloping basal lamina. Contrary to earlier statements elsewhere, the endothelium of this hypophysial microvascular bed does not phagocytose, and therefore should not be included in the reticuloendothelial system. As is generally the case, accompanying pericytes do phagocytose upon intense stimulation. The venous drainage of the pituitary occurs through **hypophysial veins** leading from the anterior and posterior lobes to the cavernous sinus.

Adenohypophysis

The anterior lobe consists of loose cords of cells surrounded by a rich network of large capillaries (sinusoids). The cells vary in size but are generally round or polygonal. (Fig. 20-3) Intercellular spaces are often wide. The cell cords are enveloped by a thin parenchymal basal lamina and a thin network of delicate collagenous and reticular fibrils. The epithelial cells vary in size and shape and there is great variation in their content of secretory granules. Seven hormones have been identified as being secreted by the adenohypophysis, and several of these hormones have been positively traced to specific epithelial cells. It should be remembered that many years of work based on a variety of staining techniques for light and electron microscopy have resulted in the following account of the architecture of the epithelial cells of the adenohypophysis. The old classification of acidophils, basophils, and chromophobes has been maintained here so that the present description can be used in conjunction with other text references.

ACIDOPHILS (ALPHA CELLS)

Among cells with acidophilic secretory granules are the somatotrophs and the mammotrophs. On the average, the acidophils make up about 40% of the cells of the anterior lobe.

Somatotrophs. These cells secrete growth hormone (STH) which influences the growth of chondroblasts in the epiphyseal cartilage of long bones. The cells are medium-sized, round or oval. The nucleus is round and large. There are a few round or oval mitochondria, a well-developed Golgi zone, a rather extensive granular endoplasmic reticulum with long, narrow cisternae, and an abundance of free ribo-

Fig. 20-5. Survey of several types of epithelial cells in the adenohypophysis. Rat. E.M. X 5300. At this magnification, cell types can be recognized more readily than in Fig. 20-4, based on the size, shape and number of secretory granules. **1.** Nucleus of capillary endothelial cell. **2.** Capillary lumen. **3.** Intercellular space. **4.** Nuclei of somatotrophs. **5.** Nucleus of mammotroph. **6.** Nuclei of thyrotrophs. **7.** Nuclei of adrenocorticotrophs. **8.** Nuclei of chromophobe precursor cells.

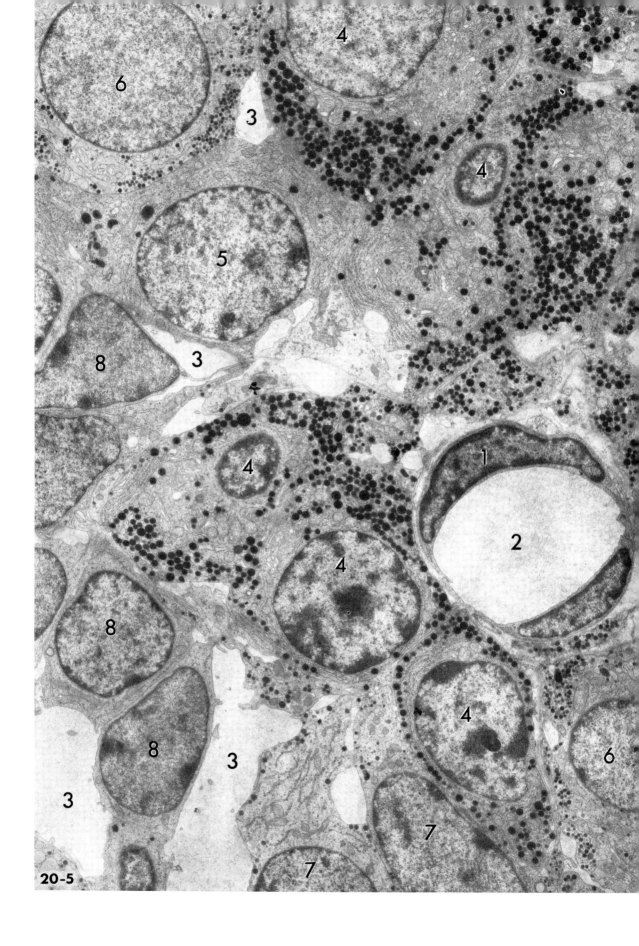

20-5

somes. The secretory granules are very numerous, spherical, and generally of equal size, ranging from 3000 Å to 3500 Å. (Fig. 20-6) The core of the granule is highly electron-dense, and enveloped by a tight fitting membrane.

Mammotrophs. These cells secrete a lactogenic hormone (prolactin, LTH) which initiates and maintains the secretion of milk in the mammary gland after pregnancy. It also stimulates the secretion of progesterone by the corpus luteum of the ovary. The cells occur mostly in the posterolateral parts of the anterior lobe and are greatly increased in number during and after pregnancy. They are small and round, and occasionally indented by another cell to give a U-shaped outline. The Golgi zone is small and mitochondria are few. The granular endoplasmic reticulum is sparse, occurring in short, flat profiles. The secretory granules are sparse, electron-dense, eliptic, with diameters ranging between 6000 Å and 9000 Å. (Fig. 20-7)

BASOPHILS (BETA CELLS)

The basophil cells are generally larger than the acidophil. There are only about 10% basophils. The secretory granules are basophilic and periodic-acid-Schiff (PAS) positive. To this group belong the gonadotrophs and the thyrotrophs.

Gonadotrophs. These cells secrete two hormones, the follicle stimulating hormone (FSH) and the luteinizing hormone (LH). The former stimulates, in females, the growth and maturation of ovarian follicles, and in males the spermatogenesis in the seminiferous tubules of the testis. The luteinizing hormone in females causes ovulation by rupturing the follicle and stimulating the development of a functional corpus luteum in the ovary. In males, this hormone stimulates the interstitial Leydig cells of the testis to produce testosterone, which in turn, stimulates growth and secretion of cells in the prostate, seminal vesicles, preputial glands, kidney, and skin. It is presently not fully established if there are two cell types or

only one secreting the two hormones. The analysis of the fine structural architecture has not established a difference, with the exception of the nucleus, which is round in the FSH-cells and infolded in the LH-cells. The gonadotrophic cells are among the largest of the anterior lobe. These cells have a rounded shape. The Golgi zone is well developed, and the granular endoplasmic reticulum predominates the cytoplasm with its many small, rounded or irregular cisternae with a relatively dense content. Secretory granules are numerous, highly electron-dense, round and with great variation in size, ranging from 1000 Å to 3000 Å. (Fig. 20-8)

Thyrotrophs. These cells secrete thyrotrophic hormone (TSH), stimulating all phases of thyroxin synthesis, storage, and release. The cell is fairly large, with a polygonal, irregular, almost stellate, shape. The nucleus is large, the Golgi zone compact, and the mitochondria relatively wide and abundant. The granular endoplasmic reticulum is sparse but increases considerably after thyroidectomy. The

Fig. 20-6. Detail of somatotrophs. Adenohypophysis. Rat. E.M. X 9500. **1.** Nucleus. **2.** Cell membranes. **3.** Granular endoplasmic reticulum with narrow cisternae. **4.** Mitochondria. **5.** Secretory granules (3000 Å–3500 Å).

Fig. 20-7. Detail of mammotroph. Posterolateral lobe of adenohypophysis. Rat. E.M. X 9000. **1.** Nucleus. **2.** Cell membranes. **3.** Granular endoplasmic reticulum. **4.** Mitochondria. **5.** Golgi complex. **6.** Secretory granules (6000 Å–9000 Å).

Fig. 20-8. Detail of gonadotroph. Adenohypophysis. Rat. E.M. X 9000. **1.** Nucleus. **2.** Cell membranes. **3.** Granular endoplasmic reticulum with dilated cisternae. **4.** Mitochondria. **5.** Golgi complex. **6.** Presecretory granules. **7.** Secretory granules (1000 Å–3000 Å).

Fig. 20-9. Detail of thyrotrophs. Adenohypophysis. Rat. E.M. X 9000. **1.** Nuclei of thyrotrophs. **2.** Cell membranes. **3.** Granular endoplasmic reticulum. **4.** Mitochondria. **5.** Golgi complex. **6.** Secretory granules (1000 Å–1600 Å). **7.** Nucleus of precursor cell.

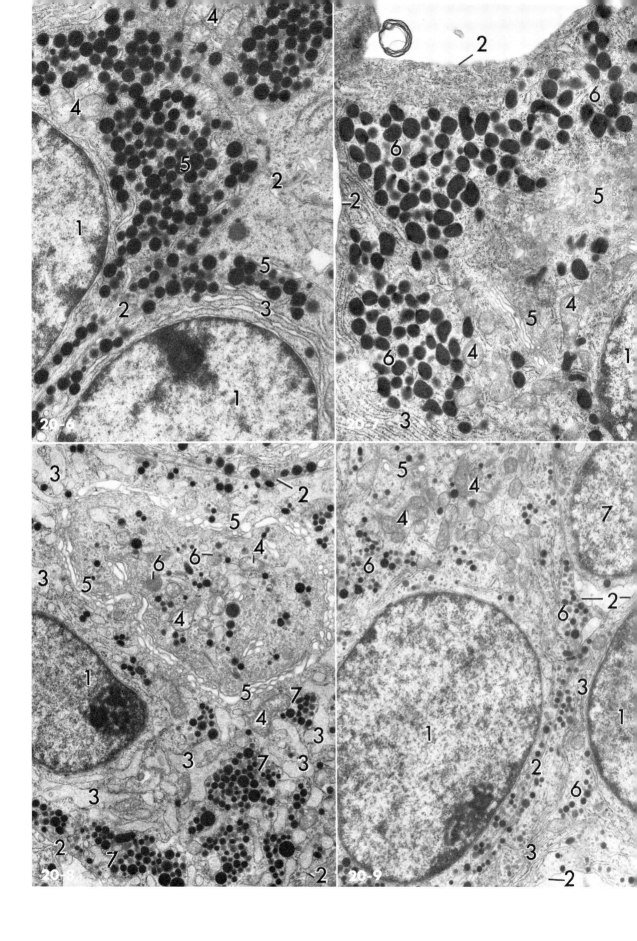

granules are fairly numerous, arranged mainly in a wide band around the cell periphery. They are moderately electron-dense. Most granules have a tightly adhering limiting membrane but some have a "haloed" appearance. They are among the smallest in the anterior lobe, ranging from 1000 Å to 1600 Å. (Fig. 20-9) The cells are quite similar to the ACTH-cells with some exceptions.

CHROMOPHOBES

These cells are generally small with little cytoplasm and a very small number of secretory granules which can be seen only with the electron microscope. To this group belong: 1) adrenocorticotrophic cells which are relatively large; and 2) small cells which are considered resting cells or stem cells (precursors) for any cell within the anterior lobe.

Corticotrophs. The cells secrete adrenocorticotrophic hormone (ACTH) which stimulates the release of glucocorticoids from the zona fasciculata of the adrenal cortex. The cells are large, irregular or stellate-shaped with long ramifying cytoplasmic processes which reach far and generally terminate near or on the wall of sinusoids. The cytoplasm is exceptionally pale and electron-lucent. The mitochondria are small and sparse. The Golgi zone is well developed and scattered throughout the cell. The granular endoplasmic reticulum is sparse, with narrow cisternae. The secretory granules are relatively sparse, and occur in a single layer subjacent to the cell membrane. The granules average 2000 Å in diameter. (Fig. 20-10)

Precursor cells. To this category belong a variety of small cells with little cytoplasm in which only a few and very small granules can be seen under the electron microscope. (Fig. 20-5) At the moment, the knowledge of lines of differentiation is insufficient to warrant a detailed discussion.

PARS INTERMEDIA

This part of the adenohypophysis is poorly developed in man but is retained better in many mammals. A melanocyte stimulating hormone (MSH) which is chemically closely related to ACTH has been identified in man. It influences the production of melanin. It is presently not known if the cells of the pars intermedia or the corticotrophs secrete this hormone. In the rat, pars intermedia is composed of densely packed polygonal cells which contain many secretory granules, averaging 2000 Å in diameter. (Fig. 20-11)

SECRETORY PROCESS

The hormones of the adenohypophysis are either non-carbohydrate proteins (STH, prolactin, ACTH, MSH) or glycoproteins (TSH, FSH, LH). Their synthesis requires therefore both granular endoplasmic reticulum and Golgi membranes. Generally, the precursor secretory granules appear within the Golgi membranes and vesicles (Fig. 20-12), and subsequently aggregate in the peripheral cytoplasm.

Fig. 20-10. Detail of corticotroph. Adenohypophysis. Rat. E.M. X 9000. **1.** Nucleus of corticotroph. **2.** Nuclei of precursor cells. **3.** Cell membranes. **4.** Granular endoplasmic reticulum. **5.** Mitochondria. **6.** Golgi complex. **7.** Marginated layer of secretory granules (2000 Å).

Fig. 20-11. Detail of cell in pars intermedia of the pituitary. Rat. E.M. X 9000. **1.** Nuclei. **2.** Cell membranes. **3.** Mitochondria. **4.** Secretory granules (2000 Å).

Fig. 20-12. Detail of gonadotroph. Adenohypophysis. Rat. E.M. X 87,000. **1.** Mitochondria. **2.** Ribosomes. **3.** Cisternae of granular endoplasmic reticulum. **4.** Golgi complex. **5.** Presecretory granules forming within the Golgi saccules. **6.** Mature secretory granule. **7.** Limiting membrane.

Fig. 20-13. Detail of gonadotroph at the moment of discharging secretory granules. Adenohypophysis. Rat. E.M. X 86,000. **1.** Mitochondrion. **2.** Cell membrane. **3.** Secretory granules. **4.** Discharging secretory granules. **5.** Basal lamina of cell cords. **6.** Capillary (sinusoidal) lumen. **7.** Fenestrated (closed) endothelium of capillary (sinusoid). **8.** Capillary basal lamina. **9.** Intercordal space with fine collagenous fibrils.

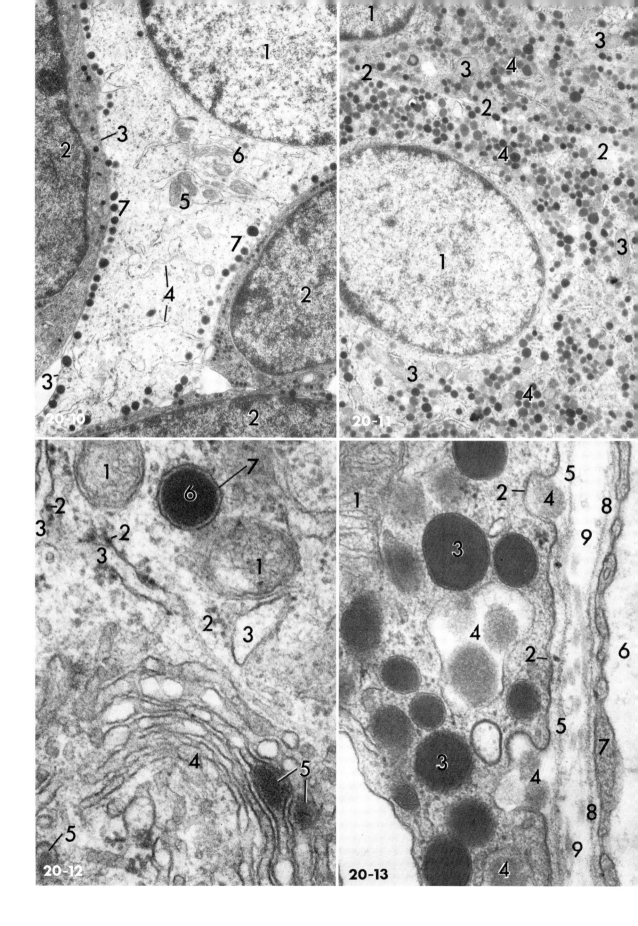

The release of the secretory granules occurs by a fusion of the limiting membrane of the granule with the cell membrane. (Fig. 20-13) It is believed that the cells have a cyclic secretory activity of synthesis, storage, and release, reflected in the great variation in number and size of secretory granules that can be observed at any time. However, cellular granularity is not necessarily an exact index of secretory activity, since the number of granules depends upon the balance between the rate of production and the rate of discharge.

Neurohypophysis

The neurohypophysis consists of the median eminence, the infundibular stem, and the posterior lobe (pars nervosa of the pituitary). All parts contain a multitude of nerve fibers, capillaries, some connective tissue stroma, particularly around the microvascular bed, and the characteristic cells of the neurohypophysis, the pituicytes. (Figs. 20-14, 20-15, 20-16)

The **nerve cells** are located in the hypothalamus, and more specifically, in the paraventricular nuclei, the supraoptic nuclei, and the tuber cinereum. The nerve **fibers** terminate at various levels in the neurohypophysis mostly near the capillaries. The nerve cells and the fibers form a system which functions as a **neurosecretory organ.** Neurosecretory (elementary) granules, 1000 Å–3000 Å wide, are synthesized by the Nissl substance in the perikaryon and passed peripherally through the nerve fibers. (Fig. 20-17) Huge accumulations of granules along the nerve fiber are recognized as **Herring bodies.** (Fig. 20-18) The granules contain the specific polypeptide hormones of the neurohypophysis, the **oxytocin** and the **vasopressin** (antiduretic hormone; ADH) which are bound to the carrier protein neurophysin in the granules. The speed and actual mechanism of transport of the granules along the nerve fibers are not fully understood. These nerve cells seem to represent a mixture of elongated glandular cells and nerve cells which have become specialized for secretion. The nerve fibers contain numerous microtubules, and it is possible that these tubules facilitate the transport of the granules in the same way that it takes place in the cytoplasmic processes of invertebrate chromatophores in which the pigment granules are transported back and forth by means of microtubules. The mechanism of **hormone release** is also not fully understood. It is conceivable that the release can occur at any place along the nerve process. Upon stimulation, the dense core of the neurosecretory granules becomes less dense or disappears, leaving behind essentially a vesicle. The release of the core must occur through a diffusion of the liberated hormones, since no merger of the granule-limiting membrane with the cell membrane has been observed. The hormones diffuse out of the nerve processes into the extracellular space and from there to the capillaries.

The **pituicytes** represent glial cells, the cytoplasm of which embraces nerve fibers, Herring bodies, and nerve terminals. Their cytoplasm contains numerous free ribosomes, some particulate glycogen, and a varying number of lipid droplets. (Fig. 20-20) In the rat pituicytes, there are no secretory granules.

At the moment, it is not known if vasopressin and oxytocin are secreted by the same cell or different cells. There are structural differences among the nerve

Fig. 20-14. Detail of the posterior lobe (pars nervosa) of the pituitary. Human. L.M. X 180. **1.** Capillaries (sinusoids). **2.** Meshwork of interweaving nerve processes, pituicytes and Herring bodies.

Fig. 20-15. Detail of the base of the neurohypophysis, fixed by intravascular perfusion. Rat. E.M. X 560. **1.** Capillary (sinusoids) with the lumen open. **2.** Meshwork of nerve fibers and pituicytes.

Fig. 20-16. Detail of the neurohypophysis. Same area and fixation as in Fig. 20-15. Rat. E.M. X 1900. **1.** Capillaries (sinusoids). **2.** Endothelial nuclei. **3.** Nuclei of pituicytes. **4.** Nuclei of fibroblasts. **5.** Nerve processes. **6.** Herring bodies.

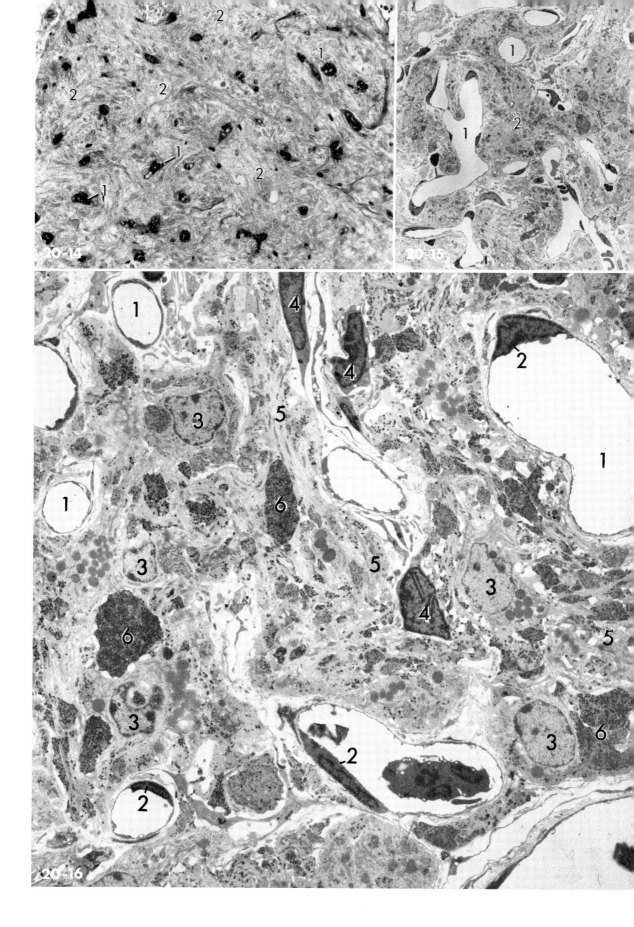

fibers, especially at their terminations. Some have a multitude of small, 400 Å wide, clear or dense vesicles; others have a mixture of vesicles and secretory granules, whereas still others contain only secretory granules. The functional significance of this is not known. The effect of oxytocin is on uterine smooth muscle and on the myoepithelial cells of the mammary gland, causing a contraction of both. The vasopressin (ADH) contracts the smooth muscle of blood vessels and also has an antidiuretic effect.

Releasing factors. The nerve cells and their fibers of the neurohypophysis also secrete hormones which stimulate the synthesis and release of STH, TSH, ACTH, and LH in the adenohypophysis. The releasing factors are probably discharged within the stalk of the pituitary and carried by the hypophysial portal system to the anterior lobe cells.

References

ADENOHYPOPHYSIS

Coates, P. W., Ashby, E. A., Krulich, L., Dhariwal, A. P. S. and McCann, S. M. Morphologic alterations in somatotrophs of the rat adenohypophysis following administration of hypothalamic extracts. Am. J. Anat. *128*: 389–412 (1970).

Dekker, A. Electron microscopic study of somatotropic and lactotropic pituitary cells of the Syrian hamster. Anat. Rec. *162*: 132–136 (1968).

Heath, E. Cytology of the pars anterior of the bovine adenohypophysis. Am. J. Anat. *127*: 131–158 (1970).

Herlant, M. The cells of the adenohypophysis and their functional significance. Int. Rev. Cytol. *17*: 299–381 (1964).

Mikami, S. Light and electron microscopic investigations of six types of glandular cells of the bovine adenohypophysis. Z. Zellforsch. *105*: 457–482 (1970).

Paiz, C. and Hennigar, G. R. Electron microscopy and histochemical correlation of human anterior pituitary cells. Am. J. Path. *59*: 43–73 (1970).

Siperstein, E. R. and Miller, K. J. Further cytophysiologic evidence for the identity of the cells that produce adrenocorticotrophic hormone. Endocrinology *86*: 451–486 (1970).

Wislocki, G. B. The vascular supply of the hypophysis cerebri of the rhesus monkey and man. *In*: The Pituitary Gland, pp. 48–68. Williams & Wilkins, Baltimore, 1938.

NEUROHYPOPHYSIS

Barer, R. and Lederis, K. Ultrastructure of the rabbit neurohypophysis with special reference to the release of hormones. Z. Zellforsch. *75*: 201–239 (1966).

Bargmann, W. Neurosecretion. Int. Rev. Cytol. *19*: 183–201 (1966).

Bodian, D. Herring bodies and neuroapocrine secretion in the monkey. An electron microscopic study of the fate of the neurosecretory product. Bull. Johns Hopkins Hosp. *118*: 282–326 (1966).

Dellmann, H. D. and Rodriguez, E. M. Herring bodies; an electron microscopic study of local degeneration and regeneration of neurosecretory axons. Z. Zellforsch. *111*: 293–315 (1970).

Heller, H. (Ed.). The Neurohypophysis. Academic Press, New York, 1957.

Lederis, K. An electron microscopical study of the human neurohypophysis. Z. Zellforsch. *65*: 847–868 (1965).

Sawyer, C. H. Brain-endocrine interactions. A symposium presented at the 83rd session of the American Association of Anatomists. Am. J. Anat. *129*: 193–246 (1970).

Scharrer, E. Principles of Neuroendocrine Integration. Endocrines and the Central Nervous System, *43*: 1–35 (1966).

Scharrer, E. and Scharrer, B. Neurosekretion. *In*: Handbuch der mikroskopischen Anatomie des Menschen. (Eds. W. von Möllendorff and W. Bargmann), Vol. 6, part 5, pp. 953–1066. Springer, Berlin, 1954.

Scharrer, E. and Scharrer, B. Neuroendocrinology. Columbia Univ. Press, New York, 1963.

Fig. 20-17. Detail of neurohypophysis. Rat. E.M. X 37,000. **1.** Longitudinally sectioned nerve processes with microtubules. **2.** Neurosecretory granules being passed along the nerve processes. **3.** Part of pituicyte.

Fig. 20-18. Detail of neurohypophysis. Rat. E.M. X 9000. **1.** Local accumulation of numerous neurosecretory granules, referred to as Herring body. **2.** Nerve processes.

Fig. 20-19. Detail of neurohypophysis. Rat. E.M. X 36,000. **1.** Cross-sectioned nerve processes with few or no neurosecretory granules. **2.** Microtubules. **3.** Club-shaped nerve ending with neurosecretory granules and vesicles. **4.** Basal lamina. **5.** Intercellular (extracellular) space.

Fig. 20-20. Detail of neurohypophysis. Rat. E.M. X 9000. **1.** Nucleus of pituicyte. **2.** Particulate glycogen. **3.** Lipid droplets. **4.** Nerve processes. **5.** Nerve ending. **6.** Capillary endothelium. **7.** Capillary lumen.

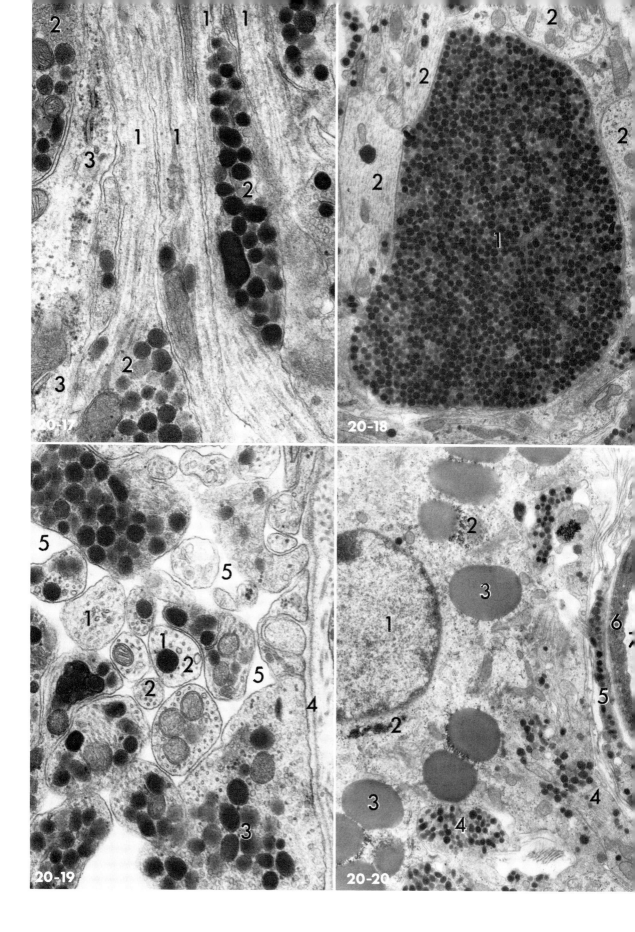

21 Thyroid gland

The thyroid gland is an endocrine gland which secretes its iodine-rich hormones **thyroxine** and **tri-iodothyronine** into small cysts, the **follicles**. The hormones are stored in the follicles and passed on, across the wall of the follicle, to the dense plexus of perifollicular capillaries. The thyroid hormones accelerate general and specific metabolic processes of the body by an increase in oxygen consumption and heat production. Among other things they influence the rate of intestinal absorption, carbohydrate metabolism, and are related to processes of growth and maturation.

Different cells occurring singly or in small groups amongst the follicles are the **parafollicular** cells. They are seemingly unrelated functionally to the follicles and secrete the hormone **calcitonin** which enters the blood stream and reduces high levels of calcium in plasma. Its action seems to be on the osteogenic cells of bone tissue, stimulating them to become osteoblasts, which manufacture the intercellular substance of bone. This process requires calcium, and since it is taken from the blood stream, it lowers the blood calcium level.

STRUCTURE

The thyroid gland is the largest endocrine organ in man. It consists of right and left lateral lobes joined by a connecting isthmus, and is located on either side of the lower part of the larynx and the upper end of the trachea. Embryologically, it is formed as a medial endodermal downgrowth from the tongue, and it is later disconnected from the oral cavity.

The gland is surrounded by an **outer capsule**, which is continuous with the deep fascia of the neck, and an **inner**, true **capsule**. The latter penetrates the glandular tissue as trabeculae and septa, giving rise to incomplete, partially enclosed areas or **lobules**. The septa contain collagenous and elastic connective tissue elements and conduct blood vessels, lymphatics, and nerves to and from the gland.

The main structural and functional unit of the thyroid parenchyma is the **follicle**. (Figs. 21-1, 21-2) The secondary unit is represented by the **parafollicular cells**. There are 20–30 million follicles in the human thyroid gland. The follicles are oval or spherical closed sacs formed by a wall of simple **cuboidal epithelium** and a central cavity filled with a viscous fluid, the **colloid**. (Fig. 21-3) Occasionally, the follicles branch or communicate with one another. The size of the follicles ranges from 0.05 to 0.5 mm. Each follicle is surrounded by a basal lamina, a network of fine reticular fibrils, and an extensive microvascular bed of arterioles, capillaries, and venules. The capillaries, as a rule, indent the epithelial cells in the wall of the follicle, establishing a very intimate relationship between the capillary wall and the base of the epithelial cell.

The **epithelial cells** which form the wall of the follicle are generally of cuboidal shape, arranged in a simple epithelial sheath. A certain variation in the height of the epithelium may reflect differences in cellular activity. In highly active glands the cells are tall columnar. In greatly distended follicles the cells become low cuboidal or squamous, possibly indicating a resting or storage phase of the thyroid follicle activity. The epithelial cell has large amounts of free ribosomes and widely branching granular endoplasmic reticulum, generally with the cisternae dilated to varying degree. (Fig. 21-4) The

Fig. 21-1. Segment of thyroid gland. Human. L.M. X 23. **1.** Lobules. **2.** Septa. **3.** Follicles.

Fig. 21-2. Survey of thyroid gland. Rat. E.M. X 600. **1.** Large follicles. **2.** Small follicles. **3.** Connective tissue septa. **4.** Parafollicular cells. **5.** Arteriole. **6.** Venule. **7.** Lymphatic capillary. **8.** Blood capillaries.

Fig. 21-3. Detail of thyroid follicle. Rat. E.M. X 1800. **1.** Colloid in center of follicle. **2.** Nuclei of follicular epithelial cells. **3.** Perifollicular capillaries. **4.** Perifollicular bundles of collagenous fibrils. **5.** Nuclei of fibroblasts.

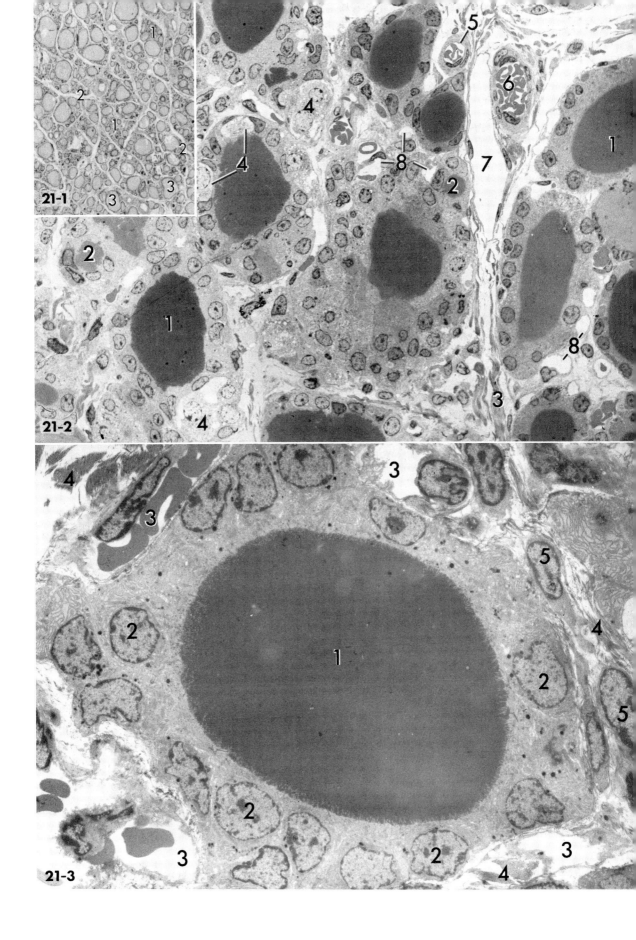

21-1

21-2

21-3

Golgi zone is in a supranuclear or paranuclear position and is relatively extensive with lots of small and medium-size vesicles and secretory granules (Fig. 21-5), the latter often referred to as **colloid droplets.** Microtubules extend between the Golgi zone and the upper part of the cell. Mitochondria and lipid droplets are small in number but lysosomes occur relatively abundantly. The nucleus is large. The lateral surfaces of the cells have small processes which interdigitate, and the intercellular space is often slightly distended with the exception of the area of cellular attachment, recognized as a junctional complex near the surface toward the follicular cavity. This cellular surface is provided with a fair number of short and slender microvilli, projecting into the colloid. The upper part of the cell is filled with small, medium-dense granules, usually referred to as **apical vesicles.** Small pinocytotic invaginations occur at this surface.

The **parafollicular cells** (clear cells or C-cells) often lie within the confines of the follicular basal lamina, but they do not abut on the follicular cavity. (Fig. 21-6) They are extremely rich in membrane-bound, highly electron-dense, argyrophilic granules averaging $0.15\,\mu$ in width. (Fig. 21-7) Mitochondria and Golgi zone are rather prominent but granular endoplasmic reticulum is largely missing. The cells present the ultrastructural architecture of a pituitary endocrine cell.

The **perifollicular capillaries** are characterized by a highly fenestrated endothelium in which the fenestrae are invariably closed by a diaphragm.

The **secretory process** of the follicular epithelium involves several steps. The steps are related to the synthesis, the storage and the release of the thyroid hormones. The colloid contains **thyroglobulin,** which is the storage form of the hormones. The thyroglobulin is a glycoprotein to which are bound several iodinated amino acids of which tyrosine is one.

The **synthesis** of thyroglobulin seems to follow the general pathway of protein synthesis. The polypeptide portion of the thyroglobulin is synthesized in the granular endoplasmic reticulum, aggregated in the Golgi zone, and transferred to the cell surface in small secretory vesicles, the apical vesicles, which in turn, deliver the glycoprotein to the colloid pool. Iodide in the blood is readily absorbed by the epithelial cells. It is oxidized to iodine, probably at the apical cell surface, and passed on to the colloid where it becomes incorporated into the thyroglobulin.

The **release** of the active components of the thyroglobulin from the colloid may occur through the hydrolytic action of a proteolytic enzyme present in the colloid and/or by a pinocytotic uptake of colloid at the apical surface which in turn is followed by lysosomal activity. In either case, the end result is that thyroxin and tri-iodothyronine are set free and leave the confines of the follicle. All phases of thyroxin synthesis and release are controlled by the thyrotrophic hormone (TSH) of the anterior lobe of the pituitary.

Fig. 21-4. Detail of epithelial cell of thyroid follicle. Rat. E.M. X 22,000. **1.** Nucleus. **2.** Colloid in center of follicle **3.** Microvilli. **4.** Cell membranes. **5.** Intercellular space. **6.** Endothelium of blood capillary. **7.** Capillary lumen. **8.** Basal laminae. **9.** Mitochondria. **10.** Golgi complex. **11.** Cisternae of granular endoplasmic reticulum. **12.** Secretory granules (colloid droplets).

Fig. 21-5. Enlargement of the central part of epithelial cell of thyroid follicle. Center of follicle to the left, base of epithelial cell to the right. Rat. E.M. X 47,000. **1.** Mitochondria. **2.** Ribosomes. **3.** Cisternae of granular endoplasmic reticulum. **4.** Vesicles, membranes, and flattened sacs of the Golgi complex. **5.** Secretory granules (colloid droplets). **6.** Primary lysosomes. **7.** Microtubule.

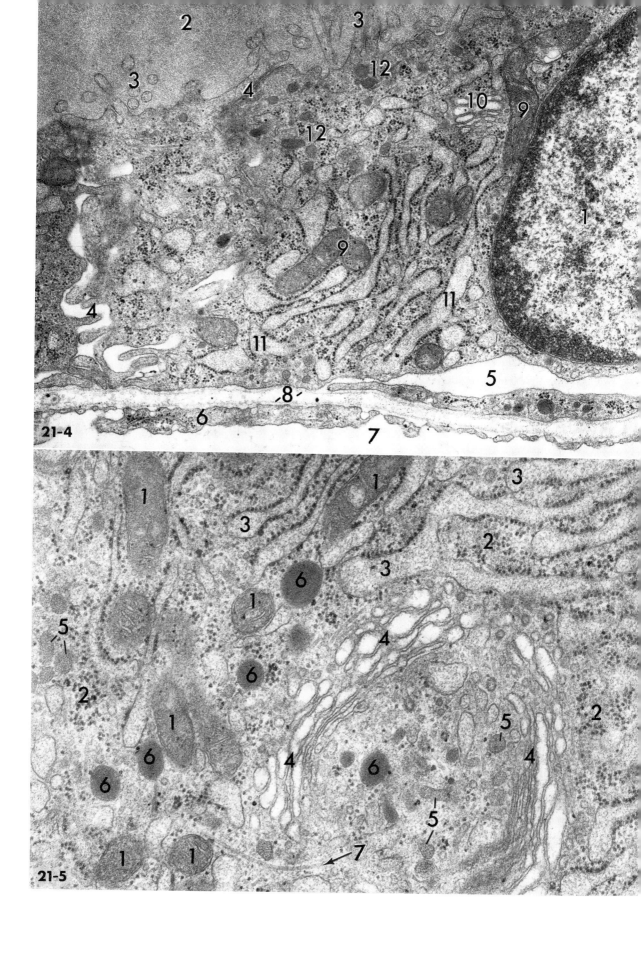

References

PRINCIPAL FOLLICULAR CELLS

Ekholm, R. Thyroid gland. *In* Electron Microscopic Anatomy (Ed. S. M. Kurtz), pp. 221–238. Academic Press, New York, 1964.

Ekholm, R. and Sjöstrand, F. S. The ultrastructural organization of the mouse thyroid gland. J. Ultrastruct. Res. *1*: 178–199 (1957).

Ekholm, R. and Strandberg, U. Thyroglobulin biosynthesis in the rat thyroid. J. Ultrastruct. Res. *20*: 103–110 (1967).

Heimann, P. Ultrastructure of human thyroid. Acta Endocrinologica *53*: Suppl. 110, 1–102 (1966).

Klinck, G. H. Structure of the thyroid. *In* The Thyroid (Eds. J. B. Hazard and D. E. Smith), pp. 1–31. Williams & Wilkins, Baltimore, 1964.

Klinck, G. H., Oertel, J. E. and Winship, T. Ultrastructure of normal human thyroid. Lab. Investig. *22*: 2–22 (1970).

Lupulescu, A. and Petrovici, A. Ultrastructure of the thyroid gland. Williams & Wilkins, Baltimore, 1968.

Nunez, E. A. and Becker, D. Secretory processes in follicular cells of the bat thyroid. Am. J. Anat. *129*: 369–398 (1970).

Seljelid, R. Endocytosis in thyroid follicle cells. I. Structure and significance of different types of single membrane-limited vacuoles and bodies. J. Ultrastruct. Res. *17*: 195–219 (1967).

Seljelid, R.: Endocytosis in thyroid follicles. II. A microinjection study of the origin of colloid droplets. J. Ultrastruct. Res. *17*: 401–420 (1967).

Seljelid, R. Endocytosis in thyroid follicle cells. III. An electron microscopic study of the cell surface and related structures. J. Ultrastruct. Res. *18*: 1–24 (1967).

Seljelid, R. Endocytosis in thyroid follicle cells. IV. On the acid phosphatase activity in thyroid follicle cells, with special reference to the quantitative aspects. J. Ultrastruct. Res. *18*: 237–256 (1967).

Seljelid, R. Endocytosis in thyroid follicle cells. V. On the redistribution of cytosomes following stimulation with thyrotropic hormone. J. Ultrastruct. Res. *18*: 479–488 (1967).

Whur, P., Herscovics, A. and Leblond, C. P. Radioautographic visualization of the incorporation of galactose-³H and mannose-³H by rat thyroids in vitro in relation to the stages of thyroglobulin synthesis. J. Cell Biol. *43*: 289–311 (1969).

Wissig, S. L. The anatomy of secretion in the follicular cells of the thyroid gland. I. The fine structure of the gland in the normal rat. J. Biophys. Biochem. Cytol. 7: 419–432 (1960).

Wissig, S. L. The anatomy of secretion in the follicular cells of the thyroid gland. II. The effect of acute thyrotrophic hormone stimulation on the secretory apparatus. J. Cell Biol. *16*: 93–117 (1963).

PARAFOLLICULAR CELLS

Chan, A. S. and Conen, P. E. Ultrastructural observations on cytodifferentiation of parafollicular cells in the human fetal thyroid. Lab. Investig. *25*: 249–259 (1971).

Ekholm, R. and Ericson, L. E. The ultrastructure of the parafollicular cells of the thyroid gland in the rat. J. Ultrastruct. Res. *23*: 378–402 (1968).

Ericson, L. E. Subcellular localization of 5-hydroxytryptamine in the parafollicular cells of the mouse thyroid gland. An autoradiographic study. J. Ultrastruct. Res. *31*: 162–177 (1970).

Gershon, M. D., Belshaw, B. E. and Nunez, E. A. Biochemical, histochemical and ultrastructural studies of thyroid serotonin, parafollicular and follicular cells during development in the dog. Am. J. Anat. *132*: 5–20 (1971).

Nonidez, J. F. The origin of the parafollicular cell, a second epithelial component of the thyroid gland of the dog. Am. J. Anat. *49*: 479–505 (1932).

Strum, J. M. and Karnovsky, M. J. Cytochemical localization of endogenous peroxidase in thyroid follicular cells. J. Cell Biol. *44*: 655–666 (1970).

Teitelbaum, S. L., Moore, K. E. and Shiebler, W. C-Cell follicles in the dog thyroid: demonstration by in vivo perfusion. Anat. Rec. *168*: 69–78 (1970).

Fig. 21-6. Detail of the wall of thyroid follicle. Rat. E.M. × 10,000. **1.** Nucleus of parafollicular cell. **2.** Nucleus of principal follicular cell. **3.** Lumen of follicle. **4.** Lumen of perifollicular capillary. **5.** Fenestrated (closed) endothelium. **6.** Basal lamina of thyroid follicle. **7.** Close association of parafollicular cell and blood capillary. **8.** Golgi complexes. **9.** Dilated cisternae of the granular endoplasmic reticulum. **10.** Mitochondria. **11.** Secretory granules of parafollicular cell. **12.** Lysosomes. **13.** Collagenous fibrils of perifollicular connective tissue.

Fig. 21-7. Enlargement of area similar to rectangle in Fig. 21-6. Secretory granules of parafollicular cell. Thyroid. Rat. E.M. × 47,500. **1.** Mitochondria. **2.** Cisternae of granular endoplasmic reticulum. **3.** Ribosomes. **4.** Very dense-core secretory granule. **5.** Secretory granule with medium-dense core. **6.** Secretory granule with very light center. These granules are structurally rather similar to some of the cisternae of the nearby granular endoplasmic reticulum. The variation in core density represents intermediate stages of either hormone release or synthesis.

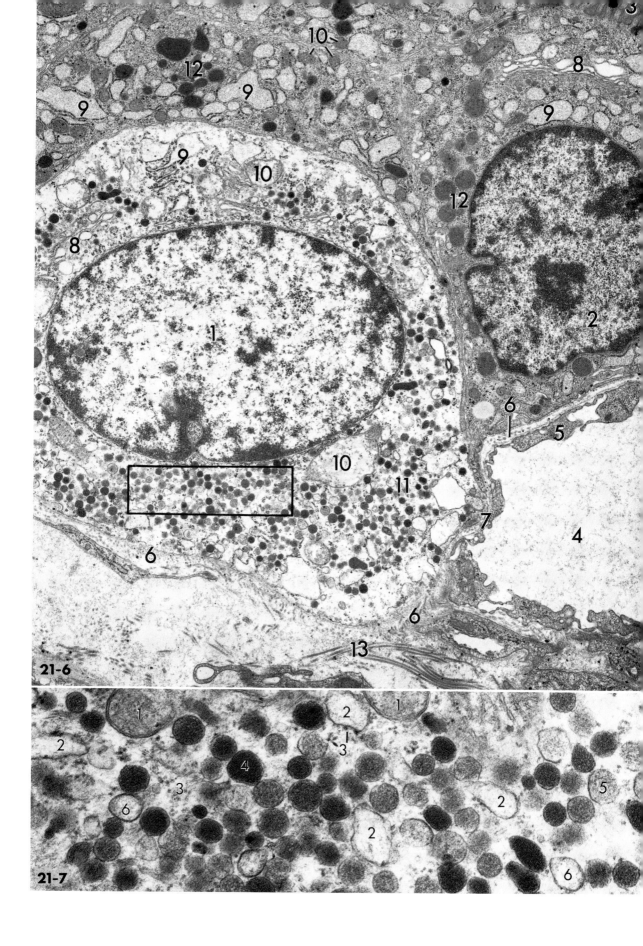

22 Parathyroid glands

The parathyroids are endocrine glands which secrete **parathyroid hormone** (parathormone). This hormone regulates the calcium and phosphorus metabolism of the body by mobilizing calcium from the bones and by increasing the excretion of phosphate by the kidney. The hormone inhibits the reabsorption of phosphate from the kidney tubules, thereby lowering the plasma level of phosphate with consequent rise in the level of the ionized calcium in the blood. The action of the hormone is related to its ability to transform osteogenic bone cells into osteoclasts which in turn set free calcium and phosphate from the organic intercellular substance of the bone.

STRUCTURE

The parathyroid glands, usually four in number, each the size of an apple seed, are situated two on each side behind the thyroid gland. They are derived from local thickenings of the endoderm of the third and fourth pharyngeal pouches, migrating downward and forward to become embedded in the outer capsule or the parenchyma of the thyroid gland. The glands are surrounded by a delicate capsule which penetrates and divides the parenchyma of the gland into incomplete lobules. The connective tissue of the capsule and the septa are rich in fat cells, and with increasing age the adipose tissue permeates and takes over increasingly larger portions of the parenchyma. (Fig. 22-1) Blood vessels, lymphatics, and nerves are abundant in the septa.

The **parenchyma** consists of densely packed epithelial cells arranged in a loose network of widely anastomosing cords or plates. (Fig. 22-3) Only rarely in young individuals are the cells arranged to form occasional follicles, similar to those which make up the thyroid gland. The epithelial cells are of two categories, the more common **chief** (principal) **cells** and the less abundant **oxyphil cells**. The chief cells are present throughout life but the oxyphil cells appear after the first decade.

The two cell types are either mixed irregularly, or the oxyphil cells may occur in scattered groups. (Fig. 22-4) The chief cells are small, whereas the oxyphil cells are large. The nuclei of both cells are small, spherical, and widely spaced in the clusters of large oxyphil cells but closely together in areas occupied only by the small chief cells. The cords of cells are enveloped by an external (basal) lamina and a network of fine reticular fibrils.

The **capillary bed** of the epithelial cell cords is much less extensive than around the follicles of the thyroid gland. The capillaries travel mostly in the delicate connective tissue septa but they also anastomose here and there across the epithelial cords and plates. Contrary to earlier reports, many epithelial cells do not abut on a capillary. The capillaries are of the fenestrated, closed variety, and the endothelial tube is enveloped by a basal lamina of its own.

The **chief cells** are small polyhedral cells. The cell borders are straight and closely applied to those of adjacent cells, occasionally attached by desmosomes or peg-in-socket intercellular arrangements. The nucleus occupies a major part of the cell. The cytoplasm contains small scattered mitochondria, groups of stacked membranes of the granular endoplasmic

Fig. 22-1. Parathyroid gland. Human. L.M. X 24. **1.** Glandular tissue. **2.** Adipose tissue. **3.** Capsule. **4.** Connective tissue septa with blood vessels.

Fig. 22-2. Enlargement of area similar to rectangle in Fig. 22-1. Parathyroid gland. Human. L.M. X 260. **1.** Fat cells. **2.** Chief cells. **3.** Oxyphil cells. **4.** Blood capillaries.

Fig. 22-3. Survey of cords of cells in parathyroid gland. Human. E.M. X 570. **1.** Fat cells. **2.** Chief cells. **3.** Oxyphil cells. **4.** Blood capillaries. **5.** Connective tissue septa.

Fig. 22-4. Detail of parathyroid gland. Human. E.M. X 4500. **1.** Nuclei of chief cells. **2.** Oxyphil cell, crowded with mitochondria. **3.** Large accumulations of particulate glycogen. **4.** Lipid droplets. **5.** Mitochondria. **6.** Cell borders. **7.** Lumen of blood capillary. **8.** Circles indicate possible secretory granules.

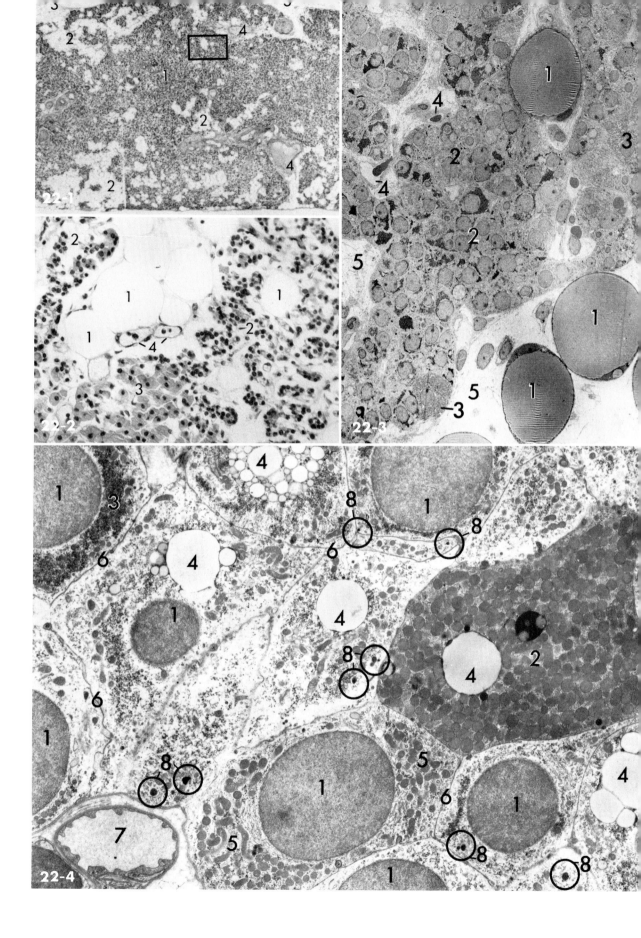

reticulum (Fig. 22-5), a Golgi zone, generally a limited number of 0.2 μ-wide, highly electron-dense granules, bounded by a membrane, vast accumulations of various-sized lipid droplets (Fig. 22-6) and particulate glycogen. A certain variation in the amount of glycogen and small dense granules has lead to the hypothesis that there exist mainly two types of chief cells, reflecting different stages of activity. The **light chief cells** (often referred to as clear cells) have huge amounts of glycogen and few electron-dense granules and may represent a resting phase, whereas the **dark chief cells** with little glycogen and relatively many small granules may represent an active, secretory phase.

The **oxyphil cells** are large polyhedral cells, also with a straight cell border. The cytoplasm is crowded with small mitochondria (Fig. 22-7), the internal membranes of which have a lamellar arrangement. The Golgi zone is rudimentarily small. Generally, the small amount of cytoplasm left between the mitochondria is filled with particulate glycogen. Large accumulations of lipid droplets admixed with densely packed particulate glycogen are common.

Little is known about the function of the two cell types and the **secretory mechanism** of hormone synthesis and release. According to current beliefs, the parathormone, a polypeptide hormone, is synthesized by the granular endoplasmic reticulum of the dark chief cells, appearing ultrastructurally as small, dense secretory granules within the Golgi zone. The granules are subsequently discharged at the cell surface into the intercellular space and the pericapillary connective tissue space. They subsequently enter the capillary endothelium and are stored there for various periods before being released into the blood stream. The light chief cells with the large amounts of glycogen reflect a stage of secretory inactivity or presecretory preparation. The vast accumulations of lipid droplets have been interpreted as signs of cellular aging, representing a con-glomeration of lipofuscin granules. The function of the oxyphil cell is still unexplained. One has hypothesized that it reflects an end-stage of cellular development, since intermediate cells occur between the chief cells and the oxyphil cells. There is a possibility that some oxyphil cells are capable of production of parathyroid hormone since apparent secretory granules have been demonstrated in parathyroid adenomas.

References

Capen, C. C. and Rowland, G. N. The ultrastructure of the parathyroid glands of young cats. Anat. Rec. *162*: 327–340 (1968).

Fetter, A. W. and Capen, C. C. The ultrastructure of the parathyroid glands of young pigs. Acta Anat. *75*: 359–372 (1970).

Munger, B. L. and Roth, S. I. The cytology of the normal parathyroid glands of man and Virginia deer. J. Cell Biol. *16*: 379–400 (1963).

Nakagima, K., Yamazaki, Y. and Isunoda, Y. An electron microscopic study of the human fetal parathyroid gland. Z. Zellforsch. *85*: 89–95 (1968).

Nunez, E. A., Whalen, J. P. and Krook, L. An ultrastructural study of the natural secretory cycle of the parathyroid gland of the bat. Am. J. Anat. *134*: 459–480 (1972).

Fig. 22-5. Detail of chief cell. Parathyroid gland. Human. E.M. X 34,000. **1.** Mitochondria. **2.** Ribosomes. **3.** Flattened cisternae of granular endoplasmic reticulum. **4.** Accumulation of particulate glycogen. **5.** Partly collapsed small lipid droplet.

Fig. 22-6. Detail of chief cell. Parathyroid gland. Human. E.M. X 34,000. **1.** Large lipid droplets. **2.** Small lipid droplets. **3.** Mitochondria.

Fig. 22-7. Detail of oxyphil cell. Parathyroid gland. Human. E.M. X 17,000. **1.** Nucleus. **2.** Mitochondria. **3.** Particulate glycogen. **4.** Accumulation of lipid droplets of various sizes.

Fig. 22-8. Detail of mitochondria in oxyphil cell. Parathyroid gland. Human. E.M. X 87,000. **1.** Mitochondrial external envelope. **2.** Mitochondrial cristae. **3.** Mitochondrial matrix. **4.** Glycogen particles.

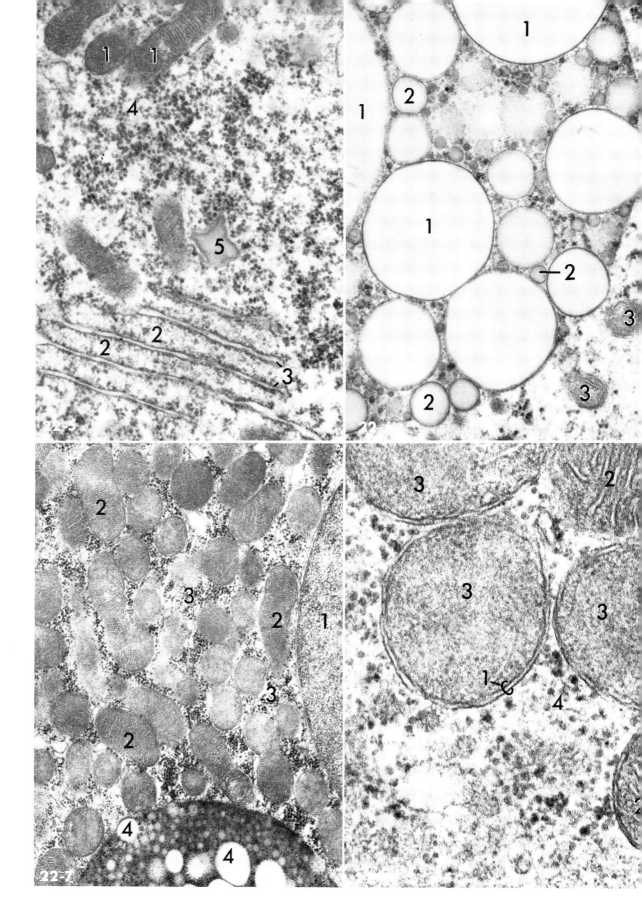

23 Adrenal (suprarenal) glands

The adrenal glands are organs which contain two structurally and functionally diffent tissues, the **cortex** and the **medulla.** (Fig. 23-1) Hormones which are synthesized in the cortex are called corticosteroids. They are of three kinds: mineralocorticoids, glucocorticoids, and androgenic corticoids. They participate in the regulation of salt and water metabolism, in the metabolism of carbohydrates and influence secondary sex characteristics. The several hormones are probably synthesized in distinctly different parts of the adrenal cortex. The medullary hormones, epinephrine and norepinephrine, generally make the vascular smooth muscle contract, and prepare the individual for the so-called fight and flight reaction. This involves a faster heart beat, increased blood pressure, rerouting of blood from the intestines and the spleen to the skeletal muscles. It should be noted that the action of the two medullary hormones differs considerably.

GENERAL

The adrenal glands are small, angular organs, resting on the upper pole of each kidney. They are embedded in the retroperitoneal tissue. Each gland is surrounded by a **capsule** containing fibroelastic tissue, in which primitive smooth muscle cells are present in addition to fibroblasts. Blood vessels, nerves, and some lymphatics enter and leave at the **hilus** of the gland, which faces the spinal column.

The cortex occupies the major part of the glands. (Fig. 23-2) The average width of the parenchyma of the cortex is 5 mm. The medulla is a small central cell mass with a thickness of about 5 mm.

BLOOD SUPPLY

On an average, three **adrenal arteries** enter the gland at the hilus. They break up into a plexus of arteries in the capsule. From this plexus emerge essentially three categories of arterial branches. **Capsular arteries** supply the capsule with a rich network of capillaries. **Cortical arteries** course between the capsule and the cortical parenchyma, and give off directly straight capillaries which traverse the entire cortex in an interconnected capillary plexus. These capillaries empty into the medullary microvascular bed. The third category are the **medullary arteries,** a limited number of arteries which go directly to the medulla across the cortex. Once they reach the medulla they give rise to a rich capillary network. Throughout the adrenal gland the **capillaries** are of the fenestrated, closed type. A basal lamina is lacking, or if present only occurs as small segments around the cortical capillaries. The basal lamina is constantly present throughout in relation to the capsular and the medullary capillaries.

The venous drainage of the gland takes

Fig. 23-1. Section of entire adrenal gland. Monkey. L.M. X 12. **1.** Capsule. **2.** Cortex. **3.** Medulla.

Fig. 23-2. Enlargement of rectangle in Fig. 23-1. Adrenal gland. Monkey. L.M. X 53. **1.** Capsule. **2.** Zona glomerulosa of cortex. **3.** Zona fasciculata of cortex. **4.** Zona reticularis of cortex. **5.** Adrenal medulla. **6.** Large medullary vein.

Fig. 23-3. Enlargement of area similar to rectangle (A) in Fig. 23-2. Adrenal gland. Rat. E.M. X 725. **1.** Capsule. **2.** Capsular arteriole. **3.** Capillaries of the zona glomerulosa. **4.** Capillaries of the zona fasciculata. Arrows indicate direction of blood flow. **5.** Approximate border between zona glomerulosa and zona fasciculata. **6.** Cords of glandular epithelial cells.

Fig. 23-4. Enlargement of area similar to rectangle (B) in Fig. 23-2. Adrenal gland. Rat. E.M. X 725. **1.** Capillaries of the zona fasciculata. **2.** Capillaries of the zona reticularis. **3.** Approximate border between fasciculata and reticularis. **4.** Adrenal medulla. **5.** Cell cords.

Fig. 23-5. Enlargement of area similar to rectangle in Fig. 23-3. Zona fasciculata. Adrenal cortex. Rat. E.M. X 5200. **1.** Lumina of capillaries. **2.** Nucleus of endothelial cell. **3.** Fenestrated (closed) endothelium. **4.** Subendothelial space. **5.** Nucleus of epithelial cell. **6.** Lipid droplets within the cell. **7.** Lipid droplets discharging at the cell surface. **8.** Mitochondria. **9.** Glycogen accumulations. **10.** Crystal.

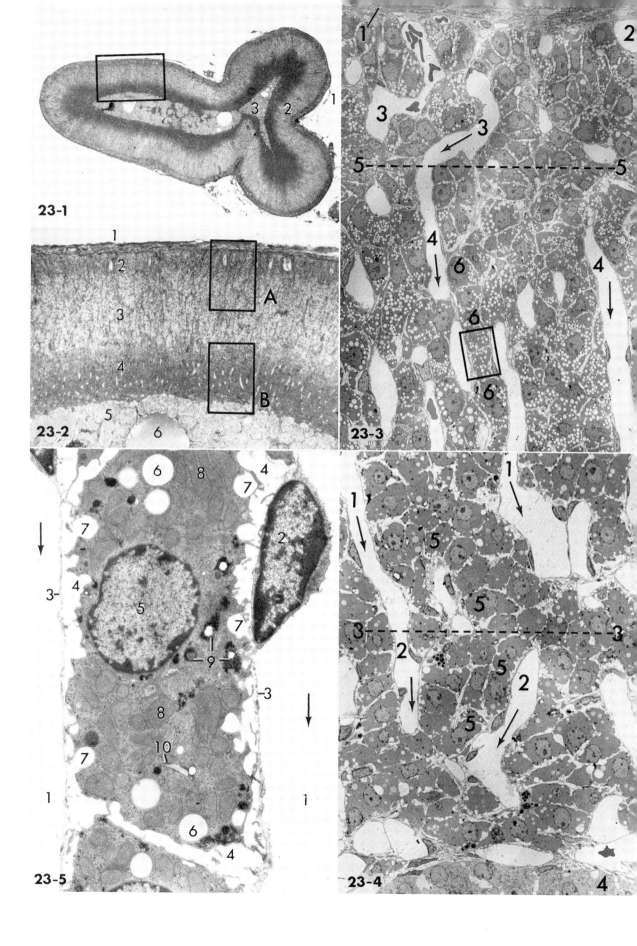

23-1

23-2

23-3

23-4

23-5

place from the center of the medulla, and to a small extent from the capsule. The medulla receives a large amount of venous blood from the cortical capillaries which are drained by large thin-walled **venules.** The medullary capillaries also empty into these venules which all eventually form the **adrenal vein.** This vein has longitudinally arranged smooth muscle cells.

ADRENAL CORTEX

The adrenal cortex is made up of cords or cylinders of epithelial cells which embryologically are derived from mesenchymal cells near the root of the dorsal mesentery. The architecture of the cell cords varies within the cortex, and based on this architecture, three zones are recognized: 1) zona glomerulosa; 2) zona fasciculata; and 3) zona reticularis. The borders between the zones are not distinctly marked.

Zona glomerulosa. The zona glomerulosa is the most peripheral area in which the cell cords form irregular, arch-like structures. This zone occupies one-tenth of the height of the cortex in the normal adult. The epithelial cells are polyhedral or columnar. (Fig. 23-3) The capillaries of this zone follow the convoluted arrangement of the epithelial cells. Most epithelial cells abut on a capillary. A basal lamina may surround the most superficial capillaries but it disappears almost completely as the capillaries reach the deeper zones of the cortex. The endothelium is of the fenestrated, closed variety throughout. The cytoplasm of the epithelial cells is filled with equally sized, 0.5 μ-wide lipid droplets. There are relatively few mitochondria. They have tubular cristae and a dense mitochondrial matrix. There is a limited number of vesicular profiles, forming the agranular endoplasmic reticulum, and a small Golgi zone. The nucleus is large, free ribosomes are abundant, but profiles of the granular endoplasmic reticulum are scarce. The cell surface is irregular and some microvilli project into the rather large intercellular space.

Zona fasciculata. The zona fasciculata occupies roughly six-tenths of the center of the adrenal cortex. The cell cords form straight columns, accompanied by equally straight capillaries which anastomose freely through short branches. Almost invariably, all epithelial cells make contact with at least one capillary. (Fig. 23-5) The fine structure of the capillary is similar to that seen in the zona glomerulosa. The epithelial cells are mostly polyhedral and larger than in the zona glomerulosa. They are filled with lipid droplets of various sizes. The number of droplets varies greatly according to the stress to which the individual is subjected at the time that the adrenal specimens are obtained. The greater the stress, the smaller the number of lipid droplets. Mitochondria are numerous, spherical, and relatively large. The mitochondrial cristae are predominantly vesicular, and the matrix is light. The agranular endoplasmic reticulum is vesicular or branched tubular, arranged largely in layers around lipid droplets and mitochondria. (Fig. 23-7) Granular endoplasmic reticulum does not occur. Particulate glycogen and free ribosomes are abundant. The Golgi zone is medium-sized.

Fig. 23-6. Detail of cell from zona fasciculata. Adrenal cortex. Rat. E.M. X 60,000.
1. Nucleus. **2.** Mitochondria with vesicular cristae. **3.** Golgi membranes. **4.** Tubular agranular endoplasmic reticulum, some profiles enlarging to form minute lipid droplets. **5.** Small lipid droplet. **6.** Large lipid droplets with center of lipid matrix slightly dissolved during preparation. **7.** Tangential section of large lipid droplet. **8.** Primary lysosome. **9.** Ribosomes.

Fig. 23-7. Detail of cell from zona fasciculata. Adrenal cortex. Rat. E.M. X 60,000.
1. Intercellular space. **2.** Cell membrane. **3.** Mitochondria with vesicular cristae. **4.** Lipid droplets with matrix well preserved. **5.** Interface lipid droplet/cytoplasm. **6.** Profiles of agranular endoplasmic reticulum adhering to interface membrane of lipid droplet. **7.** Particulate glycogen. **8.** Free ribosomes. **9.** Profiles of agranular endoplasmic reticulum free in the cytoplasm.

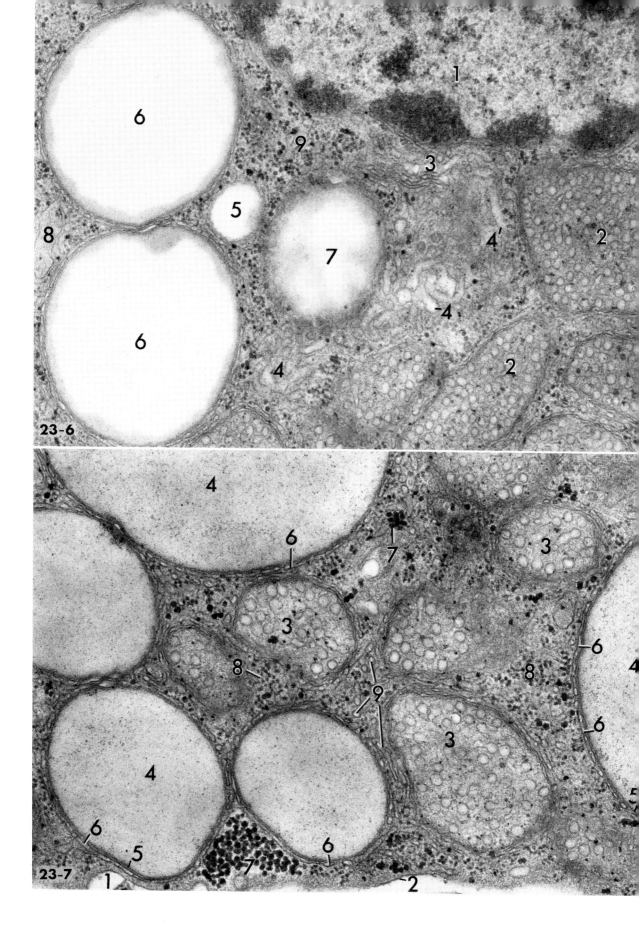

(Fig. 23-6) Lysosomes are small and often contain rectangular bodies, which probably represent cholesterol crystals.

Zona reticularis. The zona reticularis forms the innermost layer of the adrenal cortex, bordering on the medulla into which it sometimes sends aberrant clusters of cortical cells. The zone occupies about three-tenths of the cortex. The cell cords and the accompanying capillaries form a loose network. (Fig. 23-4) The capillaries tend to merge and form postcapillary venules of slightly larger diameters than in the zona fasciculata but with identical ultrastructural architecture. The epithelial cells are small, polyhedral or cuboidal. Lipid droplets are limited in number, fairly large, and highly electron-dense. Mitochondria are large and of irregular shape. The cristae are both of the tubular and the vesicular variety. The agranular endoplasmic reticulum is vesicular and abundant. There are many lysosomes, both primary and secondary, the latter collectively being referred to as pigments or lipofuscin granules. The nucleus is small. Macrophages occur in the subendothelial space in this zone. The cells of the adrenal cortex, particularly those of the zona reticularis, are very sensitive to postmortal changes. Only investigations based on adrenals preserved through an intravascular perfusion of fixatives can be considered to give acceptable results.

Hormone synthesis and release. It is generally accepted that mineralocorticoids are synthesized in the zona glomerulosa, glucocorticoids in the zona fasciculata, and the androgenic corticoids in the zona reticularis. The **synthesis** of these steroid hormones is probably accomplished by a cooperation of the agranular endoplasmic reticulum, the mitochondria, and the lipid droplets. Many of the enzymes required for this synthesis are located in the mitochondria and the agranular endoplasmic reticulum, whereas the cholesterol, the cholesterol esters, and possibly some of the intermediate hormone precursors are localized in the lipid droplets. The intimate contact between the agranular endoplasmic reticulum, the lipid droplets, and the mitochondria facilitates the exchange of enzymes and intermediate products in this synthesis. (Fig. 23-8) The mechanism of corticoid hormone **release** is not fully understood. It has been assumed that a simple process of diffusion through the cell membrane could occur, since the corticosteroid hormones are composed of small molecular-size structures. Another mechanism of release has been suggested to occur by a discharge of the content of the lipid droplets at the cell surface, since it has been found that the envelope of agranular endoplasmic reticulum that surrounds the lipid droplets, at one point merges with the surface cell membrane.

Fig. 23-8. Lipid droplet approaching the cell surface. Zona fasciculata. Adrenal cortex. Rat. E.M. $\times$ 116,000. From: Rhodin, J. Ultrastruct. Res. 34: 23 (1971). **1.** Matrix of large lipid droplet. **2.** Small lipid droplet. **3.** Subendothelial space. **4.** Cell surface membrane. **5.** Bilaminar casing of merged profiles of agranular endoplasmic reticulum. **6.** Interface lipid droplet/cytoplasm appears as a thin, 40 Å boundary membrane. **7. Asterisks:** thin sheath of cytoplasm interposed between lipid droplet and extracellular space. **8.** Mitochondrion with vesicular cristae. **9.** Mitochondrial envelope. **10.** Bilaminar casing of merged profiles of agranular endoplasmic reticulum surrounds the mitochondrion. **11.** Ribosomes. **12.** Glycogen particle.

Fig. 23-9. Lipid droplet at the moment of presumed release of the droplet matrix. Zona fasciculata. Adrenal cortex. Rat. E.M. X 120,000. From: Rhodin, J. Ultrastruct. Res. 34: 23 (1971). **1.** Center of droplet. **2.** Droplet boundary membrane, partly collapsed. **3.** Peripheral membrane of bilaminar endoplasmic casing has fused with surface cell membrane. **4.** Subendothelial space. **5.** Grazing section through edge of cytoplasmic opening. **6.** Intact central membrane of endoplasmic reticulum casing. **7.** Occasional continuity between peripheral and central membranes. **8.** Peripheral membrane of endoplasmic reticulum casing. **9.** Mitochondria. **10.** Agranular endoplasmic reticulum. **11.** Accumulation of glycogen particles.

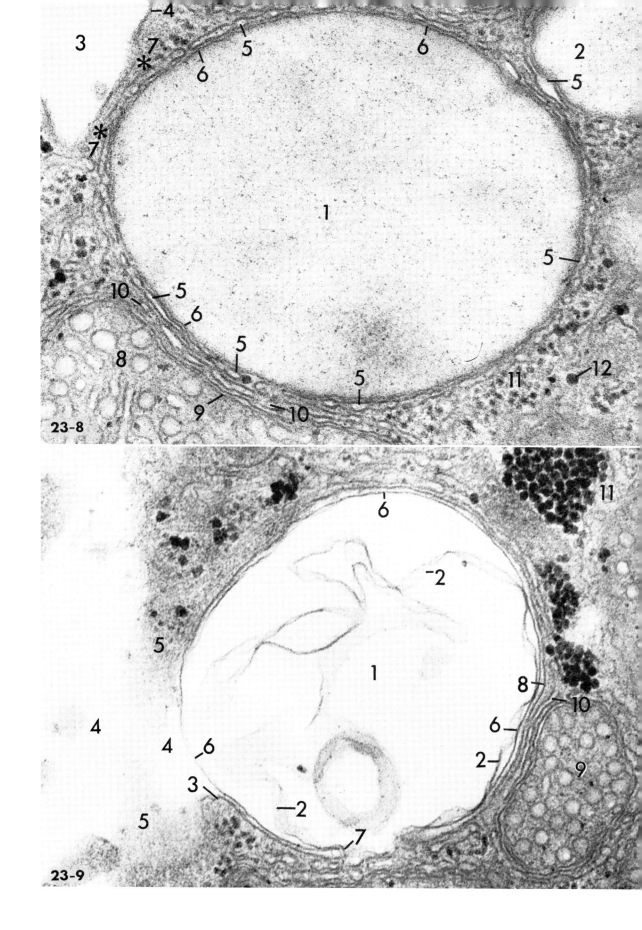

23-8

23-9

(Figs. 4-25, 23-9) In the zona fasciculata, this process can be speeded up by administration of adrenocorticotrophic hormone (ACTH), and delayed by an increase of the concentration of glucocorticoids in the blood by administration of a synthetic glucocorticoid.

Once outside the cortical epithelial cell, the steroids are bound to a protein carrier in the blood. The mineralocorticoids regulate the sodium and potassium balance by inducing a retention of sodium by the kidney tubules. Indirectly, they thereby control water retention. The glucocorticoids primarily stimulate a conversion of proteins to carbohydrates, thereby increasing the supply of energy for a "stepped-up" activity of the body in a stress situation. The androgenic corticoids influence the development of male and female secondary sex characteristics.

ADRENAL MEDULLA

The adrenal medulla consists of polyhedral cells, arranged in a loose network of cords around capillaries and venules. (Figs. 23-10, 23-11) The medullary cells originated from the ectodermal neural crest and migrated together with cells destined to become sympathetic ganglia. In similarity with ganglion cells, the mature adrenal medullary cells receive preganglionic sympathetic nerve fibers (Fig. 23-15) which make terminal contacts with the cells. (Fig. 23-16) In most mammals there are two kinds of medullary cells in addition to a small number of autonomic ganglion cells. Both cell types contain secretory granules. (Fig. 23-12) The **epinephrine** cell is the most common. There are many, medium electron-dense granules. They are membrane-bound and about 0.2μ wide. (Fig. 23-14) The Golgi zone is large, the mitochondria small and few in number, whereas free ribosomes and particulate glycogen accumulations are numerous. The **norepinephrine** cells are less common and occur in clusters. Their ultrastructure is similar to that of the epinephrine cell with the exception of the secretory gran-

ules which are extremely electron-dense. (Fig. 23-13) In the monkey and some other mammals, including man, the adrenal medulla contains only one cell type. However, two types of secretory granules are present. The majority of granules have a highly electron-dense core, the others have a light core.

Hormone synthesis and release. The synthesis of catecholamines involves successive changes in the amino acid tyrosine via dihydroxyphenylalanine (DOPA) to dopamine, and then to norepinephrine, which is converted into epinephrine by a methylation process. Since a regular protein synthesis is not involved, granular endoplasmic reticulum is probably not required. The granules first appear in the Golgi zone, subsequently aggregating in

Fig. 23-10. Adrenal gland. Medulla. Human. L.M. X 133. **1.** Cords of medullary cells. **2.** Lumen of large medullary vein. **3.** Smooth muscle cells arranged longitudinally in the wall of the vein. **4.** Area of collapsed capillaries and venules.

Fig. 23-11. Enlargement of area similar to rectangle in Fig. 23-10. Adrenal medulla. Rat. E.M. X 650. **1.** Medullary capillaries and venules. **2.** Cords of epinephrine cells. **3.** Clusters of norepinephrine cells.

Fig. 23-12. Enlargement of area similar to rectangle in Fig. 23-11. Adrenal medulla. Rat. E.M. X 4500. **1.** Nucleus of epinephrine cell. **2.** Nucleus of norepinephrine cell. **3.** Corner of cell belonging to zona reticularis. **4.** Capillary lumen. **5.** Endothelial nucleus. **6.** Subendothelial space. **7.** Intercellular space. **8.** Nerve endings.

Fig. 23-13. Detail of norepinephrine cell. Adrenal medulla. Rat. E.M. X 32,500. **1.** Nucleus. **2.** Golgi complex. **3.** Mitochondria. **4.** Secretory granules (inadequately preserved). **5.** Circle: particulate glycogen. **6.** Cell membrane. **7.** Parenchymal external (basal) lamina. **8.** Mitochondria in nerve ending.

Fig. 23-14. Detail of epinephrine cell. Adrenal medulla. Rat. E.M. X 27,000. **1.** Secretory granules of varied size and density. **2.** Circle: particulate glycogen. **3.** Secretory granule on the verge of being extruded. **4.** Cell membrane. **5.** Parenchymal basal (external) lamina. **6.** Capillary basal lamina. **7.** Capillary endothelium. **8.** Capillary lumen.

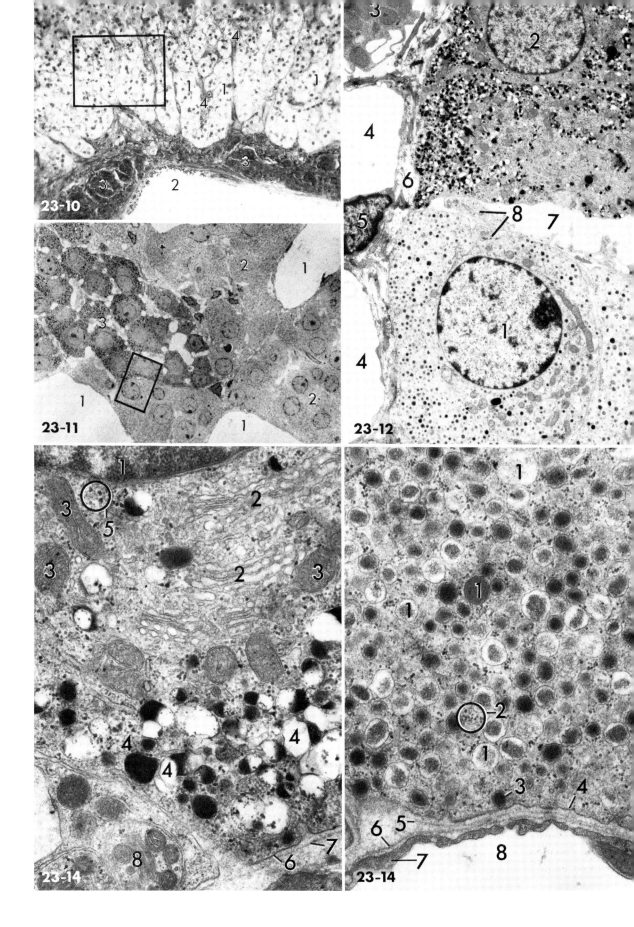

23-10

23-11

23-12

23-14

23-14

the peripheral cytoplasm, enveloped by a Golgi membrane. The core of the granule is released into the wide intercellular spaces and the subendothelial space, as the granule membrane fuses with the cell membrane. The norepinephrine cells seem to lack the methylating properties of the epinephrine cell.

Paraganglia

The cells of the adrenal medulla can be identified by their affinity for chromates. Small aggregations of chromaffin cells occur elsewhere in the body, here referred to as **paraganglia**. Most paraganglia are located retroperitoneally near the chain of sympathetic ganglia, but small groups of similar cells occur in organs such as the heart, the lungs, and the kidneys. The cells contain small, membrane-bound granules, similar to those in the cells of the adrenal medulla. The function of these cells is not known. They may secrete catecholamines. It is also possible that they secrete a variety of polypeptide hormones and that they should be included in the category of cells identified by their amine precursor decarboxylating properties, to which belong some of the enterochromaffin cells of the gastrointestinal tract and the cells of the carotid and aortic bodies. Consult the review by Dawson for further information.

References

ADRENAL CORTEX

Bennett, H. S. The life history and secretion of the cells of the adrenal cortex of the cat. Am. J. Anat. *67*: 151–228 (1940).

Bloodworth, J. M. B. and Powers, K. L. The ultrastructure of the normal dog adrenal. J. Anat. *102*: 457–476 (1968).

Brenner, R. M. Fine structure of adrenocortical cells in adult male rhesus monkeys. Am. J. Anat. *119*: 429–453 (1966).

Ford, J. K. and Young, R. W. Cell proliferation and displacement in the adrenal cortex of young rats injected with tritiated thymidine. Anat. Rec. *146*: 125–138 (1963).

Friend, D. S. and Brassil, G. E. Osmium staining of endoplasmic reticulum and mitochondria in the rat adrenal cortex. J. Cell Biol. *46*: 252–266 (1970).

Giacomelli, F., Wiener, J. and Spiro, D. Cytological alterations related to stimulation of the zona glomerulosa of the adrenal gland. J. Cell Biol. *26*: 499–522 (1965).

Idelman, S. Ultrastructure of the mammalian adrenal cortex. Int. Rev. Cytol. *27*: 181–281 (1970).

Long, J. A. and Jones, A. L. The fine structure of the zona glomerulosa and the zona fasciculata of the adrenal cortex of the opossum. Am. J. Anat. *120*: 463–488 (1967).

Long, J. A. and Jones, A. L. Observations on the fine structure of the adrenal cortex of man. Lab. Investig. *17*: 355–370 (1967).

Luse, S. Fine structure of adrenal cortex. *In:* The Adrenal Cortex (Ed. A. B. Eisenstein), pp. 1–60. Little, Brown, Boston, 1967.

Pauly, J. E. Morphological observations on the adrenal cortex of the laboratory rat. Endocrinology *60*: 247–264 (1957).

Penney, D. P. and Brown, G. M. The fine structural morphology of adrenal cortices of normal and stressed squirrel monkeys. J. Morph. *134*: 447–466 (1971).

Rhodin, J. A. G. The ultrastructure of the adrenal cortex of the rat under normal and experimental conditions. J. Ultrastruct. Res. *34*: 23–71 (1971).

Sheridan, M. N. and Belt, W. D. Fine structure of the guinea pig adrenal cortex. Anat. Rec. *149*: 73–98 (1964).

Zelander, T. The adrenal gland. *In:* Electron Microscopic Anatomy (Ed. S. M. Kurtz), pp. 199–220. Academic Press, New York, 1964.

Wood, J. G. Identification of and observation on epinephrine and norepinephrine containing cells in the adrenal medulla. Am. J. Anat. *112*: 285–303 (1963).

ADRENAL MEDULLA

Al-Lami, F. Light and electron microscopy of the adrenal medulla of macaca mulata monkey. Anat. Rec. *164*: 317–332 (1969).

Fig. 23-15. Relationship between nerves and endocrine cells of the adrenal medulla. Rat. E.M. X 10,000. **1.** Axon of myelinated nerve. **2.** Myelin sheath. **3.** Schwann cell cytoplasm. **4.** Axons of non-myelinated nerves. **5.** Nuclei of Schwann cells. **6.** Nerve axons near cell membrane of endocrine cell. **7.** Cell membrane of epinephrine cell. **8.** Intercellular space. **9.** Mitochondria. **10.** Secretory granules.

Fig. 23-16. Terminal contacts of nerve endings. Adrenal medulla. Rat. E.M. X 36,000. **1.** Nerve endings with numerous clear vesicles. **2.** Dense-core vesicles in nerve ending. **3.** Mitochondria. **4.** Synaptic junctions. **5.** Cell membrane of norepinephrine cell. **6.** Particulate glycogen. **7.** Secretory granules. **8.** Mitochondrion.

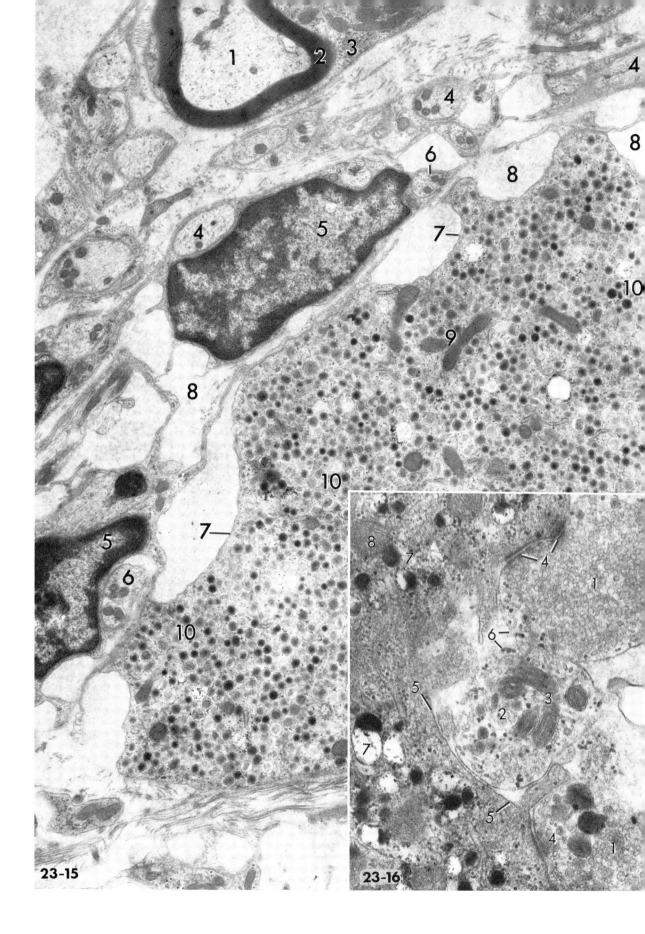

23-15

23-16

Bennett, H. S. Cytological manifestations of secretion in the adrenal medulla of the cat. Am. J. Anat. *69*: 333–383 (1941).

Brown, W. J., Barajas, L. and Latta, H. The ultrastructure of the human adrenal medulla: with comparative studies of white rat. Anat. Rec. *169*: 173–184 (1971).

Coupland, R. E. Electron microscopic observations on the structure of the rat adrenal medulla. I. The ultrastructure and organization of chromaffin cells in the normal adrenal medulla. J. Anat. *99*: 231–254 (1965).

Coupland, R. E. Electron microscopic observations on the structure of the rat adrenal medulla. II. Normal innervation. J. Anat. *99*: 255–272 (1965).

Coupland, R. E. and Weakley, B. S. Electron microscopic observations on the adrenal medulla and extra-adrenal chromaffin tissue of the postnatal rabbit. J. Anat. *106*: 213–231 (1970).

D'Anzi, F. A. Morphological and biochemical observations on the catecholamine-storing vesicles of rat adrenomedullary cells during insulin-induced hypoglycemia. Am. J. Anat. *125*: 381–398 (1969).

Elfvin, L. G. The development of the secretory granules in the rat adrenal medulla. J. Ultrastruct. Res. *17*: 45–62 (1967).

PARAGANGLIA

Böck, P. Die Feinstruktur des paraganglionären Gewebes im Plexus suprarenalis des Meerschweinchens. Z. Zellforsch. *105*: 389–404 (1970).

Dawson, I. The endocrine cells of the gastrointestinal tract. Histochem. J. *2*: 527–549 (1970).

24 Pineal body

GENERAL CONSIDERATIONS

The pineal body (synonyms: pineal gland, corpus pineale, epiphysis cerebri) develops from the neural ectoderm as a dorsal outgrowth of the caudal diencephalon. In lower vertebrates, it serves as a photoreceptor organ. In mammals, its function as an endocrine organ has only recently become more evident. It probably serves as one source of serotonin and melatonin, the latter probably acting as an antigonadal hormone, at least in rats and hamsters. The functional significance of the pineal body in man is presently not known.

The pineal body is a small, flat conical structure in the roof of the third ventricle, about 7 mm long and 4 mm wide. It is connected to the roof via a stalk which is hollow, the pineal recess of the third ventricle, lined by ependymal cells. The pineal body is surrounded by a thin connective tissue capsule which descends into the pineal body as septa, dividing the parenchyma of the gland into irregular lobules. (Fig. 24-1) The amount of connective tissue elements increases with age. The pineal body consists of: 1) pinealocytes; 2) neuroglial cells; 3) blood vessels; 4) connective tissue; and 5) nerves.

PINEALOCYTES

The pinealocytes (synonyms: parenchymal cells, chief cells, epithelioid cells) predominate in the parenchyma. (Figs. 24-3, 24-4) They are round or irregularly shaped cells with narrow, ramifying cell processes, some of which terminate as bulbous endings in the connective tissue around blood vessels. In the species used to illustrate this chapter (rat), most of the pinealocytes have an overall electron-dense appearance. (Fig. 24-5) In some species, pinealocytes are reported to have an electron-lucent cytoplasm. The possibility exists that there are functional differences reflected by the variation in cytoplasmic density, particularly since a highly electron-dense cytoplasm usually contains more ribo-

somes per square unit than does an electron-lucent cytoplasm. (Fig. 24-6)

The nucleus is large and round with a great deal of peripheral dense heterochromatin. There are many free ribosomes and polysomes, some short profiles of granular endoplasmic reticulum, and many vesicular and interconnected tubular profiles of the agranular endoplasmic reticulum. (Fig. 24-7) The Golgi apparatus is well developed as stacks of flattened saccules with peripheral vesicles and vacuoles. Mitochondria vary in size and appearance among species. In rat, they tend to be large with an electron-lucent matrix and tubular cristae. Both primary and secondary lysosomes occur. Dense granules, reminiscent of primary lysosomes and often referred to as **grumose bodies,** are present near the Golgi apparatus (Fig. 24-7), along the cell processes, and in the terminals. Some lipid droplets may occur. Glycogen particles are generally not present. Cytoplasmic filaments are extremely scarce in pinealocytes (as opposed to pineal neuroglial cells) but microtubules

Fig. 24-1. Pineal body. Human. L.M. X 168. **1.** Lobules of parenchyma. **2.** Connective tissue septa. **3.** Concretion.

Fig. 24-2. Pineal body concretion. Human. L.M. X 780. Concentric lamellae of hydroxy apatite, calcium carbonate apatite and organic matrix.

Fig. 24-3 & 24-4. Pineal body. Human. L.M. X 315. **1.** Connective tissue septa. **2.** Lumen of blood vessel. **3.** Parenchyma. Difference in cell types is not discernable. **4.** Cell shrinkage enhances the elongated shape of the cell processes and their allegedly club-shaped termination toward the connective tissue septa.

Fig. 24-5. Pineal body. Enlargement of area similar to rectangle in Fig. 24-4. Rat. E.M. X 2300. **1.** Nuclei of pinealocytes. **2.** Nuclei of pineal neuroglial cells (astrocytes). Note that differences in cell types have been verified at higher magnifications and are not discernible at this magnification. **3.** Dashed line indicates level of external (basal) lamina which surrounds the parenchymal lobule. **4.** Connective tissue septum. **5.** Lumen of capillary.

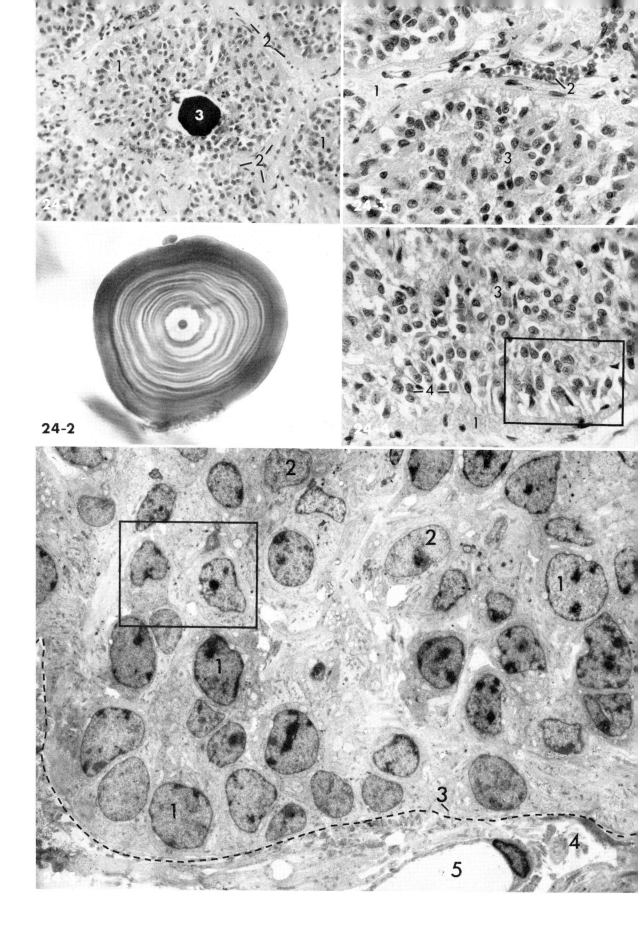

abound. The pinealocyte **processes** contain many microtubules and irregular, tubular elements of the agranular endoplasmic reticulum. (Fig. 24-9) The **terminals** of pinealocyte processes are larger and more irregular in shape than adjacent sympathetic nerve endings. They are clustered near one another in the perivascular area. They contain a varied amount of small vesicles, most of which have an electron-lucent, clear center, whereas some may be of the dense-cored variety. Larger granules with small dense particles (grumose bodies) also occur in the bulbous terminals of the pinealocyte processes.

PINEAL NEUROGLIAL CELLS

The pineal neuroglial cells (synonyms: interstitial cells, supportive cells) are stellate astrocytes. They are vastly outnumbered by the pinealocytes, and generally appear paler. (Fig. 24-6) Based on their ultrastructure, it is obvious that they are astroglial cells with a varied amount of cytoplasmic filaments. The presence of fibrillar elements makes it possible positively to identify this cell type as a glial cell rather than a pinealocyte. Differences in nuclear shape, chromatin density, and distribution are not sufficiently obvious to be used as criteria.

The pineal neuroglial cell is provided with long cytoplasmic processes or extensions which surround pineal cells and their processes, as well as sympathetic nerves and nerve endings. Many glial processes terminate at the surface of the parenchymal lobules beneath the investing external (basal) lamina. In this position, the cell membrane of the process often appears slightly thickened, its cytoplasmic aspect provided with a dense network of fine filaments.

The granular endoplasmic reticulum is more abundant in these cells than in the pinealocytes, consisting of short scattered profiles. Free ribosomes are relatively scarce. The Golgi apparatus occurs in several areas as dictyosomes. The mitochondria are small, provided with membranous cristae and a dense matrix. Primary and secondary lysosomes abound, and numerous glycogen particles of the beta-type are scattered throughout the cytoplasm. Microtubules are not very prominent, but many 50–60 Å-thick filaments occur, mostly in bundles to form fibrils. (Fig. 24-8) They are present both in the perinuclear region and in the processes.

BLOOD VESSELS

In man, most blood vessels and capillaries are present in the connective tissue septa, but in lower mammals, the parenchyma is also permeated by a rich capillary network. The capillary endothelium is of the thin, fenestrated type.

CONNECTIVE TISSUE

The capsule and the septa of the pineal body consists of a medium dense connective tissue. There is more connective tissue in pineal bodies of old people than in young ones.

In man, small concretions start to form

Fig. 24-6. Parenchymal cells. Pineal body. Enlargement of area similar to rectangle in Fig. 24-5. Rat. E.M. X 8400. **1.** Nuclei of pinealocytes. **2.** Nucleus of pineal neuroglial cell (astrocyte). **3.** Initial segment of two pinealocyte processes. **4.** Cross-sectioned pinealocyte processes. **5.** Electron-dense cytoplasm of pinealocyte. **6.** Electron-lucent cytoplasm of astrocyte. **7.** Large electron-lucent mitochondria. **8.** Small electron-dense mitochondria. **9.** Cross-sectioned sympathetic nerve process (enlarged further in Fig. 24-8, inset). **10.** Longitudinally sectioned sympathetic nerve processes. **11.** Large secondary lysosome. **12.** Glial cell membrane facing connective tissue space and external (basal) lamina.

Fig. 24-7. Detail of pinealocyte. Enlargement of area similar to rectangle (A) in Fig. 24-6. Pineal body. Rat. E.M. X 56,000. **1.** Nucleus. **2.** Nuclear membrane. **3.** Mitochondria with tubular cristae. **4.** Golgi saccules. **5.** Golgi vesicles. **6.** Condensing Golgi vacuoles. **7.** Primary lysosomes and/or grumose bodies. **8.** Ribosomes. **9.** Agranular endoplasmic reticulum. **10.** Microtubules. **11.** Cell membrane.

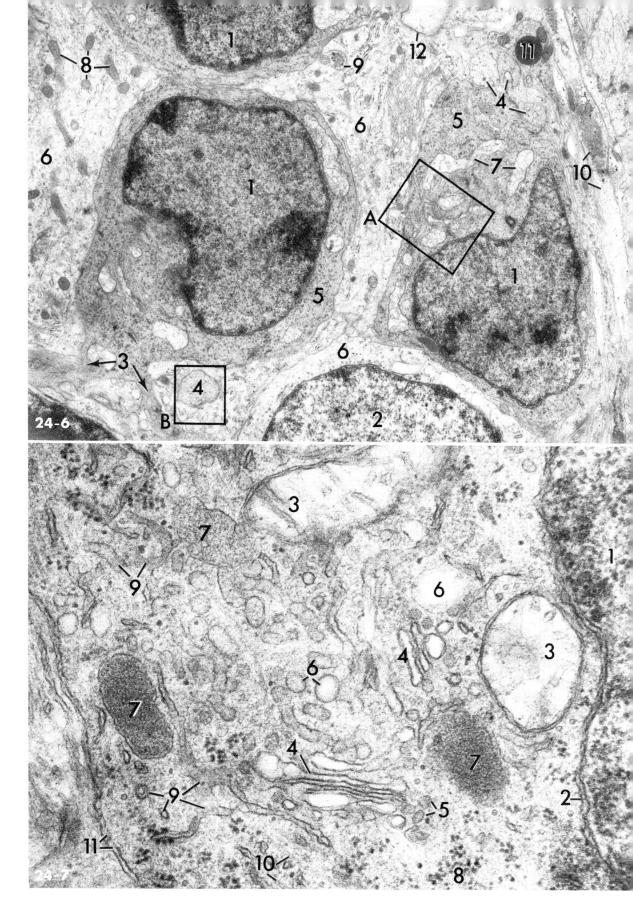

at the age of 17 years in relation to the connective tissue elements of the pineal body. The **concretions** (synonyms: brain sand; corpora arenacea; acervuli cerebri) are lamellated bodies (Fig. 24-2) formed of concentric layers of hydroxy apatite, calcium carbonate apatite, and an unknown organic matrix. The concretions increase gradually in size and number, and are quite numerous in old age. The cause and mechanism of their formation is not known.

NERVES

Some of the nerve processes present in the pineal body are myelinated, but most are non-myelinated. Some nerve fibers occur among the parenchymal cells, but the majority are present in the perivascular zones in a position peripheral of the lobular external (basal) lamina. (Fig. 24-10)

The myelinated fibers are derived from the habenular and posterior commissures, whereas the non-myelinated nerve processes come from sympathetic fibers originating in the superior cervical ganglia. The beaded non-myelinated nerves and their endings contain accumulations of two sizes of dense-core vesicles, one averaging 300 Å and the other 1000 Å. These vesicles contain norepinephrine and serotonin (5-hydroxytryptamine) and become depleted as a result of experimental reserpin administration.

FUNCTIONS

The pineal body has high concentrations of serotonin, norepinephrine, and melatonin. The **norepinephrine** is present in the sympathetic nerves and their endings. It is a neurotransmitter substance which is released by exocytosis upon the arrival of a nerve impulse. **Serotonin** (5-hydroxytryptamine) has been demonstrated in the nerve endings as well as in the terminal portion of the pinealocytic processes. **Melatonin** is an amine, synthesized from serotonin through an N-acetylation and O-methylation. There is some evidence

that melatonin is present in the pinealocytes, and that it may be the specific hormone of the pineal gland. Melatonin aggregates pigment granules in melanophores of the amphibian skin, an effect opposite to that of the melanocyte stimulating hormone of the hypophysis. In some rodents, it is known to have a reducing effect on the weight of the ovaries, and it also alters the estrus cycle. The synthesis of melatonin is influenced by light, probably via the sympathetic nervous system. In hamsters kept in the dark, the terminal processes of the pinealocytes contain an increased number of vesicles which has been interpreted as evidence of a possible secretory function of the pinealocytes.

Although very little is known of the specific function of the pineal body in man, it is presently believed, based on observations mostly in rodents, that this organ serves as a neuroendocrine transducer in many species. External stimuli of the visual, and perhaps, also olfactory

Fig. 24-8. Detail of pineal neuroglial cell (astrocyte). Pineal body. Rat. E.M. X 60,000. **1.** Nucleus. **2.** Lysosomes. **3.** Mitochondrion with membranous cristae. **4.** Golgi apparatus. **5.** Longitudinally sectioned bundle of cytoplasmic filaments. **6.** Cross-sectioned bundle of filaments. **7.** Ribosomes. **8.** Profiles of granular endoplasmic reticulum. **9.** Glycogen particles (beta type). **10.** Inset: cross-sectioned sympathetic nerve fiber, surrounded by astrocytic cytoplasm, containing clear vesicles, small and large dense-core vesicles.

Fig. 24-9. Cross-sectioned process of pinealocyte. Enlargement of area similar to rectangle (B) in Fig. 24-6. Pineal body. Rat. E.M. X 54,000. **1.** Mitochondria. **2.** Tubular elements of agranular endoplasmic reticulum. **3.** Clear vesicles. **4.** Microtubules.

Fig. 24-10. Detail of perivascular area. Pineal body. Rat. E.M. X 54,000. **1.** Cytoplasmic filaments in pineal neuroglial astrocyte. **2.** Cell membrane. **3.** External (basal) lamina of parenchymal lobule. **4.** Terminations of nerve endings. **5.** Small dense-cored vesicles. **6.** Large dense-core vesicles. **7.** Endothelium of postcapillary venule. **8.** Venular lumen.

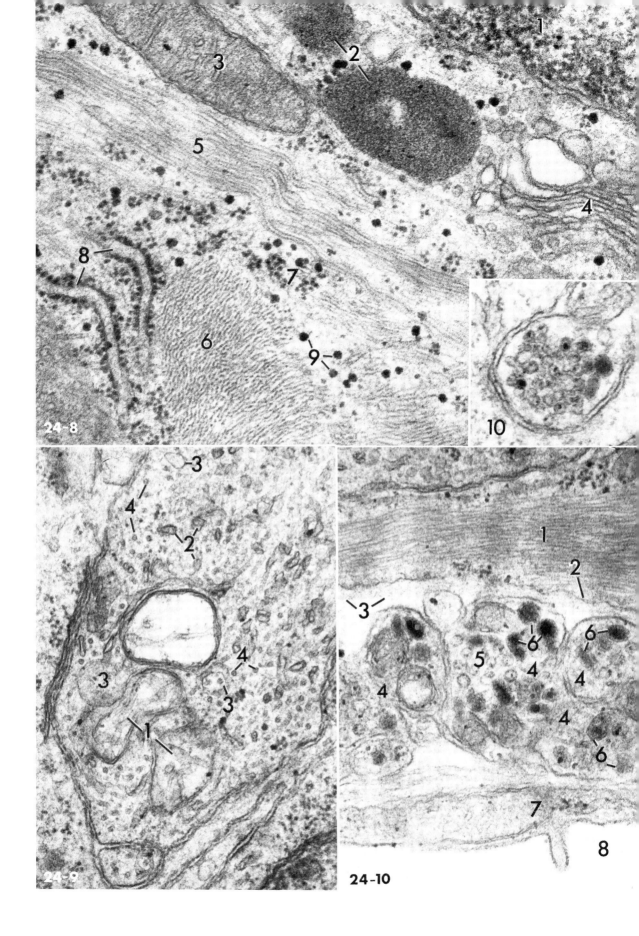

systems are relayed to the pineal body via the autonomic nervous system. As a result, changes in synthesis and release of melatonin in the pinealocytes modify the functions of some endocrine organs, primarily the gonads, but perhaps also the hypophysis, the thyroid, and the adrenal cortex.

References

Anderson, E. The anatomy of bovine and ovine pineals. Light and electron microscopic studies. J. Ultrastruct. Res. Suppl. 8 (1965).

Bertler, A., Falck, B. and Owman, Ch. Studies on 5-hydroxytryptamine stores in pineal gland of rat. Acta Physiol. Scand. 63, Suppl. 239 (1964).

Clabough, J. W. Ultrastructural features of the pineal gland in normal and light deprived golden hamsters. Z. Zellforsch. 114: 151–164 (1971).

Duffy, P. E. and Markesbery, W. R. Granulated vesicles in sympathetic nerve endings in the pineal gland: observations on the effect of the pharmacological agents by electron microscopy. Am. J. Anat. 128: 97–116 (1970).

Duncan, D. and Micheletti, G. Notes on the fine structure of the pineal organ of cats. Texas Report Biol. Med. 24: 576–587 (1966).

Hoffman, R. A. and Reiter, R. J. Pineal gland influence on gonads of male hamsters. Science 148: 1609–1611 (1965).

Kappers, J. A. The mammalian pineal organ. J. Neuro-Visceral Relations. Suppl. 9, 140–184 (1969).

Kappers, J. A. and Schadé, J. P. (Eds.). Structure and function of the epiphysis cerebri. Progr. in Brain Res. 10: 1–694 (1965).

Lederis, K. An electron microscopical study of the human neurohypophysis. Z. Zellforsch. 65: 847–868 (1965).

Lues, G. Die Feinstruktur der Zirbeldrüse normaler, trächtiger und experimentell beeinflusster Meerschweinchen. Z. Zellforsch. 114: 38–60 (1971).

Reiter, R. J. and Fraschini, F. Endocrine aspects of the mammalian pineal gland: a review. Neuroendocrinology 5: 219–255 (1969).

Sano, Y. and Mashimo, T. Elektronenmikroskopische Untersuchungen an der Epiphysis Cerebri beim Hund. Z. Zellforsch. 69: 129–139 (1966).

Sheridan, M. N. and Reiter, R. J. The fine structure of the hamster pineal gland. Am. J. Anat. 122: 357–376 (1968).

Sheridan, M. N. and Reiter, R. J. Observations on the pineal system in the hamster. II. Fine structure of the deep pineal. J. Morph. 131: 163–178 (1970).

Wartenberg, H. The mammalian pineal organ: electron microscopic studies on the fine structure of pinealocytes, glial cells, and on the perivascular compartment. Z. Zellforsch. 86: 74–97 (1968).

Wolstenhome, G. E. and Knight, J. (Eds.). The Pineal Gland. Ciba Foundation Symposium, Churchill, London, 1971.

Wurtman, R. J. and Axelrod, J. The formation, metabolism and physiological effects of melatonin in mammals. Progr. Brain Res. 10: 520–529 (1965).

25 Skin and appendages

The skin and associated structures, derived from the ectoderm, are collectively referred to as the **integumentum.** The appendages of the skin include hair, sebaceous glands, sweat glands, and nails. The integumentum functions in protecting the body surface, in regulating body temperature, in excretion, and in serving as a sense organ for touch, pressure, temperature, and pain.

Skin

The skin consists of a superficial layer of stratified squamous keratinizing epithelium, the **epidermis,** and a deep fibroelastic layer, the **dermis,** rich in vasculature and nerves. Under the dermis is a layer of connective and adipose tissues, the **hypodermis.** (Fig. 25-1) Generally, this is not considered a part of the skin, but it is functionally nevertheless quite important in connecting the dermis to underlying structures. Depending on the location, the thickness of the epidermis and the dermis varies considerably. The skin is particularly **thick** on the volar surface of hands and the plantar surface of feet. (Fig. 25-2) In these areas, the surface is characterized by ridges and grooves arranged in spiral and concentric patterns, typical for each individual and known as fingerprints. Hair follicles are not present in these areas. The **thin** skin covers areas such as the abdomen and the flexor surfaces of the arms. (Fig. 25-3) The epidermis of this skin has a very thin layer of keratinized cells, and the dermis is also very thin. Hair follicles are present, but superficial ridges and grooves are missing. Instead, a pattern of wrinkles and lines characterizes each area of the body. In areas such as the extensor surfaces of the arm, the back, and the legs, the skin shows great variation in thickness, surface pattern, and hair distribution.

EPIDERMIS

The epidermis is a stratified squamous keratinizing epithelium in which the number of cell layers varies greatly. As in all epithelia, the cells of the basal layer, through mitoses, give rise to new cells which subsequently differentiate and change structurally and functionally as they move toward the epithelial surface. (Fig. 25-4) In the epidermis, the fully keratinized superficial cells fulfill some of the main functions of the skin, namely, to protect the body against bacterial invasion, slight physical trauma, or penetration of water, as well as to prevent an abnormal evaporation of tissue fluid. The structural changes that the epidermal cells undergo are all part of a keratinization process, although many aspects of these changes are poorly understood. However, there are both genetic and environmental factors that determine whether the structural changes of the cells will ultimately lead to keratinization. Examples of this are readily observed in the stratified squamous epithelium of the mouth, pharynx, and larynx where abrasive forces will

Fig. 25-1. Section through thick skin of palm of hand. Human. L.M. X 33. **1.** Epidermis with thick stratum corneum. **2.** Dermis. **3.** Connective tissue septa of hypodermis. **4.** Subcutaneous fat tissue. **5.** Sweat glands. **6.** Ducts of sweat gland. **7.** Pacinian corpuscle. **8.** Artery. **9.** Vein.

Fig. 25-2. Thick skin of palmar surface of finger. Monkey. L.M. X 85. **1.** Ridges. **2.** Grooves. **3.** Stratum disjunctum. **4.** Stratum corneum. **5.** Stratum lucidum. **6.** Stratum granulosum. **7.** Stratum germinativum. **8.** Epidermal pegs and/or ridges. **9.** Dermal papillae.

Fig. 25-3. Thin skin of dorsal surface of hand. Human. L.M. X 210. **1.** Stratum disjunctum. **2.** Stratum corneum. **3.** Thin stratum granulosum. **4.** Stratum germinativum. **5.** Level of basal lamina. **6.** Papillary layer of dermis. **7.** Reticular layer of dermis.

Fig. 25-4. Epidermis. Enlargement of area similar to rectangle in Fig. 25-3. Axilla. Human. E.M. X 1900. **1.** Stratum corneum. Separation of layers accentuated by fixation and embedding procedures. **2.** Stratum granulosum (thin). **3.** Stratum spinosum. **4.** Stratum basale. **5.** Level of basal lamina. **6.** Collagenous fibrils of papillary layer. **7.** Fibroblasts.

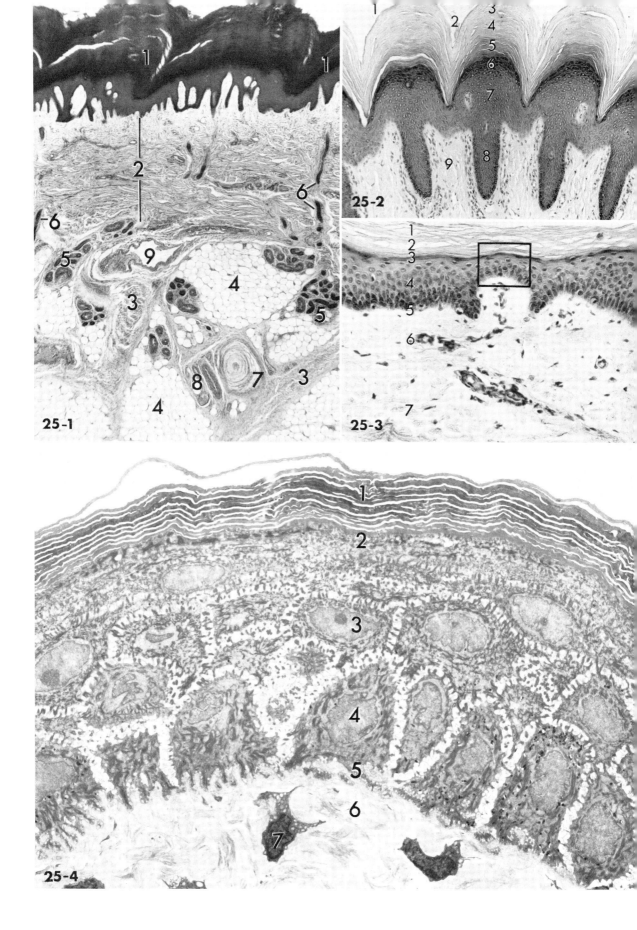

25-1

25-2

25-3

25-4

bring about keratinization in an area that otherwise would have only a non-keratinizing stratified squamous epithelium. A response by the epidermis to abrasive forces is indicated by the presence of thin and thick skin. In the case of the thick skin, the wear-and-tear stimulation results in a continuous keratinization process and the presence of a thick layer of keratinized cells. In the thin skin, this stimulation is less pronounced, leading to a thin layer of keratinized cells and periods of epidermal rest. If these differences are understood, it should be clear that the keratinization process basically is similar in thick and thin skin.

From within outward, the layers of the epidermis are as follows: 1) stratum germinativum; 2) stratum granulosum; 3) stratum lucidum; and 4) stratum corneum.

Stratum germinativum. The several basal layers of the epidermis are collectively referred to as stratum germinativum (or Malpighian layer). Mitotic activity occurs throughout but is especially high near the dermis in the **stratum basale.** (Fig. 25-7) This is a single layer of cuboidal or cylindrical cells resting on a thin **basal lamina.** The latter separates the epidermis from the dermis. (Fig. 25-8) The cells of the stratum basale have a large oval nucleus that occupies the major part of the cell. The cell border is irregular with short and thin cytoplasmic processes projecting into a narrow intercellular space, contacting similar processes of a neighboring cell. A limited number of small desmosomes secure these intercellular contacts. The base of the basal cells is extremely irregular and the cell membrane facing the basal lamina contains many **half-desmosomes.** Ribosomes are numerous, but mitochondria and profiles of the granular endoplasmic reticulum are scarce. The Golgi complex is rudimentary if at all present. Groups of short, fine tonofilaments are scattered throughout the cell, forming the tonofibrils of light microscopy. The tonofilaments average 75 Å in width and represent one of the earliest keratin precursors

that can be identified ultrastructurally in the basal stem cells of this keratinizing epithelium. Keratin is a fibrous protein and the ribosomes are clearly responsible for the synthesis of the tonofilaments. Above the basal layer is the **stratum spinosum,** the upper part of the stratum germinativum, which consists of two to ten layers of polyhedral cells. (Fig. 25-5) The mitotic activity is not as high among these cells as among the basal cells. They have round nuclei and an abundant cytoplasm. Prominent cytoplasmic processes (spines) extend to similar structures in adjacent cells, making contact via numerous large desmosomes. (Fig. 25-6) The intercellular space is the largest observed in the epidermis. Bundles of **tonafilaments,** forming tonofibrils, are larger and more numerous than in the basal cells, extending across the cell in many directions, and as a rule, originate from and terminate at **desmosomes.** Ribosomes abound, and a fair number of small membrane-bound spherical or oval bodies are present in these cells. The bodies have been described in many of the keratin-producing epithelia, including epidermis, oral and esophageal epithelia (Fig. 26-11) and have been assigned various names

Fig. 25-5. Epidermis. Detail of stratum spinosum. Rat. E.M. X 9600. **1.** Nucleus. **2.** Intercellular space. **3.** Cytoplasm.

Fig. 25-6. Stratum spinosum of epidermis. Enlargement of area similar to rectangle in Fig. 25-5. Rat. E.M. X 30,000. **1.** Free ribosomes. **2.** Bundles of tonofilaments. **3.** Cytoplasmic processes. **4.** Desmosomes. **5.** Intercellular space.

Fig. 25-7. Epidermis. Detail of stratum basale. Rat. E.M. X 9000. **1.** Nucleus of basal cell. **2.** Nucleus of cell in stratum spinosum. **3.** Intercellular space. **4.** Basal lamina.

Fig. 25-8. Stratum basale of epidermis. Enlargement of area similar to rectangle in Fig. 25-7. Rat. E.M. X 29,000. **1.** Nucleus. **2.** Ribosomes. **3.** Mitochondria. **4.** Bundles of tonofilaments. **5.** Hemidesmosomes. **6.** Basal lamina. **7.** Collagenous fibrils in papillary layer of dermis. **8.** Nerve axons. **9.** Schwann cell cytoplasm.

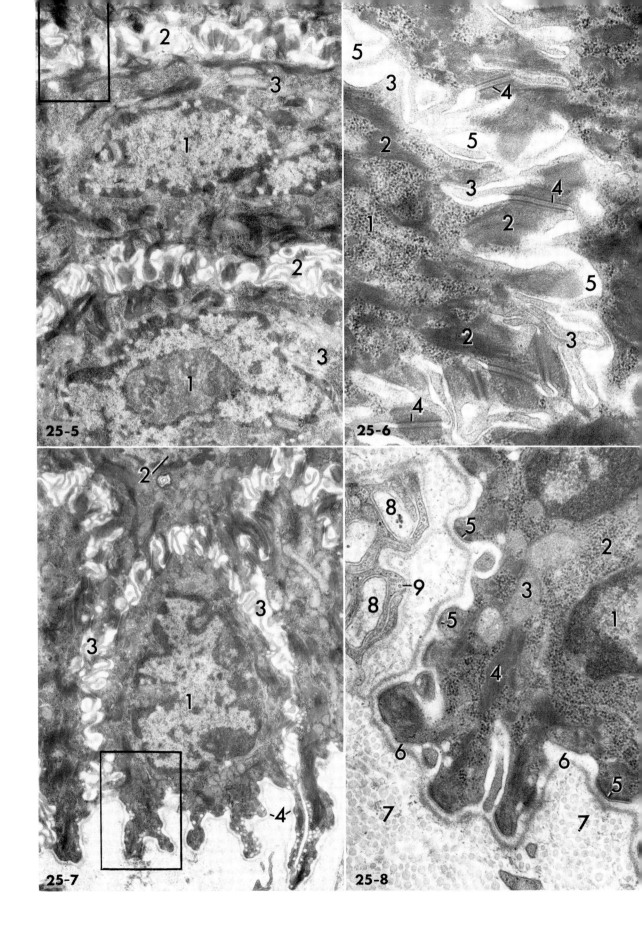

25-5

25-6

25-7

25-8

such as keratinosomes, multilamellar bodies, and **membrane-coating granules.** Their role remains to be clarified. It has been suggested that they become discharged into the intercellular space of the more superficial, squamous cell layers, and that they contribute to the intercellular material observed between the squamous cells. The membrane-coating granules may also be responsible for the thickening of the cell membrane by a deposition of dense material onto the cytoplasmic face of the inner leaflet of the cell membrane. This is discussed further on p. 482.

Stratum granulosum. As the cells of the stratum spinosum are pushed toward the surface of the epidermis, they gradually become flattened and elongated. Simultaneously, irregularly shaped **keratohyalin granules** start to appear in the cytoplasm. In thick skin, the stratum granulosum is composed of two or three layers of flattened, polyhedral cells. In thin skin, the stratum granulosum consists of only scattered cells, forming an incomplete layer above the stratum spinosum. (Fig. 25-9) The cell borders have lost the spiny cytoplasmic processes, the number of desmosomes is smaller, and the intercellular space is reduced to a 250 Å-wide gap. The keratohyalin granules are not bounded by a membrane. (Fig. 25-10) Their origin is not known. They are dense, homogeneous or finely granular structures containing proline and amino acids rich in sulfhydryl groups. Tonofilaments abound, and are closely associated with the keratohyalin granules.

Stratum lucidum. This layer is present only in thick skin, where it consists of one or two layers of extremely flattened cells. The nucleus, ribosomes, and mitochondria are obscured or replaced by the densely packed tonofibrils which are arranged parallel to the surface of the skin and more orderly than in the cells of the stratum granulosum. The keratohyalin granules have disappeared, and presumably their content is distributed among the tonofilaments as one of the last steps be-

fore the cells become fully keratinized. The failure to demonstrate a stratum lucidum in thin skin could reflect an inability to properly preserve and capture this step. However, it may also imply that the keratinization process can follow several paths in achieving a cornification. Other examples of this relate to the formation of hair and nails which occurs without the presence of keratohyalin granules. The cell membrane of the cells in the stratum lucidum has increased in thickness, here averaging 120 Å. The intercellular gap is filled largely by an extension of the material normally present between apposing desmosomes, possibly derived from discharged membrane-coating granules. (Fig. 25-12)

Fig. 25-9. Epidermis. Rat. E.M. X 12,000. **1.** Nucleus of squamous cell in layer above stratum spinosum. **2.** Nucleus of cell in stratum granulosum. **3.** Stratum corneum. **4.** Stratum disjunctum. The cytoplasm of these cells is loosened up as part of a shedding process. **5.** Keratohyalin granules.

Fig. 25-10. Epidermis. Enlargement of area similar to square (A) in Fig. 25-9. Rat. E.M. X 31,000. **1.** Ribosomes. **2.** Masses of merging keratohyalin granules and tonofilaments. **3.** Desmosomes.

Fig. 25-11. Epidermis. Enlargement of area similar to square (B) in Fig. 25-9. Rat. E.M. X 32,000. **1.** Nucleus of cell in stratum granulosum. **2.** Squamous cells of stratum corneum. **3.** Ribosomes. **4.** Keratohyalin granules. **5.** Bundles of tonofilaments. **6.** Membrane-coating granules. **7.** Desmosomes.

Fig. 25-12. Epidermis. Enlargement of area similar to rectangle (A) in Fig. 25-11. Human. E.M. X 99,000. **1.** Cytoplasm of cell in stratum granulosum. **2.** Cells in stratum corneum. **3.** Multilamellar bodies (membrane-coating granules) at the moment of discharge. **4.** Intercellular space. **5.** Desmosomes.

Fig. 25-13. Epidermis. Stratum Corneum. Enlargement of area similar to rectangle (B) in Fig. 25-11. Rat. E.M. X 96,000. The fully keratinized cells of the epidermis are made up of bundles of densely packed keratin filaments. **1.** Cross-sectioned keratin filaments (80 Å). **2.** Longitudinally sectioned keratin filaments.

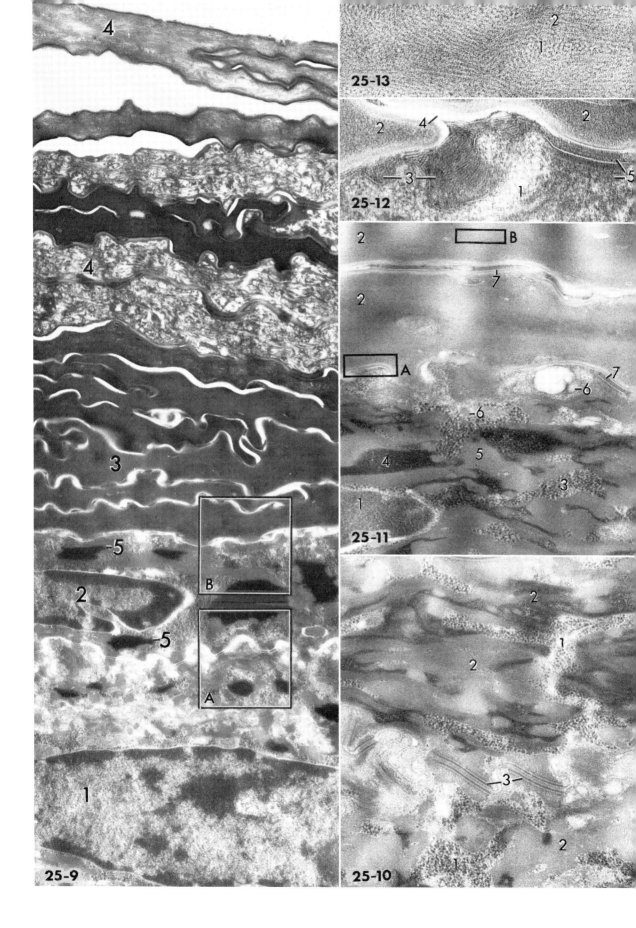

25-9

25-13

25-12

25-11

25-10

Stratum corneum. This is also called the horny layer and it is composed of fully keratinized, squamous cells with very low water content. (Fig. 25-11) In thin skin, there is only one or two layers, but in thick skin there can be up to several hundred layers. The cells contain extremely densely packed **keratin filaments,** 70–90 Å in diameter, probably derived from the tonofilaments. (Fig. 25-13) The keratin filaments are embedded in an electron-dense substance, presumably derived from the keratohyalin granules. The cell membrane of these cells is thicker than elsewhere in the epidermis and remnants of desmosomes may be present. One of the final steps in the **keratinization process** is the formation of disulfide bonds. However, it is not known how this fits in with the fine structural organization of the fully keratinized cells. Keratin is tough and resilient, as well as hard and elastic, contributing to the protective qualities of the epidermis. The thickened cell membranes and their close juxtaposition with intercellular material probably account for the high degree of water resistance of the skin. The most superficial layer is called **stratum disjunctum** because of its tendency to become detached. (Fig. 25-9) The time required for one cell to develop from a basal to a fully keratinized cell varies in humans from 30 to 90 days. In rats, the time required may be less than 20 days. However, great variations exist within the same species, and the process is greatly speeded up after epidermal injuries. Furthermore, mitotic activity in the stratum germinativum is said to be higher at night, supposedly due to a higher level of blood sugar during this time.

DERMIS

The dermis is a fibroelastic layer that contributes greatly to the toughness and pliability of the skin. It is generally thick in relation to epidermal areas with a thick stratum corneum, and conversely, it is thin in relation to thin epidermal areas.

The dermis has a superficial papillary layer and a deep, reticular layer. (Fig. 25-14)

Papillary layer. This layer is formed by numerous dermal papillae, conical eminences ascending into similar impressions on the basal surface of the epidermis. (Fig. 25-15) The papillae consist of a loosely and irregularly arranged network of fine bundles of mostly collagenous and some elastic fibrils. This connective tissue is relatively rich in cells, most of which are fibroblasts. Macrophages occur regularly but plasma cells and fat cells are rarely present. Occasional lymphocytes can be identified. The papillary layer contains a rich capillary network consisting of loops arranged perpendicularly to the skin surface, nourishing the epidermis, which is avascular, and serving as heat regulators. Venules form a bed below the bases of the dermal papillae. Nervous end organs, particularly the tactile bodies, are located in some of the dermal papillae.

Reticular layer. A dense network of irregularly arranged thick bundles of collagenous fibrils forms this layer (Fig. 25-16) which, because of its toughness in some animals, is widely used for making leather goods. Some elastic fibers are also present. There are fewer cells than in the

Fig. 25-14. Survey of dermis. Rat. E.M.X 590. **1.** Stratum germinativum of epidermis. **2.** Epidermal pegs. **3.** Dermal papillae. **4.** Papillary layer of dermis. **5.** Reticular layer of dermis with blood vessels and nerves. **6.** Hypodermis with blood vessels and nerves.

Fig. 25-15. Detail of papillary layer of dermis. Rat. E.M. X 1700. **1.** Stratum basale of epidermis. **2.** Capillary in dermal papilla (luminal diameter 11 μ). **3.** Fibroblasts. **4.** Bundles of collagenous fibrils. **5.** Nonmyelinated nerves.

Fig. 25-16. Skin. Nerve-vascular bundle in the region between dermis and hypodermis. Rat. E.M. X 1900. **1.** Small artery. **2.** Arteriole, lumen 23 μ. **3.** Capillaries, lumen approx. 8 μ. **4.** Venule lumen 30 μ. **5.** Myelinated nerves. **6.** Fibroblasts. **7.** Mast cells. **8.** Macrophages. **9.** Bundles of collagenous fibrils.

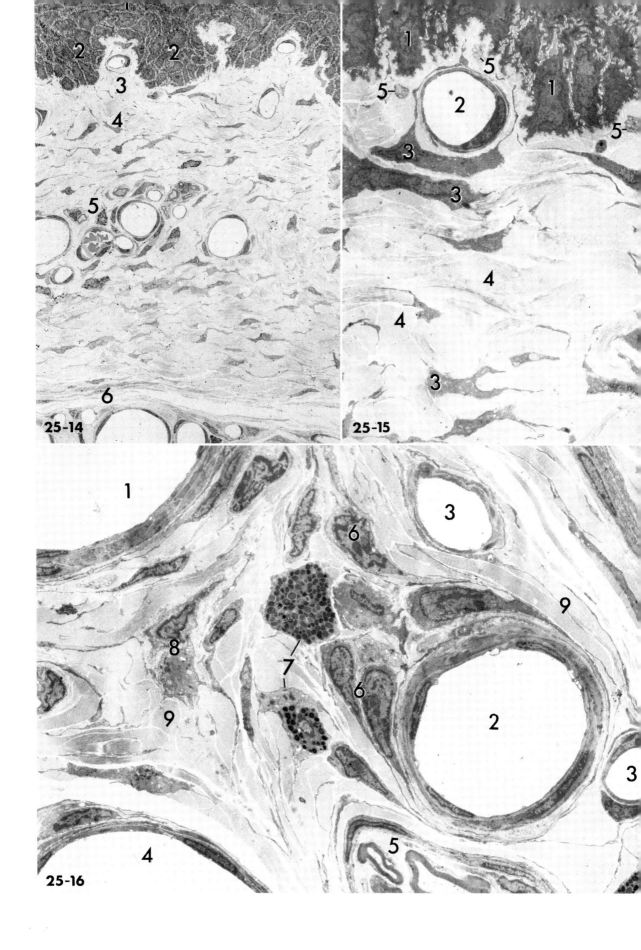

25-14

25-15

25-16

papillary layer, and those present are mostly resting fibrocytes. Capillaries are scarce except in relation to skin appendages. Smooth muscle cells occur in this layer in specific areas such as the scrotum, penis, labia majora, and the nipples.

HYPODERMIS

The deep part of the dermis borders on the subcutaneous tissue which is referred to as hypodermis or tela subcutanea. It is composed of a loose connective tissue which is rich in fat cells, particularly in the deeper parts where an abundance of adipose tissue may be accumulated to form a **panniculus adiposus**, a fat-pad. The hypodermal connective tissue allows for movement of the skin in relation to underlying structures such as muscle fasciae and periosteum. The more superficial region of the hypodermis harbors parts of hair follicles and sweat glands. The hypodermis in general contains the larger blood vessels and main nerve bundles of the skin.

SKIN COLOR

The intrinsic color of the skin is slightly yellow, but it is modified by the red blood in the capillaries of the papillary layer of the dermis. However, the specific color of the skin relates also to the amount of pigments present at any one time.

Within the stratum basale of the epidermis are present special pigment-containing cells, **melanocytes.** (Fig. 25-17) These cells are derived from the ectoderm of the neural crest. They have a small central cell body containing the nucleus, and numerous long, thin, and branching cytoplasmic processes (Fig. 25-18) that reach up in between the cells of the stratum spinosum. Desmosomes are not associated with their cell membranes. The Golgi zone is large and the granular endoplasmic reticulum is well developed. The cytoplasm contains several large mitochondria and a few cytoplasmic filaments and some ribosomes, but the paucity of the last two organelles makes the melanocytes

appear less electron-dense than the other cells of the stratum germinativum. The melanocytes contain specific pigment granules, the **melanosomes.** These are membrane-bound, ovoid bodies, the length averaging about 0.7μ and the width about 0.3μ. (Figs. 25-19, 25-20) The melanosomes are derived from Golgi vacuoles which gradually accumulate a dense core. The mature melanosome contains sheets of highly electron-dense material arranged concentrically around its long axis. The synthesis of the brown pigment in man involves the conversion of the amino acid tyrosine to **melanin** by the enzyme tyrosinase. This synthesis is stimulated by the ultra-violet rays of the sun. Melanocytes and melanosomes are present also in albinos, individuals with light skin and white hair, but here, the melanosomes lack the electron-dense material. Melanosomes occur also in the epidermal cells of the stratum basale, and in blacks also

Fig. 25-17. Epidermis from axilla. Human. Negro. E.M. × 1800. **1.** Stratum corneum. **2.** Stratum granulosum. **3.** Stratum spinosum. **4.** Stratum basale. **5.** Basal lamina. **6.** Collagenous fibrils of papillary layer of dermis. **7.** Fibroblast. **8.** Melanocyte. **9.** Langerhans' cell (melanocyte without melanosomes.).

Fig. 25-18. Melanocyte. Epidermis. Human. Negro. E.M. × 10,000. **1.** Nucleus of melanocyte. **2.** Adjacent basal cells in the epidermis. **3.** Basal lamina. **4.** Collagenous fibrils. **5.** The "tail" of the melanocyte may indicate that the cell is in the process of moving from dermis to epidermis. **6.** Intercellular space. **7.** Narrow processes of melanocyte with melanosomes.

Fig. 25-19. Detail of melanocyte. Epidermis. Human. Negro. E.M. × 58,000. **1.** Nucleus of melanocyte. **2.** Cell membrane. **3.** Basal lamina of epidermis. **4.** Mitochondrion. **5.** Mature melanosomes. **6.** Pre-melanosomes in various stages of maturation. Each pre-melanosome is surrounded by a single trilaminar boundary membrane.

Fig. 25-20. Epidermis. Detail of basal cell. Human. Negro. E.M. × 60,000. **1.** Ribosomes. **2.** Bundles of tonofilaments. **3.** Mature melanosomes. Boundary membrane obscured by melanin pigmentation.

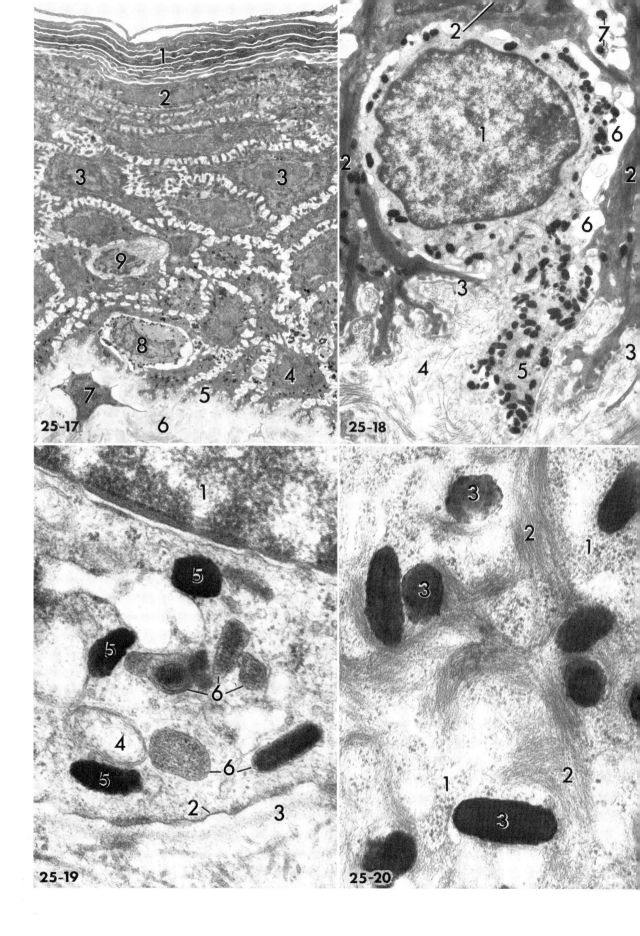

25-17

25-18

25-19

25-20

in other strata of the epidermis. It is believed that these melanosomes have been transferred from the cytoplasmic processes of the melanocyte to the epidermal cells, but the mechanism for the transfer is not known.

Occasional melanocytes may occur in the dermis. However, it is not clear if their origin is mesodermal or ectodermal. Macrophages in the papillary layer of the dermis may also contain melanosomes but these have been phagocytosed from aging or disintegrating melanocytes.

Hair

The hairs emanate from deep cylindrical invaginations of the epidermis, the hair follicles, which extend down to the hypodermis. (Fig. 25-21) The hair is composed of cells which contain a hard fibrous keratin. The cells are tightly held together and do not desquamate as the neighboring keratinized cells of the epidermis which contain a soft fibrous keratin. Hairs are present throughout the surface of the body except for a few places such as the volar surface and sides of the hand and fingers, and the plantar surface and sides of the foot and toes. Over the hairy surfaces, there is a great variation in arrangement and grouping of hairs as well as in number of hairs per unit area and in the degree of development of individual hairs. Much of this is controlled by hormones.

DEVELOPMENT

The **hair follicle** begins as a thickening of the epidermis which grows down into the dermal connective tissue as a solid cord of cells. The lower end enlarges to form a bulb, the future **hair papilla,** and connective tissue elements enter the papilla from beneath to form the **dermal papilla** of the hair. The epidermal cells in the center of the papilla gradually develop strata among which can be recognized cells similar to those in the stratum spinosum of the epidermis, as well as cells

with keratohyalin granules, hyalin cells, and fully keratinized cells. However, there is a more elaborate layering than the simple one of the epidermis. From the germinative **matrix** of the hair papilla, the central cells form the hair proper, and the peripheral cells form three strata which are structurally different. From within outward, these strata are: the **cuticles,** the **inner root sheath,** and the **outer root sheath.** As the multiplication

Fig. 25-21. Thick section of facial skin. Monkey. Preparation shows distribution of hairs and blood vessels. L.M. X 30.
1. Capillaries of papillary layer.
2. Subpapillary arterial plexus.
3. Cutaneous arterial plexus. **4.** Hair shaft.
5. Hair follicle **6.** Hair papilla.

Fig. 25-22. Thin section of skin. Scalp. Human. L.M. X 43. **1.** Epidermis. **2.** Dermis.
3. Hypodermis. **4.** Hair shaft. **5.** Hair follicle.
6. Hair papilla. **7.** Resting hair follicles.
8. Club-hairs.

Figs. 25-23 to 25-25. Longitudinal sections of human hair: **Fig. 25-23** (L.M. X 200) corresponds to rectangle (A) in Fig. 25-22; **Fig. 25-24** (L.M. X 140) corresponds to rectangle (B); and **Fig. 25-25** (L.M. X 140) corresponds to rectangle (C). **1.** Dermal papilla. **2.** Hair papilla. **3.** Hair matrix.
4. Hair medulla. **5.** Hair cortex. **6.** Inner root sheath. **7.** Outer root sheath.
8. Connective tissue sheath. **9.** Epidermis.

Fig. 25-26 to 25-29. Cross sections of human hair. L.M. X 145: **Fig. 25-26** corresponds to level A in Fig. 25-23; **Fig. 25-27** corresponds to level B in Fig. 25-24; **Fig. 25-28** corresponds to level C in Fig. 25-25; and **Fig. 25-29** corresponds to level D in Fig. 25-25. Legends to numerals 1–9 are identical to those in Fig. 25-25.

Fig. 25-30. Cross section of hair shaft at approximately the same level as Fig. 25-27. Vibrissa. Rat. E.M. X 1800. **1.** Hair cortex.
2. Hair cuticle. **3.** Remnants of keratinized inner root sheath. **4.** Stratum granulosum of outer rooth sheath. **5.** Stratum germinativum.

Fig. 25-31. Detail of cross-sectioned hair shaft. Enlargement of area similar to rectangle in Fig. 25-30. Vibrissa. Rat. E.M. X 39,000. **1.** Cells of hair cortex fully keratinized (hard keratin). Individual keratin filaments are not resolved. **2.** Cells of hair cuticle, fully keratinized. **3.** Cell membranes with intercellular substance.

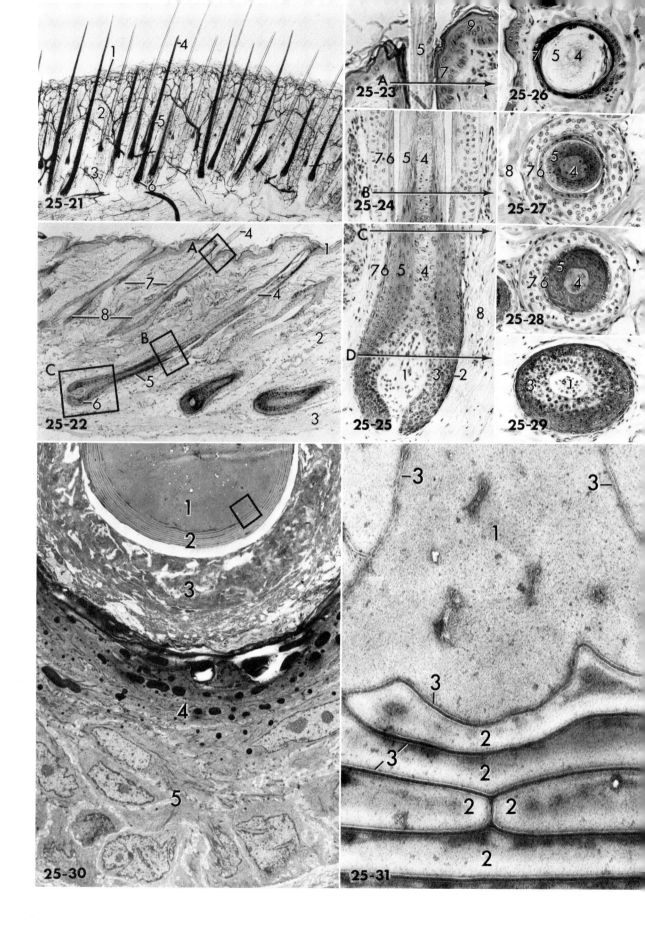

25-21

25-22

25-23 A

25-24 B

25-25 C D

25-26

25-27

25-28

25-29

25-30

25-31

of cells continues in the matrix of the hair papilla, the keratinized center of the epidermal down-growth is gradually pushed toward the surface of the skin and eventually emerges as the free, expelled **hair.**

STRUCTURE OF THE HAIR

The hair consists of the shaft and the papilla. (Fig. 25-22) The **shaft** has a free, expelled part and an intrafollicular part situated below the surface of the skin, generally referred to as the **root** of the hair. The more superficial part of the root is fully keratinized, but the lower part is only partly keratinized and merges with the cells of the cylindrical hair follicle in the **matrix** of the **hair papilla.** The hair shaft is composed of a thin, superficial hair cuticle, a thick cortex and a narrow medulla. (Figs. 25-23 through 25-29)

Cuticle of the hair. This consists of a thin layer of overlapping, transparent scales with their free edge facing up. These are fully keratinized, non-nucleated cells which are tightly held together by an intercellular dense substance. (Fig. 25-31) They contain a fibrous, hard keratin which does not require keratohyalin granules for the completion of the keratinization process.

Cortex of the hair. This consists of concentrically arranged, elongated, spindle-shaped, non-nucleated cells which are also held together tightly by an intercellular substance. The cells are completely filled by a fibrous, hard keratin in which the keratin filaments are oriented parallel to the long axis of the hair. (Figs. 25-31, 25-35) As in the hair cuticle, the cells of the hair cortex become keratinized without the presence of keratohyalin and membrane-coating granules. The difference in the **keratinization** processes leading to hard and soft keratin is poorly understood. In both instances, sulfhydryl groups are oxidized to disulfide groups, but hard keratin seems to contain more sulfur than soft keratin. During the formation of hard keratin, keratohyalin granules (or tricho-

hyalin granules as they are often referred to in the hair) are not present. Still, the fine structure of the final product in the cells of hard and soft keratin is similar, being composed of densely packed filaments (α-filaments) 60 Å thick, embedded in a highly electron-dense interfilamentous substance. However, there are obvious physical differences, since hard keratin does not desquamate, it is permanent, very solid, and must be cut in order to be removed, whereas soft keratin is resilient, although tough, and does desquamate.

Medulla of the hair. The medulla of the hair is not present in all hairs, and if present, it generally does not extend through the entire length of the hair. The medulla consists of cuboidal cells which contain soft keratin. (Fig. 25-32) Their precursor cells near the hair matrix contain keratohyalin granules.

Color of the hair. The color of the hair is determined by the number of melanin granules in the cortical cells. Melanocytes are present in the matrix of the papilla, and they synthesize melanosomes as in the epidermis. Subsequently, the melanosomes are transferred to the cortical and medul-

Fig. 25-32. Survey of hair root and papillae. Scalp. Human. L.M. X 320. **1.** Dermal papilla. **2.** Basal lamina. **3.** Hair matrix. **4.** Hair medulla. **5.** Hair cortex. **6.** Hair cuticles. **7.** Inner root sheath. **8.** Outer root sheath. **9.** Glassy membrane (basal lamina). **10.** Connective tissue sheath.

Fig. 25-33. Enlargement of area similar to rectangle in Fig. 25-32. Vibrissa. Rat. E.M. X 740. **1.** Dermal papilla. **2.** Basal lamina. **3.** Hair matrix. **4.** Hair cortex. **5.** Hair cuticle. **6.** Cuticle of inner root sheath. **7.** Huxley's layer. **8.** Henle's layer. **9.** Outer root sheath. **10.** Glassy membrane. **11.** Connective tissue sheath.

Fig. 25-34. Enlargement of area similar to rectangle in Fig. 25-33. Vibrissa. Rat. E.M. X 4500. **1.** Nuclei of cells forming the hair cuticle. **2.** Nuclei of cells forming cuticle of inner root sheath. **3.** Two layers of cells constitute Huxley's layer at this level. **4.** Trichohyalin granules. **5.** Cells of Henle's layer. **6.** Cells of outer root sheath. **7.** Basal lamina (glassy membrane).

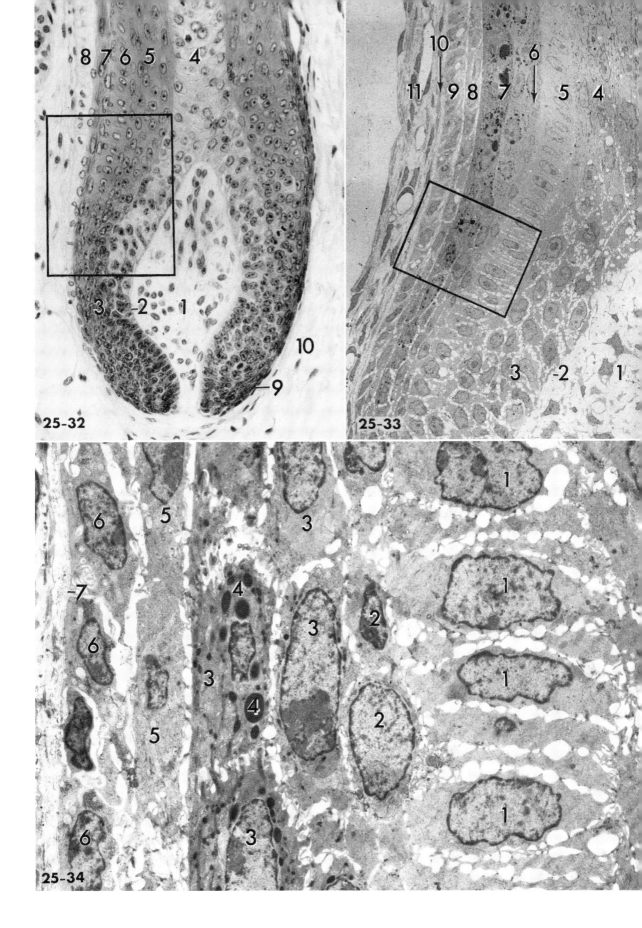

25-32

25-33

25-34

lary cells of the hair. Blonde and gray hairs do not contain melanosomes, but gray hair contains a varying amount of air between the cells contributing to the gray or white color.

HAIR FOLLICLE

The hair follicle is a cylindrical formation, derived from the epidermis, with the hair root in the center. (Fig. 25-32) The deepest part of the follicle is the papilla which contains an aggregation of poorly differentiated stem cells, collectively referred to as the **matrix**. These cells give rise to both the hair itself and to the inner root sheath of the hair. The hair follicle consists of two major strata: 1) inner epithelial root sheath; 2) outer epithelial root sheath. (Fig. 25-33)

Inner root sheath. This sheath is present from the hair papilla to the level where the sebaceous glands discharge their secretion into the hair follicle. From within outward, the inner root sheath consists of three strata: 1) cuticle of the inner root sheath; 2) Huxley's layer; and 3) Henle's layer. (Fig. 25-35) The **cuticle** of the inner root sheath consists of a single layer of flat, overlapping cells with their free edge facing down, interdigitating with and meeting the corresponding edges of the cells of the cuticle of the hair which face upward. The cells that make up the cuticle of the inner root sheath of the hair contain a soft keratin, and the partially keratinized cells near the hair papilla contain both keratohyalin granules and tonofibrils. The **layer of Huxley** contains several strata of cells. The cells change from polyhedral to elongated flattened as they move up along the hair and become keratinized. Their cytoplasm is filled with large keratohyalin (trichohyalin) granules and thick bundles of tonofibrils. The fully keratinized cells contain a soft keratin. The **layer of Henle** is made up of a single layer of cuboidal cells which early become fully keratinized and flattened out. They also contain soft keratin, and this layer is largely reminiscent of

the stratum lucidum of the epidermis of thick skin, since the cells have a hyaline or "clear" appearance. Upon reaching a complete keratinization, the inner root sheath desquamates at the level of the sebaceous glands. The function of the inner root sheath has not been adequately explored. It probably plays a certain role in the maturation and keratinization process of the hair itself, since it disappears at a level where the cells of the hair cortex have completed their keratinization process.

Fig. 25-35. Cross section of hair follicle at approximately the same level as Fig. 25-28. Vibrissa. Rat. E.M. X 1700. **1.** Center of hair. Medullary cells are not present in this particular hair. **2.** Hair cortex. Intensely black areas are cross-sectioned bundles of tonofibrils. Lighter areas are nuclei of hair cells. **3.** Layers of thin squamous hair cuticle cells. Dark lines represent beginning of keratinization. **4.** One thin layer of cells constitutes the cuticle of the inner root sheath. **5.** Huxley's layer is several cells deep. Abundant black trichohyalin granules indicate an approaching soft keratinization process. **6.** Cells of Henle's layer are keratinized at this level (soft keratin). Remnants of nuclei in some cells. **7.** Stratified epithelium of outer root sheath. Cells rich in particulate glycogen.

Fig. 25-36. Detail of cell in Huxley's layer. Enlargement of area similar to rectangle (A) in Fig. 25-35. Vibrissa. Rat. E.M. X 57,000. **1.** Trichohyalin granules. **2.** Cross-sectioned tonofilaments. **3.** Ribosomes.

Fig. 25-37. Detail of cells in hair cuticle. Enlargement of area similar to rectangle (B) in Fig. 25-35. Vibrissa. Rat. E.M. X 59,000. **1.** Cell borders. **2.** Amorphous keratin. **3.** Ribosomes.

Fig. 25-38. Detail of cell in hair cortex. Enlargement of area similar to rectangle (C) in Fig. 25-35. Vibrissa. Rat. E.M.X 59,000. **1.** Cell border. **2.** Cross-sectioned bundles of tonofibrils. **3.** Ribosomes.

Fig. 25-39. Detail of tonofibrillar bundle. Enlargement of area similar to rectangle in Fig. 25-38. Vibrissa. Rat. E.M. X 237,000. Each bundle of tonofibrils is composed of densely packed keratin filaments, referred to as α-filaments. Each filament is about 70 Å wide and has a lighter center with a dense filamentous subunit.

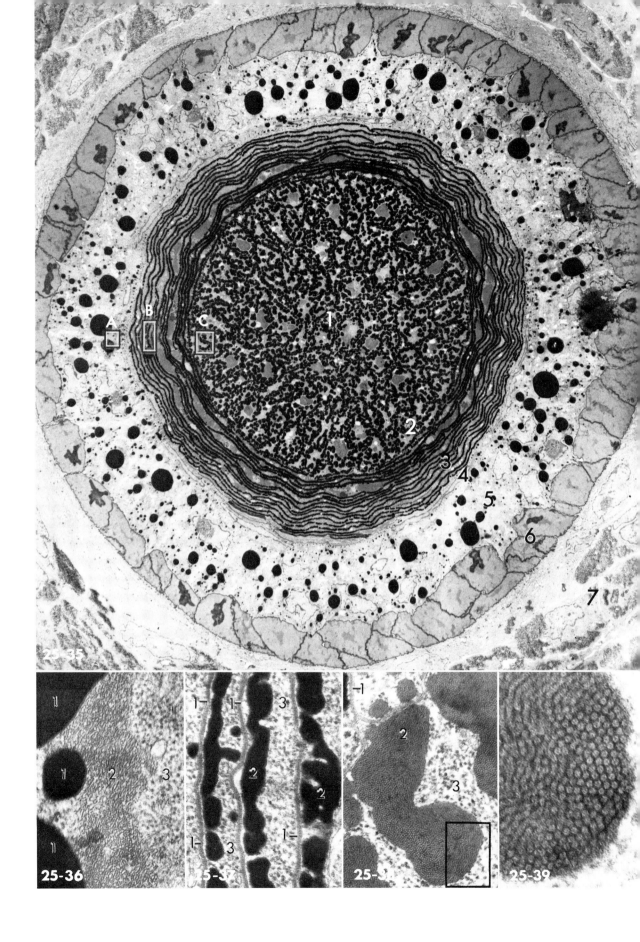

25-35

25-36

15-37

25-38

25-39

Outer root sheath. The outer root sheath consists of cells which correspond to those of the epidermis, and are considered as a direct continuation and down-growth of the epidermis. (Fig. 25-32) The stratum corneum of the outer root sheath extends from the surface of the skin to the level of the sebaceous glands. The stratum granulosum continues a short distance deeper, and the stratum germinativum continues all the way down to, and forms a functionally essential part of the papilla of the hair, blending with the cells of the hair matrix.

The basal lamina of the epidermis is continuous with a somewhat thicker **glassy membrane** that surrounds the outer root sheath and separates it from the dermal and subdermal connective tissue. It also separates the cells of the hair matrix from the dermal papilla.

A **connective tissue sheath** surrounds the hair follicle. It consists of three indistinct layers made up of thick bundles of collagenous fibers and fibroblasts derived from the dermis.

The **muscle of the hair** consists of several long, spindle-shaped smooth muscle cells, arranged to form a bundle, the **arrector pili** muscle. The hairs are set at a certain angle to the surface of the skin. The arrector pili muscle is located on the side of the hair which faces down. It originates from the subepithelial connective tissue of the skin and splits up into several bundles each of which inserts in the connective tissue sheath around the hair follicle slightly above its mid-point. On their way to the point of insertion, the smooth muscle bundles pass on the outside of the sebaceous glands. Upon contraction, the arrector pili pulls the hair to a more erect position, and it also pulls the skin down locally at the point of origin of the muscle, giving rise to the so-called "goose pimple." It also depresses slightly the sebaceous glands, aiding in the expulsion of sebum.

REPLACEMENT OF HAIR

The growth of a hair is continuous over long periods, until it stops at a certain point, that particular hair having reached its ultimate length. The cessation of hair growth and the subsequent shedding of the hair is initiated at the moment cell division stops in the matrix of the hair papilla. This is followed by a keratinization of all cells in the hair papilla, except those of the matrix, leading to the formation of a so-called club-hair. Subsequently, the matrix cells divide, but without differentiation. This forces the club-hair outward, and the movement is aided by a shrinking process within the outer root

Fig. 25-40. Section of scalp. Human. L.M. X 31. **1.** Epidermis. **2.** Hair follicles (hair shafts have fallen out during preparation). **3.** Sebaceous glands. **4.** Dermis. **5.** Subcutaneous fat.

Fig. 25-41. Section of scalp. Human. L.M. X 261. **1.** Hair shaft. (cross-sectioned). **2.** Outer root sheath. **3.** Alveoli of sebaceous glands. **4.** Sebum ready to be discharged. **5.** Duct of gland. **6.** Peripheral stem cells. **7.** Arrector pili muscle (cross-sectioned).

Fig. 25-42. Sebaceous gland. Enlargement of area similar to rectangle in Fig. 25-41. Monkey. E.M. X 1900. **1.** Nucleus of undifferentiated peripheral stem cell. **2.** Nuclei of cells with a limited number of droplets. **3.** Nucleus of a more central cell. Cytoplasm crowded with lipid droplets. **4.** Desmosomes along cell borders.

Fig. 25-43. Detail of secretory cell of sebaceous gland. Enlargement of area similar to rectangle in Fig. 25-42. Monkey. E.M. X 9300. **1.** Nucleus. **2.** Lipid droplets. Clear space and central dense mass indicate that some components have been removed in processing the tissue for microscopy. **3.** Mitochondria. **4.** Small Golgi zone. **5.** Free ribosomes. **6.** Cytoplasm filled with tubular profiles of the agranular endoplasmic reticulum.

Fig. 25-44. Enlargement of area similar to rectangle in Fig. 25-43. Monkey. E.M. X 92,000. **1.** Clear part of sebaceous droplet. **2.** Boundary membrane at interface of cytoplasm and sebaceous droplet. **3.** Cross-sectioned profiles of tubular agranular endoplasmic reticulum. **4.** Mitochondrion. **5.** Ribosomes.

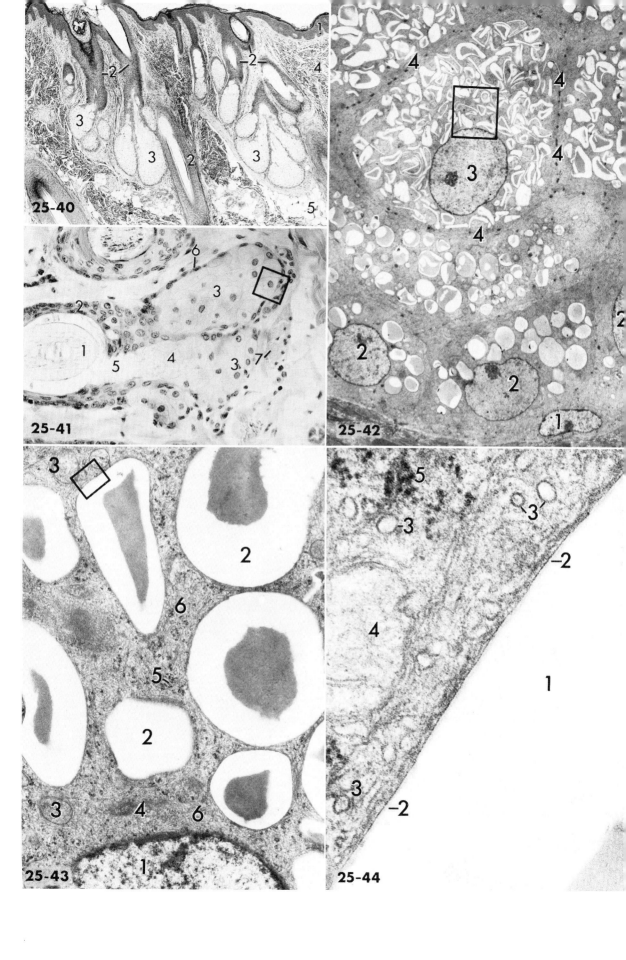

25-40

25-41

25-42

25-43

25-44

sheath. At a later stage, cells of the same epithelial bed proliferate again to form a cord of epithelial cells, and a new hair is formed in the same way outlined on p. 486 for the early development of the hair. The new hair gradually forces the old club-hair toward the skin surface and ultimately replaces it.

Sebaceous Glands

Sebaceous glands are derived from the epidermis. Most sebaceous glands are associated with hair follicles and they discharge their secretions into the distal part of the hair follicle. (Fig. 25-40) In some instances, the hairs are poorly developed or absent as in the skin of the forehead, nose, and external ear. Sebaceous glands in these locations are larger than elsewhere and often referred to as sebaceous follicles. Some sebaceous glands are not associated with hair follicles and open directly onto the skin surface. Such sebaceous glands are located in the eye lids (Meibomian glands), vermilion border of the lips, areolae of the nipple, labia minora, inside of the prepuce, and the glans penis.

STRUCTURE

In all locations throughout the body, the structure of the sebaceous glands is essentially the same. The glands are of the simple branched acinar (saccular) type with short excretory ducts. (Fig. 25-41) The ducts are generally lined by a stratified squamous epithelium which may be keratinized. The acini are masses of epithelial cells surrounded by a thin basal lamina. The most peripheral cells are undifferentiated and represent stem cells. (Fig. 25-42) Through mitosis, these cells give rise to cells which gradually become more differentiated as they are pushed toward the center of the gland. The differentiation process entails a synthesis and accumulation of lipid droplets. (Fig. 25-43) The droplets contain cholesterol, cho-

lesterol esters, phospholipids, and triglycerides. The end product, the **sebum,** represents a mixture of shed, disintegrated, and fully differentiated cells, completely filled with lipid droplets, which are delivered onto the surface of the skin in a process termed **holocrine secretion.**

The structure of the stem cells is similar to that of the basal cells of the stratum germinativum of the epidermis. There is a gradual increase in the amount of agranular endoplasmic reticulum as the cells become active in lipogenesis. Small lipid droplets appear within the Golgi region. As these droplets increase in size, they become surrounded by a large number of short, flattened tubular and vesicular profiles of the agranular endoplasmic reticulum. In many of the droplets appear angular crystals, probably reflecting the high content of cholesterol and cholesterol esters. While the cells are pushed toward the center of the gland, the lipid

Fig. 25-45. Section through thick skin of palmar surface of finger. Monkey. L.M. X 55. **1.** Body of ordinary (eccrine) sweat gland in hypodermis. **2.** Excretory duct traversing dermis. **3.** Duct traversing stratum germinativum of epidermis. **4.** Ducts traversing stratum corneum.

Fig. 25-46. Ordinary (eccrine) sweat glands. Enlargement of area similar to rectangle in Fig. 25-45. Human. L.M. X 350. **1.** Sections of coiled body of ordinary sweat gland. **2.** Sections of excretory duct. The duct cells are smaller and stain more darkly than the cells of the gland itself. **3.** Connective tissue cells.

Fig. 25-47. Survey of ordinary (eccrine) sweat gland and excretory duct. Axilla. Human. E.M. X 600. **1.** Lumen of gland. **2.** Lumen of duct lined by a stratifed epithelium. **3.** Capillary. **4.** Connective tissue. **5.** Tangential section of gland in which the spread of the myoepithelial cells is clearly seen.

Fig. 25-48. Section of body of ordinary (eccrine) sweat gland. Axilla. Human. E.M. X 1700. **1.** Lumen. **2.** Intercellular canaliculi. **3.** Dark (mucoid) cells. **4.** Clear cells. **5.** Myoepithelial cells. **6.** Basal lamina (unusually thick). **7.** Connective tissue. **8.** Capillary.

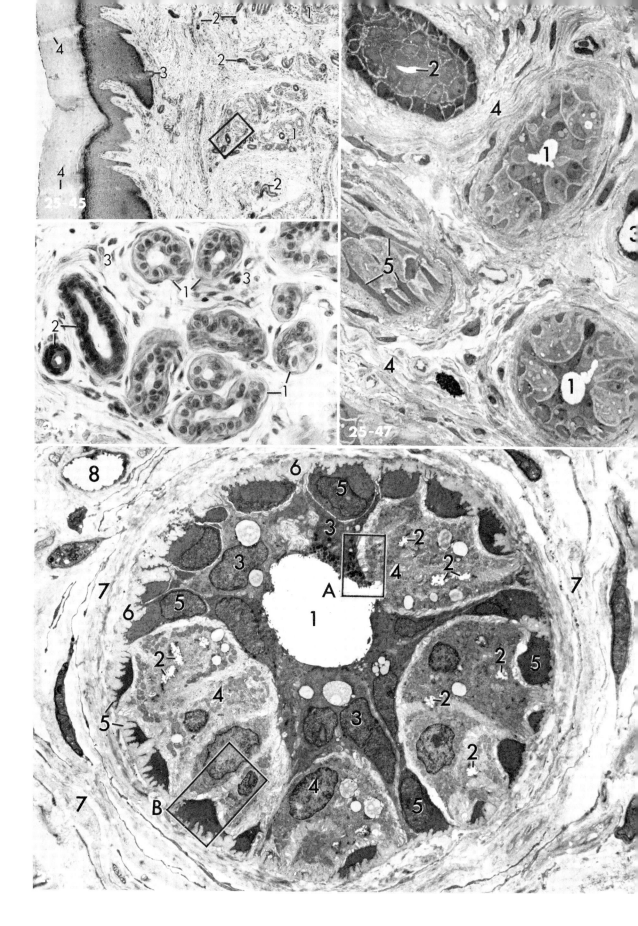

droplets enlarge and fuse to form huge sebum vacuoles. The cell nuclei remain unchanged until the terminal stage of cell differentiation, at which point they become irregularly shaped and finally disintegrate.

FUNCTION

The sebum lubricates skin and hair, protects the skin against epidermal cracking in hot temperatures, and plays a certain role in the conservation of body temperature. It may also have a bacteriostatic action. Some investigators maintain that sebum is useless and that sebaceous glands are obsolete appendages to the vestigial hairs of the human body.

Sweat Glands

Sweat glands are derivatives of the epidermis. They are coiled tubular glands with their secretory portion located deep in the dermis and a long, straight excretory duct discharging the secretion at the skin surface. (Fig. 25-45) Sweat glands are abundant in humans, monkeys, donkeys, and horses, but rare in most other mammals. Their secretion is watery and rich in sodium and chloride. Based on the fact that some sweat glands, especially those of the external genitalia and the axilla, produce a thicker and stronger smelling secretion than those of the rest of the body, one divides sweat glands into two categories: 1) ordinary (eccrine) sweat glands; and 2) odoriferous (apocrine) sweat glands. (Figs. 25-46, 25-47)

ORDINARY SWEAT GLANDS

In humans, ordinary (eccrine) sweat glands are present everywhere except in a few places such as the skin of the nipple and the margins of the lips. There are only few sweat glands on the eye lids, an average number on the legs, numerous on palms and soles, and an extreme abundance on fingertips. The ordinary sweat glands are small compared to the odoriferous sweat glands. The secretory body of the ordinary sweat gland is highly coiled and located deep in the dermis or in the hypodermis. A relatively straight excretory duct ascends to the epidermis, and here spirals through the epidermis as a canal between the epidermal cells and keratinized layers.

Figs. 25-49 & 25-50. Ordinary (eccrine) sweat gland. Secretion granules of dark (mucoid) cells. Human. E.M. X 62,000. **1.** Secretion granules of some dark cells contain a highly electron-dense core and a loosely fitted boundary membrane. **2.** Other secretion granules are more electron-lucent with a tightly fitted boundary membrane. **3.** Ribosomes.

Fig. 25-51. Detail of ordinary (eccrine) sweat gland. Enlargement of area similar to rectangle (A) in Fig. 25-48. Human. E.M. X 9300. **1.** Lumen of sweat gland. **2.** Intercellular canaliculi. **3.** Dark (mucoid) cell with dense secretory granules. **4.** Light cells. **5.** Microvilli.

Fig. 25-52. Detail of ordinary (eccrine) sweat gland. Enlargement of area similar to rectangle (B) in Fig. 25-48. Human. E.M. X 9300. **1.** Nuclei of light cells. **2.** Intercellular space with numerous small cytoplasmic processes. **3.** Mitochondria. **4.** Myoepithelial cell (nucleus not in plane of section). **5.** Thick basal lamina.

Fig. 25-53. Cross section of excretory duct of sweat gland. Axilla. Human. E.M. X 1500. **1.** Lumen. **2.** Nuclei of cells in stratified epithelium. **3.** Intercellular space is wide in basal cell layer. **4.** Connective tissue.

Fig. 25-54. Apical part of cells in duct of sweat gland. Enlargement of area similar to rectangle in Fig. 25-53. Human. E.M. X 9300. **1.** Cytoplasm of cells bordering on duct lumen is filled with ribosomes, particulate glycogen, and scattered tonofilaments. **2.** Desmosomes hold cells together. **3.** This area has been referred to as "cuticle" in ordinary light microscopy.

Fig. 25-55. Enlargement of area similar to rectangle in Fig. 25-54. Human. E.M. X 62,000. **1.** The "cuticle" consists of numerous short and densely packed microvilli. **2.** Core of each villus contains microfilaments which descend into the apical cytoplasm. **3.** Small vacuole or vesicle.

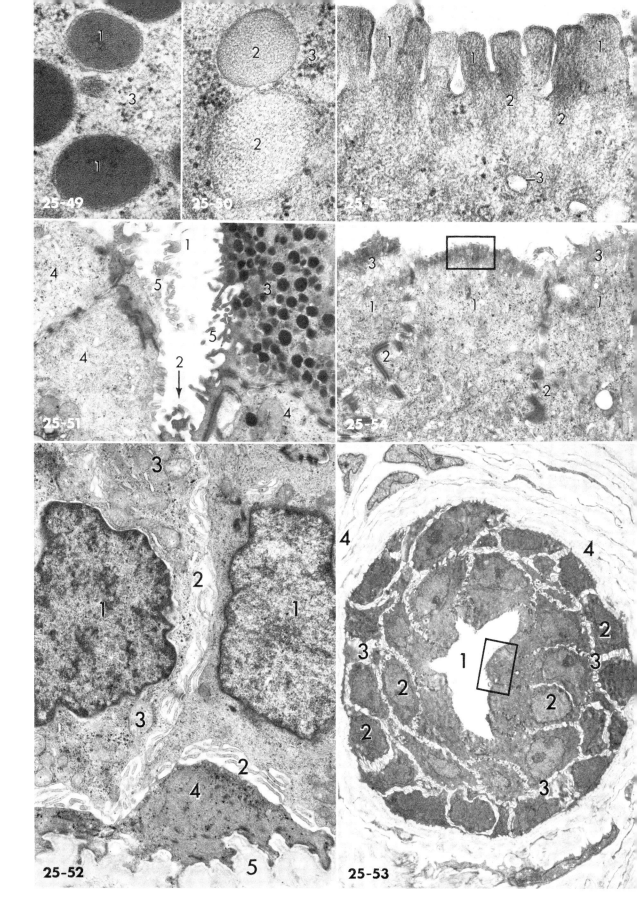

25-49

25-50

25-55

25-51

25-54

25-52

25-53

Body of gland. This is composed of a layer of small, irregularly arranged low, columnar or cuboidal **epithelial cells,** centered on a narrow, slit-like lumen. (Fig. 25-48) Some of the epithelial cells are referred to as **dark cells** or mucoid cells. They contain an abundance of ribosomes as well as dense secretory granules (Figs. 25-49, 25-50) containing mucoproteins and mucopolysaccharides. The releasing mechanism for the secretory granules is similar in all respects to the release of zymogen and mucous granules whereby the granule boundary membrane fuses with the surface membrane. Other epithelial cells are called **clear cells.** They are rich in particulate glycogen, but have few ribosomes. When two clear cells abut one another, they form between them an intercellular canaliculus. (Fig. 25-51) The cell membranes of adjacent cells interdigitate to form numerous short and narrow cell processes. The clear cells are believed to participate in transepithelial fluid and ion transport. Both cell types have a round nucleus in the center of the cell. Peripheral to the secretory cells, are spindle-shaped **myoepithelial cells,** arranged in parallel rows a few microns apart, and spiralling around the secretory tubule. (Fig. 25-52) These cells contain numerous myofilaments, and they aid in expelling the secretion by contraction. A **basal lamina** envelops the secretory tubule.

Excretory duct. This is lined by small cuboidal epithelial cells arranged in two or more layers. (Fig. 25-53) The cells appear very dense under the light microscope in contrast to the cells of the secretory portion of the gland. The apical part of the cells bordering on the lumen contains numerous tonofilaments. This zone was described earlier as representing a cuticle. (Fig. 25-54) The diameter of the duct and the lumen is small. A basal lamina surrounds the duct, but myoepithelial cells are absent.

Function. Heat is the prime physiological stimulus for the ordinary sweat glands. The glands give off a watery fluid as part of a thermo-regulating mechanism to cool the body. However, emotional stimuli can also bring about profuse sweating.

ODORIFEROUS SWEAT GLANDS

In humans, the odoriferous (apocrine) sweat glands are located in the skin of the axilla, around the nipples, scrotum, labia majora, pubic region, as well as the perineal and circumanal regions. To this category belong also the ceruminous glands of the external auditory meatus and the glands of Moll in the margin of the eye lids. As a rule, the odoriferous sweat glands are larger than the ordinary sweat glands (Fig. 25-56) but are similarly divided into a secretory, coiled portion, located in the hypodermis, and a straight ascending excretory duct that opens in or near the epidermal orifice of the hair follicle.

Fig. 25-56. Odoriferous (apocrine) sweat glands. Axilla. Human. L.M. X 57. **1.** Sections of coiled body of odoriferous sweat gland. **2.** Ordinary sweat glands. Cross-sectional diameter is far less than that of an odoriferous sweat gland. **3.** Connective tissue. **4.** Fat cells.

Fig. 25-57. Cross section of odoriferous (apocrine) sweat gland. Enlargement of area similar to rectangle in Fig. 25-56. Human. E.M. X 600. **1.** Lumen. **2.** Secretory, columnar cells. **3.** Myoepithelial cells. **4.** Connective tissue.

Fig. 25-58. Odoriferous (apocrine) sweat gland. Enlargement of area similar to rectangle in Fig. 25-57. Human. E.M. X 5600. **1.** Nuclei of epithelial cells. **2.** Myoepithelial cells. **3.** Thin basal lamina. **4.** Large Golgi zone. **5.** Mitochondria. **6.** Secondary lysosomes (or secretion granules). **7.** Apex of cell.

Fig. 25-59. Odoriferous sweat gland. Enlargement of area similar to rectangle (A) in Fig. 25-58. Human. E.M. X 60,000. **1.** Microvilli. **2.** Secretion droplets (granules).

Fig. 25-60. Odoriferous sweat gland. Enlargement of area similar to square (B) in Fig. 25-58. Human. E.M. X 60,000. **1.** Lysosomes (or secretion granules) with numerous small spheres or micelles inside. **2.** Boundary membrane. **3.** Ribosomes. **4.** Precursor of secretory granule (or primary lysosome).

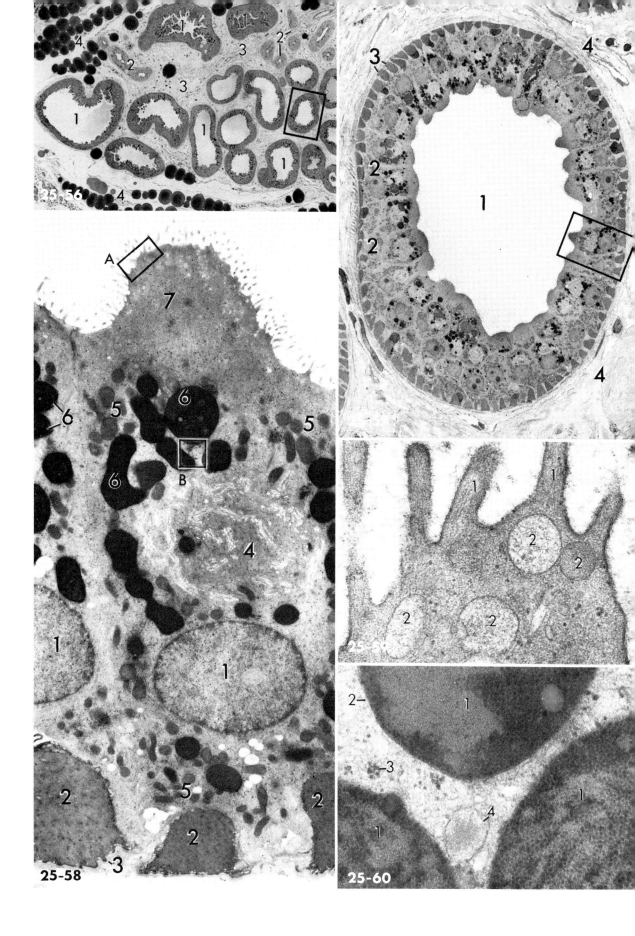

25-56

25-58

25-50

25-60

Body of gland. The odoriferous sweat glands are coiled and branched tubules, often derived from hair follicles. The secretory part of the gland is composed of a single layer of cuboidal or truncated columnar **epithelial cells** with the apex of the cell protruding into a wide tubular lumen. (Fig. 25-57) Only one cell type is present, and clear cells cannot be identified. The nucleus is round and located in the center of the cell. The cytoplasm contains many mitochondria, some of which are unusually large, and with a paucity of mitochondrial cristae. In addition, there is an abundance of secondary lysosomes, some of which represent the lipofucsin pigment granules identified with the light microscope. (Fig. 25-58) The apical cytoplasm contains numerous vacuoles which are assumed to contain mucopolysaccharides. (Fig. 25-59) The luminal cell surface is provided with many small protuberances and microvilli. According to an old theory, the apex of the cell is cast off in an apocrine secretion similar to the segregation of fat globules during the secretion of milk in the mammary gland. Recent investigations have not been able to confirm this, and it is believed that the homogeneous fluid seen in the glandular lumen is derived from a **merocrine** secretion, and that the releasing mechanism is similar to that occurring in mucous and serous glandular cells. Myoepithelial cells are present and resemble those of ordinary sweat glands.

Excretory duct. This is lined by several layers of small cuboidal cells, surrounded by a basal lamina. Myoepithelial cells are not present. The duct lumen is narrow.

Function. Emotional and sensory stimuli such as fear, apprehension, pain, and sexual excitement initiate apocrine sweating. The secretion of the apocrine sweat glands is odorless. However, odor is produced by skin bacteria through a decomposition of the apocrine sweat, leading to acrid odors.

Nails

The nails are areas of modified stratum corneum of the epidermis which protect the dorsal surface of the distal phalanges of fingers and toes. They contain hard keratin, and the keratinization process is structurally similar to the formation of the hair cortex.

The nail consists of a rectangular, slightly curved body, the **nail plate.** The plate rests on a modified epidermis, the **nail bed.** (Fig. 25-61) The proximal edge, the **nail root** is embedded in a fold of the epidermis, the **nail fold.** (Fig. 25-62) The

Fig. 25-61. Longitudinal section of finger tip. Monkey L.M. X 8. **1.** Nail plate. **2.** Nail bed. **3.** Nail root. **4.** Eponychium. **5.** Hyponychium. **6.** Bone of phalanx. **7.** Epidermis.

Fig. 25-62. Topography of proximal nail fold. Enlargement of rectangle in Fig. 25-61. Monkey. L.M. X 30. **1.** Stratum corneum of epidermis. **2.** Stratum germinativum of epidermis. **3.** Dermis. **4.** Eponychium. **5.** Epidermal nail fold. **6.** Nail matrix. **7.** Nail plate. **8.** Nail bed.

Fig. 25-63. Survey of claw matrix. Enlargement of area similar to rectangle in Fig. 25-62. Claw. Rat. E.M. X 630. **1.** Stem cells of nail (claw) matrix. Nuclei round. **2.** A continuous proliferation of stem cells make earlier generations of cells and their nuclei flatten out and move in the direction of the arrow. **3.** Cells become keratinized at this point. **4.** An increasing number of cells become keratinized and are added gradually to those previously keratinized. **5.** Beginning of nail (claw) plate. **6.** Cells of nail (claw) bed do not contribute to nail plate keratinization. **7.** Epidermal cells of nail (claw) fold give rise to eponychium (soft keratin).

Fig. 25-64. Enlargement of area similar to rectangle (A) in Fig. 25-63. Claw. Rat. E.M. X 5000. **1.** Cells with an increasingly large number of tonofibrils. **2.** Nucleus. **3.** Fully keratinized cells of claw (hard keratin).

Fig. 25-65. Enlargement of area similar to rectangle (B) in Fig. 25-63. Claw. Rat. E.M. X 5000. **1.** Squamous cells filled with tonofibrils just prior to becoming fully keratinized. **2.** Nucleus. **3.** Fully keratinized cells. **4.** Substance between cells remains unstained in this preparation.

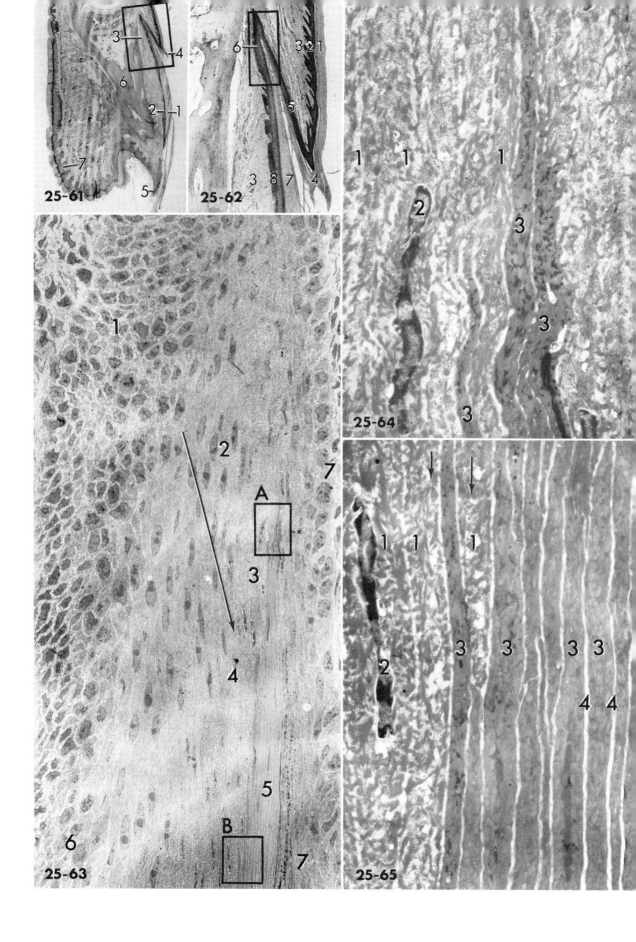

25-61

25-62

25-63

25-64

25-65

lateral edges of the nail are similarly bordered by epidermal folds. The keratinized layers of the dorsal epidermis grow out over the proximal part of the nail plate. This is the **eponychium,** or (the lay term) cuticle. The **hyponychium** is an epidermal thickening under the free edge of the nail plate. The nail bed is thicker than elsewhere beneath the nail root. This is referred to as the **nail matrix** since the nail is formed from this area by a continuous proliferation and growth of matrix cells. (Fig. 25-63) The nail plate is translucent except in the area above the nail matrix, **the lunula.** This area stands out as a white, opaque crescent because of the large number of prekeratinous fibrils in the proliferating cells of the matrix.

STRUCTURE OF THE NAIL

Nail bed. The nail plate rests on several layers of epidermal cells. These layers correspond to the stratum germinativum of the epidermis. However, they do not contribute to the formation of the nail plate except in the root of the nail. Their function elsewhere is not clear, but they participate somehow in affixing the nail plate to the nail bed while the nail slowly moves across it during the growth process. A thin basal lamina separates the cells of the nail bed from the dermis. The **dermis** forms parallel, longitudinal ridges and grooves of dense connective tissue which firmly attach the nail bed to the periosteum of the distal phalanx.

Nail matrix. This is the thickened proximal part of the nail bed. It consists of an actively proliferating stratum germinativum. Newly formed cells are being added to the nail root by a continuous keratinization process. (Fig. 25-64) The cells acquire, gradually, large amounts of tonofibrils. Keratohyalin granules are not present and the process is typical of the formation of hard keratin. As the cells keratinize, they flatten out and become firmly attached to each other through an increased thickness of the cell membranes, and through the possible discharge of membrane-coating granules into the intercellular space. The addition of newly keratinized cells to the nail root brings about a slow movement of the nail plate over the nail bed at a pace of about 0.5 mm per week.

Nail plate. The nail plate consists of many layers of thinly flattened, fully keratinized cells. (Fig. 25-65) They are firmly held together and do not desquamate. The free edge of the nail plate must therefore be trimmed from time to time. The nail plate is translucent and the dermal capillaries and microvessels can readily be observed here for diagnostic purposes. If the nail plate is removed, it will grow out again only if the nail matrix is left behind.

References

Bell, M. A comparative study of sebaceous gland ultrastructure in subhuman primates. I. Anat. Rec. *166*: 213–224 (1970).

Bell, M. A comparative study of sebaceous gland ultrastructure in subhuman primates. III. Anat. Rec. *170*: 331–342 (1971).

Breathnach, A. S. The cell of Langerhans. Int. Rev. Cytol. *18*: 1–28 (1965).

Breathnach, A. S. An Atlas of the Ultrastructure of Human Skin. J. & A. Churchill, London, 1971.

Brody, I. An electron microscopic study of the fibrillar density in the normal human stratum corneum. *J.* Ultrastruct. Res. *30*: 209–217 (1970).

Brody, I. The ultrastructure of the tonofibrils in the keratinization process of normal human epidermis. J. Ultrastruct. Res. *4*: 264–297 (1960).

Brody, I. Variations in the differentiation of the fibrils in the normal human stratum corneum as revealed by electron microscopy. J. Ultrastruct. Res. *30*: 601–614 (1970).

Charles A. and Ingram, J. T. Electron microscope observations of the melanocytes of the human epidermis. J. Biophys. Biochem. Cytol. *6*: 41–44 (1959).

Chapman, R. E. and Gemmell, R. T. Stages in the formation and keratinization of the cortex of the wool fiber. J. Ultrastruct. Res. *36*: 342–354 (1971).

Ellis, R. A. Fine structure of the myoepithelium of the eccrine sweat glands of man. J. Cell Biol. *27*: 551–563 (1965).

Farbman, A. I. Plasma membrane changes during keratinization. Anat. Rec. *156*: 269–282 (1966).

Fukuyama, K., Wier, K. A. and Epstein, W. L. Dense homogeneous deposits of keratohyalin granules in newborn rat epidermis. J. Ultrastruct. Res. *38*: 16–26 (1972).

Hashimoto, K. Demonstration of the intercellular spaces of the human eccrine sweat gland by lanthanum. J. Ultrastruct. Res. *37*: 504–520 (1971).

Hashimoto, K. The ultrastructure of the skin of human embryos. VIII. Melanoblast and intrafollicular melanocyte. J. Anat. *108*: 99–108 (1971).

Hashimoto, K. Ultrastructure of the human toenail. J. Ultrastruct. Res. *36*: 391–410 (1971).

Hibbs, R. G. Electron microscopy of human axillary sebaceous glands. J. Investig. Derm. *38*: 329–336 (1962).

Jessen, H. Two types of keratohyalin granules. J. Ultrastruct. Res. *33*: 95–115 (1970).

Lavker, R. M. and Matoltsy, A. G. Formation of horny cells. The fate of organelles and differentiation products in ruminal epithelium. J. Cell Biol. *44*: 501–512 (1970).

Martinez, I. R. and Peters, A. Membrane-coating granules and membrane modifications in keratinizing epithelia. Am. J. Anat. *130*: 93–120 (1971).

Matoltsy, A. G. Membrane-coating granules of the epidermis. J. Ultrastruct. Res. *15*: 510–515 (1966).

Matoltsy, A. G. Keratinization of the avian epidermis. An ultrastructural study of the newborn chick skin. J. Ultrastruct. Res. *29*: 438–458 (1969).

Matoltsy, A. G. and Matoltsy, M. N. The chemical nature of keratohyalin granules of the epidermis. J. Cell Biol. *47*: 593–603 (1970).

Matoltsy, A. G. and Parakkal, P. F. Membrane-coating granules of keratinizing epithelia. J. Cell Biol. *24*: 297–307 (1965).

Matoltsy, A. G. and Parakkal, P. K. Keratinization. *In* Ultrastructure of Normal and Abnormal Skin. (Ed. A. Zelickson), pp. 76–104. Lea & Febiger, Philadelphia, 1967.

Menton, D. N. and Eisen, A. Z. Structure and organization of mammalian stratum corneum. J. Ultrastruct. Res. *35*: 247–264 (1971).

Millward, G. R. The substructure of α-keratin microfibrils. J. Ultrastruct. Res. *31*: 349–355 (1970).

Montagna, W. The Structure and Function of the Skin, 2nd ed. Academic Press, New York, 1962.

Munger, B. L. The cytology of apocrine sweat glands. 2. Human. Z. Zellforsch. *68*: 837–851 (1965).

Munger, B. L. and Brusilow, S. W. The histophysiology of rat plantar sweat glands. Anat Rec. *169*: 1–22 (1971).

Odland, G. F. A submicroscopic granular component in human epidermis. J. Invest. Derm. *34*: 11–15 (1960).

Odland, G. and Ross, R. Human wound repair. I. Epidermal regeneration. J. Cell Biol. *39*: 135–151 (1968).

Rawles, M. E. Origin of melanophores and their role in development of color pattern in vertebrates. Physiol. Rev. *28*: 383–408 (1948).

Rhodin, J. A. G. and Reith, E. J. Ultrastructure of keratin in oral mucosa, skin, esophagus, claw and hair. *In* Fundamentals of Keratinization, (Eds. E. O. Butcher and R. F. Sognaes), pp. 61–94. AAAS, Publication No. 70, Washington, D.C., 1962.

Robins, E. J. and Breathnach, A. S. Fine structure of the human foetal hair follicle at hair-peg stages of development. J. Anat. *104*: 553–569 (1969).

Robins, E. J. and Breathnach, A. S. Fine structure of bulbar end of human foetal hair follicle at stage of differentiation of inner root sheath. J. Anat. *107*: 131–146 (1970).

Roth, S. I. Hair and nail. *In* Ultrastructure of Normal and Abnormal Skin (Ed. A. Zelickson), pp. 105–131. Lea & Febiger, Philadelphia, 1967.

Roth, S. I. and Jones, W. A. The ultrastructure of epidermal maturation in the skin of the boa constrictor (Constrictor constrictor). J. Ultrastruct. Res. *32*: 69–93 (1970).

Snell, R. S. The fate of epidermal desmosomes in mammalian skin. Z. Zellforsch. *66*: 471–487 (1965).

Terzakis, J. A. The ultrastructure of monkey eccrine sweat glands. Z. Zellforsch. *64*: 493–509 (1964).

Ugel, A. R. Studies on isolated aggregating oligoribonucleoproteins of the epidermis with histochemical and morphological characteristics of keratohyalin. J. Cell Biol. *49*: 405–422 (1971).

Wier, K. A., Fukuyama, K. and Epstein, W. L. Nuclear changes during keratinization of normal human epidermis. J. Ultrastruct. Res. *37*: 138–145 (1971).

Wise, G. E. Origin of amphibian premelanosomes and their relation to microtubules. Anat. Rec. *165*: 185–196 (1969).

Zelickson, A. S. (Ed.). Ultrastructure of normal and abnormal skin. Lea & Febiger, Philadelphia, 1967.

26 Digestive system— mouth

Digestion entails processes by which foods are converted into substances that can be absorbed and used by the cells of the body. The **breakdown** of the food is done both mechanically and chemically. The **absorption** requires special enzymes. The work of **elimination** of certain non-usable substances in the food terminates the handling of the foods by the digestive system. The anatomical components of the digestive system consist of the **mouth, pharynx, esophagus, stomach, small** and **large intestines, rectum,** and the **anal canal.** The mechanical breakdown, by the aid of a multitude of enzymes, starts in the mouth to a limited extent and culminates in the stomach and first part of the small intestine. The food is absorbed mainly in the small intestine, whereas the elimination process of substances in the food that cannot be utilized by the body occurs in the large intestine. The number and quantities of enzymes required for the breakdown and absorption of the food are enormous. These enzymes are synthesized in small glands located in the walls of the digestive canal, as well as in special large, extramural glands, the **salivary glands,** the **pancreas,** and the **liver,** all of which form a functionally important part of the digestive system.

Mouth

The oral cavity is formed by the lips, cheeks, hard and soft palate, and the floor of the mouth. (Fig. 26-1) The architecture of these boundary structures, and that of the pharynx, differ from the other parts of the alimentary tract. The mouth and pharynx are irregular in their shape, whereas the rest of the digestive tract is formed as a tube with largely the same basic structures. Special structures in the oral cavity include the **tongue** and the **teeth.** The mouth is designed to perform several important initial tasks in the digestive process. A testing of objects takes place through the sensation of **taste,** regis-

tered by nerve endings in the taste buds of the tongue. In addition, the mouth, lips and tongue play an important role in the formation of **speech.** The food is mechanically broken down by the action of the teeth. It is moistened and partially digested through the influence of the **saliva.** There are three important aspects of the walls of the mouth to consider: 1) the structural differentiation of the surface epithelium; 2) the lamina propria; 3) the nature of the intramural salivary glands.

ORAL SURFACE EPITHELIUM

The epithelium is, throughout, of the **stratified squamous** type, but it varies in reference to whether or not it is keratinized. Although many mammals have extensive areas of keratinized oral epithelium, this is not the case in humans. Depending on the location and functional

Fig. 26-1. Frontal section through oral cavity. Human fetus. L.M. X 6. **1.** Oral cavity. **2.** Nasal cavity. **3.** Palate. **4.** Tongue. **5.** Mandible. **6.** Floor of mouth with tongue muscles. **7.** Cheeks. **8.** Maxilla.

Fig. 26-2. Vertical section through lower lip. Human. L.M. X 5. **1.** Cutaneous area with hairs. **2.** Red border (vermilion). **3.** Oral surface. **4.** Orbicularis muscle.

Fig. 26-3. Enlargement of area similar to rectangle (A) in Fig. 26-2. Red border of lip. Human. L.M. X 110. **1.** Stratified squamous, non-keratinized epithelium. **2.** Deep connective tissue papillae.

Fig. 26-4. Enlargement of area similar to rectangle (B) in Fig. 26-2. Zone of transition between epidermis and red border. Lip. Human. L.M. X 190. **1.** Epidermis. **2.** Stratum corneum. **3.** Vermilion (red border) lacking stratum corneum. **4.** Connective tissue.

Fig. 26-5. Sagittal section through soft palate. Monkey. L.M. X 23. **1.** Oral surface. **2.** Nasal surface. **3.** Muscles. **4.** Salivary glands. **5.** Uvula.

Fig. 26-6. Enlargement of rectangle in Fig. 26-5. Oral epithelium of soft palate. Monkey. L.M. X 260. **1.** Oral cavity. **2.** Stratified squamous non-keratinized epithelium. **3.** Connective tissue. **4.** Excretory duct of salivary glands. **5.** Rectangle enlarged in Fig. 26-10.

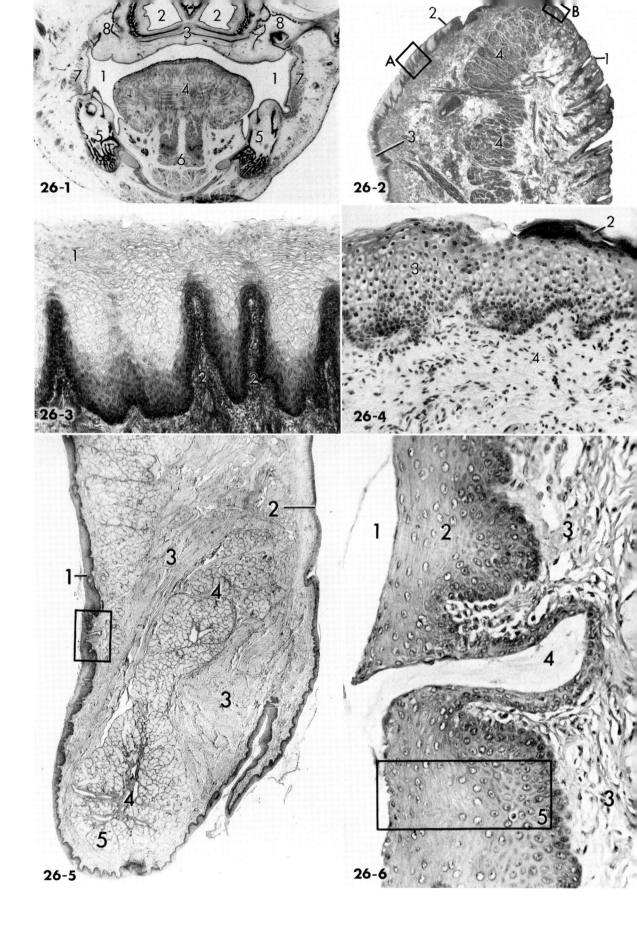

26-1

26-2

26-3

26-4

26-5

26-6

stresses, the changes in the oral epithelium may go in two directions. If subjected to strong abrasive forces, the epithelium becomes keratinized, whereas it remains non-keratinized in less stressed areas.

Non-keratinized epithelium covers the inside of the lips (Fig. 26-5), cheeks, soft palate (Figs. 26-2, 26-3, 26-4), floor of the mouth, lower surface of the tongue, and tonsils. With some exceptions, the structure of this epithelium is characterized by a layering similar to that in the epidermis. (Fig. 26-10) There is a **basal layer** of small polyhedral cells, typified by high mitotic activity and resting on a thin **basal lamina**. The basal cells change in shape as they move through the **spinous layer** to the **superficial squamous layers**. The cells of the uppermost layers are less squamous. They become detached and are shed into the oral cavity (Figs. 26-10, 26-12) where they appear in the saliva as flattened epithelial elements. The superficial layers correspond to the stratum granulosum, stratum lucidum, and stratum corneum of the skin, but they cannot be so classified because of differences in ultrastructural architecture. In the oral non-keratinized epithelium, a small number of **tonofilaments** occur in the basal and spinous layers. They become slightly more abundant in the superficial squamous layers. Keratohyalin granules are missing throughout, but small **membrane-coating granules** occur in the superficial layers. (Fig. 26-11) These granules are thought to be related to the slight increase in the thickness of the cell membrane that takes place in the superficial cells. (Fig. 26-12) **Desmosomes** are present in the basal and spinous layers (Fig. 26-11), but disappear in the superficial layers. The cohesion of cells in these layers depends upon an interlocking of short cell processes and an amorphous intercellular cement. **Glycogen** particles are abundant throughout. In contradistinction to keratinized epithelium, the **nuclei** remain in the cells of the superficial layers, although a slight pyknosis may occur. Since the superficial cells of a non-keratinizing epithelium do not contain keratohyalin granules and do not accumulate keratin filaments, it is concluded that keratohyalin granules are essential in the normal process of soft keratinization. (See p. 482)

Keratinized epithelium. This covers the hard palate (Fig. 26-9), gingiva, (Fig. 27-22), and parts of the dorsal surface of the tongue. The keratinization process in the hard palate and gingiva is considered by some to be incomplete and is referred to as parakeratinization. From an ultrastructural point of view, the epithelium of the hard palate and the gingiva is fully keratinized and similar to that of the epidermis. On the dorsal surface of the tongue, the filiform papillae display both the hard and soft variety of keratinization.

Epithelium of transitional zone (vermilion border, lip red) of the lips is a variation of a keratinized epithelium. (Fig. 26-4) It has a highly developed stratum lucidum which is thicker than elsewhere in the epidermis, whereas the stratum corneum is very thin. These factors, in addition to dermal papillae with a rich capillary network penetrating deeply into the epidermis of the lip, contribute to giving the lips their red color.

Fig. 26-7. Frontal section of hard palate. Kitten. L.M. X 23. **1.** Oral cavity. **2.** Nasal cavity. **3.** Lateral palatine processes (bone tissue). **4.** Nasal septum. **5.** Dense connective tissue and salivary glands.

Fig. 26-8. Enlargement of area similar to rectangle in Fig. 26-7. Hard palate. Kitten. L.M. X 200. **1.** Dense connective tissue. **2.** Level of basement membrane. **3.** Stratified squamous epithelium of hard palate. **4.** Stratum corneum.

Fig. 26-9. Enlargement of area similar to rectangle in Fig. 26-8. Stratified squamous keratinized epithelium. Hard palate. Cat. E.M. X 820. **1.** Subepithelial dense connective tissue. **2.** Capillary. **3.** Stratum basale. **4.** Stratum spinosum. **5.** This layer corresponds to stratum granulosum in the epidermis. However, keratohyalin granules are not present in this oral keratinized epithelium. **6.** Stratum corneum.

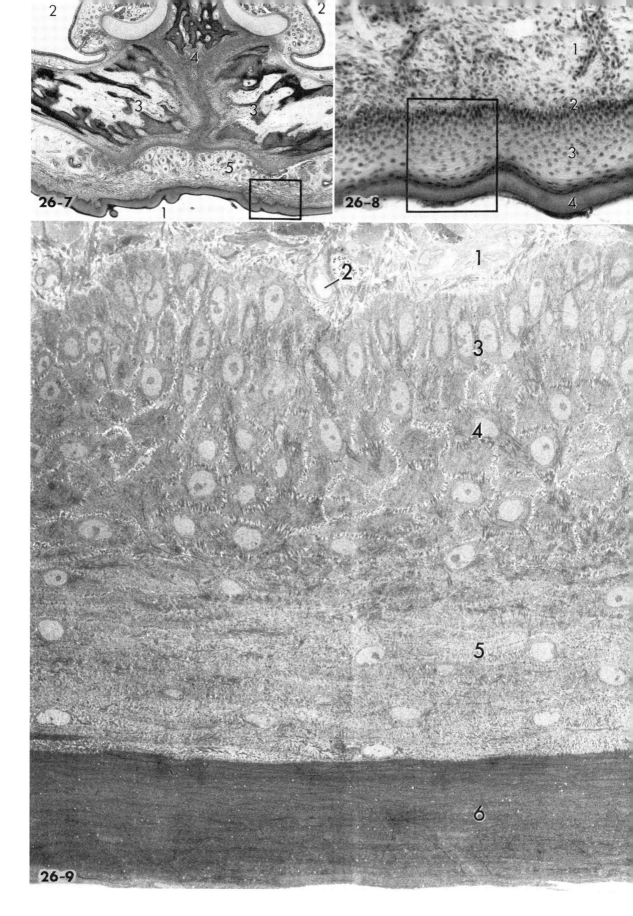

26-7

26-8

26-9

LAMINA PROPRIA

The connective tissue underlying the oral epithelium also varies according to location. Under the non-keratinized epithelium, the lamina propria is characterized by a loose connective tissue, whereas it is dense and irregular in the hard palate and gingiva where bone is the supporting tissue. Striated muscle fibers occur in the lamina propria of lips and soft palate.

SALIVARY GLANDS

The saliva is secreted by glands which open up at the oral surface epithelium. The glands are either intramural or extramural. The **extramural** glands are the parotid, sublingual, and submandibular glands. These are described on p. 520. The **intramural** glands are the labial, buccal, palatine, and lingual glands. The intramural glands discharge a predominantly mucous secretion, but they also give off a serous or a seromucous secretion. Their structure and ultrastructure is discussed together with that of the extramural glands on p. 520.

Tongue

The main, freely movable part of the tongue, the **body**, is located in the mouth proper, whereas the **base** (root) of the tongue is attached at the floor of the mouth, forming part of the pharynx. Along the **dorsum** (back) of the tongue runs a **median sulcus**, starting near the **apex** (tip) of the tongue and terminating at the **foramen caecum** of the V-shaped **sulcus terminalis**. The terminal sulcus separates the oral two-thirds of the tongue from the pharyngeal one-third. The tongue is covered by a stratified squamous **epithelium** which is entirely non-keratinized on the lower surface of the tongue. The upper surface is provided with numerous **lingual papillae** of varying shapes, and covered by a stratified squamous epithelium which is keratinized only in relation to the filiform papillae. The main core of the tongue is made up of **lingual muscles** of the striated skeletal type. The **extrinsic** muscles genioglossus, hyoglossus, styloglossus, and palatoglossus have their origin external to the body of the tongue and their insertion within. The intrinsic muscles, subdivided into longitudinal, transverse, and vertical, have both their origin and insertion within the tongue. (Fig. 26-17) The muscle cells are generally more slender than ordinary skeletal muscle fibers. Their ultrastructural organization is similar. The muscles attach to, and are surrounded by, the **lingual fascia**. This fascia is in direct contact with the **lamina propria** of the surface epithelium, since there is no submucosa present in the tongue. The lingual fascia is reinforced as a vertical **lingual septum**, dividing the tongue into two complete lateral halves. The septum is traversed only by occasional blood vessels and nerves.

Fig. 26-10. Enlargement of area similar to rectangle (5) in Fig. 26-6. Stratified squamous non-keratinized epithelium. Soft palate. Cat. E.M. X 1800. **1.** Nuclei of basal cells. **2.** Nuclei of cells in stratum spinosum. **3.** Nuclei of cells becoming increasingly elongated as the cells move toward the epithelial surface. The elongated cells correspond to those forming the stratum granulosum in the epidermis. **4.** The more superficial cells become extremely long and flat. **5.** The most superficial cells tend to swell and lose their cytoplasmic density. **6.** Oral cavity.

Fig. 26-11. Enlargement of area similar to rectangle (A) in Fig. 26-10. Soft palate. Cat. E.M. X 31,000. **1.** Nucleus **2.** Cytoplasm with densely packed tonofilaments. **3.** Intercellular space. **4.** Desmosomes. **5.** Rectangle: membrane-coating granule. **6.** Inset: membrane-coating granule. Matrix finely granular. Boundary membrane 30 Å. X 186,000.

Fig. 26-12. Enlargement of area similar to rectangle (B) in Fig. 26-10. Soft palate. Cat. E.M. X 62,000. **1.** Part of cell with densely packed tonofilaments. **2.** Cells with loosely arranged tonofilaments. **3.** Intercellular space. **4.** Remnants of detached desmosomes. **5.** Inset: cell membrane of superficial cell. Of the two laminae forming the cell membrane, the innermost is greatly thickened. X 186,000.

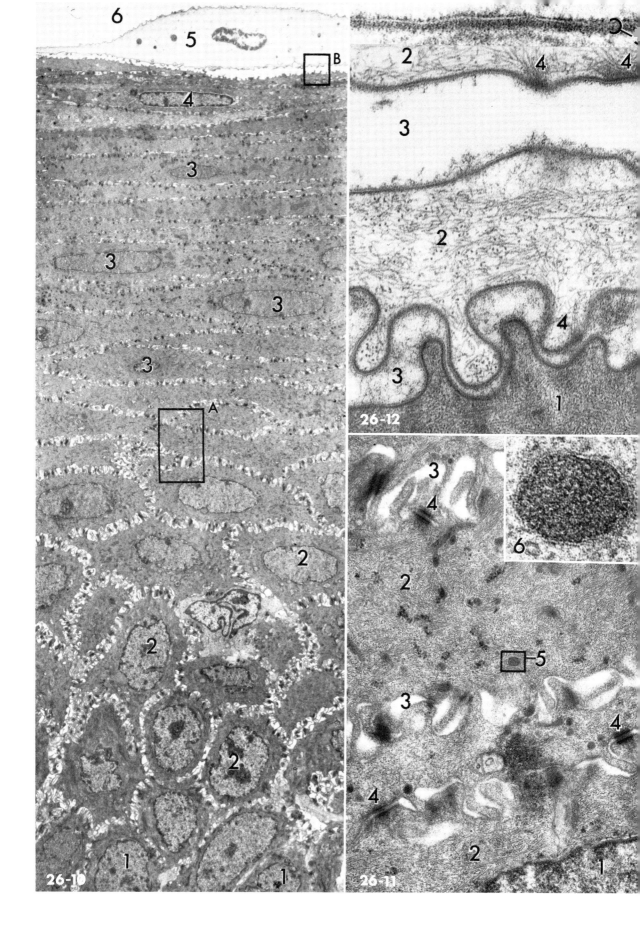

6

5

B

4

3

3

3

3

3

A

2

2

2

2

1

1

26-10

2

4

4

3

2

4

3

1

26-12

3

4

6

2

5

3

4

4

2

1

26-11

Lingual papillae. Papillae are present on the upper and lateral lingual surfaces (Fig. 26-13) and only on the part of the tongue which is in front of the sulcus terminalis. One distinguishes between filiform, fungiform, circumvallate, and foliate papillae. The **filiform** papillae are the most numerous (Fig. 26-14), distributed throughout the tongue mostly in straight rows parallel to the sulcus terminalis. Each papilla is made up of a connective tissue core and a cover of stratified squamous epithelium which, in most cases, is keratinized in man. (Fig. 26-15) In some mammals these papillae have hard keratin on one side and soft keratin on the other, probably in response to variations in abrasive stresses on the papillae during mastication (Fig. 26-16) The **fungiform** papillae are less numerous and scattered singly over the back of the tongue. They are slightly raised above the level of the lingual surface. (Fig. 26-19) They have a massive core of connective tissue and are covered by a stratified squamous epithelium which is not as completely keratinized as that on the filiform papillae. The epithelium is similar to that which covers the lips, and because of the thin stratum corneum, the rich capillary network of the connective tissue core makes the fungiform papillae stand out as small lightly red points. There may be a small number of taste buds associated with the upper surface of these papillae. The **circumvallate** papillae are few in number. In man, about ten such papillae are located in a single row just in front of the sulcus terminalis. Each papilla penetrates deeply beneath the surface epithelium of the tongue, being surrounded by a moat-like furrow. (Fig. 26-20) The connective tissue core is large. The surface epithelium is non-keratinized and contains a large number of taste buds, most of which face the cylindrical cleft. The **foliate papillae** are rudimentary in man, but well developed in some mammals, especially the cat and the rabbit. (Fig. 26-21) If present, they are located along the posterolateral borders.

Taste buds are numerous in relation to these papillae. The surface epithelium is generally not keratinized.

TASTE BUDS

Groups of taste buds are concentrated in the lingual papillae. (Fig. 26-22) Isolated taste buds are present in the palate, pharynx, and epiglottis. Each taste bud is composed of 20–30 spindle-shaped epithelial cells, most of which extend from the basal lamina to the surface of the stratified squamous epithelium. (Fig. 26-23) The tips of these cells converge upon the **taste pore** (or pit), a small recess in the surface epithelium. In the classical description, two cell types were recognized: **sustentacular** cells and **gustatory** cells. More recently, at least three cells types have been identified: basal cells, dark cells, and light cells. The **basal** cell is small and located near the base or at the periphery of the taste bud. Its fine structure is similar to that of other

Fig. 26-13. Tongue. Cross section of lateral half. Monkey. L.M. X 13. **1.** Dorsal surface. **2.** Lower surface. **3.** Lateral edge. **4.** Intrinsic muscles. **5.** Fungiform papillae.

Fig. 26-14. Enlargement of area similar to rectangle (A) in Fig. 26-13. Monkey. L.M. X 89. **1.** Stratified squamous non-keratinized epithelium. **2.** Filiform papillae. **3.** Subepithelial connective tissue. **4.** Connective tissue papillae.

Fig. 26-15. Enlargement of area similar to rectangle in Fig. 26-14. Rat. E.M. X 620. **1.** Keratinized tips of filiform papillae. **2.** Cells of stratum intermedium. **3.** Basal cells.

Fig. 26-16. Enlargement of rectangle in Fig. 26-15. E.M. X 1900. **1.** Cells undergoing soft keratinization in the direction of the arrow. **2.** Cells undergoing hard keratinization in the direction of arrow. **3.** Keratohyalin granules. **4.** Bundles of tonofilaments.

Fig. 26-17. Bundles of intrinsic striated muscles of tongue. Monkey. L.M. X 100. **1.** Cross-sectioned bundles. **2.** Longitudinally sectioned bundles. **3.** Connective tissue core of tongue.

Fig. 26-18. Lower surface of tongue. Enlargement of area similar to rectangle (B) in Fig. 26-13. Monkey. L.M. X 430. **1.** Stratified squamous non-keratinized epithelium. **2.** Connective tissue papillae.

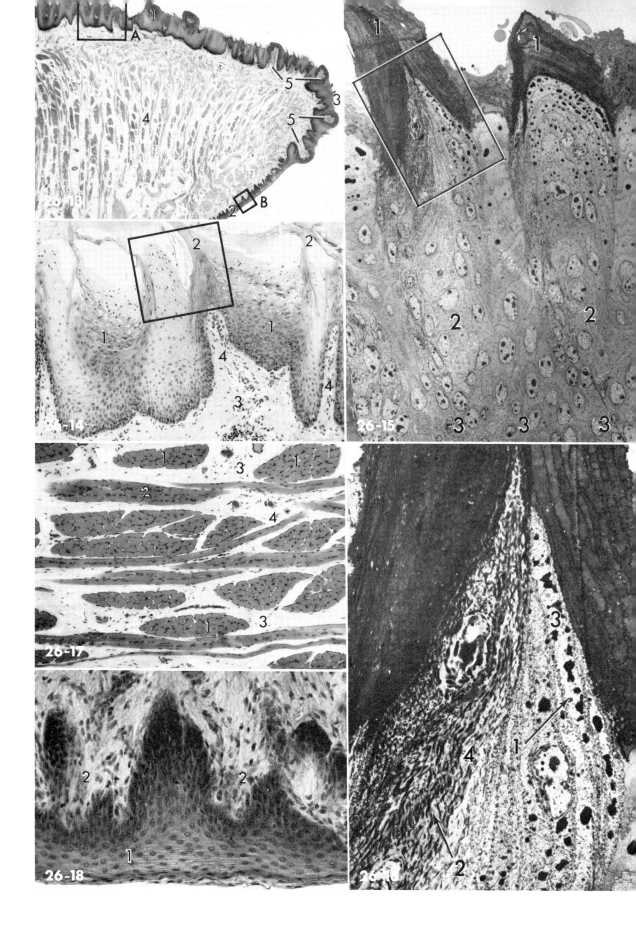

basal cells in the oral epithelium. It serves as a stem cell. The **dark** cell corresponds most closely to the classical sustentacular cell. Its cytoplasm contains free ribosomes, granular endoplasmic reticulum, Golgi complexes, and to a varying degree, dense secretory granules. Long apical microvilli with many intracytoplasmic filaments project into the taste pit. This cell is believed to have mainly a secretory function. The dense granules are probably discharged into the taste pit (Fig. 26-24), representing precursors of the mucopolysaccharide substance that bathes the microvilli in the pit. The **light** cell, of which there may be two categories, corresponds to the gustatory cell. The overall light appearance is due to a scarcity of free ribosomes and granular endoplasmic reticulum. The cells contain several primary and secondary lysosomes, and there are numerous empty vesicles present throughout the cell. The apical microvilli project into the taste pit. (Fig. 26-24) They are generally shorter than those of the dark cell, but this seems to vary according to the species. The light cells are presumed to act as the principal gustatory transducers. Non-myelinated intragemmal nerve fibers of the 7th and 9th cranial nerves surround all cells in the taste bud. The nerves are beaded and terminate as club-shaped nerve endings. The axoplasm contains occasional small, empty vesicles, some microtubules, filaments, and mitochondria. The nerves contact all cell types in the bud (Fig. 26-25) but make deep impressions only in the light cells where a synaptic-like arrangement exists with presynaptic vesicles in the light cell, thickened pre- and postsynaptic membranes and an aggregation of vesicles within the postsynaptic axoplasm.

FUNCTIONAL CONSIDERATIONS

The cells making up the taste buds are continually replaced. The life span of each cell is about seven days. It is possible that the basal cells are differentiated into dark cells, and that these in turn develop into light cells. The ultimate fate of the light cells is not known, but they probably undergo a gradual autolysis by action of their own lysosomes. On the other hand, there may exist at least two independent well-differentiated cell lines (dark and light) which may develop from the basal (stem) cell. Both may be replaced, but at different rates, since dark cells disappear more rapidly than light cells in a degenerating taste bud. It has been demonstrated that the presence of nerves is necessary for the normal development and maintenance of the taste buds (neurotrophic action). However, dark cells are more dependent on nerve processes for their survival than light cells, and they seem to have a shorter life-span and a more rapid turnover than light cells. It is not clear how the **receptor potential** is initiated. The microvilli of the light and dark cells are exposed to the stimulating substances, and it cannot be excluded that both the dark and the light cells function in transduction. Once the

Fig. 26-19. Tongue. Dorsal surface. Monkey. L.M. X 43. **1.** Connective tissue core of fungiform papilla. **2.** Solitary taste bud. **3.** Filiform papillae. **4.** Partly keratinized surface epithelium.

Fig. 26-20. Tongue. Monkey. L.M. X 41. **1.** Connective tissue core of circumvallate papilla. **2.** Moat-like furrow. **3.** Numerous taste buds. **4.** Non-keratinized surface epithelium.

Fig. 26-21. Tongue. Monkey. L.M. X 41. **1.** Connective tissue core of foliate papillae. **2.** Clefts. **3.** Numerous taste buds. **4.** Non-keratinized surface epithelium. **5.** Lingual (mixed) salivary glands.

Fig. 26-22. Enlargement of area similar to rectangle in Fig. 26-21. Circumvallate papilla. Rat. E.M. X 660. **1.** Moat-like furrow. **2.** Taste buds. **3.** Superficial squamous cells of non-keratinized epithelium.

Fig. 26-23. Survey of a taste bud. Rat. E.M. X 2700. **1.** Furrow. **2.** Taste pore. **3.** Squamous surface epithelium. **4.** Nucleus of light cell. **5.** Nuclei of dark cells. **6.** Nuclei of basal (lateral) cells. **7.** Nucleus of tongue surface epithelial cell.

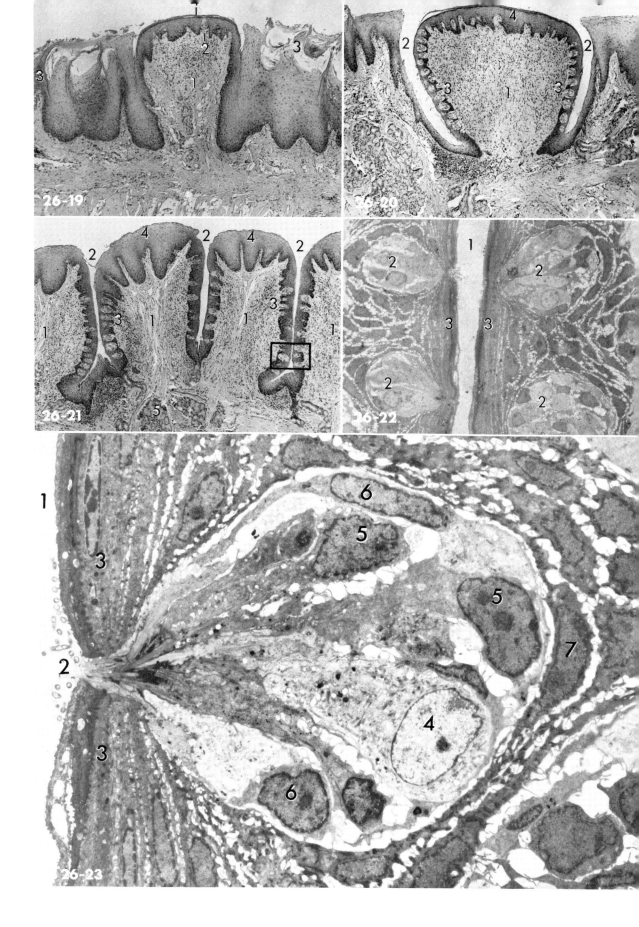

receptor potentials are initiated, impulses are generated in the taste fibers, probably across the synaptic-like regions. A given stimulus being recorded by the gustatory cells results in an impulse pattern peculiar to that substance. There are generally four taste sensations: **sweet** is recorded by the taste buds of the apical fungiform papillae; **salt** by the fungiform papillae throughout the tongue; **bitter** by the circumvallate papillae; and **sour** on lateral sides of the tongue by the fungiform papillae or foliate papillae, if present. Structurally there does not seem to be a difference between taste buds in the various locations.

LINGUAL NERVES

The **sensory** innervation of the tongue as it relates to **touch** and **temperatures** is supplied by the lingual branch of the trigeminal nerve (5th) in the anterior two-thirds of the tongue, and by the glosso-pharyngeal nerve (9th) in the posterior one-third of the tongue. As it relates to **taste,** the chorda tympani of the facial nerve (7th) innervates the taste buds of the anterior portion of the tongue, and the glossopharyngeal nerve (9th) supplies the taste buds of the circumvallate papillae. The **motor** innervation of the tongue is supplied by the hypoglossal nerve (12th).

Lingual glands. Among the muscle fibers of the tongue are present a relatively large number of small salivary glands. **Mucous** glands are located near the root. They empty their secretion in conjunction with the lingual tonsils behind the sulcus terminalis. **Serous** glands are concentrated in the body of the tongue. They open up in front of the sulcus terminalis in relation to the circumvallate papillae. **Mixed** glands are generally located near the lingual apex, discharging at the lower surface of the tongue. The histological and ultrastructural character-istics of these glands are described on p. 520.

Pharynx

The pharynx (throat) is a musculofibrous sac which serves as a passageway for both air and food. The upper part, **nasophar-ynx,** is connected to the nasal cavities via the choanae. These parts are lined by a pseudostratified ciliated columnar epithe-lium (see p. 608). The middle part, **oro-pharynx,** is connected to the oral cavity via the isthmus faucium which is formed by the soft palate, palatine arches, and pharyngeal part of the back of the tongue. It is lined by a non-keratinized, stratified squamous epithelium. The lower part, **laryngopharynx,** is tube-like and connects with the esophagus. In the anterior wall is the entrance to the larynx, covered by the epiglottis. The epithelium is of the non-keratinized stratified squamous type. The wall of the pharynx contains a strong fibrous submucosa and several skeletal muscles which serve during deglutition (swallowing).

Tonsils

In close relationship to the pharynx are accumulations of lymphoid tissue, the **lin-gual, palatine,** and **pharyngeal** tonsils. The lymphoid cells infiltrate both the epi-thelium and the lamina propria. The ton-sils form a functionally important part of the lymphatic system, and are described in detail on p. 376

Fig. 26-24. Survey of structures forming the pit of a taste bud. Rat. E.M. X 31,000. **1.** Taste pit with darkly stained mucopolysaccharide substance. **2.** Villi of dark cells. **3.** Villi of light cells. **4.** Intracytoplasmic filaments. **5.** Secretory granules. **6.** Small vesicles. **7.** Intercellular space.

Fig. 26-25. Survey of the basal region of taste bud. Rat. E.M. X 43,000. **1.** Basal (lateral) cell. **2.** Dark cell. **3.** Light cells. **4.** Nerve endings. **5.** Intercellular space. **6.** Nucleus. **7.** Mitochondria. **8.** Ribosomes. **9.** Granular endoplasmic reticulum. **10** Lysosome.

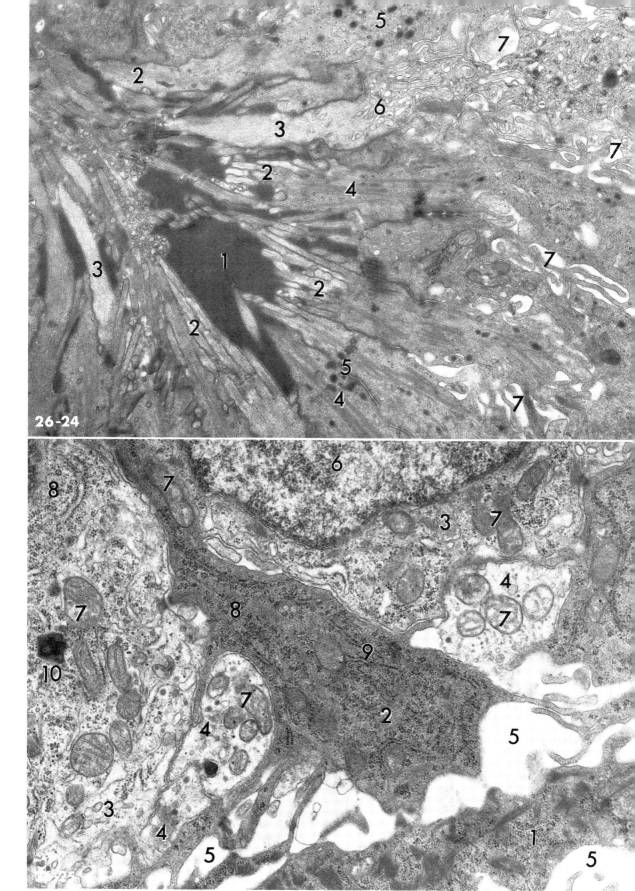

26-24

References

ORAL MUCOSA

Farbman, A. I. Electron microscope study of a small cytoplasmic structure in rat oral epithelium. J. Cell Biol. *21*: 491–495 (1964).

Farbman, A. I. Morphological variability of keratohyalin. Anat. Rec. *154*: 275–286 (1966).

Farbman, A. I.: Plasma membrane changes during keratinization. Anat. Rec. *156*: 269–282 (1966).

Farbman, A. I. The dual pattern of keratinization in filiform papillae on rat tongue. J. Anat. *106*: 233–242 (1970).

Frithiof, L. Ultrastructural changes in the plasma membrane in human oral epithelium. J. Ultrastruct. Res. *32*: 1–17 (1970).

Hashimoto, K. Fine structure of horny cells of the vermilion border of the lip compared with skin. Arch. Oral Biol. *16*: 397–410 (1971).

Hashimoto, K., DiBella, R. J. and Shklar, G. Electron microscopic studies of the normal human buccal mucosa. J. Investig. Derm. *47*: 512–525 (1966).

Listgarten, M. A. The ultrastructure of human gingival epithelium. Am. J. Anat. *114*: 49–69 (1964).

Martinez, I. R., Jr. and Peters, A. Membrane-coating granules and membrane modifications in keratinizing epithelia. Am. J. Anat. *130*: 93–120 (1971).

Meyer, J. and Gerson, S. J. A comparison of human palatal and buccal mucosa. Periodontics *2*: 284–291 (1964).

Rhodin, J. A. G. and Reith, E. J. Ultrastructure of keratin in oral mucosa, skin, esophagus, claw and hair. *In* Fundamentals of Keratinization (Eds. E. O. Butcher and R. F. Sognaes), pp. 61–94. AAAS, Publication No. 70, Washington, D.C. 1962.

Scaletta, L. J. and MacCallum, D. K. A fine structural study of divalent cation-mediated epithelial union with connective tissue in human oral mucosa. Am. J. Anat. *133*: 431–454 (1972).

Silverman, S. Jr. Ultrastructure studies of oral mucosa. I. Comparison of normal and hyperkeratotic human buccal epithelium. J. Dent. Res. *46*: 1433–1443 (1967).

Silverman, S. Jr., Barbosa, J. and Kearns, G. Ultrastructural and histochemical localization of glycogen in human normal and hyperkeratotic oral epithelium. Arch. Oral Biol. *16*: 423–434 (1971).

Stern, I. B. Electron microscopic observations of oral epithelium. I. Basal cells and basement membrane. Periodontics *3*: 224–238 (1965).

Weinmann, J. P. The keratinization of the human oral mucosa. J. Dental Res. *19*: 57–71 (1940).

TASTE BUDS

Farbman, A. I. Fine structure of the taste bud. J. Ultrastruct. Res. *12*: 328–350 (1965).

Farbman, A. I. Fine structure of degenerating taste buds after denervation. J. Embryol. Exp. Morph. *22*: 55–68 (1969).

Fujimoto, S. and Murray, R. G. Fine structure of degeneration and regeneration in denervated rabbit vallate taste buds. Anat. Rec. *168*: 393–414 (1970).

Murray, R. G. and Murray, A. Fine structure of taste buds of rabbit foliate papillae. J. Ultrastruct. Res. *19*: 327–353 (1967).

Oakley, B. and Benjamin, R. M. Neural mechanisms of taste. Physiol. Rev. *46*: 173–211 (1966).

Scalzi, H. W. The cytoarchitecture of gustatory receptors from the rabbit foliate papillae. Z. Zellforsch. *80*: 413–435 (1967).

Uga, S. A study on the cytoarchitecture of taste buds of rat circumvallate papillae. Arch. Histol. Japan. *31*: 59–72 (1969).

27 Digestive system— salivary glands and teeth

Salivary Glands

The **large** salivary glands, parotid, sub-mandibular, and sublingual, are paired structures, located outside of the oral cavity, and provided with long duct systems. The **small** salivary glands, labial, buccal, palatine, and lingual, are situated in the walls of the oral cavity and the tongue. They have short ducts. Salivary glands discharge a secretion which normally contains 90% water, several carbohydrate-splitting enzymes as well as mucins. The **glandular cells** are of two kinds: **serous** and **mucous**. Depending on the predominance of one or the other cell type, salivary glands are divided into solely serous, solely mucous, and mixed serous and mucous. The glandular cells are arranged in tubes and acini (sometimes also called alveoli). The **duct system** of the large salivary glands is composed of several, differently structured segments, the cells of which exert an influence on the ionic concentration of the primary fluid during its passage to the oral cavity through **intercalated** ducts, **striated intralobular** (secretory, salivary) ducts, and **interlobular** (excretory) ducts.

SEROUS SALIVARY GLANDS

To this group belong the small Ebner's glands of the root of the tongue and the parotid glands. The **parotid** glands (Fig. 27-1) are located in front of the ear, folded around each ramus of the mandible. Each gland is drained by the parotid duct (Stensen's) which empties into the mouth opposite the second upper molar tooth. The glands are invested by a dense fibro-elastic capsule, continuous with the deep cervical fascia. Connective tissue septa arise from the capsule and subdivide the glandular parenchyma into lobes and lobules. (Fig. 27-2) The septa contain the larger ducts, blood vessels, lymphatics, and nerves. Some fat cells occur in the septa but are more frequently scattered singly or in groups within the glandular parenchyma. (Fig. 27-1) Pyramidal **serous gland cells** make up the acini which are relatively long and tortuous, often branched and forked. The cells border on a narrow lumen, but this space is often so small that it cannot be seen with the light microscope. (Fig. 27-3) The nuclei are round, not flattened, and located near the center of the serous gland cell. The basal half of the cell contains an abundance of granular endoplasmic reticulum, free ribosomes, and scattered mitochondria. (Fig. 27-4) Above the nucleus is a large Golgi zone, and the upper half of the cell is filled with numerous presecretory granules. (Fig. 27-5) These are synthesized by the endoplasmic reticulum and the Golgi zone and discharged at the cell surface as described on p. 86. The acinar serous cells rest on a thin **basal lamina**. Between the base of the cells and this lamina are located **myoepithelial** (basket) **cells**. Their cytoplasm is differentiated into long

Fig. 27-1. Parotid (serous) gland. Human. L.M. X 28. **1.** Lobules with serous acini and fat cells (empty round spaces). **2.** Septa with ducts.

Fig. 27-2. Enlargement of rectangle in Fig. 27-1. Parotid. Human. L.M. X 200. **1.** Interlobular (excretory) duct. **2.** Intralobular (secretory) duct. **3.** Connective tissue septum. **4.** Fat cells. **5.** Serous acini.

Fig. 27-3. Survey of lingual (serous) gland. Rat. E.M. X 2500. **1.** Intralobular duct. **2.** Serous acini. **3.** Blood capillaries.

Fig. 27-4. Detail of serous acinus. Lingual gland. Rat. E.M. X 30,000. **1.** Nucleus of myoepithelial cell. **2.** Myofilaments. **3.** Mitochondria. **4.** Basal lamina. **5.** Cell borders. **6.** Ribosomes. **7.** Granular endoplasmic reticulum. **8.** Mitochondria. **9.** Golgi complex. **10.** Early secretory granule. **11.** Mature secretory granule.

Fig. 27-5. Detail of apical part of serous cell. Lingual salivary glands. Rat. E.M. X 61,000. **1.** Mature secretory granules approaching the apical cell surface. **2.** Secretory granule at the moment of discharge. **3.** Lumen of acinus with discharged content of secretory granules. **4.** Surface cell membrane. **5.** Boundary membrane of discharging secretory granule. **6.** Submembranous fine filaments. **7.** Ribosomes. **8.** Granular endoplasmic reticulum.

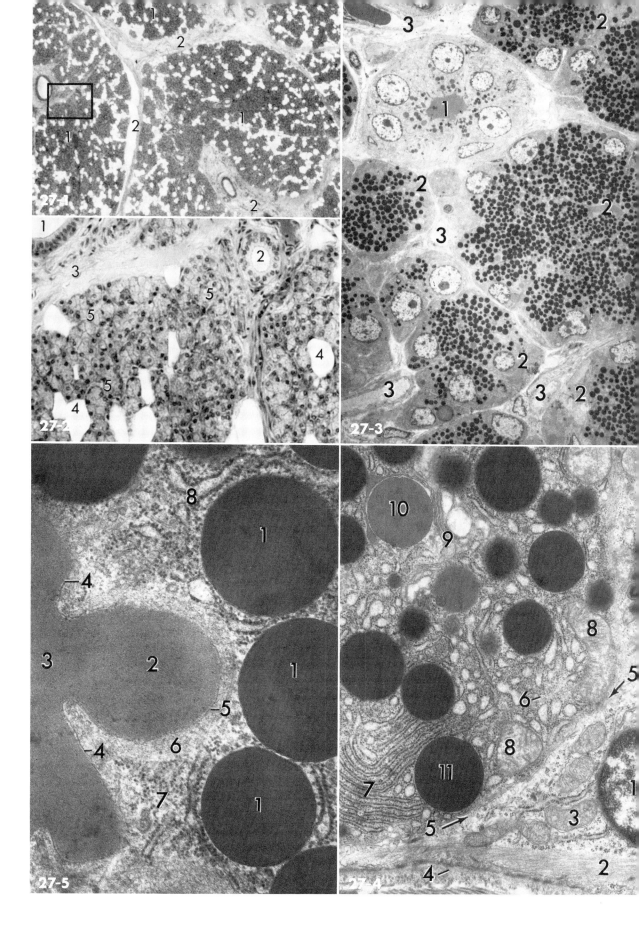

slender cell processes which contain numerous contractile filaments. (Fig. 27-4) These cells aid in expelling the secretion from the acinar lumen to the **duct system.** The ducts are highly complex in the parotid as well as in the other two large salivary glands. They are described on p. 524.

The salivary glands of Ebner in the root of the tongue are much smaller than the parotid glands. They have less connective tissue components and their ducts are shorter. The structure of the acinar gland cells is similar to that in the parotid.

MUCOUS SALIVARY GLANDS

There are very few solely mucous salivary glands in man. Some are located in the tongue, a few in the lips (Fig. 27-6) and soft palate. Among the large salivary glands, the **sublingual** consists mostly of mucous acini, although some serous cells may be present. The **mucous gland cells** are pyramidal and form the acini around a central lumen. The nucleus is flattened and located near the base of the cell. Most of the cell is occupied by the mucous presecretory droplets many of which are partly coalesced. (Fig. 27-9) The remaining cytoplasm is restricted to thin basal and lateral zones containing granular endoplasmic reticulum, Golgi complexes and mitochondria. The mechanism of mucous droplet synthesis and release was described on p. 88. The **duct system** of the mucous salivary glands, and particularly that of the sublingual gland, is shorter and simpler than in the parotid. The intercalated ducts may be absent and the striated ducts are short or may only appear as patches of basally striated cells. There are 8–20 excretory ducts opening up on either side of the frenulum linguae.

MIXED SALIVARY GLANDS

To this group belong most of the small salivary glands in the walls of the oral cavity and the tongue. Of the larger glands, the **submandibular** gland is clearly mixed (Fig. 27-7), whereas the **sublingual gland** contains mostly mucous and very few serous acini. The term "mixed" relates to the occurrence of both serous and mucous acini in a gland. In addition, the term "mixed gland" can refer to the structural arrangement where the tubules and acini are composed of mucous cells, but where their terminal ends are capped by 5–10 serous cells which in a section appear as a **demilune.** (Fig. 27-8) The structure of the mucous as well as of the serous gland cells is similar to what was described earlier. In the case of the serous demilunes, the cells often do not border on the lumen of the acinus. The secretion then reaches the lumen via intercellular spaces or intracellular canaliculi. **Myoepithelial** cells are numerous in mixed salivary glands (Fig. 27-9), being interposed between the base of the acinar cells and the **basal lamina** of the acinus.

The **submandibular** glands are situated in the submandibular triangles. Capsule and connective tissue stroma are well developed, subdividing each gland into lobes and lobules. There are generally more fat cells than in the parotid, both in the connective tissue septa and in the parenchyma. The intercalated ducts are short and narrow. The striated ducts are longer and more numerous than in the parotid. The submandibular (excretory) ducts (Wharton's) open by a narrow orifice on

Fig. 27-6. Labial salivary (mucous) gland. Human. L.M. X 110. **1.** Mucous acini. **2.** Excretory duct. **3.** Connective tissue septum.

Fig. 27-7. Submandibular salivary (mixed) gland. Human. L.M. X 333. **1.** Serous acinus. **2.** Mucous acinus. **3.** Serous demilune. **4.** Striated ducts. **5.** Fat cell.

Fig. 27-8. Sublingual salivary (mixed) gland. Rat. E.M. X 580. **1.** Mucous acini. **2.** Serous demilunes. **3.** Intercalated duct. **4.** Lumen of striated ducts. **5.** Capillaries.

Fig. 27-9. Detail of a mixed acinus. Sublingual salivary gland. Rat. E.M. X 4700. **1.** Lumen of acinus. **2.** Mucous droplets. **3.** Nuclei of mucous cells. **4.** Cells of serous demilunes with secretory granules and granular endoplasmic reticulum. **5.** Nucleus of myoepithelial cell. **6.** Nucleus of small lymphocyte. **7.** Periacinar connective tissue.

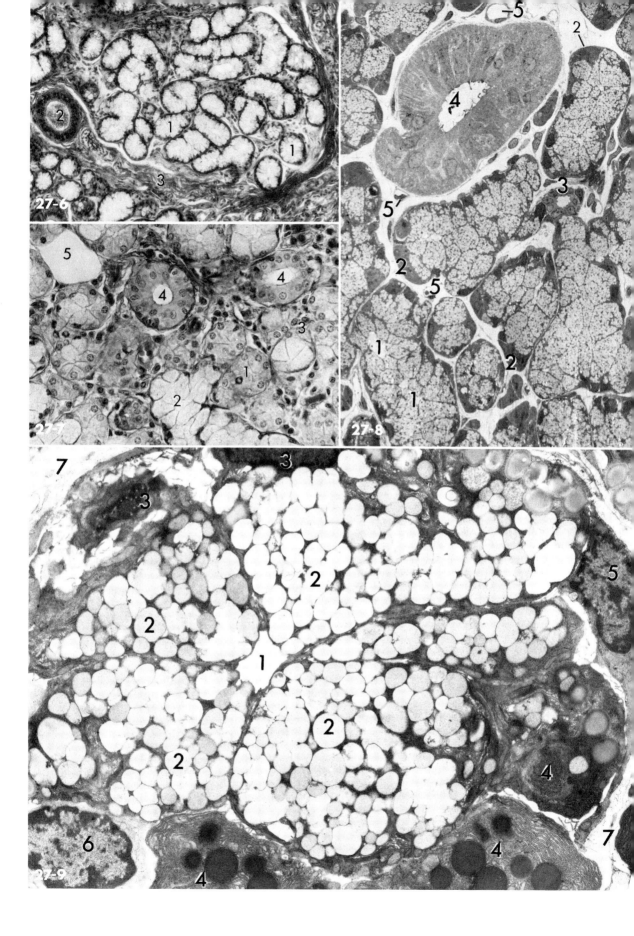

the summit of a small papilla on either side of the frenulum linguae. The **sublingual** glands are groups of small mixed salivary glands in the anterior and lateral parts of the floor of the mouth, resting on the surface of the mylohyoid muscles. A distinct capsule is missing but fine connective tissue septa subdivide the glandular parenchyma. Several ducts drain the glands. There are some 15 minor ducts emptying along the sublingual plica, and one major duct opening near the submandibular duct.

DUCT SYSTEM OF SALIVARY GLANDS

The duct system varies according to the type of salivary gland. The small oral glands have short ducts, whereas the **parotid gland** has a long and complex system of ducts which is described here. Exceptions to this general description are indicated in relation to the description of respective glands. Subsequent to the acinus are the **intercalated ducts** which are long in the parotid. They have a small diameter and are composed of small, low cuboidal cells (Fig. 27-10), some of which may contain secretory granules of both mucous and serous type. The nucleus is large, occupying the major part of the cytoplasm. Myoepithelial cells are usually part of the intercalated duct. In the sublingual and submandibular glands, the intercalated ducts often contain purely mucous secreting cells mixed in with the duct cells. The intercalated ducts are followed by the **striated ducts** which are also termed intralobular secretory or salivary ducts. They vary in length, but always have a diameter several times larger than that of an intercalated duct. They are composed of tall columnar or prismatic cells with a central nucleus. (Figs. 27-11, 27-12) The apical cytoplasm contains small vacuoles and occasional small dense granules. (Fig. 27-14) It is not known if these structures are engaged in secretion, absorption, or both. The cell surface is provided with short microvilli. The basal part of the cells is invaginated by deep folds of

the cell membrane (Fig. 27-15), and resulting cytoplasmic processes interdigitate with similar processes of neighboring cells. The cytoplasmic processes hold rod-shaped mitochondria, oriented perpendicularly to the base of the cell. This structural organization is the basis for the term "striated" duct. Myoepithelial cells do not occur in the striated ducts. The distal part of the striated duct becomes non-striated as it leaves the lobule and connects with the **interlobular ducts** (excretory ducts) in the connective tissue septa of the gland. Gradually the epithelium changes from a simple columnar to a stratified columnar type. (Fig. 27-13) The basal cells are small, polyhedral, and interdigitate with the superficial columnar cells. The interlocking cytoplasmic processes are narrow and contain only occasional mitochondria. Small microvilli are present at the cell surface.

Fig. 27-10. Cross section of intercalated duct. Sublingual mixed salivary gland. Rat. E.M. X 4500. **1.** Lumen. **2.** Nuclei of lining cells; cytoplasm devoid of secretory granules. **3.** Myoepithelial cells.

Fig. 27-11. Cross section of striated duct. Sublingual mixed salivary gland. Rat. E.M. X 750. **1.** Lumen. **2.** Nuclei of lining cells. **3.** Blood capillaries.

Fig. 27-12. Detail of striated duct. Sublingual mixed salivary gland. Rat. E.M. X 4800. **1.** Lumen. **2.** Nucleus. **3.** Basal lamina. **4.** Mitochondria. **5.** Aggregation of particulate glycogen.

Fig. 27-13. Detail of transition between a striated duct and an excretory (interlobular) duct. Sublingual mixed salivary gland. Rat. E.M. X 4500. **1.** Lumen. **2.** Nuclei of columnar surface cells. **3.** Basal cell. **4.** Basal lamina. **5.** Interdigitations of surface cells and basal cells.

Fig. 27-14. Enlarged detail of area similar to rectangle (A) in Fig. 27-12. Rat. E.M. X 9300. **1.** Lumen of striated duct. **2.** Dense granules (whether secretory or absorptive is uncertain). **3.** Apical portion of duct cells. **4.** Microvilli.

Fig. 27-15. Enlarged detail of area similar to rectangle (B) in Fig. 27-12. Rat. E.M. X 39,000. **1.** Mitochondria. **2.** Narrow interdigitating cytoplasmic processes. **3.** Basal lamina. **4.** Connective tissue.

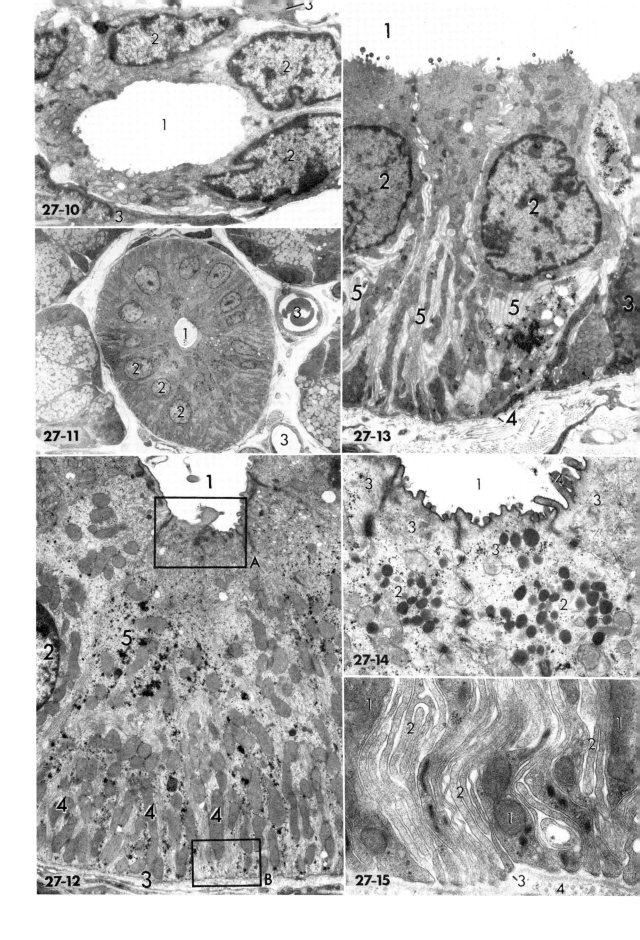

NERVES

Non-myelinated nerves make contact with both serous and mucous cells of salivary glands, whereas nerves have not been demonstrated as being in contact with epithelial cells of any part of the duct system. The secretory parasympathetic nerves are derived from the glossopharyngeal (9th) nerve. Their stimulation results in a thin serous secretion. The stimulation of the secretory sympathetic nerves from the thoracic outflow produces a thick mucous secretion.

FUNCTIONAL CONSIDERATIONS

It is generally accepted that the mucous acini secrete sialomucins and sulfomucins. The serous acini secrete mainly amylase in the highly watery, primary secretion, which also contains considerable amounts of sodium chloride. There is some evidence that the demilunes may produce a seromucous secretion containing a mucin mixed with protein. From micropuncture studies of serous salivary glands it is known that the intercalated ducts contain a fluid which becomes modified during its further passage along the duct system. The primary fluid is plasma-like in osmolarity and in sodium and potassium concentrations. The modification of the fluid occurs most likely to the largest extent in the striated ducts, consisting in a resorption of sodium and secretion of potassium. Participating in these processes are the basal infoldings of the plasma membrane, the large accumulation of mitochondria, and the apical granules and vacuoles.

Teeth

In humans, there are two sets of teeth, **permanent** and **deciduous**. The adult has 32 permanent teeth. Of the 8 teeth per quadrant in both upper and lower jaws, there are 2 incisors, 1 canine, 2 bicuspids, and 3 molars of which the third molar may not erupt. A child has 20 diciduous teeth. Of the 5 teeth per quadrant, there are 2 incisors, 1 canine, and 2 molars. Of the deciduous teeth, the central incisors erupt as the first teeth when the infant is six weeks old. The second molars erupt as the last teeth when the child is 2 years old. Of the permanent teeth, the central incisors are the first to erupt at the age of 7 years, and the second molars erupt last at the age of 24 years.

Each tooth consists of the **root** attached to a socket in the alveolar bone of the jaw; the free part, the **crown**; and a narrow region between the two, the **neck**. (Fig. 27-16) The shape of the crown varies according to location: from chisel-shaped to conical or broad with several tubercles or **cusps**. (Fig. 27-21) The incisors, canines, and bicuspids, have one root; molars two or three. All teeth have a central **pulp cavity**, continuous from crown to root. (Fig. 27-17) Each root has an **apical foramen** through which blood vessels and nerves to the **dental pulp** enter. (Fig. 27-19) The core of the tooth is made up of a bony structure, the **dentin**. (Fig. 27-18) The dentin of the crown is covered by an extremely hard ivory structure, the **enamel**, reaching down to the neck of the tooth. The root is covered by the **cementum**, a thin layer of bonelike tissue. (Fig. 27-20) The root is attached to the socket of the jaw by a tough ligament, the **periodontal membrane**.

Fig. 27-16. Ground, longitudinal section of incisor. Human. L.M. X 6. **1.** Crown. **2.** Neck. **3.** Root. **4.** Pulp cavity. **5.** Apex of root. The lines and areas that appear black contain air-filled channels in this ground specimen.

Fig. 27-17. Detail of crown of incisor. Human. L.M. X 13. **1.** Enamel. **2.** Dentin. **3.** Pulp cavity. **4.** Neck. **5.** Erosion in enamel.

Fig. 27-18. Enlargement of area similar to rectangle in Fig. 27-17. Ground section. Human. L.M. X 300. **1.** Dentin. **2.** Dentino-enamel junction. **3.** Enamel. **4.** Dentinal tubules. **5.** Enamel prisms.

Fig. 27-19. Detail of root in Fig. 27-16. Human. L.M. X 23. **1.** Dentin. **2.** Radical pulp cavity. **3.** Apical foramen. **4.** Acellular cementum. **5.** Cellular cementum.

Fig. 27-20. Enlargement of rectangle in Fig. 27-19. L.M. X 220. **1.** Dentin. **2.** Dentino-enamel junction. **3.** Cementum. **4.** Dentinal tubules. **5.** Air-filled lacunae with canaliculi for cementocytes and their processes.

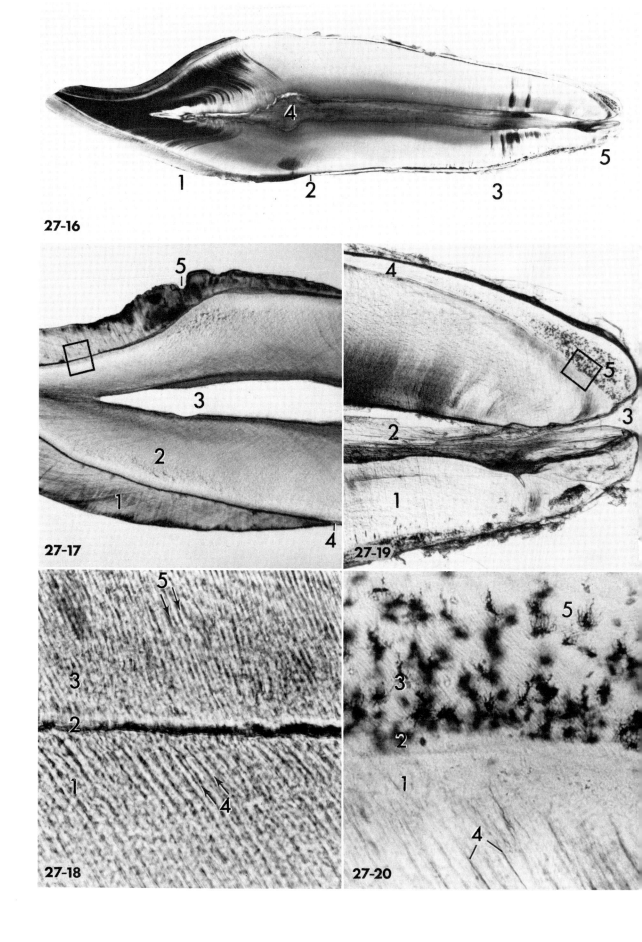

27-16

27-17

27-19

27-18

27-20

DENTIN

Dentin is harder than bone, containing 67% inorganic material, 20% organic components and 13% water. Dentin is composed of a matrix of collagenous fibrils which is mineralized by apatite crystals in similarity with bone tissue. The hard core is perforated by numerous, about 3 μ-wide tunnels, the **dentinal tubules,** which are equally spaced and arranged in parallel, stretching from the pulp cavity to the dentino-enamel junction. (Fig. 27-18) The pulpal surface of the dentin is lined by one or several layers of cylindrical cells, the **odontoblasts.** (Fig. 27-23) Each cell sends one **odontoblastic process** through the entire length of a dentinal tubule. Since the dentin is completely avascular, it is nourished through these processes and the extracellular fluid in the narrow space between the odontoblastic process and the wall of the dentinal tubule.

ENAMEL

Enamel is harder than dentine, containing 96% inorganic material, 0.5% organic components, and 3.5% water. The enamel is completely compact and acellular. It is organized in the form of long **prisms** (rods) which run from the amelodentinal junction to the enamel surface. (Fig. 27-18) Their course is slightly wavy in the inner half, whereas they lie at right angles to the enamel surface in the outer half. The rods are surrounded by interprismatic areas, small spaces containing less calcified cementine substance. Each prism is about 4 μ wide. It contains **crystallites** arranged preferentially in relation to the long axis of the prism. Each crystallite is about 0.1 μ long and has a cross-sectional diameter of 30 Å by 60 Å. Each enamel prism is formed before tooth eruption by a series of **segments** secreted by a layer of ameloblasts. Each ameloblast forms one prism in its entirety.

CEMENTUM

Cementum is an extremely thin covering of the root. It begins at the level where the enamel terminates and continues to the apex, sometimes also lining the apical root canal for a short distance. The cementum is a bone tissue which has an acellular matrix in its relation to the upper third of the tooth and contains matrix and cells, **cementocytes** (Fig. 27-20), in its lower portions. The cells occupy lacunar spaces interconnected by canaliculi in the cementum. They are derived from mesenchymal cells of the dental connective tissue sac, and thus have a similar origin as that of odontoblasts. The function of the cementum is to serve as an attachment structure for the periodontal membrane. It is formed continually throughout life.

PERIODONTAL MEMBRANE

Periodontal membrane is the dense fibrous connective tissue surrounding the root of the tooth. It is a reinforcement of the periosteum of the tooth socket in the alveolar process. There is an abundance of dense collagen bundles and some elastic fibers, fibroblasts, and a rich capillary net-

Fig. 27-21. Bicuspid in alveolar process. Decalcified. Monkey. L.M. X 35. **1.** Dissolved enamel. **2.** Dentin. **3.** Dental pulp. **4.** Bony socket. **5.** Bone marrow. **6.** Periodontal membrane.

Fig. 27-22. Detail of upper rectangle (A) in Fig. 27-21. Monkey. L.M. X 81. **1.** Dentin. **2.** Dissolved enamel. **3.** Epithelial attachment of gingiva. **4.** Free gingiva. **5.** Lamina propria. **6.** Oral cavity. **7.** Cementum.

Fig. 27-23. Enlargement of rectangle (B) in Fig. 27-21. L.M. X 420. **1.** Dental pulp. **2.** Blood vessels. **3.** Odontoblasts. **4.** Dentin. **5.** Odontoblastic processes in dentinal tubules.

Fig. 27-24. Detail of apex of root. Enlargement of area corresponding to rectangle (C) in Fig. 27-21. Monkey. L.M. X 72. **1.** Dentin. **2.** Cementum. **3.** Apical foramina. **4.** Periodontal membrane. **5.** Bony socket. **6.** Blood vessels.

Fig. 27-25. Detail of rectangle (D) in Fig. 27-21. L.M. X 260. **1.** Dentin. **2.** Acellular cementum. **3.** Principal collagenous fibers of periodontal membrane. **4.** Small blood vessel. **5.** Bone.

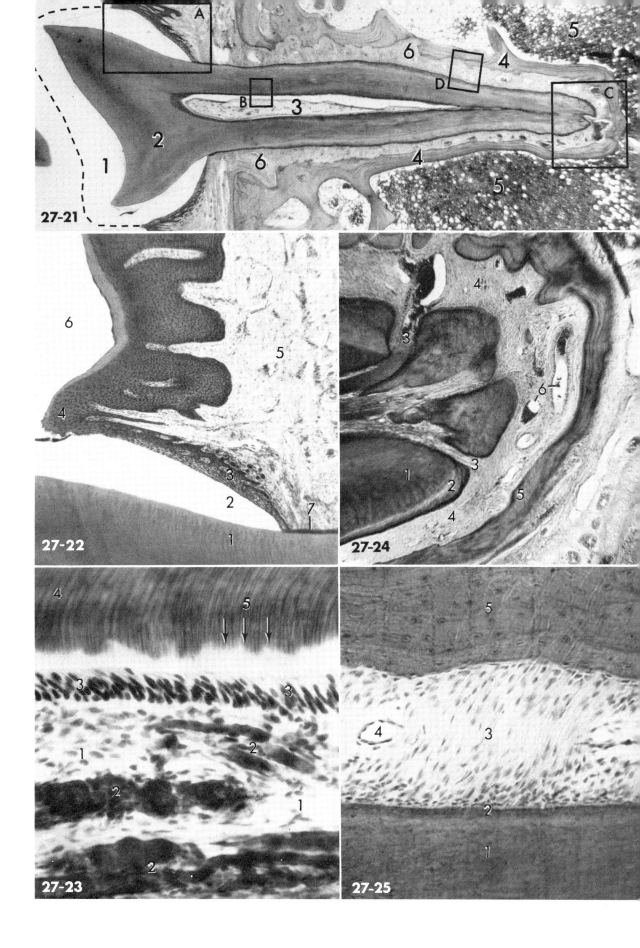

27-21

27-22

27-23

27-24

27-25

work. (Fig. 27-25) Some of the principal collagen bundles (Sharpey's fibers) are anchored in the matrix of the bone and in the cementum. The main function of the periodontal membrane is to suspend the tooth and secure its position in the alveolus.

PULP

The dental pulp is composed of loose connective tissue in which stellate fibroblasts form a framework for reticular and fine collagenous fibers. One or several layers of columnar odontoblasts establish the border between the pulp proper and the dentin. (Fig. 27-23) Other cells in the pulp are macrophages and pericytes. On an average, one arteriole and two venules supply the vast capillary bed of the pulp which extends in between the odontoblasts. Non-myelinated nerves are associated with the vascular bed. Small myelinated sensory nerves terminate as free endings among the odontoblasts. The dental pulp is essential for the nourishment and upkeep of the dentin.

DEVELOPMENT OF THE TEETH

The enamel develops from a bud-like down-growth of oral ectoderm, whereas the dentin is produced by mesenchymal cells subjacent to the ectodermal down-growth. The epithelial bud first assumes the shape of a two-layered cap, the **enamel organ** (Fig. 27-26), the innermost layer of which develops into **ameloblasts.** The enamel organ later changes to a bell-shaped structure (Fig. 27-27), partly enclosing a mesenchymal condensation, the **dental papilla,** from which develop the **odontoblasts** and the dental pulp. Mesodermal cells also surround the enamel organ to form the **dental capsule** (sac), from which develop the periodontal membrane and the cementum. (Fig. 27-28) It is in the zone between the layers of ameloblasts and odontoblasts that predentin and dentin are first formed, followed by the formation of enamel. The formation of dentin starts at the coronal end of the

tooth germ and proceeds in widening conical layers toward the root. Enamel production extends only to the neck of the tooth. The double layer of enamel epithelium, the **sheath of Hertwig,** continues to grow downward, surrounding the enlarging dental papilla. Subsequently, predentin and dentin of the root is formed. Shortly after eruption of the tooth, cementum is laid down by the fibroblasts of the dental capsule.

ODONTOBLASTS

The odontoblasts form a layer of highly polarized cells. (Fig. 27-30) They synthesize predentin by incorporating amino acids into dental collagen and bring about a mineralization and crystallization to form the dentin. Like osteoblasts, the odontoblasts are of mesenchymal origin and their ultrastructure is similar. The

Fig. 27-26. Formation of enamel organ. Cap stage. Human embryo. L.M. X 40. **1.** Oral cavity. **2.** Oral epithelium. **3.** Dentinal lamina. **4.** Enamel organ in cap stage. **5.** Dental papilla.

Fig. 27-27. Formation of tooth germ. Bell stage of enamel organ. Kitten. L.M. X 40. **1.** Outer enamel epithelium. **2.** Stellate reticulum (enamel pulp). **3.** Inner enamel epithelium (ameloblasts). **4.** Odontoblasts. **5.** Dental papilla. **6.** Dental capsule (sac). **7.** Bony socket.

Fig. 27-28. Formation of tooth. Developing crown. Kitten. L.M. X 36. **1.** Outer enamel epithelium. **2.** Stellate reticulum. **3.** Ameloblasts. **4.** Enamel. **5.** Dentin. **6.** Odontoblasts. **7.** Dental papilla (future pulp). **8.** Epithelial root sheath (of Hertwig). **9.** Dental sac (capsule). **10.** Calcification front of dentin.

Fig. 27-29. Enlargement of rectangle in Fig. 27-28. L.M. X 180. Explanation, see Fig. 27-30.

Fig. 27-30. Area similar to Fig. 27-29. Rat molar. E.M. X 700. **1.** Stellate reticulum. **2.** Stratum intermedium. **3.** Ameloblasts. **4.** Enamel. **5.** Dentin. **6.** Predentin. **7.** Odontoblasts. **8.** Dental papilla with fibroblasts. **9.** Capillary. **10.** Attachment zone of odontoblasts. **11.** Calcification front of dentin.

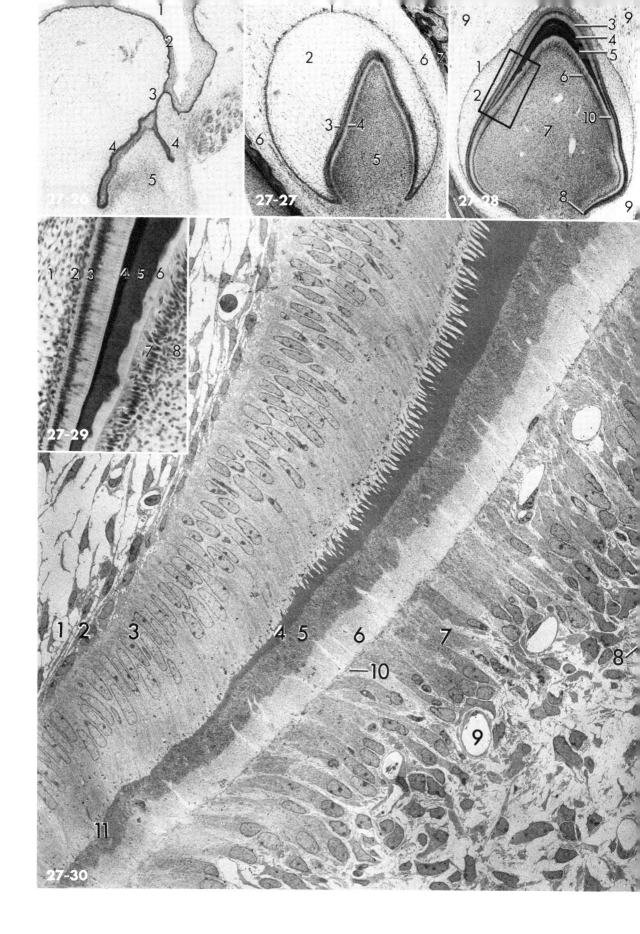

odontoblast has a cylindrical cell body with one end differentiated to a long, odontoblastic process (Tomes') which is wide in the region of the predentin but narrow in the mineralized region. Cells are held together by junctional complexes at the predentin border. (Fig. 27-33) The nucleus is in the pulpal (basal) end of the cell. In the cell body, profiles of granular endoplasmic reticulum and mitochondria are numerous, in addition to a large Golgi complex, many lysosomes and coated vesicles. The odontoblastic process contains mainly coated vesicles and microtubules in its broad segment. (Fig. 27-34) Within the mineralized dentin, the narrow process contains microvesicles and filaments. It is surrounded by a non-mineralized space in the dentinal tubule, the **sheath of Neumann.**

Dentinogenesis entails activities by the odontoblast along the lines indicated in the description of bone formation. The odontoblast synthesizes the collagen precursors, probably as a joint effort by the granular endoplasmic reticulum and the Golgi complex. The smallest collagenous fibrils are located near the base of the odontoblastic process, increasing in size toward the narrow part of the process. This organic framework is **predentin.** Dentin is formed on this by a calcification process. The odontoblast becomes displaced in toward the pulp during dentinogenesis, and the odontoblastic process elongates.

Ameloblasts. The ameloblasts form a single layer of cylindrical cells. (Fig. 27-30) The nucleus is in the basal region and in man, mitochondria are located mostly distally, together with profiles of the granular endoplasmic reticulum. There is a prominent Golgi complex and a peculiar, short attenuated cytoplasmic process (Tomes') in the distal end of the cell. (Fig. 27-31) It contains microtubules and small secretory granules which are formed in the Golgi region. The content of the granules is discharged at the cell surface to form the matrix of the enamel. The matrix occupies a narrow space between the mineralizing front of the dentin and the cell membrane of the process. (Fig. 27-32) The matrix is finely granular and represents the organic matrix of the enamel or its precursor.

Amelogenesis include several stages of cellular activity. As a first stage, the cells at the coronal end of the tooth synthesize and discharge the organic matrix which is rich in proteins, mineral salts, and sulfur. This matrix becomes mineralized immediately to form enamel prisms made up of short, needle-like crystallites. Only one Tomes' process is involved in orienting one enamel prism, but the matrix precursors forming any given rod may be secreted by several neighboring ameloblasts. The enamel subsequently undergoes a maturation process under the influence of the most coronal ameloblasts. There is a loss of organic material and water, and an increase in mineralization occurs. The crystallites increase in size and change their shape from needles to narrow plates.

Fig. 27-31. Detail of ameloblasts. Rat molar at the same stage of development as in Fig. 27-30. E.M.X 1800. **1.** Nuclei of ameloblasts. **2.** Distal ends of cells with granular endoplasmic reticulum. **3.** Ameloblastic processes. **4.** Enamel.

Fig. 27-32. Enlargement of an area similar to the rectangle in Fig. 27-31. Rat molar. E.M. X 28,000. **1.** Ameloblastic processes. **2.** Granular endoplasmic reticulum. **3.** Secretory granules. **4.** Discharging secretory granules. **5.** Extracellular space with pre-enamel matrix. **6.** Mineralized enamel prisms.

Fig. 27-33. Detail of odontoblasts from Fig. 27-30. Rat molar. E.M. X 1800. **1.** Nuclei of odontoblasts. **2.** Level of junctional complexes. **3.** Odontoblastic processes (wide part). **4.** Predentin. **5.** Odontoblastic processes (narrow part) in dentinal tubule. **6.** Dentin.

Fig. 27-34. Enlargement of an area similar to rectangle in Fig. 27-33. Rat molar. E.M. X 29,000. **1.** Odontoblastic processes (wide part). **2.** Coated vesicles. **3.** Collagenous fibrils in predentin. **4.** Odontoblastic processes (narrow part) in dentinal tubule. **5.** Mineralized dentin (decalcified specimen).

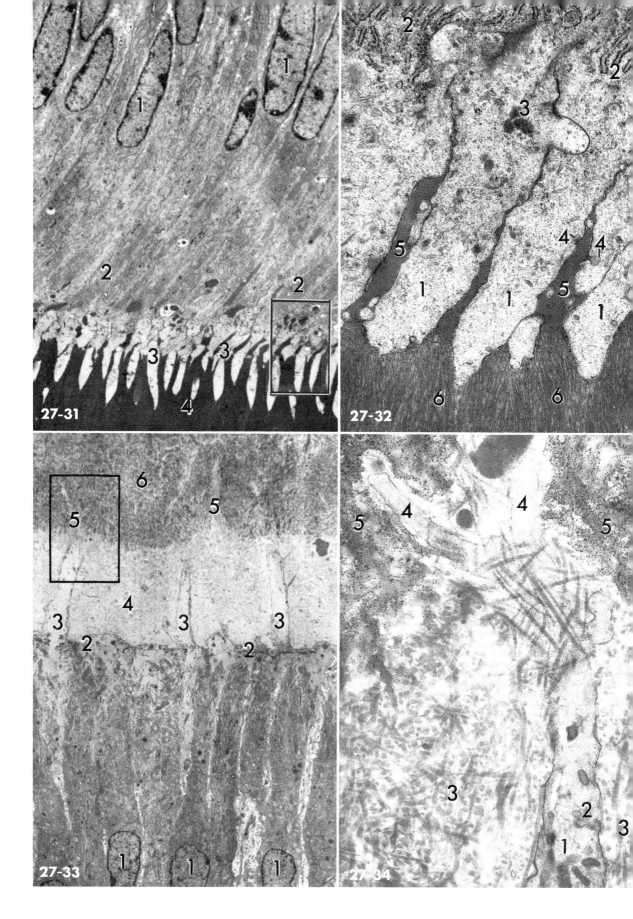

References

SALIVARY GLANDS

Amsterdam, A., Ohad, I. and Schramm, M. Dynamic changes in the ultrastructure of the acinar cells of the rat parotid gland during the secretory cycle. J. Cell Biol. *41*: 753–773 (1969).

Cowley, L. H. and Shackleford, J. M. An ultrastructural study of the submandibular glands of the squirrel monkey, Saimiri sciureus. J. Morph. *132*: 117–136 (1970).

Enomoto, S. and Scott, B. L. Intracellular distribution of mucosubstances in the major sublingual gland of the rat. Anat. Rec. *169*: 71–96 (1971).

Hand, A. R. The fine structure of von Ebner's gland of the rat. J. Cell Biol. *44*: 340–353 (1970).

Hand, A. R. Morphology and cytochemistry of the Golgi apparatus of rat salivary gland acinar cells. Am. J. Anat. *130*: 141–158 (1971).

Heap, P. F. and Bhoola, K. D. Ultrastructure of granules in the submaxillary gland of the guinea-pig. J. Anat. *107*: 115–130 (1970).

Hollmann, K. H. and Verley, J. M. La glande sous-maxillaire de la souris et du rat. Etude au microscope électronique Z. Zellforsch. *68*: 363–388 (1965).

Kagayama, M. The fine structure of the monkey sub-mandibular gland with a special reference to intraacinar nerve endings. Am. J. Anat. *131*: 185–196 (1971).

Parks, H. F. Morphological study of the extrusion of secretory materials by the parotid glands of mouse and rat. J. Ultrastruct. Res. *6*: 449–465 (1962).

Rutberg, U. Ultrastructure and secretory mechanism of the parotid gland. Acta Odontol. Scand. *19*: Suppl. 30, 1–68 (1961).

Shackleford, J. M. and Wilborn, W. H. Ultrastructural aspects of calf submandibular glands. Am. J. Anat. *127*: 259–280 (1970).

Shackleford, J. M. and Wilborn, W. H. Ultrastructural aspects of cat submandibular glands. J. Morph. *131*: 253–276 (1970).

Tandler, B., Denning, C. R., Mandel, I. D. and Kutscher, A. H. Ultrastructure of human labial salivary glands. I. Acinar secretory cells. J. Morph. *127*: 382–408 (1969).

Tandler, B., Denning, C. R., Mandel, I. D. and Kutscher, A. H. Ultrastructure of human labial salivary glands. III. Myoepithelium and ducts. J. Morph. *130*: 227–246 (1970).

Yohro, T. Nerve terminals and cellular junctions in young and adult mouse submandibular glands. J. Anat. *108*: 409–417 (1971).

TEETH

Elwood, W. K. and Bernstein, M. H. The ultrastructure of the enamel organ related to enamel formation. Am. J. Anat. *122*: 73–94 (1968).

Garant, P. R., Szabo, G. and Nalbandian, J. The fine structure of the mouse odontoblast. Arch. Oral Biol. *13*: 857–876 (1968).

Harris, R. Fine structure of nerve endings in the human dental pulp. Arch. Oral Biol. *13*: 773–778 (1968).

Jande, S. S. and Bélanger, L. F. Fine structural study of rat molar cementum. Anat. Rec. *167*: 439–464 (1970).

Kallenbach, E. Cell architecture in the papillary layer of rat incisor enamel organ at the stage of enamel maturation. Anat. Rec. *157*: 683–698 (1967).

Kallenbach, E. Fine structure of rat incisor enamel organ during late pigmentation and regression stages. J. Ultrastruct. Res. *30*: 38–63 (1970).

Lester, K. S. The unusual nature of root formation in molar teeth of the laboratory rat. J. Ultrastruct. Res. *28*: 481–506 (1969).

Lester, K. S. The incorporation of epithelial cells by cementum. J. Ultrastruct. Res. *27*: 63–68 (1970).

Lester, K. S. On the nature of "fibrils" and tubules in developing enamel of the opossum, Didelphis marsupialis. J. Ultrastruct. Res. *30*: 64–77 (1970).

Levy, B. M. and Bernick, S. Studies on the biology of the periodontium of marmosets: II. Development and organization of the periodontal ligament of deciduous teeth in marmosets (Callithrix jacchus). J. Dental Res. *47*: 27–33 (1968).

Listgarten, M. A. Electron microscopic study of the gingivo-dental junction of man. Am. J. Anat. *119*: 147–178 (1966).

Matthiessen, M. E. and Bülow, F. A. von. The ultrastructure of human fetal odontoblasts. Z. Zellforsch. *105*: 569–578 (1970).

Moe, H. Morphological changes in the infranuclear portion of the enamel-producing cells during their life cycle. J. Anat. *108*: 43–62 (1971).

Reith, E. J. The ultrastructure of ameloblasts from the growing end of rat incisors. Arch. Oral Biol. *2*: 253–262 (1960).

Reith, E. J. The ultrastructure of ameloblasts during matrix formation and the maturation of enamel. J. Biophys. Biochem. Cytol. *9*: 825–840 (1961).

Reith, E. J. The early stage of amelogenesis as observed in molar teeth of young rats. J. Ultrastruct. Res. *17*: 503–526 (1967).

Reith, E. J. Collagen formation in developing molar teeth of rats. J. Ultrastruct. Res. *21*: 383–414 (1968).

Reith, E. J. The stages of amelogenesis as observed in molar teeth of young rats. J. Ultrastruct. Res. *30*: 111–151 (1970).

Reith, E. J. and Cotty, V. F. The absorptive activity of ameloblasts during the maturation of enamel. Anat. Rec. *157*: 577–588 (1967).

Stern, I. B. An electron microscopic study of the cementum, Sharpey's fibers and periodontal ligament in rat incisors. Am. J. Anat. *115*: 377–387 (1964).

Ten Cate, A. R., Melcher, A. H., Pudy, G. and Wagner, D. The non-fibrous nature of the von Korff fibres in developing dentine. A light and electron microscope study. Anat. Rec. *168*: 491–524 (1970).

Warshawsky, H. The fine structure of secretory ameloblasts in rat incisors. Anat. Rec. *161*: 211–230 (1968).

Warshawsky, H. A light and electron microscopic study of the nearly mature enamel of rat incisors. Anat. Rec. *169*: 559–584 (1971).

Watson, M. L. The extracellular nature of enamel in the rat. J. Biophys. Biochem. Cytol. *7*: 489–492 (1960).

Weinstock, A. and Leblond, C. P. Elaboration of the matrix glycoprotein of enamel by the secretory ameloblasts of the rat incisor as revealed by radio-autography after galactose-³H injection. J. Cell Biol. *51*: 26–51 (1971).

28 Digestive system— esophagus and stomach

Esophagus

GENERAL FEATURES OF TUBULAR ALIMENTARY CANAL

Beginning with the esophagus and continuing through the stomach, the intestines, the rectum, and the anal canal, the wall of this largely tubular digestive tract consists of four primary layers. (Fig. 28-1) Innermost is the **lamina mucosae** consisting of an epithelium, a lamina propria, and a lamina muscularis mucosae. Outside these layers follow the **lamina submucosae, lamina muscularis externa,** and the **adventitia** or serosa. There is a slight structural variation of these layers in the different parts of the digestive tract, since these parts are adapted to the breaking down of the food, its absorption, as well as the elimination of residual, undigestible elements.

Structure of esophagus. The esophagus is a muscular tube connecting the pharynx with the stomach. The food is transported along the esophagus by contractions of strong muscular coats which are composed of striated skeletal muscle fibers in the upper part, and of smooth muscle fibers in the lower part. Little or no absorption takes place in the esophagus.

The **lamina mucosae** (mucous membrane) is lined by a thick stratified squamous **epithelium** which normally is not keratinized in man. (Fig. 28-2) The fine structure of this epithelium is similar to that of the oral cavity. (Fig. 28-4) The epithelium rests on a thin **basal lamina.** The **lamina propria** of the mucous membrane is composed of a relatively thick layer of interwoven fine collagenous and elastic fibrils beneath the level of the epithelium. The connective tissue also invaginates the epithelium as tall, narrow papillae, always being separated from the basal cells by the thin basal lamina. The connective tissue of the lamina propria is less cellular than in other parts of the alimentary tract, but it contains a diffuse infiltration of lymphocytes in addition to fibroblasts and macrophages. A plexus of blood vessels and lymphatics permeates the connective tissue. Small, branched tubular mucous glands, **esophageal cardiac glands** are located in the lamina propria at the level of the cricoid cartilage and near the junction with the stomach. They are structurally identical to the cardiac glands of the stomach. The **lamina muscularis mucosae** is missing in the upper part of the esophagus and begins as patches of longitudinally arranged smooth muscle cells at the level of the cricoid cartilage. It gradually becomes a thick layer in the lower parts. Through its contractions, the mucosa is thrown into longitudinal folds. The **lamina submucosae** is formed by coarse collagenous and elastic fibers which give great flexibility to the esophageal wall. It contains small blood vessels, nerves, and some mucous glands, the **esophageal glands proper,** which structurally are similar to the oral mucous glands. The **lamina muscularis externa** is com-

Fig. 28-1. Cross section of mid-portion of esophagus. Cat. L.M. X 15. **1.** Lumen with heavily folded mucous membrane. **2.** Lamina mucosae. **3.** Stratified squamous epithelium. **4.** Lamina propria. **5.** Muscularis mucosae. **6.** Submucosa. **7.** Muscularis externa: inner circular layer. **8.** Muscularis externa: outer longitudinal layer. **9.** Adventitia.

Fig. 28-2. Esophageal mucous membrane. Enlargement of area similar to rectangle (A) in Fig. 28-1. Cat. L.M. X 200. **1.** Lumen. **2.** Stratified squamous non-keratinized epithelium. **3.** Lamina propria. **4.** Connective tissue papillae.

Fig. 28-3. Esophageal musculature: lamina muscularis externa. Enlargement of area similar to rectangle (B) in Fig. 28-1. Middle third of esophagus. Cat. L.M. X 820. **1.** Nuclei of smooth muscle cells. Cell borders are not seen. **2.** Striated skeletal muscle cell. **3.** Connective tissue.

Fig. 28-4. Stratified squamous non-keratinized epithelium. Enlargement of area similar to rectangle in Fig. 28-2. Esophagus. Cat. E.M. X 1700. **1.** Basal cell nucleus. **2.** Spinous cell nucleus. **3.** Nucleus of cell which has started to become squamous. **4.** Nuclei of squamous cells. **5.** Superficial squamous cells in the process of being sloughed. **6.** Bacteria on the epithelial surface. **7.** Lumen of esophagus.

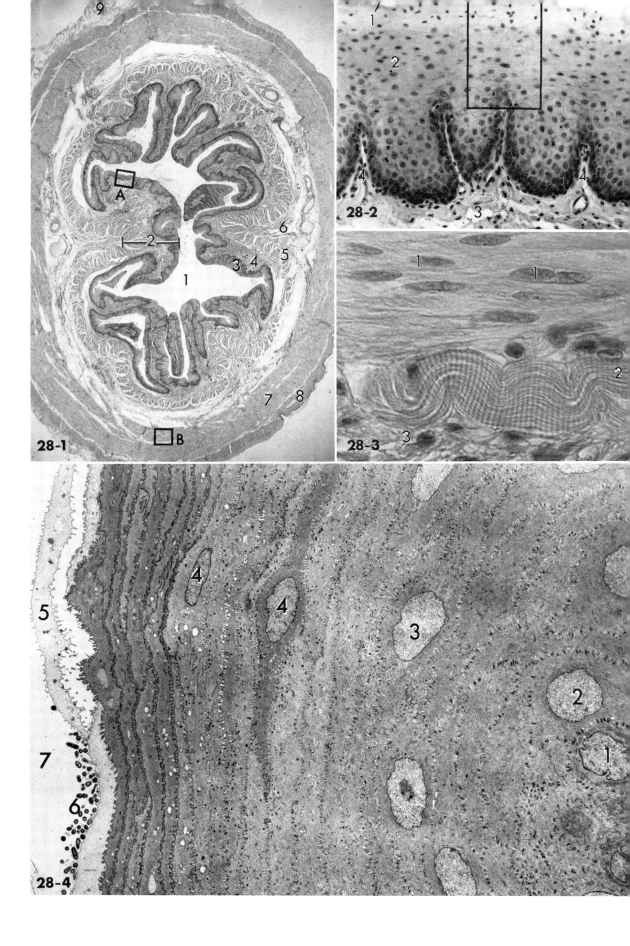

28-1

28-2

28-3

28-4

posed of an inner circular and an **outer longitudinal** layer. The upper third is made up of striated skeletal muscle cells, the middle third of a mixture of striated and smooth muscle (Fig. 28-3), and the lower third of only smooth muscle cells. The **adventitia** consists of a loose fibro-elastic connective tissue layer.

Stomach

The stomach is a sac-like dilatation of the tubular digestive tract in which food is compressed, churned, and mixed with gastric juice and mucus to form a pulp-like mass, the **chyme.** The gastric juice contains mainly protein-splitting enzymes and hydrochloric acid. Some absorption of water takes place in addition to many other fluids such as alcohol and drugs. Anatomically, the stomach can be divided into: 1) **cardiac portion,** the part at the cardio-esophageal junction; 2) **fundus,** which is the portion above the level of the cardiac orifice; 3) **body;** 4) **pyloric antrum;** and 5) **pyloric channel**—with the pyloric orifice connecting the stomach with the first part of the small intestine, the duodenum. Physiologically, the cardiac portion includes the entire part of the mucosa that contains cardiac mucous glands. The fundic portion is provided with gastric glands proper (fundic glands), which includes practically the entire stomach with the exception of the pylorus, which contains the pyloric mucous glands. The stomach is slightly curved, with a **lesser curvature** and a **greater curvature.**

The wall of the stomach contains the same four layers present in the esophagus, but the mucosa and the muscularis externa are thicker. (Fig. 28-8) The mucous membrane is thrown into longitudinal folds or ridges, **rugae,** along the lesser curvature, but the folds resemble a honeycomb elsewhere, giving rise to a pebbled or mammillated pattern, the **gastric areas.** The ridges are not permanent and include the submucosa but not the muscularis ex-

terna. Numerous small invaginations, **gastric pits** (Fig. 28-9) or foveolae, are present throughout the stomach. Villi, typical for the small intestine, do **not** occur in the stomach.

In spite of the absence of an obvious sphincter muscle, the esophago-gastric junction is able to sustain rather high pressures from below before the cardia opens. An overhanging mucosal flap (Fig. 28-5) acts as a valve in preventing a reflux of gastric content back into the esophagus.

The entire pyloric channel is surrounded by a thickening of the circular muscle layer of the muscularis externa of the stomach, which acts as a pyloric sphincter.

LAMINA MUCOSAE

The mucous membrane consists of a simple **epithelium;** a **lamina propria** crowded with short gastric glands; and a **muscularis mucosae.**

Surface epithelium. The surface of the mucosa and the gastric pits is lined by a simple columnar epithelium made up of tall mucus-producing cells, resting on a thin basal lamina. (Fig. 28-10) The nu-

Fig. 28-5. Longitudinal section of cardia. Monkey. Esophagogastric junction. L.M. X 15. **1.** Lumen of esophagus. **2.** Lumen of stomach. **3.** Mucosal flap (fold). **4.** Esophageal epithelium. **5.** Cardiac mucosa. **6.** Submucosa. **7.** Lamina muscularis externa. **8.** Adventitia.

Fig. 28-6. Enlargement of rectangle in Fig. 28-5. L.M. X 74. **1.** Stratified squamous epithelium of esophagus. **2.** Simple columnar surface epithelium of cardia. **3.** Cardiac pits. **4.** Cardiac glands. **5.** Lamina propria.

Fig. 28-7. Enlargement of rectangle in Fig. 28-6. L.M. X 300. **1.** Lumina of cardiac mucous glands. **2.** Mucous cells with flattened nuclei at the base of the cells. **3.** Lamina propria.

Fig. 28-8. Section of entire wall of stomach (body). Monkey. L.M. X 48. **1.** Lumen of stomach. **2.** Lamina mucosae. **3.** Submucosa. **4.** Lamina muscularis externa. **5.** Serosa.

Fig. 28-9. Enlargement of rectangle in Fig. 28-8. L.M. X 210. **1.** Surface epithelium. **2.** Gastric pit. **3.** Gastric gland proper. **4.** Muscularis mucosae. **5.** Submucosa.

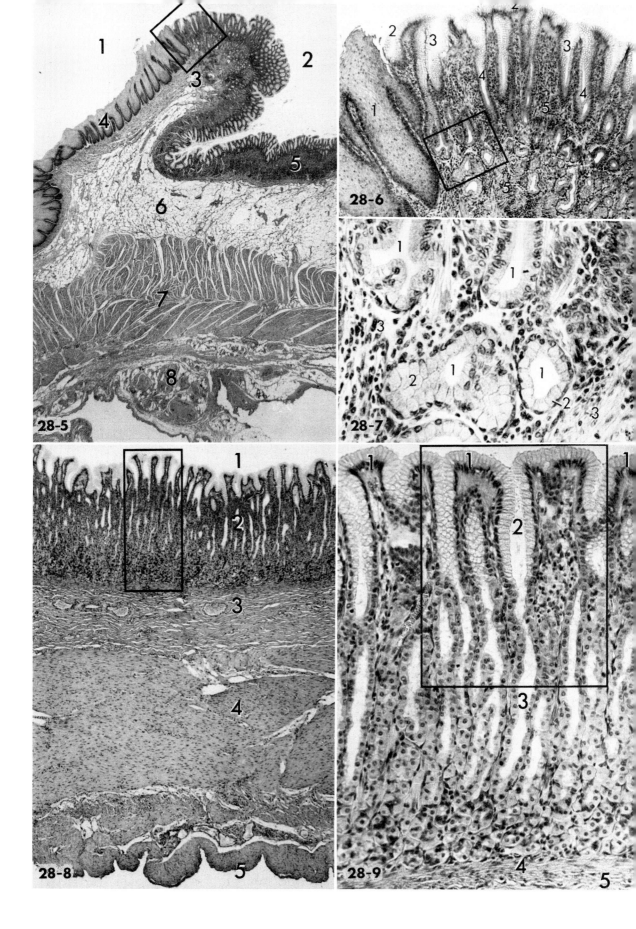

cleus is near the base of the epithelial cell. The base is often tapered, leaving an intercellular space of varying width in well-preserved specimens. (Fig. 28-11) The part above the nucleus is occupied by numerous, spherical, or ovoid, electron-dense droplets (Fig. 28-12), each bounded by a trilaminar membrane. (Fig. 28-14) The cells are ordinarily not goblet-shaped, since every cell in the surface epithelium is a mucus-producing cell. The luminal surface of the cell does not have the prominent, long microvilli of the small intestine, but only a small number of very short microvilli. The luminal aspect of the cell membrane is lined by a microfilamentous material, possibly representing a glycocalyx. The Golgi complex is small, and located above the nucleus. There is an abundance of free ribosomes, but only a small number of granular endoplasmic reticulum profiles and mitochondria. Bundles of tonofilaments permeate the cytoplasm. Several lysosomes occur near the Golgi complex. From a **functional** point of view, it is conceivable that the mucoid droplets are formed from the Golgi complex, although they are rarely seen to come off at the edge of the complex as are mucoid droplets in ordinary goblet cells. The mechanism of release of the droplets is also not clearly understood, since a discharge of droplets either singly or in bulk has not been recorded at the cell surface. (Fig. 28-13) It has been suggested that the mucoid material may leave the cell by a diffusion process to form a protective barrier against high concentrations of hydrochloric acid and pepsin in the stomach. This mucus represents the neutral mucopolysaccharides of the stomach. The epithelial cells are gradually sloughed at the gastric surface, and the epithelium is completely replaced every three days by cells moving up from the bottom of the gastric pits. The precursor cells have not been positively identified but could conceivably be mucous neck cells.

Gastric mucosal glands. The gastric mu-

cosal glands represent tubular downgrowths of epithelium from the gastric pits into the lamina propria, stopping short of the muscularis mucosae. There are three kinds of glands: 1) cardiac; 2) gastric glands proper (fundic glands); and 3) pyloric glands.

Cardiac glands are restricted to a small area near the cardiac orifice of the stomach. They are tubular, branched, slightly twisted glands, lined solely by columnar, mucus-producing cells. (Figs. 28-6, 28-7) The nucleus is flattened and located at the base of the cell. The mucous droplets and the cell organelles are structurally quite similar to those in the cells of the mucous esophageal glands, in the mucous neck cells of the gastric glands proper, and in the cells of the pyloric glands. Parietal cells are not present. The cardiac glands

Fig. 28-10. Gastric mucosa (body of stomach). Enlargement of rectangle in Fig. 28-9. Monkey. L.M. X 363. **1.** Lumen of stomach. **2.** Gastric pit. **3.** Lumina of gastric glands. **4.** Neck of glands. **5.** Surface mucous epithelium. **6.** Lamina propria. **7.** Mucous neck cells.

Fig. 28-11. Enlargement of area similar to rectangle in Fig. 28-10. Body of stomach. Cat. E.M. X 610. **1.** Lumen. **2.** Entrances to gastric pits. **3.** Simple columnar mucous epithelium. **4.** Lamina propria. **5.** Level of basal lamina. **6.** Capillary. **7.** Smooth muscle cells. **8.** Epithelial cells of pits sectioned tangentially.

Fig. 28-12. Surface mucous cell. Enlargement of area similar to rectangle in Fig. 28-11. Stomach. Cat. E.M. X 8900. **1.** Lumen. **2.** Nucleus. **3.** Intercellular space. **4.** Accumulation of highly electron-dense mucous droplets. **5.** Junctional complexes.

Fig. 28-13. Surface of mucous cell. Enlargement of area similar to rectangle in Fig. 28-12. Stomach. Cat. E.M. X 92,000. **1.** Glycocalyx. **2.** Trilaminar cell membrane. **3.** Ground substance of the cytoplasm. **4.** Mucous droplets with dense matrix. **5.** Trilaminar boundary membrane.

Fig. 28-14. Mucous neck cell. Gastric gland proper. E.M. X 92,000. **1.** Mucoid droplets with light matrix. **2.** Trilaminar boundary membrane. **3.** Small vacuoles, probably precursors of mucoid droplets.

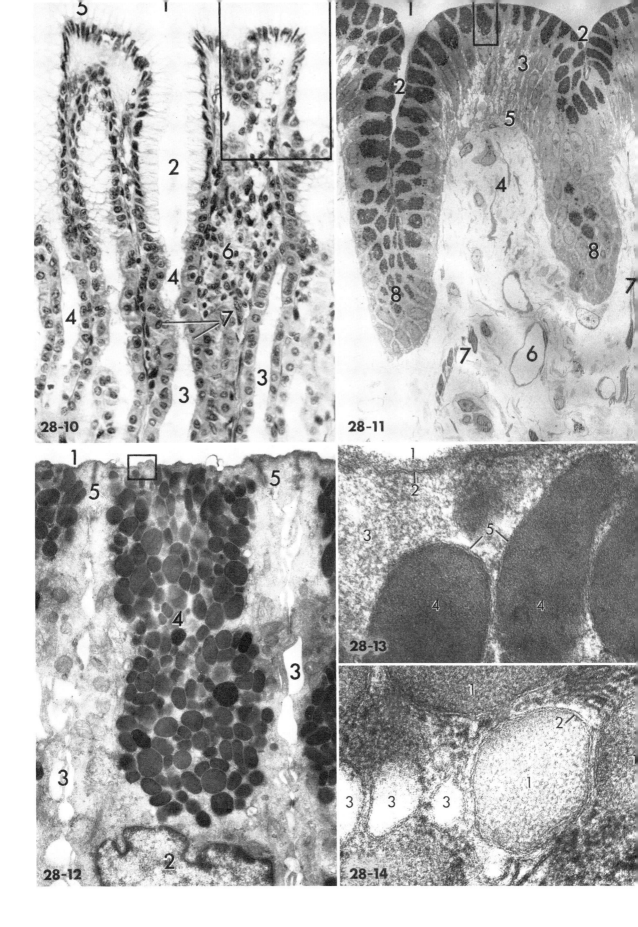

28-10

28-11

28-12

28-13

28-14

also secrete electrolytes such as calcium phosphate, sodium and potassium bicarbonates, and sodium and potassium chlorides, which are incorporated into the mucous secretion.

Gastric glands proper are also referred to as fundic glands. There are several emanating from one gastric pit. They occur throughout the fundus and the body of the stomach as straight, sometimes branched, tubules running parallel to each other and at right angles to the muscularis mucosae. (Fig. 28-9) The major part of each gland, the **body,** is connected via the **neck** to the gastric pit. (Fig. 28-10) Generally, four cell types line the glands: 1) mucous neck cells; 2) chief (zymogenic) cells; 3) parietal (oxyntic) cells; and 4) enterochromaffin (argentaffin) cells.

Mucous neck cells. These cells line the neck of the glands but occur also singly along the body of the gland. The cell is columnar or flask-shaped with a narrow apex and a broad base. The ultrastructural architecture is very similar to that of the cells of the cardiac and pyloric glands. The presecretory mucous droplets are bounded by a trilaminar membrane. They are less electron-dense than the mucous droplets of the gastric surface epithelium but are almost identical to the prezymogen granules of neighboring chief cells. The droplets of the mucous neck cells are strongly PAS-positive, a reaction which is negative in relation to the prezymogen granules. The mucous droplets contain acid mucopolysaccharides. The function of the mucous neck cells is not clear. They have a life span of about six days. There is a possibility that they move up into the pits to form the source of replacement for the surface epithelial cells. This is denied by some workers who claim that the mucous neck cells represent precursors of parietal and chief cells. A third possibility is that they represent precursor cells for both surface epithelial cells and cells of the gastric glands proper. Recently, morphologically undifferentiated cells have been found in the human stom-ach at the base of the pits, bordering on the uppermost mucous neck cells. Intermediate forms were also present which suggested the transformation of undifferentiated cells into both surface epithelial cells in the pits and mucous neck cells.

Chief (zymogenic) cells. These cells predominate in the body of the glands and intermingle with parietal and mucous neck cells toward the neck region. (Fig. 28-15) The structure of the chief cell is quite similar to that of other zymogenic cells such as serous salivary cells (p. 520) and pancreatic acinar cells (p. 596). There is a wealth of free ribosomes and granular endoplasmic reticulum but relatively few mitochondria. The Golgi complex is prominent (Fig. 28-17) and prezymogen granules are present within or near its membranes and vesicles; each granule is surrounded by a trilaminar membrane. The content of the secretory granule is discharged at the apical end of the pyramidal chief cell by fusion of its limiting membrane with the luminal cell mem-

Fig. 28-15. Longitudinal section of gastric glands proper. Stomach. Monkey. L.M. × 560. **1.** Lumen of glands. **2.** Bases of glands. **3.** Lamina propria. **4.** Muscularis mucosae. **5.** Parietal cells. **6.** Zymogenic (chief) cells.

Fig. 28-16. Gastric gland proper. Enlargement of area similar to rectangle in Fig. 28-15. Cat. E.M. × 2000. **1.** Nuclei of parietal cells. **2.** Zymogenic (chief) cells. **3.** Lumen of gastric gland proper is in this general area, but not in the plane of section. **4.** Nucleus of endocrine cell. **5.** Lamina propria. **6.** Lumen of capillary. **7.** Level of the basal lamina surrounding the gastric gland proper. **8.** Parietal cells of neighboring gastric gland.

Fig. 28-17. Detail of gastric gland proper. Stomach. Cat. E.M. × 10,500. **1.** Nucleus of parietal cell. **2.** Nucleus of chief (zymogenic) cell. **3.** Intercellular canaliculi. **4.** Junctions of adjoining cells. **5.** Intracellular canaliculi of parietal cell. **6.** Mitochondria. **7.** Zymogen granules. **8.** Golgi complex. **9.** Granular endoplasmic reticulum. **10.** Basal lamina. **11.** Inset: enlargement of area similar to rectangle. × 48,000. **12.** Vesicles bounded by a trilaminar membrane. **13.** Cell surface membrane.

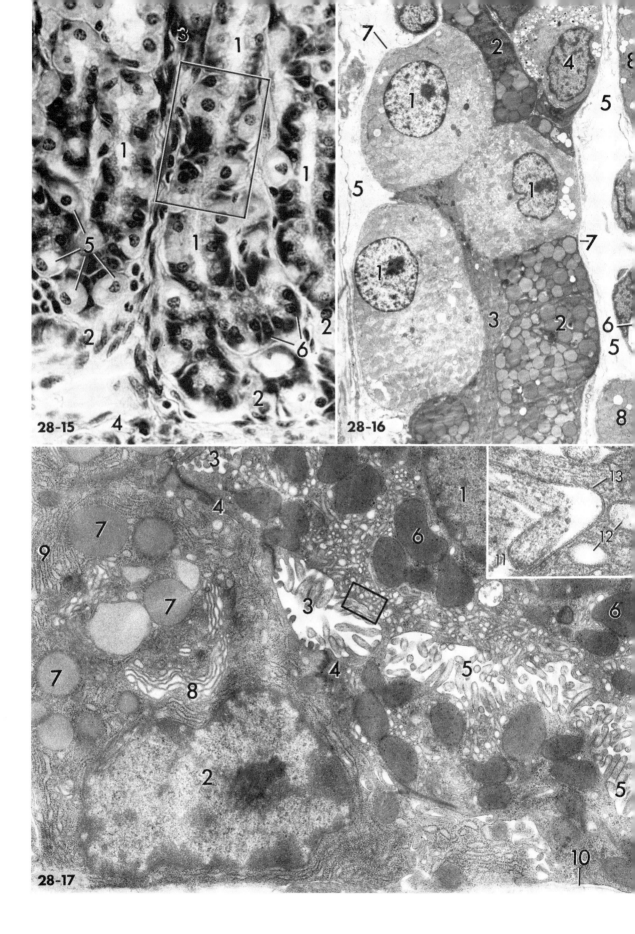

brane. The secretion contains **pepsinogen** and probably also other **proteolytic pro-enzymes.** In rat, they produce the gastric intrinsic factor as well. The pepsinogen is activated to pepsin by hydrochloric acid and digests native proteins to polypeptides. The intrinsic factor mediates the absorption of vitamin B_{12}. The proteolytic enzyme **rennin** which digests milk protein is synthesized by the chief cells in calves, but does not exist in man. Here, pepsin has this action.

Parietal (oxyntic) cells. These cells are concentrated mainly in the central half of the gland. They are larger than the chief cells and are pyramidal or oval-shaped with the base against the thin basal lamina. (Fig. 28-16) The nucleus is located in the center and the cytoplasm is transsected by several 1–$2\,\mu$ wide **secretory canaliculi** which communicate with the lumen of the gastric gland proper. (Fig. 28-17) Numerous short microvilli project into the canaliculi. The cytoplasm is filled with a multitude of relatively large, rounded mitochondria which internally have numerous densely packed cristae of the membranous variety in addition to many small dense mitochondrial matrix granules. Granular endoplasmic reticulum and free ribosomes are scarce, but the agranular endoplasmic reticulum is represented by a varying number of small vesicles and short tubules. Numerous tubulovesicular profiles (Fig. 28-17, inset) are present throughout the cytoplasm and around the intracellular canaliculi. They may not be part of the agranular endoplasmic reticulum since they are bounded by a trilaminar membrane of the same dimensions as the surface cell membrane. The Golgi complex is poorly developed. The basal cell surface is increased by shallow invaginations and microvillous projections. From a **functional** point of view, it is accepted that the parietal cells produce **hydrochloric acid,** and in man, probably also the gastric **intrinsic factor.** The mechanism of HCl formation is not fully explored. In the resting cell, the tubulo-

vesicular profiles are numerous, whereas they are greatly reduced in number and clustered about the intracellular canaliculi during active acid secretion in response to histamine, insulin, and direct electrical vagal stimulation. It has been suggested that the tubulovesicular profiles actively transport chloride ions across the cell, obtaining the energy required for this process from the numerous mitochondria. It has also been suggested that hydrogen ions are formed within the cell from a reaction which produces carbonic acid. This reaction is catalyzed by the enzyme carbonic anhydrase, abundantly present in the parietal cell. The hydrogen ions then cross the cell membrane by an active transport mechanism and combine with the chloride ions in the intracellular canaliculi to form hydrochloric acid.

Pyloric glands are restricted to the pyloric antrum. They are mucus-secreting tubular glands which are shorter than the gastric glands proper, but longer than the cardiac glands. (Fig. 28-18) They open up into the pits of the pyloric antrum which are deeper than in any other region of the stomach. The glands are composed of

Fig. 28-18. Section of pyloric mucosa. Stomach. Monkey. L.M. X 127. **1.** Lumen of pyloric channel. **2.** Lumina of pyloric glands. **3.** Lamina propria. **4.** Muscularis mucosae.

Fig. 28-19. Enlargement of area similar to rectangle in Fig. 28-18. Stomach. Cat. E.M. X 580. **1.** Lumen of cross-sectioned pyloric gland. **2.** Lumen of arteriole. **3.** Lamina propria. **4.** Muscularis mucosae. **5.** Capillary.

Fig. 28-20. Cross-sectioned pyloric gland. Stomach. Cat. E.M. X 1800. **1.** Lumen of pyloric gland. **2.** Nuclei of mucous cells. **3.** Nuclei of endocrine cells. The upper endocrine cell borders on the lumen of the gland. **4.** Lamina propria.

Fig. 28-21. Detail of pyloric gland. Stomach. Cat. E.M. X 9200. **1.** Nucleus of mucous cell. **2.** Nucleus of endocrine (argyrophil) cell, probably Type V, synthesizing gastrin or histamine. **3.** Lumen of pyloric gland. **4.** Microvilli. **5.** Basal lamina. **6.** Mitochondria. **7.** Secretory granules. **8.** Mucous droplets. **9.** Golgi zone. **10.** Lipid droplets. **11.** Lysosomes.

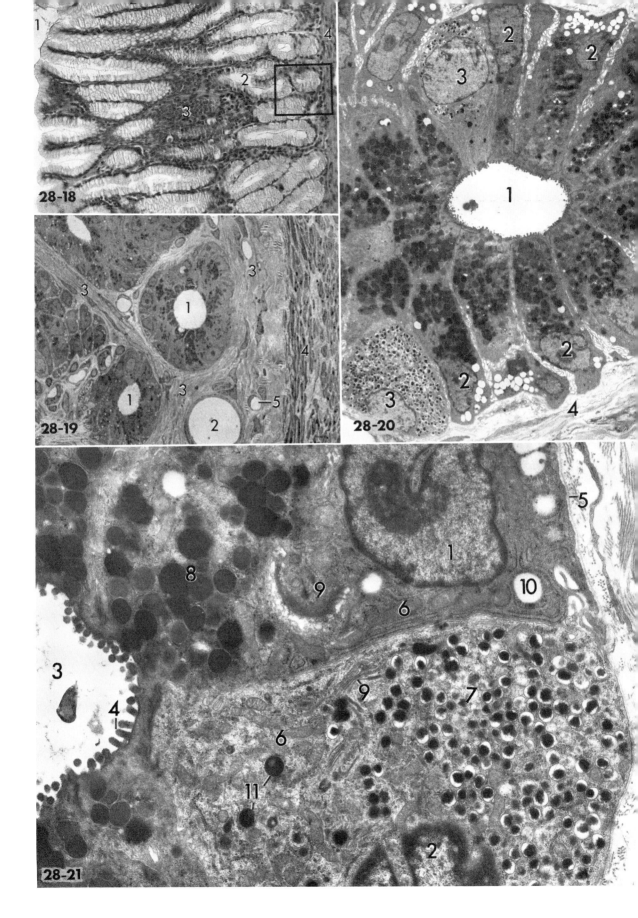

28-18

28-19

28-20

28-21

mucous cells and endocrine cells. (Fig. 28-20) Chief cells are not present and parietal cells are very rare.

Mucous cells. These cells resemble the cardiac mucous cells and also the mucous neck cells of the gastric glands proper. (Fig. 28-21) The nucleus is flattened against the base of the cell and the remainder of the cell is filled with a large number of mucous droplets. The Golgi complex is large, and there are many short microvilli at the luminal surface. Functionally, these cells may secrete a **pyloric protease** in addition to the mucosubstances. They also secrete electrolytes similar to those given off by the cardiac glands.

Endocrine cells. Yet another cell type is present in the glands of the stomach and also throughout the small and large intestines. It contains numerous small granules which can be made visible by impregnation with osmium, chrome, or silver. Recent investigations indicate that these cells have an endocrine function. Based on impregnation techniques, two kinds of cells are generally recognized: 1) enterochromaffin (argentaffin) cells; and 2) argyrophil cells.

The **enterochromaffin (argentaffin) cells** have granules which reduce alkaline silver solutions to metallic silver after formaldehyde fixations, and couple with suitable diazonium salts to yield insoluble colored azo dyes. The cells occur sparsely in the gastric glands proper but are fairly numerous in the small and large intestines. The cells are located either between the bases of other gastrointestinal gland cells, or they extend from the basal lamina to the lumen of the gland. The cytoplasmic granules are electron dense with a tightly fitted membrane. (Fig. 28-21) There is a small Golgi complex and a poorly developed granular endoplasmic reticulum. The granules are believed to contain **5-hydroxytryptamine (serotonin)** which is synthesized and/or stored by the cells. It is probably released by diffusion to reach the blood stream or the gastrointestinal wall. It has a contractile action on intestinal and vascular smooth muscle cells by serving as a neurotransmitter substance, stimulating the neuromuscular apparatus.

The **argyrophil cells** have granules which, after formaldehyde fixation, reduce silver salts only after exposure to an extraneous reducing agent. In the stomach, the cells are particularly numerous in the pyloric glands, whereas they have a similar distribution as the enterochromaffin cells in the small and large intestines. The cells sometimes do not reach the luminal surface in the intestine of rats but do so more often in the human pyloric glands. The cytoplasmic granules are less electron-dense than those in the enterochromaffin cells, and the boundary membrane is fitted loosely. The Golgi complex is prominent. There are many free ribosomes and mitochondria, and the granular endoplasmic reticulum is conspicuous. The granules are derived from the Golgi complex and

Fig. 28-22. Survey of the middle layers of the wall of the stomach. Cat. E.M. X 680. **1.** Bases of gastric glands proper. **2.** Lamina propria. **3.** Lamina muscularis mucosae. **4.** Submucosa. **5.** Part of lamina muscularis externa. **6.** Arteriole. **7.** Terminal arterioles. **8.** Precapillary sphincters. **9.** Blood capillaries. **10.** Postcapillary venule. **11.** Lymphatic capillary. **12.** Lymphatic vessel.

Fig. 28-23. Topography of lamina muscularis mucosae. Enlargement of rectangle in Fig. 28-22. Stomach. Cat. E.M. X 1600. **1.** Lumen of slightly constricted arteriole; luminal diameter 18 μ. **2.** Endothelial nucleus. **3.** Nucleus of vascular smooth muscle cells. **4.** Nucleus of adventitial fibroblasts. **5.** Bundles of fine collagenous fibrils of lamina propria. **6.** Fibroblasts. **7.** Macrophages. **8.** Eosinophil leukocytes. **9.** Lumen of lymphatic capillary. **10.** Part of smooth muscle cells ascending the lamina propria. **11.** Cross-sectioned non-myelinated nerve. **12.** Lamina muscularis mucosae is composed of a loose skein of delicate smooth muscle cells. The muscle cells contact each other via thin cytoplasmic processes. There is a large amount of collagenous fibrils between the smooth muscle cells of the muscularis mucosae. **13.** Connective tissue of the submucosa.

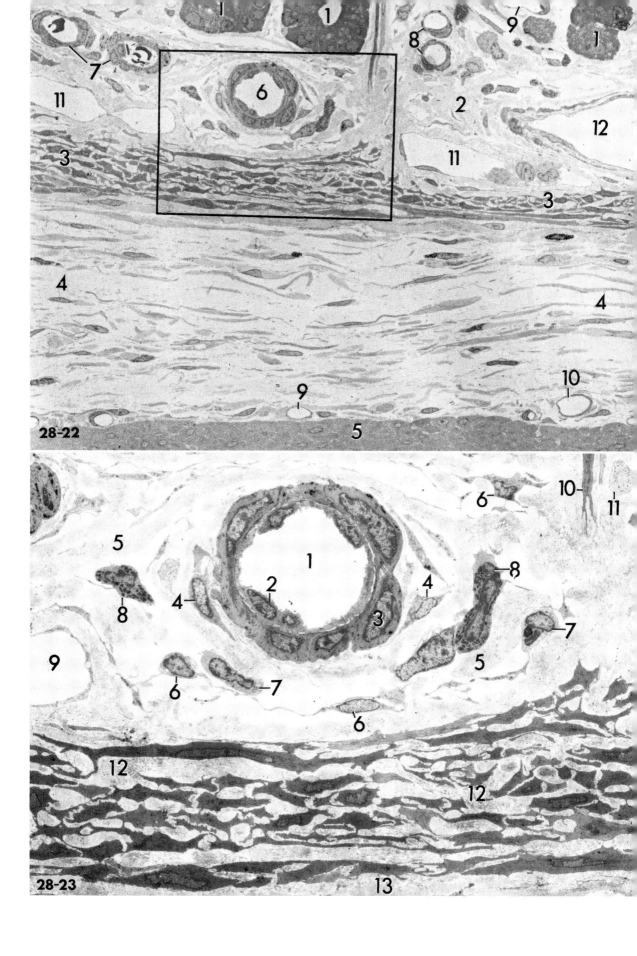

28-22

28-23

are considered as secretory granules containing **gastrin,** a polypeptide hormone which stimulates the parietal cells of the gastric glands to secrete hydrochloric acid. The distention of the stomach and the presence of partly digested protein act as a stimulus on the argyrophil cells, probably via their luminal microvilli, to release the gastrin by diffusion to the blood stream through which it ultimately reaches the parietal cells. The argyrophil cells have also been shown to contain **histamine** which acts as a local chemical stimulus on the parietal cell. The cells which secrete serotonin are also referred to as **type I cells,** and those assumed to synthesize gastrin or histamine are called **type V cells.** (Fig. 28-21) This is discussed further on p. 562).

LAMINA PROPRIA

The lamina propria of the gastric mucosa is restricted to the small area underneath the surface epithelium and to the very narrow space between the gastric mucosal glands. (Fig. 28-23) It consists of loose connective tissue dominated by narrow bundles of collagenous fibrils, a small number of fibroblasts, some macrophages and a network of blood capillaries and lymphatics. Thin strands of long smooth muscle cells ascend between the glands from the muscularis mucosae. Functionally, the lamina propria nourishes and supports the cardiac surface epithelium and the glands. In contrast to the lamina propria of the intestine, it does not contain the same rich, general distribution of lymphocytes and plasma cells, although aggregations of lymphocytes occur to form nodular regions, particularly in the pyloric area.

MUSCULARIS MUCOSAE

The muscularis mucosae consists essentially of two layers of smooth muscle cells, an inner circular and an outer longitudinal. Muscle fibers extend from the inner layer into the lamina propria between the gastric glands. (Fig. 28-23) The smooth muscle cells are thin and thread-like. They

are spaced relatively far apart, invested individually by a thin external (basal) lamina and bundles of collagenous fibrils. Contractions of the muscularis mucosae aid in emptying the gastric glands.

SUBMUCOSA

The lamina submucosae consists of an irregular connective tissue with a denser arrangement of the collagen bundles than in the lamina propria. It serves as a support for blood vessels, lymphatics, and the submucous nerve plexus, all of which supply the mucous membrane. (Fig. 28-22) The submucosa does not contain glands. In the folding and shifting of the gastric mucosa during digestion, the submucosa participates in forming the rugae and the gastric areas.

MUSCULARIS EXTERNA

The muscularis externa of the stomach is the heaviest muscular coat of the gastrointestinal tract with the exception of the rectum. It consists of three layers of smooth muscle cells: 1) inner oblique; 2) middle circular; and 3) outer longitudi-

Fig. 28-24. Survey of outer part of wall of stomach. Monkey. L.M. X 60. **1.** Bases of gastric glands proper. **2.** Muscularis mucosae. **3.** Submucosa. **4.** Muscularis externa: inner oblique layer. **5.** Muscularis externa: middle circular layer. **6.** Muscularis externa: outer longitudinal layer. **7.** Visceral peritoneum. **8.** Peritoneal cavity. **9.** Small vein. **10.** Small artery. **11.** Venule. **12.** Thin connective tissue septum.

Fig. 28-25. Enlargement of area similar to rectangle (A) in Fig. 28-24. Stomach. Cat. E.M. X 4700. **1.** Nuclei of smooth muscle cells in outer longitudinal layer of muscularis externa. **2.** Nucleus of Schwann cell. **3.** Nucleus of mesothelial cell. **4.** Bundles of densely packed collagenous fibrils. **5.** Non-myelinated nerves. **6.** Microvilli. **7.** Peritoneal cavity.

Fig. 28-26. Enlargement of area similar to rectangle (B) in Fig. 28-24. Stomach. Cat. E.M. X 1900. **1.** Densely packed smooth muscle cells in middle circular layer of muscularis externa. **2.** Nuclei of smooth muscle cells. **3.** Connective tissue septa. **4.** Lumen of venule. **5.** Non-myelinated nerve fibers.

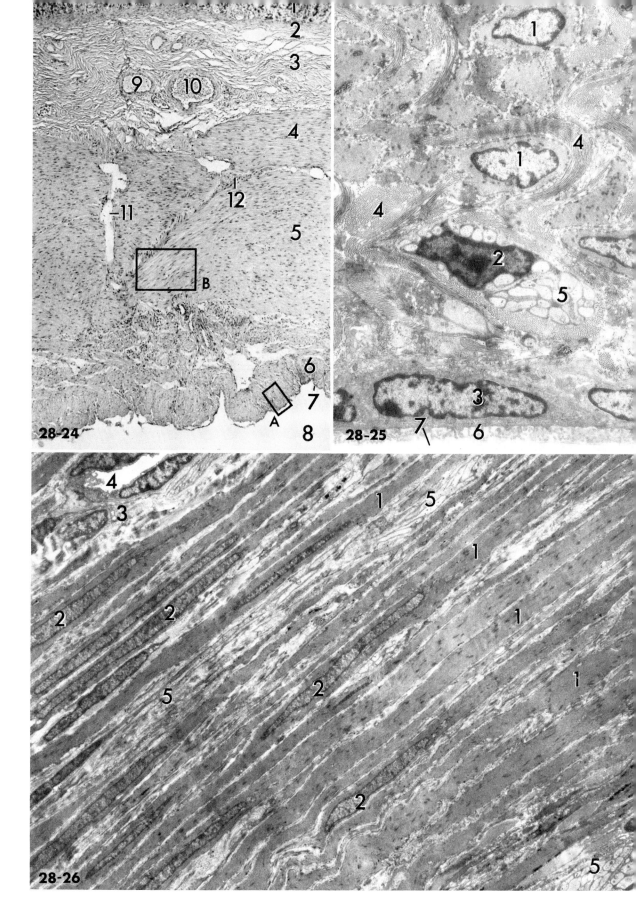

nal. (Fig. 28-24) The layers are united by thin connective tissue septa. The **inner oblique** fibers are most numerous near the cardia, scanty over the major part of the body, and are absent in relation to the pyloric channel. The **middle circular** layer is the thickest. It is equally distributed throughout the stomach (Fig. 28-26) with reinforcements in relation to the cardiac and pyloric orifices, where it forms sphincter-like structures. The **outer longitudinal** fibers are abundant along the lesser curvature and around the pyloric channel. The smooth muscle cells are larger and more densely packed than in the muscularis mucosae. The contractions of the muscle fibers aid in dividing, macerating, and homogenizing the food, and in emptying the stomach. Waves of contraction start in the area of the fundus and spread downward. In the pyloric antrum, contraction waves are stronger and mostly independent.

SEROSA

The serous coat of the stomach is formed by a thin layer of connective tissue and the mesothelium, the latter a single layer of squamous cells. (Fig. 28-25)

BLOOD VESSELS

The stomach is supplied by several large arteries which break up to form a large, anastomosing latticework of vessels in the subserosa, submucosa, and lamina propria. Many arteriovenous shunts exist in the submucosa. The architecture of the gastric microcirculation facilitates the transfer of blood from one point to another in the wall of the stomach.

NERVES

These are discussed on p. 574 as part of the nerves to the gastrointestinal tract.

References

ESOPHAGUS

Goetsch, E. The structure of the mammalian esophagus. Am. J. Anat. *10*: 1–40 (1910).

Johns, B. A. E. Developmental changes in the oesophageal epithelium in man. J. Anat. *86*: 431–442 (1952).

Mottet, N. K. Mucin biosynthesis by chick and human oesophagus during ontogenic metaplasia. J. Anat. *107*: 49–66 (1970).

Parakkal, P. F. An electron microscopic study of esophageal epithelium in the newborn and adult mouse. Am. J. Anat. *121*: 175–196 (1967).

Rhodin, J. A. G. and Reith, E. J. Ultrastructure of keratin in oral mucosa, skin, esophagus, claw and hair. *In*: Fundamentals of Keratinization (Eds. E. O. Butcher and R. F. Sognaes), pp. 61–94. AAAS, Publication No. 70, Washington, D.C., 1962.

STOMACH

Corpron, R. E. The ultrastructure of the gastric mucosa in normal and hypophysectomized rats. Am. J. Anat. *118*: 53–90 (1966).

Forssmann, W. G. and Orci, L. Ultrastructure and secretory cycle of the gastrin-producing cell. Z. Zellforsch. *101*: 419–432 (1969).

Forssmann, W. G., Orci, L., Pictet, R., Renold, A. E. and Rouiller, C. The endocrine cells in the epithelium of the gastrointestinal mucosa of the rat. An electron microscope study. J. Cell Biol. *40*: 692–715 (1969).

Hammond, J. B. and LaDeur, L. Fibrovesicular cells in the fundic glands of the canine stomach: evidence for a new cell type. Anat. Rec. *161*: 393–412 (1968).

Hayward, A. F. The ultrastructure of developing gastric parietal cells in the foetal rabbit. J. Anat. *101*: 69–81 (1967).

Hayward, A. F. The fine structure of gastric epithelial cells in the suckling rabbit with particular reference to the parietal cell. Z. Zellforsch. *78*: 474–483 (1967).

Helander, H. F. Ultrastructure of fundus glands of the mouse gastric mucosa. J. Ultrastruct. Res. *4*: 1–123 Suppl. (1962).

Helander, H. F. Ultrastructure of gastric fundus glands of refed mice. J. Ultrastruct. Res. *10*: 160–175 (1964).

Helander, H. F. Ultrastructure and function of gastric mucoid and zymogen cells in the rat during development. Gastroenterology *56*: 53–70 (1969).

Ito, S. Anatomic structure of the gastric mucosa. *In*: Handbook of Physiology, Alimentary Canal, Secretion (Eds. C. F. Code and W. Heidel). American Physiol. Soc., Washington, D.C. Sect. 6, *2*: 705–741 (1967).

Ito, S. and Winchester, R. J. The fine structure of the gastric mucosa in the bat. J. Cell Biol. *16*: 541–577 (1963).

Jacobson, E. D. The circulation of the stomach. Progress in Gastroenterology *48*: 85–109 (1965).

Johnson, F. R. and McMinn, R. M. H. Microscopic structure of pyloric epithelium of the cat. J. Anat. *107*: 67–86 (1970).

Lillibridge, C. B. The fine structure of normal human gastric mucosa. Gastroenterology *47*: 269–290 (1964).

Pfeiffer, C. J. Surface topology of the stomach in man and the laboratory ferret. J. Ultrastruct. Res. *33*: 252–262 (1970).

Rohrer, G. V., Scott, J. R., Joel, W. and Wolf, S. The fine structure of human gastric parietal cells. Am. J. Dig. Dis. *10*: 13–21 (1965).

Rubin, W. Enzyme cytochemistry of gastric parietal cells at a fine structure level. Cytochemical separation of the endoplasmic reticulum from the "tubulovesicles." J. Cell Biol. *42*: 332–338 (1969).

Rubin, W. Endocrine cells in the normal human stomach. A fine structural study. Gastroenterology *62*: 784–800 (1972).

Rubin, W., Ross, L. L., Sleisenger, M. H. and Jeffries, G. H. The normal human gastric epithelia. A fine structural study. Lab. Investig. *19*: 598–626 (1968).

Sedar, A. W. The fine structure of the oxyntic cell in relation to the functional activity of the stomach. Ann. N.Y. Acad. Sci. *99*: 9–29 (1962).

Sedar, A. W. Stomach and intestinal mucosa. *In*: Electron Microscopic Anatomy (Ed. S. M. Kurtz), pp. 123–148. Academic Press, New York, 1964.

Sedar, A. W. Fine structure of the stimulated oxyntic cell. Fed. Proc. *24*: 1360–1367 (1965).

Sedar, A. W. Electron microscopic demonstration of polysaccharides associated with acid-secreting cells of the stomach after "inert dehydration." J. Ultrastruct. Res. *28*: 112–124 (1969).

Sedar, A. W. and Friedman, M. H. F. Correlation of the fine structure of the gastric parietal cell (dog) with functional activity of the stomach. J. Biophys. Biochem. Cytol. *11*: 349–363 (1961).

29 Digestive system— intestines

Small Intestine

The small intestine is the longest part of the digestive tube, connecting the pylorus with the large intestine. Based on structural and topographical differences, the small intestine can be divided into a short segment, **duodenum,** 20 cm (11 inches) long; the **jejunum** which is about 275 cm (9 feet) long; and the **ileum,** measuring about 425 cm (14 feet) in length. Throughout the small intestine there is a continued digestion and a selective absorption of food. In the duodenum, the gastric chyme is mixed with the pancreatic and biliary secretions, and there is a passage of water and electrolytes in both directions across the wall. The main absorption of iron and calcium occurs here in addition to large quantities of sugars and amino acids. In the jejunum, small intestinal enzymes are added to the chyme, and here is the main site of homogenization and mixing of the chyme. The majority of sugars, amino acids, and fats are absorbed in the jejunum. In the ileum, additional digestive enzymes are added to the chyme, and absorption of vitamin B_{12}, bile acids and the remaining amino acids and fats takes place here.

The wall of the intestine is thick in the duodenum and thin in the jejunum and ileum. It is composed of four layers: **mucosa, submucosa, muscularis externa,** and **serosa.** The absorptive surface of the small intestine is increased greatly by two kinds of structures: 1) plicae circulares; and 2) villi intestinales.

The **plicae circulares** (valves of Kerckring) are mucosal and submucosal, permanent shelf-like folds, arranged circularly or spirally, extending to about two-thirds of the circumference. (Fig. 29-3) The plicae are absent in the proximal part of the duodenum and the distal part of the ileum. They are low and broad as they first appear in the duodenum and they become increasingly taller toward the middle of the jejunum and the proximal

part of the ileum where secondary and tertiary folds are also present. The plicae gradually decrease in height and complexity in the middle portion of the ileum.

The **villi intestinales** are finger-shaped structures which project about 0.5 mm above the surface level of the intestine. The villi are most numerous in the duodenum (Fig. 29-1), where they are broad and shaped like tongues or leaves. In the jejunum, they are shorter with a conical or rounded shape. (Fig. 29-1) In the ileum their shape is club-like. (Fig. 29-2) They are fewer than elsewhere and they become progressively lower and more scattered toward the distal part of the ileum. The villi are covered by a simple columnar epithelium, and they contain a core of highly cellular, loose connective tissue, the lamina propria of the mucosa. (Fig. 29-5) This core contains a rich network of blood capillaries forming loops which lie close to the basal surface of the intestinal epithelium. There is also a central lymphatic vessel, the lacteal, which starts at the tip of the villus as a blind, sac-like structure. Smooth muscle cells extend into the villus core from the muscularis mucosae. They are located along the sides of the lacteal.

Fig. 29-1. Duodenum. Cross section. Cat. L.M. X 8. **1.** Lumen. **2.** Mucosa. **3.** Brunner's glands in submucosa. **4.** Muscularis externa (exceptionally thick in cat). **5.** Plica circularis, obliquely cut. **6.** Villi intestinales. **7.** Pancreas. **8.** Pancreatic duct.

Fig. 29-2. Ileum. Cross section. Monkey. L.M. X 16. **1.** Lumen. **2.** Mucosa. **3.** Submucosa. **4.** Muscularis externa. **5.** Plicae circulares. **6.** Villi intestinales. **7.** Aggregated nodules (Peyer's patch).

Fig. 29-3. Jejunum. Longitudinal section. Human. L.M. X 18. **1.** Lumen. **2.** Villi intestinales. **3.** Submucosa. **4.** Muscularis externa (inner circular layer). **5.** Muscularis externa (outer longitudinal layer). **6.** Primary plicae circulares. **7.** Secondary fold. **8.** Tertiary fold.

Fig. 29-4. Jejunum. Cross section. Kitten. L.M. X 81. **1.** Lumen. **2.** Intestinal villus. **3.** Intestinal glands. **4.** Lamina propria. **5.** Muscularis mucosae. **6.** Submucosa. **7.** Muscularis externa.

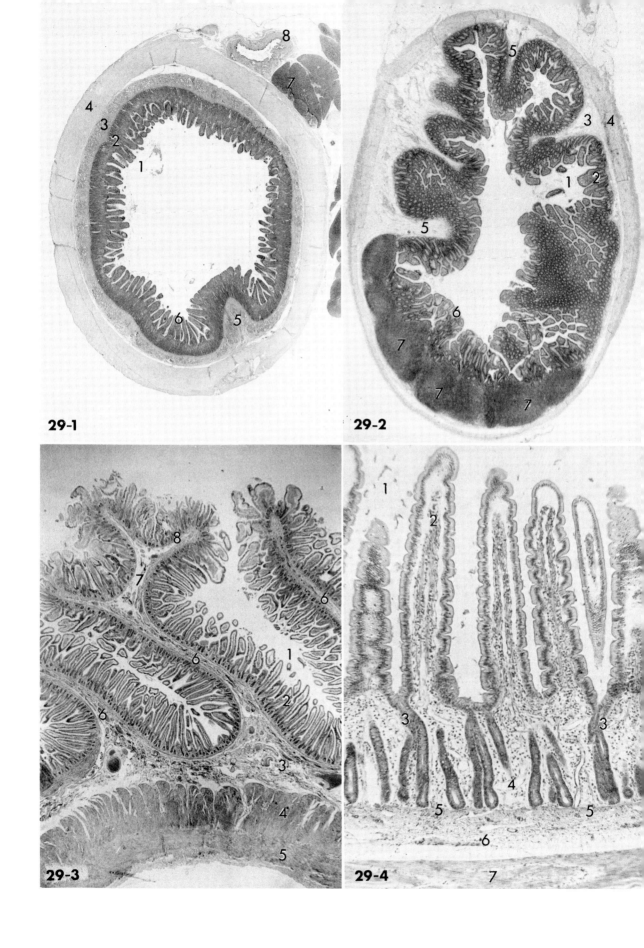

29-1

29-2

29-3

29-4

By contractions, these muscle cells aid in shortening and moving the villus back and forth, as well as in emptying the lacteal of its milky content, the chyle, which contains digested and absorbed fats.

MUCOUS MEMBRANE

The mucous membrane of the small intestine is characterized by several structures, all of which are peculiar to this long digestive tube: 1) intestinal villi; 2) intestinal glands; 3) lamina propria; 4) muscularis mucosae.

INTESTINAL VILLI

The villi are covered by a simple columnar **epithelium** which is composed of absorptive cells with scattered mucous cells (goblet cells) and occasional small lymphocytes en route through the epithelium. (Fig. 29-5) The **mucous cells** increase progressively in number in the small intestine with few in the duodenum and many in the ileum. They have the general structure described on p. 80. The mucous droplets are formed by the Golgi complex and accumulate in the apical part of the cell where they tend to coalesce and expand the cell to form the shape of a wine glass (goblet). The discharge of mucus occurs through a fusion of the membrane surrounding one or several mucous droplets with the goblet cell surface membrane. This is in contradistinction to the discharge of mucus from the surface epithelium of the stomach, where a diffusion process is believed to take place. Once the discharge by the intestinal goblet cell has occurred, the mucus synthesis may start again. The cell, therefore, goes through cycles of synthesis, accumulation, and dicharge. According to some authors, the goblet cells probably pass through only one secretory cycle under physiological conditions. Mucous cells are replaced but at a slower rate than absorptive cells. They move with the absorptive cells to the tip of the villus where they are continually shed. The discharged mucus represents an essential part of the intestinal

juice. It consists of glycoproteins and sulfated aminopolysaccharides. It protects the surface epithelium against abrasion by coarse intestinal material, lubricates the lumen, and helps to form the feces.

The **absorptive cells,** as well as the mucous cells, are separated from the core of the villus by a thin basal lamina. (Figs. 29-6, 29-8) The base of the cells rests on this basal lamina, and the apical parts of neighboring cells are held together by junctional complexes. The absorptive cells originate from undifferentiated cells in the intestinal glands and at the base of the villus. From here, they migrate up along the villus, continually replacing older cells which are being shed at the tip of the villus toward the end of their life span which is about 2–4 days. The intercellular space is wide near the base of the absorptive cells. It is believed that this route is used in passing water and electrolytes across the intestinal epithelium. The luminal surface of the absorptive cells is provided with numerous **microvilli,** about 2000 per cell, with an average height of $1\ \mu$ and a width of $0.1\ \mu$. (Figs. 29-7, 29-9) In man, the microvilli are increasingly taller along the villus, attaining their greatest length and number toward the tip of the villus. The microvillus contains a core of 40–50 straight, parallel, nonbranching **filaments.** (Fig. 29-10) The filaments penetrate about $0.5\ \mu$ into the api-

Fig. 29-5. Intestinal villus from duodenum. Tip region. Longitudinal section through the middle of the core. Rat. E.M. X 860.
1. Intestinal lumen. **2.** Nuclei of absorptive cells in the surface epithelium. **3.** Basal lamina. **4.** Mucous (goblet) cells.
5. Intercellular space. **6.** Nuclei of absorptive cells, apparently being shed into the intestinal lumen. **7.** Cross section of ateriole.
8. Blood capillaries. **9.** Postcapillary venules. **10.** Lymphatic capillary (lacteal). **11.** Smooth muscle cells. **12.** The core of the villus (lamina propria) is made up of loose connective tissue with a multitude of assorted cell elements. **13.** Lymphocytes en route through the surface epithelium.
14. Endocrine cell (argyrophil cell).

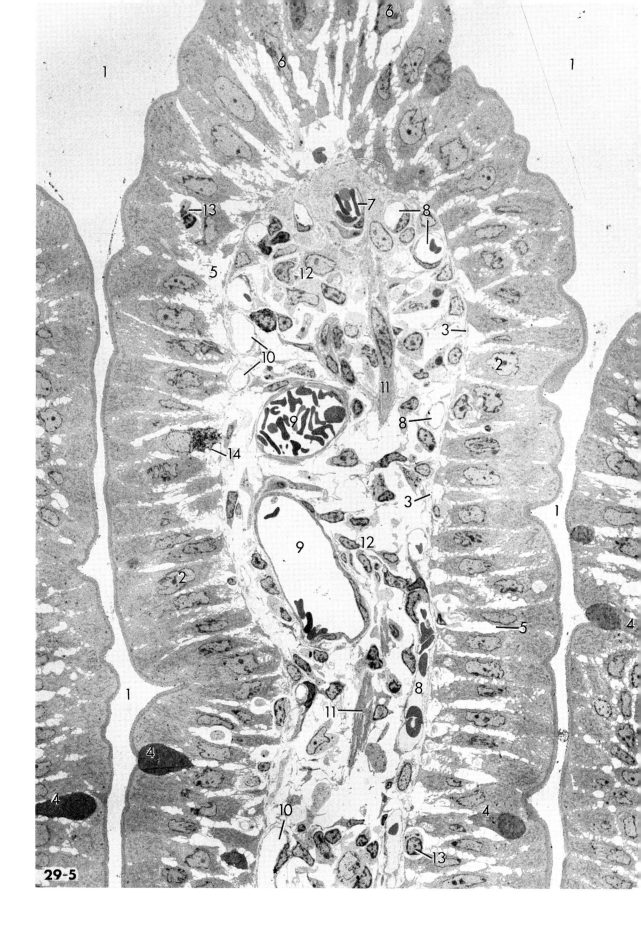

cal cytoplasm, where they form a **rootlet** which terminates abruptly at, and is embedded in, a finely fibrillar network, the **terminal web.** (Fig. 29-7) This is a 0.5 μ wide zone, parallel to the luminal surface and laterally connected to the cell membrane at the level of the apical junctional complex. The core of filaments, the rootlets and the terminal web probably function as stabilizers at the surface of the cell. The core of filaments may also aid in absorptive processes, either as a source of enzymes or as preferential guiding structures. There is no evidence in support of contractile properties as in ciliary microfilaments, although this cannot be ruled out entirely. Each microvillus is covered by a trilaminar cell membrane, 90 Å thick, the exterior surface of which is provided with thin, branching filaments oriented perpendicularly to the surface. They collectively form a layer called **glycocalyx** because of its presumed polysaccharide nature. This layer is difficult to preserve. Furthermore, it varies greatly in thickness, being of large dimensions on the tips of the microvilli, and of small dimensions between the villi where often it emerges as an embedding material for the microvilli, particularly as seen in a cross section of the microvilli. Between the bases of the microvilli are **pits,** shallow invaginations of the cell surface. Coated **vesicles** and membrane-bound canaliculi are also present beneath the bases of the villi. (Fig. 29-11) All of these structures are apparently involved in the process of absorption, dealing particularly with large molecular substances. **Mitochondria** are scattered throughout the absorptive cell, and may also occur in large numbers grouped beneath the nucleus. **Lysosomes** are present and generally become more numerous in the older cells near the tip of the villus. Granular and agranular **endoplasmic reticulum** and free **ribosomes** are present in limited number. A medium-sized **Golgi** complex is located near the nucleus on its luminal side.

Functional considerations. The surface epithelial cells are directly involved in the absorption of carbohydrates, proteins, and fats from the lumen of the small intestine. Although not fully understood, some of the processes are relatively well explored as they relate to the cell structures. **Carbohydrates** are absorbed mainly as monosaccharides. The microvilli contain enzymes which dephosphorylate and split disaccharides into monosaccharides, and it is possible that these enzymes reside in the cell membrane or in the core of the microvillus. If they are present in the cell membrane, the absorption of some carbohydrates involves enzymatic activity as they pass through the cell membrane. Once inside the cell, they may be passed on to the intercellular space, and from there reach the capillaries of the villi. **Proteins** are absorbed as amino acids or low mo-

Fig. 29-6. Surface epithelium of intestinal villus. Duodenum. Rat. E.M. X 1830. **1.** Intestinal lumen. **2.** Nuclei of absorptive cells. **3.** Basal part of mucous cell. **4.** Lymphocytes. **5.** Microvilli. **6.** Mitochondria. **7.** Intercellular space. **8.** Blood capillaries in lamina propria. **9.** Lymphatic capillary. **10.** Many cells in the connective tissue cannot be identified at this magnification.

Fig. 29-7. Enlargement of area similar to rectangle in Fig. 29-6. Duodenum. Rat. E.M. X 6000. **1.** Lumen. **2.** Microvilli. **3.** Rootlets in terminal web. **4.** Mitochondria. **5.** Granular endoplasmic reticulum. **6.** Lateral cell borders. **7.** Secondary lysosome.

Fig. 29-8. Detail of basal part of surface epithelium. Duodenum. Rat. E.M. X 4900. **1.** Base of absorptive cell with mitochondria. **2.** Intercellular space. **3.** Lymphocyte. **4.** Basal lamina. **5.** Thin collagenous fibrils. **6.** Blood capillary. **7.** Part of macrophage.

Fig. 29-9. Longitudinally sectioned microvilli of absorptive cells in duodenal intestinal villus. Rat. E.M. X 52,000. **1.** Lumen. **2.** Filaments in core of microvillus. **3.** Rootlets. **4.** Pits.

Fig. 29-10. Cross section of microvilli at level (A) in Fig. 29-9. Rat. X 86,000. **1.** Filaments in core of microvillus. **2.** Surface coat (glycocalyx). **3.** Trilaminar cell membrane.

Fig. 29-11. Cross section of rootlets at level (B) in Fig. 29-9. Rat. X 70,000. **1.** Rootlets. **2.** Pits. **3.** Coated vesicle.

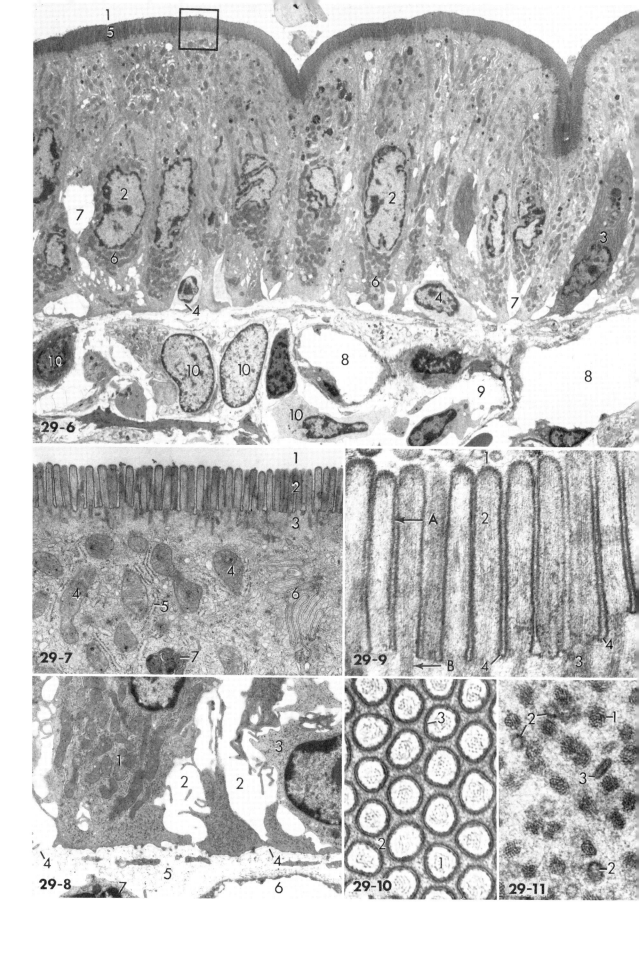

29-6

29-7

29-9

29-8

29-10

29-11

lecular weight peptides. It is known that pyridoxyl phosphate participates in transporting the amino acids across the intestinal absorptive cell, but little is known about routes used and structures involved. **Fats** are actively passed through the cell membrane in a molecular or micellar form, utilizing adenosine triphosphate for this energy-requiring process. In the intestinal lumen, first a process of emulsification occurs, which entails a combination of monoglycerides, free fatty acids, phospholipids, and bile salts to form water-soluble micelles which provide a large area for the enzyme activity required to pass the micelles through the cell membrane. Enzymes within the cell reassemble fatty acids and glycerol and coat the molecule with a lipoprotein which permits it to pass to the capillaries and the lacteals of the core of the intestinal villus. The structures involved in these processes are not known, but there are indications that in the absorption of some fats, the small surface invaginations, the coated vesicles, the agranular endoplasmic reticulum, and even the Golgi complex are used at one phase or another of the passage.

INTESTINAL GLANDS

The intestinal glands, or crypts of Lieberkühn, are short, simple tubular structures. (Fig. 29-12) They begin with pore-like openings between the bases of the villi, and their base extends to the muscularis mucosae. The glands are relatively long in the duodenum and become shorter in the jejunum and ileum. The glands appear to be concerned with the secretion of digestive enzymes and of some hormones. The glands are lined by: 1) undifferentiated cells; 2) absorptive cells; 3) Paneth cells; 4) mucous cells; and 5) endocrine cells.

The **undifferentiated cells** serve as a source of replacement for other cell types, both in the intestinal gland and on the villi. Mitotic figures are numerous in the crypts as a result of a rapid multiplication of undifferentiated cells. During mitosis,

the cell is drawn up from the basal lamina, and the plane of division is at right angles to the long axis of the cell. After mitosis the daughter cells acquire characteristics which make it possible to classify them as **absorptive cells.** These cells are similar to those covering the villi, with the exception that the absorptive cells in the crypts are narrower and have a minimum of cytoplasmic organelles as well as short and few microvilli. (Fig. 29-13) The **Paneth cells** are generally located near the base of the intestinal glands. They occur throughout the small intestine but are missing in the large intestine. They occur in man, rat, and mouse, but are absent in dog and cat. Paneth cells constitute a stable cell population with a longer life span than undifferentiated cells and mucous cells in the crypts. The Paneth cell has a pyramidal shape with the base resting against the basal lamina of the intestinal gland. (Fig. 29-14) The ultrastructural architecture is characteristic of cells engaged in exocrine secretion. The basal

Fig. 29-12. Survey of the deep part of the intestinal wall. Jejunum. Rat. E.M. X 580. **1.** Lumen of intestinal gland. **2.** Lamina propria. **3.** Muscularis mucosae. **4.** Ascending smooth muscle cells. **5.** Blood capillaries. **6.** Lymph vessels. **7.** Submucosa. **8.** Ganglion cell (plexus of Meissner). **9.** Connective tissue cells. **10.** *Asterisks:* mitoses among undifferentiated cells in glandular epithelium.

Fig. 29-13. Enlargement of area similar to rectangle (A) in Fig. 29-12. Rat. X 4800. **1.** Nuclei of undifferentiated cells. **2.** Nucleus of apparent absorptive cell. **3.** Mucous cells. **4.** Lumen. **5.** Basal lamina.

Fig. 29-14. Enlargement of area similar to rectangle (B) in Fig. 29-12. Rat. E.M. X 4800. **1.** Nucleus of Paneth cell. **2.** Presecretory granules. **3.** Mature secretory granules. **4.** Microvilli. **5.** Lumen. **6.** Paneth precursor cells. **7.** Smooth muscle cells of muscularis mucosae.

Fig. 29-15. Detail of Paneth cell. Jejunum. Rat. X 26,000. **1.** Granular endoplasmic reticulum. **2.** Vesicular (small) Golgi complex. **3.** Vacuole. **4.** Presecretory granule. **5.** Maturing secretory granules with distinct boundary membrane and dense core.

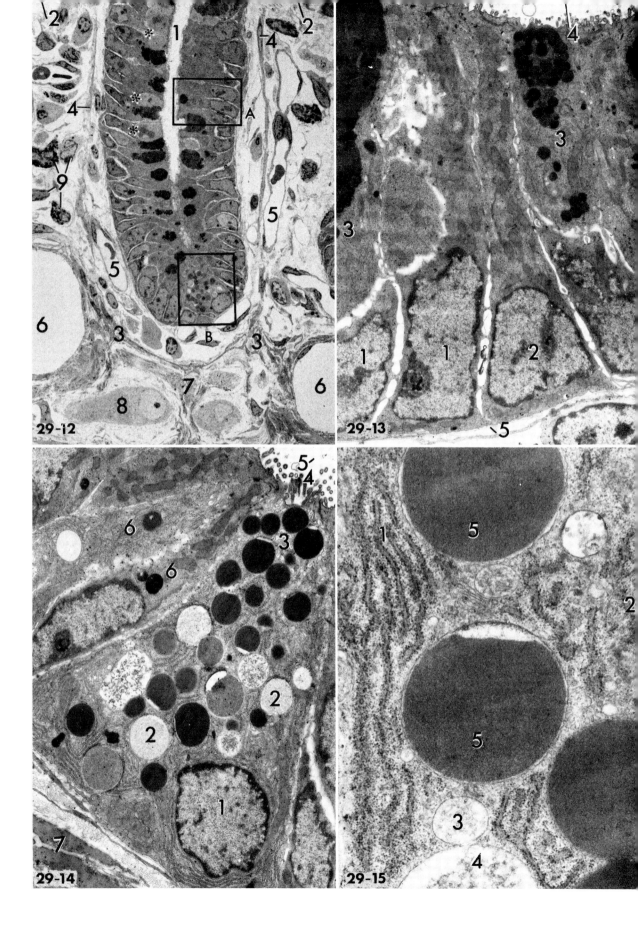

part of the cell contains numerous profiles of granular endoplasmic reticulum. The Golgi complex above the nucleus is large, and the apical part of the cell is occupied by large secretory granules. The presecretory granules emerge from the Golgi complex as membrane-bound clear vacuoles. They gradually acquire a dense core (Fig. 29-15) which is discharged at the luminal cell surface when the secretory granules reach the end stage of their maturation. The discharge occurs through a fusion of the granule membrane with the luminal cell membrane. The cells are also rich in free ribosomes and lysosomes but mitochondria are scarce. From a functional point of view, it is assumed that the Paneth cells secrete peptidases which are required for the splitting of various peptides into absorbable amino acids, since a high content of dipeptidase can be demonstrated in the deepest part of the intestinal mucosa. Furthermore, zinc has been demonstrated histochemically in the Paneth cells, and it is considered that zinc functions as a specific activator for peptidases and is also an essential component of other enzymes. However, many peptidases seem to be derived from the surface epithelial cells of the intestinal villi, and the function of the Paneth cell as the only source of intestinal peptidases is therefore questioned. Another enzyme formed by the intestinal glands, but of unknown cellular origin, is **lipase,** which acts on fats. The **mucous cells** of the intestinal glands are cylindrical or barrel-shaped (Fig. 29-12) and generally do not acquire the extreme goblet shape of the mucous cells on the intestinal villi.

However, intermediate stages between undifferentiated cells and the mucous cells do occur in the intestinal crypts. The undifferentiated mucous cell is ultrastructurally similar to that of the columnar absorptive cells except that the mucous precursor cell has a distinctly larger Golgi complex. It is assumed that most intestinal mucous cells originate from the intestinal crypts and that they migrate up

on the villi to be shed at the tip of the villus toward the end of their four-day life span. Some authors claim that mucous cells and absorptive cells are mutually interconvertible, or that mucous cells may go into resting periods during which they resemble absorptive cells. There is no recent evidence in support of this hypothesis.

Endocrine cells are present in the intestinal glands as well as on the villi. As described in connection with the gastric glands (p. 546), two kinds of endocrine cells can be identified on the basis of their differences in affinity for chrome and silver stains: enterochromaffin (argentaffin) and argyrophil cells. The human intestine contains twice as many argyrophil cells as enterochromaffin. Based on ultrastructural differences, it has recently been suggested that there are perhaps as many as five different endocrine cells throughout the gas-

Fig. 29-16. Detail of intestinal crypt. Jejunum. Rat. E.M. X 17,000. **1.** Nucleus of endocrine cell (type I). **2.** Nucleus of undifferentiated cell. **3.** Undifferentiated cell in mitosis. **4.** Basal lamina. **5.** Secretory granules.

Fig. 29-17. Enlargement of area similar to rectangle in Fig. 29-16. Endocrine cell (type I). Jejunum. Rat. E.M. X 48,000. **1.** Mitochondria. **2.** Ribosomes. **3.** Cell membrane. **4.** Pinocytotic invagination. **5.** Oval and irregularly shaped secretory granules with tightly fitted boundary membrane and ⸗ highly electron-dense core. Based on the appearance of the secretory granules, this cell is referred to as type I, and it is suggested that the secretory granules contain serotonin (5-hydroxytryptamine) or its precursor.

Fig. 29-18. Detail of gastric gland proper. Stomach. Rat. E.M. X 18,000. **1.** Nucleus of endocrine cell (type IV). **2.** Cytoplasm of neighboring chief cell. **3.** Mitochondria. **4.** Granular endoplasmic reticulum.

Fig. 29-19. Enlargement of area similar to rectangle in Fig. 29-18. Endocrine cell (type IV). Stomach. Rat. E.M. X 93,000. **1.** Ribosomes. **2.** Granule boundary membrane. **3.** Core of spherical secretory granule. Based on the appearance of the secretory granules, this cell is referred to as type IV, and it is suggested that the secretory granules contain noradrenaline or its precursor.

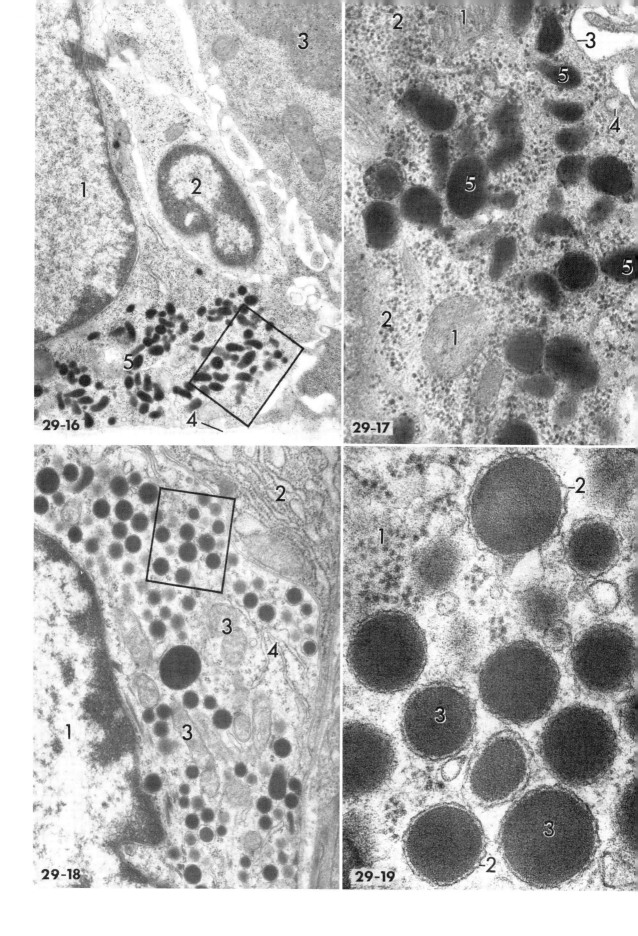

trointestinal mucosa. Of these, only one cell type has been identified solely in the gastric mucosa, referred to here as **type V cell** or the **gastrin cell,** since it is assumed to be concerned with the synthesis and release of the hormone gastrin. The intestinal endocrine cells are either pyramidal or rounded, lodged between the deep portions of the surrounding epithelial cells. Some have a thin apical prolongation reaching the lumen of the intestinal gland. These bottle-shaped cells are provided with microvilli on their free surface. The classification of the intestinal endocrine cells into at least four cell types is based on the number and ultrastructural characteristics of the secretory granules. The cells are generally well filled with small, round or oval, membrane-bound granules with great variation in electron density of their core substance. There is presently no general agreement as to the identification of specific cell types and the assignment of specific functions to the various cells. However, there are indications that the most common, **type I cell,** with large oval granules (Fig. 29-16), may produce **serotonin** (5-hydroxytryptamine) which stimulates the contraction of smooth muscle cells. **Type II** and **type III cells** may represent the same cell type at different functional stages. Based on the ultrastructural similarity between their granules and those of the pancreatic islet cells, type A and B, it has been suggested that they may produce either a glucagon-like hormone or **secretin,** the latter stimulating the exocrine pancreas to secrete a watery juice, high in bicarbonates but poor in enzymes. The **type IV cell** contains granules with a small, dense core and a loosely fitted boundary membrane. (Fig. 29-18) Because of their ultrastructural resemblance to the cells of the adrenal medulla, these cells are believed to contain catecholamines, probably **noradrenaline.** The origin of the hormone cholecystokinin which acts to induce the flow of bile, is not known, and could very well be secreted by one or the other of the

four cell types. Obviously, extensive experimental investigations are required to verify these hypotheses and to answer other questions related to the endocrine cells of the gastrointestinal mucosa. Consult the review by Dawson for further information.

LAMINA PROPRIA AND
LYMPHATIC TISSUE

The lamina propria of the intestinal mucosa is far more extensive and cellular than the lamina propria of the stomach. It is a loose connective tissue which forms the core of the intestinal villi and surrounds the intestinal glands. (Fig. 29-22) Fibroblasts and macrophages, as well as reticular and collagenous fibrils, make up the framework, in the meshes of which occur a variety of the cells which are typical of those found in loose connective tissue as described on p. 162. However, since many

Fig. 29-20. Diffuse lymphocyte aggregation. Jejunum. Cat. L.M. X 60. **1.** Intestinal lumen. **2.** Intestinal villi with normal amount of scattered lymphocytes in the lamina propria. **3.** Villus with diffuse lymphocyte aggregation. **4.** Intestinal glands. **5.** Muscularis mucosae. **6.** Lymphocyte aggregation obliterating intestinal glands and muscularis mucosae.

Fig. 29-21. Solitary lymphatic nodule. Appendix. Human. L.M. X 120. **1.** Lumen. **2.** Intestinal gland. **3.** Germinal center. **4.** Muscularis mucosae is obliterated.

Fig. 29-22. Survey of longitudinal section of intestinal villus. Area similar to rectangle in Fig. 29-20. Jejunum. Rat. E.M. X 640. This demonstrates the general architecture of loose connective tissue in the intestinal lamina propria. Identification of specific cell types is difficult at this magnification but is greatly aided by the use of a hand lens. **1.** Surface epithelium. **2.** Loops of blood capillaries. **3.** Central lacteal. **4.** Smooth muscle cells. **5.** Plasma cells.

Fig. 29-23. Enlargement of area similar to rectangle in Fig. 29-22. Core of intestinal villus. Jejunum. Rat. E.M. X 4700. **1.** Nuclei of capillary endothelial cells. **2.** Nuclei of fibroblasts. **3.** Nuclei of macrophages. **4.** Phagocytosed lymphocyte. **5.** Eosinophil leukocytes. **6.** Mast cell nucleus. **7.** Dividing lymphocyte.

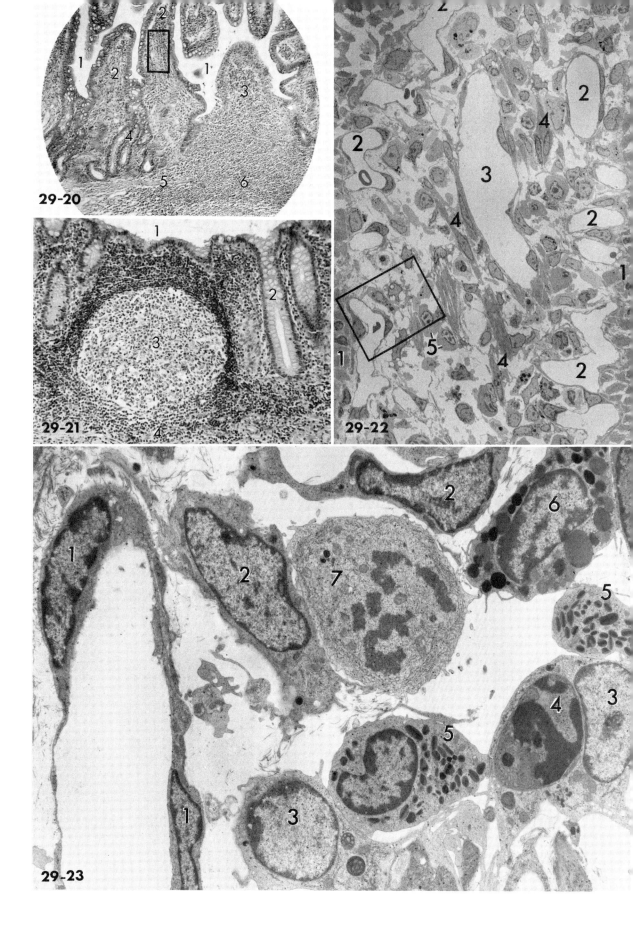

29-20

29-21

29-22

29-23

more lymphoid elements are present in the intestinal lamina propria than in the loose connective tissue in other regions of the body, it is appropriate to consider the intestinal lamina propria as a potential site for accumulation of lymphoid elements in response to the immunological challenge represented by the invasion of many foreign proteins (antigens) either as a result of normal absorptive processes or the invasion of bacteria and viruses. The accumulation of lymphoid elements in the intestinal lamina propria may assume several structural forms: 1) scattered lymphocytes throughout the lamina propria; 2) diffuse lymphocyte aggregation; 3) lymphatic solitary and aggregated nodules.

Scattered lymphocytes are common throughout the lamina propria, and they also invade the epithelium. Plasma cells, mast cells, as well as eosinophil and basophil leukocytes are equally common. Mitotic divisions often occur among the lymphocytes, probably in response to the invasion of foreign proteins. Gradually, through cell multiplication and tissue invasion of cells from the vascular system, a **diffuse lymphocyte aggregation** takes place (Fig. 29-20), leading to a situation where small and medium-size lymphocytes dominate over other cell types. (Fig. 29-23) If the lymphocytes of the diffuse tissue aggregations become mitotically very active, and if large lymphocytes also appear, this results in the appearance of a **solitary lymphatic nodule**, indicated by the presence of a germinal center. (Fig. 29-21) Further activity by this tissue leads to the accumulation of several nodules (Fig. 29-2) into **aggregated nodules** (Peyer's patches). Both solitary and aggregated nodules may invade the submucosa; and intestinal glands as well as villi may be obliterated in the region about a Peyer's patch. The nodules become progressively more abundant distally in the small intestine, and Peyer's patches are located chiefly in the lower ileum where as many as 20–30 may be present.

MUSCULARIS MUCOSAE

The muscularis mucosae consists of two thin layers of smooth muscle cells which, at times, may be arranged in an outer longitudinal and an inner circular layer. Other smooth muscle cells ascend from these layers into the core of the villus. Contractions of these muscle cells aid in emptying the intestinal glands.

SUBMUCOSA

The submucosa forms the core of the permanent plicae circulares. It consists of irregular, rather dense connective tissue in which nerves, blood vessels, and lymphatic vessels travel. In the duodenum, the submucosa is occupied by the **duodenal glands** (Brunner's glands). These are branched, tubular coiled glands which open up into the intestinal glands through short ducts penetrating the muscularis mucosae. (Fig. 29-24) Brunner's glands are less frequent in the distal third of the duodenum and may not be present at the distal end. At times they may continue

Fig. 29-24. Duodenum. Cross section. Monkey. L.M. X 94. **1.** Intestinal lumen. **2.** Intestinal villi. **3.** Intestinal glands. **4.** Muscularis mucosae. **5.** Submucosa with duodenal (Brunner's) glands. **6.** Muscularis externa (inner circular layer). **7.** Muscularis externa (outer longitudinal layer).

Fig. 29-25. Enlargement of area similar to rectangle in Fig. 29-24. Duodenum. Rat. E.M. X 600. **1.** Lumen of duodenal (Brunner's) gland. **2.** Cross-sectioned excretory duct of Brunner's gland. **3.** Thin strands of muscularis mucosae. **4.** Lamina propria. **5.** Connective tissue of submucosa. **6.** Blood capillaries. **7.** Lymphatic capillaries. **8.** Muscularis externa.

Fig. 29-26. Enlargement of area similar to rectangle in Fig. 29-25. Duodenum. Rat. E.M. X 5000. **1.** Nuclei of secretory cells of Brunner's gland. **2.** Basal lamina. **3.** Lumen of gland. **4.** Apical accumulation of secretory droplets.

Fig. 29-27. Enlargement of secretory cells of Brunner's gland. Duodenum. Rat. E.M. X 40,000. **1.** Lumen of gland. **2.** Granular endoplasmic reticulum and free ribosomes. **3.** Golgi complexes. **4.** Mitochondria. **5.** Lysosome. **6.** Secretory droplets (their boundary membrane is poorly defined).

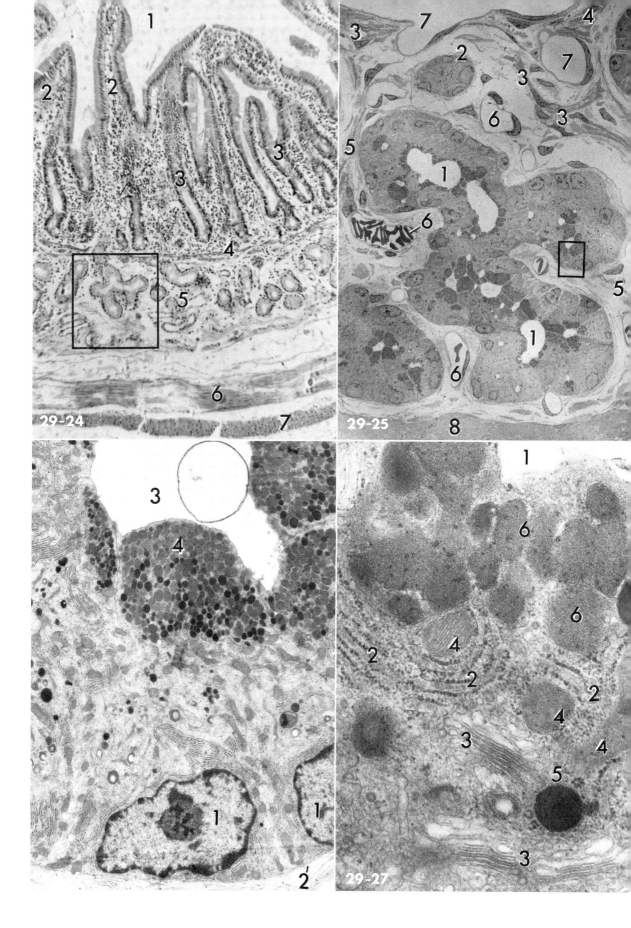

29-24

29-25

29-27

into the jejunum, and occasionally they are totally absent throughout. The secretory end pieces and the ducts are lined with a simple columnar epithelium. The secretory cells have a structure similar to that of the pyloric glands with a rich granular endoplasmic reticulum, a large Golgi complex, and numerous secretory droplets in the apical part of the cell. (Fig. 29-26) The fine structure of the secretory droplets varies greatly with the species. (Fig. 29-27) In humans they display the structure of mucous droplets, whereas in the cat they have a structure similar to both mucous and serous secretory granules. It is generally accepted that the duodenal (Brunner's) glands secrete a **mucus,** the function of which is to protect the intestinal epithelium against pancreatic enzymes and erosion by the gastric juice through the high bicarbonate content of the mucus. The secretion probably also contains a **proteolytic enzyme** which is activated by gastric hydrochloric acid, as well as **enterokinase** which activates the pancreatic trypsinogen to trypsin. However, the function or functions of the duodenal glands are by no means solved.

The submucosa in the mid-duodenum is perforated by the bile duct and the pancreatic duct which end at an orifice at the summit of the **duodenal papilla.** The muscularis mucosae reinforces the sphincter muscle which surrounds the end piece of the two ducts.

MUSCULARIS EXTERNA

The muscularis externa is composed of two complete, distinctly separate layers of long, slender, spindle-shaped, smooth muscle cells: 1) inner circular layer; 2) outer longitudinal layer. There is little connective tissue separating the individual cells, except for a thin external (basal) lamina which invests each smooth muscle cell.

SEROSA

A serosa completely surrounds all parts of the small intestine, except for a minor part of the duodenum. It consists of a squamous mesothelium and submesothe-lial connective tissue. It is described further on p. 576 in connection with the mesentery.

Large Intestine

The large intestine connects the ileum with the anus. It has a length of about 180 cm (5 feet), a width larger than the small intestine, and is divided into several, structurally different parts: **colon, appendix, rectum,** and the **anal canal.** In the proximal part of the large intestine, water and electrolytes are absorbed from the chyme. Fecal matter is temporarily stored in a continuous process of eliminating non-usable substances. A great deal of decomposition by bacterial action takes place in the large intestine, and a

Fig. 29-28. Cross section of colon. Cat. L.M. X 3. **1.** Lumen. **2.** Mucous membrane. **3.** Muscularis externa. **4.** Teniae coli. **5.** Solitary lymphatic nodules.

Fig. 29-29. Enlargement of area similar to rectangle in Fig. 29-28. Colon. Cat. L.M. X 36. **1.** Lumen. **2.** Mucous membrane. **3.** Submucosa. **4.** Muscularis externa, circular layer. **5.** Muscularis externa: one band (tenia coli) of longitudinal fibers. **6.** Solitary lymphatic nodule.

Fig. 29-30. Enlargement of area similar to rectangle in Fig. 29-29. Colon. Monkey. L.M. X 148. **1.** Lumen. **2.** Surface epithelium. **3.** Intestinal glands (crypts of Lieberkühn). **4.** Lamina propria. **5.** Muscularis mucosae.

Fig. 29-31. Survey of two intestinal glands. Colon. Rat. E.M. X 660. **1.** Lumen. **2.** Surface epithelium. **3.** Entrance to lumen of intestinal gland. **4.** Lamina propria. **5.** Venule.

Fig. 29-32. Enlargement of area similar to rectangle (A) in Fig. 29-31. Colon. Rat. E.M. X 4900. **1.** Lumen. **2.** Columnar absorptive cells. **3.** Mucous (goblet) cell. **4.** Microvilli. **5.** Intercellular space. **6.** Base of absorptive cells. **7.** Basal lamina.

Fig. 29-33. Enlargement of area similar to rectangle (B) in Fig. 29-31. Apical part of columnar cell in intestinal gland. Colon. Rat. E.M. X 28,000. **1.** Lumen. **2.** Microvilli. **3.** Secretory granules.

Fig. 29-34. Enlargement of rectangle in Fig. 29-32. Colon. Rat. E.M. X 74,000. **1.** Microvilli with central core of filaments. **2.** Rootlets. **3.** Surface coat (glycocalyx).

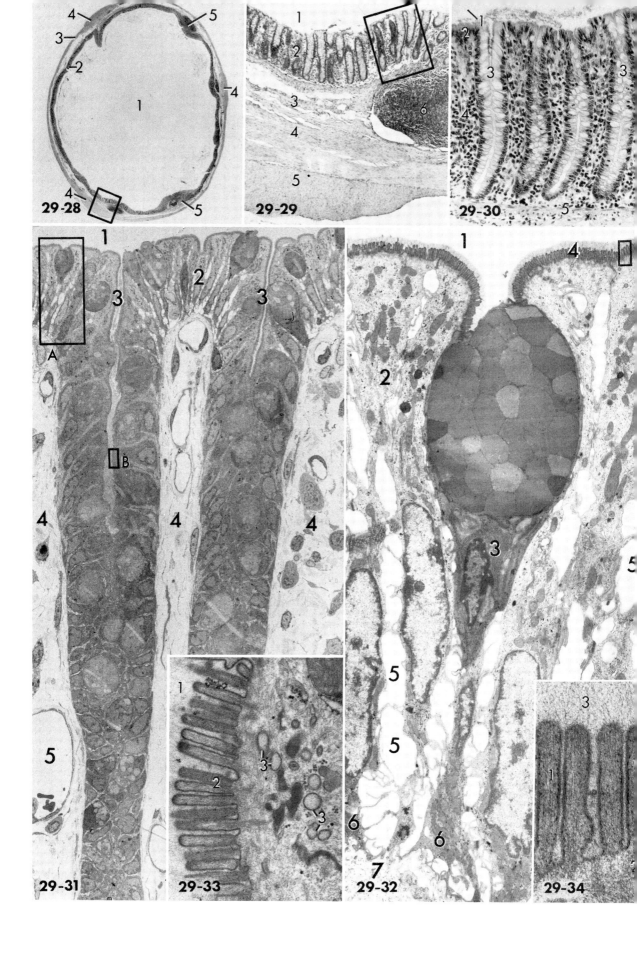

29-28

29-29

29-30

29-31

29-33

29-32

29-34

considerable amount of mucus is added as a protective lubricant. The architecture of the wall of the large intestine varies according to location, but the four principal layers of the digestive tube are retained throughout: 1) mucosa; 2) submucosa; 3) muscularis externa; and 4) serosa.

Mucosal plicae occur only in the rectum. In the colon there is a succession of transverse folds, **plicae semilunares,** formed by the entire thickness of the intestinal wall, giving rise to bulges between the folds, the **haustrae coli.** These folds are not permanent, since they are caused by local contractions of the inner circular layer of the muscularis externa. The outer part of the muscularis externa is concentrated in three evenly spaced longitudinal bands, the **teniae coli.** (Fig. 29-28) There are **no** villi in the large intestine, except in the fetus, but **intestinal glands** (crypts of Lieberkühn) occur throughout.

Colon

This part of the large intestine is subdivided into: 1) cecum; 2) ascending colon; 3) transverse colon; 4) descending colon; and 5) sigmoid colon. All parts have the same general structure. Peculiar to the colon are the teniae coli, the semilunar folds, the haustrae coli, and the **appendices epiploicae,** the last being short, serosal processes containing fat tissue.

LAMINA MUCOSAE

The mucous membrane has a smooth surface which lacks villi. It is covered by a simple columnar **surface epithelium,** composed of **absorptive** and **mucous cells** of the same ultrastructural architecture as that in the small intestine. (Fig. 29-32) The **intestinal glands** (crypts of Lieberkühn) dip directly in from the luminal surface of the colon as straight, densely packed, non-branching tubules. (Fig. 29-30) The intestinal glands are lined mostly by mucous cells, some columnar epithelial

cells, **undifferentiated cells,** and **endocrine cells.** The apical cytoplasm of the columnar cells contains a large number of small granules, probably secretory in nature (Fig. 29-33), which apparently discharge their core at the cell surface. It has been suggested that, based on histochemical, immunohistochemical, and ultrastructural methods of investigation, the granules contain immunoglobulins, and that they probably participate in the elaboration of the immunoglobulin-containing surface coat (glycocalyx) as part of an intestinal defense mechanism. The lamina propria is similar to that of the small intestine. Diffuse lymphocyte aggregation and scattered, solitary lymphatic nodules are numerous. The **muscularis mucosae** is well developed and usually has two layers: an inner circular and an outer longitudinal. The **submucosa** is composed of irregular

Fig. 29-35. Cross section of appendix. Human. L.M. X 9. **1.** Lumen. **2.** Lamina mucosae. **3.** Submucosa. **4.** Muscularis externa. **5.** Serosa. **6.** Mesoappendix.

Fig. 29-36. Cross section of appendix. Human. L.M. X 35. **1.** Lumen. **2.** Intestinal glands. **3.** Lymphatic nodule. **4.** Submucosa.

Fig. 29-37. Longitudinal section of rectum and anal canal. Monkey. L.M. X 7. **1.** Lumen of rectum proper. **2.** Anal canal. **3.** Anus (cutaneous zone of anal canal). **4.** Plicae transversales. **5.** Lymphatic nodules in submucosa. **6.** Muscularis externa. **7.** Inner anal sphincter (smooth muscle). **8.** Outer anal sphincter (striated muscle).

Fig. 29-38. Enlargement of part of Fig. 29-37. Monkey. L.M. × 23. **1.** Mucosa. **2.** Lymphatic follicles. **3.** These folds correspond to the anal valves in human. **4.** Intermediate zone of anal canal. **5.** Cutaneous zone of anal canal. **6.** Inner sphincter muscle. **7.** Outer sphincter muscle.

Fig. 29-39. Rectal lamina mucosae. Enlargement of area similar to rectangle. (A) in Fig. 29-38. Monkey. L.M. X 148. **1.** Lumen. **2.** Columnar surface epithelium. **3.** Intestinal gland. **4.** Lamina propria. **5.** Muscularis mucosae.

Fig. 29-40. Enlargement of rectangle (B) in Fig. 29-38. L.M. × 40. **1.** Lumen. **2.** Columnar surface epithelium. **3.** Stratified cuboidal epithelium. **4.** Subepithelial connective tissue.

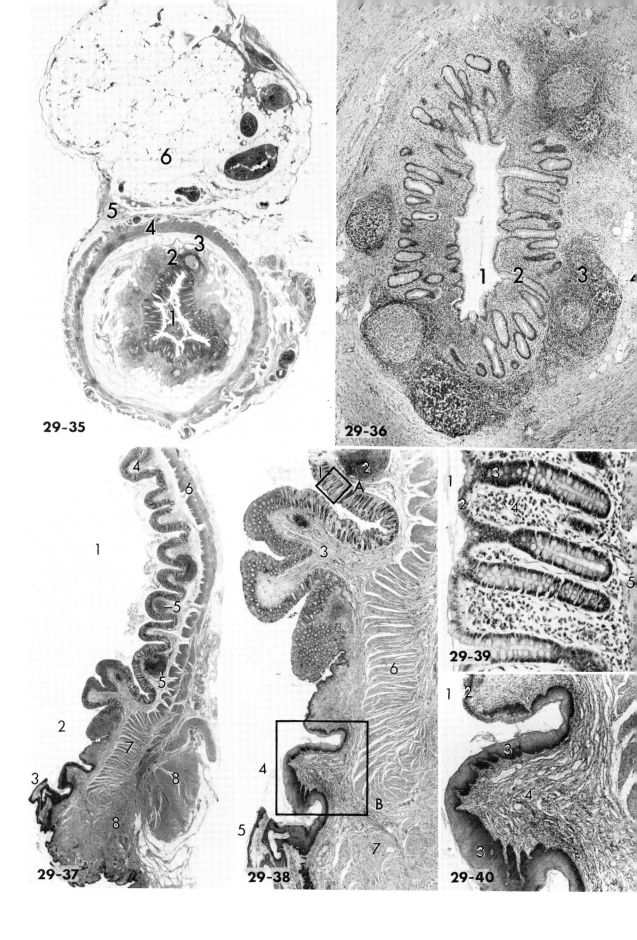

29-35

29-36

29-37

29-38

29-39

29-40

connective tissue, nerves, and blood vessels. It does not contain special glands, but at times, large fat accumulations. The **muscularis externa** has a thick, continuous inner layer of circular smooth muscle fibers, whereas the outer layer is concentrated in three longitudinal bands, the teniae coli. The **serosa** is similar to that of the small intestine, except for the large accumulations of fat tissue, the appendices epiploicae.

Appendix

The appendix, or vermiform process, is a narrow intestinal rudiment, extending from the first part of the colon, the cecum. The wall of the appendix is rather thick. (Fig. 29-35) It contains the four major tunics of the digestive tube, but the lumen is narrow and there is a predominance of lymphoid tissue. The **mucous membrane** is similar to that of the large intestine. Villi are missing, and the intestinal glands are embedded in a **lamina propria** extremely rich in diffusely scattered lymphoid elements and solitary nodules. (Fig. 29-36) The surface epithelium and the intestinal glands are lined mostly by mucous (goblet) cells, some absorptive cells and occasional Paneth cells at the bottom of the glands. Endocrine cells are regularly present in large numbers. The **muscularis mucosae** is thin. The **submucosa** is thick with fat cells, nerves, and blood vessels embedded in a loose connective tissue. The **muscularis externa** has two complete muscle layers, similar to the situation in the small intestine. The serosa surrounds and affixes the appendix by a fold of the mesentery, the meso-appendix.

Rectum

The rectum can be divided into an upper part, rectum proper, and a lower part, the anal canal. In the rectum proper, the

mucous membrane, the submucosa, and some circular fibers of the muscularis externa are thrown into several transversal folds, **plicae transversales,** extending partly around the rectum. (Fig. 29-37) Numerous intestinal glands are present in the mucous membrane, and there is a fair number of solitary lymphatic nodules. The muscularis externa has two complete layers, an inner circular and an outer longitudinal.

Anal Canal

The anal canal can be divided into three parts: 1) zona columnaris; 2) zona intermedia; and 3) zona cutanea. The mucous membrane makes several longitudinal folds, **rectal columns,** in the zona columnaris of the anal canal. These unite in the zona intermedia to form a few transverse, semilunar folds, the **anal valves.** The surface epithelium of the columnar zone is stratified cuboidal. Intestinal glands are not present, but **circumanal glands** occur in the cutaneous area. These are modified

Fig. 29-41. Survey of peripheral segment of intestinal wall. Cross section. Jejunum. Rat. E.M. X 600. **1.** Base of intestinal glands. **2.** Lamina propria. **3.** Muscularis mucosae. **4.** Submucosa. **5.** Muscularis externa: inner circular layer. **6.** Muscularis externa: outer longitudinal layer. **7.** Serosa with mesothelium. **8.** Peritoneal cavity. **9.** Ganglion cells of myenteric (Auerbach's) nerve plexus. **10.** Ganglion cell of submucous (Meissner's) nerve plexus. **11.** Arteriole. **12.** Venule. **13.** Lymphatic vessel. **14.** Blood capillaries.
Fig. 29-42. Detail of submucosa. Jejunum. Rat. E.M. X 1800. **1.** Chain of cross-sectioned smooth muscle cells in the muscularis mucosae. **2.** Collagenous bundles in the submucosa. **3.** Fibroblasts. **4.** Ganglion nerve cell in Meissner's plexus. **5.** Plasma cell. **6.** Macrophage. **7.** Lymphocyte in lymphatic capillary (lacteal). **8.** Lumen of arteriole; diameter 30 μ. **9.** Nucleus of endothelial cell. **10.** Nucleus of smooth muscle cells. **11.** Non-myelinated, sympathetic and parasympathetic, nerve fibers. **12.** Schwann cell nucleus.

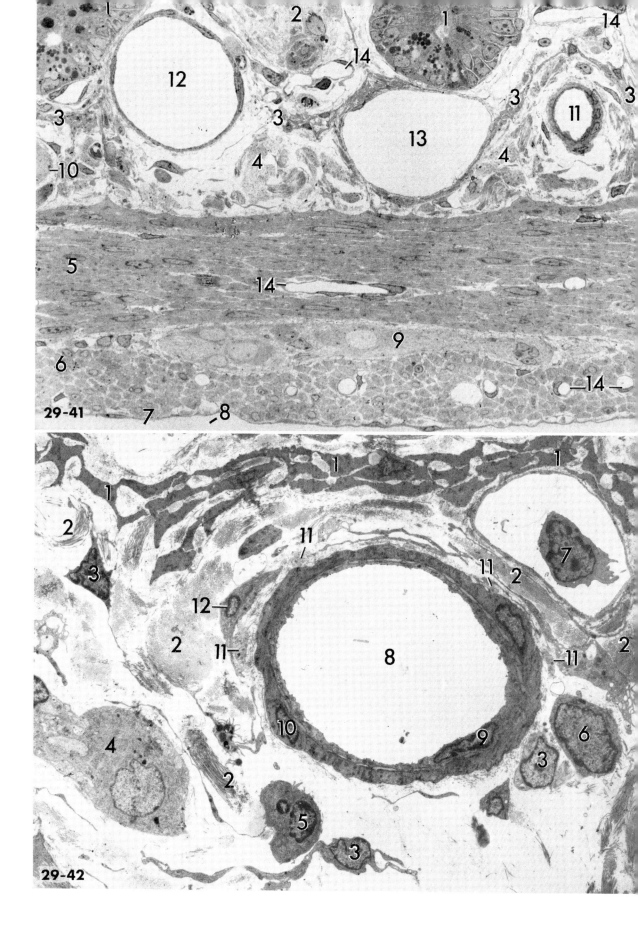

29-41

29-42

skin glands, reminiscent of apocrine sweat glands and sebaceous glands. The surface epithelium is stratified squamous, non-keratinized in the intermediate zone of the anal canal (Fig. 29-40), and keratinized in the cutaneous zone. Dilated veins are present in the lamina propria of the rectal columns. These may give rise to hemorrhoids. The inner circular layer of the muscularis externa terminates around the anus where it is enlarged to form the **inner anal sphincter** which is composed of smooth muscle cells. An external anal sphincter also exists, but it is made up of striated muscle cells.

NERVES OF THE INTESTINES

Sympathetic nerve fibers from the superior mesenteric plexus join with **parasympathetic** prolongations of the vagus nerve to form branches which travel through the mesentery into the serosa of the small and large intestines. The sympathetic nerve fibers are postganglionic, originating from paravertebral and prevertebral ganglia. The parasympathetic nerve fibers are preganglionic and synapse with ganglion nerve cells in the wall of the intestine. These ganglia are located between the circular and longitudinal layers of the muscularis externa, and in the submucosa. (Fig. 29-41) The nerves and the ganglia form an interconnected **myenteric plexus** (Auerbach's) within the muscularis externa, and a **submucous plexus** (Meissner's) in the submucosa. (Fig. 29-42) There are multiple connections between the two plexuses. Branches from the plexuses supply the smooth muscle cells of the intestinal wall, the vasculature, and the cells of the intestinal villi and the intestinal glands. Afferent, sensory nerve fibers travel from the intestinal wall to the spinal cord together with the efferent nerves. **Stimulation** of the **parasympathetic** nerve fibers causes a contraction of the musculature, initiates secretion, and dilates the blood vessels. Stimulation of the **sympathetic** nerve fibers inhibits contraction of intestinal musculature, inhibits

secretion, and constricts the blood vessels to the intestine. In general terms, higher centers control the motility of and the secretion within the intestines through **extrinsic reflexes** via sympathetic and parasympathetic nerves. Intrinsic reflexes play a major role in the mixing and transport of the chyme. Some of the more important are the **myenteric** and the **peristaltic reflexes** which function through local stretching of the smooth muscle cells, and the coordination of relaxation and contraction by the intrinsic nerve plexuses.

BLOOD VESSELS AND LYMPHATICS

Blood vessels. Branches of the mesenteric **arteries** approach the intestines

Fig. 29-43. Mesentery of the large intestine. Rat. L.M. X 64. **1.** Intestinal mucosa. **2.** Muscularis externa. **3.** Core of mesentery. **4.** Peritoneal cavity. **5.** Artery. **6.** Vein. **7.** Adipose tissue. **8.** Small vein.

Fig. 29-44. Enlargement of area similar to rectangle (A) in Fig. 29-43. Large intestine. Rat. E.M. X 4600. **1.** Peritoneal cavity. **2.** Visceral peritoneum. **3.** Muscularis externa. **4.** Nucleus of mesothelial cell. **5.** Bundles of collagenous fibrils in connective tissue part of serosa. **6.** Nucleus of smooth muscle cell. **7.** Microvilli.

Fig. 29-45. Enlargement of rectangle (B) in Fig. 29-43. Mesentery of the large intestine. Rat. E.M. X 610. **1.** Lumen of artery. **2.** Muscular media of artery. **3.** Loose connective tissue core of mesentery. **4.** Sheet of serous membrane. **5.** Peritoneal cavity. **6.** Cross-sectioned non-myelinated nerve bundles. **7.** Blood capillaries. **8.** Lymph capillary.

Fig. 29-46. Enlargement of area similar to rectangle in Fig. 29-45. Mesentery of large intestine. Rat. E.M. X 1800. **1.** Mesothelium. **2.** Elastic membrane. **3.** Bundles of collagenous fibrils. **4.** Cytoplasmic strands of fibroblast. **5.** Lymphocyte.

Fig. 29-47. Enlargement similar to rectangle in Fig. 29-46. Detail of mesenterial surface. Large intestine. Rat. E.M. X 61,000. **1.** Peritoneal cavity. **2.** Mesothelial cell cytoplasm. **3.** Basal lamina. **4.** Collagenous fibrils in submesothelial connective tissue. **5.** Microvilli. **6.** Junctional complex. **7.** Mitochondrion. **8.** Granular endoplasmic reticulum. **9.** Ribosomes. **10.** Micropinocytotic vesicles.

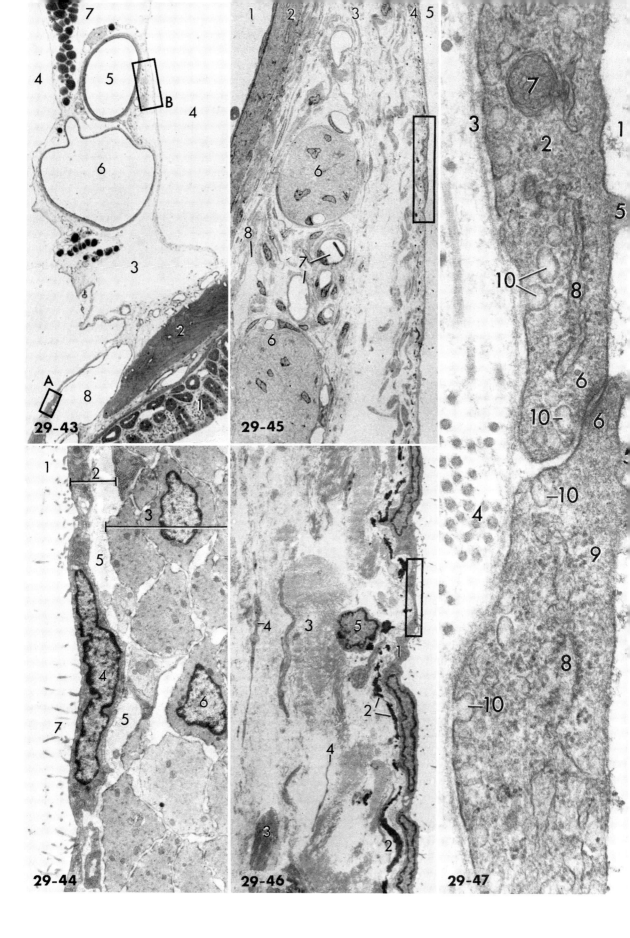

through the mesentery. They travel along the subserous connective tissue, sending branches to the muscularis externa and the submucosa. (Fig. 29-42) As they continue parallel to the long axis of the intestine, they give off, intermittently, small branches to the lamina propria. These arteries give rise to a **subvillous capillary plexus** around the intestinal glands. Other arterioles ascend through the cores of the intestinal villi, breaking up into a rich **villous capillary plexus.** The capillaries of the lamina propria have an endothelium which is thin and fenestrated, the fenestrae being bridged by a thin, single-layered membrane. The lamina propria is rich in venous capillaries, **venules,** and small **veins.** The last follow the pattern of the arterial vessels in returning the blood from the intestinal wall to veins in the mesentery where they collectively form the portal system.

Lymphatics. The lymphatic vessels start as blind capillaries in the core of the intestinal villi and around the glands. In the villi, they form a **central lacteal,** and in both the small and large intestines, they merge in the submucosa to form large lymphatic vessels. Subsequently, they leave the intestinal wall and travel within the mesentery. The fine structure of the lymphatics is similar to that described on p. 372.

SEROSA AND MESENTERY

The **serous membrane** (serosa) lines the body walls of the abdomen as **parietal peritoneum,** and it surrounds partly or entirely the gastrointestinal tract as the **visceral peritoneum.** Two sheets of the serous membrane come together to form the **mesentery** (Fig. 29-43) and **omentum,** attaching the gastrointestinal tract to the dorsal wall.

The serosa is composed of a layer of mesothelial cells, a thin basal lamina, and submesothelial connective tissue. The **mesothelium** consists of a single layer of large squamous cells attached by junctional complexes. (Fig. 29-47) The cells are provided with numerous long microvilli on the peritoneal surface. Micropinocytotic vesicles abound throughout the cytoplasm and at all cell surfaces. They are structural evidence for the high degree of a two-way fluid exchange which takes place across the mesothelium. Other cell organelles are scarce in these cells. The loose **connective tissue** of the serosa and the mesentery contains a limited number of collagenous and elastic fibers (Figs. 29-45, 29-46), some fibroblasts, and a wealth of mast cells, particularly along the many vascular channels that use this connective tissue core to reach the intestinal wall.

References

Atkins, A. M., Schofield, G. C., and Reeders, T. Studies on the structure and distribution of immunoglobulin A-containing cells in the gut of the pig. J. Anat. *109:* 385–395 (1971).

Baradi, A. F. and Hope, J. Observations on ultrastructure of rabbit mesothelium. Exp. Cell Res. *34:* 33–44 (1964).

Behnke, O. and Moe, H. An electron microscope study of mature and differentiating Paneth cells in the rat, especially of their endoplasmic reticulum and lysosomes. J. Cell Biol. *22:* 633–652 (1964).

Bennett, G. Migration of glycoprotein from Golgi apparatus to cell coat in the columnar cells of the duodenum epithelium. J. Cell Biol. *45:* 668–673 (1970).

Bonneville, M. A. and Weinstock, M. Brush border development in the intestinal absorptive cells of Xenopus during metamorphosis. J. Cell Biol. *44:* 151–171 (1970).

Brunser, O. and Luft, J. H. Fine structure of the apex of absorptive cells from rat small intestine. J. Ultrastruct. Res. *31:* 291–311 (1970).

Cardell, R. R., Jr., Badenhausen, S. and Porter, K. R. Intestinal triglyceride absorption in the rat. An electron microscopic study. J. Cell Biol. *34:* 123–155 (1967).

Cheng, H., Merzel, J. and Leblond, C. P. Renewal of Paneth cells in the small intestine of the mouse. Am. J. Anat. *126:* 507–526 (1969).

Cornell, R. and Padykula, H. A. A cytological study of intestinal absorption in the suckling rat. Am. J. Anat. *125:* 291–316 (1969).

Cotran, R. S. and Karnovsky, M. J. Ultrastructural studies on the permeability of the mesothelium to horseradish peroxidase. J. Cell Biol. *37:* 123–137 (1968).

Dawson, I. The endocrine cells of the gastrointestinal tract. Histochemical J. *2:* 527–549 (1970).

Deschner, E. E. Observations on the Paneth cell in human ileum. Exp. Cell Res. *47:* 624–628 (1967).

Dobbins, W. O., III and Rollins, E. L. Intestinal mucosal lymphatic permeability: an electron microscopic study of endothelial vesicles and cell junctions. J. Ultrastruct. Res. *33*: 29–59 (1970).

Forsmann, W. G., Orci, L., Pictet, R., Renold, A. E. and Rouiller, C. The endocrine cells in the epithelium of the gastrointestinal mucosa of the rat. J. Cell Biol. *40*: 692–715 (1969).

Freeman, J. A. Goblet cell fine structure. Anat. Rec. *154*: 121–148 (1966).

Freeman, J. A. and Geer, J. C. Intestinal fat and iron transport, goblet cell mucus secretion, and cellular changes in protein deficiency observed with the electron microscope. Am. J. Digest. Dis. *10*: 1004–1023 (1965).

Friend, D. The fine structure of Brunner's glands in the mouse. J. Cell Biol. *25*: 563–576 (1965).

Hertzog, A. J. The Paneth cell. Am. J. Path. *13*: 351–360 (1937).

Hollmann, K. H. Über den Feinbau des Rectumepithels. Z. Zellforsch. *68*: 502–542 (1965).

Ingelfinger, F. J. Gastrointestinal absorption. Nutrition Today *2*: 2–10 (1967).

Ingelfinger, F. J. For want of an enzyme. Nutrition Today *3*: 2–10 (1968).

Ito, S. The enteric surface coat on cat intestinal microvilli. J. Cell Biol. *27*: 475–491 (1965).

Jersild, R. A., Jr. A time sequence study of fat absorption in the rat jejunum. Am. J. Anat. *118*: 135–162 (1966).

Johnson, F. R. and Young, B. A. Undifferentiated cells in gastric mucosa. J. Anat. *102*: 541–551 (1968).

Krause, W. J. and Leeson, C. R. Studies of Brunner's glands in opossum. I. Adult morphology. Am. J. Anat. *126*: 255–274 (1969).

Lacy, D. and Taylor, A. B. Fat absorption by epithelial cells of the small intestine of the rat. Am. J. Anat. *110*: 155–186 (1962).

Ladman, A. J., Padykula, H. A. and Strauss, E. W. A morphological study of fat transport in the normal human jejunum. Am. J. Anat. *112*: 387–394 (1963).

Laguens, R. and Briones, M. Fine structure of the microvillus of columnar epithelial cells of human intestine. Lab. Investig. *14*: 1616–1623 (1965).

Leeson, T. S. and Leeson, C. R. The fine structure of Brunner's glands in man. J. Anat. *103*: 263–276 (1968).

Meader, R. and Landers, D. Electron and light microscopic observations on relationships between lymphocytes and intestinal epithelium. Am. J. Anat. *121*: 763–774 (1967).

Merzel, J. and Leblond, C. P. Origin and renewal of goblet cells in the epithelium of the mouse small intestine. Am. J. Anat. *124*: 281–306 (1969).

Moe, H. The ultrastructure of Brunner's glands of the cat. J. Ultrastruct. Res. *4*: 58–72 (1960).

Moe, H. The goblet cells, Paneth cells, and basal granular cells of the epithelium of the intestine. Int. Rev. Gen. Exp. Zool. *3*: 241–287 (1968).

Mukherjee, T. M. and Staehelin, L. A. The fine-structural organization of the brush border of intestinal epithelial cells. J. Cell Sci. *8*: 573–599 (1971).

Palay, S. L. and Karlin, L. J. An electron microscopic study of the intestinal villus. II. The pathway of fat absorption. J. Biophys. Biochem. Cytol. *5*: 373–384 (1959).

Palay, S. L. and Revel, J. P. The morphology of fat absorption. *In* Proceedings of an International Symposium on Lipid Transport (Ed. H. C. Meng). Charles C. Thomas, Springfield, pp. 33–43 (1964).

Pratt, S. A. and Napolitano, L. Osmium binding to the surface coat of intestinal microvilli in the cat under various conditions. Anat. Rec. *165*: 197–210 (1969).

Reynolds, D. S., Brim, J. and Sheehy, T. W. The vascular architecture of the small intestinal mucosa of the monkey (Macaca mulatta). Anat. Rec. *159*: 211–218 (1967).

Schofield, G. C. Columnar cells with secretory granules in the large intestine of the macaque (Cynamolgus iris). J. Anat. *106*: 1–14 (1970).

Schofield, G. C. and Atkins, A. Secretory immunoglobulin in columnar epithelial cells of the large intestine. J. Anat. *107*: 491–504 (1970).

Schofield, G. C. and Silva, D. The fine structure of enterochromaffin cells in the mouse colon. J. Anat. *103*: 1–13 (1968).

Singh, I. On argyrophile and argentaffin reactions in individual granules of enterochromaffin cells of the human gastro-intestinal tract. J. Anat. *98*: 497–500 (1964).

Staley, T. E., Jones, E. W. and Marshall, A. E. The jejunal absorptive cell of the newborn pig: an electron microscopic study. Anat. Rec. *161*: 497–516 (1968).

Strauss, E. W. Electron microscopic study of intestinal fat absorption in vitro from mixed micelles containing linolenic acid, monoolein, and bile salt. J. Lipid Res. *7*: 307–323 (1966).

Thrasher, J. D. and Greulich, R. C. The duodenal progenital population. III. The progenitor cell cycle of principal, goblet and Paneth cells. J. Exp. Zool. *161*: 9–19 (1966).

Toner, P. G. Cytology of intestinal epithelial cells. Int. Rev. Cytol. *24*: 233–243 (1968).

Toner, P. G. and Ferguson, A. Intraepithelial cells in the human intestinal mucosa. J. Ultrastruct. Res. *34*: 329–344 (1971).

Trier, J. S. Studies on small intestinal crypt epithelium. I. The fine structure of the crypt epithelium of the proximal small intestine of fasting humans. J. Cell Biol. *18*: 599–620 (1963).

Trier, J. S. Morphology of the epithelium of the small intestine. *In* Handbook of Pyhsiology: Sect. 6. Alimentary Canal, Vol. 32 (Ed. C. F. Code), American Physiological Society, Washington, D.C. pp. 1125–1175 (1968).

Trier, J. S., Lorenzsonn, V. and Groehler, K. Pattern of secretion of Paneth cells of the small intestine of mice. Gastroenterology *53*: 240–249 (1967).

Troughton, W. D., and Trier, J. S. Paneth and goblet cell renewal in mouse duodenal crypts. J. Cell Biol. *41*: 251–268 (1969).

Vassallo, G., Solcia, E. and Capella, C. Light and electron microscopic identification of several types of endocrine cells in the gastrointestinal mucosa of the cat. Z. Zellforsch. *98*: 333–356 (1969).

Wissig, S. L. and Graney, D. O. Membrane modifications in the apical endocytic complex of ileal epithelial cells. J. Cell Biol. *39*: 564–579 (1968).

30 Liver and pancreas

The liver and the pancreas are the two largest glands of the human body. Functionally, they form an important part of the digestive system and are closely related to many metabolic processes.

Liver

Embryologically, the liver is derived from the intestinal tract, and it maintains its connection with the gastrointestinal system in adult life through the bile duct. The main exocrine product of the liver is the bile. It is discharged via the bile duct to the duodenum of the small intestine. The bile is required in the intestine for the emulsification of fats during their absorption across the intestinal epithelium. The liver has a great capacity for storing blood, since it has an extremely rich network of sinusoidal blood capillaries. These sinusoids receive the blood from the portal vein, which in turn, drains the intestines, stomach, spleen, and pancreas. Arterial blood is also discharged into the sinusoids via hepatic arteries, which are derived from the aorta. The sinusoids are drained by hepatic veins which empty into the inferior vena cava. Therefore, from the vascular point of view, the liver is interposed in the venous pathway between the gastrointestinal tract and the inferior vena cava. This interposition is to great advantage in view of some other liver functions. The liver stores fats and carbohydrates, and it maintains the blood sugar level through its involvement in carbohydrate metabolism. It synthesizes fats, several kinds of proteins, and urea, and it activates many chemicals and detoxifies several poisons. In the embryo, it also serves as one site of hemopoiesis. A more detailed account of the liver functions as they are known to relate to hepatic cells and organelles is given on p. 588.

MICROANATOMY OF THE LIVER

The liver is the largest gland of the body. It is located in the upper right quadrant of the abdominal cavity. Surrounded by a thin connective tissue **capsule,** it consists of four indistinct **lobes** of unequal size. The hepatic parenchyma is made up of polyhedral **hepatic cells,** joined to form irregularly shaped plates, 1–2 cells thick. The plates are branching and anastomosing laminae, arranged radially around small venules to form anatomical units, referred to as **hepatic lobules.** (Fig. 30-1) These are small polyhedrons, roughly hexagonal in shape, and about 1–2 mm in diameter (Fig. 30-2), numbering about one million. The space between the converging plates of hepatic cells is occupied by **hepatic sinusoids,** and each peripheral angle of the hexagonal lobule is occupied by a **portal area** (synonym: portal canal) containing branches of the portal vein,

Fig. 30-1. Liver. Human. L.M. X 10. **1.** Capsule. **2.** Rectangle: hepatic lobule. **3.** Portal areas. **4.** Central venules. **5.** Sublobular hepatic vein.

Fig. 30-2. Hepatic lobule. Cross section. Enlargement of area similar to rectangle in Fig. 30-1. Liver. Human. L.M. X 130. **1.** Portal areas. **2.** Hepatic sinusoids. **3.** Plates of hepatic cells. **4.** Central venule. **5.** Sublobular vein.

Fig. 30-3. Hepatic lobule. Longitudinal section. Liver. Rat. L.M. X 253. **1.** Plates of hepatic cells. Nuclei of hepatic cells stained black. **2.** Hepatic sinusoids. **3.** Central venule. Arrows indicate direction of blood flow.

Fig. 30-4. Diagram of cross-sectioned hepatic lobules. **1.** Portal areas. **2.** Central venules. **3.** Hexagonal, classical **hepatic lobule.** Lines depict plates of hepatic cells and sinusoids converging on the central venule. **4.** Triangular **portal lobule. 5.** Diamond-shaped **liver acinus.**

Fig. 30-5. Three-dimensional diagram of the classical hepatic lobule. (Redrawn and modified from L. C. Junqueira & J. Carneiro, Histologia Basica, 2nd Ed., Guanabara Koogan, S.A., Rio de Janeiro, 1971). **1.** Interlobular portal veins. **2.** Interlobular hepatic arteries. **3.** Hepatic sinusoids. **4.** Plates of hepatic cells. **5.** Central venule. **6.** Sublobular hepatic vein. Arrows indicate direction of blood flow. **7.** Bile canaliculi. **8.** Bile ductules. **9.** Bile ducts. Arrows indicate direction of bile flow. **10.** Perilobular surfaces of adjoining hepatic lobules.

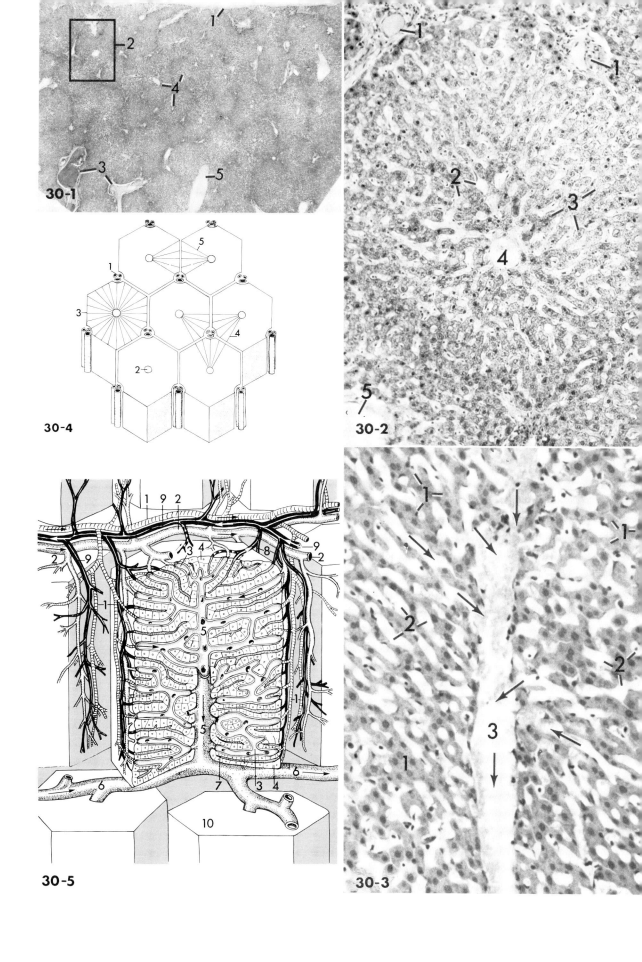

hepatic artery, bile duct, lymphatics, and nerves embedded in connective tissue trabeculae and septa. (Fig. 30-6) By **portal triad** is usually meant the portal vein, hepatic artery, and bile duct, these being the major constituents of the portal area. **Bile canaliculi** (synonym: bile capillaries) are small, almost submicroscopic channels between adjacent hepatic cells, formed by narrow grooves in the cell surface of apposed cells. They represent a system of intercellular tubules, into which the bile is secreted. At the periphery of the hepatic lobule, the bile canaliculi empty into narrow, **interlobular bile ductules,** which accompany the blood vessels of the portal area, and leave the liver as the **right** and **left hepatic bile ducts.**

The microanatomy of the liver, as outlined briefly here, does not emerge clearly and easily in histological sections. The plates of hepatic cells usually appear as rows of cells, and were earlier erroneously referred to as "cords." The hepatic sinusoids are collapsed in routine preparations and therefore difficult to discern. The anatomic unit, the **hepatic lobule,** is seen very clearly in the pig liver, but is less obvious in man and rat. In the latter species, adjacent hepatic lobules merge, and a regular distribution of portal areas is not seen at the periphery of the lobule.

Because of these structural differences between species, and based on recent analyses of functional, histopathological, and pathophysiological data, it has been suggested that the functional unit of the liver be referred to as **liver acinus.** (Fig. 30-4) As such, a liver acinus is the oval or diamond-shaped hepatic parenchyma which surrounds the terminal branches of the portal vein and hepatic artery (interlobular veins and arteries). Yet another way of looking at the subdivision of the hepatic parenchyma is the **portal lobule,** a triangular zone which has the portal area in the center, and includes parts of several adjacent hepatic lobules, with a central venule peripherally in several corners.

Each of these concepts offers a different viewpoint on the structure and function of the liver parenchyma. They are not mutually exclusive or conflicting, and are helpful in explaining and understanding the architecture of the liver and its multitude of functions.

BLOOD VESSELS AND LYMPHATICS

Distribution. Blood vessels and lymphatics enter and leave the hepatic parenchyma together with autonomic nerve fibers and bile ducts at the **hepatic portal,** where the liver capsule has considerable thickness. The hepatic blood circulation bathes the hepatic cells by flowing through the hepatic sinusoids, which form an extensive **microvascular bed** around and across the hepatic plates. The flow occurs **from** the periphery of the hepatic lobule **to** the central venule. (Fig. 30-5)

There are essentially three systems of blood vessels in the liver: 1) portal vein; 2) hepatic artery; and 3) hepatic vein. The **portal vein,** carrying blood from the intestines, stomach, spleen, and pancreas, upon entering the liver divides into **lobar** and **segmental** portal veins. These rapidly give rise to numerous **interlobular** veins, which travel in the portal area at the periphery of the hepatic lobule. Smaller branches, sometimes referred to as **inlet venules,** feed the blood into the **hepatic**

Fig. 30-6. Portal area. Liver. Rat. E.M. X 640.
  1. Portal vein. **2.** Small hepatic artery.
  3. Peribiliary blood capillaries. **4.** Bile duct.
  5. Lymphatic capillaries. **6.** Bile ductules.
  7. Inlet venule. *Arrows* indicate direction of blood flow. **8.** Hepatic sinusoids, some with erythrocytes. **9.** Nuclei of hepatic cells.
  10. Nuclei of sinusoidal endothelial cells. Rectangle (A) is enlarged in Fig. 30-8 and rectangle (B) is enlarged in Fig. 30-16.
Fig. 30-7. Central part of hepatic lobule. Liver. Rat. E.M. X 640. **1.** Hepatic sinusoids. *Arrows* indicate direction of blood flow.
  2. Central venule with numerous erythrocytes and connecting hepatic sinusoids. **3.** Nuclei of sinusoidal endothelial cells. **4.** Nuclei of hepatic cells.

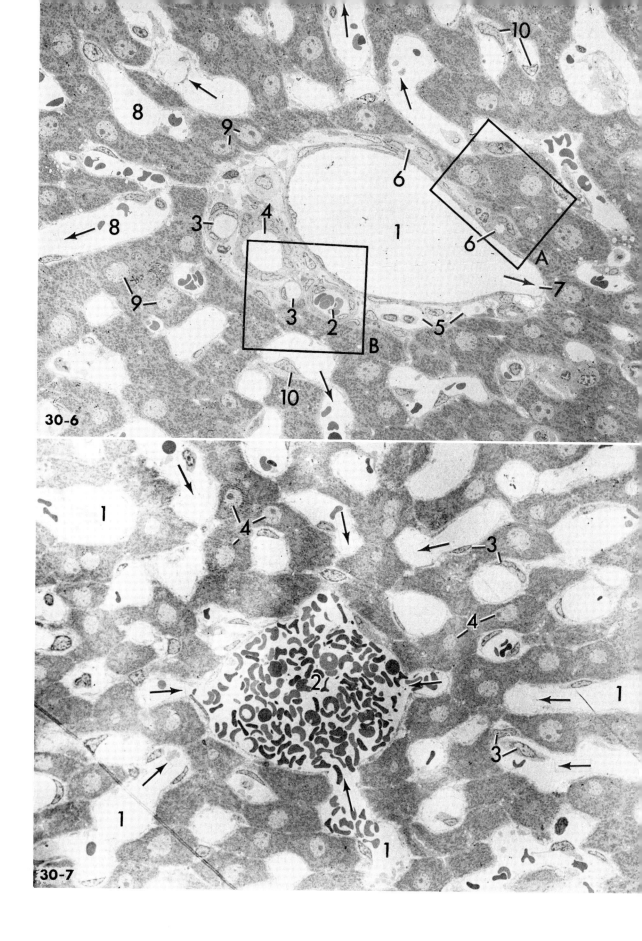

30-6

30-7

sinusoids, the terminal branches of the portal veins.

The **hepatic artery** follows largely the just mentioned branches of the portal vein and terminates as **interlobular arterioles** which deliver the blood partly to **stromal** and **peribiliary capillaries**, partly to the interlobular veins and hepatic sinusoids. Of the total hepatic blood flow, about three-fourths is supplied by the portal vein, and one-fourth by the hepatic artery.

The hepatic sinusoids converge to form the **central venule** (synonym: terminal hepatic venule) in the center of the hepatic lobule. (Figs. 30-3 and 30-7) **Sublobular veins** (synonyms: collecting veins, intercalated veins) drain the hepatic lobule. They course through the parenchyma alone and gradually merge to form increasingly larger stems of the **hepatic veins** which empty into the inferior vena cava.

The **lymphatic capillaries** emanate from within the perilobular connective tissue (Fig. 30-6), where they merge to form increasingly larger lymphatic vessels in the portal area. Lymphatic capillaries have not been demonstrated among the plates of hepatic cells in the lobules. However, the extracellular space of the liver plates, especially the perisinusoidal space (of Disse) is the major source of hepatic lymph, since the endothelium of the sinusoids is highly permeable. Large volumes (up to 50% of the total volume) of protein rich lymph is derived from the liver.

Structure. The **portal vein** and its ramifications have a thin intima without valves. The media consists of only a few smooth muscle layers, and the adventitia blends with the rather heavy accumulation of portal area connective tissue elements. (Fig. 30-8) The **inlet venules** have endothelial cells which seem to be able to change their shape (contractile?), thereby controlling the flow into the sinusoids.

The **hepatic sinusoids** average $9-12\ \mu$ in luminal width. They are extremely thin-walled with only one layer of lining cells. (Fig. 30-9) The lining cells consist of endothelial cells and Kupffer cells. The **endothelial cells** are extremely thin, squamous cells with an electron-lucent cytoplasm. The nucleus is small. The cytoplasm contains a limited amount of granular endoplasmic reticulum but a wealth of micropinocytotic vesicles, many of which are of the "bristle-coated" variety. There are numerous open endothelial fenestrations and large holes in the endothelium. (Fig. 16-38)

The **Kupffer cells** (stellate cells) are very active, fixed macrophages which line the sinusoids side by side with regular endothelial cells. Cell processes from Kupffer cells often extend across the sinusoidal lumen. The nucleus is large, and the Kupffer cell cytoplasm contains many profiles of the granular endoplasmic reticulum, lysosomes, and phagosomes. (Fig. 30-8) The cells are also fenestrated and provided with large gaps in the cytoplasm. Most investigators believe that the endothelial cells and the Kupffer cells belong to the same cell line, and that their different appearance reflects different functional states. Some investigators have expressed doubts that the sinusoidal endothelial cells can develop into Kupffer cells. However, it is a fact that both cell types have a great capacity for phagocytosis.

Fig. 30-8. Survey of part of perilobular area and peripheral portion of hepatic lobule. Enlargement of rectangle (A) in Fig. 30-6. Liver. Rat. E.M. X 1900. **1.** Lumen of portal vein lined by a squamous endothelium. **2.** Lumen of bile ductule, lined by low cuboidal epithelial cells. **3.** Nuclei of hepatic cells. **4.** Nucleus of sinusoidal endothelial (Kupffer) cell. **5.** Lumen of hepatic sinusoids. **6.** Longitudinally sectioned bile canaliculi. **7.** Cross-sectioned bile canaliculi. **8.** Perisinusoidal space of Disse. **9.** Mitochondria. **10.** Lysosomes (peribiliary dense bodies). **11.** Lymphocyte. **12.** Bundle of collagenous fibrils. **13.** Nucleus of endothelial cell lining the inlet venule. **14.** Numerous lysosomes in endothelial and Kupffer cells.

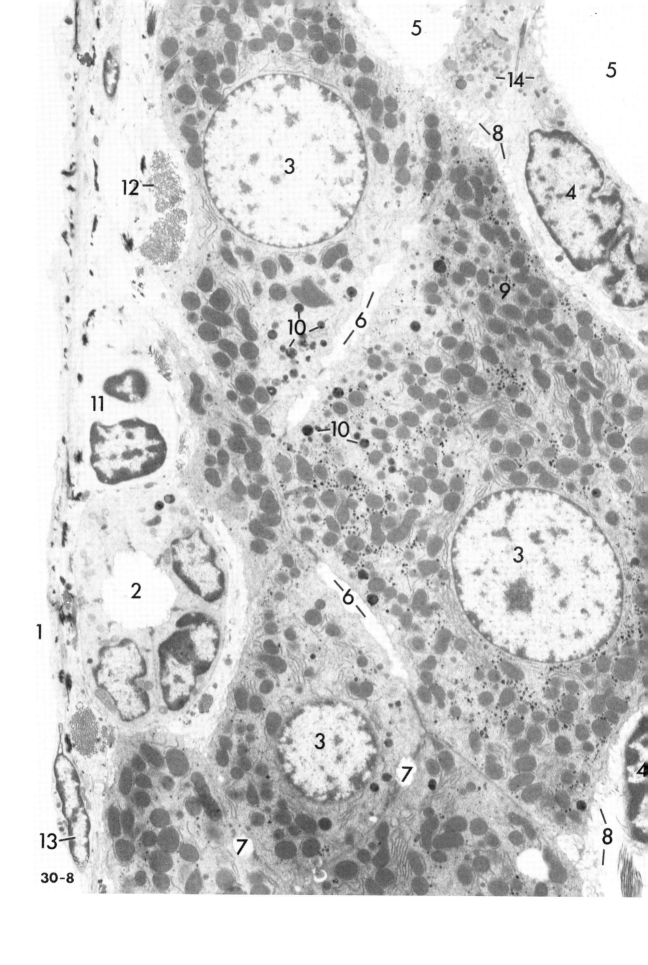

Because of this function and the large number of these cells in the liver, they represent a major part of the so-called **reticuloendothelial system** (p. 000).

A **basal lamina** is **absent** in most mammalian species. The **space of Disse** is a narrow perisinusoidal space into which project short microvilli from the hepatic cells. (Fig. 30-9) This space contains occasional bundles of reticular fibrils and occasional cells, referred to as **lipocytes** (synonyms: fat-storing cells, cells of Ito). These cells probably represent poorly differentiated mesenchymal cells which may develop into fat cells, and which may be looked upon as resting stem cells for blood cells, since erythropoiesis does occur within this area in the fetus. Fibroblasts do not occur here under normal conditions, but the lipocytes could possibly also serve as precursors for fibroblasts under pathological conditions.

The **central venule** of the hepatic lobule consists only of a thin endothelium. (Fig. 30-7) Connective tissue elements are not associated with these blood vessels to a large extent except for delicate bundles of collagenous fibrils.

The **interlobular arterioles** of the hepatic arteries retain a thin investment of smooth muscle cells within the precapillary sphincter area (Fig. 30-16), terminating at the point where these arterioles become peribiliary capillaries. They may also merge with interlobular veins, inlet venules or, occasionally, with hepatic sinusoids.

NERVES

The nerves of the liver are part of the autonomic nervous system. They follow the portal areas (Fig. 30-16) and accompany the blood vessels and the bile ducts, and as such, they represent vasomotor nerves. Efferent motor nerve endings related to the hepatic cells have not been positively identified with contemporary histological and electron microscopical techniques. Afferent, sensory nerve fibers exist as part of the vascular nerve plexus.

HEPATIC STROMA

Capsule. The liver is surrounded by a thin capsule (of Glisson) made up of dense fibrous connective tissue. (Fig. 30-1) The capsule is thicker in relation to the hepatic portal, where nerves, vasculature, and bile ducts enter and leave the liver parenchyma. A **serous membrane,** consisting of peritoneal mesothelium and associated connective tissue elements invests the greater portion of the liver capsule.

Intrahepatic stroma. The connective tissue capsule accompanies the bile ducts and the vasculature in the portal areas as **trabeculae** and **septa** (Figs. 30-6, 30-16). This connective tissue framework is also often referred to as the capsule of Glisson. The **perilobular** septa surround the hepatic lobules in the pig and the camel, but are incomplete in man, and confined to the minute areas between the adjacent angles of the lobules. **Intralobular** connective tissue is limited to a small amount of reticular fibrils in the perisinusoidal space of Disse. (Fig. 30-9)

HEPATIC PARENCHYMA

The hepatic parenchyma is made up of polyhedral **hepatic cells** (Fig. 30-10), arranged to form laminae, 1–2 cells thick, and grouped radially around a central venule, establishing the anatomical unit called **hepatic lobule.** (Fig. 30-5) The hepatic cell presents at least two sides to an hepatic sinusoid, and apposed sides of

Fig. 30-9. Cross section of hepatic sinusoid. Liver. Rat. E.M. X 12,000. **1.** Lumen of sinusoid. Distance between *asterisks* is 10 μ. **2.** Nucleus of sinusoidal endothelial cell. **3.** Squamous endothelium. **4.** Endothelial gaps. **5.** Perisinusoidal space of Disse. **6.** Bundles of collagenous fibrils. **7.** Bases of hepatic cells with microvilli projecting into the space of Disse. **8.** Mitochondria. **9.** Lipid droplets. **10.** Lysosomes. **11.** Chylomicron. Lipids, absorbed by the intestinal mucosa, are passed on to intestinal lacteals and capillary network of the core of the intestinal villus. The lipids, referred to as chylomicra, reach the liver via the portal vein.

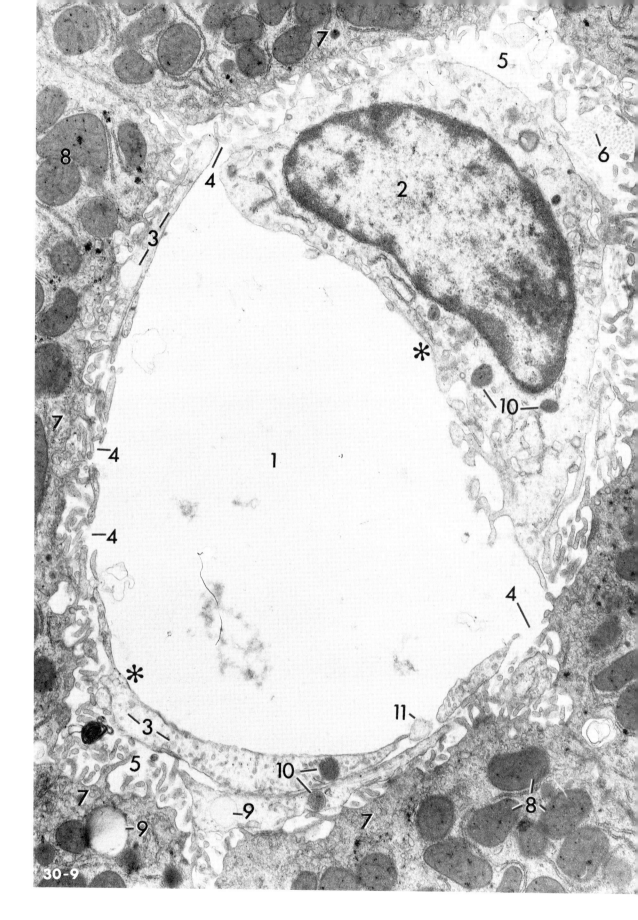

neighboring hepatic cells form a bile canaliculus between them. (Fig. 30-8)

Hepatic cell surface. The cell surface of the hepatic cells is smooth with only few lateral interdigitations. Short **microvilli** project into the bile canaliculi and to the space of Disse. **Junctional complexes** occur near the bile canaliculus. (Fig. 30-11) Desmosomes, intermediate junctions and gap-junctions have been reported. Micropinocytotic **invaginations,** the cytoplasmic aspect of their membrane often coated, and round **coated vesicles** are present at the cell membrane which borders on the perisinusoidal space of Disse. (Fig. 30-14) These two cell membrane differentiations serve processes of uptake and discharge of high molecular weight substances by the hepatic cell.

Nucleus. The nucleus is usually large, spherical, and centrally located. Two nuclei often occur in one cell. There is a large amount of light euchromatin, scattered areas of dense heterochromatin, and a distinct **nucleolus.** The nuclear membrane is well defined, containing many nuclear pores. As a rule, few mitoses are seen in routine histological sections of normal liver parenchyma. In spite of this, the regeneration ability of the liver is excellent.

HEPATIC CELL CYTOPLASM

The cytoplasm has a granular appearance in light microscope preparations. Although the hepatic cells are part of the largest gland of the body, they do not contain secretory droplets similar to those encountered in the serous cells of the pancreas or the cells of mucous glands. The granular appearance is mostly due to a large number of relatively small, round or elongated **mitochondria.** (Fig. 30-8) They have an electron-dense matrix, containing mostly tubular cristae and some dense mitochondrial granules. **Lysosomes** form a second, granular organelle, concentrated largely in the cytoplasm around the bile canaliculi. (Fig. 30-8) Before their positive identification, these structures were re-

ferred to as "peribiliary dense granules." The lysosomes of the hepatic cells are extremely pleomorphic (Fig. 30-11), and to this group belong hemosiderin granules, lipofuscin granules and multivesicular bodies, all somehow related to the digestive and lytic functions of the hepatic cell in the process of bile formation, urea synthesis, detoxification, and inactivation of chemicals. **Microbodies** (synonym: peroxisomes) are also common, often containing a core or crystalloid made up of delicate microtubules and lamellae. (Fig. 2-55) The microbodies are assumed to participate in gluco-neogenesis, metabolism of purines, break-down of cholesterol and disposition of hydrogen peroxide. **Lipid droplets,** averaging 1μ in diameter, occur in varied numbers under normal conditions. (Fig. 30-10) They are often invested by tubules of the agranular endoplasmic reticulum, and are surrounded by a thin interface membrane. The lipid droplets arise in the cells by an esterification of free fatty acids, and serve as stores for neutral lipids.

The liver functions as an important source of plasma triglycerides. Fat depots in the body release free fatty acids into the blood plasma. Hepatic cells remove them, re-esterifying them as triglycerides and incorporating the triglycerides into lipoproteins which are secreted to the blood and returned to adipose tissue. Probably as part of this process, so-called very low density lipoproteins rich in

Fig. 30-10. Detail of hepatic cell. Liver. Mouse. E.M. X 26,000. **1.** Lumen of hepatic sinusoid. **2.** Cytoplasm of endothelial (Kupffer) cell. **3.** Endothelial gaps. **4.** Perisinusoidal space of Disse. **5.** Microvilli. **6.** Mitochondria. **7.** Microbodies (peroxisomes). **8.** Golgi zone. **9.** Lipid droplets. **10.** Lysosomes (peribiliary dense bodies). **11.** Bile canaliculus (bile capillary). **12.** Junctional complexes. **13.** Glycogen particles. **14.** Agranular endoplasmic reticulum. **15.** Granular endoplasmic reticulum. **16.** Free monoribosomes and polysomes. **17.** Nucleus. **18.** Vacuoles with amorphous granules of "very low density lipoproteins." **19.** Micropinocytotic invagination.

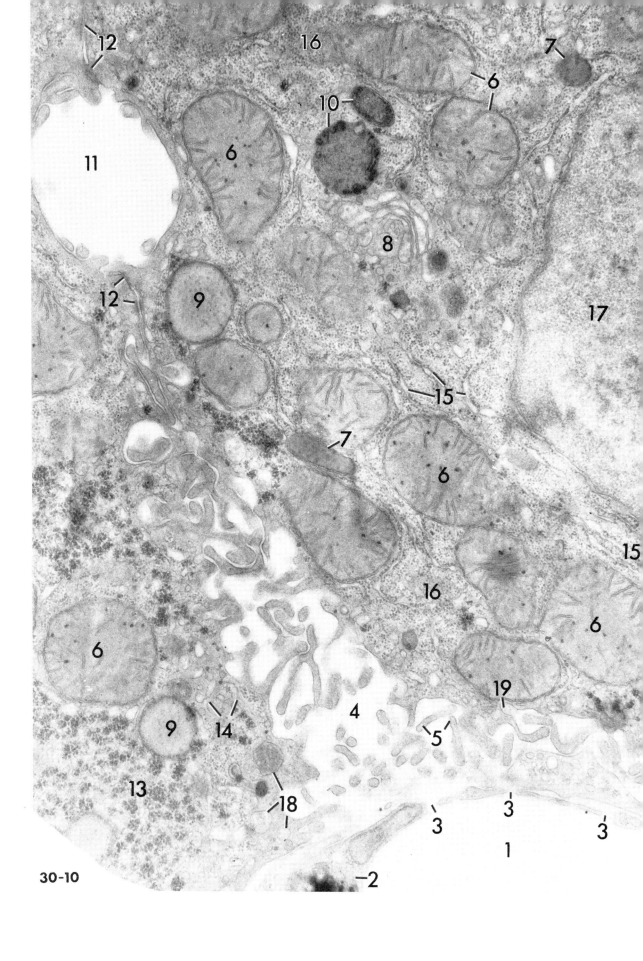

30-10

triglycerides have been identified ultra-structurally as electron-dense **amorphous granules,** ranging from 300 Å to 800 Å in diameter. They first appear within the tubules of the agranular endoplasmic reticulum. From here, they are channeled to Golgi saccules (Fig. 30-13), where they become aggregated in bulbous dilatations of the saccules. Subsequently, the bulbous dilatations become sequestered as small vacuoles and apparently move to the perisinusoidal cell surface, fuse with the cell membrane, and discharge the amorphous granules into the space of Disse in a process of exocytosis.

Membrane systems. The hepatic cells contain a fairly large amount of endoplasmic reticulum of both the granular and agranular variety. The **granular endoplasmic reticulum** occurs in groups of 5–10 parallel cisternae. (Fig. 30-10) Their occurrence and location vary greatly among cells within the same lobular region, and also with reference to cells located near the portal area as opposed to cells near the central venule of the hepatic lobule. Free **ribosomes** occur both as monoribosomes and as polysomes in addition to those attached to the membranes of the granular endoplasmic reticulum. (Fig. 30-10) These organelles are engaged in protein synthesis, the end products being blood albumin and fibrinogen. Direct continuities exist between the cisternae of the granular endoplasmic reticulum, and the **agranular endoplasmic reticulum.** The latter consists of a meshwork of branching and anastomosing tubules and irregularly shaped vesicles. (Fig. 30-12) Amount and location vary from cell to cell. The tubules may provide a site for the location of enzymes involved in glycogen metabolism. In addition, it has been suggested that they are engaged in cholesterol biosynthesis, and perhaps serve as carriers for bilirubin and other bile constituents. The **Golgi** zone consists of stacks of flat, slightly curved saccules with dilated bulbous ends, often containing small amorphous, medium electron-dense granules. A varied number of different size vesicles are associated with the Golgi saccules. (Fig. 30-13) Several Golgi zones (dictyosomes) are present, some located near the nucleus, others near the bile canaliculi.

Glycogen. Glycogen particles are often closely associated with the intertubular space of the agranular endoplasmic reticulum. The glycogen occurs both as single β-**particles,** averaging 300 Å in diameter, and as clusters or "rosettes", referred to as α-**particles,** averaging 900 Å in diameter. (Fig. 30-12) The deposition of glycogen in the hepatic cells and its removal occurs over a time span of 1–3 hours following a meal, and follows a certain pattern. It is first deposited in the peripheral zone of the hepatic lobule, and last in the hepatic cells near the central venule. On the other hand, glycogen is first removed from the central cells, and last from the peripheral. Virtually all the reactions of intermediary carbohydrate metabolism can take place in the hepatic cells, and one of the main functions of the liver is the maintenance

Fig. 30-11. Peribiliary region. Hepatic cell. Liver. Rat. E.M. X 70,000. **1.** Bile canaliculus with microvilli projecting into it. **2.** Junctional complex. **3.** Lysosomes (peribiliary dense bodies). **4.** Part of microbody (peroxisome). **5.** Cisterna of granular endoplasmic reticulum. **6.** Part of multivesicular body.

Fig. 30-12. Central region. Hepatic cell. Liver. Rat. E.M. X 83,000. **1.** Tubules of agranular endoplasmic reticulum. **2.** Glycogen particles (beta particles). **3.** Glycogen particles (alpha particles). **4.** Mitochondrion.

Fig. 30-13. Golgi region. Hepatic cell. Liver. Rat. E.M. X 75,000. **1.** Saccules of Golgi zones. **2.** Dilated, bulbous ends of Golgi saccules, containing very low density lipoprotein granules. **3.** Cisterna of granular endoplasmic reticulum. **4.** Mitochondria. **5.** Microbody (peroxisome).

Fig. 30-14. Perisinusoidal region. Hepatic cell. Liver. Rat. E.M. X 83,000. **1.** Part of sinusoidal endothelial cell. **2.** Perisinusoidal space of Disse. **3.** Microvilli. **4.** Coated micropinocytotic invaginations. **5.** Tubules of agranular endoplasmic reticulum among ribosomes and glycogen particles. **6.** Mitochondria. **7.** Lumen of sinusoid.

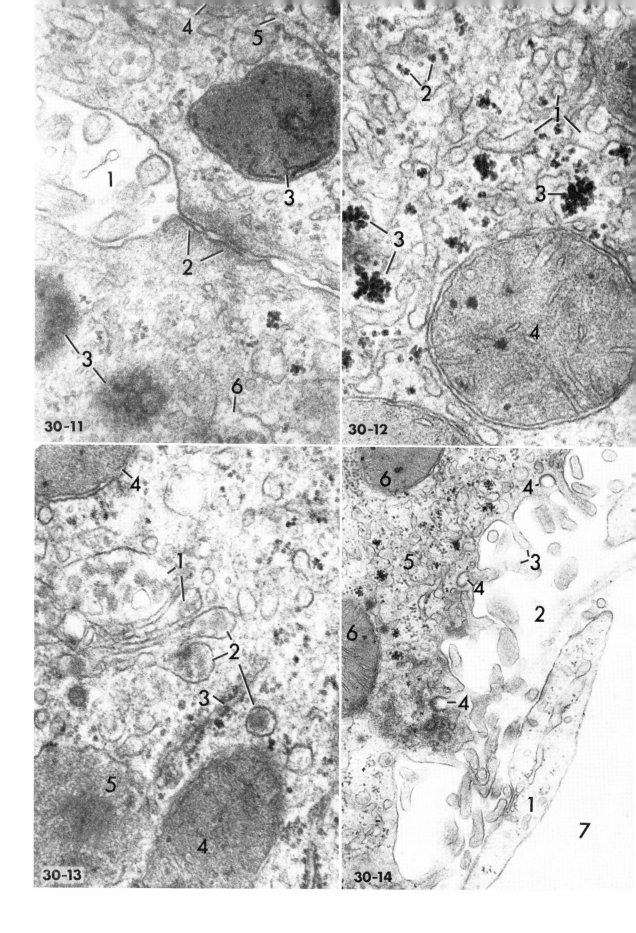

30-11

30-12

30-13

30-14

of the normal glucose concentration of the blood plasma.

As indicated by the description above, the hepatic cells have great structural and functional diversity. Yet, all cells probably have the same functions. The formation and excretion of bile in the liver are not fully understood from an ultrastructural point of view. As indicated earlier in this chapter (p. 588), secretory droplets or secretory granules in the classical sense do not occur. Bilirubin is formed through the breakdown of hemoglobin by macrophages in the spleen and the Kupffer cells of the liver, whereas the excretion of the bile pigment is done by the hepatic cells.

INTRAHEPATIC BILIARY SYSTEM

The intrahepatic biliary system consists of: 1) bile canaliculi; 2) bile ductules; and 3) bile ducts.

Bile canaliculi. The bile canaliculi (synonym: bile capillaries) are $0.1–0.2\ \mu$ wide channels formed by apposing hepatic cells. (Fig. 30-10) They have no wall of their own, but rather represent grooves in the cell surface of apposed hepatic cells. The cytoplasmic zone of the hepatic cell adjacent to the bile canaliculi is largely devoid of cell organelles except for a few vesicles, microtubules, and finely fibrillar material. Microvilli of the hepatic cell project into the lumen of the bile canaliculus, and junctional complexes secure the attachment of the hepatic cells around these canaliculi. (Fig. 30-11) The bile canaliculi form a wide system of interconnected submicroscopic channels which direct the bile from the central parts of the hepatic lobule to the peripheral parts.

Bile ductules. Near the periphery of the hepatic lobule, the bile canaliculi empty into small, narrow tubes, the bile ductules. They may originate within the lobule as **cholangioles** (intralobular bile ductules), or within the portal area as **perilobular ductules.** (Fig. 30-8) In either case, the ductules are lined by a single layer of very small cuboidal cells, held together near the luminal surface by junctional com-

plexes. The electron-lucent cytoplasm contains a small number of mitochondria, some profiles of granular endoplasmic reticulum, ribosomes, and occasional lysosomes. The ductules are invested by a thin basal lamina.

Bile ducts. The perilobular bile ductules empty into interlobular bile ducts (Fig. 30-16), which originate as narrow tubes, lined by a simple cuboidal epithelium. Gradually, the interlobular bile ducts merge and increase in diameter (Fig. 30-15) as they travel with branches of the hepatic artery and portal vein in the connective tissue of the portal area, emerging from the liver as right and left hepatic bile ducts at the hepatic portal. The epithelium changes gradually from a cuboidal to a columnar type. The cells display the same general ultrastructure as the cells of the bile ductules. A **basal lamina** invests the ducts. Smooth muscle cells are not associated with the walls of the intrahepatic bile ducts.

EXTRAHEPATIC BILIARY SYSTEM

The extrahepatic biliary system consists of: 1) right and left hepatic bile ducts;

Fig. 30-15. Large portal area. Liver. Rat. L.M. X 160. **1.** Portal vein. **2.** Hepatic artery. **3.** Hepatic arteriole. **4.** Lymphatics. **5.** Biliary duct. **6.** Portal area connective tissue. **7.** Hepatic sinusoids and plates of hepatic cells.

Fig. 30-16. Small portal area. Enlargement of rectangle (B) in Fig. 30-6. Liver. Rat. E.M. X 4700. **1.** Lumen of portal vein. **2.** Nuclei of endothelial cells. **3.** Vascular smooth muscle cells. **4.** Lumen of small hepatic artery. **5.** Erythrocytes. **6.** Lumen of precapillary arteriole. **7.** Lumen of interlobular biliary duct. **8.** Nuclei of epithelial duct cells. **9.** Non-myelinated nerve fibers (require higher magnification for positive identification). **10.** Nucleus of lymphocyte. **11.** Nucleus of fibroblast. **12.** Bundles of collagenous fibrils. **13.** Mitochondria in hepatic cells. **14.** Cross-sectioned bile canaliculi. **15.** Lumen of hepatic sinusoid. **16.** Part of plasma cell with dilated cisternae of the granular endoplasmic reticulum.

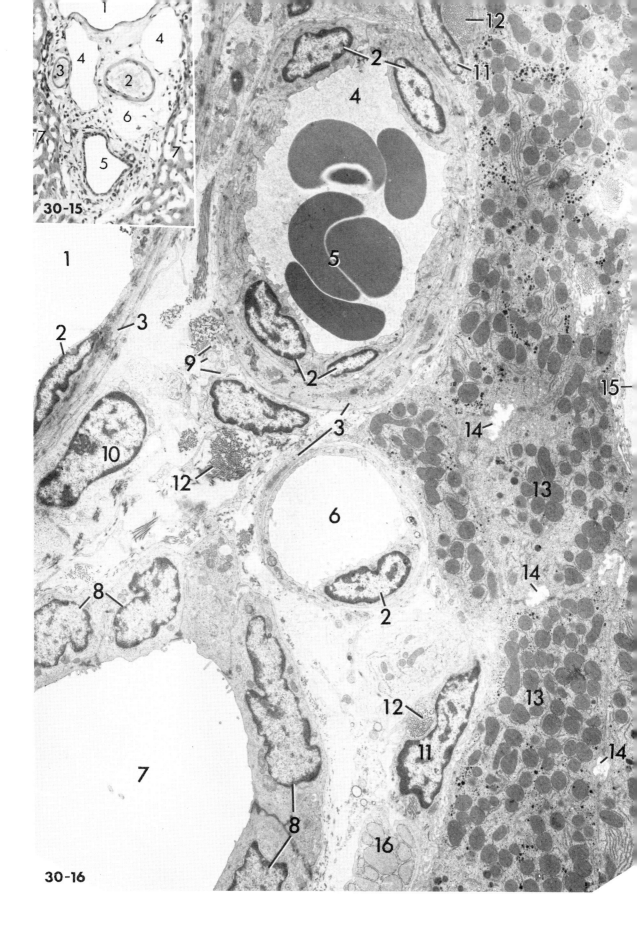

2) cystic duct; 3) common bile duct; and 4) gallbladder.

The **right** and **left** hepatic **bile ducts** join with the **cystic duct** from the gallbladder to form the **common bile duct** which terminates in the small intestine at the duodenal papilla, often jointly with the pancreatic duct. A tall, simple columnar epithelium lines the extrahepatic bile ducts. The left and right bile ducts, and the cystic duct have a small number of smooth muscle cells. Only in relation to the common bile duct are there several layers of smooth muscle cells peripheral to the epithelium.

Gallbladder. The gallbladder is a small, elongated pear-shaped sac located near the anterior border of the liver. It is connected to the common bile duct via the cystic duct.

The wall of the gallbladder is thin. It consists of: 1) mucous membrane; 2) lamina muscularis; and 3) adventitia. The **mucous membrane** is thrown into a system of deep folds with many pocket-like recesses. (Fig. 30-17) A tall, simple columnar epithelium lines the luminal surface. (Fig. 30-18) The **epithelial cells** are provided with short microvilli, and the apical part of the cells contains a varied number of small, membrane-bound, medium electron-dense granules (droplets) which are assumed to contain mucoid substances. (Fig. 30-20) Lipid droplets often occur near the base of the cell. There is a small number of mitochondria, a small Golgi zone, but relatively many profiles of granular endoplasmic reticulum and few ribosomes. The lateral contact surfaces have many cell to cell interdigitations (Fig. 30-19), and junctional complexes occur near the apex of the cell. Mucous cells of the goblet type do not occur in the gallbladder, except in the neck near the cystic duct. The epithelium rests on a thin **basal lamina** beneath which is a relatively wide zone of **stroma** (synonym: lamina propria) consisting of loose connective tissue. Glands and a muscularis mucosae of the type present in the intestinal tract are missing. Irregularly arranged smooth muscle cells make up the thin **lamina muscularis.** (Fig. 30-18) The perimuscular layer of loose connective tissue, often referred to as **adventitia,** contains many blood vessels (Fig. 30-17), lymphatics, and nerves. The portion of the gallbladder which does not face the liver is covered by a **serous membrane,** similar to that which surrounds the liver and the intestines.

With regard to the **functions** of the gallbladder, it stores the bile in anticipation of a fatty meal, when the bile is discharged into the duodenum in response to release of the hormone cholecystokinin from the intestinal glands. While in the gallbladder, the bile is concentrated by an absorption of excess water, and a mucoid substance is added to the bile.

Pancreas

The pancreas is a large gland, located in the upper part of the abdominal cavity behind the stomach in a retroperitoneal position. It is primarily an **exocrine** gland.

Fig. 30-17. Gallbladder. Monkey. L.M. X 56.
 1. Lumen. **2.** Mucous membrane. **3.** Lamina muscularis. **4.** Adventitia. **5.** Blood vessels. **6.** Serosa.
Fig. 30-18. Gallbladder. Enlargement of rectangle in Fig. 30-17. L.M. X 315.
 1. Lumen. **2.** Simple columnar epithelium. **3.** Stroma of connective tissue ("lamina propria"). **4.** Venule. **5.** Smooth muscle cells of lamina muscularis.
Fig. 30-19. Gallbladder epithelium. Enlargement of area similar to rectangle in Fig. 30-18. Rat. E.M. X 7,000. **1.** Lumen of gallbladder. **2.** Microvilli. **3.** Cell borders. **4.** Junctional complexes. **5.** Basal body of cilium. **6.** Centriole. **7.** Mitochondria. **8.** Nuclei. **9.** Basal lamina. **10.** Collagenous fibrils of stroma. **11.** Accumulation of glycogen particles.
Fig. 30-20. Surface of epithelial cells. Gallbladder. Enlargement of area similar to rectangle in Fig. 30-19. Rat. E.M. X 34,000. **1.** Lumen of gallbladder. **2.** Microvilli. **3.** Junctional complex. **4.** Cell to cell interdigitations. **5.** Mucoid granules.

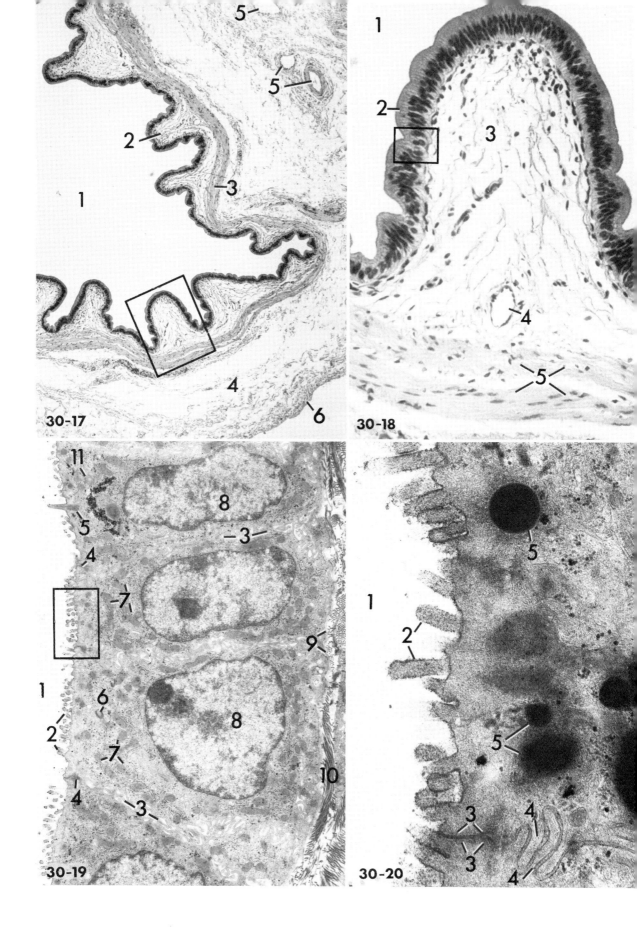

30-17

30-18

30-19

30-20

The secretions are carried via the pancreatic main duct (of Wirsung) to the duodenum where they participate in the latter stages of enzymatic breakdown of proteins, fats, and carbohydrates. **Endocrine** cells, synthesizing hormones involved in carbohydrate metabolism, are aggregated in small clumps, the islets of Langerhans. (Fig. 30-21) Like other endocrine glands, the secretions of the pancreatic islets are picked up by the microvascular bed and circulated through the cardiovascular system.

EXOCRINE PORTION OF PANCREAS

The exocrine portion of the pancreas is a compound acinar gland, which means that the serous secreting endpieces are pear-shaped, and that the secretory products are collected by a widely branching system of ducts. The pancreas is structurally very similar to the parotid gland (p. 520).

Stroma. The pancreas is surrounded by a thin, indistinct **capsule** of loose fibrous connective tissue. The parenchyma of the gland is divided by thin connective tissue **septa** into primary and secondary **lobules.** (Fig. 30-21) These septa contain excretory ducts, blood vessels, lymphatics and nerves. Extremely delicate connective tissue septa subdivide the lobules into acini (Fig. 30-22), each of which is invested by a thin basal (external) lamina.

Acini. The pear-shaped acini (synonym: alveoli) are arranged quite irregularly. They are composed of tall, irregularly columnar or pyramidal **acinar epithelial cells** with one or two nuclei in the basal end of the cell, the cytoplasm of which is strongly basophilic (Fig. 30-23). The apex of the cell is filled with numerous, highly refractive, eosinophilic secretory droplets. The cell apex borders on the **acinar lumen,** often referred to as secretory capillary. This lumen occasionally originates either as an intracellular or an intercellular canaliculus. Protruding partly into the acinar lumen in a telescoping fashion are so-called **centroacinar cells.** (Fig. 30-23)

These are small flattened epithelial cells which represent the beginning of the duct system.

Acinar epithelial cells. The acinar epithelial cells are serous-type glandular cells. (Fig. 30-24) The luminal surface is provided with a small number of delicate and short microvilli which protrude into the 0.1–0.2 μ wide acinar lumen. The latter often contains a homogeneous, medium electron-dense secretion. Adjoining cells are held together by junctional complexes near the lumen. The lateral and basal cell borders are relatively straight with few cell to cell interdigitations. The **nucleus** is round with a distinct peripheral zone of dense heterochromatin. One or two **nucleoli** are also present with prominent strands of nucleolonema.

The basal two-thirds of the cell is occupied by a dense aggregation of flat cisternae of the **granular endoplasmic reticulum** (Fig. 30-24), and numerous free monoribosomes and polysomes. Some oval and elongated **mitochondria** with mem-

Fig. 30-21. Pancreas. Human. L.M. X 12.
1. Thin capsule. **2.** Septa. **3.** Lobes. **4.** Lobules.
5. Islets of Langerhans.

Fig. 30-22. Pancreas. Enlargement of area similar to rectangle in Fig. 30-21. Monkey. L.M. X 305. **1.** Arterioles. **2.** Acini (alveoli). **3.** Interlobular duct. **4.** Intralobular duct.

Fig. 30-23. Two acini and interlobular connective tissue septum. Enlargement of area similar to rectangle in Fig. 30-22. Pancreas. Rat. E.M. X 1800. **1.** Nuclei of acinar epithelial cells. **2.** Lumen (secretory capillary) of acinus, surrounded by intracellular zymogen (secretory) granules. **3.** Centroacinar cells. **4.** Lumen of intralobular (intercalated) duct, lined by low cuboidal duct cells. *Arrow* indicates position of duct cells which connect centroacinar cells with intercalated (intralobular) duct. **5.** Lumina of blood capillaries. **6.** Nucleus of Schwann cell with associated non-myelinated nerve fibers. **7.** Nuclei of lymphocytes. **8.** Connective tissue fibrils and fibroblasts of interlobular septum. **9.** Delicate interacinar connective tissue septum. **10.** Lumen of arteriole. **11.** Lumen of interlobular duct. **12.** Epithelial duct cells. Area corresponding to rectangle is enlarged in Fig. 30-24.

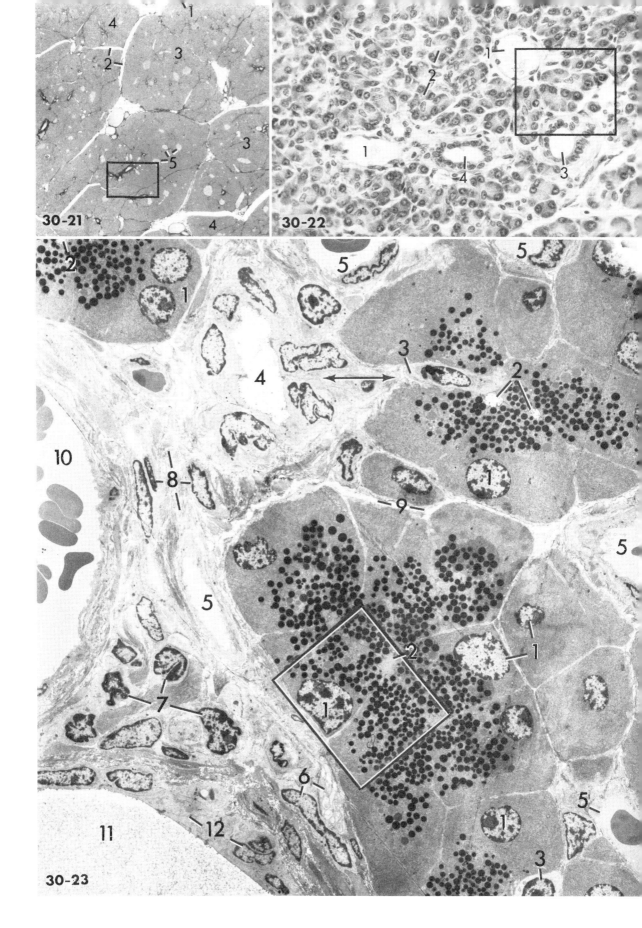

30-21

30-22

30-23

branous cristae also occur here. The **Golgi zone** is located on the luminal side of the nucleus. It is extensive, consisting of vesicles, vacuoles, and flat saccules containing medium electron-dense amorphous material. Arising from the Golgi vacuoles appear condensing, membrane-bound **prezymogen vacuoles** and **granules.** Their matrix is less dense, and their bordering membrane more distinct than corresponding structures in the nearby accumulations of numerous zymogen granules. The mature **zymogen granules** are spherical. The boundary membrane is difficult to resolve because of the high electron density of the matrix. (Fig. 30-25) There is no apparent ultrastructural difference between the zymogen granules of the same cell or of different cells. They vary in size, but it is presently assumed that each granule contains several enzymes or precursors of enzymes which participate in proteolytic, lipolytic and carbohydrate breakdown processes in the intestine.

The ultrastructural basis for the synthesis, maturation and discharge of secretory granules was described in Chapter 4, p. 86. To re-emphasize part of this process, the discharge of the content of the zymogen granules occurs through a process of exocytosis, whereby the boundary membrane of the zymogen granule fuses with the luminal cell membrane and the matrix of the granule is extruded into the lumen of the pancreatic acinus.

Among other cell organelles found in the acinar cells are **lysosomes** to a limited extent, 1–2 **centrioles,** and occasional **lipid droplets.** The acinus is invested by a delicate **basal lamina.** Myoepithelial cells are not present in relation to acini in the pancreas. A rich **capillary network** surrounds the pancreatic acini and lobules.

Ducts. The duct system begins with the flat or low cuboidal **centroacinar cells.** Their cytoplasm is electron-lucent (Fig. 30-26) and contains few organelles except ribosomes, some mitochondria, lysosomes, and lipid droplets. **Intercalated ducts** (synonym: intralobular ducts) establish a

direct continuation of the centroacinar cells. In man, they are long, slender and extremely branching tubules, also lined with low cuboidal epithelial cells (Fig. 30-23). The intercalated ducts connect with **interlobular ducts** which are located in the connective tissue septa. They are lined with a simple cuboidal (Fig. 30-23) or columnar epithelium, the height depending on the diameter of the duct; the larger the duct, the taller the epithelium. The cells contain more mitochondria than the cells of the preceding duct segments, but the orderly arrangement of long mitochondria between infoldings of the basal cell membrane present in the salivary glands (striated ducts) does not occur in the pancreas. Myoepithelial cells or ordinary smooth muscle cells are absent from the ducts just described. However, in the main **pancreatic duct** (of Wirsung), smooth muscle cells form a peripheral layer around the epithelium. The pan-

Fig. 30-24. Acinar epithelial cells. Enlargement of area corresponding to rectangle in Fig. 30-23. Pancreas. Rat. E.M. X 9000. **1.** Nucleolus. **2.** Euchromatin. **3.** Heterochromatin. **4.** Granular endoplasmic reticulum. **5.** Mitochondria. **6.** Golgi zones. **7.** Prezymogen granules. **8.** Zymogen granules. **9.** Centriole. **10.** Acinar lumen filled with dense secretory material. **11.** Cell border. **12.** Basal lamina. **13.** Non-myelinated nerve fibers. **14.** Lumen of blood capillary.

Fig. 30-25. Secretory granules. Acinar cell. Enlargement of area similar to rectangle in Fig. 30-24. Pancreas. Rat. E.M. X 62,000. **1.** Saccule of Golgi zone containing medium electron-dense amorphous material. **2.** Condensing Golgi vacuoles. **3.** Prezymogen granule. **4.** Zymogen granule. **5.** Vacuolar profile of granular endoplasmic reticulum. **6.** Transfer vesicle.

Fig. 30-26. Center of acinus. Pancreas. Rat. E.M. X 8000. **1.** Lumen of acinus with flocculent secretory material. **2.** Microvilli. **3.** Apices of acinar cells. **4.** Zymogen granules. **5.** Nuclei of centroacinar cells. **6.** Mitochondria. **7.** Lipid droplets in cytoplasm of centroacinar cells. **8.** Basal lamina. **9.** Interacinar connective tissue fibrils. **10.** Basal cytoplasm of acinar cells in adjacent acinus.

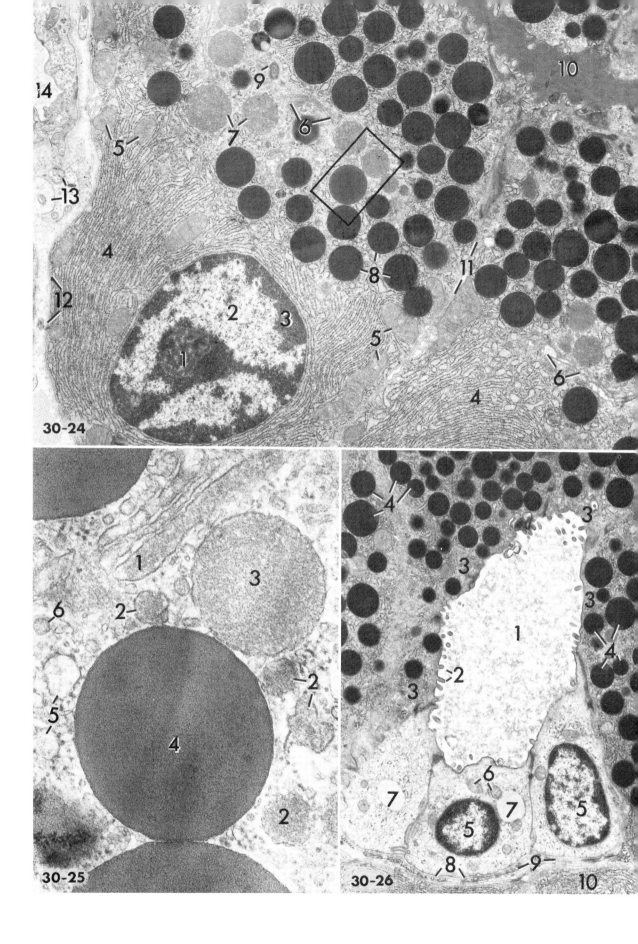

30-24

30-25

30-26

creatic duct is lined by a tall, simple columnar epithelium with occasional mucus producing goblet cells mixed in. A considerable amount of dense fibrous connective tissue surrounds the main pancreatic duct.

NERVES

Nerves are derived from the sympathetic and parasympathetic (vagus) system. Numerous parasympathetic ganglia occur in the connective tissue septa of the pancreas. The nerve fibers supply the vascular walls. In addition, a delicate network of efferent, denuded nerve fibers are present around the acini. (Fig. 30-24) They also penetrate the basal lamina and terminate upon the acinar secretory cells.

FUNCTIONS

The acinar cells synthesize several enzymes. Proteolytic enzymes identified are trypsinogen, chymotrypsin and carboxypeptidase. Fat-splitting enzymes present are lipase and lecithinase. Ribonuclease and deoxyribonuclease have also been demonstrated, as well as amylase which acts on glycogen and starch. The intestinal hormones pancreozymin and secretin are released from intestinal glands in response to the presence of chyme in the duodenum. Pancreozymin initiates the discharge of zymogen granules from the pancreatic acinar cells, whereas secretin brings on an outpouring of water and mineral constituents from the pancreas. Stimulation of the vagus nerve initiates a discharge of secretions rich in pancreatic enzymes.

ENDOCRINE PORTION OF PANCREAS

The islets of Langerhans represent the endocrine portion of the pancreas. There are two hormones secreted by the islet cells, insulin and glucagon, both involved in carbohydrate metabolism.

The islets vary in size and shape, but are generally spherical, the width being about 0.2 mm. (Fig. 30-27) In the human pancreas, they are more abundant in the tail than in the head of the gland. The islets are not surrounded by a true connective tissue capsule but are enveloped by a thin network of delicate collagenous fibrils and a basal (external) lamina. The islets are made up of irregular cords or masses of polygonal **epithelial cells** (Fig. 30-28) which, in routine histological preparations, stain less intensely than the exocrine part of the pancreas. The cords are surrounded and penetrated by a very rich capillary network. The capillaries are of the fenestrated type, with the fenestrae closed by a thin diaphragm.

There are two main cell types, the alpha (A) cells and the beta (B) cells. A third less common cell type is the delta (D) cell, and a fourth, very rare cell is the C-cell.

Alpha (glucagon) cells. The alpha cells make up about 20% of the islet cells, and are usually located in the periphery of the islet. (Fig. 30-29) They have a small number of long slender mitochondria, a small Golgi zone, and a varied number of short profiles of the granular endoplasmic reticulum. The secretory granules are generally numerous, but the amount varies greatly from cell to cell. They are uniform in size, averaging 3000 Å in width. A boundary membrane surrounds a core which has a highly electron-dense center, and an outer less dense mantle. In preserving the granules for light microscopy, they are alcohol resistant but water soluble.

Beta (insulin) cells. The beta cells are

Fig. 30-27. Islet of Langerhans. Pancreas. Human. L.M. X 190. **1.** Cords of cells in islet. **2.** Collapsed blood capillaries.
3. Acini of exocrine portion of pancreas.
4. Plane of section to obtain Fig. 30-28.
Fig. 30-28. Edge of islet of Langerhans. Plane of section indicated by 4—4 in Fig. 30-27. Pancreas. Rat. E.M. X 4500.**1.** Lumina of blood capillaries. **2.** Nuclei of endothelial cells. **3.** Nucleus of pericyte. **4.** Nuclei of fibroblasts. **5.** Bundles of collagenous fibrils.
6. Nuclei of alpha (glucagon) cells.
7. Nuclei of beta (insulin) cells. **8.** Nucleus of delta cell. **9.** Nuclei of C-cells.
Identification of cell types is based on analysis of this field at higher magnifications.

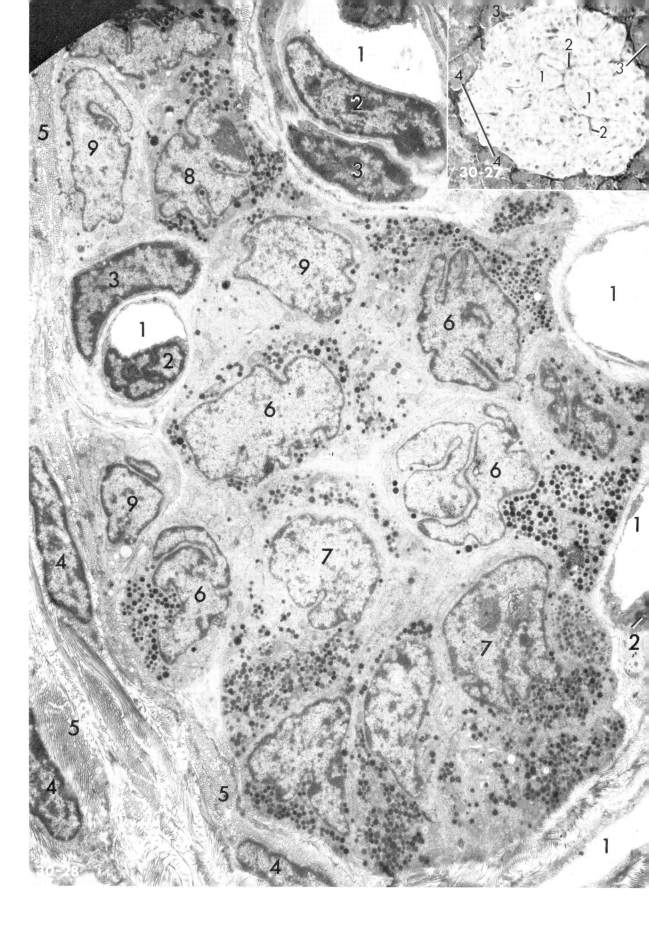

numerous and occupy the interior of the islet. (Fig. 30-30) The mitochondria are large, rounded and more numerous than those of the alpha cells. The Golgi zone is large with many stages of immature, presecretory granules. The granular endoplasmic reticulum is unobtrusive with short and usually vesicular cisternae. The secretory granules are numerous and variable in size and shape. The average width is about 2000 Å. In man and dog, the granules consist of a loose fitting boundary membrane and a core of one or several rectangular or polygonal crystals, embedded in a flocculent substance. A regularly repeated linear substructure characterizes the crystals. In preserving the beta cells for light microscopy, their granules are alcohol soluble.

Delta cells. In man and dog, the delta cells can be distinguished ultrastructurally from the alpha cells on the basis of their lower electron density and the larger secretory granules. The delta cells are always located among the alpha cells, and are generally larger. (Fig. 30-31) The secretory granules have less distinct inner and outer zones than the alpha cell granules, and the central core lacks high electron density. Other cell organelles also appear less distinct.

C-Cells. The C-cells have been described in the guinea pig and may be found also in rat and man. Their cytoplasm is electron-lucent. In size, number and distribution, cell organelles are similar to what is recorded in the beta cells. Small secretory granules may be present in limited number (Fig. 30-32), or they are totally absent.

SYNTHESIS AND FUNCTIONS OF HORMONES

It is generally recognized that the beta cells secrete insulin and that the glucagon is secreted by the alpha cells. Both hormones are polypeptides and their synthesis therefore probably occurs by action of the granular endoplasmic reticulum and the Golgi membranes. The release of the hormones may occur through a diffusion across the cytoplasm and cell membrane,

although discharge of secretory granules can be recorded in rare instances. There is mounting evidence that the C-cells are undifferentiated precursor cells, probably responsible for the regeneration of both alpha and beta cells. The delta cell most likely represents a functional variation of the alpha cell. Its ultrastructural appearance indicates that it is engaged in either presecretory synthetic build-up of secretory granules, or hormonal release by diffusion, since the secretory granules have a low electron density.

Insulin stimulates the conversion of glucose to glycogen and increases the glucose uptake by cells, especially the liver and skeletal muscle, thereby lowering blood sugar levels. The effect of glucagon is opposite that of the insulin, since it brings about a breakdown of liver glycogen, elevating blood sugar concentration. It also inhibits protein synthesis in general. There are indications that a hormone in the anterior lobe of the pituitary, probably the growth hormone (STH) has a pancreotrophic influence, particularly on the insulin release.

Fig. 30-29. Detail of alpha (glucagon) cell. Islet of Langerhans. Pancreas. Rat. E.M. X 17,000. **1.** Nucleus. **2.** Mitochondria. **3.** Secretory granules with loosely fitting boundary membrane. **4.** Cell membrane. **5.** Collagenous fibrils. **6.** Capillary endothelium. **7.** Capillary lumen. **8.** Inset: secretory granules; X 60,000. **9.** Discharging secretory granule, boundary membrane fused with surface membrane.

Fig. 30-30. Detail of beta (insulin) cell. Islet of Langerhans. Pancreas. Rat. E.M. X 17,000. **1.** Nucleus. **2.** Mitochondria. **3.** Secretory granules with angular core. **4.** Inset: secretory granule with rectangular crystalline core; X 60,000.

Fig. 30-31. Detail of delta cell. Islet of Langerhans. Pancreas. Rat. E.M. X 17,000. **1.** Nucleus. **2.** Mitochondria. **3.** Dense secretory granule. **4.** Electron-lucent secretory granules.

Fig. 30-32. Detail of C-cell. Islet of Langerhans. Pancreas. Rat. E.M. X 17,000. **1.** Nucleus. **2.** Mitochondria. **3.** Golgi zone. **4.** Limited number of small secretory granules. **5.** Lysosome.

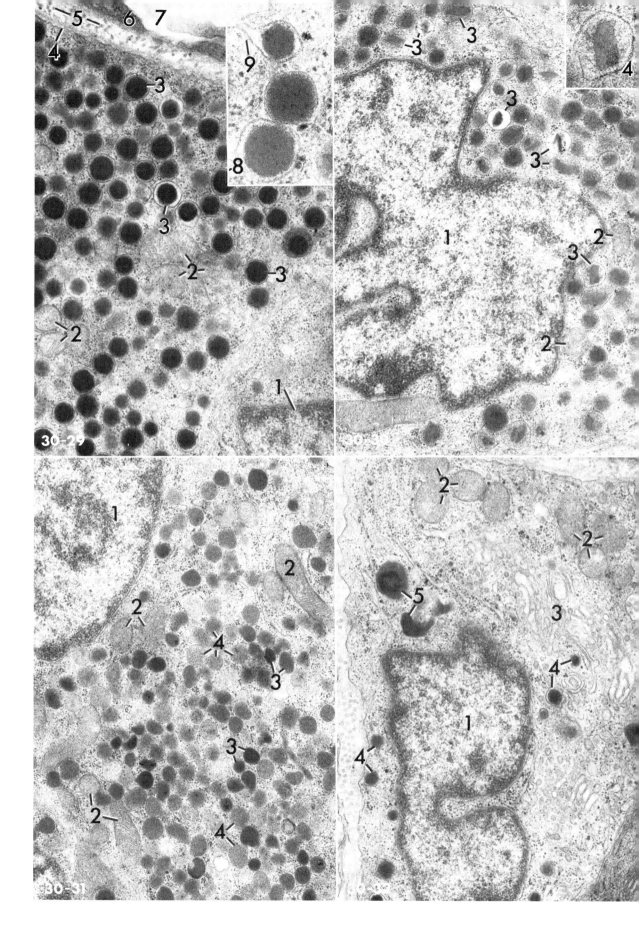

References

LIVER

Amakawa, T. Electron microscopic studies on lysosomes in human hepatic parenchymal cells. J. Electron Micr. *16*: 154–168 (1967).

Bassi, M., Cajone, F. and Bernelli-Zazzera, A. Agranular endoplasmic reticulum in liver cells during glycogen loss and glycogen accumulation. J. Submicr. Cytol. *1*: 143–158 (1969).

Biempica, L. Human hepatic microbodies with crystalloid cores. J. Cell Biol. *29*: 383–386 (1966).

Boler, R. K. Fine structure of canine Kupffer cells and their microtubule-containing cytosomes. Anat. Rec. *163*: 483–496 (1969).

Brown, W. R., Grodsky, G. M. and Carbone, J. V. Intracellular distribution of tritiated bilirubin during hepatic uptake and excretion. Am. J. Physiol. *207*: 1237–1244 (1965).

Bruni, C. and Porter, K. R. The fine structure of the parenchymal cell of the normal rat liver. Am. J. Path. *46*: 691–755 (1965).

Burkel, W. E. The fine structure of the terminal branches of the hepatic arterial system of the rat. Anat. Rec. *167*: 329–350 (1970).

Burkel, W. E. and Low, F. N. The fine structure of rat liver sinusoids, space of Disse and associated tissue space. Am. J. Anat. *118*: 769–784 (1966).

Cardell, R. R., Jr. Action of metabolic hormones on the fine structure of rat liver cells. I. Effects of fasting on the ultrastructure of hepatocytes. Am. J. Anat. *131*: 21–54 (1971).

Chapman, G. B., Chiarodo, A. J., Coffey, R. J. and Wieneke, K. The fine structure of mucosal epithelial cells of a pathological human gallbladder. Anat. Rec. *154*: 579–616 (1966).

Cossel, L. Die menschliche Leber im Elektronenmikroskop. Gustav Fischer, Jena, 1964.

DeMann, J. C. H. and Blok, A. P. R. Relationship between glycogen and agranular endoplasmic reticulum in rat hepatic cells. J. Histochem. Cytochem. *14*: 135–146 (1966).

Elias, H. Liver morphology. Biological Reviews *30*: 263–310 (1955).

Elias, H. and Sherrick, J. C. Morphology of the Liver. Academic Press, New York, 1969.

Essner, E. Endoplasmic reticulum and the origin of microbodies in fetal mouse liver. Lab. Investig. *17*: 71–87 (1967).

Fawcett, D. W. Observations on the cytology and electron microscopy of hepatic cells. J. Nat. Cancer Inst. *15*: Supp. 1475–1503 (1955).

Flaks, B. Observations on the fine structure of the normal porcine liver. J. Anat. *108*: 563–577 (1971).

Fox, H. Ultrastructure of the human gallbladder epithelium in cholelithiasis and chronic cholecystitis. J. Path. *108*: 157–164 (1972).

Goldfischer, S., Novikoff, A. B., Albala, A. and Biempica, L. Hemoglobin uptake by rat hepatocytes and its breakdown within lysosomes. J. Cell Biol. *44*: 513–529 (1970).

Grubb, D. J. and Jones, A. L. Ultrastructure of hepatic sinusoids in sheep. Anat. Rec. *170*: 75–80 (1971).

Hamilton, R. L., Regen, D. M., Gray, M. E. and LeQuire, V. S. Lipid transport in liver. I. Electron microscopic identification of very low density lipoproteins in perfused rat liver. Lab. Investig. *16*: 305–319 (1967).

Hampton, J. C. Liver. *In* Electron Microscopic Anatomy. (Ed. S. M. Kurtz), Chapter 2, pp. 41–58, Academic Press, New York, 1964.

Hayward, A. F. The fine structure of the gallbladder epithelium of the sheep. Z. Zellforsch. *65*: 331–339 (1965).

Hayward, A. F. The structure of gallbladder epithelium. Int. Rev. Gen. Exp. Zool. *3*: 205–239 (1968).

Ito, T. and Nemoto, M. Über die kupfferschen Sternzellen und die "Fettspeicherungszellen" in der Blutkapillarwand der menschlichen Leber. Okajimas Folia Anat. Japan. *24*: 243–258 (1952).

Ito, T. and Nemoto, M. Über die kupfferschen Sternthe hepatic sinusoidal wall and the fat-storing cells in the normal human liver. Arch. Histol. Japon. *29*: 137–192 (1968).

Kaye, G. I., Wheeler, H. O., Whitlock, R. T. and Lane, N. Fluid transport in rabbit gallbladder. J. Cell Biol. *30*: 237–268 (1966).

Kugler, J. H. Correlation of the glycogen concentration in rat liver and the appearance of glycogen and agranular endoplasmic reticulum. J. Roy. Microsc. Soc. *86*: 285–296 (1966).

Laschi, R. and Casanova, S. Fenestrae closed by a diaphragm in the endothelium of liver sinusoids. J. Microscopie *8*: 1037–1040 (1969).

Leeson, T. S. and Melax, H. Fine structure of the common bile duct in adult rats. Can. J. Zool. *47*: 33–35 (1969).

Loud, A. V. A quantitative stereological description of the ultrastructure of normal rat liver parenchymal cells. J. Cell Biol. *37*: 27–46 (1968).

Luciano, L. Die Feinstruktur der Gallenblase und der Gallengänge. I. Das Epithel der Gallenblase der Maus. Z. Zellforsch. *135*: 87–102 (1972).

Luciano, L. Die Feinstruktur der Gallenblase und der Gallengänge. II. Das Epithel der extrahepatischen Gallengänge der Maus und der Ratte. Z. Zellforsch. *135*: 103–114 (1972).

McCuskey, R. S. A dynamic and static study of hepatic arterioles and hepatic sphincters. Am. J. Anat. *119*: 455–477 (1966).

McCuskey, R. S. Dynamic microscopic anatomy of the fetal liver. I. Microcirculation. Angiology *18*: 648–653 (1967).

Ma, M. H. and Biempica, L. The normal human liver cell. Am. J. Path. *62*: 353–376 (1971).

Nicolescu, P. and Rouiller, C. Beziehungen zwischen den Endothelzellen der Lebersinuoside und den von Kupfferschen Sternzellen. Z. Zellforsch. *76*: 313–338 (1967).

Novikoff, A. B. and Essner, E. The liver cell; some new approaches to its study. Am. J. Med. *29*: 102–131 (1960).

Novikoff, A. B. and Shin, W. Y. The endoplasmic reticulum in the Golgi zone and its relations to microbodies, Golgi apparatus and autophagic vacuoles in rat liver cells. J. Microscopie *3*: 187–206 (1964).

Oudea, P. and Domart-Oudea, M.-C. L'ultrastructure hépatique. I. Le foie normal. Rev. fr. Étud. Clin. biol. *12*: 527–543 (1967).

Parks, H. F. On the uptake of chylomicrons by hepatic cells of mice. Anat. Rec. *142*: 320 (1962).

Parks, H. F. An experimental study of microscopic and submicroscopic lipid inclusions in hepatic cells of the mouse. Am. J. Anat. *120*: 253–280 (1967).

Parks, H. F. Notes on membrane-enclosed lipid spherules in hepatic cells of the mouse. Anat. Rec. *151*: 397 (1965).

Rappaport, A. M. Acinar units and the pathophysiology of the liver. *In* The Liver, Morphology, Biochemistry, Physiology (Ed. C. Rouiller). Vol. 1, pp. 265–328. Academic Press, New York, 1965.

Rhodin, J. A. G. Ultrastructure and function of liver sinusoids. Proc. IV. Intern. Symp. of R. E. S. Kyoto, Japan, pp. 108 –124. 1964.

Riches, D. J. and Palfrey, A. J. The ultrastructure of the bile duct epithelium of the rat. J. Anat. *100*: 429–430 (1966).

Rouiller, C. and Jezequel, A. M. Electron microscopy of the liver. *In* The Liver, Morphology, Biochemistry, Physiology (Ed. C. Rouiller), Vol. I, pp. 195–264. Academic Press, New York, 1965.

Steiner, J. W. and Carruthers, J. S. Studies on the fine structure of the terminal branches of the biliary tree. I. The morphology of normal bile canaliculi, bile pre-ductules (ducts of Hering) and bile ductules. Am. J. Path. *38*: 639–661 (1961).

Sternlieb, I. Electron microscopic study of intrahepatic biliary ductules. J. Microscopie *4*: 71–80 (1965).

Sternlieb, I. Mitochondrion desmosome complexes in human hepatocytes. Z. Zellforsch. *93*: 249–253 (1969).

Svoboda, D., Grady, H. and Azarnoff, D. Microbodies in experimentally altered cells. J. Cell Biol. *35*: 127–152 (1967).

Trotter, N. L. A fine structure study of lipid in mouse liver regeneration after partial hepatectomy. J. Cell Biol. *25*: 233–244 (1964).

Vrensen, G. F. J. M. and Kuyper, Ch. M. A. Involvement of rough endoplasmic reticulum and ribosomes in early stages of glycogen repletion in rat liver. J. Microscopie *8*: 599–614 (1969).

Weibel, E. D., Stäubli, W., Gnägi, H. R. and Hess, F. A. Correlated morphometric and biochemical studies on the liver cell. I. Morphometric model, stereologic methods, and normal morphometric data for rat liver. J. Cell Biol. *42*: 68–91 (1969).

Widman, J.-J., Cotran, R. S. and Fahimi, H. D. Mononuclear phagocytes (Kupffer cells) and endothelial cells. Identification of two functional cell types in rat liver sinusoids by endogenous peroxidase activity. J. Cell Biol. *52*: 159–170 (1971).

Willis, E. J. Crystalline structures in the mitochondria of normal human liver parenchymal cells. J. Cell Biol. *24*: 511–514 (1965).

Wisse, E. An electron microscopic study of the fenestrated endothelial lining of rat liver sinusoids. J. Ultrastruct. Res. *31*: 125–150 (1970).

Wisse, E. An ultrastructural characterization of the endothelial cell in the rat liver sinusoid under normal and various experimental conditions, as a contribution to the distinction between endothelial and Kupffer cells. J. Ultrastruct. Res. *38*: 528–562 (1972).

Wisse, E. and Daems, T. Fine structural study on the sinusoidal lining cells of rat liver. *In* Mononuclear Phagocytes (Ed. R. van Furth), pp. 200–210. Blackwell Scientific Publications, Oxford, 1970.

Wood, R. L. Evidence of species differences in the ultrastructure of the hepatic sinusoid. Z. Zellforsch. *58*: 679–692 (1963).

Wood, R. L. Development of peribiliary dense bodies in embryonic rat. Anat. Rec. *166*: 635–658 (1970).

Yamada, E. The fine structure of the gallbladder epithelium of the mouse. J. Biophys. Biochem. Cytol. *1*: 445–458 (1955).

Yamada, K. Aspects of the fine structure of the intrahepatic bile duct epithelium in normal and cholecystectomized mice. J. Morph. *124*: 1–22 (1968).

Yamada, K. Fine structure of rodent common bile duct epithelium. J. Anat. *105*: 511–523 (1969).

PANCREAS

Caramia, F., Munger, B. L. and Lacy, P. E. The ultrastructural basis for the identification of cell types in the pancreatic islets. I. Guinea pig. Z. Zellforsch. *67*: 533–546 (1965).

Caro, L. G. and Palade, G. E. Protein synthesis, storage, and discharge in the pancreatic exocrine cell. J. Cell Biol. *20*: 473–495 (1964).

Ekholm, R. and Edlund, Y. Ultrastructure of the human endocrine pancreas. J. Ultrastruct. Res. *2*: 453–481 (1959).

Ekholm, R., Zelander, T. and Edlund, Y. The ultrastructural organization of the rat exocrine pancreas. 1. Acinar cells. J. Ultrastruct. Res. *7*: 61–72 (1962).

Ekholm, R., Zelander, T. and Edlund, Y. The ultrastructural organization of the rat exocrine pancreas. 2. Centroacinar cells. Intercalary and intralobular ducts. J. Ultrastruct. Res. *7*: 73–83 (1962).

Greider, M. H., Bencosme, S. A. and Lechago, J. The human pancreatic islet cells and their tumors. I. The normal pancreatic islets. Lab. Investig. *22*: 344–354 (1970).

Ichikawa, A. Fine structural changes in response to hormonal stimulation of the perfused canine pancreas. J. Cell Biol. *24*: 369–385 (1965).

Jamieson, J. D. and Palade, G. E. Condensing vacuole conversion and zymogen granule discharge in pancreatic exocrine cells: metabolic studies. J. Cell Biol. *48*: 503–522 (1971).

Jamieson, J. D. and Palade, G. E. Intracellular transport of secretory proteins in the pancreatic exocrine cell. I. Role of the peripheral elements of the Golgi complex. J. Cell Biol. *34*: 577–596 (1967).

Jamieson, J. D. and Palade, G. E. Intracellular transport of secretory proteins in the pancreatic exocrine cell. II. Transport to condensing vacuoles and zymogen granules. J. Cell Biol. *34*: 597–615 (1967).

Jamieson, J. D. and Palade, G. E. Intracellular transport of secretory proteins in the pancreatic exocrine cell. III. Dissociation of intracellular transport from protein synthesis. J. Cell Biol. *39*: 580–588 (1968).

Jamieson, J. D. and Palade, G. E. Intracellular transport of secretory proteins in the pancreatic exocrine cell. IV. Metabolic requirements. J. Cell Biol. *39*: 589–603 (1968).

Kern, H. F. and Ferner, H. Die Feinstruktur des exokrinen Pankreasgewebes vom Menschen. Z. Zellforsch. *113*: 322–343 (1971).

Lacy, P. E. Electron microscopy of the islets of Langerhans. Diabetes *11*: 509–513 (1962).

Lacy, P. E. The pancreatic beta cell. Structure and function. New Eng. J. Med. *276*: 187–195 (1967).

Lacy, P. E. and Greider, M. H. Ultrastructural organization of mammalian pancreatic islets. *In* Handbook of Physiology, Section 7, Vol. I, Digestion, 1970, pp. 77–000.

Like, A. A. The ultrastructure of the secretory cells of the islets of Langerhans in man. Lab. Investig. *16*: 937–951 (1967).

Merlini, D. and Caramia, F. G. Electron microscopic study of the cells of the human pancreatic islets. Rev. Int. Hepat. *16*: 687–694 (1966).

Munger, B. L., Caramia, F. and Lacy, P. E. The ultrastructural basis for the identification of cell types in the pancreatic islets. II. Rabbit, dog and opossum. Z. Zellforsch. *67*: 776–798 (1965).

Palade, G. E., Siekevitz, P. and Caro, L. G. Structure, chemistry and function of the pancreatic exocrine cell. Ciba Foundation Symp. Exocrine Pancreas, pp. 23–55 (1963).

Sjöstrand, F. S. and Hanzon, V. Membrane structures of cytoplasm and mitochondria in exocrine cells of mouse pancreas as revealed by high resolution electron microscopy. Exp. Cell Res. *7*: 393–414 (1954).

Sjöstrand, F. S. and Hanzon, V. Ultrastructure of Golgi apparatus of exocrine cells of mouse pancreas. Exp. Cell Res. *7*: 415–429 (1954).

31 Respiratory system

The respiratory system in man is designed to facilitate the exchange of oxygen and carbon dioxide between blood and air. This exchange occurs in the respiratory portion of the system across the blood-air barrier, a thin 0.1 μ-membrane which forms an essential part of the pulmonary alveoli or air sacs, of which each lung contains about 150 million. The conducting portion of the respiratory system prepares the air for this exchange by making it warm and moist, and by trapping some of the air-borne dust particles along the way. This portion consists of the nasal cavities, pharynx, larynx, bronchi, and bronchioles, most of which are lined by a special respiratory mucous membrane.

Nasal Cavities

The nasal cavities have several distinctly different regions: 1) vestibular region; 2) respiratory region; 3) olfactory region; and 4) paranasal sinuses.

VESTIBULAR REGION

The vestibular region is restricted to a narrow zone inside the nostrils. It is lined by a thin stratified, squamous epithelium which is only moderately keratinized. The region contains coarse hairs (vibrissae) as well as sebaceous and sweat glands.

RESPIRATORY REGION

This region includes the major part of the nasal cavities with the exception of the upper one-third. Its respiratory mucosa lines the nasal septum, the floor of the nasal cavity and the lateral walls, including the two lower nasal conchae. The respiratory mucosa is composed of: 1) epithelium and 2) lamina propria.

Epithelium. The epithelium is of the pseudostratified ciliated columnar type. This epithelium, with minor modifications, exists throughout the conducting portion of the respiratory system. It is composed of ciliated cells, goblet cells, basal cells, and some intermediate cells.

(Fig. 31-3) The histological and ultrastructural details are described below under the trachea (p. 618). In the nasal cavity, the pseudostratification is less pronounced than in the trachea because of a smaller epithelial height in the nose. The cilia of the nasal mucosa beat and move surface secretions toward the nasopharynx. The epithelium rests on a basement membrane, composed of a thin basal lamina and a network of reticular and collagenous fibrils.

Lamina propria. The lamina propria is unusually thick, being composed of a loose fibroelastic connective tissue. There are no muscle fibers. The lamina propria, especially of the nasal conchae, is richly endowed with large venous plexuses. Their primary function is to warm the air as it passes by. They may become engorged as part of an allergic reaction, or during a nasal infection leading to a

Fig. 31-1. Frontal section of olfactory region of the nasal cavity. Cat. L.M. X 25. 1. Nasal septum. 2. Nasal cavities. 3. Nasal conchae (cat has several more than man). 4. Respiratory epithelium. 5. Olfactory epithelium.

Fig. 31-2. Section of nasal concha. Enlargement of rectangle in Fig. 31-1. Cat. L.M. X 235. 1. Respiratory epithelium. 2. Lamina propria. 3. Bone. 4. Olfactory epithelium. 5. Olfactory nerve bundle.

Fig. 31-3. Transition between respiratory and olfactory epithelia. Enlargement of area similar to rectangle (A) in Fig. 31-2. Cat. E.M. X 1600. 1. Cilia. 2. Nuclei of ciliated cells in respiratory epithelium. 3. Basal cell. 4. Basal lamina. 5. Lamina propria. 6. Sinusoidal capillary. 7. Nuclei of sustentacular cell in olfactory epithelium. 8. Nuclei of olfactory bipolar nerve cells.

Fig. 31-4. Olfactory epithelium. Enlargement of area similar to rectangle (B) in Fig. 31-2. Cat. E.M. X 580. 1. Level of nuclei of sustentacular cells. 2. Nuclei of olfactory bipolar nerve cells. 3. Basal cells. 4. Level of basal lamina. 5. Lamina propria. 6. Olfactory nerve bundle. 7. Bowman's glands. 8. Lumen of excretory duct of Bowman's gland. 9. Postcapillary venule. 10. Lymphatic capillary.

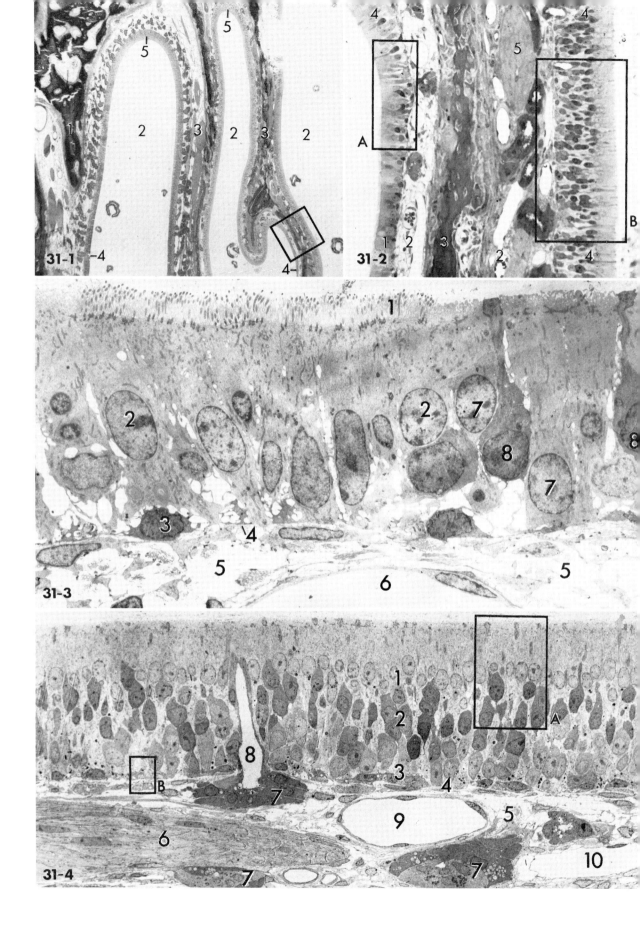

31-1   1   5   2   3   2   3   2   4   4

31-2   A   4   5   1   2   3   2   4   B   4

31-3   1   2   2   7   8   7   3   4   5   6   5

31-4   1   2   8   3   4   7   9   5   6   7   10   7   A   B

swelling of the mucous membrane and a restriction of air passage. There are numerous mixed (seromucous) glands in the lamina propria. These glands are controlled by autonomic nerves, whereas the goblet cells of the epithelium discharge as a result of local stimulation.

OLFACTORY REGION

The olfactory region comprises the roof of the nasal cavity, the upper third of the nasal septum, and the superior nasal concha. (Fig. 31-1) This region is lined by a very high pseudostratified columnar olfactory epithelium and by a vascularized lamina propria rich in olfactory nerve bundles and the special seromucous glands of this region, the Bowman's glands.

Olfactory epithelium. The olfactory pseudostratified columnar epithelium is twice as high as the respiratory epithelium, averaging about 60 μ in height. (Fig. 31-2) Normally, it has a slight yellow color because of an accumulation of pigment granules in some of the cells. It is composed of: 1) olfactory bipolar nerve cells; 2) sustentacular cells; and 3) basal cells. (Fig. 31-4)

The **olfactory cells** are true bipolar neurons. The nuclei of neighboring olfactory nerve cells are situated at different levels within the lower half of the epithelium, giving it the typical appearance of a pronounced crowding of nuclei. (Fig. 31-5) A peripheral, thin **dendritic process** extends to the surface of the epithelium where it terminates as a club-shaped swelling, the **olfactory vesicle.** Ten to fifteen very long non-motile cilia extend laterally from this vesicle above and parallel to the epithelial surface. (Figs. 31-7, 31-8) They contain the typical 9 + 2 pattern of longitudinally arranged microtubules, originating from a basal body. The outer two-thirds of each cilium are greatly reduced in diameter and contain only two or three single microtubules. The olfactory vesicle and the dendritic process contain many mitochondria, microtubules and neurofilaments. Below the

nucleus of the olfactory cell, the cytoplasm forms a thin, 0.1 μ-wide thread-like **central process** (axon) which perforates the basal lamina and joins up with similar processes from other olfactory cells to form bundles of non-myelinated olfactory nerves. (Fig. 31-10) They perforate the lamina cribriformis of the ethmoid bone as fila olfactoria and synapse with a second neuron in the olfactory bulbs.

The **sustentacular cells** are tall columnar cells with a tapering base resting on the basal lamina. Their nuclei form the most superficial layer of nuclei in the epithelium. Numerous long and slender microvilli extend from their apical surface, forming an entangled network of olfactory cilia and microvilli from other sustentacular cells. (Fig. 31-6) The cytoplasm of the sustentacular cells contains many tubular profiles of the agranular

Fig. 31-5. Olfactory epithelium. Enlargement of area similar to rectangle (A) in Fig. 31-4. Cat. E.M. $\times$ 1900. **1.** Nuclei of sustentacular cells. **2.** Nuclei of olfactory bipolar nerve cells. **3.** Peripheral dendritic processes of olfactory bipolar nerve cells. **4.** Olfactory vesicle. **5.** Microvilli of sustentacular cells.

Fig. 31-6. Detail of free surface of sustentacular cell of olfactory epithelium. Enlargement of area similar to rectangle (A) in Fig. 31-5. Cat. E.M. X 80,000. **1.** Thin, branching microvilli. **2.** Cross-sectioned peripheral parts of cilia from adjacent olfactory bipolar nerve cells containing two or three microtubules. **3.** Profiles of agranular endoplasmic reticulum. **4.** Mitochondrion.

Fig. 31-7. Detail of olfactory vesicle. Enlargement of area similar to rectangle (B) in Fig. 31-5. Cat. E.M. X 48,000. **1.** Parts of sustentacular cells. **2.** Junctional complexes. **3.** Mitochondria in olfactory vesicle. **4.** Basal bodies. **5.** Olfactory cilia. **6.** Microvilli. **7.** Mitochondria in sustentacular cell. **8.** Microtubules.

Fig. 31-8. Cross section of olfactory vesicle (sectioned parallel to the epithelial surface). Rat. E.M. X 87,000. **1.** Center of olfactory vesicle. **2.** Basal bodies. **3.** Olfactory cilia **4.** Longitudinally sectioned peripheral parts of olfactory cilia from adjacent olfactory vesicles. **5.** Cross-sectioned microvilli ascending from sustentacular cells.

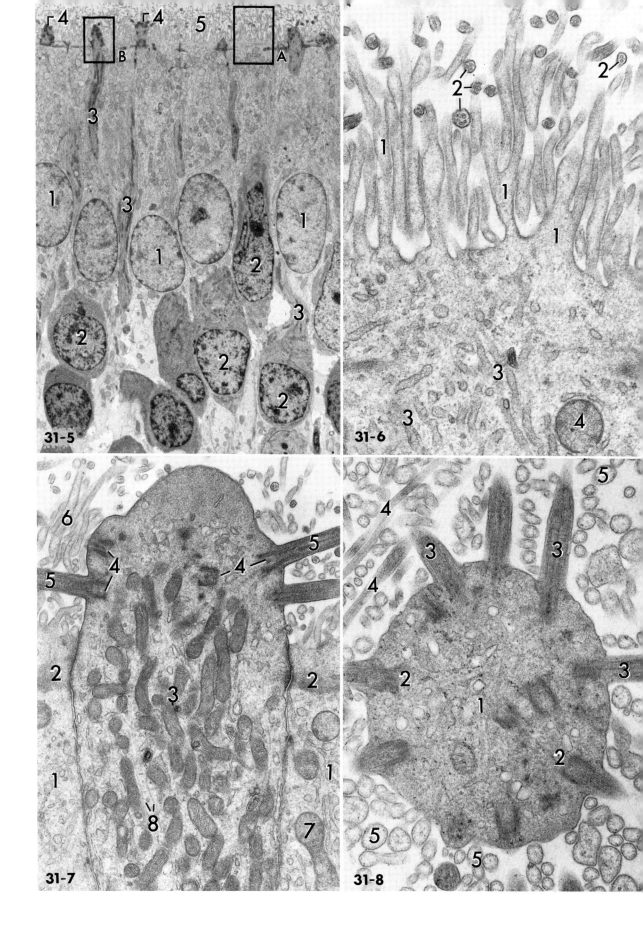

endoplasmic reticulum, but also some tonofilaments and a wealth of mitochondria, lysosomes, and lipofuscin granules (pigments). Junctional complexes and terminal webs make the contact firm between sustentacular cells and bipolar olfactory neurons.

The **basal cells** are small and few in number. They probably represent stem cells which may develop into sustentacular cells. (Fig. 31-11)

The **basal lamina** is extremely thin, and cannot be seen under the light microscope, mainly because reticular and collagenous fibrils are not present to enhance its thickness. (Fig. 31-10)

Lamina propria. In similarity with the respiratory region of the nasal cavity, it contains a loose network of fibroelastic connective tissue. The vascularization is rich but the large venous plexuses are less prominent. There are many large glands, specific for this region, the glands of Bowman. The acini of these glands contain both serous and mucus-producing cells. (Fig. 31-12) The cytoplasm of the serous cells contains an extremely large amount of concentrically arranged profiles of agranular endoplasmic reticulum. Mixed in with the secretory granules of these cells are numerous lysosomes and lipofuscin granules, and it has been assumed that this is also a source of the yellow pigmentation of the olfactory region.

Function. The cilia of the olfactory bipolar nerve cells undoubtedly represent the part that reacts with the air-borne scent particles and brings about a change in cell membrane potential, initiating the nerve impulse. The secretions of the Bowman's glands probably serve as mediators in this process by dissolving the odor-producing chemicals. It is uncertain what role the sustentacular cells play in this process. There is a possibility that they moderate the viscosity of the mucous layer by absorption, but it is more likely that they establish a lateral support and represent a means of intraepithelial ionic com-munication through their junctional association with the olfactory bipolar neurons.

PARANASAL SINUSES

These include the maxillary, ethmoid, frontal, and sphenoid sinuses. Lining the sinuses is a pseudostratified ciliated columnar epithelium similar to the epithelium of the respiratory region of the nasal cavities. However, in man, this epithelium is often of the simple columnar ciliated type with few goblet cells. The cilia beat toward the nasal ostium of the sinus. The lamina propria is very thin and blends with the periosteum. Only very few and small seromucous glands are present.

Fig. 31-9. Detail of basal part of olfactory epithelium. Enlargement of area similar to rectangle (B) in Fig. 31-4. Cat. E.M. X 39,000. **1.** Nucleus of olfactory bipolar nerve cell. **2.** Basal part of sustentacular cells. **3.** Tonofibrils. **4.** Central processes (axons) of bipolar nerve cells. **5.** Basal lamina. **6.** Bundle of olfactory nerves in lamina propria. **7.** Collagenous fibrils. **8.** Lipofuscin granules.

Fig. 31-10. Detail of basal part of olfactory epithelium. Enlargement of area similar to rectangle in Fig. 31-9. Cat. E.M. X 128,000. **1.** Cytoplasm of sustentacular cell. **2.** Cytoplasmic processes of basal cells. **3.** Cross-sectioned central processes (axons) of olfactory bipolar nerve cells. **4.** Microtubules. **5.** Mitochondria. **6.** Desmosomes. **7.** Basal lamina. **8.** Collagenous fibrils in lamina propria.

Fig. 31-11. Olfactory epithelium. Enlargement of duct of Bowman's gland seen in Fig. 31-4. Cat. E.M. X 1200. **1.** Lumen of duct. **2.** Nuclei of secretory cells of Bowman's gland. **3.** Nucleus of secretory duct cell. **4.** Nucleus of squamous duct cell. **5.** Nuclei of basal cells. **6.** Nuclei of olfactory bipolar nerve cells.

Fig. 31-12. Olfactory epithelium. Detail of Bowman's gland in lamina propria. Cat. E.M. X 25,000. **1.** Nuclei of serous cells. **2.** Nucleus of mucous cell. **3.** Mucous droplets. **4.** Discharging mucous droplets containing a dense granular substance. **5.** Lumen of gland. **6.** Golgi zone. **7.** Serous secretory granules. **8.** Granular endoplasmic reticulum. **9.** Agranular endoplasmic reticulum.

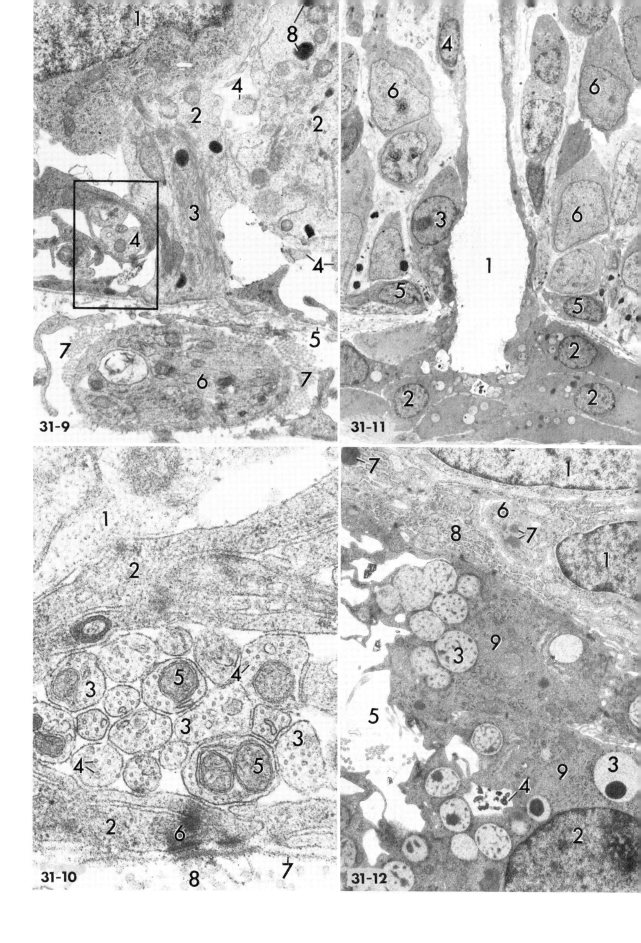

31-9

31-11

31-10

31-12

Nasopharynx

The pharynx is generally divided into nasopharynx, oropharynx, and hypopharynx (or laryngeal pharynx). The nasal cavities and the auditory (Eustachian) tubes open into the nasopharynx, which is the uppermost part of the pharynx. The nasopharynx is lined by the same respiratory pseudostratified ciliated columnar epithelium found in the nasal cavities. The lamina propria contains fibroelastic connective tissue and lymphocytes of which many are aggregated to form the pharyngeal tonsils in the roof of the nasopharynx. Seromucous glands are present in the lamina propria. A thick coat of striated muscle fibers forms a muscularis externa. It consists of an inner longitudinal layer (levator) and an outer circular layer (constrictor). There is no distinct borderline where the respiratory epithelium of the nasopharynx changes to the stratified squamous epithelium of the oropharynx. However, the change of epithelium is generally seen in the area where the uvula and the soft palate touch the posterior and lateral walls of the pharynx during the act of swallowing. Both the oropharynx and the laryngeal pharynx are lined by stratified squamous non-keratinized epithelium of the same type which covers the major part of the oral cavity (p. 506).

Larynx

The larynx is interposed between the pharynx above and the trachea below. In this position, it is part of the conducting portion of the respiratory system and it also serves as an important part of the organ of voice in the production of sound. The larynx is composed of three single and three paired cartilages, several striated muscles, and a laryngeal cavity lined by a mucous membrane.

LARYNGEAL CARTILAGES

The three single cartilages are the epiglottis, the thyroid, and the cricoid. The **epiglottis** is spoon-shaped and made of elastic cartilage (Fig. 31-13), whereas the **thyroid** and the **cricoid cartilages** are ring-shaped and consist of a hyaline type of cartilage which has a tendency of becoming calcified and even ossified early in life. The paired cartilages, smaller and irregularly shaped, are the **arytenoid, corniculate,** and **cuneiform cartilages.** The major part of the arytenoid cartilages consists of hyaline cartilage, but their tips and the entire corniculate and cuneiform cartilages are elastic in type.

Fig. 31-13. Frontal section of epiglottis. Monkey. L.M. X 15. **1.** Hypopharynx. **2.** Cartilage of epiglottis. **3.** Vestibule of laryngeal cavity. **4.** Pharyngeal tonsils. **5.** Stratified squamous non-keratinized epithelium.

Fig. 31-14. Epiglottis. Enlargement of rectangle in Fig. 31-13. Monkey. L.M. X 105. **1.** Stratified squamous non-keratinized epithelium. **2.** Lamina propria with elastic fibers. **3.** Mucous glands. **4.** Elastic cartilage of epiglottis. **5.** Single taste bud.

Fig. 31-15. Frontal section of larynx. Monkey. L.M. X 10. **1.** Vestibule. **2.** Ventricles. **3.** Rima glottidis. **4.** Infraglottic cavity. **5.** Ventricular folds (false vocal cords). **6.** Vocal folds (true vocal cords). **7.** Vocal (thyroarytenoid) muscle. **8.** Thyroid cartilage. **9.** Cricoid cartilage.

Fig. 31-16. Enlargement of larynx in Fig. 31-15. Monkey. L.M. X 31. **1.** False cords. **2.** Laryngeal ventricle. **3.** Vocal muscle. **4.** Vocal ligament. **5.** Mucous glands. **6.** Lymph nodule.

Fig. 31-17. Stratified squamous non-keratinized epithelium. Vocal folds. Larynx. Enlargement of rectangle (A) in Fig. 31-16. Monkey. L.M. X 600. **1.** Lamina propria. **2.** Basal lamina. **3.** Stratum germinativum. **4.** Nuclei are retained in squamous superficial layers.

Fig. 31-18. Stratified or pseudostratified columnar epithelium. Ventricle of larynx. Enlargement of rectangle (B) in Fig. 31-16. Monkey. L.M. X 600. **1.** Diffuse lymphoid infiltration in lamina propria. **2.** Basal lamina. **3.** Basal cells. **4.** Columnar non-ciliated cells.

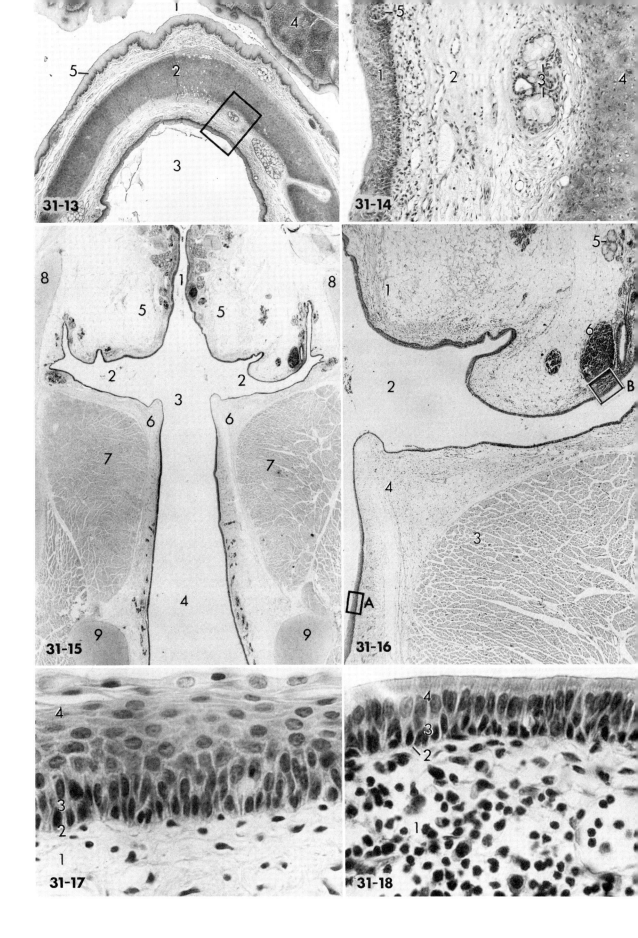

31-13

31-14

31-15

31-16

31-17

31-18

LARYNGEAL MUSCLES

There are nine **extrinsic** muscles. They originate in structures other than the larynx, and their function is to move the larynx as a whole, which is necessary during swallowing. The **intrinsic** muscles, of which there are also nine, originate from and insert on the laryngeal cartilages. These muscles move the laryngeal cartilages in relation to each other, and thereby change the laryngeal cavity and modulate the sounds produced as the air passes through the rima glottidis. The muscles consist of delicate striated skeletal muscle fibers. The intrinsic muscles, except for one, receive their motor innervation from the recurrent laryngeal nerve.

LARYNGEAL CAVITY

The laryngeal cavity consists of the vestibule, the ventricles, and the infraglottic cavity. (Fig. 31-15) This subdivision of the cavity is based on two pairs of lateral folds which extend in an anterior-posterior direction. These are uppermost the **ventricular folds** (synonyms: vestibular folds; false vocal cords); and beneath, the **vocal folds** (true vocal cords). The vocal cords limit the **rima glottidis** which is the central laryngeal opening. The vocal cords and the rima glottidis constitute the **glottis**. The **vestibule** extends from the entrance of the larynx to the ventricular folds. The right and left **laryngeal ventricles** are situated between the ventricular folds and the true vocal cords. (Fig. 31-16) The **infraglottic cavity** is located beneath the true vocal cords and is continuous with the lumen of the trachea. The laryngeal cavity is lined by a mucous membrane which consists of a surface epithelium and a lamina propria. Generally, one recognizes also a submucosa.

Epithelium. The epithelium varies according to its location. The entire pharyngeal surface of the epiglottis, the upper half of the laryngeal surface, a portion of the ventricular folds, and the true vocal cords are lined by a stratified squamous, non-keratinized epithelium. (Fig. 31-17)

Including the lower half of the laryngeal surface of the epiglottis, the rest of the laryngeal cavity is lined by a respiratory pseudostratified ciliated columnar epithelium with goblet cells. In the narrow zones of transition between these two kinds of epithelia, there often occurs a stratified columnar epithelium which may be ciliated. (Fig. 31-18) Throughout the larynx, the cilia beat and move the superficial blanket of mucus toward the pharynx.

Lamina propria. The lamina propria contains a large number of elastic fibrils. The true vocal cords have a concentration of elastic fibers referred to as **vocal ligaments** (thyroarytenoid ligaments). In relation to the laryngeal ventricles are numerous lymphocytes, often aggregated to form solitary nodules. (Fig. 31-16) Mucous and seromucous glands are abundant in the lamina propria of the ventricles and the ventricular folds. Peripheral to the elastic vocal ligaments lie the intrinsic thyroarytenoid muscles which control the ten-

Fig. 31-19. Cross section of trachea. Monkey. L.M. X 10. **1.** Lumen. **2.** Mucous membrane. **3.** C-shaped cartilage. **4.** Adventitia. **5.** Trachealis muscle. **6.** Fibroelastic membrane. This part of the trachea faces posteriorly. **7.** Part of adjacent esophagus.

Fig. 31-20. Wall of trachea. Enlargement of area similar to rectangle in Fig. 31-19. Monkey. L.M. X 80. **1.** Lumen. **2.** Epithelium. **3.** Lamina propria. **4.** Submucosa. **5.** Mucous glands. **6.** Fibrous perichondrium. **7.** Hyaline tracheal cartilage. **8.** Outer fibroelastic membrane.

Fig. 31-21. Wall of trachea. Enlargement of area similar to rectangle in Fig. 31-20. Human. E.M. X 320. **1.** Lumen of trachea. **2.** Pseudostratified, columnar ciliated (respiratory) epithelium. **3.** Level of basement membrane. **4.** Lamina propria. **5.** Blood vessel. **6.** Submucosa.

Fig. 31-22. Pseudostratified, columnar ciliated (respiratory) epithelium. Trachea. Human. E.M. X 1800. **1.** Lumen of trachea. **2.** Cilia. **3.** Nuclei of ciliated cells. **4.** Nuclei of goblet (mucous) cells. **5.** Nuclei of intermediate cells. **6.** Nuclei of basal cells. **7.** Basement membrane. **8.** See Fig. 31-25.

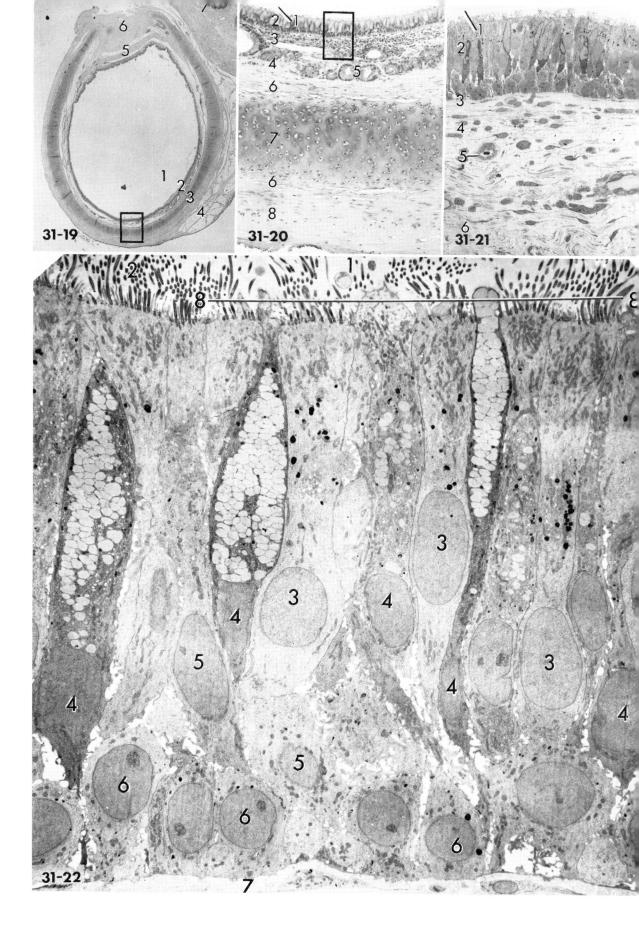

31-19

31-20

31-21

31-22

sion of the true vocal cords and, therefore, often are referred to as the **vocal muscles.**

Submucosa. The submucosa consists of a layer of connective tissue fibers which are more loosely arranged than those of the lamina propria. The seromucous glands are often situated in the submucosa. Peripherally, the submucosa merges with the fibroelastic membranes which connect the thyroid, cricoid, and arytenoid cartilages to one another.

Trachea and Primary Bronchi

The trachea and the two primary (main) bronchi which are smaller tubes, establish the main and longest extrapulmonary conducting portion of the respiratory system. Their structural organization is similar, consisting of a mucous membrane, a fibroelastic membrane, and rings of cartilage. (Fig. 31-19) The structures aid in ensuring the permanent patency of these tubes which is required to pass air to and from the lungs.

MUCOUS MEMBRANE

The mucous membrane lines the lumen of the trachea and primary bronchi, presenting slight longitudinal folds. It consists of a respiratory epithelium and a lamina propria. (Fig. 31-21) A lamina muscularis mucosae, a characteristic structure of the mucosa of the digestive tube, is lacking in the trachea but is present in the bronchi. (Fig. 31-33)

Epithelium. This is a **typical respiratory** pseudostratified ciliated columnar epithelium. The height is slightly larger in the trachea and smaller in the main bronchi, averaging about 30 μ. It is composed of ciliated cells, goblet cells, basal cells, intermediate cells, and some brush cells. (Fig. 31-22)

The **ciliated cells** predominate. Above the nucleus the cell is columnar; below, it may taper off as it touches the basement membrane. The nuclei of adjacent cells may be located at different levels, giving the false impression of a stratification of cells. The cells contain numerous mitochondria, most of which are clustered in the apical part of the cell. There is a large Golgi zone, some profiles of granular endoplasmic reticulum, many ribosomes and lysosomes, both primary and secondary. Occasional bundles of tonofilaments occur. Small desmosomes along the lateral cell borders attach the ciliated cells to neighboring cells in addition to junctional complexes near the epithelial surface. Short, slender microvilli and long cilia extend from the luminal surface of the ciliated cells. (Fig. 31-23) There are about 250 cilia per cell (Fig. 31-25), averaging 5μ in length. Each cilium contains longitudinally arranged microtubules: two single in the center and nine double in the periphery. The latter emanate from nine

Fig. 31-23. Detail of free surface of ciliated cells. Respiratory epithelium. Trachea. Human. E.M. X 7000. **1.** Lumen. **2.** Cilia. **3.** Short microvilli. **4.** Basal bodies. **5.** Junctional complexes. **6.** Cell borders. **7.** Mitochondria. **8.** Lysosomes.

Fig. 31-24. Detail of respiratory epithelium Trachea. Human. E.M. X 15,000. **1.** Cytoplasm of ciliated cell. **2.** Cytoplasm of mucous (goblet) cell. **3.** Cell borders. **4.** Intercellular space. **5.** Nucleus. **6.** Mitochondria. **7.** Lysosomes.

Fig. 31-25. Cross section of cilia and mucous cells at the level indicated by line 8–8 in Fig. 31-22. Trachea. Human. E.M. X 15,000. **1.** Domes of mucous cells with secretory droplets, protruding above surface level of adjacent ciliated cells. **2.** The line indicates the group of cilia (about 250) that belongs to one ciliated cell. The demarcation lines of groups of cilia indicating other cells are more difficult to see. They are indicated by incompletely drawn dotted lines.

Fig. 31-26. Cross section of cilia and basal bodies. Respiratory epithelium. Trachea. Human. E.M. X 60,000. **1.** Basal bodies with 9 triplets of microtubules. **2.** Lateral spurs. **3.** At a level above the basal bodies, the 9 triplets become 9 doublets of microtubules. **4.** At a slightly higher level, a central pair of microtubules takes its origin and runs the entire length of the cilium. See also p. 19.

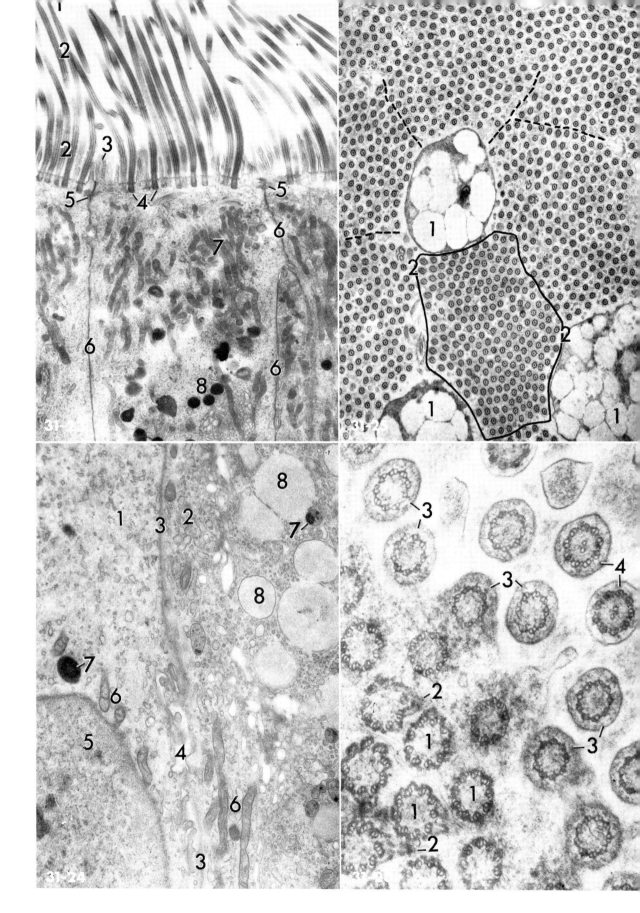

triple microtubules in the basal bodies just below the cell surface. (Fig. 31-26) The basal bodies possess short striated rootlets and often lateral spurs. The cilia beat with a rapid stroke forward while they are rigid and straight; and a slow recovery stroke when they are flaccid and bending. The beating is brought about by a sliding of the peripheral microtubules. The actual mechanism is not understood but it is believed that the different phases of the stroke originate in the basal body. The two central microtubules may have a conducting function. A thin network of cytoplasmic filaments interconnects the basal bodies in some mammalian species which may account for the synchronization of ciliary beat within restricted areas. By their beating, 22 beats/sec, the cilia move the highly viscous superficial blanket of mucus in the direction of the larynx at a pace of about 14 mm/min. The normal life span of the ciliated cells has not been determined. It is known that the cells are readily sloughed as a result of viral or bacterial infections, or as a result of abrasive forces brought on by mucous surfaces rubbing against each other. If the infection or abrasive forces persist over prolonged periods a metaplasia occurs, resulting in a stratified squamous epithelium.

The **goblet cells** are mucus-producing cells occurring singly in the respiratory epithelium. Their structure is similar to that of goblet cells in the small and large intestines (Fig. 31-24), and has been described on p. 80. The goblet cells of the respiratory epithelium discharge as a result of local stimulation. Contributing factors are the temperature and moisture, as well as the degree of dust and noxious gases in the inhaled air. The blanket of mucus has a highly viscous surface layer, touched by the tips of the cilia during the forward stroke, and a serous basal layer in which the cilia move during the recovery stroke. The viscosity of the layers is adjusted by secretory and absorptive processes, governed by the epithelium itself.

The **basal cells** are small, polyhedral cells resting on the basement membrane. The round nucleus occupies a large portion of the cell. (Fig. 31-22) The cytoplasm contains a few mitochondria, numerous free ribosomes, and bundles of tonofilaments. (Fig. 31-28) The Golgi zone is vestigial if present at all. These cells represent stem cells of the respiratory epithelium and may develop into either ciliated cells or goblet cells via the intermediate cells.

The **intermediate cells** are pyramidal cells with their broad base touching the basal lamina and the apical end wedged between ciliated and goblet cells, not quite reaching the epithelial surface. The nucleus is above the level of the basal cell nuclei. (Fig. 31-22) The cytoplasm is rich in ribosomes and tonofilaments. The intermediate cells are derived from the basal

Fig. 31-27. Survey of basement membrane. Respiratory epithelium. Trachea. Human. E.M. X 3000. **1.** Basal cells of pseudostratified columnar ciliated (respiratory) epithelium. **2.** Basement membrane is made up of densely packed fine collagenous fibrils. **3.** Nuclei of fibroblasts. **4.** Loose connective tissue of lamina propria.

Fig. 31-28. Detail of basal cell. Respiratory epithelium. Trachea. Enlargement of area similar to rectangle in Fig. 31-27. Human. E.M. X 30,000. **1.** Nucleus of basal cell. **2.** Mitochondria. **3.** Tonofilaments. **4.** Ribosomes. **5.** Basal cell membrane. **6.** Basal lamina forms a thin part of the basement membrane of the respiratory epithelium. **7.** Delicate collagenous fibrils of basement membrane.

Fig. 31-29. Posterior wall of trachea. Cross section. Monkey. L.M. X 56. **1.** Lumen of trachea. **2.** Respiratory epithelium. **3.** Lamina propria. **4.** Trachealis muscle. **5.** Fibroelastic membrane. **6.** Free ends of C-shaped tracheal cartilage. **7.** Excretory duct of tracheal glands.

Fig. 31-30. Detail of posterior wall of trachea. Monkey. L.M. X 120. **1.** Lumen of trachea. **2.** Respiratory epithelium. **3.** Lamina propria. **4.** Trachealis muscle. **5.** Perichondrium. **6.** Tracheal cartilage (hyaline). **7.** Fibroelastic membrane. **8.** Serous glands. **9.** Excretory duct.

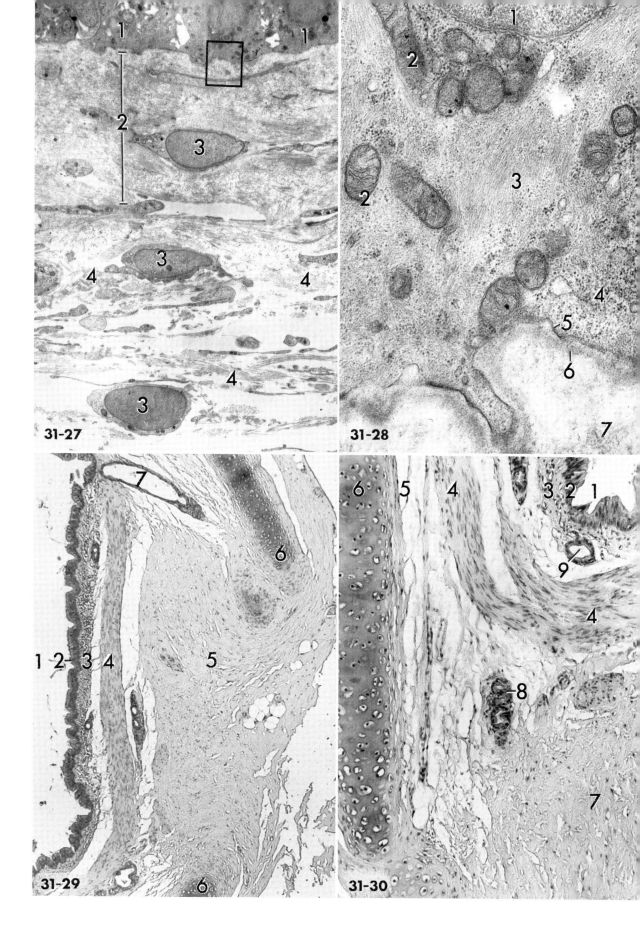

31-27

31-28

31-29

31-30

cells and represent intermediate stages of the development into either ciliated or goblet cells.

Yet another cell, termed **brush cell,** is infrequently present. It is columnar; and the luminal surface is provided with numerous microvilli, each containing longitudinally arranged, irregularly distributed filaments which do not originate from basal bodies, although they descend into the apical part of the cell. The cytoplasm contains mitochondria, ribosomes, and lysosomes. Sensory nerve endings are present near the base of the cell. The origin and function of this cell type are still largely unexplored. Suggestions relate to absorptive processes, sensory functions, and precursor or degenerative stages of either ciliated or goblet cells.

The **basement membrane** is composed of a thin basal lamina and a thick, dense network of reticular and collagenous fibrils. (Fig. 31-27) This is the best example of an epithelial basement membrane that can easily be observed by light microscopy.

Lamina propria. This includes a relatively narrow inner layer of fibrous connective tissue rich in lymphocytes, wandering blood cells, and vasculature. An outer layer consists of elastic tissue in which most of the elastic fibers are longitudinally disposed. This is often referred to as the inner **fibroelastic membrane** (Fig. 31-29), an arrangement that originates in the larynx and continues down into the secondary and tertiary intrapulmonary bronchi.

Muscularis mucosae. This layer is missing in the trachea but is present in the main bronchi where it is composed of interlacing bundles of circularly arranged smooth muscle cells. The cells form a complete muscular coat at the outermost boundary of the mucous membrane of the bronchi. (Fig. 31-33)

SUBMUCOSA

The submucosa consists of loose connective tissue. It supports the many small

mucous and **seromucous glands** which send short excretory ducts through the mucosa and empty their secretions at the epithelial surface.

CARTILAGE

There are about 20 c-shaped cartilages in the trachea and an additional 6–10 cartilages in each of the main bronchi. They are arranged at regular intervals. The gap in the incomplete rings faces posteriorly. Each cartilage, being of the hyaline type, is surrounded by a fibrous perichondrium. As a continuation of this perichondrium, an intercartilaginous, outer **fibroelastic membrane** unites the edges and the ends of adjoining cartilages. The elastic components of the trachea facilitate the stretching during breathing and swallowing. Assisting in closing the posterior gap is a **trachealis muscle,** composed of transversely and obliquely arranged smooth muscle cells, mixed in with the fibroelastic membrane. (Fig. 31-30) The muscle fibers are inserted into the perichondrium. In the posterior membranous part of the trachea and main bronchi, the mucosa and submucosa are especially thick. Here the seromucous glands are large and often situated outside of the trachealis muscle and muscularis mucosae of the bronchi.

ADVENTITIA

The adventitia, of which the cartilaginous rings often are considered an essential part, consists of loose connective tissue

Fig. 31-31. Survey of lung. Monkey. L.M. X 7. **1.** Secondary bronchi. **2.** Tertiary bronchi and their subdivisions. **3.** Bronchioles. **4.** Respiratory bronchioles. **5.** Branches of pulmonary artery. **6.** Branches of pulmonary vein. **7.** Alveolar ducts and alveoli. **8.** Pleura visceralis. *Rectangles:* **A** is enlarged in Fig. 31-32. **B** is enlarged in Fig. 31-38; it contains a bronchiole and a branch of the pulmonary artery. **C** is enlarged in Fig. 31-41; it contains bronchioles, respiratory bronchioles, alveolar ducts, and alveoli. **D** is enlarged in Fig. 31-62; it contains a branch of the pulmonary vein.

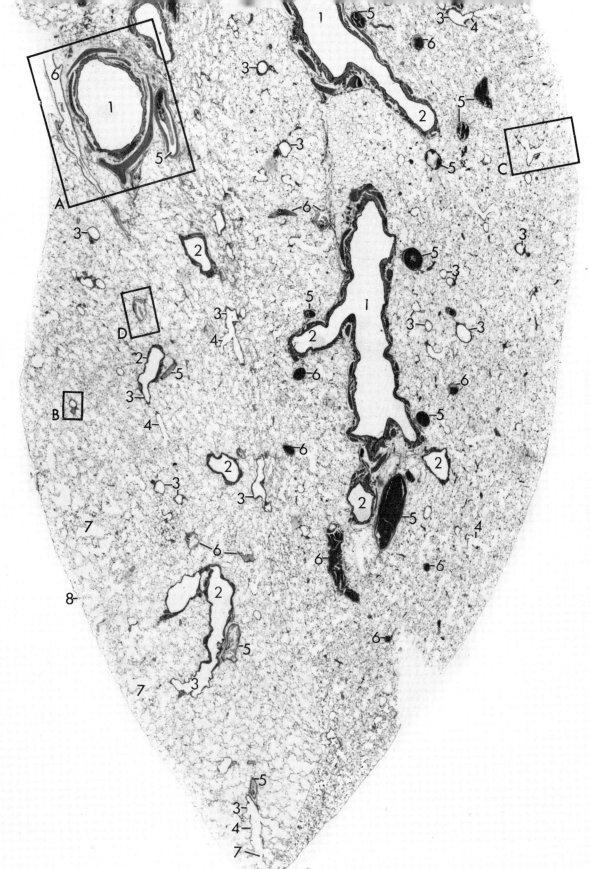

rich in adipose tissue, blood vessels, nerves, lymph nodes, and lymphatics. The loose connective tissue is continuous with the fascia of the neck and mediastinum.

Lungs

The two lungs represent the sites of exchange between the inspired air and the blood of the pulmonary capillaries. The major part of the lungs is occupied by small alveoli in which this exchange takes place. (Fig. 31-31) The rest of the lungs is made up of partly air conduits (bronchi and bronchioles), and partly of vasculature and fibroelastic connective tissue. The vascular channels of the lungs at any one time contain about half of the quantity of circulating blood available to the body.

GENERAL ORGANIZATION

Each lung rests with its **base** on the diaphragm, and reaches the inferior neck region with its **apex**. The broad outer convex **costal surface** faces the ribs, whereas the smaller inner concave **medial surface** borders on the heart and the mediastinum. The **hilus** is a central depression of the medial surface, where the primary bronchus, pulmonary artery and veins, as well as lymphatics and nerves, enter and leave the lung. These structures are collectively referred to as the **root** of the lung. The right lung is divided by **fissures** into 3 **lobes,** whereas the left lung has only 2 lobes. Each lobe receives a **secondary bronchus** (lobar). The lungs can be further subdivided into **bronchopulmonary segments.** This is based on the fact that there are 10 **tertiary bronchi** (segmental) on the right and 8 on the left, each of which provides air for a certain segment of each lung. There are no fissures between segments, nor are there obvious connective tissue septa. It is believed that intersegmental air flow can occur. The importance of pulmonary segmentation relates to the surgical removal of parts of the lung. Within the pulmonary segment, the tertiary bronchi give rise to many generations of smaller **subdivisions of bronchi,** all reinforced by small pieces of cartilage in their walls. As the diameter of the bronchi drops below 1 mm, the cartilage is no longer present in the wall. These fine branches of the air conduits are called **bronchioles.** They ramify further, and when their diameter is less than 0.5 mm, they are referred to as **terminal bronchioles,** and the pulmonary tissue they serve is called a **pulmonary lobule.** Within the lobule, the bronchioles further subdivide into **respiratory bronchioles** and **alveolar ducts,** terminating in the most peripheral part of the lung, the **alveoli.**

The **pulmonary arteries** and their branches carry deoxygenated blood to the lungs. The arterial branches closely accompany the bronchi and bronchioles. The **pulmonary veins,** carrying oxygenated blood from the lungs, largely stay away from the bronchioles and smaller bronchi as they travel through the lung, but tend to accompany the tertiary and secondary bronchi.

The lungs are surrounded by a connective tissue capsule, covered by a mesothe-

Fig. 31-32. Cross section of secondary bronchus. Enlargement of rectangle (A) in Fig. 31-31. Monkey. L.M. X 16. **1.** Lumen of bronchus, 4 mm wide. **2.** Cartilage. **3.** Bronchial glands. **4.** Pulmonary artery. **5.** Pulmonary vein.

Fig. 31-33. Cross section of tertiary bronchus (or ramification thereof). Cat. L.M. X 120. **1.** Lumen of bronchus, 0.9 mm wide. **2.** Mucous membrane. **3.** Bronchial glands. **4.** Bronchial cartilage. **5.** Branch of pulmonary artery. **6.** Bronchial artery. **7.** Fat cells. **8.** Alveoli.

Fig. 31-34. Detail of wall of tertiary bronchus. Enlargement of rectangle (A) in Fig. 31-33. Cat. E.M. X 590. **1.** Lumen. **2.** Pseudostratified columnar ciliated (respiratory) epithelium. **3.** Narrow lamina propria. **4.** Bronchial muscle. **5.** Glands. **6.** Submucosa. **7.** Perichondrium. **8.** Matrix of hyaline cartilage. **9.** Chondrocytes. **10.** Pulmonary alveoli. **11.** Arterioles in submucosa.

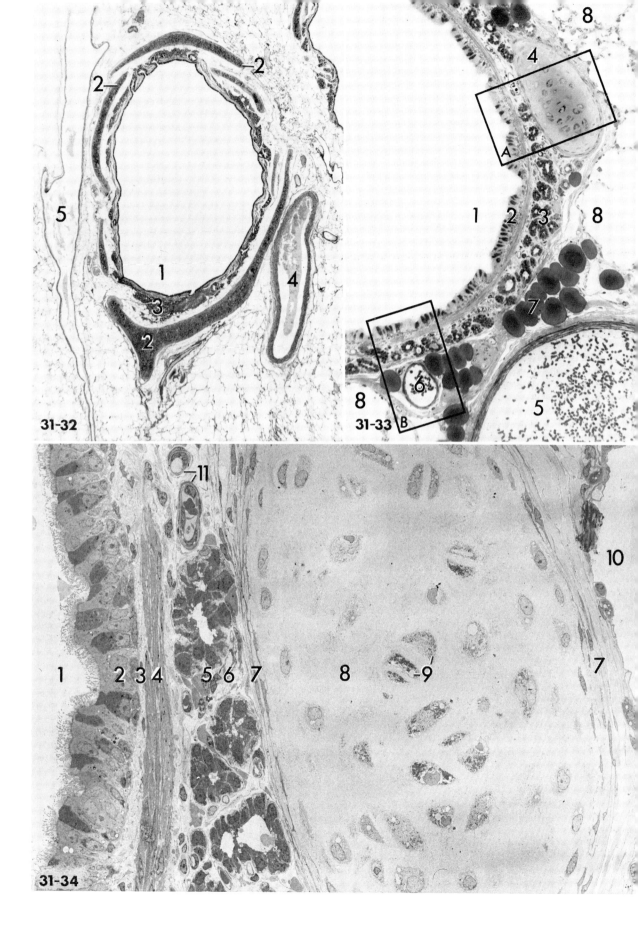

lium. This is the **visceral pleura**. There is a similar connective tissue sac lining the inner surface of the chest wall, the **parietal pleura**. The space enclosed by the two sacs is the **pleural cavity**. There is a separate set of pleurae for each lung. The visceral pleura forms a part of the interlobar fissures.

BRONCHI

The bronchi are divided into extrapulmonary and intrapulmonary bronchi. The structure of the **extrapulmonary bronchi** (primary or main bronchi) has been described on p. 618 together with the trachea. The **intrapulmonary bronchi** can be further divided into: 1) secondary bronchi (lobar); 2) teritary bronchi (segmental); and 3) subdivisions of tertiary bronchi.

Secondary bronchi. The wall of the lobar (secondary) bronchi consists of a mucous membrane, submucosa, and a fibrous adventitia with hyaline cartilages. (Fig. 31-32) The diameter of the secondary bronchi is smaller than that of the primary (main) bronchi. The mucous membrane is similar, consisting of a relatively tall, pseudostratified columnar ciliated epithelium with numerous goblet and basal cells; a lamina propria with fibroelastic tissue rich in lymphoid elements, diffuse lymphocytic infiltration, and lymph nodes; and a lamina muscularis mucosae which forms a complete layer of interwoven bundles of smooth muscle cells. The submucosa contains numerous seromucous glands. The cartilages are irregularly shaped plates with numerous interconnecting bars. The incomplete cartilagenous rings of the trachea and main bronchi do not exist here. A dense fibroelastic membrane connects the cartilagenous plates to one another and forms an essential part of the adventitial connective tissue layer.

Tertiary bronchi. The cross-sectional diameters of the segmental (tertiary) bronchi, and of their subdivisions, de-

crease gradually toward the periphery as these air conduits undergo some 50 generations of dichotomous division. Basically their walls consist of: 1) mucous membrane; 2) submucosa; 3) cartilagenous plates; and 4) adventitia. (Figs. 31-33, 31-34)

The **epithelium** of the smaller bronchi is of the simple columnar ciliated type with numerous goblet cells. (Fig. 31-37) There occur some small basal cells, which would make the epithelium a pseudostratified type. However, the basal cells disappear gradually as the bronchi become smaller. In the bronchial epithelium all non-ciliated columnar cells are mucus-secreting goblet cells with the exception of an occasional brush cell, similar to those located in the trachea. The **basement membrane** is a thin layer composed of a basal lamina and reticular fibrils. The latter merge with the **lamina propria** in which there is a predominance of longitudinal elastic fibers and a small amount of collagenous bundles. Fibroblasts are scarce. The **lamina muscularis mucosae** is thin in the tertiary bronchi (Fig. 31-34) but increases toward the periphery and becomes quite thick in the generations of

Fig. 31-35. Wall of tertiary bronchus. Lung. Cat. E.M. X 590. **1.** Lumen of bronchus. **2.** Pseudostratified columnar ciliated epithelium. **3.** Lamina propria. **4.** Submucosa. **5.** Adventitia with dense connective tissue. **6.** Edge of bronchial smooth muscle, interrupted by excretory ducts. **7.** Venule. **8.** Acini of mixed glands. **9.** Excretory ducts of serous and mucous bronchial glands.

Fig. 31-36. Detail of bronchial gland. Tertiary bronchus. Cat. E.M. $\times$ 4400. **1.** Lumen of gland. **2.** Discharged mucus. **3.** Intracellular mucous droplets. **4.** Nuclei of mucous cells. **5.** Intercellular space with narrow lateral cell processes. **6.** Thin basal lamina.

Fig. 31-37. Detail of simple columnar ciliated epithelium of small bronchus. Cat. E.M. X 4800. **1.** Lumen. **2.** Cilia. **3.** Nuclei of ciliated cells. **4.** Nuclei of mucous cells. **5.** Basal lamina. **6.** Cross-sectioned elastic fibers of lamina propria. **7.** Nucleus of fibroblast.

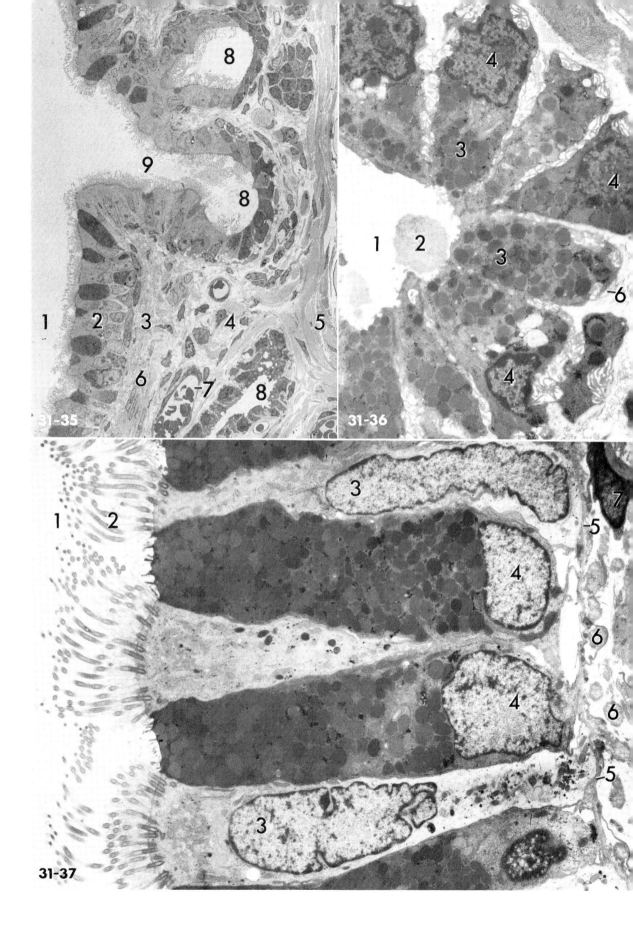

small bronchi just preceding the bronchioles. Most of the smooth muscle cells are arranged circularly or spirally around the bronchi. The **submucosa** is composed of a loose connective tissue in which numerous seromucous glands are present. (Fig. 31-36) They discharge their secretions into the bronchial lumen through excretory ducts lined by a simple cuboidal ciliated epithelium. (Fig. 31-35) The submucosa is rich in fibroblasts, lymphoid elements, and small nerves. It is permeated by a rich network of blood capillaries. The **adventitia** consists largely of bundles of collagenous fibers mixed in with some elastic fibers. Fat cells accumulate often to form adipose tissue in the adventitia. Bronchial arteries and veins as well as large nerve bundles also travel in this tissue space. The plates of hyaline **cartilage** are attached to and surrounded by the fibrous tissue of the adventitia. (Fig. 31-34) The cartilagenous plates gradually become very small and are spaced farther apart as the small bronchi approach the bronchioles. The **function** of the bronchi is similar to that of the trachea: to conduct the air; to moisten and warm it; to trap air-borne particles and transport them toward the trachea. The cartilage gives stability to the wall and helps keep the lumen open. The smooth muscle layer aids in expelling accumulated mucus but does not change the bronchial diameter to any great extent.

BRONCHIOLES

In this category belong air conduits with a diameter of 0.5 to 1 mm. There are about 20 **generations of bronchioles,** the smallest being referred to as **terminal bronchioles.** All bronchioles lack cartilagenous plates, and the small ones also lack glands, but all have a relatively well-developed muscularis mucosae. (Fig. 31-38)

The **epithelium** of the bronchioles changes from a simple columnar ciliated type with some goblet cells in the larger bronchioles, to a simple cuboidal, ciliated

and non-ciliated type without goblet cells in the terminal bronchioles. (Fig. 31-39) The **ciliated cells** are similar to those in the bronchi with the exception that lipid droplets of varying sizes (at least in the cat) become increasingly more common toward the terminal bronchioles. The **non-ciliated cells** (Clara cells) are probably secretory in nature. (Fig. 31-40) The nucleus takes up a major part of the cell. The apex of the cell forms a dome-like protrusion, provided with a few short microvilli but no cilia. Free ribosomes, mitochondria, and accumulations of particulate glycogen are numerous. The Golgi zone is prominent but profiles of the granular endoplasmic reticulum and peroxisomes (microbodies) vary greatly in number. In the apical region of the cell occur, to a varying degree, round, homogeneous, uniformly electron-dense granules that are believed to represent secretory granules, although a discharge of them has not been recorded. The **function** of the Clara cell is not known, but it has been suggested that the cell may represent the equivalent of the granular pneumocyte (type II cell) of the

Fig. 31-38. Bronchiole and pulmonary artery. Enlargement of rectangle (B) in Fig. 31-31. Monkey. L.M. X 185. **1.** Bronchiole, lumen 300 μ (0.3 mm) wide. **2.** Epithelium, its scalloped appearance caused by slightly contracted bronchial muscle. Note the absence of cartilage in the bronchiolar wall. **3.** Bronchiolar smooth muscle. **4.** Branch of pulmonary artery, lumen 120 μ wide.

Fig. 31-39. Part of bronchiole. Enlargement of area similar to rectangle in Fig. 31-38. Cat. E.M. X 600. **1.** Lumen 200 μ wide. **2.** Simple low columnar respiratory epithelium with several ciliated cells, many Clara cells, and occasional mucous cells. **3.** Lamina propria. **4.** Bronchiolar smooth muscle. **5.** Submucosa.

Fig. 31-40. Clara cell. Respiratory epithelium. Bronchiole. Enlargement of area similar to rectangle in Fig. 31-39. Cat. E.M. X 10,000. **1.** Lumen. **2.** Microvilli. **3.** Mitochondria. **4.** Small Golgi areas. **5.** Nucleus. **6.** Accumulations of particulate glycogen. **7.** Basal lamina. **8.** Cilia of adjacent ciliated cell.

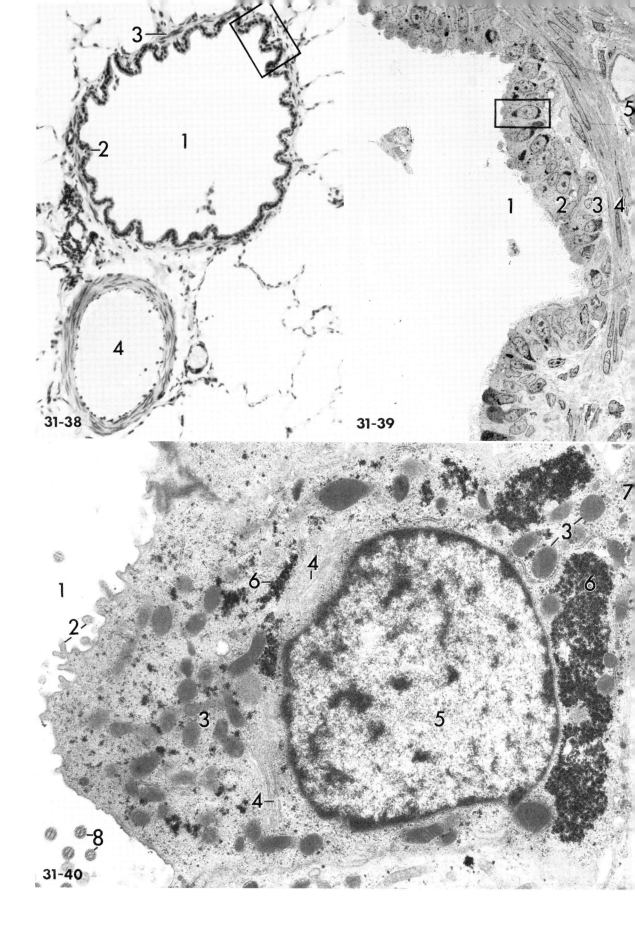

31-38

31-39

31-40

pulmonary alveolar wall, and that it is the source of the hypophase of the surfactant present in the alveoli.

The bronchiolar epithelium rests on a thin **basal lamina** bordering directly on the lamina propria. The **lamina propria** is made up of a loose connective tissue with elastic and collagenous fibrils, fibroblasts, and lymphoid cells. The **muscularis mucosae** forms complete layers of spirally or irregularly arranged smooth muscle cells in the larger bronchioles (Fig. 31-39), but the layers are incomplete in the terminal bronchioles. The fibrous **submucosa** contains a capillary network and merges with the extremely thin adventitia. Through their relatively well-developed smooth muscle layer and lack of cartilaginous plates, the bronchioles control the width of their own lumen. The best-known pathological state is the asthmatic attack, during which marked constriction of the bronchiolar smooth muscle layers occurs.

PULMONARY LOBULES

The pulmonary lobule represents the functional respiratory unit of the lungs. In mammals such as the pig it can easily be identified in sections under the light microscope through the presence of connective tissue septa, but in man septa are poorly defined. A **primary pulmonary lobule** begins where the terminal bronchioles divide and give rise to respiratory bronchioles. The primary lobule consists of: 1) respiratory bronchioles; 2) alveolar ducts; 3) alveolar sacs; and 4) alveoli. A **secondary pulmonary lobule** is composed of some 50 primary lobules; it can be seen with the naked eye. This description of a primary lobule does not follow the original made in 1947 by Miller, who claimed that a primary lobule consists of one alveolar duct and the atria, alveolar sacs and alveoli which arise from that alveolar duct. However, it seems only natural to include the respiratory bronchiole in the primary lobule since it **does** participate in the gas exchange.

Respiratory bronchioles. The respiratory bronchioles are very short and not always present in man. (Fig. 31-41) Their width varies from about 0.5 mm to 0.1 mm. They differ from terminal bronchioles by the presence of occasional outpockets, **alveoli,** along the wall. (Fig. 31-42) The alveoli are structurally similar to other pulmonary alveoli; they are described on p. 632. The **epithelium** of the respiratory bronchiole is low cuboidal and largely made up of non-ciliated Clara cells and some ciliated cells. (Fig. 31-43) The layer of smooth muscle cells is thin and incomplete.

Alveolar ducts. The respiratory bronchioles divide and give rise to 2–3 generations of alveolar ducts which have an average width of about 0.1 mm (100 μ). The alveolar duct is characterized by numerous alveoli, arranged side by side. (Fig. 31-42) There is essentially no alveolar duct wall, and therefore, the low cuboidal

Fig. 31-41. Terminal ramification of air passages. Lung. Enlargement of rectangle (C) in Fig. 31-31. Monkey. L.M. X 40. **1.** Terminal bronchiole. **2.** Respiratory bronchioles. **3.** Alveolar ducts. **4.** Alveolar sacs. **5.** Alveoli. **6.** Branch of pulmonary artery. **7.** Visceral pleura.

Fig. 31-42. Detail of terminal air passages. Lung. Monkey. L.M. X 110. **1.** Terminal bronchiole. **2.** Respiratory bronchiole. **3.** Alveolar duct. **4.** Alveoli. **5.** Wall of respiratory bronchiole. **6.** Knob-like swelling at the entrance to alveolus of an alveolar duct.

Fig. 31-43. Wall of respiratory bronchiole. Lung. Enlargement of area similar to rectangle (A) in Fig. 31-42. Cat. E.M. X 600. **1.** Lumen of respiratory bronchiole. **2.** Alveoli. **3.** Alveolar capillaries. **4.** Clara cells make up the simple cuboidal epithelium. **5.** Bronchiolar smooth muscle cells. **6.** Lymphatic capillary.

Fig. 31-44. Knob-like swelling at the entrance to alveolus of an alveolar duct. Enlargement of area similar to rectangle (B) in Fig. 31-42. Cat. E.M. X 3000. **1.** Alveoli. **2.** Pulmonary capillaries. **3.** The knob-like swelling contains smooth muscle cells. **4.** Bundles of collagen. **5.** Occasional fibroblasts. **6.** Erythrocytes. **7.** Leukocyte in capillary. **8.** Leukocyte in connective tissue.

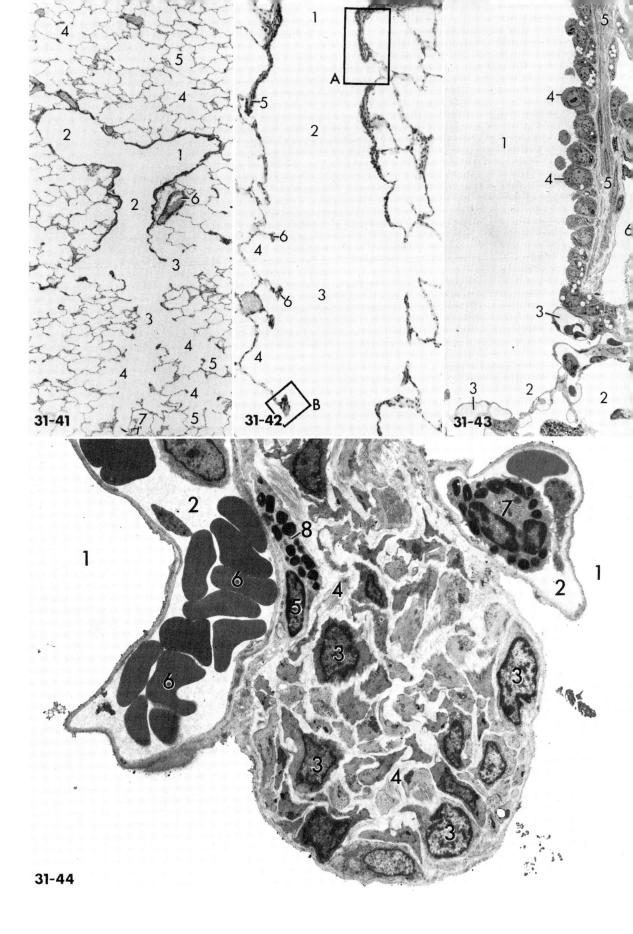

31-41

31-42

31-43

31-44

epithelium of the respiratory bronchiole has disappeared and a simple squamous epithelium lines the alveolar duct (what is left of it) and the pulmonary alveoli. Narrow bundles of smooth muscle cells encircle the entrance to each alveolus of the alveolar duct. They are the only structures remaining from the wall of the respiratory bronchiole; in sections, they are seen as small knob-like swellings of the alveolar septa. (Figs. 31-42, 31-44)

Alveolar sacs and alveoli. These are the terminations of the conducting part of the respiratory system and they also represent the functionally very important respiratory part of the lungs. An alveolar sac is a cluster of alveoli. (Fig. 31-45) Each pulmonary alveolus is a sphere with a small opening connecting it to the central space of an alveolar sac, an alveolar duct, or a respiratory bronchiole. The inside of the alveolus is lined by a very thin squamous epithelium. The outside is made up of a dense network of blood capillaries embedded in a loose fibroelastic connective tissue. Since millions of alveoli are crowded into the lung tissue, they are closely backed up against one another, and adjacent alveoli always share capillary bed and connective tissue space. (Fig. 31-46) This common wall is referred to as **alveolar septum** (alveolar wall). Local defects in this wall are referred to as alveolar pores. There are about 150 million alveoli in each lung. The alveolus has an inner diameter of about 275 μ, which varies during inspiration and expiration. The total alveolar surface area available for gas exchange is about 30 square meters in expiration and 100 square meters in deepest inspiration.

The components of the alveolar septum are: I. **Inner alveolar lining:** 1) squamous alveolar cells; 2) great alveolar cells; 3) alveolar phagocytes; and 4) basal lamina. II. **Pulmonary capillaries:** 1) endothelial cells; 2) basal lamina. III. **Interstitial connective tissue space:** 1) fibroblasts; 2) macrophages; 3) wandering blood cells; 4) collagenous and elastic fibers and fibrils.

The **squamous alveolar cell** (synonyms: type I cell; membranous pneumocyte; respiratory cell) has an extremely large, attenuated cytoplasm that may extend for about 50–100 μ. The nucleus is usually located in a niche (Fig. 31-48) and is difficult to find in a thin section, since the cell is so large, and nuclei therefore are few in number. The cytoplasm is rich in ribosomes and pinocytotic vesicles but other cell organelles are very scarce. Occasional lysosomes are present, although it is generally considered that this cell is non-phagocytic. The cells rest on a thin basal lamina. (Fig. 31-55)

The **great alveolar cell** (synonyms: type II cell; granular pneumocyte; septal cell) is cuboidal with a large rounded nucleus. These cells occur in relative abundance and are located in niches of the alveolar wall, resting on the basal lamina. (Fig. 31-48) The luminal surface has short mi-

Fig. 31-45. Pulmonary alveoli. Lung. Monkey. L.M. X 290. **1.** Alveolar sac. **2.** Alveoli. **3.** Alveolar septum (wall). **4.** Visceral pleura. **5.** Subpleural connective tissue.

Fig. 31-46. Survey of pulmonary alveolus. Lung. Enlargement of area similar to rectangle in Fig. 31-45. Cat. E.M. X 440. **1.** Entrance to pulmonary alveolus (atrium). **2.** Center of pulmonary alveoli. **3.** Alveolar septa with pulmonary capillaries. **4.** Pulmonary venule. **5.** Alveolar phagocyte in a niche of alveolar septum.

Fig. 31-47. Edge of entrance to pulmonary alveolus. Lung. Enlargement of rectangle (A) in Fig. 31-46. Cat. E.M. X 4000. **1.** Nucleus of fibroblast in core of alveolar edge. **2.** Bundles of collagenous fibrils. **3.** Elastic fibers. **4.** Nucleus of great alveolar cell (type II cell). **5.** Lumen of pulmonary capillary. **6.** Lymphocyte in mitosis. **7.** Pulmonary alveoli.

Fig. 31-48. Detail of alveolar septum. Lung. Enlargement of area similar to rectangle (B) in Fig. 31-46. Cat. E.M. X 5400. **1.** Pulmonary alveoli. **2.** Lumen of pulmonary capillary. **3.** Nuclei of capillary endothelial cells. **4.** Nucleus of squamous alveolar cell (type I cell). **5.** Nucleus of great alveolar cell. This particular cell borders on both pulmonary alveoli. **6.** Leukocyte in lumen of pulmonary capillary.

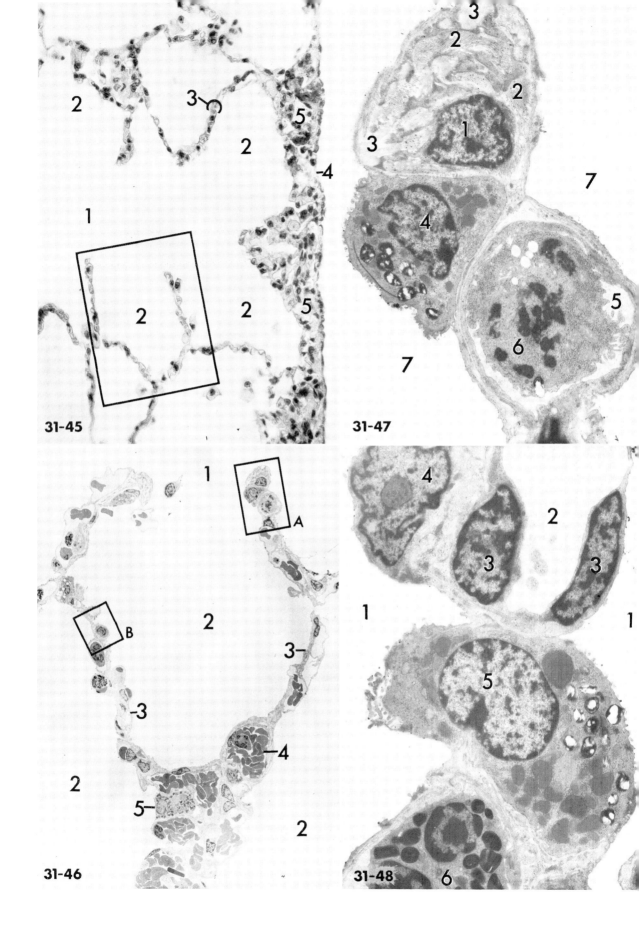

31-45

31-47

31-46

31-48

crovilli. In the cytoplasm are numerous mitochondria, ribosomes, and a few lysosomes and some profiles of the granular endoplasmic reticulum. In addition, numerous peculiar round and oval, highly electron-dense bodies are present. (Fig. 31-49) These are termed cytosomes or **lamellar bodies** because of the alternating light and dark lamellae in their interior. (Fig. 31-50) It is not known from where the cytosomes develop, but both mitochondria and multivesicular bodies have been suggested as possible precursors. The cytosomes are bounded by a 40 Å-thick trilaminar membrane which fuses with the apical surface plasma membrane at the moment the cytosomes discharge their lipoprotein content onto the surface of the squamous alveolar cells. Because of this mechanism, the great alveolar cells are considered to be secretory in nature. It is believed that the secreted material forms an essential part of the **surfactant system** of the lungs, probably the most superficial layer. The surfactant consists of surface-active phospholipids very rich in saturated lecithin which reduces the surface tension of the alveoli, preventing a collapse. The surfactant may also have a hypophase, containing proteins, polysaccharides, and reserve phospholipids, all or some of which may be derived from the Clara cells of the nearby bronchioles, although this is only hypothetical at the moment.

The **alveolar phagocytes** (dust cells) do not form a permanent part of the inner alveolar lining and they move about on the alveolar surface of the squamous alveolar cells. Their structure is similar to that of wandering macrophages and also to monocytes and neutrophils. (Fig. 31-51) Occasional cytosomes (lamellar bodies) can be present in their cytoplasm. Their origin is obscure, but it has been suggested that they emanate from either granular pneumocytes, squamous alveolar cells, interstitial macrophages, monocytes, or neutrophils of the blood. Of these potential precursor cells, the interstitial macro-phage is the most likely candidate. Their function is to pick up air-borne particles that reach the alveolus. Ultimately, the alveolar phagocytes migrate into the connective tissue space of the alveolar septum and reach the lymphatics of the lung. They may also migrate toward the alveolar duct and respiratory bronchiole in which case they eventually will be carried by the bronchial mucous film to the trachea and larynx and become expectorated.

The alveolar **basal lamina** is thin and continuous, forming a complete separation between the inner alveolar lining and the connective tissue interstitium of the alveolar septum. (Fig. 31-56)

Fig. 31-49. Detail of great alveolar cell. Lung. Cat. E.M. X 25,000. **1.** Pulmonary alveolus. **2.** Nucleus of great alveolar cell. **3.** Mitochondria. **4.** Lamellar bodies. **5.** Lipid droplets. **6.** Multivesicular bodies.

Fig. 31-50. Lamellar body. Enlargement of rectangle in Fig. 31-49. Cat. E.M. X 85,000. **1.** Typical appearance of lamellar body in the great alveolar cell of the pulmonary alveoli. The electron-lucent areas have probably been dissolved during preparation. **2.** 40 Å-thick trilaminar boundary membrane. **3.** Part of early lamellar body. **4.** Part of multivesicular body.

Fig. 31-51. Alveolar phagocyte in pulmonary alveolus. Cat. E.M. X 4400. **1.** Nucleus **2.** Golgi region. **3.** Mitochondria. **4.** Numerous primary and secondary lysosomes.

Fig. 31-52. Lysosomes. Enlargement of rectangle in Fig. 31-51. Cat. E.M. X 58,000. **1.** Primary lysosomes. **2.** Secondary lysosomes. **3.** Trilaminar boundary membrane. **4.** Lipoprotein layering.

Fig. 31-53. Detail of connective tissue core of the alveolar septum. Lung. Cat. E.M. X 20,000. **1.** Alveolar lumen. **2.** Capillary lumen. **3.** Capillary endothelium. **4.** Alveolar epithelium. **5.** Nucleus of fibroblast (septal cell). **6.** Collagenous fibrils. **7.** Elastic fibers. **8.** Basal lamina.

Fig. 31-54. Enlargement of rectangle in Fig. 31-53. E.M. X 53,000. **1.** Cytoplasmic strand of fibroblast. **2.** Basal lamina. **3.** Cross-sectioned collagenous fibrils. **4.** Longitudinal section of collagenous fibrils. **5.** Amorphous part of elastic fiber. **6.** Filamentous part of elastic fiber. **7.** Alveolar epithelium. **8.** Alveolar lumen.

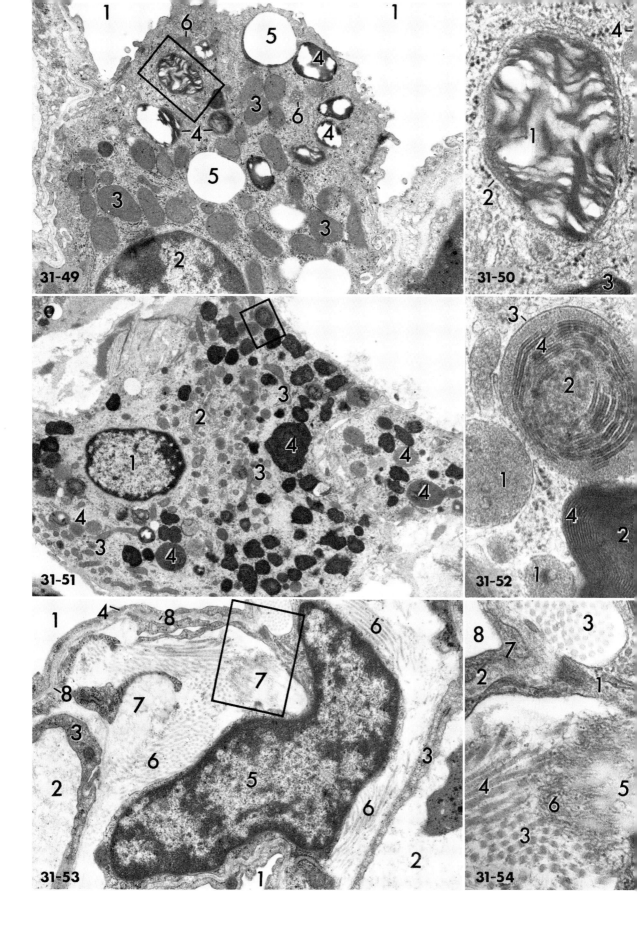

The **pulmonary capillaries** form a very dense network in the alveolar septum. The capillaries, which have an average luminal diameter of 7–10 μ, are widely interconnected, and the blood flow through this capillary bed is sheet-like, since the interstitial connective tissue space is relatively small compared with the space of the capillary lumina. To better visualize the sheet flow of the blood, the alveolar capillary bed has been compared to a large parking garage. The floor and the ceiling are the walls of the capillaries; the pillars extending between them represent the interstitial connective tissue. Upon entering the alveolar capillary bed, the blood quickly flows through the capillary spaces, the only hindrance being the pillar-like connective tissue areas. The capillaries are lined by a squamous **endothelium** which is surrounded by its own **basal lamina**. The endothelial cytoplasm is thinly attenuated without fenestrations, but contains many micropinocytotic vesicles. (Fig. 31-55) The area of the endothelial cell facing the alveolus makes close contact with the squamous alveolar cell, and the basal laminae of the alveolar cell and endothelium often fuse. This area of close contact represents the **blood-air barrier** (Fig. 31-56), measuring about 0.1–0.2 μ in thickness. Endothelial cells are held together by gap-junctions.

The **interstitial connective tissue space** of the alveolar septum is made up of bundles of **collagenous fibrils** and **elastic fibers** forming an intricate network around the alveoli and in the alveolar septum. (Fig. 31-53) The connective tissue fibers are particularly prominent in the wall at the entrance to each alveolus. Although earlier accounts indicated that smooth muscle cells are present here, electron microscopy has demonstrated that this is not the case, and that only the entrance to alveoli of alveolar ducts and respiratory bronchioles contains smooth muscle cells. During ordinary breathing, the elastic fibers do not undergo much linear extension. Their role is to serve as protection

against shock to the inextensible collagenous fibers if some of them should rupture during coughing or sneezing. The main interstitial cell is a **fibroblast** (Fig. 31-53) (also referred to as **septal cell**, although this term has been used mostly in reference to the great alveolar cell). In addition to its typical cytoplasmic organelles, the fibroblast contains accumulations of small lipid droplets. This cell is largely responsible for the synthesis and maintenance of the collagenous and elastic fibers. The fibroblast and adjacent connective tissue fibers form the pillarlike areas between the alveolar capillaries. Other cells in this space are macrophages and occasional **wandering blood cells** such as lymphocytes and granulocytes.

Functions of the lungs. The major function of the lungs is to exchange gases such as carbon dioxide and oxygen across the blood-air barrier. The lungs have also several non-respiratory functions. Under average conditions, large amounts of water and heat are lost across the barrier, and the lung plays a part in the excretion of solutes by way of the carbon dioxide that it eliminates. All metabolites in the blood that are volatile at 37°C can traverse the barrier, enter the gas phase within the alveoli, and appear in the exhaled air. The capillaries of the alveoli act as filters

Fig. 31-55. Pulmonary capillary. Rat. E.M. X 23,000. **1.** Pulmonary alveolus. **2.** Lumina of capillaries. **3.** Nucleus of squamous alveolar cell (type I cell). **4.** Arrow marks point where the squamous cytoplasm of type I cell begins its stretch around the pulmonary capillary. **5.** Nucleus of capillary endothelial cell. **6.** Junctions of strands of endothelial cytoplasm. **7.** Basal lamina. **8.** Collagenous fibrils in connective tissue core of alveolar septum. **9.** Thin cytoplasmic strands of fibroblasts. **10.** Blood-air barrier (0.2–0.3 μ).

Fig. 31-56. Detail of blood-air barrier (0.2 μ). Lung. Mouse. E.M. X 84,000. **1.** Lumen of pulmonary capillary. **2.** Thin sheet of endothelial cytoplasm (200 Å). **3.** Basal lamina (900 Å). **4.** Thin sheet of squamous alveolar epithelial cell (900 Å). **5.** Pulmonary alveolus.

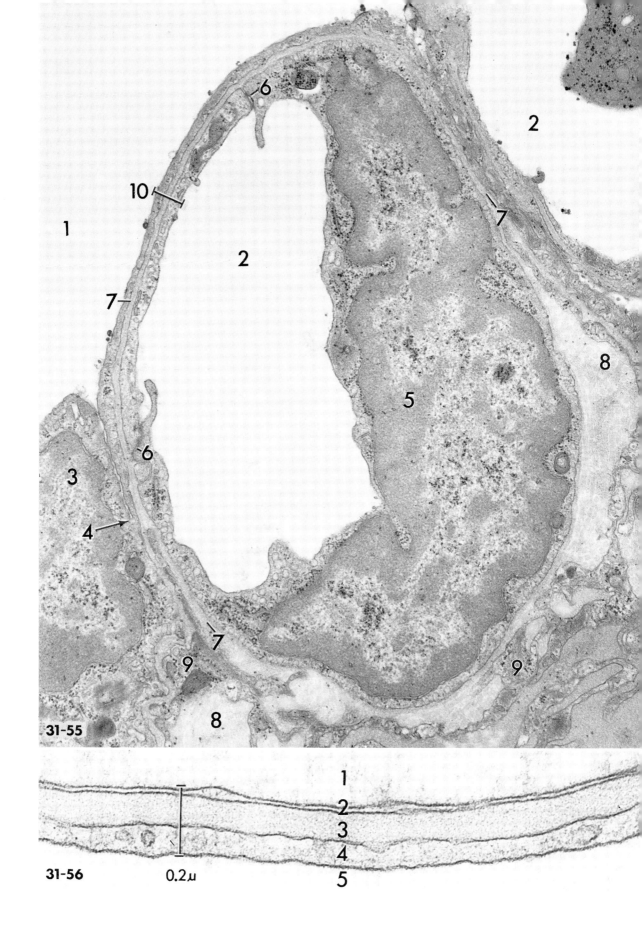

31-55

31-56   0.2µ

that rid the blood of particles such as microemboli. Some granulocytes, lymphocytes, and monocytes may also be removed from the blood as part of a mechanism to maintain a stable level of circulating leukocytes. Several vasoactive substances such as histamine, serotonin, bradykinin, and catecholamines are added to the blood as it passes through the lungs. Other substances such as prostaglandins are removed from the circulation by the lungs, indicating that the lungs, in addition to their role as an organ for external gas exchange, are also metabolically very active. The role of the several cells of the alveolar septum in these metabolic processes is largely unexplored.

BLOOD VESSELS

The blood vessels of the lungs are closely related to the respiratory function of this organ which is carried out in the extensive capillary bed of the pulmonary alveoli. The pulmonary artery and its branches carry deoxygenated blood to the capillary bed, and the pulmonary venules and veins carry oxygenated blood from the capillary bed to the left atrium of the heart. All vessels with diameters less than 30μ are part of the alveolar wall, whereas those greater than 30μ are extra-alveolar. Vessels of 100μ and larger are invested with interstitial connective tissue. The bronchial arteries and their branches originate from the aorta and supply the system of bronchi and bronchioles as well as the pleura with arterial blood. The venous blood is returned to the azygos vein via bronchial veins.

Pulmonary arteries. The pulmonary arteries accompany the bronchi and bronchioles to a point distal to the alveolar ducts, where the terminal pulmonary arterioles give off final branches to alveolar sacs and alveoli. The pulmonary arteries are of the elastic type (Fig. 31-57) until their diameter decreases to less than 1 mm, at which point they become muscular arteries. The elastic pulmonary arteries have a thin intima and a relatively thin media

consisting of alternating layers of smooth muscle cells and elastic membranes. (Fig. 31-58) The adventitia is thick. The small muscular pulmonary arteries have a distinct inner elastic membrane. The terminal arterioles in man, cat, and rat shed their smooth muscle layers gradually (Fig. 31-60), being completely devoid of these cells at luminal diameters of $30-40 \mu$, at which point they are referred to as precapillaries. No distinct precapillary sphincter is seen in these species. In relation to

Fig. 31-57. Pulmonary artery. Same artery as that in Fig. 31-32, several sections deeper. Lung. Monkey. L.M. X 25. **1.** Cartilage of nearby bronchus. **2.** Lumen of artery, 565μ wide at site indicated. **3.** Thickness of arterial wall (intima and media) is 70μ. **4.** Adventitia. **5.** Branch of pulmonary artery, 265μ wide at site indicated.

Fig. 31-58. Branch of pulmonary artery, mostly muscular type. Enlargement of area similar to rectangle (A) in Fig. 31-57. Cat. E.M. X 620. **1.** Lumen of artery, 640μ wide. **2.** Thickness of arterial wall (intima and media) is 20μ. **3.** Dense connective tissue adventitia. **4.** Pulmonary alveoli. **5.** Venule. **6.** Lymphatic vessel.

Fig. 31-59. Wall of pulmonary artery. Enlargement of area similar to rectangle in Fig. 31-58. Cat. E.M. X 8300. **1.** Lumen of artery, 640μ wide. **2.** Nucleus of endothelial cell. **3.** Internal elastic membrane. **4.** Smooth muscle cells. **5.** Central elastic membrane. **6.** Mostly collagenous fibrils in the narrow intermuscular spaces. **7.** External elastic membrane.

Fig. 31-60. Terminal ramifications of pulmonary artery. Enlargement of area similar to rectangle (B) in Fig. 31-57. Cat. E.M. X 670. **1.** Lumen of pulmonary artery, 360μ wide. **2.** Branch of pulmonary artery, entrance of which is 68μ wide at site indicated by bar. **3.** The branch rapidly decreases in size and the lumen of the pulmonary arteriole is 13μ at site indicated by bar. Observe the gradual reduction in number of smooth muscle layers with decreasing luminal diameter. Arrow indicates direction of blood flow. **4.** Terminal arterioles, luminal diameter averaging 10μ. **5.** Pulmonary capillaries. **6.** Alveoli.

Fig. 31-61. Enlargement of area similar to rectangle in Fig. 31-60. Cat. E.M. X 13,000. **1.** Lumen. **2.** Endothelium. **3.** Smooth muscle cell. **4.** Myoendothelial junctions.

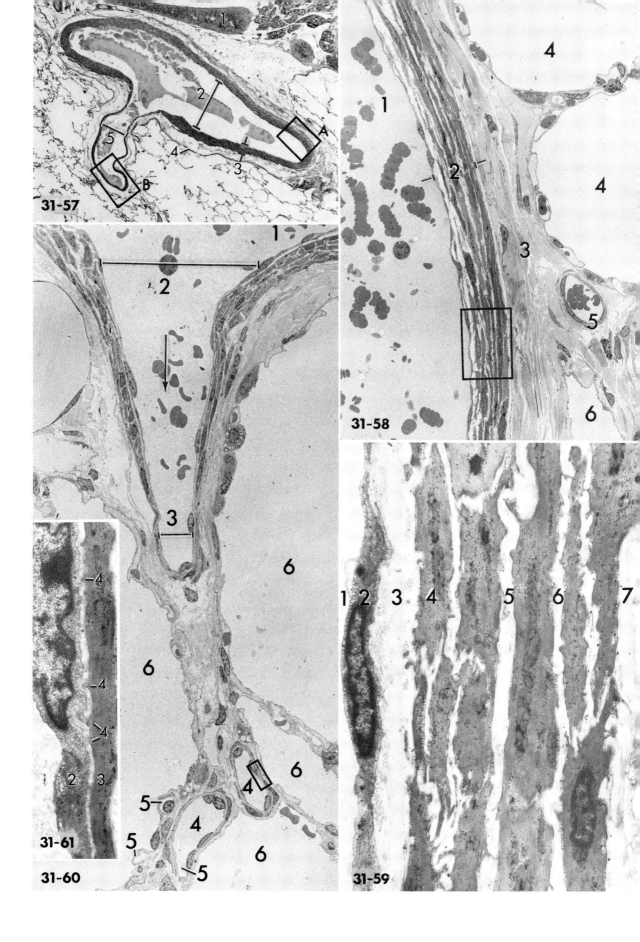

31-57

31-58

31-60

31-61

31-59

respiratory bronchioles, anastomosing may occur between branches of the pulmonary arterioles and the bronchial arterioles.

Pulmonary veins. The pulmonary venules originate from capillaries in alveoli and alveolar ducts, and also in the pleura. At some distance from the bronchiole-artery complex the venules travel in the interlobular connective tissue septa; when they join the complex they become large veins. The venules are thin-walled (Fig. 31-63) and smooth muscle cells are present only in venules larger than 100 μ. The pulmonary veins have a thin intima. The endothelium contains many specific endothelial granules (Figs. 31-66, 31-67), the function of which is obscure. The muscular media is slightly thinner than in pulmonary arteries of the same luminal diameter. Elastic membranes are missing, but small elastic fragments are scattered throughout the media. (Fig. 31-65) The adventitia is thick. In some mammals (rat) it may contain layers of cardiac muscle near the pulmonary hilus.

The **identification of pulmonary vessels** is difficult if only structural differences are taken into account. Pulmonary veins occur singly, whereas pulmonary arteries always occur together with bronchi. Pre- and postcapillary vessels are generally identifiable as such only if one can trace them back to larger vessels. Pulmonary veins in ox, pig, sheep, and rat have local accumulations of smooth muscle cells in the media which could make them look like arteries, but this is not observed in man, mouse, cat, dog, and monkey.

Bronchial vessels. The **bronchial arteries** originate from the aorta and travel in the submucosa of the bronchi. They give rise to two capillary beds, one on either side of the muscularis mucosae. There are no bronchial arterioles that supply air conduits beyond the respiratory bronchioles, but some bronchial arteries reach the pleura. The bronchial arteries are of the muscular type with distinct elastica interna. (Fig. 31-68) The

bronchial veins return along the bronchi and drain into the posterior intercostal veins, the azygos, and hemiazygos veins.

LYMPHATICS

The lung tissue contains a **superficial plexus** of lymph capillaries under the visceral pleura, and a **deep plexus,** located

Fig. 31-62. Branch of pulmonary vein. Enlargement of rectangle (D) in Fig. 31-31. Monkey. L.M. X 30. **1.** Branch of pulmonary vein. These vessels always occur singly in the pulmonary tissue. **2.** Alveolar ducts. **3.** Alveolar sacs.

Fig. 31-63. Enlargement of pulmonary vein in Fig. 31-61. Monkey. L.M. X 89. **1.** Lumen, 500 μ wide at site indicated. **2.** Thickness of venous wall (intima and media) is 12 μ. **3.** Adventitia and perivascular loose connective tissue. **4.** Pulmonary alveoli.

Fig. 31-64. Detail of branch of pulmonary vein. Enlargement of area similar to rectangle in Fig. 31-63. Cat. E.M. X 600. **1.** Lumen, 400 μ wide. **2.** Endothelial cells. **3.** Media consists of scattered smooth muscle cells. **4.** Adventitia with dense connective tissue. **5.** Lymphoid infiltration in perivascular loose connective tissue. **6.** Pulmonary alveoli.

Fig. 31-65. Wall of pulmonary vein. Enlargement of area similar to rectangle in Fig. 31-64. Cat. E.M. X 12,000. **1.** Lumen, 400 μ wide. **2.** Nucleus of endothelial cell. **3.** Fine collagenous and reticular fibrils. Note the absence of basal lamina and internal elastic membrane. **4.** Nucleus of smooth muscle cell. **5.** Bundles of medium-size collagenous fibrils. **6.** Elastic fibers form an incomplete outer elastic membrane. **7.** Myoendothelial junction.

Fig. 31-66. Wall of pulmonary vein. Enlargement of area similar to rectangle in Fig. 31-65. Rat. E.M. X 47,000. **1.** Smooth muscle cell with myofilaments sectioned longitudinally. **2.** Endothelial cell. **3.** Myoendothelial junction. In rat pulmonary veins these junctions continue for up to 20 μ or more without an interposed basal lamina. **4.** Specific endothelial granules. **5.** Mitochondrion. **6.** Granular endoplasmic reticulum. **7.** Pinocytotic vesicles. **8.** Lumen of pulmonary vein.

Fig. 31-67. Specific endothelial granules. Pulmonary vein. Rat. E.M. X 120,000. **1.** Core of granule, finely stippled. In some species, this core may contain microtubules. See Fig. 2-57 (p. 35). **2.** Single boundary membrane.

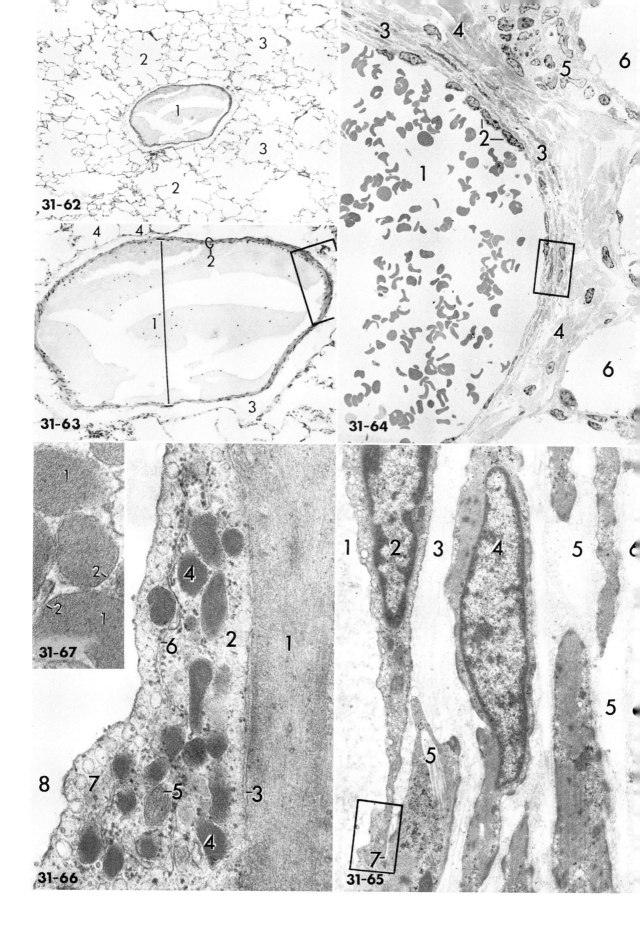

31-62

31-63

31-64

31-67

31-66

31-65

in the perivascular and peribronchial interstitia. There are no lymphatic capillaries in the alveolar septa. Both lymphatic plexuses are drained by lymphatic vessels which conduct the lymph to hilar nodes around the root of the lung. From there, the lymph reaches nodes in the mediastinum.

NERVES

Parasympathetic branches of the vagus nerve and **sympathetic** fibers from the second, third, and fourth thoracic segments of the spinal cord form plexuses which innervate the musculature and the glands of the bronchial tree. Other plexuses innervate the pulmonary and bronchial arteries as well as the pulmonary veins. Stimulation of the vagus nerve contracts the bronchial smooth muscle, whereas sympathetic stimulation causes relaxation of the bronchial smooth muscle. Near the root of the lung, the media of the pulmonary arteries contain sensory nerve endings, so-called **baro-receptors** for registration of pressure changes, and possibly also **chemoreceptors,** collectively referred to as glomus pulmonale.

PLEURA AND CONNECTIVE TISSUE

The visceral pleura (Fig. 31-69) consists of a squamous mesothelial lining, which structurally is similar to the peritoneal mesothelium (p. 576). The mesothelium is separated by a thin basal lamina (Fig. 31-71) from a layer of connective tissue, which, in man, is relatively thick, consisting of collagenous and elastic fibers in addition to occasional smooth muscle cells. In man, this connective tissue layer continues into the lung tissue as septa between the secondary lobules. In animals with thin pleura, these septa are poorly developed or missing. In all mammals, the perivascular and peribronchial interstitium represents the largest connective tissue space of the lung.

References

NASAL CAVITY

Adams, D. R. Olfactory and non-olfactory epithelia in the nasal cavity of the mouse. Am. J. Anat. *133*: 37–50 (1972).

Andres, K. H. Der Feinbau der Regio olfactoria von Makrosmatikern. Z. Zellforsch. *69*: 140–154 (1966).

Andres, K. H. Der olfaktorische Saum der Katze Z. Zellforsch. *96*: 250–275 (1969).

Breipohl, W. Licht- und elektronenmikroskopische Befunde zur Struktur de Bowmanschen Drüsen im Riechepithel der weissen Maus. Z. Zellforsch. *131*: 329–346 (1972).

Cauna, N., Hinderer, K. H. and Wentges, R. T. Sensory receptor organs of the human nasal respiratory mucosa. Am. J. Anat. *124*: 187–210 (1969).

Frisch, D. Ultrastructure of mouse olfactory mucosa. Am. J. Anat. *121*: 87–120 (1967).

Gemne, G. and Doving, K. B. Ultrastructural properties of primary olfactory neurones in fish (Lota lota L.). Am. J. Anat. *126*: 457–476 (1969).

Matulionis, D. H. and Parks, H. F. Ultrastructural morphology of the normal nasal respiratory epithelium in the mouse. Anat. Rec. *176*: 65–83 (1973).

Fig. 31-68. Survey of peribronchial space. Tertiary bronchus. Enlargement of rectangle (B) in Fig. 31-33. Cat. E.M. X 700. **1.** Lumen of bronchus. **2.** Pseudostratified columnar ciliated (respiratory) epithelium. **3.** Lamina propria. **4.** Bronchial smooth muscle. **5.** Submucosa. **6.** Mixed (seromucous) bronchial glands. **7.** Lumen of bronchial arteriole, 70 μ wide. **8.** Peribronchial dense connective tissue. **9.** Lymphatic vessel. **10.** Pulmonary alveolus. **11.** Fat cells. **12.** Non-myelinated nerve bundle. **13.** Blood capillaries.

Fig. 31-69. Periphery of lung. Cat. E.M. X 580. **1.** Pulmonary alveoli. **2.** Alveolar septa. **3.** Visceral pleura. **4.** Pleural cavity.

Fig. 31-70. Visceral pleura. Enlargement of area similar to rectangle in Fig. 31-69. Cat. E.M. X 4500. **1.** Pleural cavity. **2.** Mesothelial cell with numerous microvilli. **3.** Elastic membrane. **4.** Cytoplasmic strands of fibroblasts. **5.** Bundles of collagenous fibrils.

Fig. 31-71. Pleural mesothelium. Enlargement of area similar to rectangle in Fig. 31-70. Cat. E.M. X 60,000. **1.** Amorphous part of elastic membrane. **2.** Filamentous part of elastic membrane. **3.** Basal lamina. **4.** Nucleus of mesothelial cell. **5.** Pleural cavity. **6.** Microvilli. **7.** Junctional complex. **8.** Intercellular space. **9.** Micropinocytotic vesicles. **10.** Mitochondria. **11.** Tonofilaments. **12.** Ribosomes.

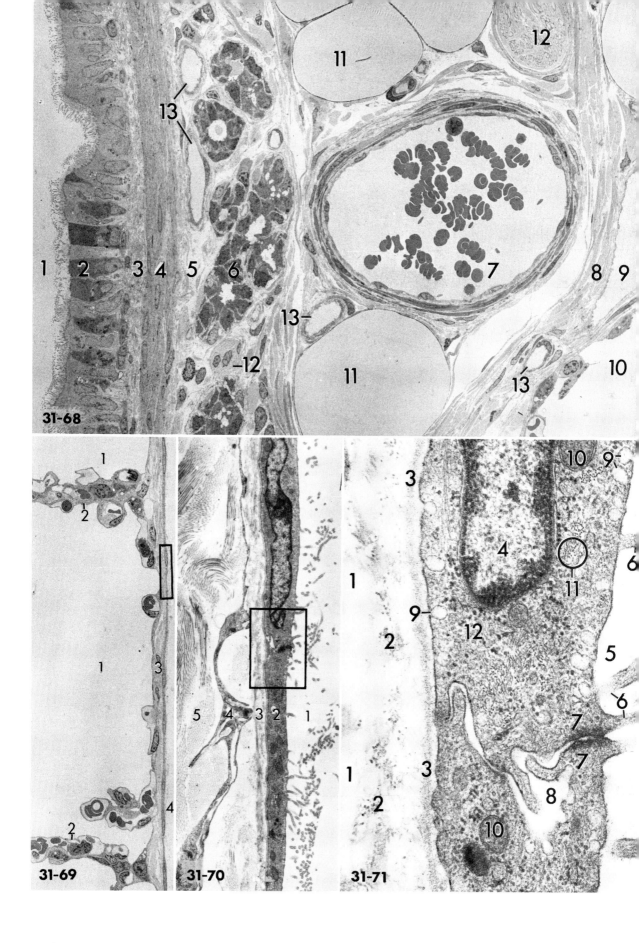

31-68

31-69

31-70

31-71

Mozell, M. M. The spatiotemporal analysis of odorants at the level of the olfactory receptor sheet. J. Gen. Physiol. *50*: 25–41 (1969).

Mulvaney, B. D. Chemography of lysosome-like structures in olfactory epithelium. J. Cell Biol. *51*: 568–574 (1971).

Okano, M., Weber, A. F. and Frommes, S. P. Electron microscopic studies of the distal border of the canine olfactory epithelium. J. Ultrastruct. Res. *17*: 487–502 (1967).

Pinching, A. J. and Powell, T. P. S. The neuropil of the periglomerular region of the olfactory bulb. J. Cell Sci. *9*: 379–409 (1971).

Price, J. L. and Powell, T. P. S. The morphology of the granule cells of the olfactory bulb. J. Cell Sci. 7: 91–123 (1970).

Thornhill, R. A. The ultrastructure of the olfactory epithelium of the lamprey Lampreta fluviatilis. J. Cell Sci. *2*: 591–602 (1967).

Zotterman, Y. (Ed.). Olfaction and Taste. Pergamon, Oxford, 1963.

TRACHEA AND BRONCHI

Baskerville, A. Ultrastructure of the bronchial epithelium of the pig. Souder. Zentra. Veter. *17*: 796–802 (1970).

Bensch, K. G., Gordon, C. B. and Miller, L. R. Studies on the bronchial counterpart of the Kultschitzky (argentaffin) cell and innervation of bronchial glands. J. Ultrastruct. Res. *12*: 668–686 (1965).

Clara, M. Histologie des Bronchialepithels. Z. mikr.-anat. Forsch. *41*: 321–347 (1937).

Cutz, E. and Conen, P. E. Ultrastructure and cytochemistry of Clara cells. Am. J. Path. *62*: 127–134 (1971).

Frasca, J. M., Auerbach, O., Parks, V. R. and Jamieson, J. D. Electron microscopic observations of the bronchial epithelium of dogs. Exp. Molec. Path. *9*: 363–379 (1968).

Hansell, M. M. and Moretti, R. L. Ultrastructure of the mouse tracheal epithelium. J. Morphol. *128*: 159–170 (1969).

Luciano, L., Reale, E. and Ruska, H. Über eine "chemorezeptive" Sinneszelle in der Trachea der Ratte. Z. Zellforsch. *85*: 350–375 (1968).

Meyrick, B. and Reid, L. Ultrastructure of cells in the human bronchial submucosal glands. J. Anat *107*: 281–299 (1970).

Miani, A., Pizzini, G. and DeGasperis, C. "Special type cells" in human tracheal epithelium. J. Submicroscop. Cytol. *3*: 81–84 (1971).

Rhodin, J. A. G. Ultrastructure and function of the human tracheal mucosa. Am. Rev. Resp. Dis. *93*: 1–15 (1966).

Rhodin, J. A. G. and Dalhamn, T. Electron microscopy of the tracheal ciliated mucosa in rat. Z. Zellforsch. *44*: 345–412 (1956).

Watson, J. H. L. and Brinkman, G. L. Electron microscopy of the epithelial cells of normal and bronchitic human bronchus. Am. Rev. Resp. Dis. *90*: 851–866 (1964).

LUNG

Askin, F. B. and Kuhn, C. The cellular origin of pulmonary surfactant. Lab. Investig. *25*: 260–268 (1971).

Basset, F., Poirier, J., Le Crom, M. and Turiaf, J. Étude ultrastructurale de l'épithelium bronchiolaire humain. Z. Zellforsch. *116*: 425–442 (1971).

Blümcke, S., Kessler, W. D., Niedorf, H. R., Becker, N. H. and Veith, F. J. Ultrastructure of lamellar bodies of type II pneumocytes after osmium-zinc impregnation. J. Ultrastruct. Res. *42*: 417–433 (1973).

Boyden, E. A. Segmental Anatomy of the Lungs. A study of the patterns of the segmental bronchi and related pulmonary vessels. The Blakiston Div. McGraw-Hill, New York, 1955.

Brooks, R. E. Ultrastructural evidence for a non-cellular lining layer of lung alveoli: a critical review. Arch. Intern. Med. *127*: 426–428 (1971).

Collet, A. J. Fine structure of the alveolar macrophage of the cat and modifications of its cytoplasmic components during phagocytosis. Anat. Rec. *167*: 277–290 (1970).

Curry, R. H., Simon, G. T. and Ritchie, A. C. An electron microscopic study of normal mouse lung and the early diffuse changes following uracil mustard administration. J. Ultrastruct. Res. *28*: 335–352 (1969).

Clements, J. A. Pulmonary surfactant. Am. Rev. Resp. Dis. *101*: 984–990 (1970).

Dermer, G. B. The fixation of pulmonary surfactant for electron microscopy. I. The alveolar surface lining layer. J. Ultrastruct. Res. *27*: 88–104 (1969).

Dermer, G. G. The fixation of pulmonary surfactant for electron microscopy. II. Transport of surfactant through the air-blood barrier. J. Ultrastruct. Res. *31*: 229–246 (1970).

Dermer, G. B. The pulmonary surfactant content of the inclusion bodies found within type II alveolar cell. J. Ultrastruct. Res. *33*: 306–317 (1970).

Divertie, M. B. and Brown, A. L. The fine structure of the normal human alveolocapillary membrane. J. A. M.A. *187*:938–41 (1964).

Gil, J. and Weibel, E. R. Extracellular lining of bronchioles after perfusion-fixation of rat lungs for electron microscopy. Anat Rec. *169*: 185–200 (1971).

Heinemann, H. O. and Fishman, A. P. Nonrespiratory functions of mammalian lung. Physiol. Rev. *49*: 1–47 (1969).

Kalifat, S. R., Dupuy-Coin, A. M. and Delarue, J. Démonstration ultrastructurale des polysaccharides dont certains acides dans le film de surface de l'alvéole pulmonaire. J. Ultrastruct. Res. *32*: 572–589 (1970).

Karrer, H. E. Electron microscopic study of bronchiolar epithelium of normal mouse lung. Exp. Cell Res. *10*: 237–241 (1956).

Kikkawa, Y. Morphology of alveolar lining layer. Anat. Rec. *167*: 389–400 (1970).

Kikkawa, Y. and Spitzer, R. Inclusion bodies of type II alveolar cells: species differences and morphogenesis. Anat. Rec. *163*: 525–542 (1969).

Krasno, J. R., Kneslon, J. H. and Dalldorf, F. G. Changes in the alveolar lining with onset of breathing. Am. J. Path. *66*: 471–476 (1972).

Lambson, R. O. and Cohn, J. E. Ultrastructure of the lung of the goose and its lining of surface material. Am. J. Anat. *122*: 631–650 (1968).

Lauweryns, J. M. and Boussauw, L. The ultrastructure of pulmonary lymphatic capillaries of newborn rabbits and of human infants. Lymphology *2*: 108–129 (1969).

Liebow, A. A. and Smith, D. E. (Eds.). The Lung.

Int. Acad. Path. Monograph, Williams & Wilkins, Baltimore, 1968.

Ludatscher, R. M. Fine structure of the muscular wall of rat pulmonary veins. J. Anat. *103*: 345–357 (1968).

Mann, P. E. G., Cohen, A. B., Finley, T. N. and Ladman, A. J. Alveolar macrophages. Structural and functional differences between nonsmokers and smokers of marijuana and tobacco. Lab. Investig. *25*: 111–120 (1971).

Meyrick, B. and Reid, L. The alveolar brush-cell in rat lung—a third pneumocyte. J. Ultrastruct. Res. *23*: 71–80 (1968).

Miller, W. S. The Lung. Charles C. Thomas, Springfield, Ill., 1947.

O'Hare, K. H. and Sheridan, M. N. Electron microscopic observations on the morphogenesis of the albino rat lung with special reference to pulmonary epithelial cells. Am. J. Anat. *127*: 181–206 (1970).

Petrik, P. Fine structural identification of peroxisomes in mouse and rat bronchiolar and alveolar epithelium. J. Histochem. Cytochem. *19*: 339–348 (1971).

Petrik, P. and Collet, A. J. Infrastructure descellules bronchiolaires non ciliées chez la souris. Rev. Canad. Biol. *29*: 141–152 (1970).

Policard, A., Collet, A. and Giltaire-Ralyte, L. Observations micro-électronique sur l'infrastructure des cellules bronchiolaires. Bronches *5*: 187–196 (1955).

Pratt, S. A., Finley, T. N., Smith, M. H. and Ladman, A. J. A comparison of alveolar macrophages and pulmonary surfactant (?) obtained from the lungs of human smokers and nonsmokers by endobronchial lavage. Anat. Rec. *163*: 497–508 (1969).

Pump, K. K. Morphology of the acinus of the human lung. Dis. Chest *56*: 126–134 (1969).

Ryan, S. F. The structure of the interalveolar septum of the mammalian lung. Anat. Rec. *165*: 467–484 (1965).

Ryan, S. F., Ciannella, A. and Dumais, C. The structure of the interalveolar septum of the mammalian lung. Anat. Rec. *165*: 467–484 (1969).

Schneeberger-Keeley, E. E. and Karnovsky, M. J. The ultrastructural basis of alveolar-capillary membrane permeability to peroxidase used as a tracer. J. Cell Biol. *37*: 781–793 (1968).

Schultz, von H. The Submicroscopic Anatomy and Pathology of the Lung. Springer-Verlag, Berlin, 1959.

Smith, U., Smith, D. S. and Ryan, J. W. Tubular myelin assembly in type II alveolar cells: freeze-fracture studies. Anat. Rec. *176*: 125–128 (1973).

Sobin, S. S., Intaglietta, M., Frasher, W. G. and Tremer, H. M. The geometry of the pulmonary microcirculation. Angiology *17*: 24–30 (1966).

Sorokin, S. P. A morphologic and cytochemical study on the great alveolar cell. J. Histochem. Cytochem. *14*: 884–897 (1967).

Verity, M. A. and Bevan, J. A. Fine structural study of the terminal effector plexus, neuromuscular and intermuscular relationships in the pulmonary artery. J. Anat. *103*: 49–63 (1968).

Wang, N. S., Huang, S. N., Sheldon, H. and Thurlbeck, W. M. Ultrastructural changes of Clara and type II alveolar cells in adrenalin-induced pulmonary edema in mice. Am. J. Pathol. *62*: 237–252 (1971).

Weibel, E. R. The ultrastructure of the alveolar-capillary membrane or barrier. *In* The Pulmonary Circulation and Interstitial Space (Eds. A. P. Fishman and H. H. Hecht), pp. 9–27. University of Chicago Press, Chicago, 1969.

Weibel, E. R. The mystery of "non-nucleated plates" in the alveolar epithelium of the lung explained. Acta Anat. *78*: 425–443 (1971).

Weibel, E. R. and Knight, B. W. A morphometric study on the thickness of the pulmonary air-blood barrier. J. Cell Biol. *21*: 367–384 (1964).

32 Urinary system

Kidney

The kidneys of the human body are bilateral organs which eliminate metabolic end-products, especially nitrogenous waste; help regulate the fluid balance of the body by retention or loss of water; and assist in maintaining an appropriate salt balance. Two main steps are involved in the processes of excretion and urine formation: first, an **ultrafiltration** of the blood plasma, proteins larger than 70,000 molecular weight being unaffected by this process; and second, a **reabsorption** of a major part of the ultrafiltrate and its components. The kidney is essentially an excretory organ in which the functional units, the **nephrons,** are closely related to an intricate and rich supply of blood vessels. The nephron is a long (50–70 mm) tubule. The ultrafiltrate (the primary urine) is formed at one end, that of the renal corpuscle. Substances and fluid are added to and subtracted from the urine as it passes along the length of the tubule. The relationship of the vascular system to the nephron, the topography of the nephron itself and its relationship to the adjacent nephrons, are central to an understanding of the functions of the kidney. For this reason, the major architectural features of the mammalian kidney will be outlined in brief.

MICROANATOMY OF THE KIDNEY

The kidneys are bean-shaped organs. The concave side is known as the hilus. Many structures enter or leave the kidney via the hilus. These include the ureter, which conducts urine to the urinary bladder, the renal artery and vein, the lymphatics, and the nerves of the kidney. The general architecture of the kidney parenchyma is best displayed in a longitudinal, frontal cut through the organ. Two main parts are evident, an outer one, the **cortex** and an inner one, the **medulla.** The human fetal kidney has 10–12 lobes comprising both cortex and medulla. Some mammalian kidneys are strictly unilobar (unipyramidal) throughout life. (Fig. 32-1) In the mature human kidney, however, the lobation remains only in the medulla. The cortex forms a non-lobated cap of renal tissue covering the medullary lobes. Each medullary lobe forms a pyramid with a slightly convex base connected to the cortical parenchyma (corticomedullary junction). Cortical parenchyma is interposed between pyramids as **interlobar columns.** These columns also contain adipose tissue, interlobar arteries, and veins. The cortex is granulated, whereas the pyramids of the medulla are striated. The striations of the pyramids continue as **medullary rays** into the cortex, where they alternate laterally with areas of granular cortical parenchyma. (Fig. 32-2) The pyramids of the medulla have a densely striated outer zone and a lightly striated inner zone. The **papillae,** or tips of pyramids, project into the **renal sinus.** This sinus is lined by the ureter, and the space thus formed is the **renal pelvis.** The renal pelvis is subdivided into major and minor **calyces.**

BLOOD VESSELS

Distribution. Blood vessels in the kidney are arranged to serve two main functions. The primary purpose is to bring arterial blood directly to the site where

Fig. 32-1. Section of unilobar kidney. Rabbit. L.M. X 14. **1.** Capsule. **2.** Cortex. **3.** Medulla. **4.** Pyramid. **5.** Papilla. **6.** Renal pelvis. **7.** Adipose tissue. **8.** Surface epithelium of ureter. See also Fig. 1-1, p. 2.

Fig. 32-2. Enlargement of rectangle in Fig. 32-1. Kidney. Rabbit. L.M. X 40. **1.** Capsule. **2.** Cortex. **3.** Cortical labyrinth. **4.** Medullary rays. **5.** Outer zone of medulla. **6.** Inner zone of medulla. Dotted lines indicate approximate levels of zonal borders.

Fig. 32-3. Enlargement of area similar to rectangle in Fig. 32-2. Kidney. Rat. E.M. X 620. **1.** Renal corpuscle. **2.** Proximal convoluted segment. **3.** Distal convoluted segment. **4.** Cortical collecting tubule. **5.** Afferent arteriole. **6.** Peritubular capillaries.

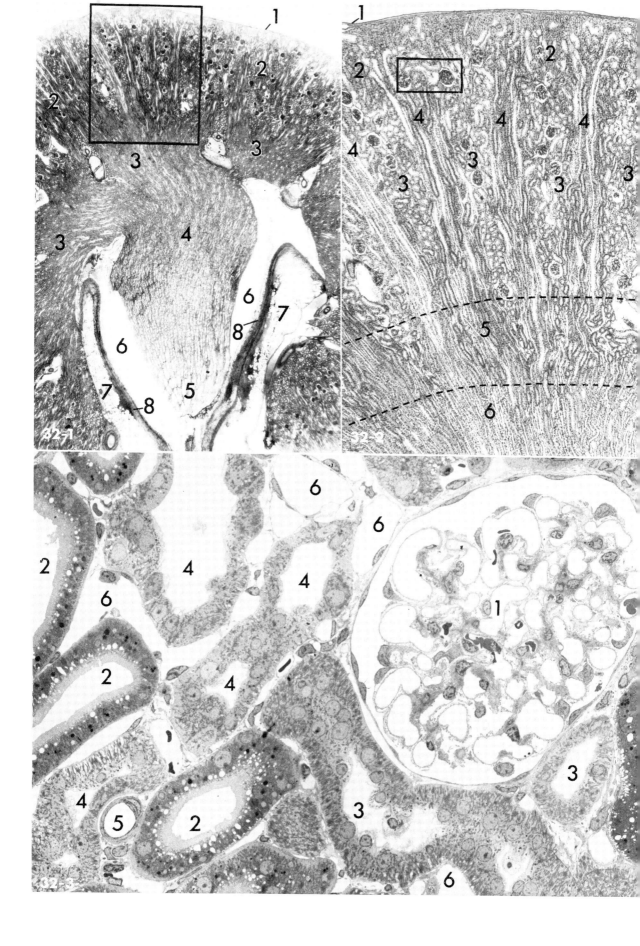

ultrafiltration occurs. This ultrafiltration occurs within the capillary network, the glomerulus, of the renal corpuscle. The second purpose is to provide a network of fine capillaries around all parts of the tubule for the reabsorptive processes occurring throughout the nephron. Reabsorbed materials are returned to the peritubular capillaries and from there to the main circulation.

The **renal artery** divides into ventral and dorsal branches upon entering the renal sinus. These branches give off several **interlobar** arteries, each of which in turn gives off several **arcuate** arteries. (Fig. 32-4) The arcuate arteries traverse the renal parenchyma at the level of the corticomedullary junction. **Interlobular** arteries emerge from the arcuate arteries and traverse the cortical parenchyma radially. (Fig. 32-5) The interlobular arteries give off **afferent arterioles** intermittently and at right angles (Fig. 32-6), and these supply the renal corpuscles. The arcuate and interlobular arteries of any one lobe are end arteries since they do not anastomose with similar arteries from an adjacent lobe.

The afferent arteriole breaks up into a network of capillaries, the **glomerulus**, within the renal corpuscle. (Fig. 32-9) The capillaries subsequently reunite to form the **efferent arteriole** which drains the glomerulus. (Fig. 32-8) The continuation of the efferent arteriole follows differing architectural patterns, depending upon the location of the renal corpuscle. Efferent arterioles from glomeruli near the medulla (juxtamedullary nephrons) turn toward the medullary pyramid as **arterial vasa recta** (spuria), and pass to varying levels of the medulla. They then turn back as **venous vasa recta** and drain into the **arcuate veins** at the corticomedullary junction. Efferent arterioles associated with glomeruli located nearer the outer surface of the kidney break up into a richly interconnected peritubular network in the cortex. This network is drained by **interlobular veins** which also empty into

the arcuate veins. Venous drainage of the cortex is further enhanced by both superficial and deep **cortical veins** which also drain into the arcuate veins.

The arterial supply of the cortex is well secured by the many interlobular arteries. The medulla, on the other hand, has a poor arterial supply, particularly to the inner zone and the papillae. Some arterial branches to the medulla arise directly from the arcuate arteries, the **vasa recta vera**, but they are relatively few.

Fine structure. The arteries of the kidney are typical muscular arteries with a

Fig. 32-4. Diagram of vasculature and nephron in a unilobular kidney. **1.** Arcuate artery. **2.** Interlobular artery. **3.** Afferent arteriole. **4.** Glomerulus. **5.** Efferent arteriole. **6.** Arterial vasa recta (spuria). **7.** Arterial vasa recta (vera). **8.** Venous vasa recta. **9.** Cortical vein. **10.** Arcuate vein. **11.** Bowman's capsule (of the renal corpuscle). **12.** Proximal convoluted segment. **13.** Straight descending limb of Henle's loop. **14.** Thin segment of Henle's loop. **15.** Thick ascending limb of Henle's loop. **16.** Distal convoluted segment. **17.** Macula densa of distal convoluted segment. **18.** Cortical collecting tubule. **19.** Straight collecting tubule. **20.** Collecting duct.

Fig. 32-5. Survey of kidney cortex. Rat. E.M. X 380. **1.** Arcuate artery (cross-sectioned). **2.** Interlobular artery. **3.** Afferent (glomerular) arteriole. Arrows indicate direction of blood flow. **4.** Arcuate vein (thin-walled in rat). **5.** Proximal convoluted segment. **6.** Distal convoluted segment. **7.** Cortical collecting tubule.

Fig. 32-6. Cross section of afferent arteriole. Kidney. Rat. E.M. X 4000. **1.** Lumen, 16 μ wide. **2.** Nucleus of endothelial cell. **3.** Nucleus of smooth muscle cell. **4.** Remnants of elastic membrane. **5.** Juxtaglomerular cell.

Fig. 32-7. Detail of efferent arteriole. Kidney. Rat. E.M. X 27,000. **1.** Lumen. **2.** Nucleus of endothelial cell. **3.** Basal lamina. **4.** Secretory granules of JG-cell. **5.** Secretory granule with crystalline core. **6.** Mitochondrion. **7.** Particulate glycogen.

Fig. 32-8. Cross section of efferent arteriole. Kidney. Rat. E.M. X 4000. **1.** Lumen. **2.** Nuclei of endothelial cells. **3.** Nuclei of smooth muscle cells. **4.** Non-myelinated nerves.

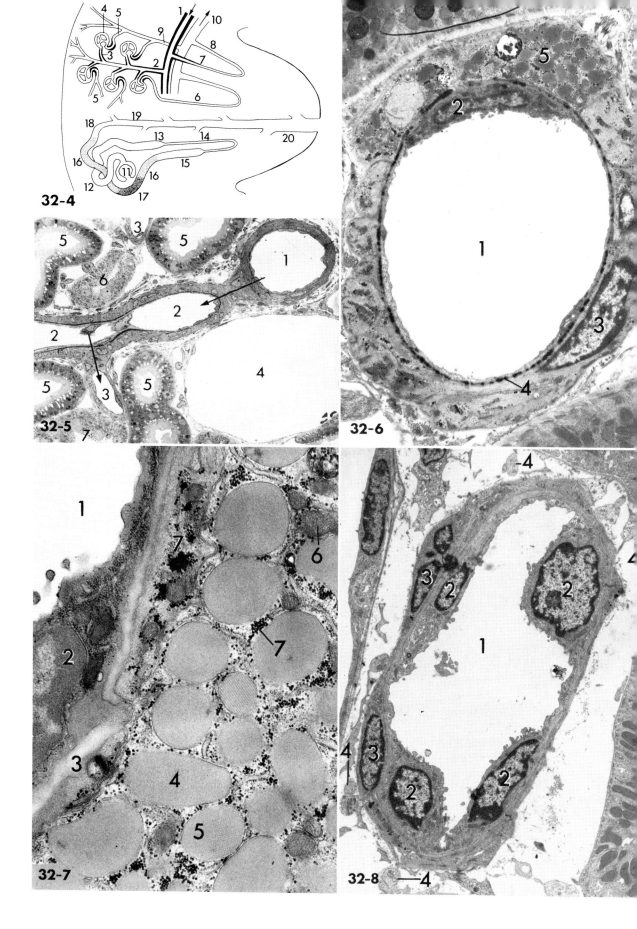

32-4

32-5

32-6

32-7

32-8

well-developed elastica interna (Fig. 16-30) up to a point about 25 μ proximal to the glomerulus. Here the smooth muscle cells of the afferent arterioles are exchanged for cells which contain large secretion granules. (Fig. 32-6) These are the **juxtaglomerular cells** (JG-cells), the granules (Fig. 32-7) of which may possibly contain precursors of renin. Renin is a hormone which acts on other blood-borne agents in a mechanism which affects vascular smooth muscle cells throughout the body and induces increase in blood pressure. The efferent arterioles have a thin smooth muscular coat. (Fig. 32-8) The cells lack secretory granules, these disappearing just distal to the glomerulus. The arteries and arterioles are rich in myoendothelial junctions and are invariably accompanied by nerves. The glomerular capillaries are mainly of the fenestrated (open) type, although capillaries of the fenestrated (closed) type are often present. The reason for this variation in fine structure is unexplained at the moment. The cortical peritubular capillaries and the venous vasa recta are invariably of the fenestrated (closed) type. The arterial vasa recta are a non-fenestrated, vesiculated type usually described in muscle tissues. The veins of the kidney are extremely thin-walled. The endothelium may be of the fenestrated (closed) type even where the luminal diameter reaches 200 μ, a most unusual feature for veins of this size.

THE NEPHRON

General. The structural and functional unit of the kidney is the nephron. It has two parts, the **renal corpuscle,** and the **tubule.** The tubule is structurally and functionally subdivided into: 1) proximal convoluted segment; 2) loop of Henle consisting of: (a) straight descending limb; (b) thin segment; (c) thick ascending limb; 3) distal convoluted segment (with its macula densa). (Fig. 32-4)

Continuous with the distal end of the nephron is the **collecting tubule,** which is derived embryologically from the ureteric

bud and joins up with the distal convoluted segment during development. The collecting tubule itself is divided into three parts: the short arched or connecting tubule; the straight collecting tubule which gradually increases in diameter; and finally the large papillary duct which opens at the papilla. Topographically, renal corpuscles, proximal and distal convoluted segments, and arched collecting tubules are all confined in their extent to the cortex. (Fig. 32-3) The loop of Henle, the straight collecting tubules, and the vasa recta leave the cortex via the medullary rays and extend into the renal pyramids. The parallel arrays of tubules and blood vessels give rise to the striations of the pyramid. The convolutions of the tubules are responsible for the granular appearance of the cortex. The juxtamedullary nephrons, the earliest to develop, have long thin segments. Nephrons with their glomeruli near the kidney surface have either short thin segments or none at all.

Renal corpuscle. The renal corpuscle is formed by tufts of glomerular capillaries invading the blind end of the tubule (the future Bowman's capsule) to form a spherical or slightly ovoid body. (Fig. 32-9) The corpuscle thus has a vascular pole at the point of origin of the glomerulus, and a urinary pole at the point of origin of the tubule. As the capillary tufts grow into the blind end of the tubule, they become

Fig. 32-9. Renal corpuscle. Kidney. Fixed by vascular perfusion. Rat. E.M. X 1200.
1. Afferent arteriole. **2.** Efferent arteriole.
3. Lumina of glomerular capillaries.
4. Glomerular filtration membrane. **5.** Urinary space of Bowman's capsule. **6.** Nuclei of cells of parietal layer of Bowman's capsule.
7. Nuclei of cells of visceral layer of Bowman's capsule; glomerular epithelial cells; podocytes. **8.** Nuclei of endothelial cells.
9. Nuclei of mesangial cells. **10.** Vascular pole of renal corpuscle. Urinary pole is not in plane of section. **11.** Cells of macula densa. **12.** Nucleus of JG-cell. **13.** Proximal convoluted segment of the nephron.
14. Peritubular capillaries.

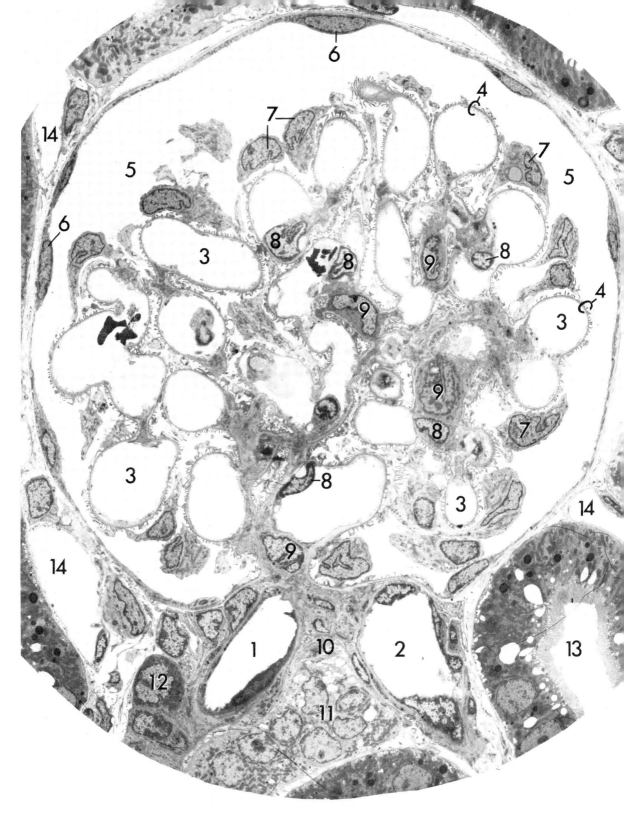

32-9

covered by attenuated epithelium of the tubule, the **visceral** layer of Bowman's capsule, in much the same fashion that the fingers of a hand on being pushed into an inflated rubber balloon, are covered by the rubber. The corpuscle has an outer wall, the **parietal** layer of Bowman's capsule. There is a space (Bowman's space) between the visceral and the parietal layers of the capsule into which urine filters.

There is a slight lobation of the capillaries within the glomerulus with one or two main capillary channels to each capillary loop. Anastomoses occur between lobules and also between capillaries of the same lobule. The inner luminal diameters of these capillaries vary from $3\,\mu$ to $10\,\mu$.

The **glomerular filtration membrane** is formed by the endothelium of the capillaries, the basal lamina, and the visceral layer of Bowman's capsule. The last is composed of cells of intricate morphology called podocytes. (Fig. 32-10) The filtration membrane has an average thickness of about $0.2\,\mu$. As a rule, the nucleus of the **endothelial** cells in the glomerular capillaries is located in that part of the capillary which is attached to or borders on the central part, or stalk, of the glomerulus. The endothelial cytoplasm is highly attenuated and perforated by fenestrations with an average width of $800\,\text{Å}$. (Fig. 32-11) The fenestrations are both of the closed and the open variety. The **basal lamina** is continuous except beneath the endothelial nuclei. Here, it breaks up into a network to surround the **mesangial** cells. These cells are few in number and represent mesenchymal cells that have retained their embryological association with the extraglomerular interstitial space throughout the development of the renal corpuscle. The mesangial cell is structurally a pericyte. Functionally, it stabilizes the capillaries both physically and chemically. It participates in the metabolic turnover of the basal lamina. **Podocytes** have a highly branched cytoplasm. The cytoplasmic extensions are of many differing shapes and sizes. The smallest extensions,

the **pedicles,** surround the capillaries and attach to the basal lamina. The pedicles, or foot processes, of one cell interdigitate with others from either the same cell or adjacent cells. A narrow, shallow intercellular space is present between the interdigitating pedicles, referred to as the **slit-pore.** (Fig. 32-11) It is bridged by a single, $50\,\text{Å}$-thick membrane. There are numerous microtubles and filaments in the cytoplasm of the pedicles and podocytes.

The function of the glomerular filtration membrane is to prevent both formed elements of the blood and proteins larger than 70,000 molecular weight from leaving the bloodstream. The actual mechanism whereby this is accomplished is unknown.

Proximal convoluted segment. This segment begins at the urinary pole of the renal corpuscle. (Fig. 32-12) It runs in the cortex for about 20 mm in a highly tortuous manner near its glomerulus before entering a medullary ray as the loop of Henle. The average diameter of the proximal tubule is about $50\,\mu$ but varies according to the rate of glomerular filtration and tubular absorption. (Fig. 32-13) One extreme is complete closure of the lumen upon cessation of blood flow in the glomerulus. The cells of the proximal convoluted segment are relatively large, only two or three nuclei being visible in a cross-

Fig. 32-10. Glomerular capillary. Kidney. Rat. E.M X 10,000. **1.** Lumen, $10\,\mu$ wide. **2.** Nuclei of endothelial cells. **3.** Nucleus of epithelial cell (podocyte). **4.** Glomerular filtration membrane. **5.** Urinary space. **6.** Nucleus of mesangial cell.

Fig. 32-11. Detail of architecture of glomerular filtration membrane. Kidney. Rat. E.M. X 20,500. **1.** Lumina of glomerular capillaries. **2.** Urinary space. **3.** Cross section of filtration membrane. **4.** Oblique to tangential section of filtration membrane. **5.** Endothelium with fenestrae. **6.** Basal lamina. **7.** Large cytoplasmic processes of podocytes. **8.** Small cytoplasmic foot processes (pedicles) of podocytes. **9.** Interlocking of pedicles. **10.** Slit-pore.

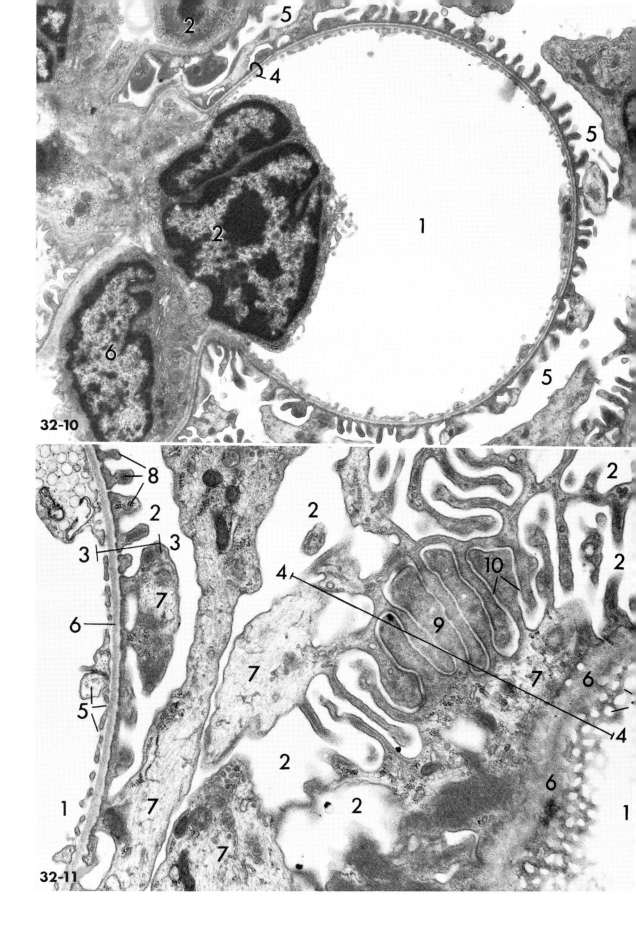

32-10

32-11

sectioned tubule. The cell boundaries are highly irregular and indefinite and cannot be identified under the light microscope in routinely stained sections. The cells have a multitude of long microvilli (collectively called a brush border) at the luminal surface. (Fig. 32-14) Short, narrow, tubular invaginations of the cell membrane are present between the bases of adjacent microvilli. Long and short mitochondria are numerous and the cells contain a wealth of pinocytotic vesicles and vacuoles, lysosomes, phagosomes, and microbodies (peroxisomes). The basal and lateral surfaces are also deeply invaginated, the clefts providing for extensive irregular interdigitations of processes from adjacent cells.

Among the major **functions** of the proximal convoluted segment are the absorption of large amounts of fluid and the reabsorption of glucose, amino acids, sodium chloride, potassium, phosphates, and sulphates. This requires energy and special enzyme systems which are provided for in the various organelles and in the cell membrane. The pathways through the cell for many of these substances are not known. The possibilities are numerous, however, as evidenced by the various structural specializations of invaginated cell membranes, brush border, intercellular clefts, and vacuoles. Sodium and glucose are reabsorbed by an active process, whereas water, chlorides, and bicarbonates traverse the cells of the proximal convoluted segment by a passive diffusion as a result of osmotic forces arising from the active absorption of sodium and glucose. The luminal, basal, and lateral cell surfaces, greatly enlarged by microvilli and foldings of the cell membrane, serve as interfaces for these active and passive processes.

Amino acids may possibly diffuse directly across the cell membrane. Low molecular weight proteins, on the other hand, are absorbed by the apical invaginations. These become detached from the luminal surface and subsequently enlarge to form apical vacuoles (phagosomes). These vacuoles probably merge with primary lysosomes to form large dense granules believed to represent secondary lysosomes. The proteins, absorbed by this process, are probably degraded in the lysosome. It cannot be excluded that some proteins are passed on to the peritubular blood capillaries, but most proteins reach the peritubular fluids after they have been digested into their constituent amino acids by the action of the lysosomal enzymes. In some instances, secondary lysosomes have been captured in a position which seems to imply that they can be discharged at the luminal surface of the cell by a process of exocytosis.

The function of the microbodies (peroxisomes) in the cells of the proximal convoluted segment is still unknown. It has been suggested that the enzymes present in the microbodies, catalase, d-amino acid oxidase, and urate oxidase, act mainly as a safety device to stem the overflow of hydrogen peroxide should the supply of hydrogen donors for peroxidative reactions fail to keep up with the production of hydrogen peroxide.

Loop of Henle. The loop of Henle con-

Fig. 32-12. Renal corpuscle. Kidney. Rat. E.M. X 300. **1.** Vascular pole. **2.** Urinary pole. **3.** Glomerular capillaries. **4.** Urinary space. **5.** Entrance to proximal convoluted segment. **6.** Lumen of proximal tubule.

Fig. 32-13. Cross section of proximal convoluted segment. Kidney. Rat. E.M. X 2500. **1.** Lumen of tubule. **2.** Nuclei of epithelial cells. **3.** Microvilli (brush border). **4.** Apical vacuole (phagosome). **5.** Mitochondria. **6.** Dense granules (secondary lysosomes). **7.** Peritubular capillaries.

Fig. 32-14. Enlargement of area similar to rectangle in Fig. 32-13. Kidney. Rat. E.M. X 12,000. **1.** Lumen of tubule. **2.** Microvilli. **3.** Tubular invaginations. **4.** Circles: junctional complexes. **5.** Apical vacuoles (phagosomes). **6.** Mitochondria. **7.** Microbodies. **8.** Primary lysosomes. **9.** Secondary lysosomes (dense granules). **10.** Nucleus. **11.** Basal lamina. **12.** Basal infoldings of cell membrane. **13.** Fenestrated endothelium of peritubular capillary.

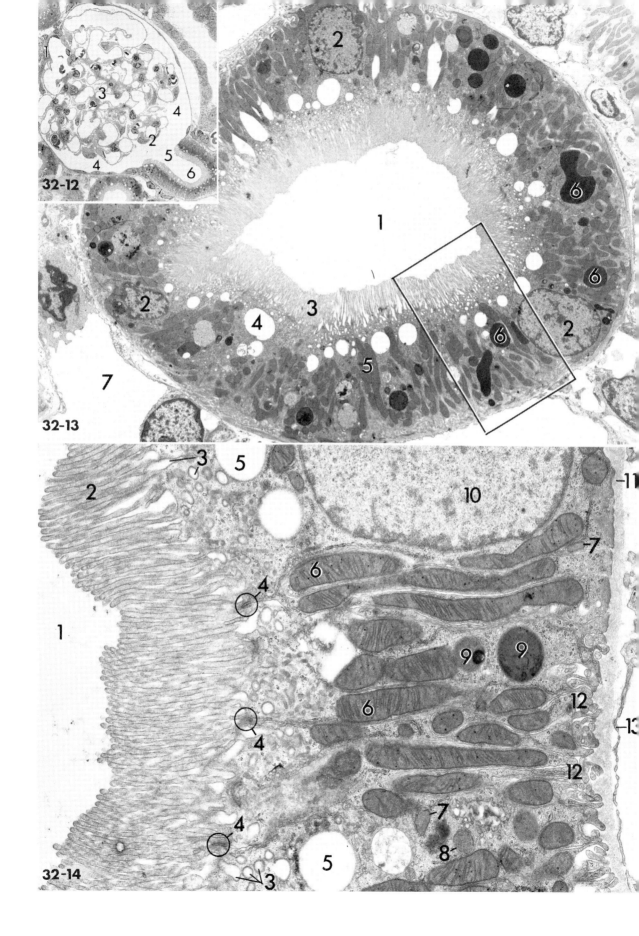

32-12

32-13

32-14

sists of three parts: 1) straight descending limb; 2) thin segment; and 3) thick ascending limb. Structurally, the straight descending limb is similar to the proximal convoluted segment of the tubule, and the thick ascending limb is identical to the distal convoluted segment. Nevertheless, one is inclined to regard the loop of Henle as a functional unit, particularly in view of the "countercurrent multiplier" system that it represents. This system involves streams moving in opposite directions and lying sufficiently close together to facilitate the mutual exchange of fluids, ions, and substances. Straight collecting tubules and arterial and venous vasa recta participate in this system. It is discussed later in this chapter on p. 664.

The convoluted tubule of the proximal segment becomes the **straight descending limb** of Henle's loop upon entering a medullary ray and continues through the cortex within the medullary ray to the medulla. The outer diameter of the straight descending tubule is similar to that of the convoluted proximal segment. The cells of the straight descending limb are of the same size as those within the convoluted part but, in contrast to these, they have fairly straight cell borders. The microvilli are rather long and the height of the brush border equals that of the cell. (Fig. 32-15) Cellular interdigitations are rare. Mitochondria are generally round or oval and relatively few. Pinocytotic vacuoles and lysosomes are scarce, whereas microbodies are numerous. This part of the tubule performs similar functions to the convoluted part. However, the scarcity of infoldings, interdigitations, mitochondria, and lysosomes suggests a lesser degree of involvement in active reabsorptive processes.

The straight descending limb becomes the **thin segment** of Henle's loop within the medulla. The actual level at which this occurs depends on the location in the cortex of the renal corpuscle of the particular nephron. Thus, juxtamedullary nephrons have long thin segments comprising both descending and ascending limbs with the hairpin turn located in close proximity to the papillae. The more superficial, cortical nephrons have short thin segments comprising only a small part of the descending portion of Henle's loop and located at varying levels within the outer medulla.

In either case, the change from straight descending limb to thin segment is abrupt. (Fig. 32-15) Both the outer and the luminal diameters decrease at this point. The cells of the thin segment are very low, almost squamous. (Fig. 32-16) Long cytoplasmic processes interdigitate with those of adjacent cells in an interlocking fashion. These long processes or arms contain occasional mitochondria and possess junc-

Fig. 32-15. Part of descending limb of Henle's loop. Kidney. Rat. E.M. X 1650. **1.** Lumen of straight descending limb. **2.** Lumen of thin segment of Henle's loop. **3.** Nuclei of epithelial cells. **4.** Microvilli. **5.** Termination of long microvilli, marking point of transition between thick descending and thin segments. **6.** Lumen of thick ascending limb. Arrows indicate direction of urine flow.

Fig. 32-16. Detail of area similar to rectangle in Fig. 32-15. Kidney. Rat. E.M. X 9000. **1.** Lumen of thin descending limb. Arrow indicates direction of urine flow. **2.** Epithelium of thin descending limb. **3.** Endothelium of peritubular capillary. **4.** Lumen of capillary. **5.** Epithelium of thick ascending limb. **6.** Mitochondria.

Fig. 32-17. Enlargement of area similar to rectangle in Fig. 32-16. Kidney. Rat. E.M. X 28,000. **1.** Lumen of thin segment. **2.** Interdigitating processes of epithelial cytoplasm. **3.** Mitochondria. **4.** Junctional complexes. **5.** Intercellular space. **6.** Basal lamina.

Fig. 32-18. Hairpin turn of Henle's loop. Kidney. Rat. E.M. X 1100. **1.** Lumen of thin segment. **2.** Lumen of thick ascending limb. **3.** Hairpin turn. Arrows indicate direction of urine flow. **4.** Nuclei of cells at point of transition between thin descending and thick ascending segments of Henle's loop. **5.** Peritubular capillaries of differing diameters. **6.** Adjoining thin segment. **7.** Cells of thick ascending limb are provided with numerous mitochondria.

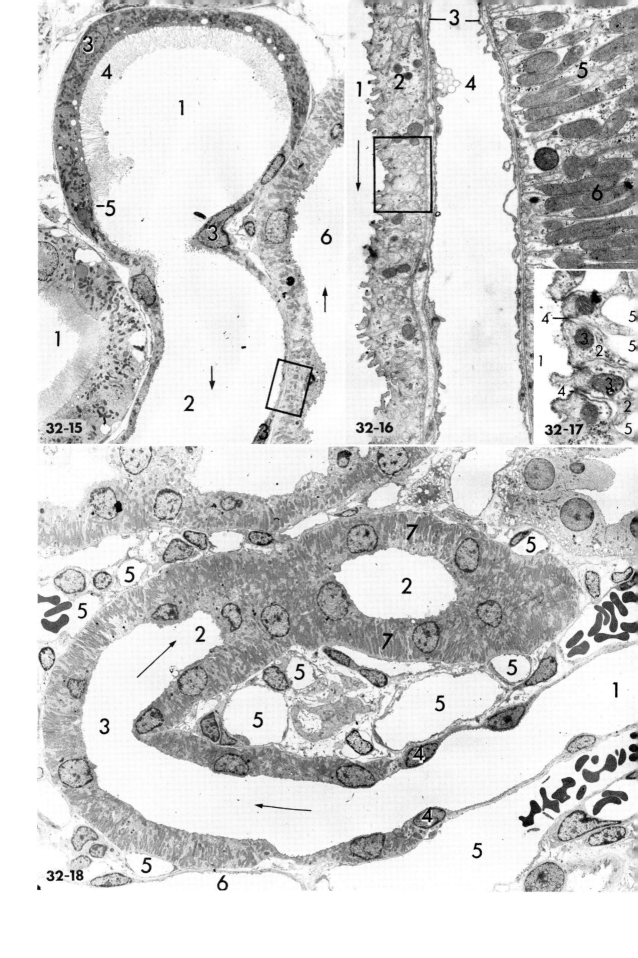

32-15

32-16

32-17

32-18

tional complexes near the luminar surface. (Fig. 32-17) The cells are provided with short microvilli.

There are structural differences between the short and the long thin segments. Species differences also exist. However, these differences are not sufficiently analyzed at the moment to permit a detailed account. It is clear nevertheless that, from a functional point of view, the cells of the thin segment offer less of a barrier to potential active and passive transport systems than do other parts of the tubule. It has therefore been concluded that the thin segment probably is permeable to sodium and water.

The thin segment changes abruptly to the **thick ascending limb.** This change occurs before the hairpin turn for cortical nephrons (Fig. 32-18) and after the turn for juxtamedullary nephrons. The transition from thin to thick segment entails an increase in both outer and luminal diameters.

Changes occur also in the tubule cells. The cells of the thick ascending limb are not as large as those of the proximal segment, several more nuclei appearing in a cross section of the former. In light microscopy, this is often used to differentiate between a proximal and a distal segment of the nephron. The cell borders are as irregular as those of the proximal segment. The cells of the thick ascending limb contain a large number of long, irregularly shaped, densely packed mitochondria oriented at right angles to the base of the cell. (Fig. 32-18) As with the thin segment, cellular interdigitation occurs from the base to the luminal surface. Numerous, closely spaced junctional complexes are associated with this. The surface of the cells of the thick ascending limb is smooth with only the occasional, very short microvillus.

Functionally, the cells are the most active within the loop of Henle. The large number of mitochondria has been taken as structural evidence for the theory that this segment of the tubule acts as an ion

pump, particularly for sodium ions which are passed across the epithelial cell from the lumen to the interstitium against an osmotic gradient.

Distal convoluted segment. The thick ascending limb returns to the cortex via a medullary ray. The tubule becomes tortuous upon leaving the ray and is then referred to as the distal convoluted segment. The latter tubule returns to the parent renal corpuscle, passing near the afferent and efferent arterioles at the vascular pole as it does so. This part of the tubule is known as the **macula densa.** The tubule continues for a short distance before connecting with the system of collecting tubules whereupon it is known as the **arched collecting tubule.** The collecting tubule system begins within the medullary rays and continues through the medulla to the area cribrosa of the papillae.

The cells of the distal convoluted segment are quite similar to those of the ascending thick limb. There are 4–6 nuclei per cross-sectioned tubule (Fig. 32-19), indicating that the cells are not as wide as those of the proximal convoluted segment. The cell borders retain the irregular interlocking pattern seen in the ascending limb. The absence of a brush border makes the lumen of this segment appear generally larger than in the proximal segment. Short, narrow microvilli occur at the luminal surface. The nuclei occupy a large part of the cell and are often located apically with a resultant bulge of the lu-

Fig. 32-19. Cross section of distal convoluted segment. Kidney. Rat. E.M. X 4500. **1.** Lumen of tubule. **2.** Nuclei of epithelial cells. **3.** Short microvilli. **4.** Vacuoles. **5.** Mitochondria. **6.** Peritubular blood capillaries.

Fig. 32-20. Enlargement of area similar to rectangle in Fig. 32-19. Kidney. Rat. E.M. X 19,000. **1.** Lumen of tubule. **2.** Very short microvilli. **3.** Junctional complexes. **4.** Mitochondria. **5.** Nucleus. **6.** Basal infoldings of cell membrane. **7.** Basal lamina. **8.** Fenestrated endothelium of peritubular capillary.

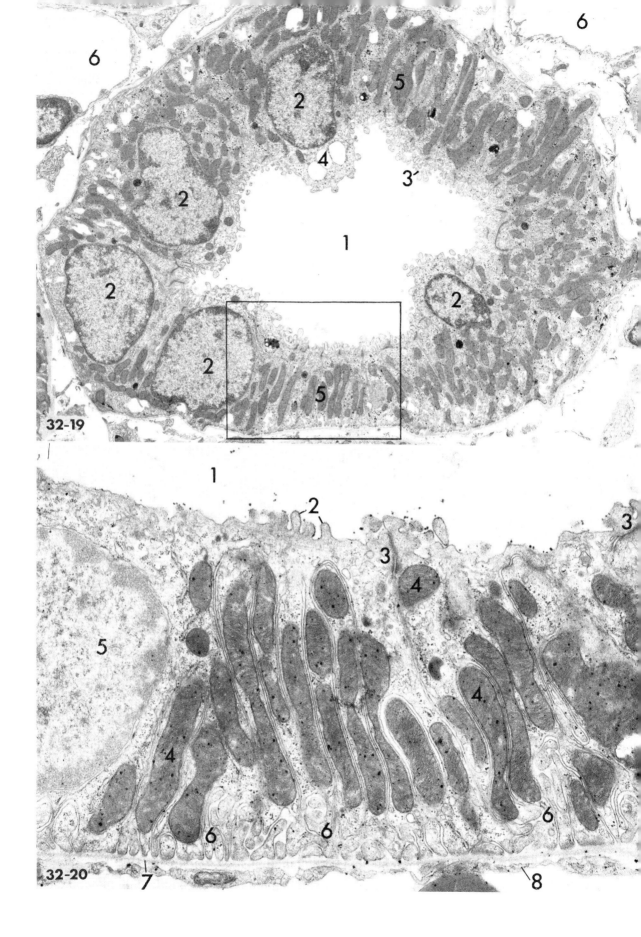

32-19

32-20

minal surface. Mitochondria are long, densely packed, and oriented perpendicularly to the cell base. (Fig. 32-20) Primary and secondary lysosomes occur less frequently than in the proximal segment. The luminal part of the cell contains small vesicles and short, rod-shaped, curved structures which increase in number toward the terminal portion of the distal convoluted segment.

The cells of the **macula densa** are essentially similar to the rest of this segment. They are recognizable, however, by the following differences. The cells are slightly narrower and the nuclei correspondingly closer together. Mitochondria and basal infoldings are fewer and there is not the same degree of interlocking of the lateral cell borders. Contrary to the descriptions based on light microscopical observations, a basal lamina does invest the macula densa part of the distal segment.

The major functions of the distal segment are related to the formation of ammonia and the acidification of the urine. The ultrastructural basis for these processes is poorly understood at the moment. The absence of a brush border makes it less well suited to absorptive functions.

Collecting tubules. The collecting tubules begin in the cortex as short **arched collecting tubules.** These extend to the medullary rays where they merge with other arched collecting tubules to form the **straight collecting tubules.** They in turn traverse the outer and inner medulla, merging as they do so with other straight collecting tubules. The diameter of the tubules gradually increases until the tubules are recognized as **papillary ducts.** These open at the tip of the papillae.

The cells of the collecting tubules gradually increase in height from low cuboidal in the early parts to high columnar in the terminal portions. The cell borders are generally straight and interdigitations are either shallow or absent.

Two cell-types are present in the arched collecting tubule. The **intercalated, dark cell** has numerous spherical mitochondria;

a wealth of small vesicles in the apical part of the cell; narrow, shallow basal infoldings at the cell membrane; and short luminal microvilli. The other cell-type, the **light cell,** has fewer of these organelles, its cytoplasm being richly endowed with particulate glycogen. This mixture of cell-types is probably a result of the embryological fusion of the nephron proper with the collecting tubule, the latter being derived from the ureteric bud.

The cells of the straight collecting tubule are structurally similar to the light cells of the arched collecting tubule. The cells of the papillary ducts (Fig. 32-23) have a few scattered mitochondria, some lipid droplets, and an abundance of ribosomes. The lateral cell surface has short finger-like processes which project into a slightly widened intercellular space.

The system of collecting tubules serves primarily as a conduit for urine. There is also a final concentrating of urine by absorption of water as it passes toward the papillae. The antiduretic hormone (ADH) of the pituitary controls this absorption, probably by acting on the junctional complex at the luminal surface.

Fig. 32-21. Longitudinal section of renal papilla. Kidney. Rat. L.M. X 30. **1.** Papilla. **2.** Tip of papilla with openings of papillary ducts. **3.** Renal pelvis. **4.** Transitional epithelium of renal pelvis.

Fig. 32-22. Survey of collecting duct. Longitudinal section. Kidney. Rat. E.M. X 720. **1.** Lumen of duct. **2.** Columnar epithelial cells. **3.** Peritubular capillaries. **4.** Connective tissue cells.

Fig. 32-23. Enlargement of area similar to rectangle (A) in Fig. 32-22. Kidney. Rat. E.M. X 9300. **1.** Lumen of duct. **2.** Short microvilli. **3.** Junctional complexes. **4.** Nuclei. **5.** Basal lamina. **6.** Mitochondria. **7.** Lipid droplets. **8.** Ribosomes form the finely stippled background. **9.** Intercellular space.

Fig. 32-24. Enlargement of area similar to rectangle (B) in Fig. 32-22. Kidney. Rat. E.M. X 9300. **1.** Nucleus of fibroblast-like cell. **2.** Matrix of connective tissue. **3.** Collagenous fibrils. **4.** External lamina. **5.** Golgi complex. **6.** Mitochondria. **7.** Lysosome. **8.** Lipid droplet. **9.** Pit-like depressions of unknown nature.

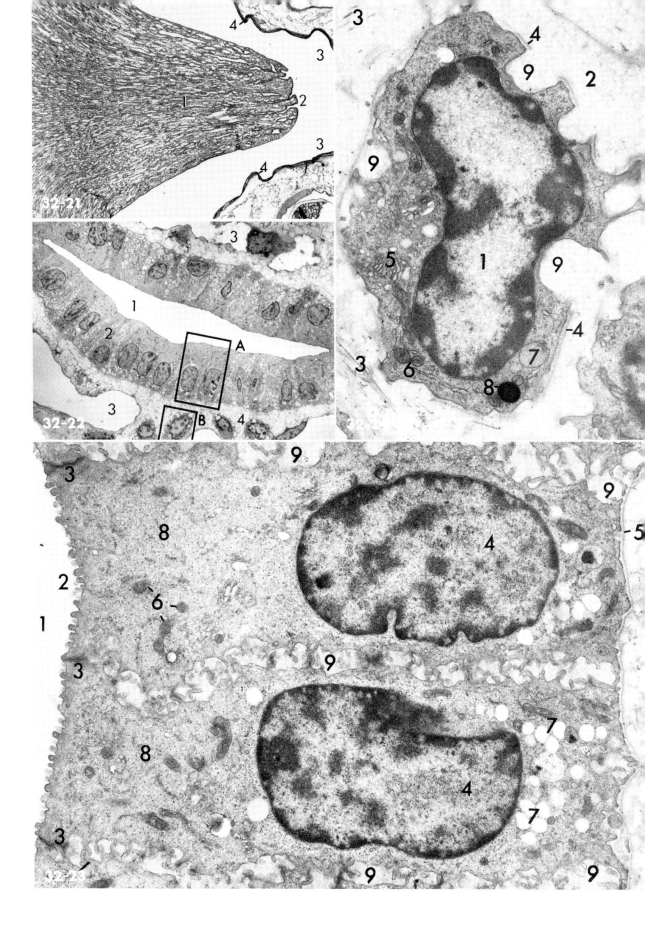

COUNTERCURRENT MULTIPLIER SYSTEM

The morphological basis for this system is the close proximity to each other of the straight members of the loop of Henle, the arterial and venous vasa recta, and the collecting tubules within the medullary rays and within the medulla. (Figs. 32-25, 32-26, 32-27) The interstitial space between these elements is very limited, the walls of the different duct systems being practically back to back. There is a tendency in the medulla for the thin segments to be accompanied by the vasa recta (Fig. 32-28), particularly the arterial vasa recta, whereas the thick ascending limbs are usually adjacent to the collecting tubules. It should be noted that this kind of morphological arrangement is easily identified in mammals with a unipyramidal kidney. Even if present in man, it may not be of equal functional significance.

A countercurrent mechanism relates to the exchange that can take place between two parallel streams, if the flow in the adjoining conduits moves in opposite directions. In principle, exchange of fluids, ions, cold, and heat can take place. In the case of the mammalian kidney, one set of countercurrent conduits is represented by the hairpin configuration of Henle's loop, the other by the arterial and venous vasa recta. The urine is hyperosmotic in the tip of the loop, in the collecting ducts, and in the interstitial fluid near the tips of the papillae, whereas the primary urine and the interstitial fluid in the renal cortex is iso-osmotic. The two systems of countercurrents maintain a high sodium concentration in the interstitium and the urine near the tip of the papilla by exchanging sodium ions between the arterial and venous vasa recta, and by a multiplication of a small concentration difference between the two columns of Henle's loop at each level along the course. By this mechanism, sodium is trapped near the papillae and prevented from leaving this region. The driving force is the epithelial cells of the thick ascending limb which actively pump sodium from the luminal fluid to the interstitium. From the interstitium, the sodium returns to the lumen of the descending limb of Henle's loop, the cells of this segment being permeable to sodium and water.

CONNECTIVE TISSUE

The kidney has a thin connective tissue capsule. Scattered collagenous fibrils and the occasional fibroblast constitute the cortical stroma. These components increase in the medulla and are prominent in the papilla. Fibroblast-like cells extend between collecting tubules and blood vessels. (Fig. 32-24) They contain lipid droplets and are surrounded partly by an external lamina. The function of these interstitial cells, apart from their collagen production, is unknown.

LYMPHATICS

Lymphatic vessels accompany the larger arteries and veins of the kidney. They cannot usually be identified beyond the interlobular arteries, although some lymphatic capillaries may be present in both cortex and medulla. The lymphatic vessels either leave together with the blood vessels at the hilus or pass through the capsule to join the lymphatic vessels in the perinephric adipose capsule.

Fig. 32-25. Longitudinal section of the renal medulla. Kidney. Rat. L.M. X 27. **1.** Cortex. **2.** Outer zone of medulla. **3.** Inner zone of medulla. **4.** Plane of section to produce Fig. 32-26.

Fig. 32-26. Cross section of the outer medullary zone in the plane indicated by 4–4 in Fig. 32-15. Kidney. Rat. L.M. X 175. **1.** Rete or bundle of vasa recta and some thin segments of Henle's loop. **2.** Mostly collecting tubules and thick ascending loops of Henle.

Fig. 32-27. Enlargement of area similar to rectangle in Fig. 32-26. Kidney. Rat. E.M. X 580. **1.** Thick ascending limbs. **2.** Straight collecting tubules. **3.** Vasa recta. **4.** Thin segments.

Fig. 32-28. Enlargement of rectangle in Fig. 32-27. Kidney. Rat. E.M. X 17,500. **1.** Thin segment. **2.** Thick ascending limb. **3.** Collecting tubule. **4.** Arterial vasa recta. **5.** Venous vasa recta. **6.** Nucleus of connective tissue cell

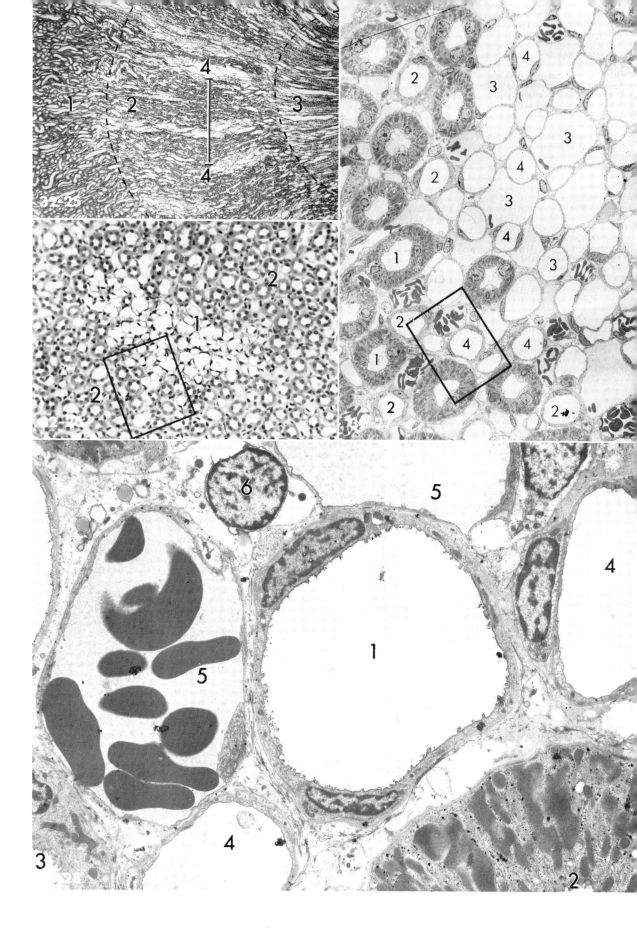

NERVES

The blood vessels are accompanied by a network of autonomic nerves, but free nerve endings are not present in relation to the tubules. Sensory fibers innervate the renal pelvis and the capsule of the kidney.

Ureter

Each ureter is a long, narrow tube, leading from the renal pelvis to the urinary bladder. The diameter averages 5–10 mm. The wall of the ureter is composed of connective tissue, smooth muscle, with a multilayered epithelium lining the lumen. (Fig. 32-29)

The **epithelium** is of the transitional type. When the ureter is collapsed, the epithelium has 3–4 cell layers. In the distended state, there may be only 2 layers since the cells become greatly flattened and stretched. The most superficial layer of cells is different from the basal layers as far as its ultrastructure is concerned. This is discussed below under urinary bladder.

A thin **basal lamina** separates the transitional epithelium from the underlying connective tissue.

The **connective tissue** is relatively densely populated with bundles of collagen. It is denser between the epithelium and smooth muscle than in the area peripheral to the smooth muscle layers.

The **smooth muscle cells** are arranged loosely in an inner longitudinal and an outer circular layer. (Fig. 32-30) Some helically arranged cells are also present. The smooth muscle moves the urine by rhythmic, peristaltic contractions. There are many neuromuscular junctions in comparison with other sites of smooth muscle, such as the intestines and arteries. Numerous points of contacts exist between smooth muscle cells, established by nexi (gap-junctions). These structural specializations facilitate greatly the spreading of contrac-

tion impulse, and make the smooth muscle of the ureter a fast-acting variety among smooth muscle aggregations.

The supply of **blood vessels** is rich both in the connective tissue and the smooth muscle. Capillaries form a rich network immediately beneath the epithelium, whereas most arteries and veins lie in the adventitial connective tissue layer together with lymphatic vessels and nerves.

Urinary Bladder

The urinary bladder is located in the lesser pelvis behind the symphysis pubis. In the male, the bladder is in front of the rectum, resting on the prostate gland. In the female, the bladder is in front of the uterus and the vagina. The two ureters connect with the posterior lateral parts of the bladder, traversing the wall at an oblique angle.

The structure of the wall of the urinary bladder is similar to that of the ureter. It is composed of four parts: the mucous membrane, the submucosa, the muscular coat, and the serous tunic. (Figs. 32-31, 32-32)

The **mucosa** of the empty bladder is heavily folded except over the trigonum vesicae. Here it closely adheres to the muscular coat, giving it a smooth and flat appearance which prevails throughout the bladder in the distended state.

Fig. 32-29. Ureter. Cross section. Human. L.M. X 26. **1.** Lumen. **2.** Transitional epithelium. **3.** Connective tissue. **4.** Smooth muscle. **5.** Loose connective tissue with adipose tissue and blood vessels.

Fig. 32-30. Enlargement of area similar to rectangle in Fig. 32-29. Ureter. Cross section. Rat. E.M. X 1860. **1.** Lumen. **2.** Nuclei of cells of transitional epithelium. **3.** Level of basal lamina. **4.** Lumina of subepithelial blood capillaries. **5.** Bundles of collagenous fibrils. **6.** Fibroblasts. **7.** Nuclei of smooth muscle cells. **8.** Lumen of capillary in smooth muscle layer. **9.** Non-myelinated nerves. **10.** Arterioles. **11.** Venule. **12.** Mast cell.

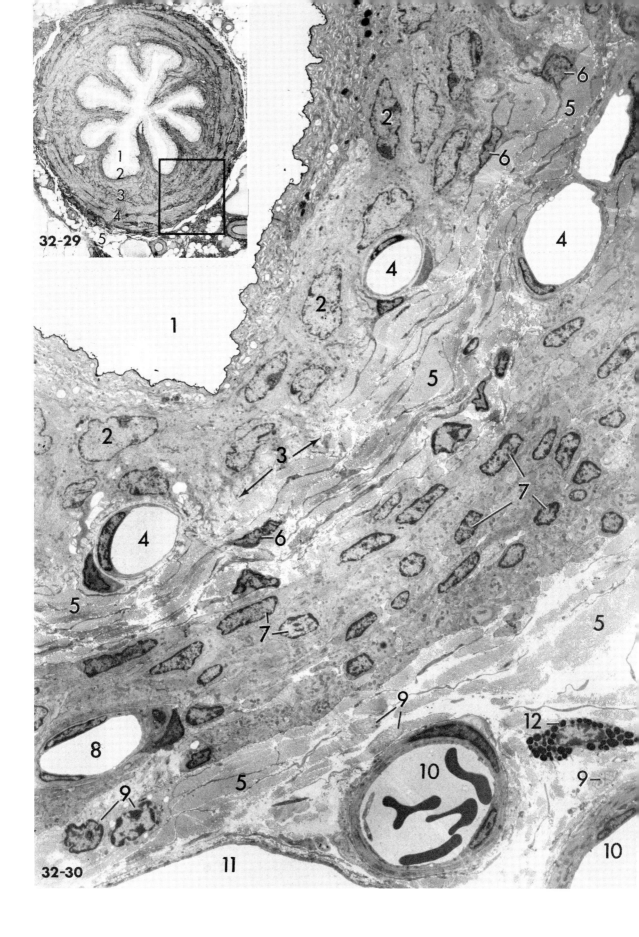

32-29

32-30

The epithelium is a modification of the stratified cuboidal type, referred to as a **transitional epithelium.** In the empty bladder, it may have 8–10 layers, whereas the distended bladder has only 2–3 layers. In the empty bladder the basal layers of the epithelium are composed of small polyhedral or spindle-shaped cells. The middle layers of the epithelium are occupied by relatively large, club-shaped cells. The superficial layer is composed of large polyhedral flattened cells with one or several nuclei. (Fig. 32-33) The cell borders are highly interdigitated throughout the epithelium. (Fig. 32-34) These infoldings help to provide for the increased epithelial surface necessary during distension of the bladder. There is a limited number of desmosomes forming a part of the cell membrane. Throughout the epithelium the cells are bordered by a conventional trilaminar cell membrane. However, the luminal cell membrane of the superficial cells is asymmetric and the leaflet adjacent to the lumen is thicker than the one facing the cytoplasm. There is some extraneous dense filamentous material adhering to the luminal cell membrane. (Fig. 32-35) It is believed that the thick asymmetric cell membrane serves as a selective barrier against a loss of intracellular ions to the hyperosmotic urine. The cells have a limited number of small mitochondria, a fair amount of tonofilaments, free ribosomes, and some particulate glycogen. The Golgi complex is of medium size. In the cells of the middle layers is present a small number of flat, discoid vesicles. (Fig. 32-35) They become more numerous in the cells located toward the surface, and they become quite prominent in the large, flat superficial cells, where lysosomes are also abundant. The flat vesicles are bounded by a trilaminar, asymmetrical membrane of the same dimensions as the cell membrane. The vesicular boundary membrane has a thick luminal leaflet and a thinner leaflet on the cytoplasmic border. There is some evi-

dence that the membranous material is synthesized from the Golgi complex. The center of the vesicles is electron lucent.

The function of these flat vesicles is not known. It has been suggested that they serve as a readily available source of cell membrane to allow a rapid increase in cell surface as the bladder dilates. Other suggestions related to their function consider them representing absorption or excretion vacuoles, removing material from the urine or excess water from the epithelial cells into the urine.

The epithelium rests on a thin **basal lamina** which cannot be resolved with the light microscope. The boundary line of the epithelium toward the submucosa is irregular. (Fig. 32-32)

The **submucosa** is quite loose and contains a rich capillary network as well as many elastic and collagenous fibers. The capillaries often indent the basal lamina and the basal cells of the epithelium.

The **muscularis** has three smooth muscle layers. The outer and the inner layers are thin and arranged longitudinally. The middle layer is relatively thin and arranged in a circular manner. This arrangement is pronounced at the base of the bladder where the middle layer forms an

Fig. 32-31. Wall of partly collapsed urinary bladder. Human. L.M. X 24. **1.** Lumen. **2.** Transitional surface epithelium. **3.** Submucosa. **4.** Cross-sectioned bundles of smooth muscle cells. **5.** Longitudinally sectioned bundles of smooth muscle cells. **6.** Serosa.

Fig. 32-32. Wall of distended urinary bladder. Rat. E.M. X 1900. **1.** Lumen. **2.** Nuclei of cells in transitional epithelium. **3.** Plane of basal lamina. **4.** Subepithelial capillaries indenting the base of the epithelium. **5.** Submucosa. **6.** Nuclei of fibroblasts. **7.** Bundles of collagen. **8.** Cross-sectioned smooth muscle cells. **9.** Bundles of collagen between layers of smooth muscle cells. **10.** Longitudinally sectioned smooth muscle cells. **11.** Submesothelial connective tissue of the serosa. **12.** Mesothelial cell nucleus. **13.** Peritoneal cavity.

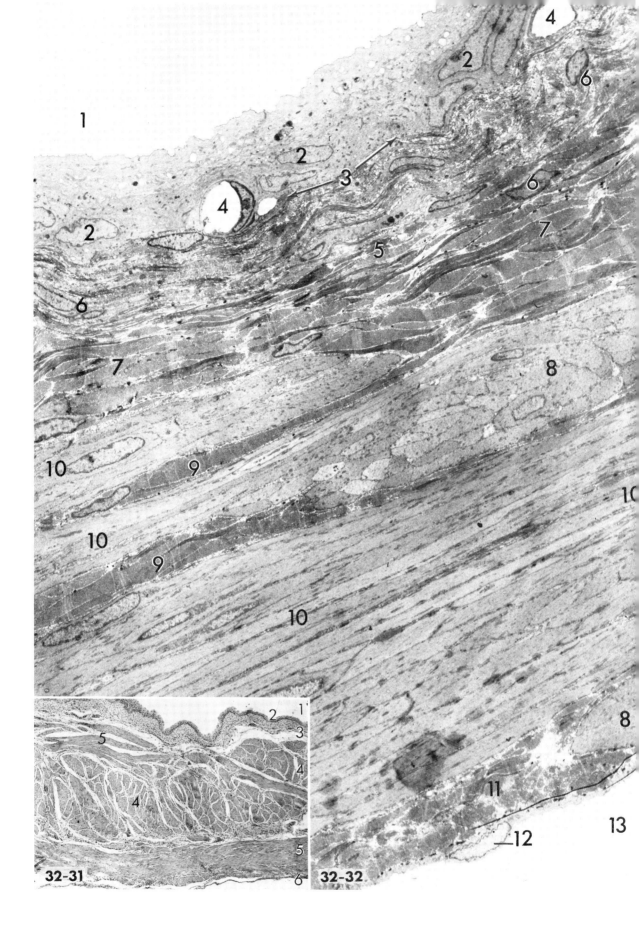

32-31

32-32

indistinct internal sphincter muscle at the place where the urethra begins. The orifices of the ureters do not have sphincters.

The **serosa** is found only in relation to the superior and upper lateral surfaces of the bladder. It contains the mesothelial lining of the peritoneum and a loose submesothelial connective tissue. This loose connective tissue surrounds the urinary bladder also in the areas not covered by the mesothelium.

Urethra

MALE

The male urethra has three distinctly different portions, depending on the location: pars prostatica, pars membranacea, and pars cavernosa (penile portion). The wall of the urethra has a mucous membrane, consisting of an epithelium and underlying connective tissue, both of which vary according to the part through which the urethra passes.

In the **pars prostatica,** the epithelium is generally of the transitional type, but both stratified cuboidal and columnar types occur. The subepithelial connective tissue is identical with the stroma of the prostate gland, being composed of a mixture of fibroblasts and smooth muscle cells. In the **pars membranacea,** the narrowest and shortest part of the male urethra, the epithelium is mostly of the stratified cuboidal or columnar type.

The layer of subepithelial connective tissue is rather thin. It is surrounded by the external sphincter muscle of the bladder. The **pars cavernosa** (penile portion) is the longest. (Fig. 32-37) The epithelium is generally of the stratified cuboidal type. (Fig. 32-41) Near the external orifice in the glans penis it changes to a stratified squamous epithelium in the part of the cavernous urethra which is referred to as the **fossa navicularis.** Throughout, the subepithelial connective tissue is relatively sparse and blends with that of the corpus cavernosum (spongiosum) urethrae.

The architecture of the **corpus spongio-** sum is essentially similar to that of the corpora cavernosa penis, being composed of **erectile tissue.** Interconnecting **trabeculae** form the framework around the **cavernae** or venous sinuses. The cavernae near the urethra are smaller than those in the periphery of the corpus spongiosum. (Fig. 32-39) The cavernae are lined by a simple squamous endothelium. The trabeculae near the urethra have a core made up mostly of fibroblasts and collagenous fibers. Farther away from the urethra, the trabecular network contains many smooth muscle cells (Fig. 32-40) arranged in bundles, in addition to fibroblasts and collagen. The corpus spongiosum is surrounded by a thin **tunica albuginea** rich in collagenous and elastic fibers. Branches from the deep arteries of the penis supply the erectile tissue of the corpus spongiosum, and special veins drain the tissue. The mechanism of filling and draining the erectile tissue is similar to that of the corpora cavernosa penis. For details see page 700.

Fig. 32-33. Transverse section of transitional epithelium. Urinary bladder. Monkey. L.M. X 550. **1.** Lumen. **2.** Superficial cells. **3.** Intermediate cells. **4.** Basal cells. **5.** Submucosa.

Fig. 32-34. Transverse section of transitional epithelium. Ureter. Rat. E.M. X 5300. **1.** Lumen. **2.** Nucleus of superficial cell. **3.** Nuclei of intermediate cells. **4.** Nuclei of basal cells. **5.** Lumen of subepithelial capillary. **6.** Collagen of submucosa. **7.** Discoid vesicles. **8.** Lysosomes.

Fig. 32-35. Enlargement of rectangle (A) in Fig. 32-34. Transitional epithelium. Ureter. Rat. E.M. X 60,000. **1.** Lumen. **2.** Surface cell membrane. Dense material attached to luminal aspect is of unknown nature. **3.** Flat discoid vesicles. **4.** Trilaminar membrane. **5.** Particulate glycogen. **6.** Ribosomes.

Fig. 32-36. Enlargement of area similar to rectangle (B) in Fig. 32-34. Detail of basal region of transitional epithelium. Ureter. Rat. E.M. X 44,000. **1.** Lumen of capillary. **2.** Basal lamina. **3.** Collagenous fibrils. **4.** Basal cell membrane. **5.** Mitochondria. **6.** Ribosomes. **7.** Particulate glycogen. **8.** Golgi complex.

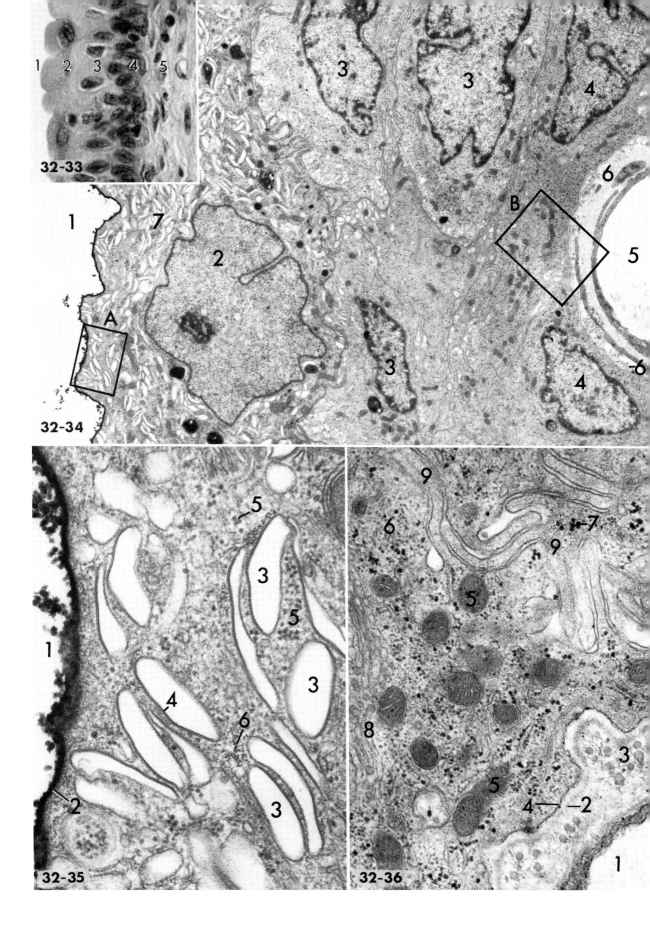

32-33

32-34

32-35

32-36

FEMALE

The female urethra is lined by an epithelium which is of the transitional type near the urinary bladder. The major part of the urethra, and especially the part near the meatus, is lined by a stratified squamous epithelium. The subepithelial connective tissue is rich in thin-walled veins, to the extent that this arrangement has been described as representing an erectile tissue. (Fig. 32-38) There are two layers of smooth muscle fibers. On their outside, they are in turn joined by a coat of striated muscle fibers from the urethral constrictor muscle, forming a sphincter near the urethral orifice.

References

KIDNEY

Bulger, R. E. The shape of rat kidney tubular cells. Am. J. Anat. *116*: 237–255 (1965).

Bulger, R. E. and Trump, B. F. Fine structure of the rat renal papilla. Am. J. Anat. *118*: 685–721 (1966).

Bulger, R. E., Tisher, C. C., Myers, C. H. and Trump, B. F. Human renal ultrastructure. II. The thin limb of Henle's loop and the interstitium in healthy individuals. Lab. Investig. *16*: 124–141 (1967).

Dieterich, H. J. Die Ultrastruktur des Gefässbündel im Mark der Rattenniere. Z. Zellforsch. *84*: 350–371 (1968).

Ericsson, J. L. E. Transport and digestion of hemoglobin in the proximal tubule. II. Electron microscopy. Lab. Investig. *14*: 16–39 (1965).

Ericsson, J. L. E. and Trump, B. F. Electron microscopic studies of the epithelium of the proximal tubule of the rat kidney. Lab. Investig. *11*: 1427–1456 (1964).

Farquhar, M. G. and Palade, G. E. Functional evidence for the existence of a third cell type in the renal glomerulus. J. Cell Biol. *13*: 55–87 (1962).

Forster, R. P. Kidney cells. In The Cell, Vol. 5 (Eds. J. Brachet and A. E. Mirsky), pp. 89–161. Academic Press, New York, 1961.

Gottschalk, C. W. and Mylle, M. Micropuncture study of the mammalian urinary concentrating mechanism: evidence for the countercurrent hypothesis. Am. J. Physiol. *196*: 927–936 (1959).

Griffith, L. D., Bulger, R. E. and Trump, B. F. Fine structure and staining of mucosubstances on "intercalated cells" from the rat distal convoluted tubule and collecting duct. Anat. Rec. *160*: 643–662 (1968).

Johnson, F. R. and Darnton, S. J. Ultrastructural observations on the renal papilla of the rabbit. Z. Zellforsch. *81*: 390–406 (1967).

Jorgensen, F. The Ultrastructure of the Normal Human Glomerulus. Munksgaard, Copenhagen, 1966.

Jorgensen, F. Electron microscopic studies of normal visceral epithelial cells (human glomerulus). Lab. Investig. *17*: 225–242 (1967).

Latta, H., Maunsbach, A. B. and Madden, S. C. The centrolobular region of the renal glomerulus studied by electron microscopy. J. Ultrastruct. Res. *4*: 455–472 (1960).

Miller, F. Hemoglobin absorption by the cells of the proximal convoluted tubule in mouse kidney. J. Biophys. Biochem. Cytol. *8*: 689–718 (1960).

Moffat, D. B. and Fourman, J. The vascular pattern of the rat kidney. J. Anat. *97*: 543–553 (1963).

Mueller, C. B. The structure of the renal glomerulus. Am. Heart J. *55*: 304–322 (1958).

Myers, C. H., Bulger, R. E., Tisher, C. C. and Trump, B. F. Human renal ultrastructure. IV. Collecting ducts of healthy individuals. Lab. Investig. *15*: 1921–1950 (1966).

Nissen, H. M. On lipid droplets in renal interstitial cells. IV. Isolation and identification. Z. Zellforsch. *97*: 274–284 (1969).

Oliver, J. New directions in renal morphology. Harvey Lectures Series *40*: 102–155 (1944–45).

Osvaldo, L. and Latta, H. Interstitial cells of the renal medulla. J. Ultrastruct. Res. *15*: 589–613 (1966).

Rhodin, J. Correlation of ultrastructural organization and function in normal and experimentally changed proximal convoluted tubule cells of the mouse kid-

Fig. 32-37. Cross section of male urethra (pars cavernosa). Child. L.M. X 40. **1.** Lumen of urethra. **2.** Subepithelial connective tissue. **3.** Trabeculae. **4.** Lacunae. **5.** Small arteries.

Fig. 32-38. Cross section of female urethra. Human. L.M. X 27. **1.** Lumen, lined by stratified squamous epithelium. **2.** Subepithelial connective tissue. **3.** Thin-walled veins. **4.** Arteries. **5.** Smooth muscle cells. **6.** Striated muscle fibers of urethral sphincter.

Fig. 32-39. Enlargement of area similar to rectangle in Fig. 32-37. Detail of male urethra and corpus cavernosum (spongiosum). Rat. E.M. X 1800. **1.** Lumen of urethra. **2.** Stratified epithelium. **3.** Subepithelial connective tissue with some capillaries. **4.** Narrow trabeculae of corpus spongiosum. **5.** Lacunae. **6.** Wide trabeculae.

Fig. 32-40. Enlargement of area similar to rectangle (A) in Fig. 32-39. Detail of a wide trabeculum of corpus spongiosum. Rat. E.M. × 1800. **1.** Lumen of lacuna. **2.** Endothelium. **3.** Fibroblasts. **4.** Smooth muscle cells. **5.** Bundles of collagen. **6.** Schwann cell nucleus.

Fig. 32-41. Enargement of area similar to rectangle (B) in Fig. 32-39. Detail of stratified epithelium. Male urethra. Pars cavernosa. Rat. E.M. X 4700. **1.** Lumen of urethra. **2.** Nuclei of cuboidal, basal cells. **3.** Nuclei of cuboidal cells in the middle of the epithelium. **4.** Squamous and/or cuboidal surface cells. **5.** Basal lamina. **6.** Particulate glycogen. **7.** Microvilli.

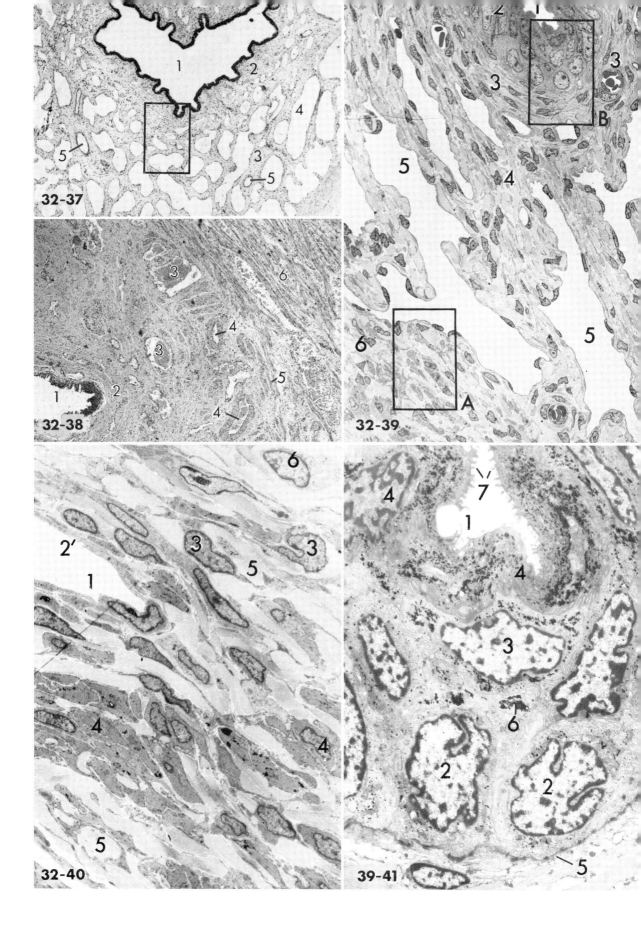

ney. Thesis. Karolinska Institutet, Stockholm. pp. 1–76, 1954.

Rhodin, J. Anatomy of kidney tubules. Int. Rev. Cytol. 7: 485–534 (1958).

Rhodin, J. Electron microscopy of the kidney. Am. J. Med. 24: 661–675 (1958).

Rhodin, J. A. G. Electron microscopy of the kidney. In Renal Disease (Ed. D. A. K. Black), pp. 117–156. Blackwell, Oxford, 1962.

Rhodin, J. A. G. The structure of the kidney. In Diseases of the Kidney (Eds. M. B. Strauss and L. G. Welt), pp. 10–55. Little, Brown, Boston, 1963.

Ross, M. H. and Reith, E. J. Myoid elements in the mammalian nephron and their relationship to other specializations in the basal part of the kidney tubule cells. Am. J. Anat. 129: 399–416 (1970).

Tisher, C. C., Bulger, R. E. and Valtin, H. Morphology of renal medulla in water diuresis and vasopressin-induced antidiuresis. Am. J. Physiol. 220: 87–94 (1971).

Tisher, C. C., Bulger, R. E. and Trump, B. F. Human renal ultrastructure. I. Proximal tubule of healthy individuals. Lab. Investig. 15: 1357–1394 (1966).

Waugh, D., Prentice, R. S. A. and Yadav, D. The structure of the proximal tubule: a morphological study of basement membrane cristae and their relationships in the renal tubule of the rat. Am. J. Anat. 121: 775–786 (1967).

URETER AND URINARY BLADDER

Dixon, J. S. and Gosling, J. A. Electron microscopic observations of the renal caliceal wall in the rat. Z. Zellforsch. 103: 328–340 (1970).

Dixon, J. S. and Gosling, J. A. Histochemical and electron microscopical observations on the innervation of the upper segment of the mammalian ureter. J. Anat. 110: 57–66 (1971).

Hicks, R. M. The fine structure of the transitional epithelium of rat ureter. J. Cell Biol. 26: 25–48 (1965).

Hicks, R. M. The function of the Golgi complex in transitional epithelium. Synthesis of the thick cell membrane. J. Cell Biol. 30: 623–643 (1966).

Monis, B. and Zambrano, D. Transitional epithelium of urinary tract in normal and dehydrated rats. Z. Zellforsch. 85: 165–182 (1968).

Porter, K. R., Kenyon, K. and Badenhausen, S. Specializations of the unit membrane. Protoplasma 63: 262–274 (1967).

Richter, W. R. and Moize, S. M. Electron microscopic observations on the collapsed and distended mammalian urinary bladder. J. Ultrastruct. Res. 9: 1–9 (1963).

33 Male reproductive system

The male reproductive system consists of: 1) two **testes** for the development of the male sexual cells, the spermatozoa, and the secretion of the male sexual hormone, testosterone; 2) **excretory ducts** (epididymis, ductus deferens, ejaculatory ducts) in which the spermatozoa are stored and given ability to move by an admixture of secretions; 3) **auxiliary glands** (seminal vesicles, prostate gland, bulbo-urethral glands); and 4) the copulatory organ, the **penis.** In addition, the urethra goes through the prostate gland and the penis, serving the purposes of conducting the urine as well as the **semen,** the latter a mixture of sperm and secretions from the auxiliary glands.

Testis

The testis develops retroperitoneally in the abdomen and gradually descends through the inguinal canal to the **scrotum,** an evaginated bag of the skin and the tela subcutanea. The wall of the scrotum also contains a thin sheath of smooth muscle, the **tunica dartos,** and the striated **cremaster muscle,** the latter corresponding to the internal oblique muscle of the abdominal wall. During the descent of the testis, the peritoneum initially covers the inside of the scrotum as the processus vaginalis. In the mature male, this process remains about the testis as the **tunica vaginalis,** having lost its connection with the peritoneal cavity.

GENERAL

The testis is a smooth ovoid body (Fig. 33-1) surrounded by a thick connective tissue capsule, the **tunica albuginea,** under which lies a richly vascularized **tunica vasculosa.** The connective tissue capsule is especially well developed toward the medial side in the testis, the **mediastinum,** where it surrounds the system of ducts carrying sperm from the testis to the epididymis. From the mediastinum radiate

connective tissue **septula,** dividing the parenchyma of the testis into about 250 **lobules.** These are pyramidal, incomplete compartments, each containing several convoluted **seminiferous tubules.** (Fig. 33-2) The tubules are long loops which begin and terminate as short **straight tubules** leading to the **rete testis.** The rete is a network of narrow channels within the mediastinum. From the rete testis, about 10–12 **efferent ductules** carry sperm to the epididymis. Between the seminiferous tubules is a small capillary network, an extremely extensive lymphatic capillary system, and the endocrine interstitial cells of Leydig.

INTERSTITIAL TISSUE

The intertubular space is occupied by a system of lymphatic capillaries, blood vessels, nerves, and the interstitial cells of Leydig. (Fig. 33-4)

The **cells of Leydig** vary greatly in number according to the species. In man they occur singly or in small groups. In rat the cells sometimes border on the lumen of the lymphatics, but mostly they abut on the lymphatic endothelium. Their cytoplasm contains an abundance of vesicular

Fig. 33-1. Section of testis. Rabbit. L.M. X 5. **1.** Testis. **2.** Efferent ductules. **3.** Head of epididymis. **4.** Tunica albuginea.

Fig. 33-2. Enlargement of area similar to rectangle in Fig. 33-1. Section of four segments of seminiferous tubules. Testis. Human. L.M. X 168. **1.** Lumen of seminiferous tubule. **2.** Stratified epithelium of spermatogenic cells. **3.** Interstitial tissue. **4.** Cells of Leydig.

Fig. 33-3. Enlargement of area similar to rectangle in Fig. 33-2. Cross section of seminiferous tubule. Testis. Rat. E.M. X 580. **1.** Lumen of seminiferous tubule. **2.** Sertoli cells. **3.** Spermatogonia type B or very early primary spermatocytes. **4.** Primary spermatocytes in the pachytene stage of chromosomal rearrangement (late prophase of meiotic division). **5.** Early spermatids. **6.** Interstitial cells of Leydig. **7.** Peritubular capillaries and venules. **8.** Arteriole. **9.** Peritubular lymphatic space.

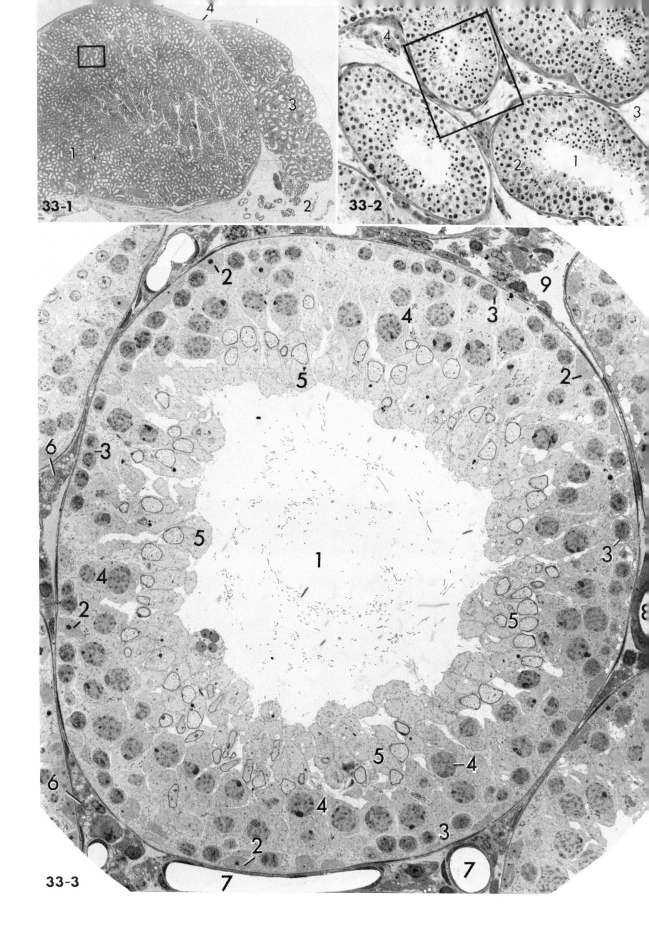

33-1

33-2

33-3

and tubular profiles of the agranular endoplasmic reticulum (Fig. 33-5); a varied number of lipid droplets; some mitochondria; a fairly large Golgi zone; and vacuoles some of which open to the cell surface. In man, protein crystals also occur. The cellular structures are typical of an endocrine organ secreting steroid hormones, in this case androgen. This hormone, also referred to as testosterone, influences secondary sexual characteristics such as the distribution of hair (chin, chest, abdomen); the pitch of the voice; and psychological characteristics of maleness.

The **connective tissue** of the intertubular space is largely composed of collagenous fibers and occasional fibroblasts, the latter particularly around blood vessels. In several mammals, including man, flat sheathlike cells are arranged in a narrow layer around the seminiferous tubules. (Fig. 33-6) In the past these cells have collectively been referred to as "lamellated connective tissue cells." These cells have ultrastructural characteristics such as numerous cytoplasmic filaments and fusiform densities attached to the cytoplasmic aspect of the cell membrane as well as occurring among the filaments. These structures justify classifying these cells as **smooth muscle cells.**

SEMINIFEROUS TUBULES

The seminiferous tubules are lined by a stratified epithelium which consists of **spermatogenic** and **supporting** (Sertoli) cells. (Fig. 33-3) The tubules are surrounded by a **basal lamina** and by the thin, squamous **smooth muscle cells,** described above, invested by their own basal (external) lamina. The connective tissue aspect of the smooth muscle cells, in turn, is covered by the thin endothelium of a vast system of large lymphatic capillaries. The lymphatic investment of the seminiferous tubule and the smooth muscle sheath represent a physiological barrier to blood-borne substances intended to reach the spermatogenic cells. The smooth muscle cells

probably contribute to the gradual movement of sperm from the seminiferous tubules to the epididymis.

The seminiferous epithelium and the spermatogenic cells go through several cycles of development, involving cellular divisions and maturations. The original cell, the **spermatogonium,** develops into **primary spermatocytes** which in turn give rise to **secondary spermatocytes.** The latter develop into **spermatids.** Finally, the spermatid develops into a **spermatozoon.** This entire process is called **spermatogenesis.** However, since the spermatogenesis encompasses about three developmental stages, each different from that preceding, it is advisable to study each step separately. The steps are: 1) spermatocytogenesis; 2) meiosis; and 3) spermiogenesis. The various typical developmental stages of the spermatogenic cells will be described under these steps. It should be remembered, however, that it is a continuous developmental process and that there occur many more intermediate stages than the few described. (Figs. 33-8, 33-9)

Fig. 33-4. Survey of the interstitial space of the testis. Rat. E.M. X 1800. **1.** Base of spermatogenic epithelium. **2.** Interstitial cells of Leydig. **3.** Capillaries and venules. **4.** Lymphatic space. **5.** Lymphatic endothelium. **6.** Lymphocyte.

Fig. 33-5. Detail of Leydig cell. Testis. Rat. E.M. X 37,000. **1.** Agranular endoplasmic reticulum. **2.** Small mitochondria. **3.** Lipid droplets. **4.** Golgi vacuoles. **5.** Ribosomes.

Fig. 33-6. Detail of the base of the seminiferous tubule and adjacent structures. Testis. Rat. E.M. X 27,000. **1.** Part of Sertoli cell. **2.** Cell membrane. **3.** Basal lamina. **4.** Part of squamous smooth muscle cell. **5.** Myofilaments. **6.** Granular endoplasmic reticulum. **7.** Basal (external) lamina surrounding smooth muscle cell. **8.** Lumen of lymphatic space. **9.** Endothelial cytoplasm. **10.** Endothelial nucleus.

Fig. 33-7. Part of Sertoli cell. Seminiferous tubule. Testis. Rat. E.M. X 15,000. **1.** Nucleus. **2.** Mitochondria. **3.** Lipid droplets. **4.** Agranular endoplasmic reticulum. **5.** Golgi zone. **6.** Basal lamina. **7.** Smooth muscle cell. **8.** Lymphatic endothelium.

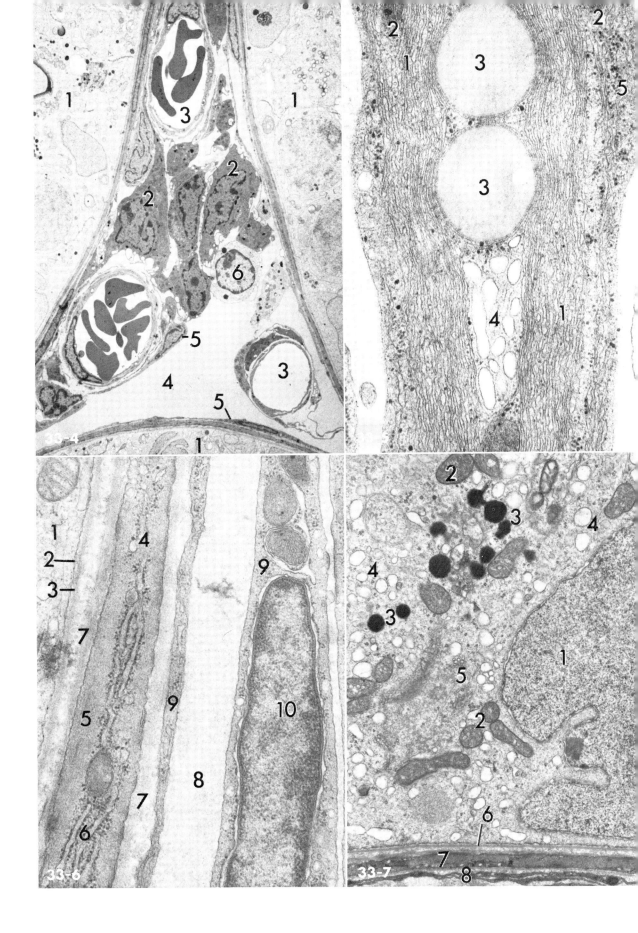

Supporting (Sertoli) cells. Before considering the development of the spermatogenic cells it should be recognized that the Sertoli cells perform a supportive and nutritive function during this developmental process. The Sertoli cells rest on the tubule basal lamina, and extend to the lumen of the tubule. (Fig. 33-7) The lateral parts of the cells harbor the spermatogenic cells in shallow and deep indentations, giving the Sertoli cell a very irregular and sometimes narrow shape. The nucleus is large, deeply indented, with a homogeneous nucleoplasm and a prominent nucleolus. The long axis of the nucleus is most often parallel to the basal lamina but sometimes perpendicular to it. The cytoplasm contains some oval mitochondria, a small Golgi zone, vesicular and tubular profiles of the **agranular endoplasmic reticulum,** some free ribosomes, lipid droplets, primary and secondary lysosomes, filaments, and microtubules. In man, **protein crystals** also occur. Where two Sertoli cells border on each other, the cell membranes display a peculiar variety of a junctional complex.

Spermatocytogenesis. This comprises the mitotic proliferation of the spermatogonia to primary spermatocytes. The spermatogonia rest on or near the tubule basal lamina. (Fig. 33-10) There are two kinds of spermatogonia, termed type A and type B.

The nuclei of **type A spermatogonia** are usually ovoid with either dark or pale nucleoplasm. (Fig. 33-11) The chromatin granules are finely dispersed, and the nucleoli are closely applied to the nuclear membrane. The cytoplasm is sparse, but electron-dense, containing only a few mitochondria, a small Golgi zone, and many free ribosomes. When type A spermatogonia divide by mitosis, about half the number of the daughter cells become type A spermatogonia (stem cells), whereas the other half become type B spermatogonia.

The **type B spermatogonia** differ from type A spermatogonia by their mostly round nuclei, heavily stained chromatin masses attached to the nuclear membrane or to the nucleoli, the latter located near the center of the nucleus. (Fig. 33-12) When the type B spermatogonia divide by mitosis, the daughter cells all differentiate to become primary spermatocytes.

Upon division of the type B spermatogonia, their daughter cells, the **primary spermatocytes,** are at first indistinguishable from their mother cell. Gradually, their nuclei and the cytoplasm enlarge, and the chromatin pattern of the nucleus rearranges typically as the chromosomes go through the various steps of reorganization. This rearrangement of the chromosomes during the prolonged prophase, preliminary to the meiotic division, is reflected somewhat in the ultrastructural architecture of the nucleus. During the leptotene and zygotene stages, the chromosomes are seen as fine and highly coiled threads. In the pachytene stage, the nucleus of the primary spermatocyte contains coarse threads because of the fusion of homologous chromosomes. (Fig. 33-13) The cytoplasm of the primary spermato-

Fig. 33-8. Cross section of seminiferous tubule. Testis. Rat. E.M. X 600. **1.** Lumen of tubule with tails of late spermatids. **2.** Sertoli cells. **3.** Primary spermatocytes (leptotene stage of prophase). **4.** Early spermatids. **5.** Middle piece of late spermatids.

Fig. 33-9. Cross section of seminiferous tubule. Testis. Rat. E.M. X 600. **1.** Lumen of tubule. **2.** Sertoli cells. **3.** Spermatogonia type B. **4.** Dividing primary spermatocytes (meiotic division). **5.** Secondary spermatocytes. **6.** Spermatids in midstage of their development.

Fig. 33-10. Survey of the stratified spermatogenic epithelium. Testis. Rat. E.M. X 1800. **1.** Smooth muscle sheath surrounding the seminiferous tubule. **2.** Sertoli cell nucleus. **3.** Type A spermatogonia with oval nuclei and a broad cytoplasmic base resting on the basal lamina. **4.** Nuclei of primary spermatocytes (leptotene stage of prophase of meiotic division). **5.** Nuclei of early spermatids with rows of marginated small mitochondria. **6.** Vesiculated vertical cytoplasm of Sertoli cell with heads of late spermatids. **7.** Vesiculated horizontal stretch of Sertoli cell cytoplasm.

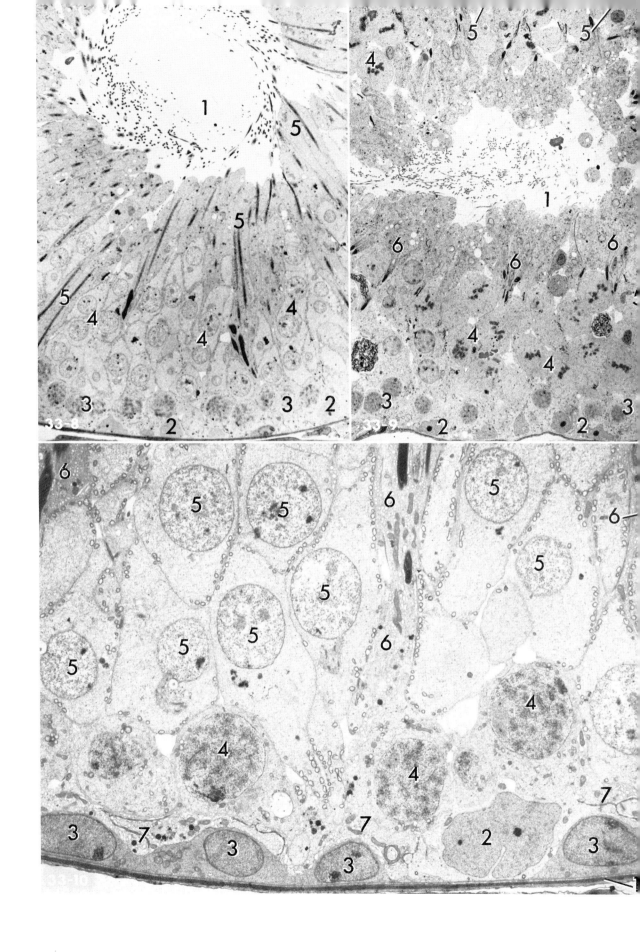

cyte is small in relation to the nucleus and contains only a few mitochondria and many free ribosomes. The development of the primary spermatocytes takes several days. Therefore, primary spermatocytes in various stages of growth are frequently seen in a section.

Meiosis (reduction division). During this phase of the development, the primary spermatocytes go through two divisions. During the **first meiotic division,** when primary spermatocytes generate secondary spermatocytes, there occurs a 50 percent reduction in the number of chromosomes. Ordinary somatic cells, as well as primary spermatocytes, contain 46 chromosomes (or 23 pairs). They have, therefore, a diploid (= double) number of chromosomes. After the first meiotic division of the primary spermatocytes which results in **secondary spermatocytes,** the nucleus of the secondary spermatocyte contains only 23 single chromosomes. It therefore has a haploid (= single) number of chromosomes. (See also p. 58)

The secondary spermatocytes are smaller than the primary spermatocytes, and are rarely observed in a section, since they rapidly divide by a regular mitosis to give rise to spermatids. This is the **second meiotic division** which does not result in a further reduction of the 23 single chromosomes of the secondary spermatocytes. During the two meiotic divisions, the daughter cells aggregate above the basal layer of spermatogonia, and the final product, the spermatids, border on the lumen of the seminiferous tubule. There is a tendency for some of the dividing generations of type B spermatogonia and spermatocytes to remain in contact through a narrow cytoplasmic bridge. This may contribute to the development of abnormal spermatozoa with dual heads or tails.

As a result of the second meiotic division, spermatids arise, each retaining 23 single chromosomes from the first meiotic division. The **early spermatid** has a medium-size pale, round, or oval nucleus

with a loose chromatin network. Mitochondria are small, spherical, and have an electron-lucent center. They are arranged in a layer along the cell membrane. There are numerous free ribosomes, vesicular profiles of the agranular endoplasmic reticulum, and a Golgi zone which is rather prominent. (Fig. 33-14) The spermatids do not divide further but go through a cytological transformation in several steps, leading to a mature spermatozoon.

Spermiogenesis. This term relates to the cytological transformation of a spermatid into a mature spermatozoon. The spermatid is a spherical cell which is transformed into an elongated structure not unlike a tadpole. Generally, the transformation encompasses: a condensation of the nuclear chromatin material into the **head** of the sperm; the formation of the head cap; the outgrowth of a cilium-like structure, the sperm **tail;** an aggregation of mitochondria around the middle piece of the sperm tail; and the shedding of the superfluous part of the spermatid cytoplasm.

Fig. 33-11. Spermatogonium type A. Seminiferous tubule. Testis. Rat. E.M. X 15,000. **1.** Oval nucleus. **2.** Nucleolus. **3.** Nuclear envelope. **4.** Circle: polysomes in dense cytoplasm. **5.** Mitochondrion. **6.** Light cytoplasm of Sertoli cell. **7.** Cell borders.

Fig. 33-12. Spermatogonium type B. Seminiferous tubule. Testis. Rat. E.M. X 18,000. **1.** Round nucleus. **2.** Chromatin masses. **3.** Circle: polysomes. **4.** Mitochondrion. **5.** Golgi zone. **6.** Granular endoplasmic reticulum. **7.** Chromatoid body. **8.** Cell borders.

Fig. 33-13. Primary spermatocyte. Seminiferous tubule. Testis. Rat. E.M. X 10,000. **1.** Nucleus in late pachytene stage of chromosomal rearrangement during prophase of first meiotic division. **2.** Nuclear envelope. **3.** Narrow rim of cytoplasm. **4.** Mitochondria. **5.** Masses of delicate granules represent chromosomes, sectioned at varied angles. **6.** Fibrillar core in chromosomes (transient structure).

Fig. 33-14. Early spermatid. Seminiferous tubule. Testis. Rat. E.M. X 10,000. **1.** Nucleus. **2.** Nuclear envelope. **3.** Large Golgi zone. **4.** Centriole. **5.** Aggregations of mitochondria.

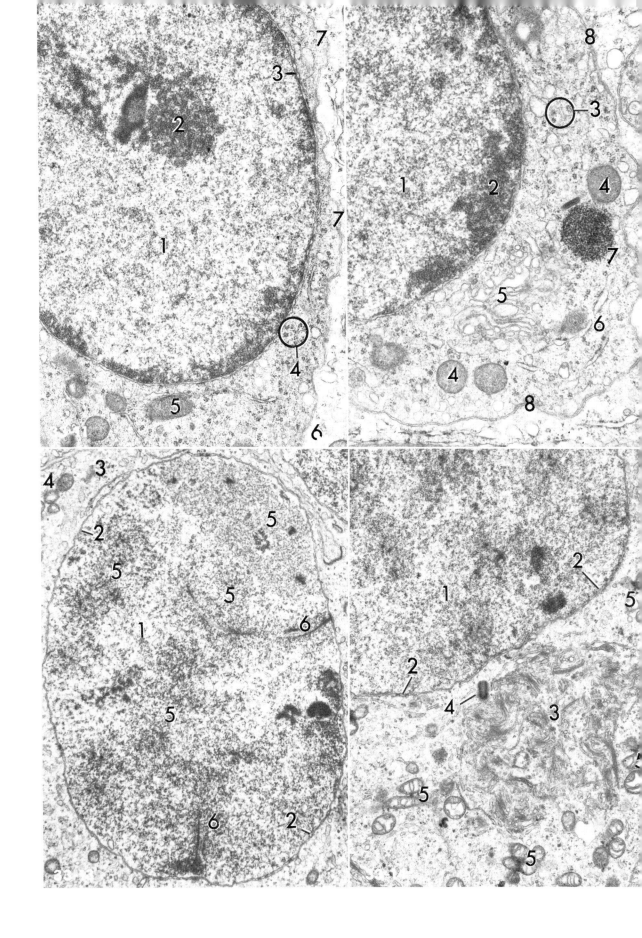

Specifically, the formation of the head cap involves the Golgi zone, in which a mucopolysaccharide material is secreted and accumulated in a membranous sac of the Golgi zone. (Fig. 33-15) Subsequently, this sac settles as a cap on the top of one pole of the nucleus. (Fig. 33-16) Ultimately, this **acrosomal cap** covers about half of the nucleus. (Fig. 33-18) This part becomes the front end of the mature spermatozoon. Simultaneously a condensation of the nucleoplasm occurs whereby the nucleus elongates, leaving the front end curved and flattening the caudal pole. The 2 centrioles of the spermatid move to the area behind the flat caudal pole (Fig. 33-17), and the more distal of the 2 centrioles grows out to become an extremely elongated flagellum, the **axoneme**, which forms the core of the sperm tail. The axoneme has the classical architecture of a cilium with 2 central single microtubules and 9 peripheral double microtubules. With the growth of the axoneme the spermatid gradually becomes elongated.

As final steps in the development, 9 thick longitudinal fibrils form peripherally of the axial microtubules. The place of the connecting piece of the future sperm is marked by the formation of segmented rings around the 2 centrioles behind the nucleus. The middle piece of the sperm is marked by the aggregation of mitochondria around the thick longitudinal fibrils, and the principal piece by the formation of a peripheral fibrous sheath around the axoneme and the thick longitudinal fibrils.

Spermatozoon. The mature spermatozoon is an extremely elongated structure, in man measuring about 65 μ. There are several structurally distinct parts: **head**; **neck** (or connecting piece); and **tail**, consisting of middle piece, principal piece, and end piece. (Figs. 33-22 to 33-25)

The shape of the **head** varies greatly with the species. In man it is almond-shaped, measuring about 5 μ in length, 3 μ in width, and 1 μ in thickness. The head contains the nucleus with its highly condensed chromatin material, and the acrosomal cap, consisting of a greatly enlarged former Golgi saccule, filled with a dense mucopolysaccharide content containing essentially the enzyme hyaluronidase. This enzyme functions as a lytic spreading factor during the penetration of the zona pellucida of the ovum during fertilization. Outermost is the cell membrane of the sperm, snugly fitted over the head cap and the free lateral and caudal parts of the nucleus.

The **neck** is the short piece that connects the head to the tail. It is about 1 μ wide and contains the proximal and the distal centrioles, surrounded by segmental fibrous rings.

Throughout, the core of the **tail** is made up of the axoneme consisting of 2 single central microtubules and a cylinder of 9 double peripheral microtubules. They participate in propelling the spermatozoon in a forward motion.

In the **middle piece** of the tail, which is about 7 μ long and 1 μ thick, there are nine additional coarse outer fibrils, oriented longitudinally. These fibrils do not have a clear center. (Fig. 33-19) Their function is not known, but they most likely participate in the contractions of the tail. The fibrils are in turn surrounded by elongated mitochondria, joined end-to-

Fig. 33-15. Early spermatid. Seminiferous tubule. Testis. Rat. E.M. X 17,000.
1. Nucleus. **2.** Nuclear envelope. **3.** Golgi zone. **4.** Acrosomal vesicle. **5.** Acrosomal granule. **6.** Point of adherence between acrosomal vesicle and nuclear envelope, marking future tip of the sperm nucleus.
Fig. 33-16. Spermatid in a developmental stage subsequent to that seen in Fig. 33-15. Seminiferous tubule. Testis. Rat. E.M. X 17,000. **1.** Nucleus. **2.** Nuclear envelope. **3.** Acrosome. **4.** Acrosomal head cap.
Fig. 33-17. Late spermatid. Seminiferous tubule. Testis. Mouse. E.M. X 16,000. **1.** Caudal, flat end of nucleus. **2.** Axoneme. **3.** Manchette: transient structure, composed of microtubules.
Fig. 33-18. Late spermatid. Seminiferous tubule. Testis. Mouse. E.M. X 30,000. **1.** Frontal end of nucleus. **2.** Acrosome. **3.** Cytoplasm of Sertoli cell. **4.** Head cap.

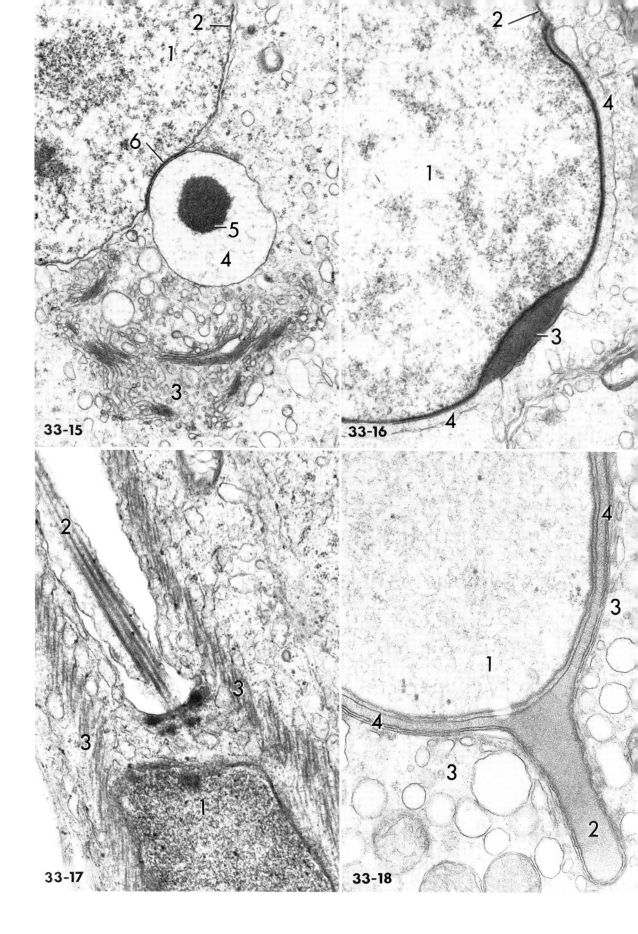

33-15

33-16

33-17

33-18

end, and arranged in a helix throughout the middle piece. The mitochondria provide the energy required for the sperm movements. A fibrous end-ring, the annulus, marks the termination of the mitochondrial helix, and the transition of the middle piece into the principal piece.

The **principal piece** of the tail is about 45 μ long. It is narrower than the middle piece, averaging 0.5 μ in width. The coarse longitudinal outer fibrils continue through the principal piece and are surrounded by a fibrous sheath, consisting of circumferentially arranged dense fibrils, reminiscent of the ribs in the thorax. (Fig. 33-20)

The tapering **end piece** is about 5 μ long and contains only the microtubules of the axoneme. (Fig. 33-21) The cell membrane closely surrounds the tail throughout. Except for the organelles described, there are none present in the normal spermatozoon.

To summarize the **functions** of the various parts of the spermatozoon: The head contains the haploid (single; 1 $\times$ 23) number of chromosomes in the highly condensed chromatin of the nucleus. The headcap carries the acrosomal substance which contains hyaluronidase, a lytic enzyme which acts as a spreading factor during the penetration of the corona radiata and zona pellucida of the ovum. The centrioles of the neck region and the microtubules of the tail are responsible for the motile activity of the spermatozoon. It has been suggested that rhythmic impulses arise at one point in the distal centriole and circulate around it, thereby propagating waves of microtubule contraction in a spiral pattern throughout the array of 9 peripheral, double microtubules. It is not clear if the microtubules actually contract. Instead, each pair may slide in relation to the neighboring pair, as suggested for ciliary movements (p. 22). To bring about bending in the tail, shortening need only amount to about 5 percent of the total microtubule. The contraction (sliding) results in a bending wave, accompanied by a relaxation (sliding) in the opposite direc-

tion. The central pair of microtubules are regarded as either conductile or supportive. The fibrous sheath and the coarse outer fibrils are believed to be supportive. The energy necessary to effect wave motion is primarily supplied by the coiled mitochondria, but components of the respiratory chain may not be limited to the mitochondrial apparatus.

BLOOD VESSELS, LYMPHATICS, AND NERVES

The **blood supply** of the testis is derived mainly from branches of the internal spermatic artery to the tunica vasculosa under the testicular capsule. Arteries enter the parenchyma via the septula and distribute arterioles and capillaries in the interstitial tissue and interstitial space. The blood capillaries are of the thin, continuous, non-fenestrated type. The venous drainage occurs to a major degree through venules and veins coursing through the mediastinum testis. To a minor degree, some veins also go toward the tunica vasculosa.

Cross and longitudinal sections of rat spermatozoon.

Fig. 33-19. Cross section of **middle piece.**
E.M. $\times$ 108,000.
Fig. 33-20. Cross sections at varied levels of **principal piece.** E.M. $\times$ 80,000.
Fig. 33-21. Cross section of **end piece.**
E.M. $\times$ 72,000.
Fig. 33-22. Longitudinal section of frontal end of **head.** E.M. $\times$ 70,000.
Fig. 33-23. Longitudinal section of **head, neck** and beginning of **middle piece.**
E.M. $\times$ 51,000.
Fig. 33-24. Longitudinal section of **principal piece.** E.M. $\times$ 64,000.
Fig. 33-25. Longitudinal section of **principal piece,** near its end. E.M. $\times$ 96,000.

1. Cell membrane. **2.** Acrosome. **3.** Acrosomal cap. **4.** Subacrosomal space. **5.** Nucleus. **6.** Nuclear membrane. **7.** Caudal end of nucleus. **8.** Modified proximal centriole. **9.** Distal centriole. **10.** Central microtubules. **11.** Peripheral microtubules. **12.** Outer dense fibrils. **13.** Longitudinal column. **14.** Rib of fibrous sheath. **15.** Mitochondrial sheath.

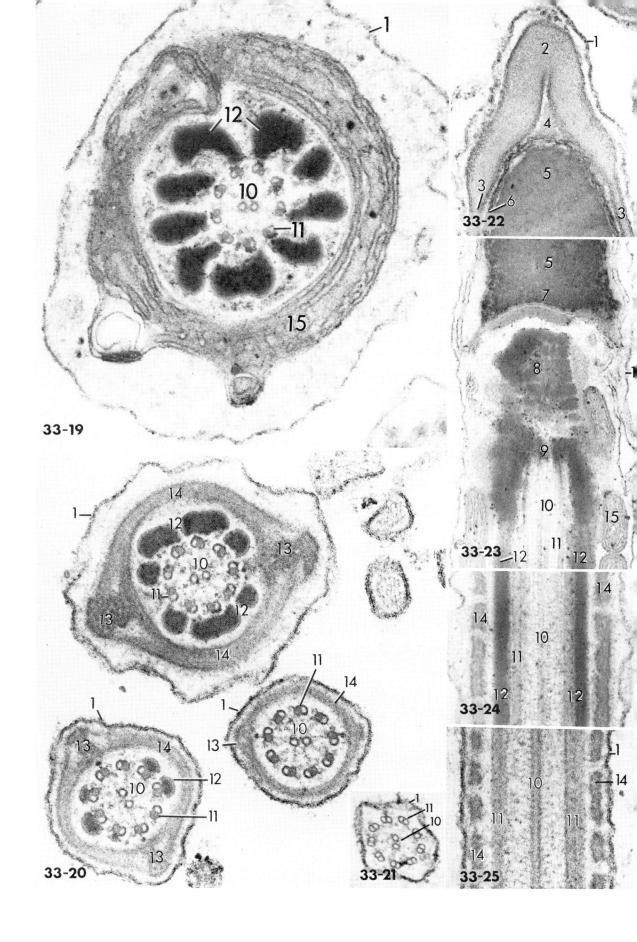

33-19

33-20

33-21

33-22

33-23

33-24

33-25

The **lymphatic** network is quite extensive in the intertubular space. Lymphatic capillaries surround all blood vessels and closely invest the interstitial aspect of the seminiferous tubules. Most of the lymphatic outflow goes via the mediastinum.

Nerves present in the testis are derived from the internal spermatic plexus. They accompany the blood vessels as fine plexuses. Nerve endings have not been identified in relation to spermatogenic cells.

Excretory Ducts

A set of relatively short ducts serve to transport the sperm from the seminiferous tubules of the testis to the epididymis. Included are the tubuli recti, the rete testis, the ductuli efferentes, the ductus epididymidis, the ductus deferens, and the ductus ejaculatorius.

Tubuli recti. From each lobule of the testis, one tubulus rectus emerges, connecting the seminiferous tubule with the rete testis. Directly following the seminiferous tubule, the tubulus rectus is lined by a columnar epithelium composed mostly of cells structurally similar to Sertoli cells. The rest of the straight tubule is lined by a cuboidal epithelium. The luminal surface of the cells is smooth and is not provided with cilia. The cells rest on a basal lamina. The tubules are not surrounded by smooth muscle cells.

Rete testis. The rete testis is a network of irregular labyrinthine spaces and interconnected tubules in the mediastinum testis. (Fig. 33-26) They are lined by a simple epithelium composed of a mixture of low columnar, cuboidal, or squamous cells. (Fig. 33-27) Their luminal surface is smooth with the exception of a single cilium on an occasional cell. There is a thin basal lamina separating the epithelium from the connective tissue of the mediastinum. This connective tissue is composed of mostly collagenous fibers and some fibroblasts. There are no smooth muscle cells present.

Ductuli efferentes. From the upper, posterior part of the mediastinum testis emerge 15–20 ductuli efferentes. They connect the rete testis with the ductus epididymidis. Each ductulus begins relatively straight, but becomes increasingly tortuous as it enters and forms part of the head of the epididymis. (Fig. 33-28) By its tortuosity, each ductulus forms a pyramid with the tip toward the rete testis and the base toward the ductus epididymidis. This formation is called a **conus vasculosus.** The ductuli efferentes are lined by a pseudostratified epithelium of varying height, giving it a folded appearance. (Fig. 33-29) It is composed of columnar and cuboidal cells with an incomplete layer of small polyhedral basal cells. There is a mixture of ciliated and non-ciliated cells. The cilia beat toward the ductus epididymidis. The non-ciliated cells are provided with short microvilli. These cells are considered to be secretory in nature, although secretory granules have not been demonstrated in man. In routine histological preparations, the apical cytoplasm of these cells is often seen to rise toward the lumen in a drop-

Fig. 33-26. General architecture of rete testis. Human. L.M. X 300. **1.** Interconnected tubules; arrows indicate direction in which sperm moves from testis to epididymis. **2.** Irregular dense connective tissue of the mediastinum testis.

Fig. 33-27. Enlargement of rectangle in Fig. 33-26. Testis. Human. L.M. X 630. **1.** Tubular lumen. **2.** Columnar epithelial cells. **3.** Cuboidal cells. **4.** Squamous cells. **5.** Dense bundles of collagenous fibrils. **6.** Nucleus of fibroblast.

Fig. 33-28. Section through head of epididymis. Human. L.M. X 42. **1.** Efferent ductules. **2.** Sections of the convoluted duct of epididymis. **3.** Loose connective tissue. **4.** Capsule of caput epididymidis.

Fig. 33-29. Enlargement of a cross-sectioned efferent ductule. Human. L.M. X 510. **1.** Lumen. **2.** Pseudostratified columnar epithelium. **3.** Area with simple cuboidal epithelium. **4.** Cilia. **5.** Secretory cell with coarse cytoplasmic processes extending into the lumen. **6.** Basal lamina. **7.** Collagenous bundles. **8.** Nuclei of fibroblasts.

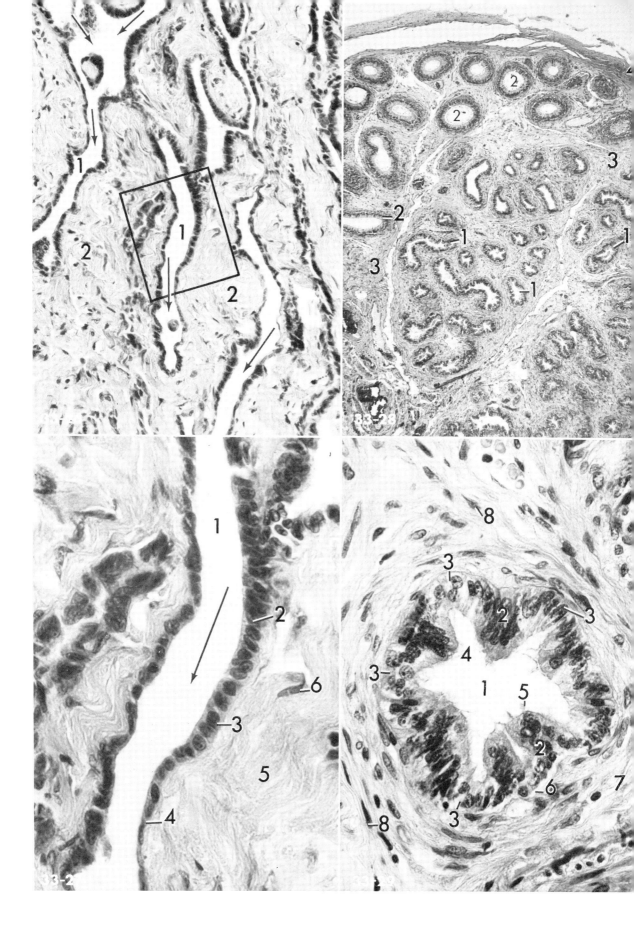

shaped formation. This has been interpreted as a sign of apocrine secretion.

The epithelium rests on a thin basal lamina. The ductules are surrounded by a thin layer of smooth muscle cells. The mechanism by which the sperm are moved from the seminiferous tubules to the ductus epididymidis is not fully understood. However, the beats of the cilia of the efferent ductules and contractions of the smooth muscle cells are believed to aid in this transport.

Epididymis

The epididymis consists of head, body, and tail. The head (caput) is located at the upper pole of the testis. (Fig. 33-30) The body (corpus) is attached to and follows the medial posterior side of the testis. The tail (cauda) is near the lower pole of the testis, connecting here with the ductus deferens.

The main component of the epididymis is the highly convoluted **ductus epididymidis**. The coni vasculosi of the ductuli efferentes form a major part of the head of the epididymis. They all empty into the beginning of the ductus epididymidis within the head region. Together with loose connective tissue, the coiled tubular duct (Fig. 33-31) forms the body and the tail of the epididymis.

The duct is lined by a pseudostratified stereociliated **epithelium** with tall columnar cells and an incomplete layer of small polygonal basal cells. (Fig. 33-32) The columnar cells are generally taller in the head of the epididymis than they are in the body or the tail. In addition, there are other marked regional variations of the duct epithelium within the head, possible reflecting a difference in the functions of the several regions. Projecting from the luminal surface of the columnar cells are found throughout numerous long and narrow microvilli, usually referred to as **stereocilia** because of their alleged lack of mobility. (Fig. 33-33) The stereocilia

often arise in a tuft-like arrangement from a luminal bulge of the apical cytoplasm. Similar to most microvilli throughout the body, the stereocilia contain a varying number of filaments. They are not arranged as regularly as in cilia, nor do they emanate from basal corpuscles, although the filaments continue down into the apical cytoplasm. Of cytoplasmic organelles, the Golgi complex and the granular endoplasmic reticulum occupy the largest part of the cell. (Fig. 33-34) Mitochondria are elongated and occur in limited numbers, whereas lysosomes, multivesicular bodies, and profiles of the agranular endoplasmic reticulum are quite numerous. In several species, including man, droplets and vacuoles occur in the apical cytoplasm. In addition, vesicular cytoplasm is often seen to be associated with the bases of some stereocilia.

The functions of the columnar cells are not completely explored and understood. Ultrastructural analyses of the epithelium under normal and experimental condi-

Fig. 33-30. Section of epididymis. Rabbit. L.M. X 14. **1.** Part of testis. **2.** Efferent ductules. **3.** Convoluted ductus epididymidis.

Fig. 33-31. Ductus epididymidis. Rat. L.M. X 170. **1.** Lumen of the duct. **2.** Pseudostratified columnar epithelium. **3.** Loose connective tissue.

Fig. 33-32. Enlargement of an area similar to rectangle in Fig. 33-31. Epididymis. Rat. E.M. X 600. **1.** Lumen of the duct. **2.** Stereocilia. **3.** Nuclei of columnar cells. **4.** Nuclei of basal cells. **5.** Nuclei of smooth muscle cells. **6.** Fibroblasts of loose connective tissue. **7.** Prominent Golgi complexes in columnar cells. **8.** Basal lamina.

Fig. 33-33. Enlargement of rectangle (A) in Fig. 33-32. Epididymis. Rat. E.M. X 8400. **1.** Mitochondria. **2.** Large and medium size secretory droplets. **3.** Vesicles. **4.** Stereocilia. **5.** Lumen. **6.** Filaments of stereocilia continue down into the cell. **7.** Vesicular cytoplasm along stereocilia.

Fig. 33-34. Enlargement of rectangle (B) in Fig. 33-32. Epididymis. Rat. E.M. X 8400. **1.** Nuclei of columnar cells. **2.** Granular endoplasmic reticulum. **3.** Mitochondria. **4.** Ribosomes. **5.** Golgi complexes. **6.** Secretory droplets.

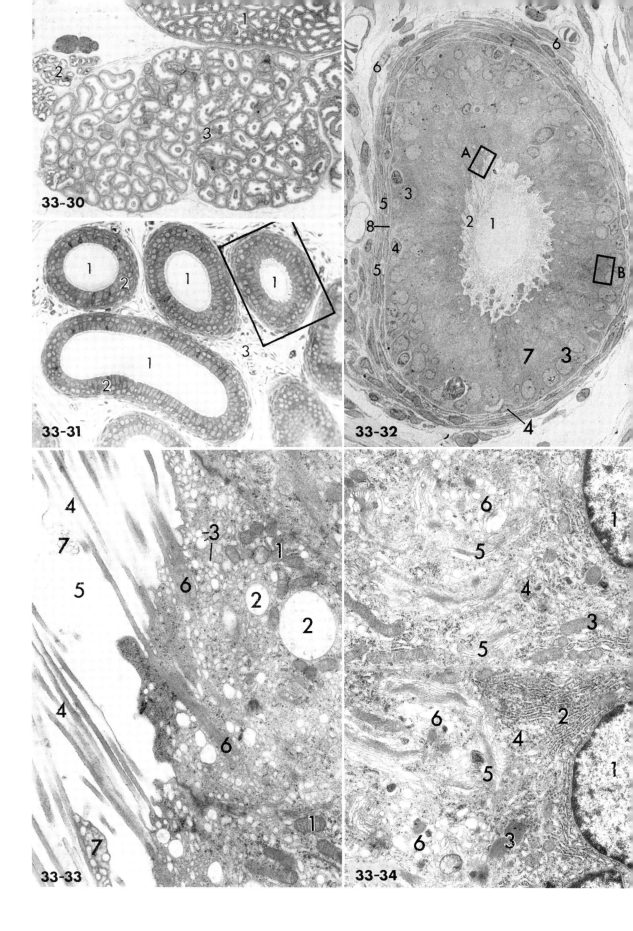

33-30

33-31

33-32

33-33

33-34

tions in several mammalian species indicate that the epithelium of the ductus epididymidis aids in both secretory and resorptive processes. The large number of vacuoles, lysosomes and multivesicular bodies points to phagocytic and eliminating functions. The vast amounts of granular and agranular endoplasmic reticulum are in support of secretory functions, possibly both exocrine and endocrine in nature. In either case the products synthesized would be secreted into the epididymidal fluid and there exert their effect on the sperm in processes involved in activating the fertilizing capacity of sperm (capacitation).

The epithelium rests on a thin **basal lamina.** Surrounding the duct are thin layers of smooth muscle cells, forming a **muscularis.** This is instrumental in forwarding the sperm to the ductus deferens by peristaltic movements.

Ductus Deferens

The duct of the epididymis continues directly into the ductus deferens at the tail of the epididymis. Initially convoluted, it gradually becomes straight and makes a sharp turn, beginning its course up toward the inguinal canal. The ductus deferens, together with spermatic arteries, convoluted veins of the pampiniform plexus, nerves, and muscular extensions of the abdominal wall, form the **spermatic cord.** There is a spindle-shaped dilatation of the ductus deferens, the **ampulla,** just before the junction of the ductus deferens and the excretory duct of the seminal vesicle. The united ducts form the **ejaculatory duct.** The ducts, one from each side, traverse the prostate gland and open up into the prostatic part of the urethra. The wall of the ductus deferens has three layers, the mucosa, the muscularis, and the adventitia or fibrosa.

The **mucosa** is composed of a pseudostratified columnar epithelium and a thin lamina propria. (Figs. 33-35, 33-36) The

mucous membrane is thrown into a few folds throughout the ductus deferens. In the ampulla, the folds are higher and more complex. In the **epithelium,** tall columnar cells predominate over the less numerous, small cuboidal basal cells. The columnar cells are provided with stereocilia. (Fig. 33-37) They have the same fine structure as those in the epididymis. There is an abundance of mitochondria and ribosomes, but a scarcity of lysosomes and profiles of granular endoplasmic reticulum. The Golgi area is small and restricted. Secretory droplets occur but are less frequent than in the epididymis. This indicates that the columnar stereociliated cells of the ductus deferens have less of a secretory function than their counterparts in the epididymis. It has been demonstrated that the epithelium of the ductus deferens in the rat functions in absorption of protein from the lumen of the duct. In the ampulla, there is an increased

Fig. 33-35. Cross-sectioned ductus deferens. Monkey. L.M. X 130. **1.** Lumen. **2.** Pseudostratified columnar epithelium. **3.** Lamina propria. **4.** Inner longitudinal smooth muscle layer. **5.** Middle circular smooth muscle layer. **6.** Outer longitudinal smooth muscle layer.

Fig. 33-36. Enlargement of area similar to rectangle in Fig. 33-35. Ductus deferens. Rat. E.M. X 640. **1.** Lumen. **2.** Pseudostratified columnar epithelium. **3.** Lamina propria. **4.** Capillaries. **5.** Inner longitudinal smooth muscle layer.

Fig. 33-37. Enlargement of rectangle (A) in Fig. 33-36. Ductus deferens. Rat. E.M. X 4300. **1.** Lumen. **2.** Stereocilia. **3.** Nuclei. **4.** Golgi complexes. **5.** Mitochondria. **6.** Lipid droplets. **7.** Secretory droplets.

Fig. 33-38. Enlargement of area similar to rectangle (B) in Fig. 33-36. Ductus deferens. Rat. E.M. X 4500. **1.** Some of the cells in the lamina propria are smooth muscle cells, representing a kind of muscularis mucosae. **2.** Collagen of lamina propria. **3.** Nucleus of Schwann cell of non-myelinated nerve. **4.** Nuclei of smooth muscle cells in the inner longitudinal layer. **5.** Cross-sectioned peripheral parts of smooth muscle cell cytoplasm.

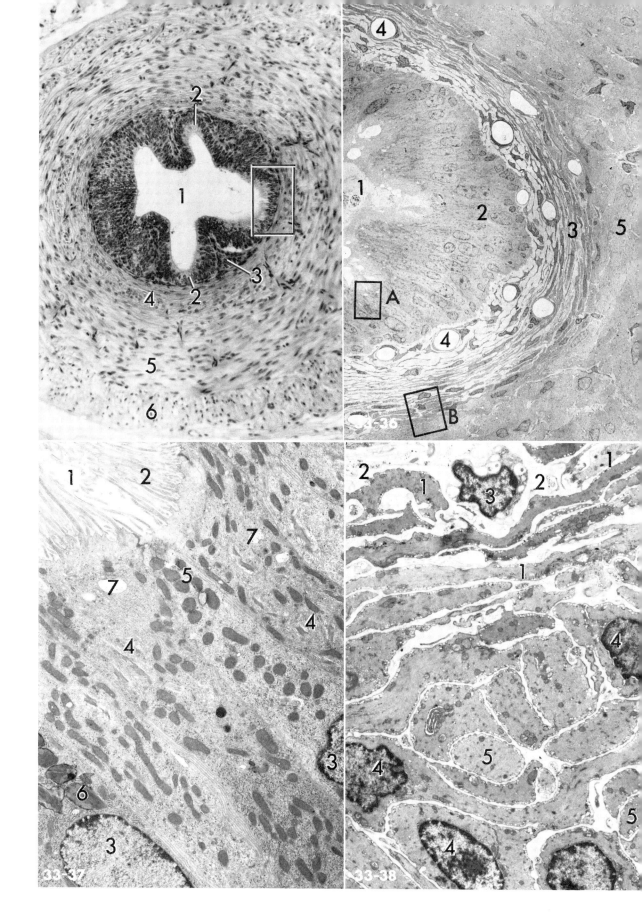

secretory activity by these cells. In the ejaculatory duct near the urethral opening the epithelium changes to a transitional type. Everywhere, the epithelium rests on a basal lamina. The **lamina propria** contains a rich capillary network, fibroblasts arranged in a lamellated pattern, and a predominance of elastic fibers over the collagenous type.

The **muscularis** consists of three smooth muscle layers: an **inner** longitudinal which is relatively thin; a **middle** circular, rather thick; and an **outer** layer, relatively thin and oriented longitudinally. (Fig. 33-38) The muscle bundles of the various layers seem to be related to one another in a spiral arrangement. There is an abundance of autonomic motor nerves mixed in with the smooth muscle cells. At the ultrastructural level, it has been confirmed that almost every smooth muscle cell has a neuromuscular junction. This explains the fast contraction of the ductus deferens during ejaculation. It is in contrast to the arrangement of smooth muscle cells elsewhere in the body with fewer nerve endings terminating directly on the muscle cell membrane. In this case the contraction is slower.

The **adventitia** contains fibroblasts, elastic and collagenous fibers, in addition to nerves, blood vessels, and lymphatics.

Seminal Vesicles

The two seminal vesicles are saccular glands (Fig. 33-39) located behind the prostate gland and lateral to each ampulla of the ductus deferens. They develop as outgrowths from the ductus deferens near the ampulla. The seminal vesicles are irregularly shaped, elongated small bodies with the front end tapering off and joining the terminal end of the ductus deferens to form one ductus ejaculatorius on either side of the prostate gland.

The wall of the seminal vesicle contains three major strata: the adventitia, the muscularis, and the mucosa. The adventitia forms a thin **capsule** of fibrous connective tissue, richly mixed in with elastic fibers. The **lamina muscularis** is relatively thick. It consists of an inner circular layer and an outer longitudinal layer of smooth muscle cells.

The **mucous membrane** has a lamina propria which contains a network of loose vascularized connective tissue. The architecture of the mucosa is relatively complicated. The entire seminal vesicle is actually a single highly coiled and convoluted tube which has many diverticula, recesses, and small crypts. The mucous membrane is arranged in many folds and tall ridges, and both secondary and tertiary folds exist. (Fig. 33-40) This arrangement increases the epithelial surface considerably but reduces simultaneously the originally large lumen of the seminal vesicle. In sections, the mucous membrane therefore has a honeycombed pattern simulating tubuloalveolar glands, although

Fig. 33-39. Cross section of ductus deferens and seminal vesicle. Monkey. L.M. X 11.
1. Ductus deferens. **2.** Lumen of the coiled tube which constitutes the seminal vesicle.
3. Capsule.

Fig. 33-40. Enlargement of rectangle in Fig. 33-39. Seminal vesicle. Monkey. L.M. X 107.
1. Main lumen. **2.** Diverticulum. **3.** Crypt.
4. Ridge covered by epithelium. **5.** Lamina muscularis.

Fig. 33-41. Enlargement of area similar to rectangle in Fig. 33-40. Seminal vesicle. Rat. E.M. X 630. **1.** Lumina of diverticuli.
2. Accumulation of secretion. **3.** Simple columnar epithelium. **4.** Connective tissue with capillaries.

Fig. 33-42. Enlargement of area similar to rectangle (A) in Fig. 33-41. Seminal vesicle. Rat. E.M. X 10,000. **1.** Nuclei of epithelial cells. **2.** Granular endoplasmic reticulum.
3. Mitochondria. **4.** Golgi complexes.
5. Secretory granules, with and without electron-dense core.

Fig. 33-43. Enlargement of area similar to rectangle (B) in Fig. 33-41. Seminal vesicle. Rat. E.M. X 32,000. **1.** Lumen.
2. Microvilli. **3.** Ribosomes. **4.** Small secretory granules. **5.** Large secretory granules with dense core. **6.** Residue of discharged dense core of secretory granule.

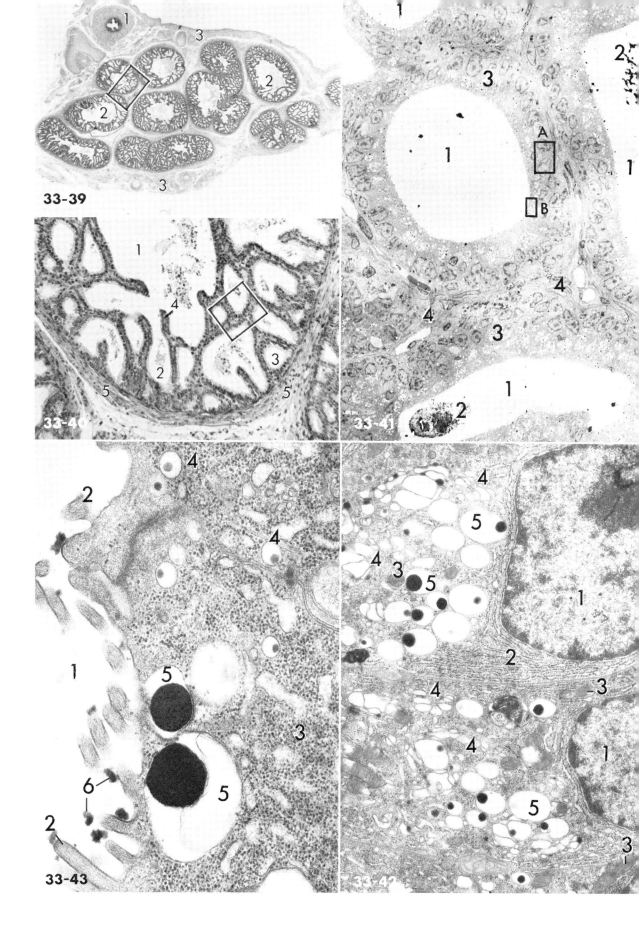

33-39

33-40

33-41

33-43

33-42

all recesses, crypts, and diverticuli are connected to the central lumen of the coiled seminal vesicle.

The **epithelium** is simple with low or high columnar cells resting on a thin basal lamina. (Fig. 33-41) The cell height is dependent upon the action of testosterone. Highly active cells are tall columnar. At times, particularly in man, a pseudostratified epithelium with some small basal cells can occur. The cells have large oval nuclei. The cytoplasm is dominated by the granular endoplasmic reticulum with mostly flattened cisternae. The Golgi zone is supranuclear (Fig. 33-42), rather large, and contains many presecretory granules. Mitochondria are small and scarce. The secretory granules have a small, electron-dense core and a peripheral, less dense halo bounded by a membrane. Lysosomes and lipofuscin granules occur. They probably represent the brownish-yellow lipochrome pigment granules, identified early by light microscopy. The secretory granules are discharged into the lumen of the gland at the apical cell surface. (Fig. 33-43)

Ordinarily, the secretion is stored in the lumen as deeply staining masses of finely granular material. The secretion is an alkaline, clear, slightly sticky gelatinous fluid of a brownish-yellow color.

The secretion contains globulin. It serves as a fluid vehicle for the spermatozoa, and it probably has some nutritive influence on them.

Prostate

The prostate is a serous gland with the size and the shape of a chestnut. Its base is attached to the inferior surface of the urinary bladder, and the urethra passes through the anterior part of the prostate. The anterior surface of the gland is directed toward the symphysis pubis. The posterior surface can be palpated through the rectum, and at the inferior part, the apex rests against the deep layer of the urogenital diaphragm. Within the prostatic urethra, the **urethral crest** forms a narrow longitudinal ridge with prostatic **sinuses** on either side. The **colliculus seminalis** is a median elevation on the crest where the slit-like openings of two **ejaculatory ducts** are situated. The **utriculus prostaticus** is a small, pocket-like indentation of the colliculus between the orifices of the ejaculatory ducts. (Fig. 33-44)

A thin **capsule** surrounds the gland and penetrates the parenchyma as septa and trabeculae to form the prostatic **stroma** of fibroelastic tissue, poor in fibroblasts but mixed in with a considerable amount of smooth muscle cells. A broad, median septum contains the urethra. The prostate is subdivided by the septa into five lobes. The left and right lateral lobes form the main part of the gland, whereas the middle, anterior, and posterior lobes are small and grouped around the prostatic urethra. The glandular **parenchyma** normally occupies about half the volume of the gland. It consists of compound tubuloalveolar

Fig. 33-44. Cross section of prostate gland. Monkey. L.M. X 5. **1.** Anterior (pubic) surface. **2.** Posterior (rectal) surface. **3.** Lateral lobes. **4.** Broad median septum. **5.** Prostatic urethra. **6.** Prostatic sinus. **7.** Colliculus seminalis of urethral crest. **8.** Capsule.

Fig. 33-45. Enlargement of area similar to circle in Fig. 33-44. Prostate. Human. L.M. X 125. **1.** Alveolar lumen. **2.** Glandular epithelium. **3.** Corpora amylacea. **4.** Connective tissue stroma. **5.** Smooth muscle cells.

Fig. 33-46. Survey of prostatic alveoli. Dorsal prostate. Rat. E.M. X 560. **1.** Alveolar lumen. **2.** Glandular epithelium. **3.** Epithelial folds. **4.** Connective tissue stroma. **5.** Smooth muscle cells.

Fig. 33-47. Enlargement of area similar to rectangle in Fig. 33-46. Dorsal prostate. Rat. E.M. X 8000. **1.** Lumen of gland. **2.** Nucleus of cuboidal epithelial cell. **3.** Nucleus of smooth muscle cell. **4.** Dilated cisternae of granular endoplasmic reticulum. **5.** Golgi complexes. **6.** Mitochondria. **7.** Lysosome. **8.** Secretory droplets. **9.** Thin basal lamina (not seen at this magnification).

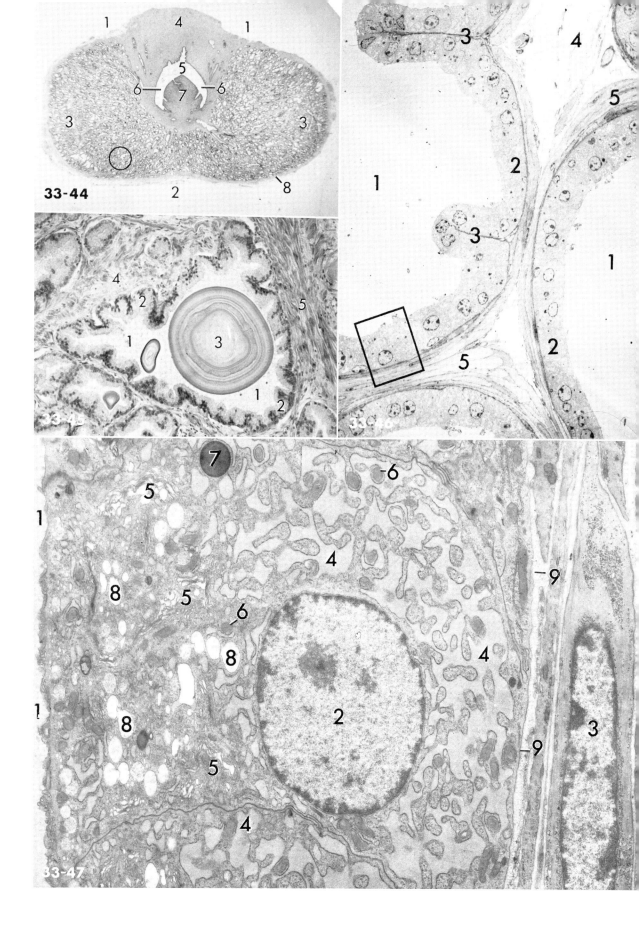

33-44

33-45

33-47

serous glands, separated by septa into about 40 indistinct lobules. They are grouped into mucosal glands in close proximity around the urethra; submucous glands in a wider ring around the urethra; and the prostatic glands proper, occupying the lateral lobes. There are about 12 main excretory ducts opening up into the prostatic sinuses. The ducts have saccular and tubular diverticula. The blind ends of the glands, the alveoli, vary in size and shape, and their lumina are large and irregular with the walls raised into folds. (Fig. 33-45) They are lined by a simple epithelium. (Fig. 33-46) The height of the cells is related to the functional state of the gland, varying from cuboidal to columnar. Pseudostratification also occurs. The epithelium rests on a thin basal lamina.

The **epithelial cells** have a structure characteristic of secretory cells. (Fig. 33-47) During active synthesis, there is a large granular endoplasmic reticulum with dilated cisternae. Mitochondria are small and, in similarity with the lysosomes, occur in small numbers. The Golgi zone, located apically of the nucleus, is large and separated into several units. Secretory granules of varying electron density arise within the Golgi and are discharged at the luminal surface by the usual mechanism in serous glands (exocytosis). The secretory material is finely granular. It is stored temporarily in the alveolar lumen or in the excretory ducts. The secretion sometimes appear as colloidal masses, **corpora amylacea,** which in older people may become calcified concretions. (Fig. 33-45) The secretion contains enzymes such as acid phosphatase, diastase, protease, and fibrinolysin. It has a milky appearance, a characteristic odor, and is alkaline. It stimulates the motility of the spermatozoa, coagulates the fluid of the seminal vesicle, and alkalizes the vaginal acidity. The secretory mechanism of the prostate gland is dependent on the stimulation of an adequate supply of androgens.

Penis

The penis is an elongated organ which consists of three cylindrical bodies: two **corpora cavernosa penis** and one **corpus cavernosum** (spongiosum) **urethrae.** (Fig. 33-48) The latter surrounds the urethra and terminates distally in the **glans penis.** All cavernous bodies contain erectile tissue. The body of the penis is covered by thin skin which turns over the glans as a fold, the **prepuce.** The glans penis is covered with thin skin firmly attached to the underlying erectile tissue. Its epithelium is thinly keratinized. Near the corona of glans penis, large sebaceous glands, the **preputial glands,** discharge an odiferous sebum, the **smegma.** Hairs are not associated with these glands, nor with the inside of the prepuce. The skin of the shaft of the penis is loosely attached to the fascia penis. It contains several types of sensory nerve endings, including Meissner's and Pacinian corpuscles, Krause's end-bulbs, and peculiar genital corpuscles.

Each of the corpora cavernosa is surrounded by a **tunica albuginea.** The tunic is thick around the penile bodies but thin in relation to the corpus spongiosum. The

Fig. 33-48. Cross section of root of penis. Newborn child. L.M. X 13. **1.** Corpora cavernosa penis. **2.** Corpus cavernosum (spongiosum) urethrae. **3.** Urethra. **4.** Tunica albuginea. **5.** Septum penis. **6.** Fascia penis. **7.** Dorsal arteries. **8.** Dorsal vein. **9.** Central arteries.

Fig. 33-49. Enlargement of area similar to rectangle in Fig. 33-48. Penis. Newborn child. L.M. X 90. **1.** Lacunae (sinuses). **2.** Trabeculae. **3.** Central artery. **4.** Helicine arteries and arterioles. **5.** Tunica albuginea.

Fig. 33-50. Enlargement of area similar to square in Fig. 33-49. Penis. Rat. E.M. X 600. **1.** Lumen of helicine artery. **2.** Lacunae (sinuses). **3.** Trabeculae. **4.** Nerve bundle (only non-myelinated axons). **5.** Smooth muscle cells in media. **6.** Trabecula with collagenous bundles. **7.** Trabecula with smooth muscle bundles. **8.** Fat cell. **9.** Nuclei of endothelial cells.

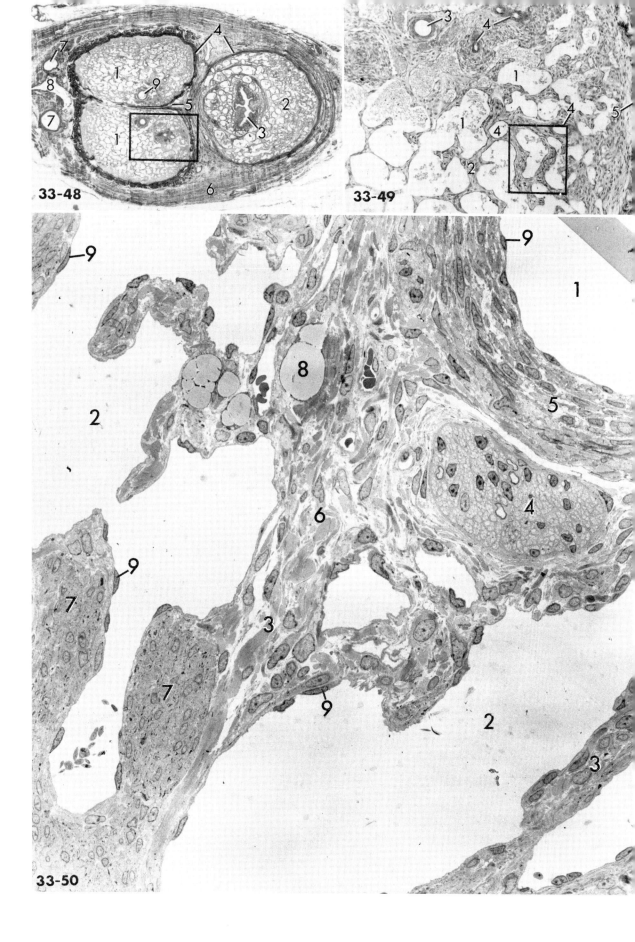

33-48

33-49

33-50

erectile tissue is composed of connective tissue septa, **trabeculae,** between which are large blood spaces, the **lacunae** or cavernous sinuses. (Fig. 33-49) The core of the trabeculae contains a mixture of collagenous and elastic fibers, fibroblasts, and smooth muscle cells. (Fig. 33-50) The latter occur singly or in bundles of varied thickness. The lacunae are lined by a thin squamous endothelium resting on a basal lamina. (Fig. 33-51) Central **deep arteries** supply the central lacunae, whereas **superficial arteries** deliver blood to the peripheral network of capillaries and venous plexuses. The deep arteries give off many branches, most of which are coiled arteries or arterioles, **helicine arteries** which empty into the lacunae. (Fig. 33-52) In the intima of most deep penile arteries and arterioles are present bundles of longitudinally arranged smooth muscle cells. (Fig. 16-28) The walls of the lacunae have similar arrangements of smooth muscle bundles, making up the core of most trabeculae. (Fig. 33-53)

In the **flaccid state** of the penis, the smooth muscle cells of the deep arteries and trabeculae are considered to be in a tonic contraction, preventing blood from entering the lacunae by bending the vessel. During this time, the penis is supplied with blood through the superficial arteries. The **turgid state** of the penis is brought about by a loss of tonus in the smooth muscle cells of the deep arterial supply and the trabeculae. The nervi erigentes carry parasympathetic vasodilator nerves from the sacral spinal cord, which probably decrease muscular tone. This straightens out the arteries and arterioles and dilates the lumina of these vessels and the lacunae, enabling the blood to rush into the erectile tissue. At the same time the venous drainage of the lacunae is almost completely blocked. This drainage occurs partly through connections between the most peripheral lacunae and the superficial venous capillary network, partly through special veins equipped with funnel-shaped valves. These veins connect the center of the erectile tissue with the periphery of the tunica albuginea. A flaccid state is resumed by an increase in the tone of the smooth muscle cells of the deep arteries and lacunae. This shuts off the inflow of blood and slowly drives out the blood from the lacunae.

References

TESTIS

Bawa, S. R. The fine structure of the Sertoli cell of the human testis. J. Ultrastruct. Res. *9:* 459–474 (1963).

Bedford, J. M. and Nicander, L. Ultrastructural changes in the acrosome and sperm membranes during maturation of spermatozoa in the testis and epididymis of the rabbit and monkey. J. Anat. *108:* 527–543 (1971).

Belt, W. D. and Cavazos, L. F. Fine structure of the interstitial cells of Leydig in the boar. Anat. Rec. *158:* 333–350 (1967).

Bishop, D. Sperm motility. Physiol. Rev. *42:* 1–59 (1962).

Burgos, M. H., Vitale-Calpe, R. and Aoki, A. Fine structure of the testis and its functional significance. *In:* The Testis. (Eds. A. D. Johnson, W. R. Gomes and N. L. Van Demark), Vol. I, pp. 551–649. Academic Press, New York, 1970.

Bröckelman, J. Fine structure of germ cells and Sertoli cells during the cycle of the seminiferous epithelium in rat. Z. Zellforsch. *59:* 820–850 (1963).

Fig. 33-51. Survey of cavernous tissue. Corpus cavernosum penis. Rat. E.M. X 1740. **1.** Lacunae (sinuses). **2.** Nuclei of endothelial cells. **3.** Trabeculae. **4.** Bundles of collagenous fibrils. **5.** Bundles of smooth muscle cells. **6.** Nuclei of singly occurring smooth muscle cells. **7.** Nuclei of fibroblasts.

Fig. 33-52. Trabecula. Corpus cavernosum penis. Rat. E.M. X 1800. **1.** Lacunae. **2.** Nuclei of endothelial cells. **3.** Lumen of cross-sectioned small helcine arteriole. Luminal diameter 10 μ. **4.** Nuclei of smooth muscle cells in a muscle bundle in the core of a trabecula. **5.** Nuclei of fibroblasts. **6.** Bundles of collagenous fibrils. **7.** Longitudinally oriented smooth muscle cells of the helicine arteriole.

Fig. 33-53. Enlargement of rectangle in Fig. 33-51. Corpus cavernosum penis. Rat. E.M. X 9000. **1.** Lacuna. **2.** Endothelium (nonfenestrated). **3.** Nucleus of smooth muscle cell. **4.** Basal lamina of endothelium. **5.** Basal (external) lamina of smooth muscle cell. **6.** Cytoplasmic strands of fibroblasts. **7.** Bundles of collagenous fibrils. **8.** Circles: cross-sectioned elastic fibrils.

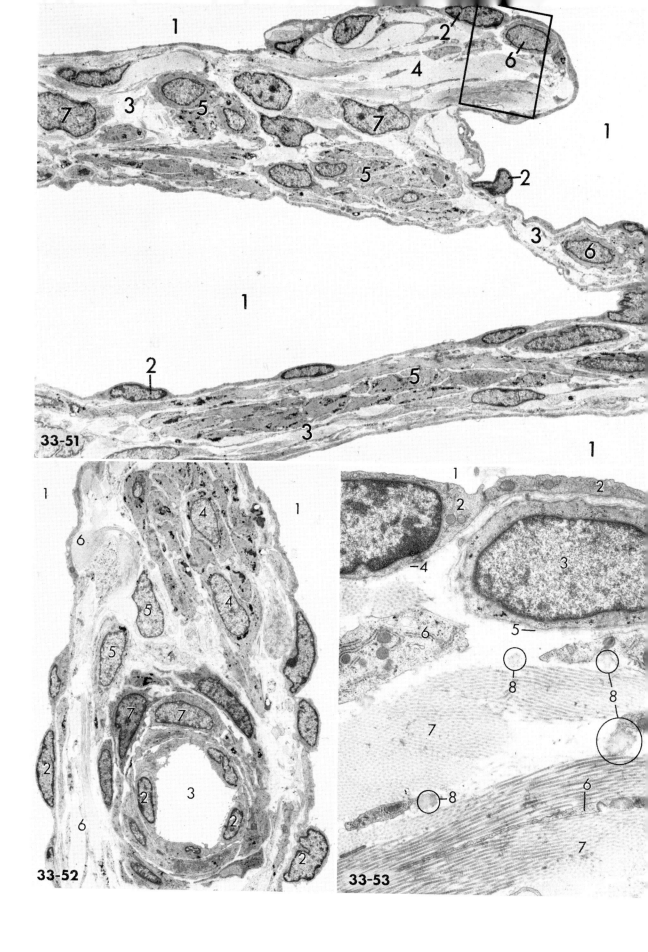

33-51

33-52

33-53

Christensen, A. K. and Fawcett, D. W. The fine structure of testicular interstitial cells in mice. Am. J. Anat. *118:* 551–572 (1966).

Clermont, Y. The cycle of the seminiferous epithelium in man. Am. J. Anat. *112:* 35–52 (1963).

de Kretser, D. M. The fine structure of the testicular interstitial cells in men of normal androgenic status. Z. Zellforsch. *80:* 594–609 (1967).

Dym, M. and Fawcett, D. W. The blood-testis barrier in the rat and the physiological compartmentation of the seminiferous epithelium. Biol. Reprod. *3:* 308–326 (1970).

Fawcett, D. W. The structure of the mammalian spermatozoon. Int. Rev. Cytol. *7:* 195–234 (1958).

Fawcett, D. W. The topographical relationship between the plane of the central pair of flagellar fibrils and the transverse axis of the head in guinea-pig spermatozoa. J. Cell Sci. *3:* 187–189 (1968).

Fawcett, D. W. and Ito, S. The fine structure of bat spermatozoa. Am. J. Anat. *116:* 567–610 (1965).

Flickinger, C. and Fawcett, D. W. The junctional specializations of Sertoli cells in the seminiferous epithelium. Anat. Rec. *158:* 207–222 (1967).

Mann, T. Biochemistry of Semen and of the Male Reproductive Tract. Wiley, New York, 1964.

Nicander, L. An electron microscopical study of cell contacts in the seminiferous tubules of some mammals. Z. Zellforsch. *83:* 375–397 (1967).

Roosen-Runge, E. C. The process of spermatogenesis in mammals. Biol. Rev. *37:* 343–377 (1962).

Ross, M. H. Contractile cells in human seminiferous tubules. Science *153:* 1271–1273 (1966).

Schmidt, F. C. Licht- und elektronenmikroskopische Untersuchungen am menschlichen Hoden und Nebenhoden. Z. Zellforsch. *63:* 707–729 (1964).

EPIDIDYMIS

Friend, D. S. Cytochemical staining of multivesicular body and Golgi vesicles. J. Cell Biol. *41:* 269–279 (1969).

Friend, D. S. and Farquhar, M. G.: Functions of coated vesicles during protein absorption in the rat vas deferens. J. Cell Biol. *35:* 357–376 (1967).

Hamilton, D. W., Jones, A. L. and Fawcett, D. W. Cholesterol biosynthesis in the mouse epididymis and ductus deferens: a biochemical and morphological study. Biol. Reprod. *1:* 167–184 (1969).

Horstmann, E. Elektronenmikroskopie des menschlichen Nebenhodenepithels. Z. Zellforsch. *57:* 692–718 (1962).

Ladman, A. J. The fine structure of the ductuli efferentes of the opossum. Anat. Rec. *157:* 559–576 (1967).

Ladman, A. J. and Young, W. C. An electron microscopic study of the ductuli efferentes and rete testis of the guinea pig. J. Biophys. Biochem. Cytol. *4:* 219–226 (1958).

Mason, K. E. and Shaver, S. L. Some functions of the caput epididymis. Ann. N.Y. Acad. Sci. *55:* 585–593 (1952).

Morita, I. Some observations on the fine structure of the human ductuli efferentes testis. Arch. Histol. Japon. *26:* 341–365 (1966).

Nicander, L. An electron microscopical study of absorbing cells in the posterior caput epididymidis of rabbits. Z. Zellforsch. *66:* 829–847 (1965).

Niemi, M. The fine structure and histochemistry of the epithelial cells of the rat vas deferens. Acta Anat. *60:* 207–219 (1965).

Orgebin-Crist, M. C. Studies on the function of the epididymis. Biol. Reprod. Suppl. 1: 155–175 (1969).

SEMINAL VESICLES

Deane, H. W. and Porter, K. R. A comparative study of cytoplasmic basophilia and the population density of ribosomes in the secretory cells of the mouse seminal vesicle. Z. Zellforsch. *52:* 697–711 (1960).

Riva, A. Fine structure of human seminal vesicle epithelium. J. Anat. *102:* 71–86 (1967).

PROSTATE

Brandes, D. The fine structure and histochemistry of prostatic glands in relation to sex hormones. Int. Rev. Cytol. *20:* 207–276 (1966).

Brandes, D. and Portela, A. The fine structure of the epithelial cells of the mouse prostate. I. Coagulating gland epithelium. J. Biophys. Biochem. Cytol. *7:* 505–510 (1960).

Brandes, D. and Portela, A. The fine structure of the epithelial cells of the mouse prostate. II. Ventral lobe epithelium. J. Biophys. Biochem. Cytol. *7:* 511–514 (1960).

Flickinger, C. J. The fine structure and development of the seminal vesicles and prostate in the fetal rat. Z. Zellforsch. *109:* 1–14 (1970).

Huggins, C. The prostatic secretion. Harvey Lectures *42:* 148–193 (1947).

PENIS

Leeson, T. S. and Leeson, C. R. The fine structure of cavernous tissue in the adult rat penis. Investig. Urology *3:* 144–154 (1965).

34 Female reproductive system

The female reproductive system consists of organs which produce female germ cells (2 ovaries); offer sites for the fertilization of the ova (2 oviducts); and the uterus which subsequently harbors the fertilized ovum during the gestation period. A canal (vagina) connects the inner reproductive organs with the exterior. Additional functionally important parts are the mammary glands for milk production (2 breasts). The activity of the entire female reproductive system is regulated to some degree by nerves, and to a high degree by hormones (gonadotrophins) from the adenohypophysis as well as from within its own system: estrogens from ovarian follicles; progesterone from the corpus luteum. A cyclic activity typifies the organs of the female reproductive system.

Ovary

There are two ovaries, each having the size and shape of a peach stone. They are located on either side of the uterus, enclosed in a fold of the peritoneum, the **mesovarium.** This fold binds one side of the ovary to the broad ligament, with the rest of the ovary projecting freely into the peritoneal cavity. The round ligament of the ovary connects the medial end with the uterus. The free surface of the ovary is covered by the so-called **germinal epithelium.** This is a misnomer since it does not give rise to oogonia as previously thought. The germinal epithelium is actually a specialization of the peritoneal mesothelium. The cells are of the low cuboidal or squamous type. Similar to other mesothelial cells, they are provided with microvilli. Among the organelles are commonly seen a small number of lipid droplets. The epithelium rests on a thin **basal lamina.** The ovary has a thin connective tissue capsule or **tunica albuginea** with a few fibroblasts and a dense arrangement of collagenous fibers. The ovary has a large cortical and a small medullary re-

gion. (Fig. 34-1) The **cortex** or the zona parenchymatosa contains the ovarian follicles and the corpora lutea. The **medulla** or the zona vasculosa carries the larger blood vessels, the lymphatics, and the nerves. Both the cortex and the medulla are made up of a stromal or **interstitial tissue.** In the cortex, this is composed of intercellular substance, collagenous fibers, and spindle-shaped, fibroblast-like cells which pervade the organ as interlacing bundles. (Fig. 34-3) Many of these cells display ultrastructural characteristics typical of both fibroblasts and smooth muscle cells. When these cells are orderly arranged around the periphery of the ovarian follicles, they are referred to as theca folliculi cells. In some mammals, particularly rabbit and rat, an additional type of interstitial cell occurs. This cell type may be related to the theca interna cells, since it contains a multitude of lipid droplets. Accumulations of these cells remain for long periods in the stroma and are referred to as "interstitial gland." In the ovarian medulla, the interstitial tissue is less dense. It contains many elastic fibers, fibroblast-like stromal cells, and bundles of true smooth muscle cells.

PRIMORDIAL FOLLICLE

There are large numbers of small primordial follicles near the cortical surface of the ovary. (Fig. 34-2) Each primordial follicle is composed of the original pri-

Fig. **34-1.** Ovary. Cat. E.M. X 11. **1.** Cortex. **2.** Medulla. **3.** Follicles. **4.** Corpora lutea.

Fig. **34-2.** Enlargement of rectangle in Fig. 34-1. L.M. X 16. **1.** Primordial follicles. **2.** Secondary follicle. **3.** Stroma. **4.** Corpus luteum. **5.** Interstitial gland.

Fig. **34-3.** Enlargement of area similar to rectangle in Fig. 34-2. Rat. E.M. X 860. **1.** Peritoneal cavity. **2.** Germinal epithelium. **3.** Tunica albuginea with interstitial fibroblasts. **4.** Primordial follicles. **5.** Oocyte of secondary follicle. Nucleus is not in plane of section. **6.** Zona pellucida. **7.** Follicular cells. **8.** Basal lamina. **9.** Theca folliculi. (interna). **10.** Theca folliculi (externa). **11.** Capillaries.

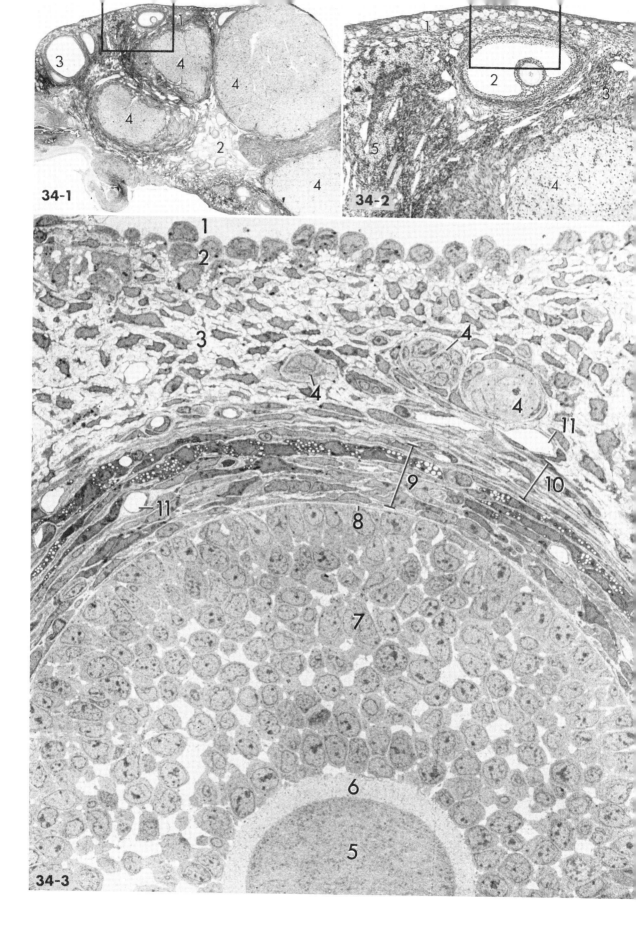

34-1

34-2

34-3

mordial germ cell, the oogonium and a thin single coat of squamous follicular cells. The primordial germ cells originate from cells in the endodermal layer of the blastodisc. During early embryonic life, the primitive germ cells multiply in the developing ovary. Subsequently, they enter the prophase of meiosis and reach a final resting stage characterized by a diplotene nucleus. Stromal cells brought into the gonad in association with blood vessels encase individual germ cells as follicular cells to produce primordial follicles.

The **oogonium** has a large nucleus and a prominent nucleolus. The cytoplasm of the oogonium (ooplasm) is limited to a narrow rim around the nucleus. (Fig. 34-4) It contains small, round mitochondria and lipid droplets, the latter corresponding to the yolk granules in some species. The Golgi complex is large, whereas the granular endoplasmic reticulum is limited to small, short profiles. Ribosomes are abundant. The surface of the oogonium is relatively smooth with only very small microvilli present in limited number.

The **follicular cells** are small and flat. In their most primitive stage, they are almost indistinguishable from the stromal cells. The nucleus is irregular and oval. The cytoplasm contains a few mitochondria. The entire primordial follicle is surrounded by a thin **basal lamina** which separates the follicle from the ovarian stroma. The primordial follicles remain quiescent for many years. They number about 400,000 in the young adult and decrease progressively in number throughout life.

PRIMARY FOLLICLE

Beginning already during the latter months of fetal life, and continuing through childhood, primordial follicles are stimulated to grow and follicles are present in various stages of development and regression. The primordial follicle first reaches the stage which is referred to as primary follicle.

In the primary follicle, the **primary** oocyte continually becomes enlarged by an increase in the volume of the ooplasm. (Fig. 34-5) The mitochondria become more abundant and have a pale matrix and a few plate-like cristae. The Golgi complex is dispersed into numerous aggregates of vesicles and tubules which migrate to the cortex of the primary oocyte, where they play an important role in the synthesis of dense cortical granules, 3000–5000 Å wide. Stacks of annulate lamellae are frequently present. They are considered a specialized form of the endoplasmic reticulum derived from the nuclear envelope. They are characteristically found in cells undergoing active growth and differentiation and represent a potential mechanism for transfer of genetic information to the cytoplasm. The surface of the primary oocyte gradually develops numerous short microvilli.

The **follicular cells** become more numerous and change from a squamous to a cuboidal shape. As the primary follicle gradually changes into a secondary follicle, the follicular cells become numerous and stratified. The follicle is surrounded by a thin **basal lamina**. Outside the follicle, the stromal cells tend to become concentrically arranged to form the **theca folliculi**.

Fig. 34-4. Primordial follicle. Ovary. Rat. E.M. X 5400. **1.** Nucleus of primordial germ cell. **2.** Nucleolus in reticular form. **3.** Ooplasm. **4.** Mitochondria. **5.** Golgi complex. **6.** Cortical granules. **7.** Slightly ruffled surface of primordial germ cell. **8.** Nuclei of follicular cells. **9.** Thin cytoplasmic sheath of follicular cells, embracing the germ cell. **10.** Stromal cells. **11.** Lumen of capillary. **12.** Nucleus of endothelial cell.

Fig. 34-5. Primary follicle. Ovary. Rat. E.M. X 4400. **1.** Nucleus of primary oocyte. The nucleolus is not in the plane of section. **2.** Nuclear envelope. **3.** Ooplasm. **4.** Mitochondria. **5.** Cortical granules. **6.** Surface of oocyte. **7.** Nuclei of cuboidal follicular cells. **8.** Basal lamina. **9.** Nuclei of stromal cells. There is no theca folliculi formed as yet. **10.** Collagen of ovarian stroma.

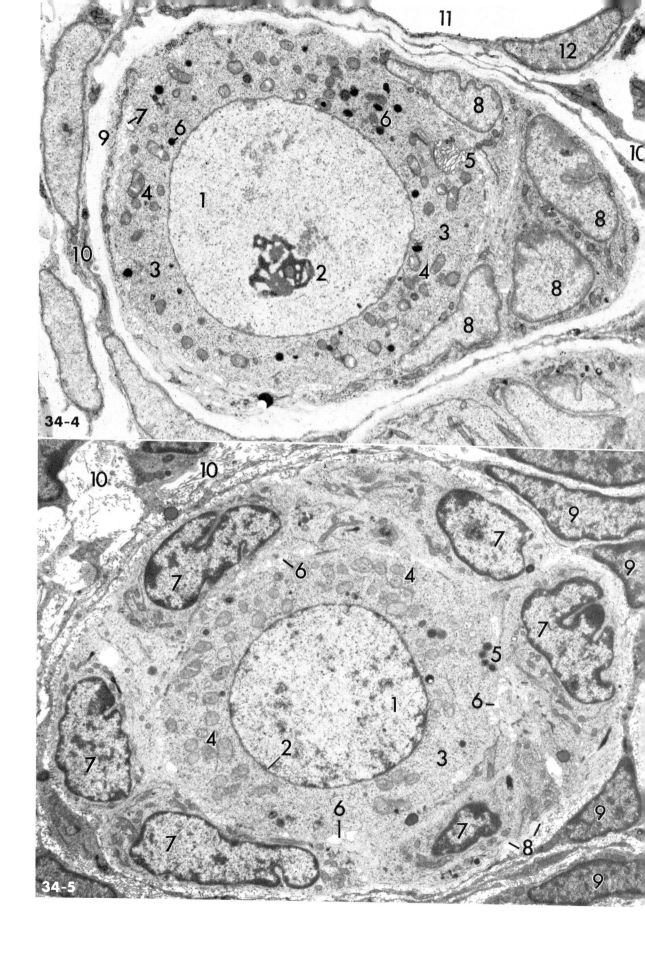

34-4

34-5

SECONDARY SOLID FOLLICLE

It should be realized that the development of the ovarian follicles from the primordial stage to the time of ovulation is gradual, and that the subdivision of this development into distinct stages is somewhat artificial. Nevertheless, it is a convenient means of identifying certain developmental stages such as secondary solid follicle, secondary vesicular follicle, and mature, Graafian follicle. The maturation of the follicular oocyte can also be distinguished schematically into three stages, namely, the quiescent stage, the stage of growth, and the meiotic stage. During the development, changes occur in three main regions: the oocyte; the follicular cells; and the theca folliculi. The most dramatic changes relate to the arrangement and number of follicular cells, and the differentiation of the theca folliculi.

The **oocyte** continues to enlarge until it reaches a size which is about three times that of the primordial germ cell. At some point, not accurately determined, it undergoes **unequal meiotic division** resulting in two daughter cells: a large **secondary oocyte** and a very small **polar body**. The **follicular cells** proliferate rapidly and form a multilayered solid mass of cells around the secondary oocyte. Simultaneously, the **zona pellucida** is gradually formed. This is an extracellular mucoprotein substance, synthesized by the follicular cells and laid down as a separating layer between the oocyte and the inner layer of follicular cells. (Fig. 34-7) In its final form, it reaches a thickness of 5–10 μ. The **basal lamina,** separating the follicular cells from the stromal cells, gradually thickens to a width of 1–2 μ, and is then called **glassy membrane.** The stromal cells near the follicle become increasingly well organized into concentrically arranged layers, the **thecae folliculi.** Near the follicle, the stromal cell layers are permeated by a rich capillary network and this part is referred to as **theca interna,** as opposed to the **theca externa** which is peripheral and poorly vascularized.

SECONDARY VESICULAR FOLLICLE

General. Follicular fluid gradually accumulates between the follicular cells. By this accumulation, intercellular spaces are created which eventually give rise to a follicular cavity, the **antrum,** transforming the ovarian follicle from a solid to a vesicular secondary follicle. (Fig. 34-6) As the antrum enlarges, the follicular cells come to lie in a stratified manner along the glassy membrane. This layer of follicular cells is called **membrana granulosa.** The oocyte is still surrounded by the follicular cells, the **corona radiata** (Fig. 34-7), and this structural entity connects with the membrana granulosa as the **cumulus oophorus.** The **mature, Graafian follicle** also has this general architecture but is very much larger than the early secondary vesicular follicle. Also, during the development of the ovarian follicles, there is first a movement from the cortex of the ovary to the medulla as the secondary follicles form. Subsequently, as the follicular maturation is reached, the Graafian follicle moves toward the ovarian surface, causing a pre-ovulatory swelling of the follicle. The follicle forms a thin-walled nipple, the **stigma,** which rises from the ovarian surface. This marks the site where the wall will burst and the oocyte with the zona pellucida and the corona radiata will be extruded.

Fig. 34-6. Early secondary vesicular follicle. Ovary. Rat. E.M. X 580. **1.** Nucleus. **2.** Secondary oocyte. **3.** Zona pellucida. **4.** Corona radiata. **5.** Antrum folliculi. **6.** Cells of membrana granulosa, many of which are in various stages of mitosis (circles). **7.** Basal lamina (glassy membrane). **8.** Thecae folliculi. **9.** Perifollicular capillaries. **10.** Ovarian stroma.

Fig. 34-7. Part of early secondary vesicular follicle. Ovary. Rat. E.M. X 1800. **1.** Nucleolus. **2.** Nucleus of secondary oocyte. **3.** Cortical granules. **4.** Surface oocyte. **5.** Zona pellucida. **6.** Nuclei of the follicular cells which make up the corona radiata. **7.** Slender cell processes from the oocyte and the corona radiata cells penetrate the zona pellucida. **8.** Antrum folliculi with precipitated liquor folliculi.

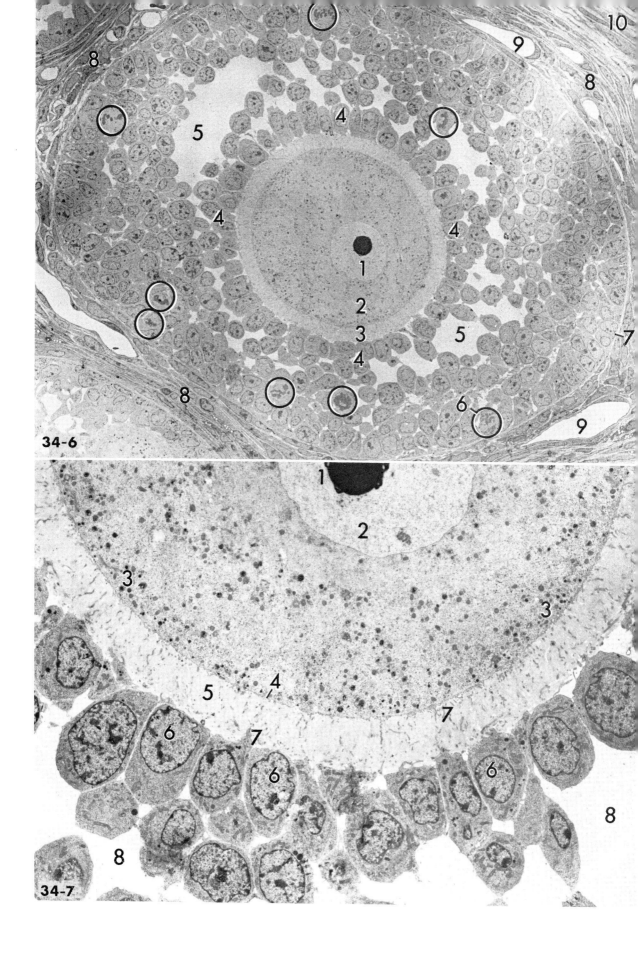

Fine structure. During the differentiation of the ovarian follicles, the various cells undergo changes which reach their first end stage at the time of the rupture of the Graafian follicle. The following is a short account of the major ultrastructural features by the time of the ovulation. The **nucleus** of the secondary oocyte contains the haploid (single; 1×23) number of chromosomes after completing the first meiotic division. The nucleus of the secondary oocyte enters the second meiotic division shortly after ovulation, but the chromosomal rearrangement is arrested in metaphase until fertilization. The second meiotic division is an ordinary mitotic cell division, although with a reduced (haploid) number of chromosomes. (See p. 58) Also, the second meiotic division gives rise to a polar body which may go through a couple of cleavages before being discarded. The nucleolus of the secondary oocyte loses its thread-like configuration as one of the earliest changes in preparation for the meiotic division. It is transformed into a compact body made up of granular material of non-uniform electron density. The **nuclear envelope** is richly endowed with pores (Fig. 34-8), and through complicated foldings gives rise to the stacks of **annulate lamellae** which are typical of both the primary and the secondary oocytes. The composition of the ooplasm is similar to what is present in the primary oocyte. Dense cortical granules are quite numerous (Fig. 34-9 inset), as are lipid droplets, lysosomes and ribosomes. Exceptionally abundant throughout the ooplasm are long and densely packed pairs or triplets of sheets, lamellae or narrow tubules, apposing each other laterally and cross-linking. A faint periodicity of about 100 Å is present with the membranes. These structures are collectively referred to as **crystalline bodies** or **plaques**. (Fig. 34-9) Their function is not known. The **microvilli** at the surface of the oocyte are quite numerous and vary greatly in length. Some may reach through the zona pellucida and make contact with the fol-

licular cells of the corona radiata. The material of the **zona pellucida** is finely filamentous and made up of gel-like neutral protein-polysaccharides. (Fig. 34-10) It is presently believed that it is chiefly the follicular cells that are involved in the synthesis and maintenance of the zona pellucida. The **follicular cells** display a high mitotic activity throughout the development of the ovarian follicles. (Figs. 2-87 through 2-94) The cytoplasm is rich in granular endoplasmic reticulum and ribosomes. (Fig. 34-11) Mitochondria are sparse. Lipid droplets and lysosomes occur but are not abundant. The cells of the corona radiata have many microvilli, some of which penetrate the zona pellucida to make membranous contacts with the oocyte membrane. It has been suggested that the follicular cells synthesize **estrogens** which may be temporarily stored

Fig. 34-8. Secondary follicle. Ovary. Rat. E.M. X 15,000. **1.** Nucleolus of oocyte is extremely electron-dense with only occasional peripheral threads. **2.** Nucleoplasm is finely granular. **3.** Nuclear envelope with numerous pores (arrows). **4.** Ooplasm. **5.** Crystalline bodies (plaques).

Fig. 34-9. Detail of the ooplasm of a secondary oocyte. Ovary. Rat. E.M. X 60,000. **1.** Mitochondria with membranous cristae. **2.** Inset: granule of the type classified as cortical granule; boundary membrane is of the single trilaminar type. (X 100,000). **3.** The majority of these dense dots are particulate glycogen; the smaller may be ribosomes. **4.** Crystalline bodies (plaques).

Fig. 34-10. Detail of secondary follicle. Ovary. Rat. E.M. X 13,000. **1.** Peripheral part of secondary oocyte. **2.** Zona pellucida with finely fibrillar substance. **3.** Nuclei of follicular cells of corona radiata. **4.** Cortical granules. **5.** Lysosome. **6.** Microvilli. **7.** Mitochondria. **8.** Granular endoplasmic reticulum.

Fig. 34-11. Detail of secondary follicle. Ovary. Rat. E.M. X 8000. **1.** Nucleus of membrana granulosa cell. **2.** Nucleus in late telophase. **3.** Intercellular space which communicates with antrum folliculi. **4.** Basal lamina. **5.** Mitochondria. **6.** Golgi complex. **7.** Granular endoplasmic reticulum. **8.** Lipid droplet.

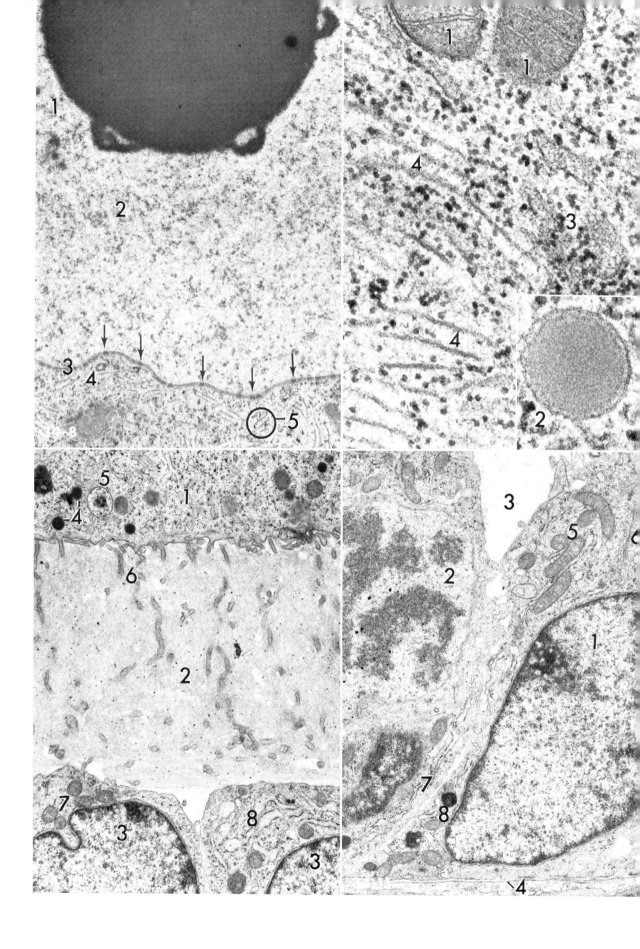

in the liquor folliculi of the antrum before they reach the bloodstream. The cells of the cumulus oophorus and the membrana are loosely arranged with generous, irregular intercellular spaces. Junctional complexes occur between follicular cells. This probably reinforces the structural integrity of the oocyte, the zona pellucida, and the corona radiata during the ovulation, since they all continue to stay together even while passing down the oviduct. The **glassy membrane** is essentially a basal lamina in lower mammals. In man its thickness is greater, augmented by an addition of collagenous and reticular fibrils.

The differentiation of the **theca folliculi** is of major importance in the development of the ovarian follicles. As indicated already, the stromal cells differentiate into two regions of circumferentially arranged cells, referred to as the theca interna and the theca externa. (Fig. 34-12) The **theca interna** is made up of layers of polyhedral or elongated cells permeated by a rich capillary network. The theca interna cells have an oval or round nucleus. There is an abundance of granular endoplasmic reticulum and free ribosomes. (Fig. 34-13) The cells also contain varying amounts of lipid droplets that gradually increase in size and number—as do the mitochondria—before ovulation. To a varying degree, filamentous material is present in the cytoplasm, rendering the cells an appearance which is reminiscent of both fibroblasts and smooth muscle cells. In the extracellular space is a small number of collagenous fibers, as well as reticular and elastic fibrils. The cells of the **theca externa** are long, narrow, and spindle-shaped. Their nucleus is also long and narrow. There is a predominance of filamentous material in the cytoplasm but cells occur which, in addition to filaments, have a fair amount of granular endoplasmic reticulum. Particulate glycogen abounds in the cells which are rich in filaments. (Fig. 34-14) The extracellular material is more prominent and fibrous

in the theca externa in comparison with the theca interna. Bundles of collagen predominate, but reticular and elastic fibrils also occur. It is quite probable that some of the cells of the theca externa in fact represent smooth muscle cells or are intermediate forms between fibroblasts and smooth muscle cells. (Fig. 34-14) The cells of the theca interna are gradually changing into cells which may be responsible for the synthesis of hormones, and it has been suggested that they produce estrogens, although this function has also been attributed to the follicular cells. Their endocrine function is proven beyond doubt by the time they are transformed into the theca lutein cells of the corpus luteum.

CORPUS LUTEUM

Upon ovulation, the follicle collapses and the membrana granulosa becomes folded. There is an initial bleeding from ruptured blood vessels into the antrum, form-

Fig. 34-12. Section of part of wall of secondary follicle. Ovary. Rat. E.M. X 1800. **1.** Nuclei of follicular cells of membrana granulosa. **2.** Dividing follicular cell. **3** Plane of basal lamina (glassy membrane). The lamina itself is not discernible at this magnification. **4.** Nuclei of the cells which make up the theca interna. **5.** These cells are also part of the theca interna; their cytoplasm is filled with lipid droplets. **6.** Capillaries in theca interna. **7.** Nuclei of cells which make up the theca externa.

Fig. 34-13. Detail of cells in the theca interna of secondary follicle. Ovary. Rat. E.M. X 29,000. **1.** Nucleus. **2.** Golgi complex. **3.** Mitochondria. **4.** Cisternae of the granular endoplasmic reticulum. **5.** Ribosomes. **6.** Slender part of an adjacent cell with thin filaments in the cytoplasm. **7.** Lysosome. **8.** Intercellular space. **9.** Collagenous fibrils.

Fig. 34-14. Detail of cells in theca externa of secondary follicle. Ovary. Rat. E.M. X 9000. **1.** Nuclei. **2.** Major part of the cytoplasm is occupied by filaments. **3.** A minor part of the cytoplasm has granular endoplasmic reticulum. **4.** Particulate glycogen. **5.** Large intercellular spaces with a network of collagenous fibrils.

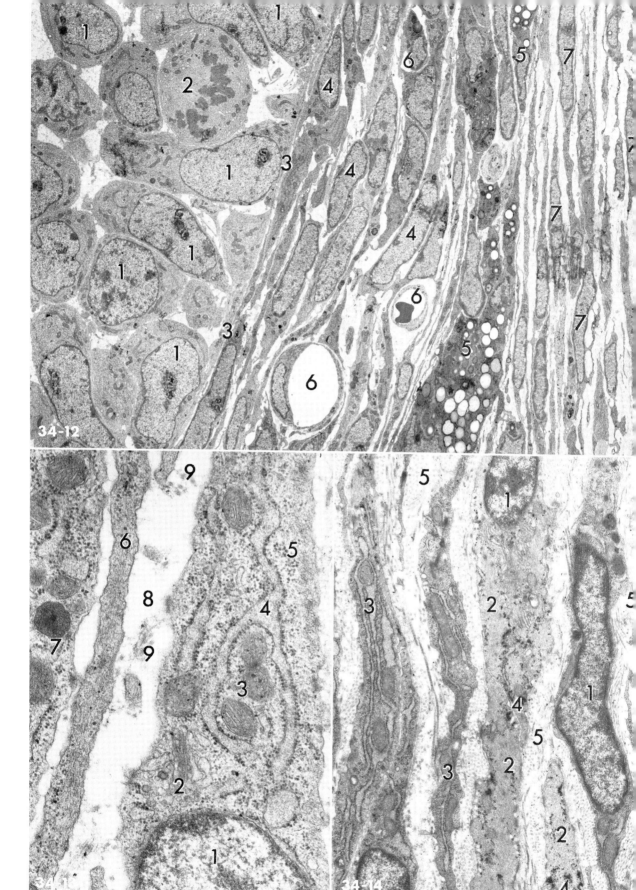

ing a blood clot in the center of the collapsed follicle. Originating from the capillary plexus of the theca interna, blood vessels start to grow through the glassy membrane toward the antrum, carrying with them pericytes and fibroblasts which transform the blood clot of the former antrum to a loose connective tissue. Simultaneously, the follicular cells hypertrophy and become arranged into cords in the multilayered, highly folded wall of the structure which now gradually develops into a **corpus luteum.** (Fig. 34-15) With the folding of the membrana granulosa, the cells of the theca interna become wedged in between the folds. (Fig. 34-16) In similarity with the granulosa cells, the theca interna cells hypertrophy, but only slightly. Both cell types accumulate lipid droplets and lipofuscin pigment granules. The pigment is yellow in man but colorless in most other mammals. The cells which are derived from the membrana granulosa, the **granulosa lutein cells,** have large spherical nuclei with a homogeneous, electron-lucent nuclear matrix. (Fig. 34-17) The mitochondria are dispersed throughout the cytoplasm. They vary in size, shape, and configuration, and their cristae are predominantly tubular. Many mitochondria have large, dense globular inclusions within their matrices. The Golgi complex is relatively small and appears as isolated regions (dictyosomes). Both the granular and the agranular endoplasmic reticulum are abundant. (Fig. 34-22) The granular variety is disposed as whorls or parallel cisternal stacks, whereas the agranular endoplasmic reticulum consists of a network of interconnecting tubules, concentric membranous whorls, and a folded membrane complex. Bundles of filaments commonly traverse the cytoplasm. Lipid droplets are numerous. (Fig. 34-18) They vary in size and electron density, and are dispersed throughout the cell singly or in clusters. The lipid droplets are closely surrounded by a casing of agranular endoplasmic reticulum. The lipofuscin pigment granules are abundant.

Their ultrastructural architecture indicates their lysosomal nature. (Figs. 34-21, 34-23)

The cells derived from the theca interna, the **theca lutein cells,** are prominent in human corpora lutea but absent in many lower animals. In man these cells are generally smaller than the granulosa lutein cells. They display generally the same ultrastructure as do the granulosa lutein cells but with some exceptions. Mitochondria are rod-shaped, and the Golgi complexes are less numerous. Whorls of agranular endoplasmic reticulum, folded-membrane complexes, and regions of fine filaments are not present.

Fig. 34-15. Corpus luteum of pregnancy. Ovary. Human. L.M. X 5.5. **1.** Folded layer of granulosa lutein cells. **2.** Former follicular cavity. **3.** Wedges of theca lutein cells. **4.** Theca externa cells. **5.** Ovarian surface.

Fig. 34-16. Enlargement of area similar to rectangle in Fig. 34-15. Corpus luteum of pregnancy. Ovary. Human. L.M. X 100. **1.** Cords of granulosa lutein cells. **2.** Wedges of theca lutein cells. **3.** Theca externa cells. **4.** Capillary. **5.** Fibroblasts and loose connective tissue in former follicular antrum.

Fig. 34-17. Enlargement of area similar to rectangle in Fig. 34-16. Corpus luteum. Ovary. Rat. E.M. X 540. **1.** Cords of granulosa lutein cells. **2.** Capillaries. **3.** Large venous capillaries. **4.** Theca externa (barely seen). **5.** Intercellular spaces.

Fig. 34-18. Enlargement of area similar to rectangle in Fig. 34-17. Ovary. Rat. E.M. X 1700. **1.** Nuclei of granulosa lutein cells. **2.** Lipid droplets. **3.** Capillaries. **4.** Nuclei of endothelial cells. **5.** Erythrocytes. **6.** Pericyte. Note that theca lutein cells are missing in rats. **7.** Intercellular spaces.

Fig. 34-19. Corpus albicans. Ovary. Human. L.M. X 43. **1.** Corpus albicans is made up of extracellular hyaline masses and some residual cells of the former corpus luteum. **2.** Ovarian stroma. **3.** Border toward the ovarian stroma is sharp and the transition abrupt.

Fig. 34-20. Corpus atreticum. Ovary. Human. L.M. X 85. **1.** Ovarian stroma. **2.** Folded, thickened remnant of the glassy membrane. **3.** Former membrana granulosa, now highly disorganized. **4.** Residue of collapsed zona pellucida.

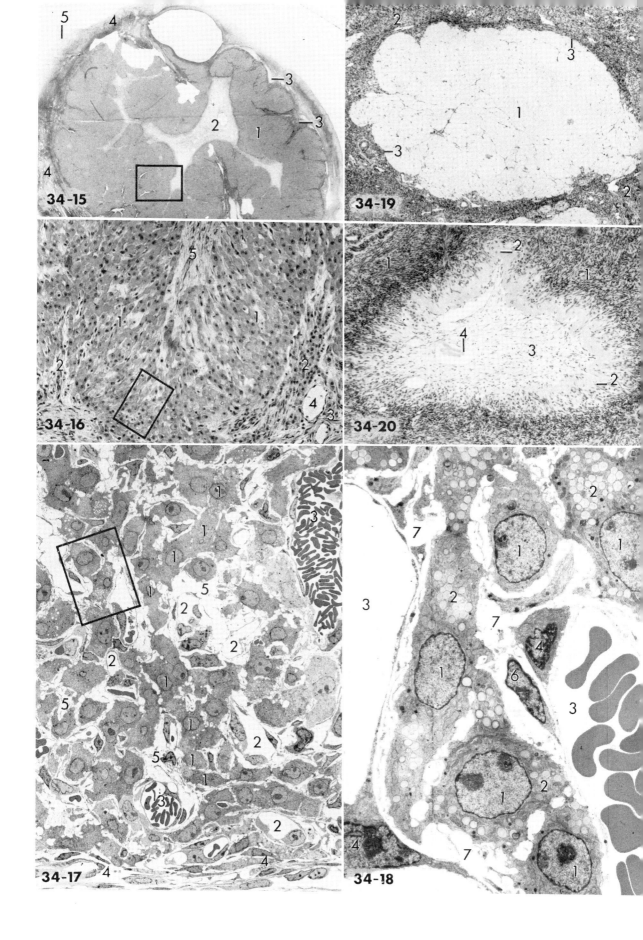

The main function of the corpus luteum is the synthesis and secretion of progesterone. Presently, it has not been determined which cell type is responsible for the synthesis, and it is safe to assume that both the granulosa lutein and the theca lutein cells are involved in the process. **Corpus luteum of menstruation** (spurium) starts to involute about two weeks after ovulation if fertilization of the ovum does not occur. The process of involution begins with an increased accumulation of lipid droplets and a high intracellular activity by the lysosomes of the lutein cells. The cells become vacuolized, reduced in size, and are finally resorbed. Gradually, the stromal and connective tissue cells of the corpus luteum also degenerate. A hyaline intercellular material accumulates and the remains of the corpus luteum are seen as a small area characterized by hyaline, non-staining white masses, the **corpus albicans.** (Fig. 34-19) If fertilization of the ovum takes place, the corpus luteum increases in size several times, and is now referred to as a **corpus luteum of pregnancy** (verum). It retains this size through the sixth month of pregnancy but degenerates gradually during the last trimester of pregnancy. The degeneration progresses rapidly after delivery and the corpus luteum of pregnancy is then transformed into a corpus albicans.

ATRESIA

The development of ovarian follicles can be interrupted at any time. This phenomenon is referred to as follicular atresia. The direct cause of the degeneration is not known, but there is an overabundance of primordial follicles considering the few that ultimately reach full maturation and ovulation (400–500). If **primary follicles** degenerate, they disappear completely from the ovary through a resorption via blood and lymphatic capillaries. Degenerating **secondary follicles** leave structures behind, **corpora atretica,** which superficially look like corpora albicantes. (Fig. 34-20) The degeneration as a rule starts in the oocyte and spreads to the follicular cells. They show pyknosis of nuclei and accumulations in the cytoplasm of lipid droplets and large conglomerations of lysosomes. The oocyte disappears and there is an admixture of fibroblasts and stromal cells in the antrum due to the collapse of the follicle and an invasion of thecal cells. The zona pellucida and the glassy membrane increase in thickness, become highly folded, and often remain for a long time in the ovarian stroma. Although corpora atretica may superficially look like corpora albicantes, the latter never contain the zona pellucida and the thickened glassy membrane.

VASCULATURE AND NERVES

Blood vessels. The ovarian blood vessels are derived from the ovarian and uterine arteries. They enter through the mesovarium and penetrate the stroma of the medulla as **helicine arteries** which give off several generations of spiral arteries, radiating toward the ovarian cortex. The arterioles are similarly coiled, and they supply the stroma and the theca folliculi with an extremely rich capillary network. There is also a vast network of venules and veins, particularly in the mature

Fig. 34-21. Fine structural organization of granulosa lutein cell. Corpus luteum. Ovary. Rat. E.M. X 14,500. **1.** Nucleus. **2.** Golgi complexes. **3.** Mitochondria. **4.** Granular endoplasmic reticulum. **5.** Lipofuscin pigment granules (secondary lysosomes). **6.** Lipid droplets. **7.** The overall "busy" cytoplasmic background is occupied by vesicular and tubular profiles of the agranular endoplasmic reticulum.

Fig. 34-22 & 34-23. Details of granulosa lutein cell. Corpus luteum. Ovary. Rat. E.M. X 58,000. **1.** Golgi complex. **2.** Mitochondria. **3.** Lipid droplets. **4.** Granular endoplasmic reticulum. **5.** Ribsosomes. **6.** Agranular endoplasmic reticulum. **7.** Lipid droplet boundary membrane. **8.** Agranular endoplasmic reticulum closely apposed to lipid boundary membrane. **9.** Microtubule. **10.** Inset: lysosome with single trilaminar boundary membrane (X 100,000).

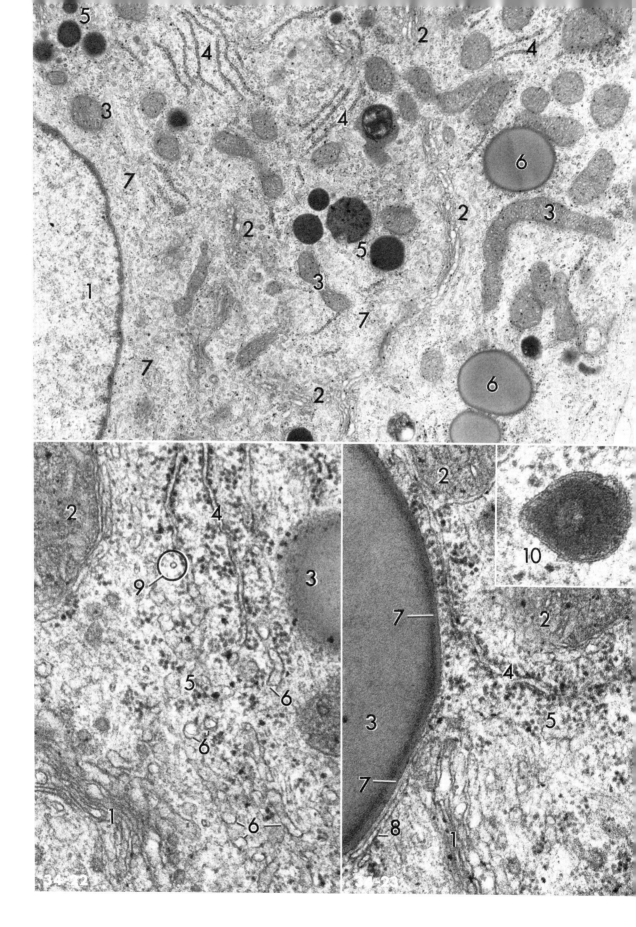

Graafian follicles and in the corpora lutea. The veins form a **pampiniform plexus** of large, thin-walled vessels in the medulla and mesovarium. The helicine arteries contain longitudinally arranged smooth muscle cells in their media in similarity with arteries of the same name in the cavernous tissue of the penis. There is a large number of myoendothelial junctions in the helicine arterioles of the ovary. A contraction of the longitudinal smooth muscle cells brings about a coiling, a relaxation, an extension of these blood vessels, actions which facilitate an adaptation to the changes that occur during normal cycles of follicular growth and regression. The rich capillary network of the ovary makes it possible for gonadotrophic hormones to reach all parts of the ovary, and to facilitate the removal of ovarian hormones. Capillaries in the thin wall of the Graafian follicles near the ovarian surface are probably related to the rupture of the follicle at ovulation, but the actual mechanism is not known.

Lymphatic capillaries are abundant in the wall of the Graafian follicles. This bed is drained by lymph vessels, converging on the medulla. These are in turn drained by large lymphatic vessels with valves, carrying the lymph to nodes in the pelvic and lumbar regions.

Nerves. The nerves encountered in the ovary are largely sympathetic in nature, derived from the ovarian plexus and uterine nerves. They innervate the smooth muscle cells of the blood vessels and of the ovarian stroma.

Oviduct

The two oviducts are tube-like structures serving as ducts for the ovum as it passes from the ovary to the uterus. The oviduct also serves as a place where fertilization of the ovum may take place and where the first cell divisions of the embryo occur.

The oviduct has a wide, trumpet-shaped opening toward the peritoneal cavity, the **infundibulum.** This is provided with **fimbriae,** extensions with a rich vascular supply. The fimbriae are covered by the same epithelium present throughout the oviduct. The infundibulum leads to the **ampulla,** the widest part of the oviduct. (Fig. 34-24) Toward the uterus, the ampulla narrows down to become the **isthmus,** and the oviduct penetrates the uterine wall as the **interstitial** or intramural portion. The wall of the oviduct has three layers: the mucosa, the muscularis, and the serosa.

The **mucosa** is composed of a columnar epithelium with a mixture of ciliated and non-ciliated cells. There is no real lamina propria. The muscularis mucosae is missing, and the subepithelial connective tissue layer is minimal. The mucosa is highly folded in the ampulla. (Figs. 34-25, 34-26) The folds and grooves decrease toward the uterus. They are very low in the isthmus, and they disappear in the intramural part of the oviduct. The **epithelium** varies in height and cellular composition in response to hormonal influence. During the proliferative phase of the endometrial cycle, the cells are tall columnar, and there is a predominance of ciliated cells. (Fig. 34-27) During the secretory phase of the endometrial cycle, the cells gradually

Fig. 34-24. Cross section of oviduct. Human. L.M. X 8. **1.** Fimbriae. **2.** Ampulla. **3.** Mesosalpinx. **4.** Peritoneal cavity. **5.** Muscularis.

Fig. 34-25. Enlargement of rectangle in Fig. 34-24. Human. L.M. X 44. **1.** Muscularis. **2.** Highly folded mucosa. **3.** Lumen of ampulla.

Fig. 34-26. Part of ampullary mucosa in oviduct. Mouse. E.M. X 560. **1.** Muscularis. **2.** Lamina propria of folded mucous membrane. **3.** Ciliated epithelium. **4.** Lumen of ampulla.

Fig. 34-27. Part of simple columnar ciliated epithelium in ampulla of oviduct. Rat. E.M. X 1750. **1.** Lumen of ampulla. **2.** Nuclei of ciliated cells. **3.** Nuclei of non-ciliated, secretory cells (peg-cells). **4.** Occasionally, basal cells occur. **5.** Cilia. **6.** Basal bodies. **7.** Microvilli. **8.** Capillary lumina. **9.** Fibroblasts in lamina propria.

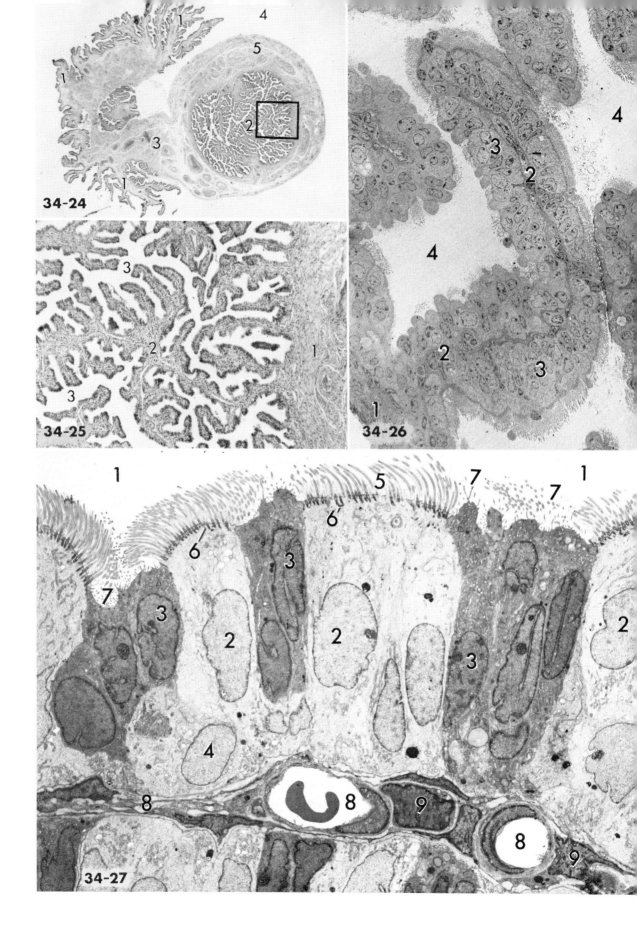

34-24

34-25

34-26

34-27

change to low columnar or cuboidal with a high number of non-ciliated cells present. The **ciliated** cells have no special fine structural characteristics that would make them different from similar cells in, for instance, the respiratory tract. The cilia beat toward the uterine opening of the oviduct, causing the fluid blanket to move. The non-ciliated cells vary in shape. At one stage, they are referred to as peg-cells because of their narrow width. All non-ciliated cells are secretory cells. It is believed that they secrete a mucoproteinaceous nutritive material. The cytoplasm is rich in granular endoplasmic reticulum and ribosomes. In the mouse, secretory granules occur which are reminiscent of mucous granules. These have not been identified in man or rat. The epithelium rests on a thin **basal lamina.**

The **muscularis** has an inner circular or spiral, and an outer longitudinal layer of smooth muscle cells. The circular layer is relatively thick and closely apposed to the thin subepithelial connective tissue. The outer muscular layer is thin, particularly in the ampulla. It becomes thicker toward the isthmus. Contractions of the muscular layers occur in peristaltic waves. They participate in forwarding the ovum from the peritoneal opening of the oviduct to the uterine opening.

The **serosa** is composed of simple squamous mesothelial cells and submesothelial connective tissue. The serosa covers the oviduct and forms a mesenteric attachment, the **mesosalpinx,** which joins the upper edge of the broad ligament.

Uterus

The uterus is a rounded, pear-shaped organ with a thick muscular wall and a narrow central cavity lined by a mucous membrane. In preparation for the reception of an ovum, the mucous membrane goes through cyclic changes of growth and degeneration, known as the menstrual cycle. This cycle is under endocrine con-

trol by hormones synthesized in the hypophysis and the ovary. Upon the arrival of a fertilized ovum, the uterus enlarges gradually to harbor the developing fetus. This process entails structural reorganization of both the mucous membrane and the muscular wall.

The uterus is situated in the pelvic cavity between the urinary bladder and rectum. The two uterine tubes connect with the upper end of the uterus, and the vagina with its lower end. The upper end, the **corpus** forms the main part of the uterus. The rounded top, the **fundus,** receives the uterine tubes, one on each side. The lower end of the uterus, the **cervix,** is a tube-like continuation of the corpus. It terminates with the **portio vaginalis** protruding slightly into the vagina. The corpus and the cervix are connected by a narrow part, the **isthmus.** In this region, the corpus is flexible in relation to the cervix, and can be bent back toward the sacrum or forward toward the symphysis pubis. However, the flexibility of the en-

Fig. 34-28. Section of wall of uterus. Proliferative phase. Human. L.M. X 7. **1.** Uterine cavity. **2.** Endometrium. **3.** Myometrium. **4.** Functionalis of endometrium. **5.** Basalis of endometrium (between levels indicated by dashed lines).

Fig. 34-29. Endometrium in proliferative phase. Uterus. Human. L.M. X 30. **1.** Uterine cavity. **2.** Endometrial stroma. **3.** Straight uterine glands in functionalis. **4.** Slightly coiled uterine glands in basalis. **5.** Myometrium.

Fig. 34-30. Enlargement of area similar to rectangle in Fig. 34-29. Uterine gland. Proliferative phase. Human. E.M. X 540. **1.** Lumen of uterine gland. **2.** Tall, columnar epithelial cells, some with short dome-like protrusions into the lumen. **3.** Epithelial cells in mitosis. **4.** Endometrial stroma.

Fig. 34-31. Enlargment of rectangle in Fig. 34-30. Detail of epithelium of uterine gland. Proliferative phase. Human. E.M. X 4500. **1.** Lumen of uterine gland. **2.** Thin basal lamina. **3.** Nuclei of columnar epithelial cells. **4.** Nuclei in late telophase of mitosis. **5.** Plane of cell separation. **6.** Mitochondria. **7.** The high background electron density is due to numerous microsomes. **8.** Microvilli.

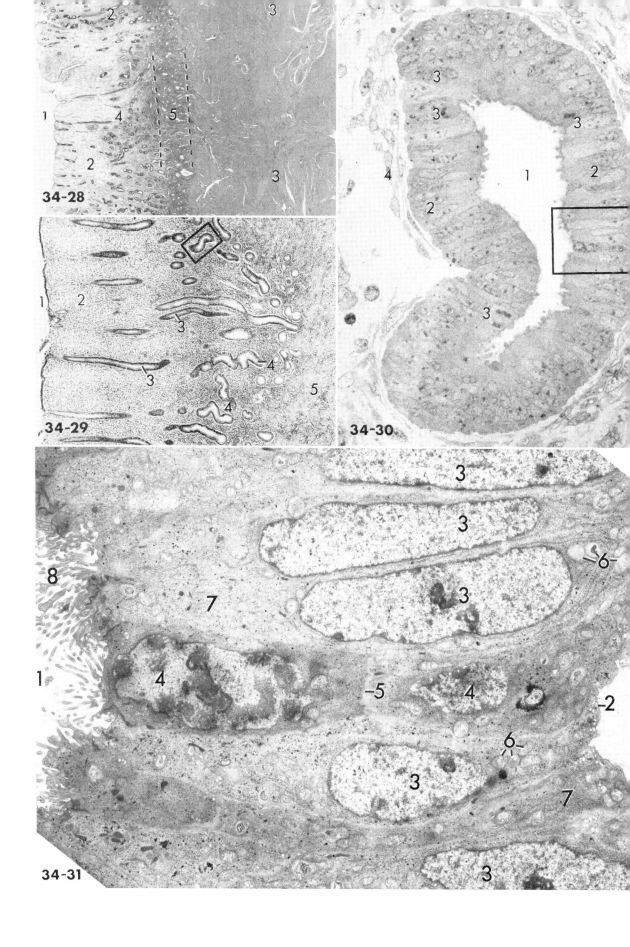

34-28

34-29

34-30

34-31

tire uterus is restricted by several ligaments which attach the uterus to the walls of the pelvis.

CORPUS

The wall of the body of the uterus consists of three layers: 1) endometrium (mucous membrane); 2) myometrium (muscle layer); and 3) perimetrium (serosa). (Fig. 34-28)

Endometrium. The endometrium is a mucous membrane, the thickness of which varies according to the age of the individual and to the phase of the menstrual cycle. It consists of an epithelial lining, uterine glands, and an endometrial stroma or lamina propria. (Fig. 34-29) The surface **epithelium** is composed of a single layer of columnar secretory cells, most of which produce mucus. Patches of ciliated cells occur. The **uterine glands** are simple, slightly branched, tubular glands, lined by cells similar to those of the surface epithelium. Ciliated cells are very rare. The highly cellular endometrial **stroma,** or the lamina propria of the mucous membrane, is composed of numerous stromal cells, an abundant mucoid matrix, and fine collagenous and elastic fibrils. In addition, the stroma contains many blood vessels and a rich capillary network.

The components of the endometrium change gradually during the progression of the menstrual cycle. (These changes will be considered shortly in relation to each phase of this cycle.) The endometrium is composed of two layers: the **basalis** (basal layer) which always remains a part of the uterine wall; and the **functionalis** (functional or decidual layer) which is sloughed at regular intervals.

Cyclic endometrial changes. The endometrium goes through cyclic changes which are brought about by hormones, synthesized by the hypophysis, the ovarian follicles, and the corpus luteum. One overt sign of these changes is menstruation, at which time the functionalis becomes detached, accompanied by a hemorrhage. Starting with the first day of menstrua-

tion, the endometrial cycle encompasses the following major steps: 1) menstruation (1st–4th day); 2) proliferation (5th–14th day); 3) secretion (15th–28th day). The rupture of an ovarian follicle and the expulsion of an ovum (ovulation) occurs, as a rule, on the 14th day of menstrual cycle.

The **endocrine control** of the endometrial changes involves the following major steps: 1) growth of primary ovarian follicles is controlled by the follicle stimulating hormone (FSH) synthesized by the adenohypophysis; 2) maturing ovarian follicles synthesize estrogens which stimulate growth of uterine glands during the proliferative phase; 3) ovulation occurs under the influence of FSH and LH (luteinizing) hormones from the adenohypophysis; 4) corpus luteum arises from the ruptured follicle through the stimulation of LH; 5) corpus luteum synthesizes estrogens and progesterone which influence the uterine glands to go into their

Fig. 34-32. Endometrium in late secretory phase. Uterus. Human. L.M. X 27. **1.** Uterine cavity. **2.** Endometrial stroma. **3.** Highly coiled uterine glands in functionalis. **4.** Slightly coiled uterine glands in basalis. **5.** Myometrium.

Fig. 34-33. Enlargement of area similar to rectangle in Fig. 34-32. Uterine gland. Late secretory phase. Human. E.M. X 480. **1.** Lumen of uterine gland. **2.** Medium high columnar epithelial cells, some with tall dome-like protrusions. **3.** Endometrial stroma.

Fig. 34-34. Enlargement of area similar to rectangle in Fig. 34-33. Detail of epithelial cell in uterine gland. Late secretory phase. Human. E.M. X 9500. **1.** Nucleus of epithelial cell in uterine gland. **2.** Junctional complexes. **3.** Mitochondria. **4.** Golgi zone. **5.** Secretory droplets. **6.** Lumen of uterine gland. **7.** Dome-like cell protrusions. **8.** Finely fibrillar masses of mucin.

Fig. 34-35. Enlargement of rectangle in Fig. 34-34. Tip of epithelial cell in uterine gland. Late secretory phase. Human. E.M. X 55,000. **1.** Secretory droplets. **2.** Particulate glycogen. **3.** Granular endoplasmic reticulum. **4.** Mitochondrion. **5.** Surface membrane. **6.** Glycocalyx or layer of mucin attached to the cell surface. **7.** Mucin free in the lumen. **8.** Microvillus.

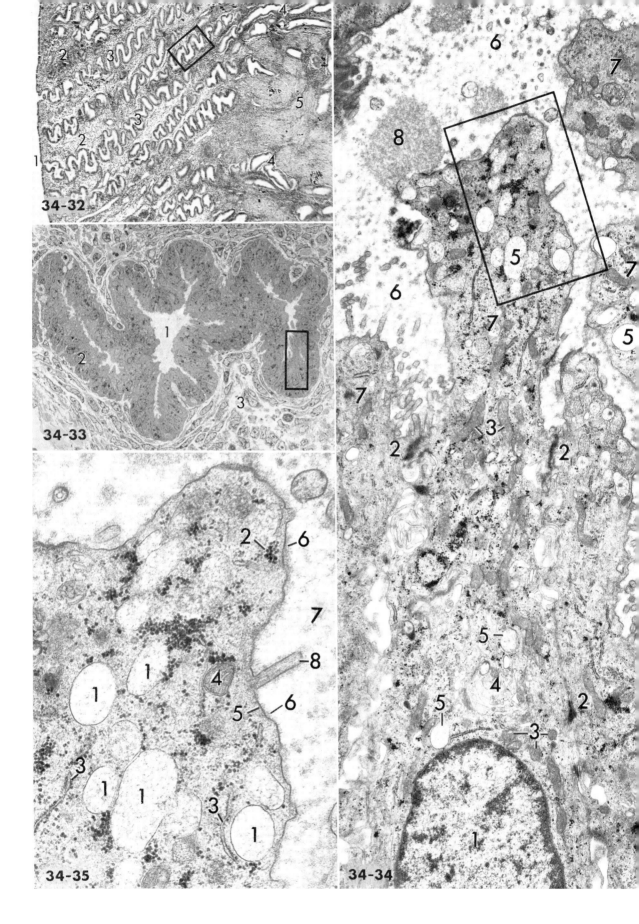

34-32

34-33

34-35

34-34

secretory phase, whereby the endometrium becomes ready to receive the ovum; 6) if the ovum does not become fertilized, corpus luteum involutes, the endometrium breaks down, and menstruation occurs; 7) if fertilization and implantation occur, chorionic gonadotrophin from the placenta keeps the corpus luteum secreting estrogens and progesterone and the endometrium is maintained in a secretory phase.

During the **proliferative phase** (synonyms: reparative; estrogenic; follicular) the endometrium increases in thickness from 1 mm to about 5 mm. (Fig. 34-29) The proliferation phase can be subdivided into an early, a mid-proliferative, and a late phase. However, as long as one remembers that the proliferation of the endometrium is gradual, one would have little difficulty in extrapolating between a proliferative and a secretory phase. The **uterine glands** are generally straight and narrow during the entire phase. There is a very active regeneration of the glandular epithelium from the glands remaining in the basalis, indicated by the numerous mitotic figures in the glandular epithelium. (Fig. 34-30) The cells progressively become taller during this phase, and there is a pseudostratification among the crowded, elongated nuclei. The cytoplasm has an abundance of ribosomes, some profiles of granular endoplasmic reticulum, and a few mitochondria. The apical part of the cell is dome-like and the luminal cell surface is provided with long microvilli. (Fig. 34-31) Some electron-lucent secretory droplets occur in the apical part of the cell. Toward the end of the late proliferative phase an irregular network of fine filaments appears on the luminal aspect of the microvilli and in the lumen between the microvilli. This luminal substance is believed to be secreted by the cells and to contain mucopolysaccharides. Accumulations of particulate glycogen appear in the basal part of the cells, particularly in the late proliferative phase. A **basal lamina** separates the epithelial cells

from the stroma. The **stroma** is rich in fibroblasts at this time. These fibroblasts are highly reminiscent of embryonic, mesenchymal cells, and mitotic figures are frequent among them. The transition from a proliferative to a secretory phase occurs shortly after ovulation while the corpus luteum develops.

During the **secretory phase** (synonyms: progravid; progestational; premenstrual; luteal), the endometrium increases by 3 mm to reach a total average thickness of 8 mm. (Fig. 34-32) The secretory phase can be subdivided into an early and a late phase. The early phase is characterized by alterations mainly in the uterine glands, whereas the endometrial stroma changes most drastically during the late secretory phase. The **uterine glands** progressively become more coiled, tortuous, and dilated. (Fig. 34-33) Mitotic figures among the epithelial cells are less frequent during the late phase of this period compared to the early phase. The profiles of the glands are scalloped. This is caused

Fig. 34-36. Endometrial stroma. Late secretory phase. Uterus. Human. L.M. X 200. **1.** Uterine cavity. **2.** Surface epithelium. **3.** Loose endometrial stroma between uterine glands (glands not shown).

Fig. 34-37. Transitional zone between endometrium and myometrium. Late secretory phase. Uterus. Human. L.M. X 220. **1.** Lumen of uterine glands in basal layer of endometrium (basalis). **2.** Dense endometrial stroma. **3.** Smooth muscle cells of myometrium.

Fig. 34-38. Enlargemeent of area similar to rectangle in Fig. 34-36. Detail of endometrial stroma. Late secretory phase. Uterus. Human. E.M. X 1800. **1.** Nuclei of fibroblast-like stromal cells. **2.** Stromal cell with large glycogen accumulations. **3.** Lymphocytes. **4.** Monocytes. **5.** Intercellular space with mucoid material.

Fig. 34-39. Detail of fibroblast-like cell (stromal or decidual cell). Endometrial stroma. Late secretory phase. Uterus. Human. E.M. X 9000. **1.** Nucleus. **2.** Mitochondria. **3.** Granular endoplasmic reticulum. **4.** Free ribosomes. **5.** Bulbous cell processes (pseudopods). **6.** Mucoid masses in extracellular space. **7.** Fine collagenous fibrils.

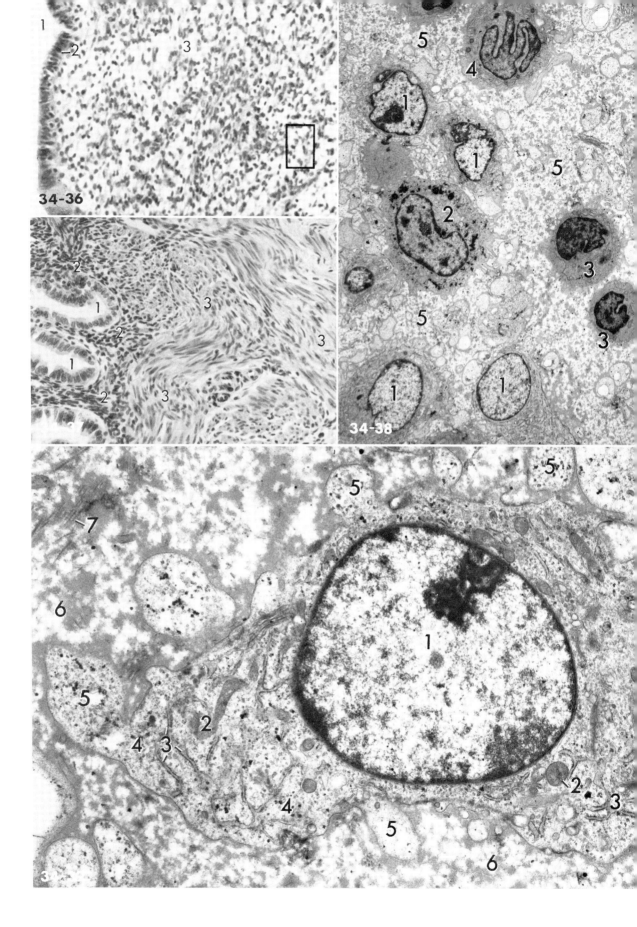

34-36

34-38

not only by the coiling of the gland but also by the unequal height and pseudo-stratification of the epithelial cells. The changes of the epithelial cells during the late proliferative and early secretory phases involve accumulation of glycogen and reorganization of the apex of the cells. Glycogen particles first accumulate in the basal part of the cells, pushing the nucleus toward the apical region. Simultaneously, secretory droplets and vacuoles, derived from the Golgi complex, appear in the apical region. (Fig. 34-35) The frothy, finely fibrillar substance now becomes quite abundant in the lumen. It is believed that the masses of glycogen particles and the Golgi vacuoles participate in the synthesis of mucopolysaccharides and mucins which subsequently are discharged and appear as the finely fibrillar substance in the glandular lumen. There is an initial predominance of glycogen in the secretion which later yields to mucus. The secretion provides nutrition for the fertilized ovum which arrives in the uterine cavity about three days after ovulation. During the late secretory phase, the dome-like protrusions of the epithelial cells may become detached and appear to float freely in the glandular lumen. (Fig. 34-34) This has been interpreted as an apocrine secretion, but is more likely an early sign of degeneration and cell death, initial to the menstrual phase, when a complete sloughing of the functionalis occurs. The endometrial **stroma** becomes progressively more loose through accumulation of extracellular fluid (edema) and increased amount of mucoid matrix, particularly toward the late secretory phase. (Fig. 34-36) The stromal, fibroblast-like cells enlarge toward the end of the menstrual cycle to become **decidual cells.** These are large, epithelial-like, polyhedral cells. (Fig. 34-39) Their cytoplasm contains numerous free ribosomes, many profiles of granular endoplasmic reticulum, and varied amounts of glycogen. The cells aggregate in large sheets around the coiled arterioles of the endometrium and be-

neath the surface epithelium. They develop further to form the decidua basalis in the event that an ovum is fertilized and implanted, and a placenta is formed. Other stromal cells present during this phase are lymphocytes, macrophages, monocytes, and the occasional polymorphonuclear leukocyte. (Fig. 34-38)

Preceding the **menstrual phase,** there is a constriction of coiled endometrial arterioles, resulting in a temporary reduction in blood flow (ischemia). This leads to a degeneration and loss of the superficial layer of the endometrium. Capillaries and arterioles rupture, the coiled arterioles relax, and a hemorrhage occurs, whereby the functionalis is shed. Since the basalis is retained, regeneration of the endometrium and proliferation of the uterine glands start a new cycle.

Myometrium. The myometrium consists of several layers of widely interlacing

Fig. 34-40. Longitudinal section of cervix uteri. Human. L.M. X 24. **1.** External cervical os. **2.** Cervical canal. **3.** Endocervix. **4.** Exocervix. **5.** Portio vaginalis. **6.** Mixture of dense connective tissue and smooth muscle fibers.

Fig. 34-41. Enlargement of the rectangle in Fig. 34-40. Endometrium. Cervix uteri. Human. L.M. X 125. **1.** Cervical canal. **2.** Surface epithelium. **3.** Branched, tubular cervical glands. **4.** Dense endometrial connective tissue. **5.** Smooth muscle cells.

Fig. 34-42. Enlargement of area similar to rectangle in Fig. 34-41. Survey of glandular epithelium. Cervix uteri. Human. E.M. X 1800. **1.** Lumen of gland. **2.** Nucleus of mucous cell. **3.** Nucleus of ciliated cell. **4.** Level of basal lamina. **5.** Nuclei of fibroblasts in stroma.

Fig. 34-43. Enlargement of area similar to rectangle in Fig. 34-42. Glandular epithelium. Cervix uteri. Human. E.M. X 4400. **1.** Nuclei. **2.** Mucigen granules. **3.** Cell borders. **4.** Cell apex.

Fig. 34-44. Enlargement of area similar to rectangle in Fig. 34-43. Apex of epithelial cell. Cervical gland. Human. E.M. X 29,000. **1.** Highly electron-dense secretory (mucigen) granules. **2.** Secretory vacuoles. **3.** Microvilli. **4.** Lumen with mucoid masses. **5.** Junctional complex.

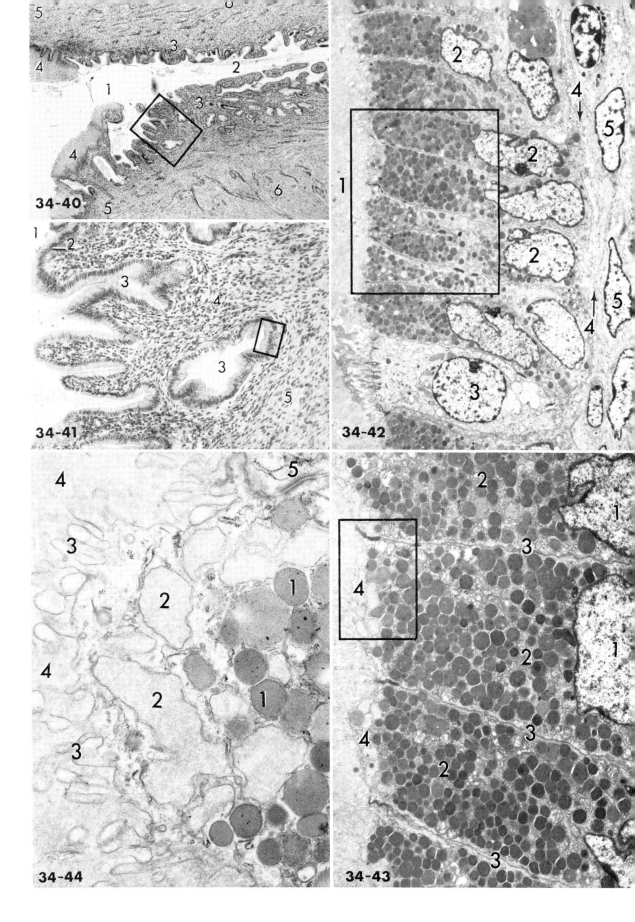

34-40

34-41

34-42

34-44

34-43

bundles of large and long smooth muscle cells. There is also an abundance of fibrous connective tissue and elastic fibers mixed in with the smooth muscle. The muscle cells are oriented chiefly in the circular direction, although bundles of longitudinally arranged cells occur subjacent to the endometrium (Fig. 34-37) and perimetrium. The smooth muscle cells increase greatly in length during pregnancy, but there is also an increase in number.

Perimetrium. The perimetrium consists of the peritoneal mesothelium and submesothelial connective tissue.

Blood supply. The uterine artery supplies the myometrium with several arcuate and spiral intramural vessels which in turn give off short, straight arteries to the basalis, and long **coiled arterioles** to the functionalis. The coiled arterioles run parallel to the uterine glands in a spiral manner. They have longitudinally arranged smooth muscle cells beneath the intima. A contraction of these cells bends the arteriole and reduces the blood flow. The coiled arterioles terminate in a capillary network beneath the surface epithelium. The capillaries are drained by a complex network of lacunar venous capillaries, venules, and veins.

CERVIX

The cervix is the tube-like lower end of the uterus. Its central cavity, **cervical canal** begins near the isthmus uteri with the internal os, and terminates with the external os at the lower end of the cervix, the **portio vaginalis.** The cervical canal is lined by a mucous membrane, the **endocervix.** The portio vaginalis is covered by its own special mucous membrane, the **exocervix,** which is continuous with the vaginal mucosa. (Fig. 34-40)

The wall of the cervix consists of endometrium, myometrium, and perimetrium. The **perimetrium,** serosa, lacks the mesothelial lining in relation to the anterior, vesical surface of the cervix. The **myometrium** contains a limited number of

smooth muscle cells and a large amount of dense connective tissue devoid of elastic fibers.

Endocervix. The endometrium of the cervix is about 2 mm thick with longitudinal folds, plicae palmatae. The surface is lined by a single layer of tall columnar, mucus-secreting cells, and some ciliated cells. (Fig. 34-42) There are large, branched tubular glands (Fig. 34-41), made up of cells with straight cell borders and a round nucleus located at the base of the cell. The apical two-thirds of the cell are filled with secretory granules of high electron density. (Fig. 34-43) The most apical part contains secretory vacuoles (Fig. 34-44) filled with the same flocculent material present in the glandular lumen, which is an alkaline mucus. Cyclic changes do not

Fig. 34-45. Wall of vagina. Human. L.M. X 30. **1.** Lumen of vagina. **2.** Stratified squamous epithelium. **3.** Lamina propria. **4.** Venous channels.

Fig. 34-46. Enlargement of rectangle in Fig. 34-45. Stratified squamous non-keratinized epithelium. Vagina. Human. L.M. X 200. **1.** Lumen with some superficial squamous cells being shed. **2.** Intermediate cells. **3.** Basal cells. **4.** Lamina propria. **5.** Connective tissue papillae.

Fig. 34-47. Enlargement of area similar to rectangle in Fig. 34-46. Stratified squamous non-keratinized epithelium. Vagina. Human. E.M. X 600. **1.** Connective tissue papilla. **2.** Cuboidal basal cells. **3.** Nuclei of cells in layers above basal cell layer. **4.** Cells in the middle of the epithelium starting to accumulate glycogen. **5.** Superficial cells with large accumulations of glycogen. These cells appear vacuolated in routine histological preparations.

Fig. 34-48. Enlargement of area similar to rectangle in Fig. 34-47. Epithelium of vagina. Human. E.M. X 10,000. **1.** Nucleus. **2.** Large glycogen accumulations. **3.** Ribosomes. **4.** Intercellular space. **5.** Desmosomes.

Fig. 34-49. Detail of cell from middle layers of stratified squamous epithelium. Vagina. Human. E.M. X 43,000. **1.** Masses of particulate glycogen. **2.** Mitochondria. **3.** Tonofilaments. **4.** Membrane-coating granules. **5.** Desmosomes. **6.** Intercellular space.

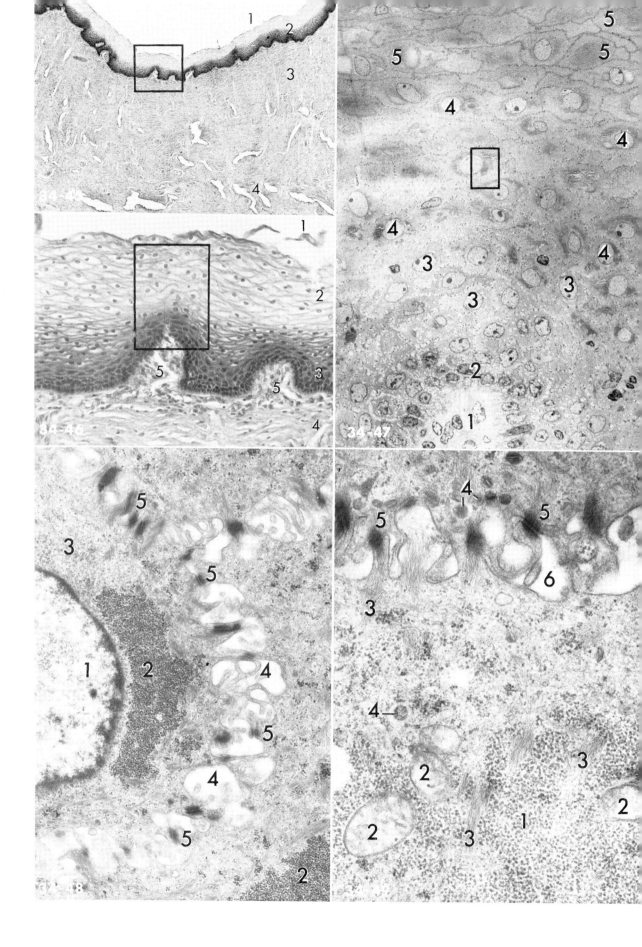

occur in the endocervix. The glandular openings often become obstructed, leading to a retention of mucus in the glands. The glands become greatly expanded and once were thought to represent small ova, referred to as ovula Nabothi. The stroma of the endocervix is a cellular, fibrous connective tissue.

Exocervix. The mucous membrane which lines the vaginal portion of the cervix is called exocervix. It consists of a stratified squamous, non-keratinized epithelium, identical in structure to the vaginal epithelium. (Figs. 34-40, 34-46) The lamina propria is fibrous and devoid of glands. Under normal circumstances, patches of endocervix may appear within the exocervix, and the stratified squamous epithelium of the exocervix may extend for varied lengths into the cervical canal.

Vagina

The vagina is a tubular organ which connects the uterus with the exterior of the body. Its wall, richly endowed with blood vessels, consists of a mucous membrane, a muscular sheath, and a fibrous adventitia. (Fig. 34-45) The mucous membrane is thrown into many transverse folds, or rugae, of which the hymen in the virgin forms an especially high fold near the external orifice. There are no glands in the wall of the vagina. The moisture present in the vagina comes from glands in the uterus, the cervix, and the vestibular glands of Bartholin. Some vaginal fluid may be derived from the abundant blood vessels in the lamina propria and the adventitia.

Mucous membrane. The mucous membrane consists of a stratified squamous epithelium and a lamina propria.

The stratified squamous **epithelium** is not keratinized in man. It has an average height of 200μ with a well-developed papillary layer. The normal thickness of the epithelium is maintained by the fe-

male sex hormones, and it becomes thin and atrophic when hormonal stimulation ceases. The epithelium is structurally similar to other non-keratinized stratified squamous epithelia with the exception of a marked accumulation of particulate glycogen in the cells, being moderate in the more basal cell layers and becoming heavy in the superficial cell layers. (Fig. 34-47) The particulate glycogen is first concentrated near the nucleus. (Fig. 34-48) As the cells move toward the surface of the epithelium, the glycogen gradually takes over larger parts of the cell and mixes with mitochondria, ribosomes, tonofilaments (Fig. 34-49), and membrane-coating vesicles. In routine histological preparations, the glycogen is dissolved away, rendering to the cells a swollen and empty appearance. There is an increase in glycogen accumulation toward the time of ovulation in response to estrogen stimulation. At the same time, keratohyalin granules and an increased number of tonofilaments may appear in the superficial

Fig. 34-50. Cross section of umbilical cord. Human. L.M. X 15. **1.** Umbilical vein. **2.** Umbilical arteries. **3.** Mucous connective tissue (Wharton's jelly). **4.** Amnion.

Fig. 34-51. Enlargement of vein in Fig. 34-50. Umbilical cord. Human. L.M. X 38. **1.** Lumen. **2.** Endothelium. **3.** Inner (thin) longitudinal layer of smooth muscle cells. **4.** Outer (thick) circular layer of smooth muscle cells. **5.** Mucous connective tissue.

Fig. 34-52. Enlargement of lower artery in Fig. 34-50. Umbilical cord. Human. L.M. X 44. **1.** Lumen. **2.** Endothelium (elastica interna missing). **3.** Inner (thick) longitudinal layer of smooth muscle cells. **4.** Outer circular layer of smooth muscle cells. **5.** Mucous connective tissue.

Fig. 34-53. Full term placenta. Human. L.M. X 6. **1.** Chorionic plate. **2.** Chorion frondosum. **3.** Surface detached from decidual (basal) plate. **4.** Main-stem villus. **5.** Cut surfaces.

Fig. 34-54. Part of placenta. Second month of gestation. Human. L.M. X 36. **1.** Chorionic plate. **2.** Main-stem villus. **3.** Terminal villi. **4.** Intervillous space. **5.** Amnion. **6.** Extra-embryonic mesoderm. **7.** Placental vein. **8.** Trophoblastic layer.

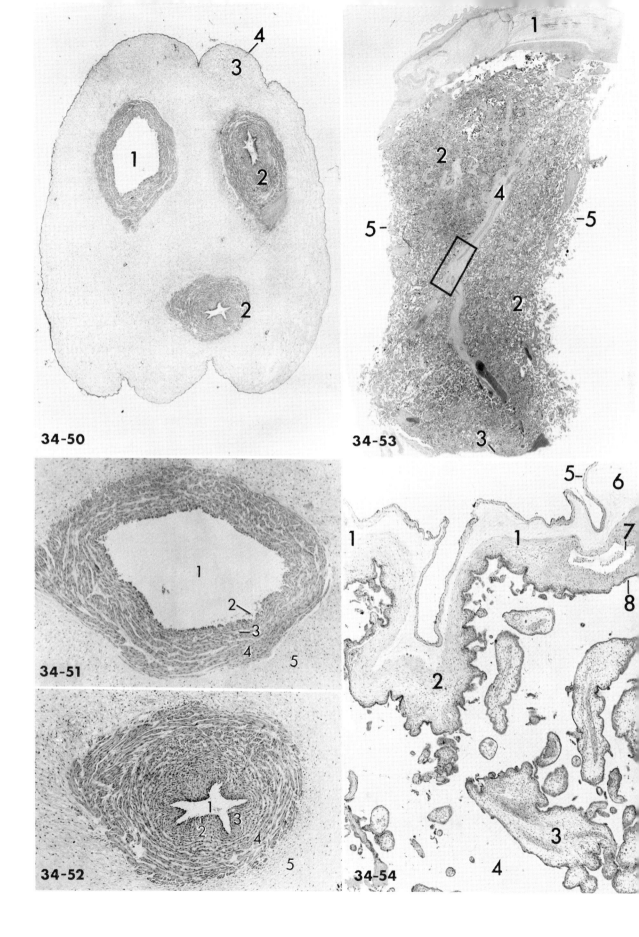

34-50

34-53

34-51

34-52

34-54

cell layers. However, true keratinization does not occur in man except as a result of vitamin A deficiency. Some of the superficial cells of the epithelium are shed during the menstruation. Cyclic changes of the epithelium are insignificant in man. They are quite prominent in guinea pigs and rats where the epithelium goes through a pre-estrus proliferation, an estrus keratinization, and a post-estrus atrophy in response to variations in hormonal stimulation. The glycogen in the vaginal epithelium may serve as nutriment for sperm cells. Bacteria in the vagina also use the glycogen by converting it to lactic acid in order to create optimal environmental conditions for normal bacterial life in the vagina.

The **lamina propria** is composed of dense connective tissue near the epithelium and it becomes more loose toward the muscularis. It contains bundles of collagen, many elastic fibers, numerous fibroblasts, and lymphocytes to the extent of a diffuse lymphoid infiltration. Many polymorphonuclear leukocytes invade the lamina propria and the epithelium before, during, and after menstruation.

Muscularis. The muscular sheath is composed of an inner layer of circular, and an outer layer of longitudinal smooth muscle cells, but the division is often indistinct. The entrance of the vagina is surrounded by a sphincter of skeletal muscle fibers.

Adventitia. The adventitia is made up of a thin layer of dense connective tissue. It contains a well-developed venous plexus which serves the function of an erectile tissue during sexual excitement.

External Genitalia

The external genitalia consist of labia majora and minor, the vestibule, and the clitoris.

The **labia majora** are thick folds of skin. The external surface is lined by keratinized, stratified squamous epithe-

lium, provided with hair follicles, as well as sweat glands and sebaceous glands. The inner surface has a thinly keratinized epithelium devoid of hair follicles but containing sebaceous and sweat glands.

The **labia minora** are thin folds of skin covered by the same epithelium as the inner surface of the labia majora. Hair follicles are missing but small sebaceous glands occur. There is a rich vascular bed in the lamina propria.

The **vestibule** forms the entrance to the vagina between the labia. It is lined by an epithelium similar to that in the vagina. This vestibular epithelium contains both small and large mucus-secreting glands. The large glands (of Bartholin) are located in the lateral walls of the vestibule, one on each side.

The **clitoris** contains cavernous tissue similar to that of the male penis. The head of the clitoris is lined by stratified squamous epithelium.

The mucous membrane of the external female genitalia is richly innervated and contains numerous sensory nerve endings such as Meissner's and Pacinian corpuscles, as well as Krause's end-bulbs.

Placenta

GENERAL

After the fertilization of the ovum and the initial cell division, a peripheral trophoblastic layer of cells develops which is instrumental in securing the fertilized ovum to the uterine wall and in the ex-

Fig. 34-55. Enlargement of rectangle in Fig. 34-53. Full term placenta. Human. L.M. X 31. **1.** Main-stem villus. **2.** Branching villus. **3.** Terminal villi. **4.** Arteries.

Fig. 34-56. Enlargement of area similar to rectangle in Fig. 34-55. Full term placenta. Human. L.M. X 130. **1.** Terminal villi of varying sizes. **2.** Intervillous space. **3.** Fetal blood vessels. **4.** Trophoblastic layers.

Fig. 34-57. Area similar to Fig. 34-56. Mid-pregnancy placenta. Human. E.M. X 600. **1.** Intervillous space. **2.** Maternal erythrocytes. **3.** Cores of terminal villi. **4.** Fetal blood vessels. **5.** Trophoblastic layers.

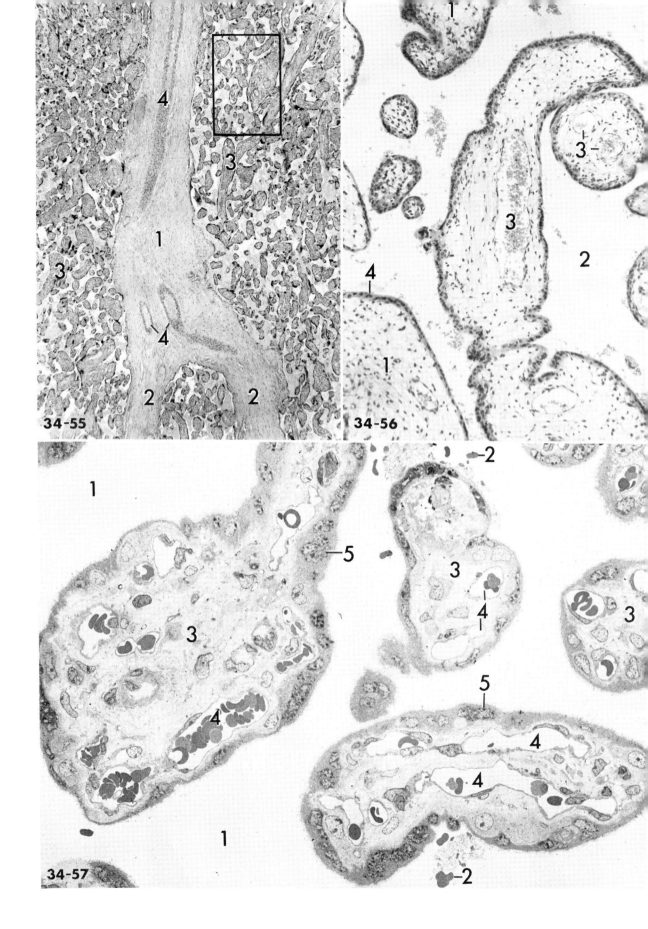

34-55

34-56

34-57

change of nutrients, wastes, and gases taking place between the developing fetus and the maternal circulation of the uterus. It is the trophoblastic layer and its spatial relationship to the uterine wall that are essential features of the **placenta.** The architecture of the fully developed placenta is more readily understood if some of the steps are first explained relating to the implantation of the blastocyst in the endometrium and the early development of the placenta.

Implantation. Following fertilization, the ovum goes through repeated mitoses, resulting first in a solid cell mass, the **morula,** and secondly in a cystic formation, the **blastocyst.** It consists of an inner solid cluster of cells which will form the embryo proper; a central, fluid-filled cavity; and surrounding the cavity and the embryo a single layer of cells, the trophoblasts. Surrounding the entire blastocyst is the zona pellucida. This layer disappears at about 6–8 days after ovulation, immediately preceding the implantation. The blastocyst penetrates the surface epithelium of the endometrium and sinks into the stroma between the uterine glands. Subsequently, the endometrial epithelium closes over the penetration site.

Early development of placenta. The trophoblastic cells proliferate rapidly and a stratification occurs. About 14 days after ovulation, the trophoblastic cells differentiate into two cell types, a superficial multinucleate **syncytiotrophoblastic** layer and a basal layer of **cytotrophoblasts** (Langhans cells). The trophoblastic layers form proliferating cell cords which invade the endometrium and destroy the walls of the coiled arterioles and veins of the endometrial stroma. The maternal blood, thus extravasated, creates irregular spaces in the trophoblastic cords. The cords come to form a three-dimensional network of trabeculae which are called **primary villi.** Fetal mesoderm soon extends from the developing blastocyst into these solid trabeculae of trophoblastic cells, creating cores of loose mesenchymal connective tis-

sue, covered by the layers of trophoblastic cells. These structures are referred to as **secondary villi.** Gradually, primitive blood vessels develop, both in the mesoderm of the embryo and in the connective tissue cores of the secondary villi. Eventually, the two sets of blood vessels unite and a circulation is established which takes the blood from the fetus to the villi of the placenta and back to the fetus. The villi which contain fetal blood vessels with circulating blood and mesenchymal connective tissue, are the **tertiary villi,** and will remain as such throughout the entire gestational period. The intervillous space is filled with maternal blood, delivered there by the coiled arterioles of the uterine endometrium, and drained by veins of the same tissue. At first the chorionic villi are present all around the implanted blastocyst, but as the fetus develops the villi become concentrated mostly toward the decidua basalis of the endometrium. Some of the larger villi, referred to as **mainstem villi** (Fig. 34-53), anchor the placentar villi to the basal endometrial stroma, the decidual (basal) plate. The attachment of the main-stem villi occurs through a rapid proliferation of cytotrophoblasts, forming columns of cells. These break through the syncytiotrophoblastic surface layer and mix with the decidual cells of the endometrial stroma, establishing the attachment of an **anchoring villus.**

MATURE PLACENTA

General. The mature placenta has a discoid shape with a diameter of about

Fig. 34-58. Cross-sectioned terminal villus. Mid-pregnancy placenta. Human. E.M. X 2100. **1.** Intervillous space. **2.** Maternal erythrocytes. **3.** Nuclei of syncytiotrophoblastic layer. **4.** Nuclei of cytotrophoblasts (Langhans cells). **5.** Fetal blood capillaries. **6.** Arterioles. **7.** Bundles of collagenous fibrils in the mesenchymal connective tissue core of the villus. **8.** Mesenchymal cells (fibroblasts). **9.** Part of macrophage (Hofbauer cell). **10.** Lymph capillary.

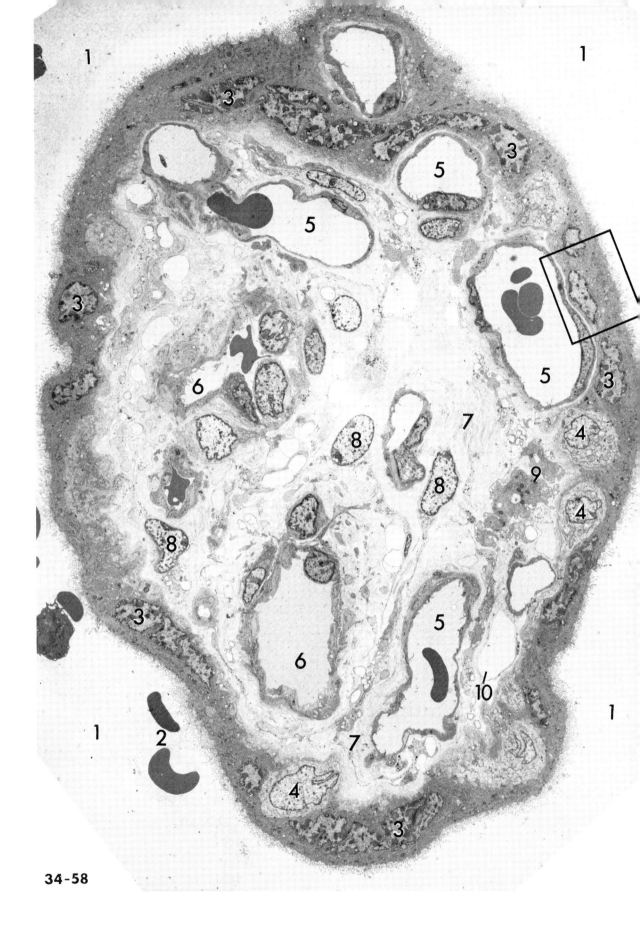

34-58

20 cm and a central thickness of about 5 cm. It is composed of the **decidual** (basal) **plate,** attaching the placenta to the uterine wall; and the **chorionic plate** which is the extra-embryonic mesoderm of the chorion, bordering on the amniotic cavity and lined by the amnion. (Fig. 34-54) The umbilical cord (Fig. 34-50) enters at the center of the chorionic plate. The **chorion frondosum** occupies the major part of the placenta (Fig. 34-53), interposed between the decidual and the chorionic plates. The chorion frondosum is made up of about 200 main-stem villi and innumerable branching terminal villi. The chorion frondosum is divided by decidual septa into cup-shaped compartments, **cotyledons.** The septa arise from the decidual plate and terminate short of the chorionic plate, thereby making it possible for maternal blood to pass from the intervillous space of one cotyledon to the next. Each cotyledon contains one main-stem villus. The **main-stem villus** constitutes the essential structural unit of the placenta. (Fig. 34-55) It is chiefly a blood vessel-transmitting structure with a core of mesenchymal connective tissue covered by the trophoblastic layers and bordering on the intervillous space. The **terminal villi** represent an extensive system of branches projecting freely in all directions into the intervillous space. (Figs. 34-55, 34-56, 34-57)

Placental circulation. The two umbilical arteries (Fig. 34-52) which carry blood rich in carbon dioxide from the fetus give rise to numerous placental arteries which radiate into the chorionic plate. From here, branches enter and follow the main-stem villi and enter the cores of the branching terminal villi, where they break up into capillaries. (Fig. 34-58) The **fetal capillaries** form a sinusoidal network which is closely applied to the basal lamina (Fig. 34-62) of the trophoblastic layers. (Fig. 34-59) The capillaries have a continuous, thick endothelium and are surrounded by a basal lamina. The endothelium contains micropinocytotic vesi-

cles, and numerous cytoplasmic filaments, possibly contractile. The luminal surface is provided with some short, slender microvilli and some short and bulbous excrescences. The oxygenated fetal blood is returned through a system of veins which accompanies the arteries and empties into the umbilical vein.

The **maternal blood** reaches the intervillous spaces through the coiled arterioles of the decidual plate. It is delivered by forceful pulsations, diffuses laterally and basally, and is drained by numerous venous outlets in the decidual plate.

Placental barrier. All chorionic villi are covered by the layers of syncytiotrophoblasts and cytotrophoblasts which represent the selective barrier between the fetal and the maternal circulations. (Fig. 34-59)

During the first trimester, the **cytotrophoblasts** (Langhans cells) form a complete basal layer of cuboidal cells, resting on a thin **basal lamina.** (Fig. 34-59) In relation to the main-stem villi, many of these cells disappear toward the end of the second trimester but some persist as isolated ovoid or flattened cells throughout gestation in the terminal villi. The cyto-

Fig. 34-59. Enlargement of area similar to rectangle in Fig. 34-58. General organization of placental barrier. Mid-pregnancy placenta. Human. E.M. X 9200. **1.** Lumen of fetal capillary. **2.** Erythrocytes. **3.** Reticulocyte. **4.** Nucleus of endothelial cell. **5.** Endothelial cytoplasm. **6.** Collagenous fibrils. **7.** Basal lamina. **8.** Nucleus of cytotrophoblast (Langhans cell). **9.** Nucleus of syncytiotrophoblastic layer. **10.** Microvilli. **11.** Club-shaped cytoplasmic protrusion. **12.** Intervillous space.

Fig. 34-60. Detail of placental barrier. Mid-pregnancy. Human. E.M. X 18,000. **1.** Basal lamina. **2.** Nucleus of cytotrophoblast. **3.** Basal cell membrane. **4.** Lateral cell membrane with narrow cytoplasmic processes. **5.** Golgi complex. **6.** Granular endoplasmic reticulum. **7.** Mitochondria. **8.** Circle: desmosome. **9.** Nucleus of syncytiotrophoblastic layer. **10.** Highly condensed chromatin. **11.** Granular endoplasmic reticulum. **12.** Primary lysosomes. **13.** Microvilli of varied shape.

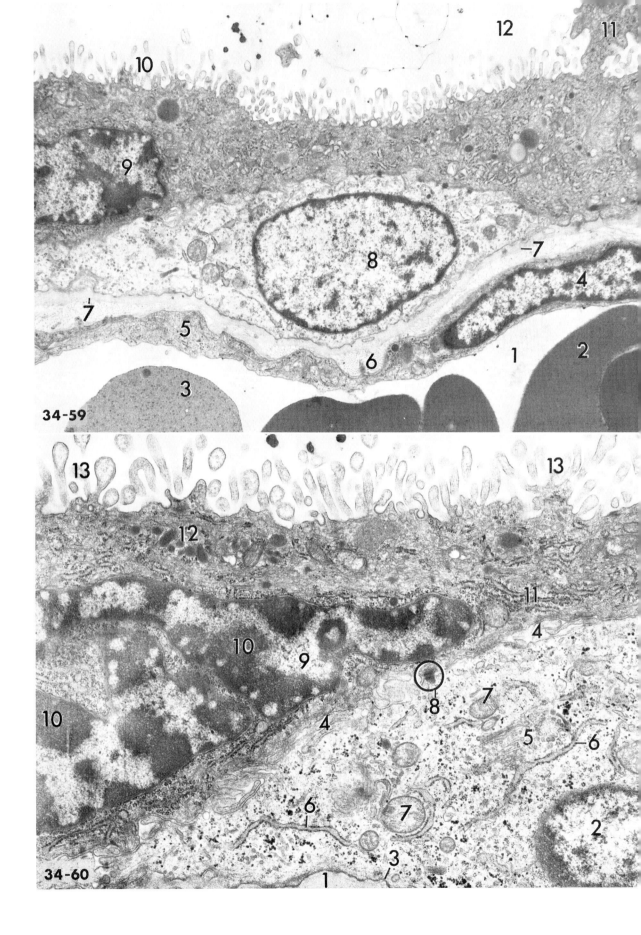

34-59

34-60

trophoblasts proliferate by mitosis. Their cytoplasm possesses only moderate electron density (Fig. 34-60) and contains a small number of free ribosomes and particulate glycogen. Profiles of granular endoplasmic reticulum are sparse, as are the mitochondria. The Golgi zone is relatively prominent. The cell membrane is slightly folded and the cell surface is provided with short and narrow cell processes. Desmosomes occur between the adjacent cytotrophoblasts and also between cytotrophoblasts and syncytiotrophoblastic layer.

The **syncytiotrophoblastic layer** is a continuous, superficial sheath of multinucleate cytoplasm, which covers all aspects of the villi and of the decidual and chorionic plates, bordering on the intervillous spaces. (Fig. 34-60) The layer arises through a fusion of cytotrophoblasts. These cells mitose continuously and add cells to the syncytiotrophoblastic layer. The nuclei are evenly distributed at first. Toward the end of pregnancy, the layer becomes thin in some areas and nuclei aggregate in local syncytial knots. The chromatin is heavily condensed in the syncytial nuclei. The cytoplasm is markedly electron-dense. Ribosomes are numerous in the second trimester and decrease in number in the third. Granular endoplasmic reticulum is extensive throughout, being composed of both short and long cisternae. Golgi zones are large and numerous. Mitochondria and profiles of tubular, agranular endoplasmic reticulum occur in moderate numbers. Primary and secondary lysosomes are numerous (Fig. 34-61), but lipid droplets vary in number from cell to cell. The free cell surface is provided with an extensive brush border, composed of short microvilli and small indentations and micropinocytotic vesicles between their bases. (Fig. 34-61)

The **core of the villi** contains a network of fine collagenous fibrils, fibroblast-like mesenchymal cells, and macrophages (Hofbauer cells). Occasional plasma cells are present. (Fig. 34-58)

The **functions** of the trophoblastic layers relate to the exchange of nutrients, wastes and gases between the fetal capillaries and the maternal blood. In addition, several hormones are synthesized here. The brush border and the pinocytotic vesicles participate in the resorption of most materials from the maternal blood in a manner similar to the cells of the proximal segment of the renal nephron. Lysosomal activity may be required for some of the processes. However, some of the cell structures may also be involved in a transport in the opposite direction, eliminating waste products from the fetal circulation. Among the hormones synthesized by the placenta are chorionic gonadotrophin, estrogen, and progesterone. Secretory granules similar to those in the adenohypophysis are not present in the trophoblastic cells. Some granules, reminiscent of small primary lysosomes may represent secretory granules. However, definite organelles associated with placental hormone synthesis and release have not been identified.

Mammary Glands

The mammary glands are derived from the epidermis and structurally represent modified sweat glands. They develop in both males and females up to the time of puberty. In the male they then atrophy, whereas in the female they continue to

Fig. 34-61. Detail of apical part of syncytiotrophoblast. Placenta. Mid-pregnancy. Human. E.M. X 40,000. **1.** Intervillous space. **2.** Microvilli. **3.** Pinocytotic invaginations. **4.** Mitochondria. **5.** Lysosomes. **6.** Granular endoplasmic reticulum. **7.** Free ribosomes.

Fig. 34-62. Detail of base of placental barrier. Mid-pregnancy. Human. E.M. X 40,000. **1.** Nucleus of cytotrophoblast (Langhans cell). **2.** Adjoining membranes of cytotrophoblast and syncytiotrophoblast. The cytoplasm is highly electron-dense in the syncytiotrophoblast, and electron-lucent in in the cytotrophoblast. **3.** Basal lamina. **4.** Mitochondria. **5.** Granular endoplasmic reticulum. **6.** Free ribosomes. **7.** Lysosomes.

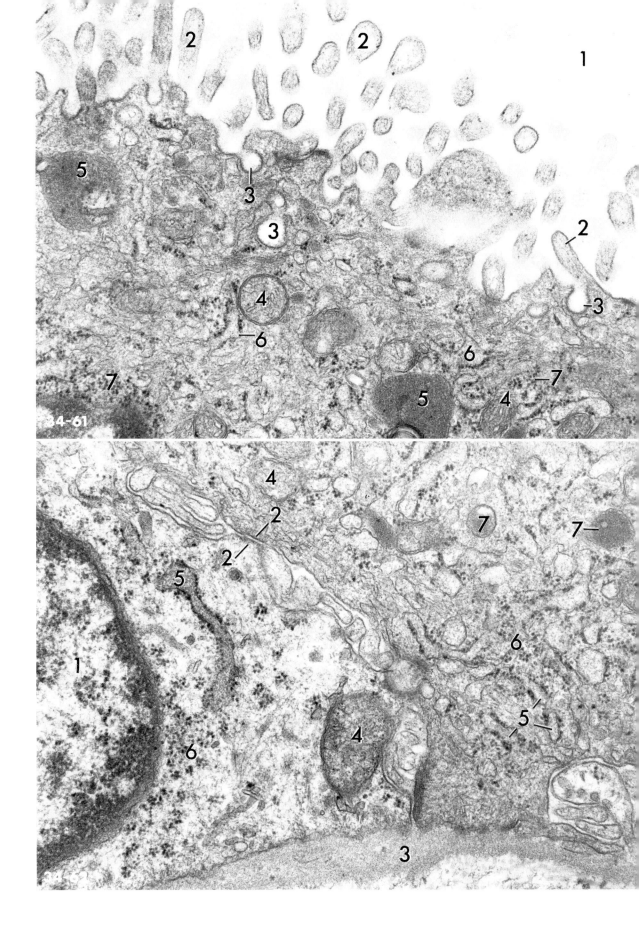

develop, reaching functional maturation after pregnancy. This development is guided by hormones. Estrogens from the ovarian follicles stimulate growth of the glandular duct system. Progesterone from the corpus luteum stimulates, together with estrogens, the development of the secretory alveoli. Prolactin is required to bring about milk secretion. This hormone is synthesized by the mammotrophs of the adenohypophysis.

GENERAL ORGANIZATION

The mammary glands form the major part of the two female breasts. The breasts also contain a rich network of connective tissue **stroma,** and a varying amount of **adipose** tissue. The **glandular** tissue is grouped into 10–20 **lobes,** separated by dense connective tissue **septa.** Each lobe is in turn subdivided into **lobules** by narrow septa. A system of **ducts** drains the glandular tissue. The smaller **intralobular** ducts merge to form **interlobular** ducts which in turn form 10–20 lactiferous ducts, opening on the surface of the **nipple** as small pores. The lactiferous ducts become slightly dilated within the nipple to form **lactiferous sinuses.** The nipple can be made to protrude above the surface of the breast to a varying degree because of a system of smooth muscle cells around the lactiferous ducts. The epidermal layer of the nipple is heavily pigmented, as is the areola, a circular area around the nipple. This pigmentation becomes even more marked during and after pregnancy. The areola contains sweat glands, sebaceous glands often without hairs, and the areolar glands of Montgomery, which are modified sweat glands. Depending upon the state of duct and glandular development, one recognizes: 1) an inactive resting phase; 2) a proliferative phase as pregnancy proceeds; and 3) a phase of active lactation after pregnancy. There are also some minor changes during the menstrual cycle. After pregnancy the mammary glands undergo regressive changes, and after the menopause atrophy of the glandular tissue occurs.

INACTIVE, RESTING GLANDS

The connective tissue elements predominate in the resting mammary glands. (Fig. 34-63) The connective tissue is generally of the dense, irregular variety, and there is a rich accumulation of adipose tissue. The glandular parenchyma, during the resting period, is reduced to essentially the system of lactiferous ducts, intralobar and interlobular ducts. The **smaller ducts** are lined by a simple **cuboidal epithelium** resting on a thin **basal lamina.** At intervals, **myoepithelial** cells are interposed between the basal lamina and the base of the duct cells. The myoepithelial cells are smooth muscle cells of ectodermal origin which serve as contractile elements in emptying the ducts. The **lactiferous ducts** are lined by a **stratified cuboidal-columnar**

Fig. 34-63. Resting mammary gland of non-pregnant adult woman. L.M. X 30. **1.** Dense irregular connective tissue. **2.** Interlobar duct. **3.** Intralobular ducts. **4.** Branches of intralobular ducts. **5.** Remaining alveolar buds; present because of possible slight proliferation during latter part of menstrual cycle.

Fig. 34-64. Proliferating mammary gland toward end of pregnancy. Human. L.M. X 30. **1.** Interlobular connective tissue septa. **2.** Adipose tissue. **3.** Intralobular duct. **4.** Proliferating intralobular ducts with some collapsed and some distended alveoli.

Fig. 34-65. Lactating mammary gland. Human. L.M. X 30. **1.** Interlobular connective tissue septum. **2.** Interlobular ducts. **3.** Dilated secretory alveoli.

Fig. 34-66. Enlargement of rectangle in Fig. 34-65. Human. L.M. X 350. **1.** Branching of terminal duct. **2.** Alveoli. **3.** Simple cuboidal epithelium. **4.** Milk droplets. **5.** Intralobular loose connective tissue. **6.** Capillary.

Fig. 34-67. Alveoli of lactating mammary gland. Mouse. E.M. X 1800. **1.** Nuclei and cytoplasm of alveolar epithelial cells. **2.** Lumina of aveoli with small milk protein particles. **3.** Lipid droplets of milk. **4.** Perialveolar capillaries in loose connective tissue. **5.** Circles: sites where a cytoplasmic process of a myoepithelial cell is located.

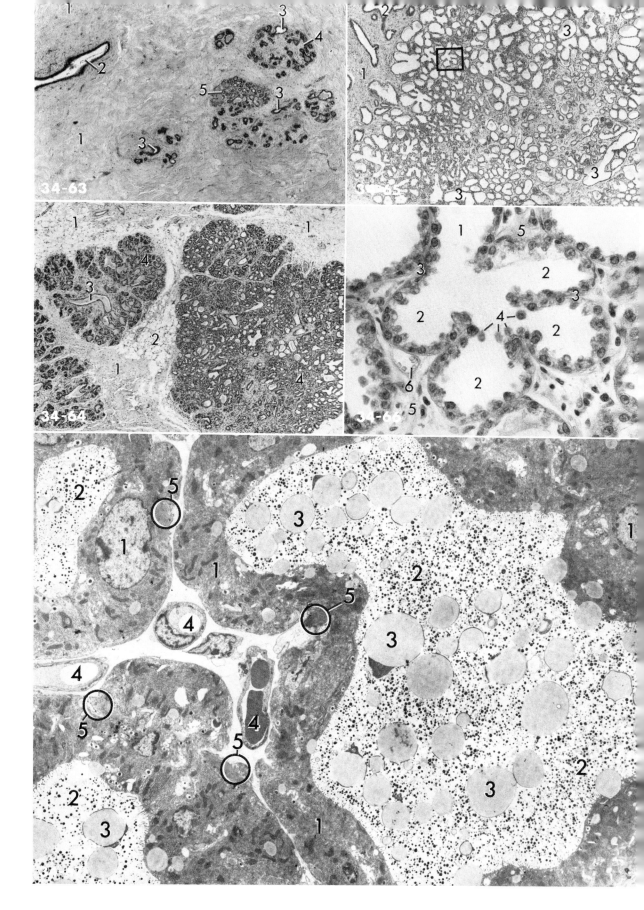

epithelium which changes to a stratified squamous epithelium near the pore at the surface of the nipple. There may be a slight growth of the duct system and the development of a few bud-like alveoli during the secretory phase of the menstrual cycle. There are great individual variations in this respect, and the gland is still considered to be in a resting state.

PROLIFERATIVE GLANDS

This stage is initiated with the onset of pregnancy and develops gradually as the pregnancy proceeds. (Fig. 34-64) The terminal portion of the ducts starts to grow, sending out new branches, some of which end in alveolar enlargements. There is a gradual replacement of the connective tissue with ducts and, budding from the ducts, an increasingly large number of small collapsed alveoli. Toward the end of pregnancy, the collapsed alveoli begin to enlarge and expand, making the mammary gland into a typical compound tubulo-alveolar gland. The alveoli are lined by a simple cuboidal epithelium. With the expansion of the glandular elements, the connective tissue is compressed into very thin septa between the alveoli.

LACTATING GLANDS

At the end of pregnancy and after parturition, the duct system and the secretory alveoli reach their state of maximum development, and the lobes and lobules with their corresponding ducts are easily recognized. (Fig. 34-65) The alveoli are lined by a **cuboidal epithelium** that is actively secreting at this point. (Figs. 34-66, 34-67) The initial secretion is called colostrum, which is rich in protein, low in fat, and contains so-called colostrum bodies which probably represent macrophages filled with lipid droplets. A few days after delivery, this secretion ceases, and the secretion of **milk** sets in. The milk is rich in fat, sugar (lactose), and protein (casein) in addition to mineral salts. The synthesis by the alveolar cells of these products has been analyzed ultrastructurally rather ex-

tensively. The **secretory cells** have a vast system of granular endoplasmic reticulum and an abundance of free ribosomes. (Fig. 34-69) Mitochondria are few in number. The Golgi complex is large and widespread. Within the saccules of the Golgi appear condensations which in the shape of small vacuoles are carried to the luminal surface of the cell. (Fig. 34-70) The core of the vacuole is discharged into the alveolar lumen by a fusion of the vacuolar membrane and the surface membrane. Most likely, these particles represent the **protein** component of the milk. (Fig. 34-71) The **fatty** components are formed and discharged in a different manner. Throughout the cytoplasm of the alveolar cells occur a large number of lipid droplets, varying in size. The origin and mode of formation of the lipid droplets are not known. Ultimately the droplets are released at the apical cell surface by a mechanism referred to as apocrine secretion. (Fig. 34-72) Upon discharge the droplet takes along a thin coating of cytoplasm and the apical cell membrane. (Fig. 34-73) The lumen of the alveolus is filled with two categories of discharged cellular products, suspended in a watery fluid. (Fig. 34-68) The alveoli are surrounded by **myoepithelial** cells.

Fig. 34-68. Survey of secretory epithelium in alveolus of lactating mammary gland. Mouse. E.M. X 9500. **1.** Lumen of alveolus. **2.** Nucleus of secretory epithelial cell. **3.** Nucleus of myoepithelial cell. The cell borders of these two cells can be seen with some difficulty at the tip of the arrows. **4.** Large milk lipid droplet suspended in luminal fluid. **5.** Small milk lipid droplets. **6.** Lipid droplets retaining detached peripheral coat of cytoplasm. **7.** Milk protein particles. **8.** Lipid droplets in cell cytoplasm. **9.** Lipid droplet near cell surface. **10.** Protein particle in a vacuole. **11.** Mitochondrion. **12.** Short profiles of granular endoplasmic reticulum. **13.** Short microvilli. **14.** Bundle of myofilaments. **15.** Basal lamina. **16.** Reticular fibrils. **17.** Loose connective tissue. **18.** Lumen of blood capillary. **19.** Endothelium. **20.** Basal lamina of capillary.

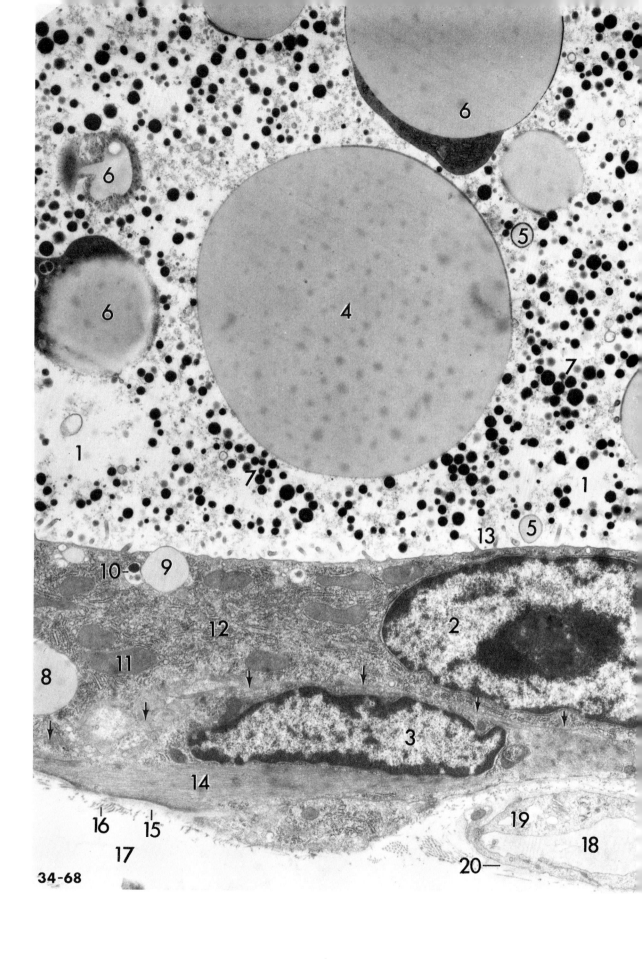

REGRESSION AND ATROPHY

Regular suckling stimulates the continuation of milk secretion. If stopped, the secretion ceases, the alveoli collapse and become absorbed, returning the gland to a resting state. After menopause, the major part of the duct system atrophies, and the gland acquires the structural appearance of the early, prepubertal state.

References

OVARY

Adams, E. C. and Hertig, A. T. Studies on guinea pig oocytes. I. Electron microsccopic observations on the development of cytoplasmic organelles in oocytes of primordial and primary follicles. J. Cell Biol. *21*: 397–427 (1964).

Adams, E. C. and Hertig, A. T. Studies on the human corpus luteum. I. Observations on the ultrastructure of development and regression of the luteal cells during the menstrual cycle. J. Cell Biol. *41*: 696–715 (1969).

Adams, E. C. and Hertig, A. T. Studies on the human corpus luteum. II. Observations on the ultrastructure of luteal cells during pregnancy. J. Cell Biol. *41*: 716–735 (1969).

Baca, M. and Zamboni, L. The fine structure of human follicular oocytes. J. Ultrastruct. Res. *19*: 354–381 (1967).

Baker, T. G., Beaumont, H. M. and Franchi, L. L. The uptake of tritiated uridine and phenylalanine by the ovaries of rats and monkeys. J. Cell Sci. *4*: 655–675 (1969).

Baker, T. G. and Franchi, L. L. The fine structure of oogonia and oocytes in human ovaries. J. Cell Sci. *2*: 213–224 (1967).

Belt, W. D., Cavazos, L. F., Anderson, L. L. and Kraeling, R. R. Fine structure and progesterone levels in the corpus luteum of the pig during pregnancy and after hysterectomy. Biol. Reprod. *2*: 98–113 (1970).

Bjersing, L. On the morphology and endocrine function of granulosa cells in ovarian follicles and corpora lutea. Acta Endocrinol. Suppl. *125*: 1–23 (1967).

Bjersing, L. On the ultrastructure of granulosa lutein cells in porcine corpus luteum. With special reference to endoplasmic reticulum and steroid hormone synthesis. Z. Zellforsch. *82*: 187–211 (1967).

Blanchette, E. J. A study of the fine structure of the rabbit primary oocyte. J. Ultrastruct. Res. *5*: 349–363 (1961).

Blanchette, E. J. Ovarian steroid cells. I. Differentiation of the lutein cells from the granulosa follicle cell during the preovulatory stage and under the influence of exogenous gonadotrophins. J. Cell Biol. *31*: 501–516 (1966).

Blanchette, E. J. Ovarian steroid cells. II. The lutein cell. J. Cell Biol. *31*: 517–542 (1966).

Cavazos, L. F., Anderson, L. L., Belt, W. D., Henricks, D. M., Kraeling, R. R. and Melampy, R. M. Fine structure and progesterone levels in the corpus luteum of the pig during the estrous cycle. Biol. Reprod. *1*: 83–106 (1969).

Crisp. T. M. and Browning, H. C. The fine structure of corpora lutea in ovarian transplants of mice following luteotrophin stimulation. Am. J. Anat. *122*: 169–192 (1968).

Crisp, T. M., Dessouky, A. D. and Denys, F. R. The fine structure of the human corpus luteum of early pregnancy and during the progestational phase of the menstrual cycle. Am. J. Anat. *127*: 37–70 (1970).

Dahl, E. Studies of the fine structure of ovarian interstitial tissue. I. A comparative study of the fine structure of the ovarian interstitial tissue in the rat and the domestic fowl. J. Anat. *108*: 275–290 (1971).

Davies, J. and Broadus, C. D. Studies on the fine structure of ovarian steroid-secreting cells in the rabbit. I. The normal interstitial cells. Am. J. Anat. *123*: 441–474 (1968).

Fig. 34-69. Detail of epithelial cells in alveolus of lactating mammary gland. Mouse. E.M. X 29,000. **1.** Nucleus. **2.** Mitochondria. **3.** Golgi membranes and saccules. **4.** Early synthesis of core of protein particle in a Golgi saccule. **5.** Protein particle in vacuole, separating from the Golgi zone. **6.** Granular endoplasmic reticulum. **7.** Cell membrane. **8.** Junctional complex. **9.** Microvilli. **10.** Lumen of alveolus.

Fig. 34-70. Detail of apical surface of lactating epithelial cell. Mammary gland. Mouse. E.M. X 59,000. **1.** Lumen of alveolus. **2.** Surface membrane. **3.** Protein particles in vacuoles. **4.** Thin sheet of cytoplasm separates boundary membrane of vacuole from surface membrane. These two membranes fuse at the moment of particle discharge. **5.** Discharged milk protein particles. **6.** Lipid droplet sectioned tangentially

Fig. 34-71. Detail of discharged milk protein particles. Mammary gland. Mouse. E.M. X 172,000. The particles are not surrounded by a membrane. They are composed of minute globules, each about 25 Å in diameter, arranged in a crystalline array.

Fig. 34-72. Detail of apical surface of lactating epithelial cell. Mammary gland. Mouse. E.M. X 62,000. **1.** Lumen of alveolus. **2.** Mitochondria. **3.** Lipid droplet elevating the cell surface in the process of discharge. **4.** Thin boundary membrane at cytoplasm/droplet interface. **5.** Thin rim of cytoplasm.

Fig. 34-73. Highly enlarged detail of part of discharged milk lipid droplet. Mammary gland. Mouse. E.M. X 129,000. **1.** Alveolar lumen. **2.** Core of lipid droplet. **3.** Superficial leaflet of surface trilaminar membrane. **4.** Fusion of inner leaflet and lipid droplet boundary membrane.

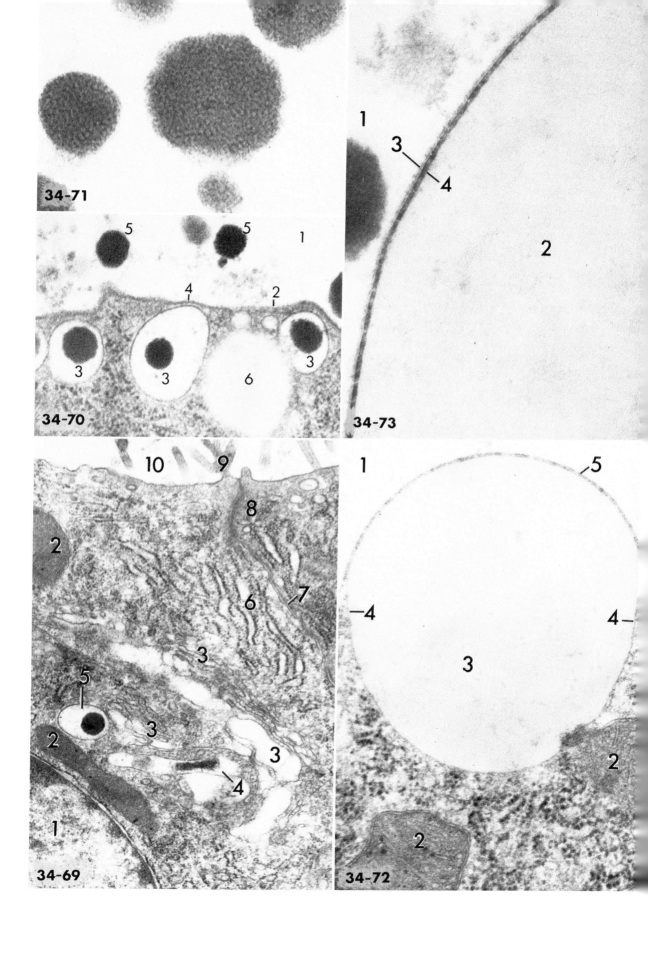

34-71

34-70

34-73

34-69

34-72

Delson, B., Lubin, S. and Reynolds, S. R. M. Vascular patterns in the human ovary. Am. J. Obstet. Gynecol. *57*: 842–853 (1949).

Enders, A. C. and Lyons, W. R. Observations on the fine structure of lutein cells. II. The effects of hypophysectomy and mammotrophic hormone in the rat. J. Cell Biol. *22*: 127–141 (1964).

Espey, L. L. Ultrastructure of the apex of the rabbit Graafian follicle during the ovulatory process. Endocrinology *81*: 267–276 (1967).

Gillim, S. W., Christensen, A. K. and McLennan, C. E. Fine structure of the human menstrual corpus luteum at its stage of maximum secretory activity. Am. J. Anat. *126*: 409–428 (1969).

Goecke, H. Die Endausbreitung des vegetativen Nervengewebes im menschlichen Ovarium und ihre Bedeutung für die Funktion des Ovariums. Arch. Gynäk. *166*: 187–189 (1938).

Hadek, R. The structure of the mammalian egg. Int. Rev. Cytol. *18*: 29–72 (1965).

Hertig, A. T. The primary human oocyte: some observations on the fine structure of Balbiani's vitelline body and the origin of the annulate lamellae. Am. J. Anat. *122*: 107–138 (1968).

Hertig, A. T. and Adams, E. C. Studies on the human oocyte and its follicle. I. Ultrastructural and histochemical observations on the primordial follicle stage. J. Cell Biol. *34*: 647–675 (1967).

Hisaw, F. L. The development of the Graafian follicle and ovulation. Physiol. Rev. *27*: 95–119 (1947).

Norrevang, A. Electron microscopic morphology of oogenesis. Int. Rev. Cytol. *23*: 114–186 (1968).

Odor, D. L. The ultrastructure of unilaminar follicles of the hamster ovary. Am. J. Anat. *116*: 493–522 (1965).

Odor, D. L. and Blandau, R. J. Ultrastructural studies on fetal and early postnatal mouse ovaries. Am. J. Anat. *124*: 163–186 (1969).

O'Shea, J. D. An ultrastructural study of smooth muscle-like cells in the theca externa of ovarian follicles in the rat. Anat. Rec. *167*: 127–140 (1970).

Osvaldo-Decima, L. Smooth muscle in ovary of the rat and monkey. J. Ultrastruct. Res. *29*: 218–237 (1970).

Papadaki, L. and Beilby, J. O. W. The fine structure of the surface epithelium of the human ovary. J. Cell Sci. *8*: 445–465 (1971).

Schlafke, S. and Enders, A. C. Cytological changes during cleavage and blastocyst formation in the rat. J. Anat. *102*: 13–32 (1967).

Short, R. V. Steroids in the follicular fluid and the corpus luteum of the mare. A "two-cell type" theory of ovarian steroid synthesis. J. Endocrin. *24*: 59–63 (1962).

Simkins, C. S. Development of the human ovary from birth to sexual maturity. Am. J. Anat. *51*: 465–505 (1932).

Szollosi, D. Development of cortical granules and the cortical reaction in rat and hamster eggs. Anat. Rec. *159*: 431–446 (1967).

Witschi, E. Migration of germ cells of human embryos from the yolk sac to the primitive gonadal folds. Contr. Embryol. *32*: 67–80 (1948).

OVIDUCT

Björkman, N. and Fredricsson, B. Ultrastructural features of the human oviduct epithelium. Int. J. Fertil. *7*: 259–266 (1962).

Clyman, M. J. Electron microscopy of the human fallopian tube. Fertil. & Steril. *17*: 281–301 (1966).

Novak, E. and Everett, H. S. Cyclical and other variations in the tubal epithelium. Am. J. Obstet. Gynecol. *16*: 499–530 (1928).

Nilsson, O. Electron microscopy of the fallopian tube epithelium of rabbit in oestrus. Exp. Cell Res. *14*: 341–354 (1958).

Snyder, F. F. Changes in the human oviduct during the menstrual cycle and pregnancy. Bull. Johns Hopkins Hosp. *35*: 141–146 (1924).

UTERUS

Albert, E. N. and Pease, D. C. An electron microscopic study of uterine arteries during pregnancy. Am. J. Anat. *123*: 165–194 (1968).

Bo, W. J., Odor, D. L. and Rothrock, M. L. The fine structure of uterine smooth muscle of the rat uterus at various time intervals following a single injection of estrogen. Am. J. Anat. *123*: 369–384 (1968).

Bo, W. J., Odor, D. L. and Rothrock, M. L. Ultrastructure of uterine smooth muscle following progesterone or progesterone-estrogen treatment. Anat. Rec. *163*: 121–132 (1969).

Borell, U., Nilsson, O. and Westman, A. The cyclical changes occurring in the epithelium lining the endometrial glands. An electron microscopic study in the human being. Acta Obstet. Gynecol. Scand. *38*: 364–377 (1959).

Cavazos, F., Green, J. A., Hall, D. G. and Lucas, F. V. Ultrastructure of the human endometrial glandular cell during the menstrual cycle. Am. J. Obstet. Gynecol. *99*: 833–854 (1967).

Colville, E. A. The ultrastructure of the human endometrium. J. Obstet. Gynaecol. Brit. Commonwealth *75*: 342–350 (1963).

Danforth, D. N. The fibrous nature of the human cervix, and its relation to the isthmic segment in gravid and non-gravid uteri. Am. J. Obstet. Gynecol. *53*: 541–560 (1947).

Daron, G. H. The arterial pattern of the tunica mucosa of the uterus in Macacus rhesus. Am. J. Anat. *58*: 349–419 (1936).

Enders, A. C. and Schlafke, S. Cytological aspects of trophoblast-uterine interaction in early implantation. Am. J. Anat. *125*: 1–30 (1969).

Enders, A. C. and Schlafke, S. Penetration of the uterine epithelium during implantation in the rabbit. Am. J. Anat. *132*: 219–240 (1971).

Goerttler, K. Die Architektur der Muskelwand des menschlichen Uterus und ihre funktionelle Bedeutung. Morphol. Jahrb. *65*: 45–128 (1930).

Gompel, C. The ultrastructure of the human endometrial cell studied by electron microscopy. Am. J. Obstet. Gynecol. *84*: 1000–1009 (1962).

Hinglais-Guillaud, N. L'ultrastructure de l'exocol normal de la femme (exocervix). Bulletin du Cancer *46*: 212–252 (1959).

Laguens, R. and Lagrutta, J. Fine structure of human uterine muscle in pregnancy. Am. J. Obstet. Gynecol. *89*: 1040–1048 (1964).

Larkin, L. H. and Flickinger, C. J. Ultrastructure of the metrial gland cell in the pregnant rat. Am. J. Anat. *126*: 337–354 (1969).

Nilsson, O. Electron microscopy of the glandular epithelium in human uterus. I. Follicular phase. J. Ultrastruct. Res. *6*: 413–421 (1962).

Nilsson, O. Electron microscopy of the glandular epithelium in human uterus. II. Early and late luteal phase. J. Ultrastruct. Res. *6*: 422–431 (1962).

Ross, R. and Klebanoff, S. J. Fine structural changes in uterine smooth muscle and fibroblasts in response to estrogens. J. Cell Biol. *32*: 155–167 (1967).

Salvatore, C. A. The growth of human myometrium and endometrium. Studies of cytological aspects. Anat. Rec. *108*: 93–109 (1950).

Sengel, A. and Stoebner, P. Ultrastructure de l'endomètre humain normal. I. Le chorion cytogène. Z. Zellforsch. *109*: 245–259 (1970).

Sengel, A. and Stoebner, P. Ultrastructure de l'endomètre humain normal. II. Les glandes. Z. Zellforsch. *109*: 260–278 (1970).

Smith, L. J. Metrial gland and other glycogen containing cells in the mouse uterus following mating and through implantation of the embryo. Am. J. Anat. *119*: 15–23 (1966).

Themann, H. and Schünke, W. The fine structure of the glandular epithelium of the human endometrium, electron microscopic morphology. pp. 99–134. *In* The Normal Human Endometrium (Ed. H. Schmidt-Matthiesen). McGraw-Hill, New York, 1963.

Terzakis, J. A. The nucleolar channel system of human endometrium. J. Cell Biol. *27*: 293–304 (1965).

Wynn, R. M. and Harris, J. A. Ultrastructural cyclic changes in the human endometrium. I. Normal preovulatory phase. Fertil. & Steril. *18*: 632–648 (1967).

Wynn, R. M., Harris, J. A. and Wooley, R. S. Ultrastructural cyclic changes in the human endometrium. II. Normal postovulatory phase. Fertil. & Steril. *18*: 721–738 (1967).

UMBILICAL CORD

Hoyes, A. D. Ultrastructure of the epithelium of the human umbilical cord. J. Anat. *105*: 149–162 (1969).

Leeson, C. R. and Leeson, T. S. The fine structure of the rat umbilical cord at various times of gestation. Anat. Rec. *151*: 183–197 (1965).

Parry, E. W. Some electron microscope observations on the mesenchymal structures of full-term umbilical cord. J. Anat. *107*: 505–518 (1970).

PLACENTA

Boyd, J. D. and Hamilton, W. J. Development and structure of the human placenta from the end of the 3rd month of gestation. J. Obstet. Gynaecol. Brit. Commonwealth *74*: 161–226 (1967).

Enders, A. C. Formation of syncytium from cytotrophoblast in the human placenta. Obstet. Gynecol. *25*: 378–386 (1965).

Enders, A. C. Fine structure of anchoring villi of the human placenta. Am. J. Anat. *122*: 419–452 (1968).

Enders, A. C. and King, B. F. The cytology of Hofbauer cells. Anat. Rec. *167*: 231–252 (1970).

Hamilton, W. J. and Boyd, J. D. Development of the human placenta in the first three months of gestation. J. Anat. *94*: 297–328 (1960).

Rhodin, J. A. G. and Terzakis, J. The ultrastructure of the human full-term placenta. J. Ultrastruct. Res. *6*: 88–106 (1962).

Terzakis, J. A. The ultrastructure of normal human first trimester placenta. J. Ultrastruct. Res. *9*: 268–284 (1963).

Wislocki, G. B. and Dempsey, E. W. Electron microscopy of the human placenta. Anat. Rec. *123*: 133–168 (1955).

VAGINA

Cooper, R. A., Cardiff, R. D. and Wellings, S. R. Ultrastructure of vaginal keratinization in estrogen treated immature Balb/cCRGL mice. Z. Zellforsch. *77*: 377–403 (1967).

Eddy, E. M. and Walker, B. E. Cytoplasmic fine structure during hormonally controlled differentiation in vaginal epithelium (mouse). Anat. Rec. *164*: 205–218 (1969).

Gregoire, A. T., Kandil, O. and Ledger, W. J. The glycogen content of human vaginal epithelial tissue. Fertil. & Steril. *22*: 64–68 (1971).

Papanicolaou, G. N. The sexual cycle in the human female as revealed by vaginal smears. Am. J. Anat. *53*: 519–637 (1933).

Smith, B. G. and Brunner, E. K. The structure of the human vaginal mucosa in relation to the menstrual cycle and to pregnancy. Am. J. Anat. *54*: 27–86 (1934).

Stegner, H. and Iwata, M. Elektronenmikroskopische Untersuchungen am Scheidenepithel der Ratte. Mikr. Anat. Forsch. *76*: 491–508 (1967).

MAMMARY GLANDS

Bargmann, W. and Knoop, A. Über die Morphologie der Milchsekretion. Licht- und elektronenmikroskopische Studien an der Milchdrüse der Ratte. Z. Zellforsch. *49*: 344–388 (1959).

Helminen, H. J. and Ericsson, J. L. E. Studies on the mammary gland involution. I. On the ultrastructure of the lactating mammary gland. J. Ultrastruct. Res. *25*: 193–213 (1968).

Hollmann, K. H. Sur des aspects particuliers des protéines élaborées dans la glande mammaire. Étude au microscope électronique chez la lapine en lactation. Z. Zellforsch. *69*: 395–402 (1966).

Kurosumi, K., Kobayashi, Y. and Baba, N. The fine structure of the mammary glands of lactating rats, with special reference to the apocrine secretion. Exp. Cell Res. *50*: 177–192 (1968).

Wooding, F. B. P. The mechanism of secretion of the milk fat globule. J. Cell Sci. *9*: 805–821 (1971).

Wooding, F. B. P. The structure of the milk fat globule membrane. J. Ultrastruct. Res. *37*: 388–400 (1971).

35 Eye

The eye is the special sense organ for light. It contains receptor cells, refractive media, and other structures necessary to form an image at the level of the photoreceptors. In the embryo the eye develops as a cup-like outpocketing of the forebrain. The cup-shaped structure develops into a sphere, the eyeball (Fig. 35-1), in the process incorporating the lens, which originates from the surface ectoderm. The **innermost layer** of the wall of the eyeball consists of neuroepithelial receptor cells, nerve cells, and nerve processes which form the retina and the optic nerve. The retina is covered by the **middle layer** of the wall of the eyeball, which is highly vascular and referred to as choroid (uveal tract). To this layer belong the ciliary body and the iris. The **outermost layer** of the eyeball consists of the sclera and the cornea. The center of the eyeball is occupied by the large vitreous body, the lens; the anterior and posterior chambers of the eye, are filled with aqueous humor.

Structures associated with the eye, and of paramount importance for the proper functioning of the eye, are the extraocular muscles, the eyelids, the lacrimal glands, and the tear ducts.

SCLERA

The sclera corresponds to the dura mater. It is a 0.3-1mm thick white, nontransparent layer of dense connective tissue which forms the posterior five-sixths of the eyeball. The **episclera** is a thin external layer of relatively loose connective tissue which contains a few blood vessels. It connects the sclera to the **capsule of Tenon,** which is a dense fibrous connective tissue capsule, bordering on the orbital fat pad. The **stroma** of the sclera consists of densely packed collagenous fibrils, which vary greatly in diameter, and scattered fibroblasts. (Fig. 35-3) There is a dearth of interfilamentous water-binding substance. This is believed to contribute to the opacity of the sclera. **Lamina fusca** is the innermost narrow zone of the sclera, which contains occa-

sional pigmented cells, that represent stray uveal melanocytes. The melanocytes reach this region by migrating through **emissaria,** the small canals present in the scleral stroma and ordinarily used by blood vessels and nerves to enter and leave the eyeball. In the region where the optic nerve fibers leave the eye, the sclera is richly perforated. This disk-shaped area is called **lamina cribrosa.**

CORNEA

The anterior one-sixth of the outer layer of the eyeball is formed by the cornea, which is the major refractive element of the eye. The cornea protrudes slightly, since it has a shorter radius of curvature than the sclera. (Fig. 35-10) It is a transparent, avascular connective tissue membrane, 0.5-1 mm thick, the inner and outer surfaces of which are covered by layers of cells. (Fig. 35-4) The sclerocorneal junction which is called **limbus;** it marks the area where the opaque sclera becomes the transparent cornea. (Fig. 35-11) Within this general region is present

Fig. 35-1. Vertical meridional section of eyeball and eyelids through pupil and optic nerve. Monkey. L.M. X 7.5. **1.** Upper eyelid (enlarged in Fig. 35-39). **2.** Lower eyelid (enlarged in Fig. 35-42). **3.** Cornea. **4.** Anterior chamber. **5.** Pupil. **6.** Iris. **7.** Lens (center of lens removed by the preparation process). **8.** Posterior chamber. **9.** Ciliary body. **10.** Vitreous body. **11.** Retina. **12.** Optic disk and papilla. **13.** Sclera. **14.** Optic nerve (enlarged in Fig. 35-32). **15.** Fornix of conjunctival sac (enlarged in Fig. 35-43).

Fig. 35-2. Principal layers of wall of eyeball. Enlargement of area similar to rectangle in Fig. 35-1. Monkey. L.M. X 168. **1.** Retina (innermost layer). **2.** Choroid (middle layer). **3.** Sclera (outermost layer).

Fig. 35-3. Choroid and sclera. Enlargement of area similar to rectangle in Fig. 35-2. Monkey. L.M. X 435. **1.** Outer segments of rods and cones. **2.** Pigmented epithelium of retina. **3.** Choriocapillaris. **4.** Heavily pigmented stroma. **5.** Blood vessel. **6.** Suprachoroidea. **7.** Collagenous bundles and nuclei of fibroblasts in sclera.

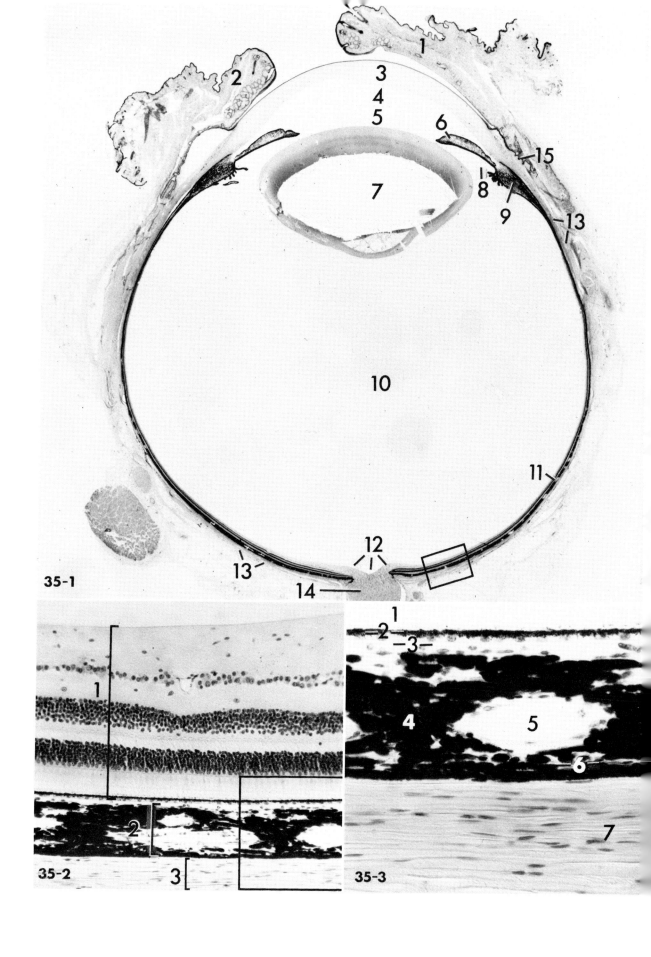

35-1

35-2

35-3

the **canal of Schlemm,** which runs in the connective tissue stroma as a leaky water pipeline around the periphery of the cornea. This channel drains the aqueous humor of the anterior chamber of the eye via the intertrabecular spaces into the neighboring system of ocular veins.

The cornea consists of: 1) epithelium; 2) Bowman's membrane; 3) stroma; 4) Descemet's membrane; and 5) endothelium.

Epithelium. The epithelium, which is continuous with that of the bulbar conjunctiva, is of the stratified squamous, non-keratinized type, averaging 50 μ in thickness. It is avascular but contains many free, non-myelinated nerve endings derived from pain fibers. The basal cells are columnar and rich in tonofilaments but poor in other organelles. (Fig. 35-5) They rest on a thin **basal lamina** and their basal cell membrane is provided with many half-desmosomes in this region. There are several layers of intermediate cells with numerous desmosomes and an increasing number of tonofilaments. These cells are often referred to as **wing cells.** The superficial squamous cells are extremely rich in tonofilaments but they do not become keratinized. Their free surface is provided with small microvilli and ridge-like folds, which presumably facilitate the maintenance of a tear film at the corneal surface.

Bowman's membrane. This is a specialized layer of corneal stroma which contains randomly distributed, delicate collagenous and reticular fibrils.

Stroma. This constitutes the major portion of the cornea; it averages 500 μ in thickness and consists of stromal lamellae, fibroblasts, and matrix. The **lamellae** consists of densely packed bundles of delicate collagenous fibrils of uniform diameter. The bundles run in different directions and are oriented obliquely in the anterior portion of the cornea and in parallel arrays in the posterior portion. (Fig. 35-6) The **fibroblasts** (keratocytes) are very scarce and mostly present as resting fibro-

cytes. Upon stimulation they become fibroblasts, actively synthesizing collagenous fibrils. The **matrix** of the stroma is rich in acid mucopolysaccharides and chondroitin sulfate, which may contribute to the transparency of the cornea, in combination with the regular stromal lamellae and the uniform fibrils.

Descemet's membrane. This is a 5–10 μ thick homogeneous elastic membrane in which occurs dense small fibrils with a periodicity of about 1000 Å. (Fig. 35-6) It is believed that they represent a unique type of collagen. The fibrils are embedded in an amorphous substance rich in mucopolysaccharides, and similar to the thin basal laminae of epithelia.

Endothelium. A single layer of flattened cuboidal cells lines the inner surface of the cornea, bordering on the membrane of Descemet. Although the layer is mostly referred to as endothelium, it is more in the nature of a mesothelium. The cells are hexagonal and joined by junctional complexes in addition to an interlocking system of adjacent cellular ridges and grooves. The cells are rich in organelles,

Fig. 35-4. Cornea. Human. L.M. X 184. **1.** Stratified squamous non-keratinized epithelium. **2.** Bowman's membrane. **3.** Stroma. **4.** Descemet's membrane. **5.** Endothelium.

Fig. 35-5. Corneal epithelium. Enlargement of area similar to rectangle (A) in Fig. 35-4. Human. E.M. X 3200. **1.** Superficial squamous cells. **2.** Wing cell with partly obscured nucleus. **3.** Nucleus of polyhedral intermediate cell. **4.** Nuclei of columnar cells. **5.** Level of basal lamina (not resolved). **6.** Bowman's membrane. **7.** Stromal connective tissue elements.

Fig. 35-6. Corneal stroma and endothelium. Enlargement of area similar to rectangle (B) in Fig. 35-4. E.M. X 10,000. **1.** Longitudinally sectioned collagenous fibrils of corneal stroma. **2.** Cross-sectioned collagenous fibrils of corneal stroma. **3.** Cytoplasmic extensions of fibroblasts (keratocytes). **4.** Border zone between corneal stroma and Descemet's membrane. **5.** Descemet's membrane with some faintly discernible periodicity. **6.** Nucleus of endothelial cell. **7.** Numerous mitochondria.

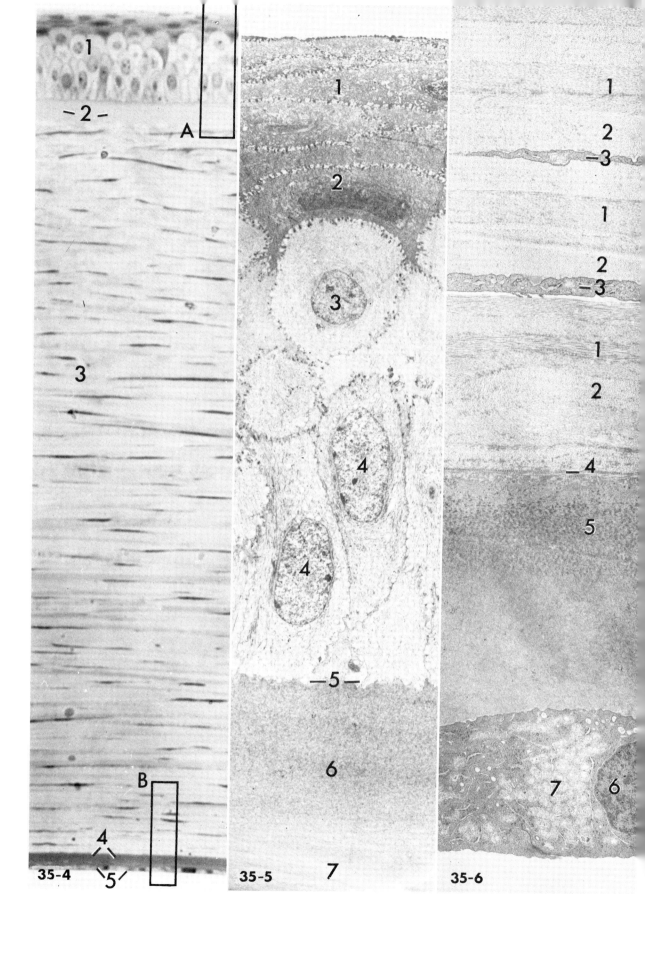

35-4

35-5

35-6

especially mitochondria and pinocytic invaginations and vesicles. (Fig. 35-6) These cells are believe to be involved in active transport of ions and fluids, as well as in the synthesis of Descemet's membrane.

CHOROID

The choroid proper forms the middle layer of the wall of the eyeball. (Fig. 35-2) It extends from the edge of the optic nerve forward to the ora serrata, which is the anterior line of termination for the optic retina. The choroid, the ciliary body, and the iris, are referred to as the **uveal tract** (or uvea). The choroid proper contains numerous blood vessels for the anterior portion of the eye and nourishes the outer parts of the retina through an extensive capillary network. The choroid consists of: 1) suprachoroidea; 2) stroma; 3) choriocapillaris; and 4) Bruch's membrane.

Suprachoroidea. This layer borders on the lamina fusca of the sclera. It is thin and contains numerous pigmented, star-shaped melanocytes distributed in a loose connective tissue containing many bundles of collagenous fibrils; it is oriented parallel to the inner surface of the sclera.

Stroma. The choroidal stroma contains many arterioles and venules embedded in a loose connective tissue rich in fibroblasts and melanocytes. (Figs. 35-3, 35-9) Mast cells and macrophages occur but are less numerous. The many blood vessels contribute to the spongy texture of the choroid proper, reminiscent of cavernous (erectile) tissue.

Choriocapillaris. This is a thin layer of capillaries with fenestrated endothelium derived from the arterioles of the choroidal stroma. (Fig. 35-7) This flat capillary network supplies the photoreceptor cells of the retina with oxygen and nutrients.

Bruch's membrane borders on the pigmented epithelium of the retina and its thin basal lamina. It is an elastic membrane, 1–2 μ thick, consisting of a central network of elastic fibers, surrounded on both sides by delicate collagenous and reticular fibrils. (Fig. 35-8)

CILIARY BODY

The ciliary body is a fibromuscular ring representing a direct continuation of the choroid. It extends forward from the choroid proper at the ora serrata to the root of the iris. It serves as attachment for the suspensory ligament of the lens and contains smooth muscle cells which control the focal power of the lens. It also contains a rich capillary network which participates in the production of the aqueous humor. In a meridional section of the eye the ciliary body has a triangular shape. (Fig. 35-10) The anterior portion, **pars plicata** (corona ciliaris), is elevated, and consists of 70–80 radiating surface folds (crests, ciliary processes) projecting into the posterior chamber of the eye. (Figs. 35-11, and 35-14) The pars plicata also contains the major portion of the ciliary muscle. The posterior portion, **pars plana** (orbiculus ciliaris), forms a wide posterior ring between the ora serrata and the ciliary processes. It contains radiating smooth muscle cells.

Fig. 35-7. Junctional area between retina and choroid. Rat. E.M. X 1900. **1.** Outer segments of rods and cones. **2.** Pigmented epithelium of retina. **3.** Nucleus of pigmented cell. **4.** Bruch's membrane. **5.** Lumina of blood capillaries of choriocapillaris. **6.** Connective tissue elements of choroid stroma.

Fig. 35-8. Bruch's membrane. Enlargement of area similar to rectangle in Fig. 35-7. Rat. E.M. X 15,000. **1.** Nucleus of pigmented epithelial cell of retina. **2.** Mitochondria. **3.** Base of epithelial cell with cell membrane folds. **4.** Basal lamina of retina. **5.** Collagenous fibrils of Bruch's membrane. **6.** Elastic fibers of Bruch's membrane. **7.** Basal lamina of blood capillary. **8.** Fenestrated endothelium. **9.** Junctional area of apposed endothelial cells. **10.** Capillary lumen. **11.** Nucleus of endothelial cell.

Fig. 35-9. Choroid stroma. Monkey. E.M. X 14,000. **1.** Melanocyte cell membrane. **2.** Melanocyte. **3.** Pigment granules. **4.** Bundles of collagenous fibrils.

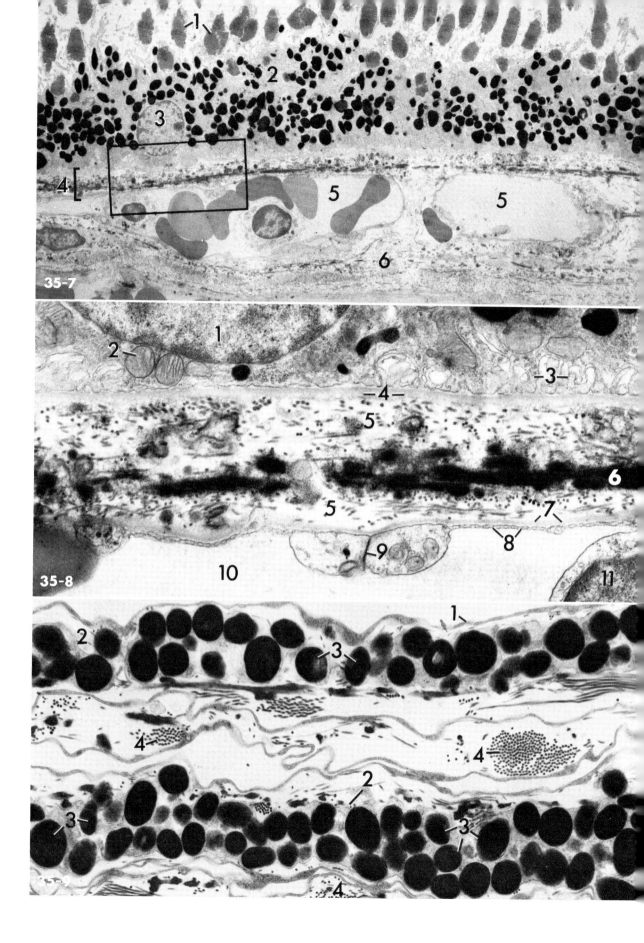

From a developmental point of view, the ciliary body consists of an outer (uveal) part, derived from the mesoderm, and an inner (retinal) part, originating from the neuroectoderm. The **outer part** consists of the ciliary muscle and the stroma; the **inner part,** of the ciliary epithelium.

Ciliary muscle. In front, smooth muscle cells are attached to the sclera in the region of the limbus (scleral spur), and behind to the stroma of the choroid proper. Early investigators identified a meridional-radial portion (Brücke's muscle) and a circular portion (Müller's muscle), but recent investigations indicate that there is considerable interweaving of smooth muscle cells from layer to layer. (Figs. 35-12, 35-13). The fibers of the suspensory ligament of the lens attach at the surface of the ciliary processes. Upon contraction, particularly of the circular muscle portion, tension in the suspensory ligament is decreased, allowing the lens to assume a more curved shape, thereby increasing its focal power, and providing accommodation for near vision. The function of the meridional-radial smooth muscle cells is not known, but it is believed that all smooth muscle cells act jointly, regardless of their orientation.

Ciliary stroma. The inner portion of the pars plicata consists of a loose connective tissue with many fibroblasts, melanocytes, and mast cells. A rich vascular bed permeates the stroma, consisting mostly of capillaries with fenestrated endothelium and venules. (Fig. 35-15) The major arterial circle is also located in this stroma.

Ciliary epithelium. The inner surface of the ciliary body which faces the posterior chamber of the eye and the vitreous body is lined by a double layer of cuboidal cells (Fig. 35-15) enclosed in a thin basal lamina, the **internal limiting membrane.** The inner cell layer, which borders on the vitreous body and the posterior chamber, consists of **non-pigmented** cells (Fig. 35-16) rich in mitochondria, granular

endoplasmic reticulum, and some profiles of the agranular endoplasmic reticulum. The cell surface is highly folded and interlocked with adjacent cells. The outer cell layer is **pigmented** and borders on the stroma of the ciliary body; it is separated from the stroma by a thin **basal lamina** in young individuals. This lamina is subject to aging changes, becoming increasingly thickened and assuming the structure of a basement membrane. (Fig. 35-15) Cells of apposing layers are held together by junctional complexes. (Fig. 35-16)

The **aqueous humor** is produced by the pars plicata of the ciliary body and accumulates in the posterior chamber. The numerous capillaries of the stroma adjacent to the pigmented epithelial layer are the main source for diffusion of fluid and ions. It is believed that an active transport of some substances (i.e. ascorbic acid) takes place across the ciliary epithelium and that the non-pigmented epithelial cells are particularly active in these processes. The aqueous humor flows from the posterior chamber via the pupil to the anterior chamber. It leaves the anterior

Fig. 35-10. Meridional section of anterior portion of the eye. Eyelids removed. Monkey. L.M. X 9. **1.** Cornea (appears dark with trichrome stain). **2.** Anterior chamber. **3.** Pupil. **4.** Lens. **5.** Iris. **6.** Ciliary body. **7.** Sclera (appears dark with trichrome stain).

Fig. 35-11. Root of iris. Enlargement of rectangle in Fig 35-10. Monkey. L.M. X 43. **1.** Posterior chamber. **2.** Iris. **3.** Anterior chamber. **4.** Cornea. **5.** Canal of Schlemm. **6.** Intertrabecular spaces. **7.** Limbus (sclerocorneal junction). **8.** Bulbar conjunctiva. **9.** Ciliary processes (pars plicata). **10.** Ciliary muscle. **11.** Sclera. **12.** Episclera.

Fig. 35-12. Ciliary muscle. Enlargement of area similar to rectangle (A) in Fig. 35-11. Monkey. L.M. X 320. **1.** Meridional-radial smooth muscle cells. **2.** Circular smooth muscle cells. **3.** Melanocytes. **4.** Small arteriole.

Fig. 35-13. Ciliary body. Pars plana. Enlargement of rectangle (B) in Fig. 35-11. Monkey. L.M. X 120. **1.** Smooth muscle cells of ciliary body. **2.** Melanocytes. **3.** Small artery. **4.** Ciliary epithelium. **5.** Zonules.

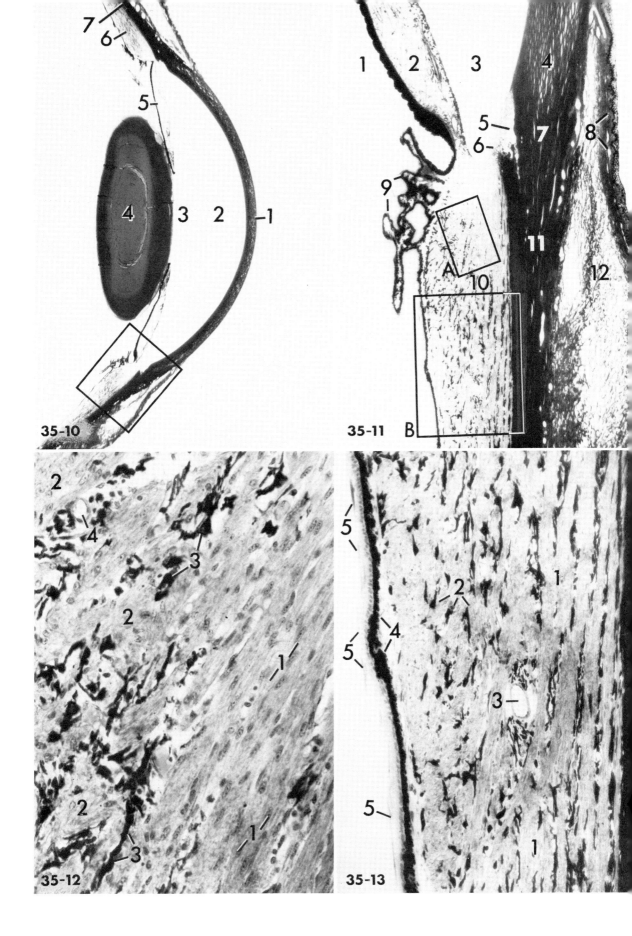

35-10

35-11

35-12

35-13

chamber via the intertrabecular spaces and the canal of Schlemm, ultimately reaching the scleral and episcleral veins.

IRIS

The iris is the most anterior part of the uveal tract (middle layer of the eyeball). It is a thin annular plate: its outer rim is attached to the ciliary body; its inner rim borders the pupil. (Figs. 35-10, 35-17) The iris plate consists of a stroma of loose connective tissue, smooth muscle tissue, melanocytes, and pigmented epithelial cells. It functions as an adjustable diaphragm which controls the amount of light that enters the interior of the eye.

Stroma. The major portion of the iris is made up of loose connective tissue consisting of fibroblasts, melanocytes, giant macrophages (clump cells), mast cells, and a delicate network of collagenous fibrils. (Fig. 35-19) The fibroblasts and the melanocytes are more densely packed near the **anterior surface** of the iris, where they are oriented parallel to the surface. This surface borders on the anterior chamber of the eye and is not lined by an epithelium but is formed by the fibroblasts and melanocytes. (Fig. 35-18) The clump cells are peculiar giant cells (70–100 μ) which represent macrophages with numerous ingested melanin granules; they are permanently lodged in lysosomal residual bodies. The number of melanocytes determines the eye color: there are many present in brown eyes, but only a few in blue eyes.

The stroma contains numerous small blood vessels and capillaries; large vessels form vascular rings near the ciliary body. The adventitial collagen is arranged in a very distinct circular pattern.

Sphincter muscle. In the stromal connective tissue near the pupillary border, smooth muscle cells are arranged circularly around the pupil in groupings of 5–10 cells, representing the sphincter muscle of the pupil. (Fig. 35-19) Individual smooth muscle cells are invested by an external lamina, except for areas of gap-

junction (nexus). Non-myelinated, autonomic nerves occur in close proximity to the smooth muscle cells.

Posterior surface. The posterior surface of the iris is lined by a double layer of pigmented epithelial cells, often called pars iridica retinae. One of these two layers the **posterior pigment epithelium,** borders on the posterior chamber of the eye. It consists of cuboidal or low columnar cells held together by junctional complexes and separated from the pos-

Fig. 35-14. Ciliary body. Pars plicata. Monkey. L.M. X 200. **1.** Posterior chamber. **2.** Posterior surface epithelium of iris. **3.** Root of iris. **4.** Ciliary processes covered by ciliary epithelium. **5.** Ciliary stroma with blood capillaries. **6.** Melanocytes.

Fig. 35-15. Ciliary process. Enlargement of area similar to rectangle in Fig. 35-14. Human. E.M. X 600. **1.** Inner non-pigmented epithelium. **2.** Outer pigmented epithelium. **3.** Basement membrane, increased in thickness as part of aging changes. **4.** Ciliary stroma. **5.** Blood capillary.

Fig. 35-16. Ciliary epithelium. Enlargement of area similar to rectangle in Fig. 35-15. Human. E.M. X 3500. **1.** Basement membrane. **2.** Nuclei of pigmented cells. **3.** Junctional complexes of apposed cell membranes. **4.** Nuclei of non-pigmented cells. **5.** Interlocking of highly folded cell membranes. **6.** Level of inner limiting membrane (basal lamina). **7.** Posterior chamber.

Fig. 35-17. Iris. Monkey. L.M. X 33. **1.** Anterior chamber. **2.** Anterior surface of iris. **3.** Stroma. **4.** Posterior surface of iris. **5.** Posterior chamber. **6.** Lens. **7.** Pupillary border of iris. **8.** Sphincter muscle.

Fig. 35-18. Iris. Anterior surface. Enlargement of area similar to rectangle (A) in Fig. 35-17. Human. E.M. X 4000. **1.** Nucleus of fibroblast. **2.** Nuclei of melanocytes. **3.** Cell processes of melanocytes in stroma. **4.** Delicate bundles of collagenous fibrils.

Fig. 35-19. Iris. Pupillary border zone. Enlargement of area similar to rectangle (B) in Fig. 35-17. Human. E.M. X 1600. **1.** Smooth muscle cells of pupillary sphincter. **2.** Nuclei of fibroblasts. **3.** Collagenous fibrils in stroma of iris. **4.** Nuclei of anterior pigmented epithelial cells. **5.** Nucleus of posterior pigmented epithelial cell. **6.** Levels of basal laminae. **7.** Posterior chamber.

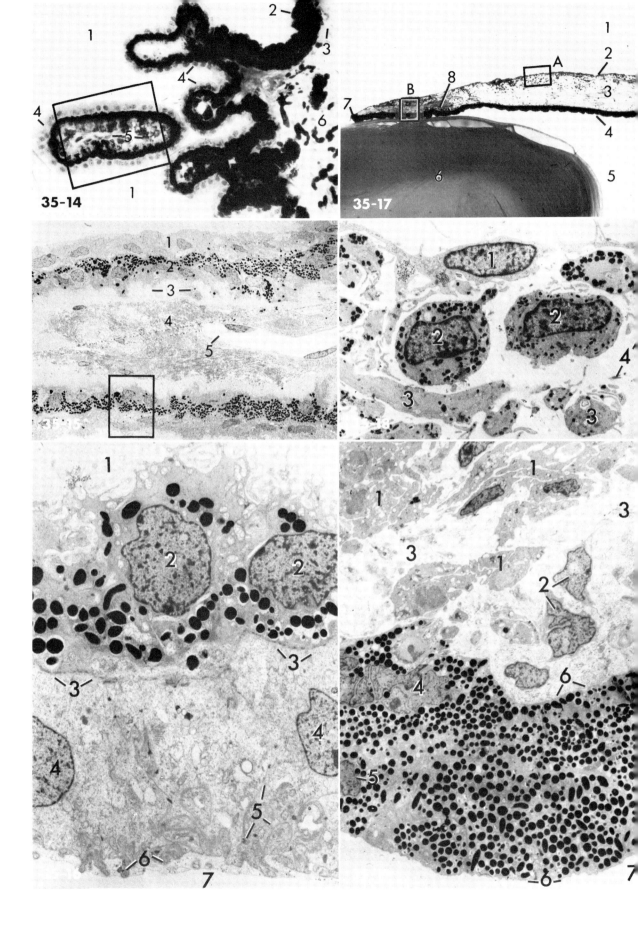

35-14

35-17

terior chamber of the eye by a thin basal lamina. (Fig. 35-19) The cells are filled with melanin granules. Together with the melanocytes of the stroma they contribute to the eye color.

The second pigmented cell layer, which borders on the stroma of the iris, consists of anterior **pigmented myoepithelial cells.** In the outer one-half of the iris, the stromal (anterior) portions of these myoepithelial cells extend radially and their cytoplasmic organization is identical to that of a smooth muscle cell. The processes are invested by an external (basal) lamina. Processes from several cells form 3–5 layers, which collectively are referred to as the **dilator muscle.** The posterior portion of these myoepithelial cells is cuboidal and contains melanin granules. In the inner one-half of the iris the pigmented myoepithelial cells are cuboidal without cytoplasmic smooth muscle processes.

RETINA

The retina is the transparent innermost layer of the wall of the eyeball. It is derived from the optic vesicle, an outpocketing of the forebrain in the embryo. The vesicle invaginates, assuming a cup-shape with two apposing layers. The outer layer of the vesicle becomes the **pigmented epithelium** of the retina, and the inner, invaginated layer of the vesicle becomes the **retina proper.** For a detailed review of further development of the retina and the eye consult textbooks of embryology. The retina contains specialized photoreceptor cells that are stimulated by light, as well as nerve cells that conduct nerve impulses to other parts of the central nervous system.

Pigmented epithelium. The pigmented epithelium extends from the edge of the optic disk to the ora serrata. It consists of cuboidal, hexagonal cells which rest on a thin basal lamina, adjacent to the elastic membrane of Bruch. (Fig. 35-7) A large spherical nucleus is situated in the basal portion of the cell. The basal cell membrane is irregularly infolded. The apical cell surface is provided with microvilli, and the tips of the photoreceptor outer segments are recessed within this apical cytoplasm between the microvilli. (Fig. 35-25) Adjacent pigmented epithelial cells are held together by junctional complexes, but there are no special attachments between the epithelial cells and the tips of the receptor cells. Separation may occur at this level, giving rise to an intraretinal space. This happens during retinal detachment. Spherical and ovoid melanin granules occur in the innermost zone of the cell near and within the microvilli. Mitochondria are more numerous near the cell base. The entire cell is pervaded by a rich network of tubular agranular endoplasmic reticulum and many free ribosomes. Lipofuscin granules are also common, representing lysosomal residual bodies.

Retina proper. Pars optica retinae (neural retina) consists of: 1) neuroepithelial photoreceptor cells; 2) bipolar neurons (1st neurons); and 3) ganglion cells (2nd neurons). The three cell types are interconnected to form a functional chain with the photoreceptor cells in an outer layer, the bipolar neurons in a middle layer, and the ganglion cells in an inner

Fig. 35-20. Retina. Rat. E.M. X 840.
Fig. 35-21. Retina. Monkey. L.M. X 200.
  1. Vitreous body. **2.** Inner limiting membrane. **3.** Nerve fiber layer. **4.** Ganglion cells. **5.** Inner plexiform (synaptic) layer. **6.** Inner nuclear layer of bipolar cells. **7.** Blood vessel. **8.** Outer plexiform (synaptic) layer. **9.** Outer nuclear layer of rods and cones. **10.** Outer limiting membrane of zonulae adhaerentes. **11.** Inner segments of rods and cones. **12.** Outer segments of rods and cones. **13.** Pigmented epithelium. **14.** Bruch's membrane. **15.** Choriocapillaris.
Fig. 35-22. Cone cell. Enlargement of area similar to rectangle in Fig. 35-20. Retina. Rat. E.M. X 6500. **1.** Nucleus of cone cell. **2.** Cytoplasm (finely filamentous). **3.** Inner cone segment (ellipsoid) filled with elongated mitochondria. **4.** Zonulae adhaerentes forming outer limiting membrane. **5.** Inner segments of rod cells.

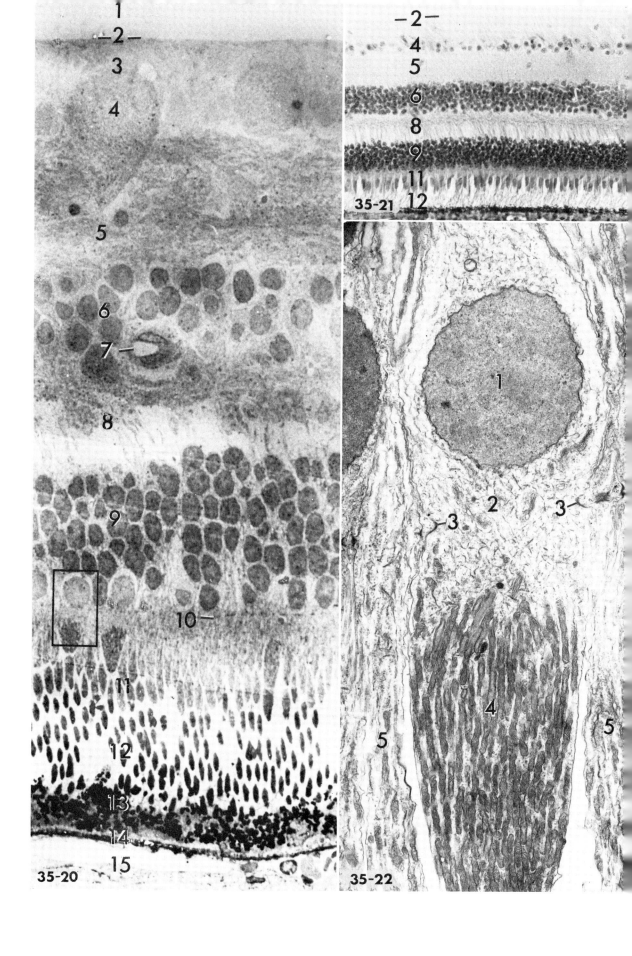

1

—2—

3

4

5

6

7—

8

9

10—

11

12

13

14

15

35-20

—2—

4

5

6

8

9

11

12

35-21

0

1

2

3

3

4

5

5

35-22

layer. A section of the retina (Fig. 35-20) demonstrates several more layers, which arise through synaptic junctions of the bipolar neurons with the photoreceptor cells (outer plexiform layer) as well as with the ganglion cells (inner plexiform layer). The central (axonal) processes of the ganglion cells form a distinct, innermost nerve fiber layer. Lateral integration of nerve impulses within the retina is provided for by so-called horizontal cells at the level of the outer synaptic layer, and by amacrine cells at the level of the inner synaptic layer. In addition, supporting (Müller) cells are joined by junctional complexes which show up as an outer limiting membrane, and there is an inner limiting membrane which borders on the vitreous body and consists of a thin basal lamina.

The neuroepithelial **photoreceptors** consist of rod cells and cone cells (rods and cones). The bodies of these cells are very thin and thread-like. The bulk of the nucleus produces the widest part of the cell. (Fig. 35-27) The nuclei of the rods and cones are aggregated at varied levels and are collectively referred to as the **outer nuclear layer.** The **rod proper** is composed of a slender **inner segment** filled with mitochondria (Fig. 35-23), and an **outer segment** made up of stacks of disk-like membranes formed by deep folds of the rod cell membrane. (Fig. 35-25) The photopigments (rhodopsin in rods, and iodopsin in cones) are present within the confines of these folds. The outer and inner segments are connected by a short cilium-like structure emerging from a basal body in the inner segment. (Fig. 35-24) The **cone proper** has an inner (ellipsoid) segment with numerous mitochondria. (Fig. 35-22) The outer segment is wider near its inner portion than the corresponding area in the rod. Otherwise, the cone proper is ultrastructurally similar to the rod proper. The central (synaptic) ending forms a dilated oval termination in the rods, the **spherule,** and a pyramidal termination in the cones, the **pedicle.** (Fig. 35-26) These make intricate synaptic contacts with several bipolar neurons and horizontal cells within the **outer plexiform layer** of the retina. The photoreceptor endings contain clear presynaptic vesicles and one or several **synaptic ribbons,** which are highly electron-dense, sickle-shaped lamellar structures. (Fig. 35-26) The specific function of the ribbon is not known. The rod outer segments contain more photopigments than the cone outer segments. The rods, therefore, contribute more to the perception of light at dusk (night vision). The cones, which are less photosensitive, are responsible for color perception. Because of the synaptic interneuronal connections at the inner and outer plexiform layers, the light sensitivity of the rods is increased through their many lateral neuronal connections. The cones have fewer interneuronal connec-

Fig. 35-23. Inner and outer segments of rods. Retina. Monkey. E.M. X 10,000. **1.** Inner segments of rods (ellipsoids) filled with long mitochondria. **2.** Outer segments. **3.** Connecting region. Section does not traverse plane of connecting cilium.

Fig. 35-24. Connecting region of inner and outer rod segments. Retina. Cat. E.M. X 19,000. **1.** Mitochondria of inner segment of rod. **2.** Basal body of cilium. **3.** Connecting cilium. **4.** Rod cell membrane. **5.** Outer segment with rod disks.

Fig. 35-25. Rod outer segment. Retina. Rat. E.M. X 31,000. **1.** Rod disks. **2.** Rod cell membrane. **3.** Microvilli of pigment epithelium. **4.** Pigment granules. **5.** Area of contact between rod outer segment and pigment epithelium.

Fig. 35-26. Pyramidal synaptic termination of cone cell (pedicle). Retina. Cat. E.M. X 28,000. **1.** Dendritic branches of bipolar neurons and horizontal cells in outer plexiform layer. **2.** Synaptic ribbons. **3.** Synaptic vesicles of cone pedicle. **4.** Mitochondria. **5.** Narrow part of cone cell, continuous with its perinuclear cytoplasm. **6.** Adjacent oval terminations of rod cells (spherules).

Fig. 35-27. Rod cell. Nuclear region. Inner nuclear layer. Retina. Rat. E.M. X 9000. **1.** Nuclei of rod cells. **2.** Perinuclear cytoplasm (perikaryon). **3.** Narrow part of rod cell cytoplasm.

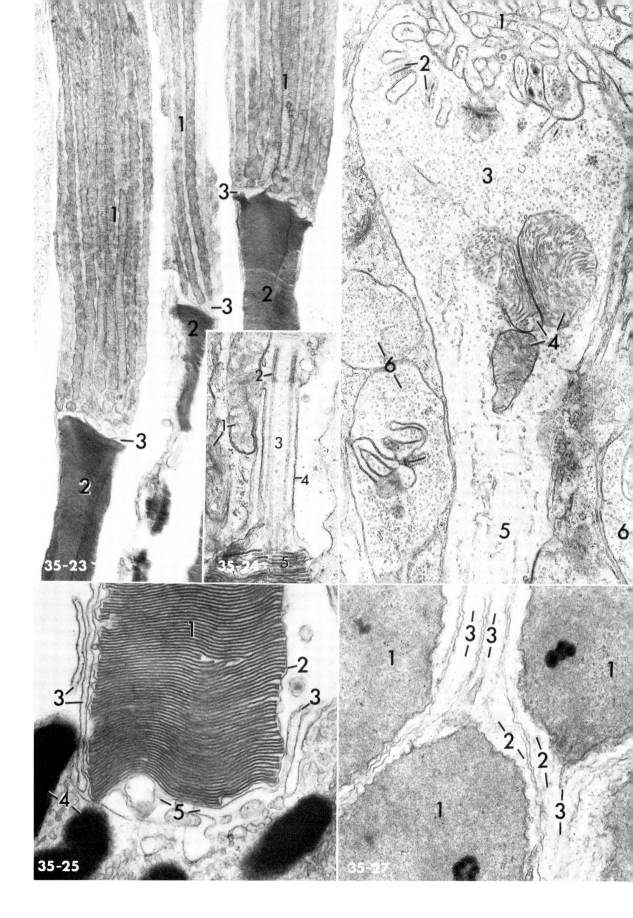

35-23

35-24

35-25

35-27

tions and therefore contribute more to visual acuity, as evidenced by their sole presence in the fovea centralis of the retina.

The nuclei of the bipolar neurons form the **inner nuclear layer** together with the nuclei of multipolar horizontal nerve cells and the large unipolar amacrine nerve cells. The **bipolar neurons** have slender dendritic processes which synapse with the rod and cone terminations in the outer plexiform layer. The axons of the bipolar cells are similarly narrow and branching (Fig. 35-29), making synaptic contacts with several ganglion cells in the **inner plexiform layer**. (Fig. 35-28)

The perikarya of the horizontal cells and the amacrine cells are situated among the cell bodies of the bipolar neurons. The **horizontal cell** processes interconnect a large number of rods and cones at the level of the outer plexiform layer. It is believed that these processes can conduct impulses in both directions along their entire length. The **amacrine cells** are basically unipolar cells with a large rounded perikaryon. The single cell process extends toward the innex plexiform layer, branching extensively and synapsing with several ganglion cells at the inner plexiform layer.

The **ganglion cells** are round multipolar neurons of varied size which form the innermost layer of nuclei together with some glial cells. The ganglion cells have an abundant cytoplasm with an ultrastructure similar to that of other sensory ganglion cells. (Fig. 35-31) Dendritic cell processes make synaptic junctions with bipolar neurons and amacrine cells in the inner plexiform layer. (Fig. 35-28) The axons form a distinct innermost **nerve fiber layer** in the retina. (Fig. 35-30) The axons are non-myelinated and run parallel to the inner surface of the retina, leaving the eyeball via the lamina cribriformis of the sclera, where they form the optic nerve. (Fig. 35-32)

The **glial cells** of the retina are starshaped astrocytes which occur mostly among the ganglion cells and the nerve fiber layer of the retina. Their ultrastructure is similar to that described for astrocytes elsewhere in the central nervous system (p. 000). The **Müller cells** are structurally and functionally related to glial cells since they have a supporting and nutritive function. They are elongated, giant cells which extend from the inner limiting membrane to the inner segments of the rods and cones. The nucleus of the Müller cell is situated among the nuclei of the bipolar neurons in the inner nuclear layer. The cytoplasm forms sheet-like processes which surround the perikarya and cell processes of rods, cones, bipolar neurons, and ganglion cells. The cytoplasm abounds in fine, 100-Å thick filaments, vesicular profiles of agranular endoplasmic reticulum, and glycogen particles. The Müller cell cytoplasm forms broad, plate-like bases (Fig. 35-30) against the inner limiting membrane of the retina, and is united to the cytoplasm of the rods and cones by zonulae adhaerentes to form the **outer limiting membrane** at the level of the inner segments of the photoreceptor cells. (Fig. 35-22) Microvilli extend from the Müller cells for a short distance beyond the level of the outer lim-

Fig. 35-28. Inner plexiform (synaptic) layer. Retina. Rat. E.M. X 19,000. **1.** Axonal endings of bipolar cells with synaptic vesicles. **2.** Ganglion cell processes. **3.** Synaptic junctions.

Fig. 35-29. Axon hillock of bipolar neuron. Retina. Rat. E.M. X 9000. **1.** Nucleus of bipolar neuron. **2.** Golgi apparatus. **3.** Mitochondria. **4.** Axon hillock. **5.** Axon.

Fig. 35-30. Nerve fiber layer. Retina. Rat. E.M. X 5000. **1.** Axons of retinal ganglion cells with mitochondria. **2.** Cytoplasm of glial cells. **3.** Cytoplasm of Müller cells. **4.** Internal limiting membrane.

Fig. 35-31. Ganglion cell. Retina. Rat. E.M. X 2700. **1.** Nerve fiber layer. **2.** Nucleus of ganglion cell. **3.** Voluminous perikaryon with numerous Nissl bodies, mitochondria and secondary lysosomes (dark bodies). **4.** Dendrite. **5.** Inner plexiform layer.

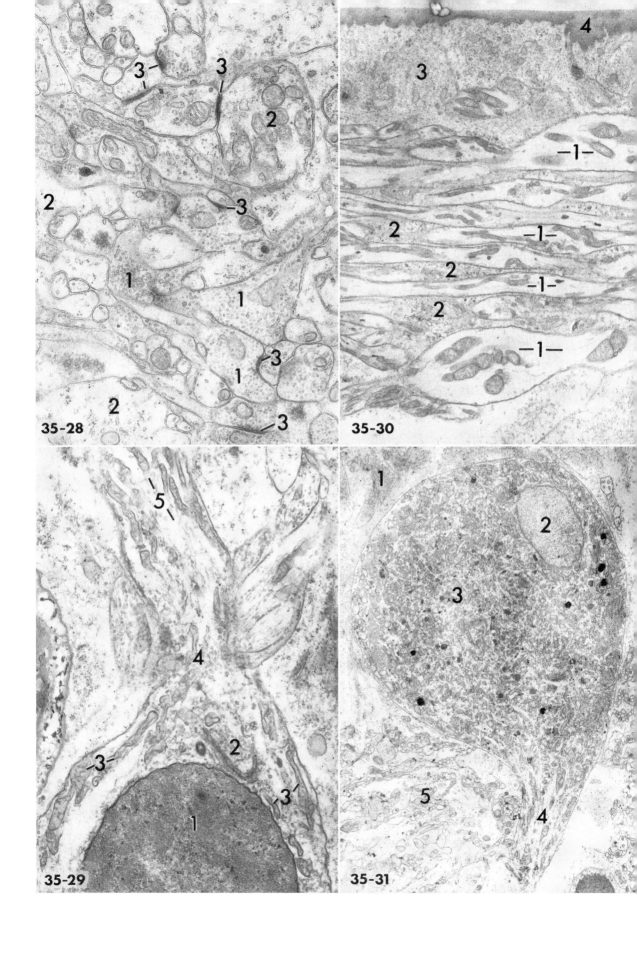

35-28

35-30

35-29

35-31

iting membrane. The **inner limiting membrane** is a basal lamina (Fig. 35-30) which separates the vitreous body from the base plates of the Müller cells and from the axons of the ganglion cells (nerve fiber layer).

The **blood vessels** of the retina (central artery and vein) enter and leave with the optic nerve and are distributed in very distinct individual patterns within the bipolar (Fig. 35-20) and ganglion cell layers. They do not reach the inner nuclear layer of photoreceptor cells. The capillaries are surrounded by glial and Müller cell processes, and their walls consist of non-fenestrated endothelial cells and pericytes (mural cells) distributed evenly along the capillary. For a detailed description of the vascular pattern of the optic disk and the fundus of the eye consult textbooks of ophthalmology.

Macula. The retina is thinned out to about one-third of its average height within the zone of greatest visual acuity at the posterior pole of the eye, and referred to as the macula. This is an area about 1.5 mm in diameter located temporal to the optic disk. The macula has an annular outer pigmented elevated ridge, the **macula lutea,** and an inner **fovea centralis,** which is the thinnest part of the retina. The ridge is caused by an accumulation of nerve cells and nerve fibers. The fovea contains only slender cones, and the internal retinal layers are reduced considerably in height.

Optic disk. The point where the nerve fibers leave the retina, and where the retinal blood vessels enter and leave, is referred to as the **optic disk** (nerve head). This area is about 1 mm wide and does not contain photoreceptor cells, bipolar neurons, or ganglion cells. It is therefore referred to as the "blind spot" of the retina. The ganglion cell axons (nerve fibers of retina) converge on the margin of the optic disk, where they pile up to form the **optic papilla,** an annular ridge surrounding the optic disk. (Fig. 35-32)

OPTIC NERVE

The nerve fibers of the retina become segregated into nerve fascicles by tubes of astrocytes in the **intraocular part** of the optic nerve. As the fibers pierce the sclera in the lamina cribrosa, these fascicles become further separated by the connective tissue elements of the sclera. Beyond the lamina cribrosa the nerve fibers become myelinated in the **orbital part** of the optic nerve, and the diameter of the nerve increases from about 1.5 mm to about 3.5 mm. (Fig. 35-33) The myelinization is derived from oligodendrocytes which are present only within the fascicles, oriented parallel to the direction of the axons. (Fig. 35-35) The optic nerve is therefore similar to a tract of the white matter of the brain.

The optic nerve is surrounded by all three **meninges** (dura, arachnoid, pia) in the orbit and the optic nerve canal. In the optic nerve the subdural and arachnoid spaces are called **vaginal spaces.** The connective tissue of the innermost meninx, the pia mater, extends into the optic nerve forming the **septal tissue,** which is continuous with the connective tissue septa of

Fig. 35-32. Meridional section of optic disk and optic nerve. Monkey. L.M. X 32. **1.** Optic disk. **2.** Optic papilla (annular ridge). **3.** Retina. **4.** Sclera. **5.** Lamina cribrosa with intraocular part of optic nerve. **6.** Orbital part of optic nerve.

Fig. 35-33. Orbital part of optic nerve. Cross section. Monkey. L.M. X 24. **1.** Meninges. **2.** Vaginal spaces. **3.** Septal tissue. **4.** Nerve fascicles. **5.** Central blood vessels.

Fig. 35-34. Optic nerve. Cross section. Enlargement of area similar to rectangle in Fig. 35-33. Rat. E.M. X 620. **1.** Pia mater. **2.** Each nerve fascicle contains numerous myelinated nerve axons. **3.** Blood vessels.

Fig. 35-35. Optic nerve. Cross section. Enlargement of area similar to rectangle in Fig. 35-34. Rat. E.M. X 1900. **1.** Blood vessel in pia mater. **2.** Capillary in nerve fascicle. **3.** Myelinated axons. **4.** Astrocytic (glial) cytoplasm. **5.** Nucleus of astrocyte. **6.** Nuclei of oligodendrocytes.

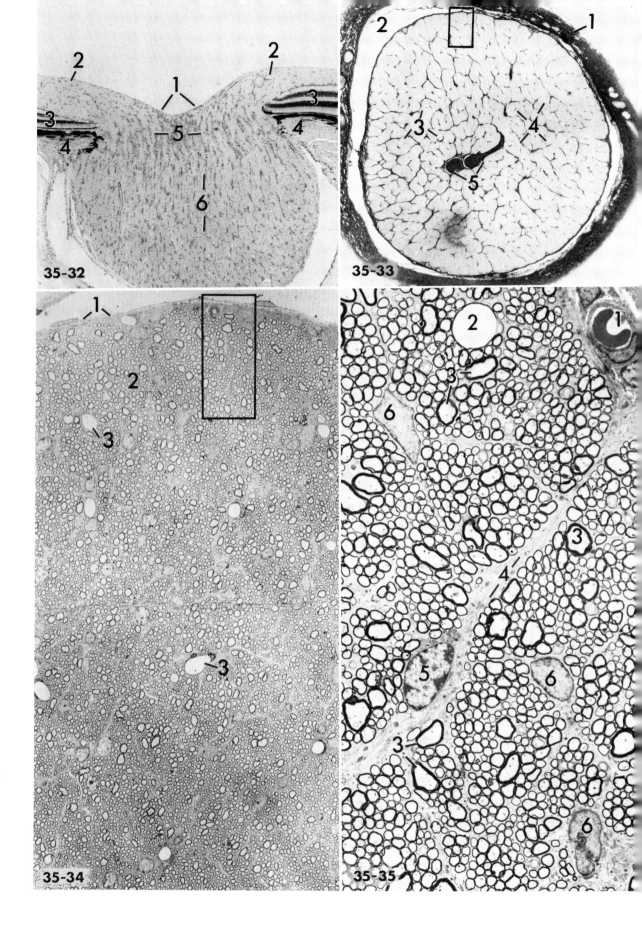

35-32

35-33

35-34

35-35

the lamina cribrosa. A mantle of astrocytes surrounds each nerve fascicle throughout the optic nerve. (Fig. 35-35)

VITREOUS BODY

The vitreous is a transparent gel-like, slightly viscid body which occupies the major central part of the eyeball. It consists of 99 per cent water, a very small amount of extracellular fibrils, an interfibrillar substance of hyaluronic acid, and some cells. There is a thin **cortex** formed of delicate collagenous fibrils, 100 Å thick and with a definite banding of about 120 Å periodicity. The **central** vitreous contains fewer fibrils, but those present are of similar size and pattern. Some cells (hyalocytes) are present in both areas, representing fibroblasts, macrophages, and possibly secretory cells. The vitreous body adheres to the retina proper, particularly in relation to the macula and the optic disk. It is not attached to the ciliary body or the lens.

LENS

The lens, a biconvex, transparent body of epidermal origin, is attached via the suspensory ligament to the ciliary body behind the iris. The anterior lens surface shows a spherical convexity, whereas the posterior is paraboloid. The lens has an inherent tendency to become spherical (Fig. 35-36), and this tendency is opposed by an increase in the tension of the zonules of the suspensory ligament. The lens consists of: 1) lens capsule; 2) epithelial cells; and 3) lens cells (fibers).

The **lens capsule** is a homogeneous, hyaline membrane which averages 100 μ in thickness at the anterior lens surface and 30–40 μ at the posterior surface. Fibrillar components with periodic banding have been demonstrated in some regions of the capsule.

The anterior and equatorial surfaces of the lens are lined by a simple **epithelium.** The cells are low columnar near the center of the lens and gradually change to cuboidal and squamous toward the equa-

tor. Their cytoplasm is finely granular and filamentous. Adjacent cells are attached to each other and to the underlying lens cells by numerous intermittent zonulae occludentes. There is no intervening basal lamina between the simple epithelium and the lens cells. At the equator of the lens the cells of the anterior epithelium elongate and enter beneath the anterior epithelial layer to form the major portion of the lens between the anterior epithelial layer and the posterior capsule. (Fig. 35-36) The elongated cells are now referred to as **lens fibers.** The nuclei of these fibers (cells) are situated at, and slightly behind, the equator of the lens. The terminations of the extremely elongated, hexagonal, prismatic lens cells (fibers) form so-called **lens sutures** as they become apposed to and interlocked with other lens fiber terminations at the anterior and posterior surfaces of the lens. (Fig. 35-37)

The lens fibers (cells) undergo cytoplasmic condensation and nuclear pyknosis as the oldest lens fibers accumulate in the center of the lens during development, growth, and aging. The processes involved are not entirely understood. The lens fibers become closely packed, intercellular spaces are reduced, and adjacent cell borders interlock and adhere through large and small zonulae occludentes. (Fig. 35-38) The cytoplasm becomes increasingly dense and filled with numerous deli-

Fig. 35-36. Lens. Mouse. Adult. L.M. X 136. **1.** Anterior lens capsule. **2.** Cuboidal epithelial cell. **3.** Lens fibers. **4.** Nuclei of lens fibers. **5.** Posterior lens capsule.

Fig. 35-37. Lens fibers (cells). Cross section. Enlargement of area similar to rectangle (A) in Fig. 35-36. Rat. E.M. X 1700. **1.** Hexagonal profiles of cross-sectioned lens fibers are quite apparent. **2.** Small dense dots represent mitochondria. **3.** Dense accumulations of fibrillar material. Nuclei are not present at level of this section.

Fig. 35-38. Lens fibers. Longitudinal section. Rat. E.M. X 20,000. **1.** Finely granular and filamentous cytoplasm. **2.** Zonulae occludentes of apposed cell membranes. **3.** Interdigitations. **4.** Mitochondria.

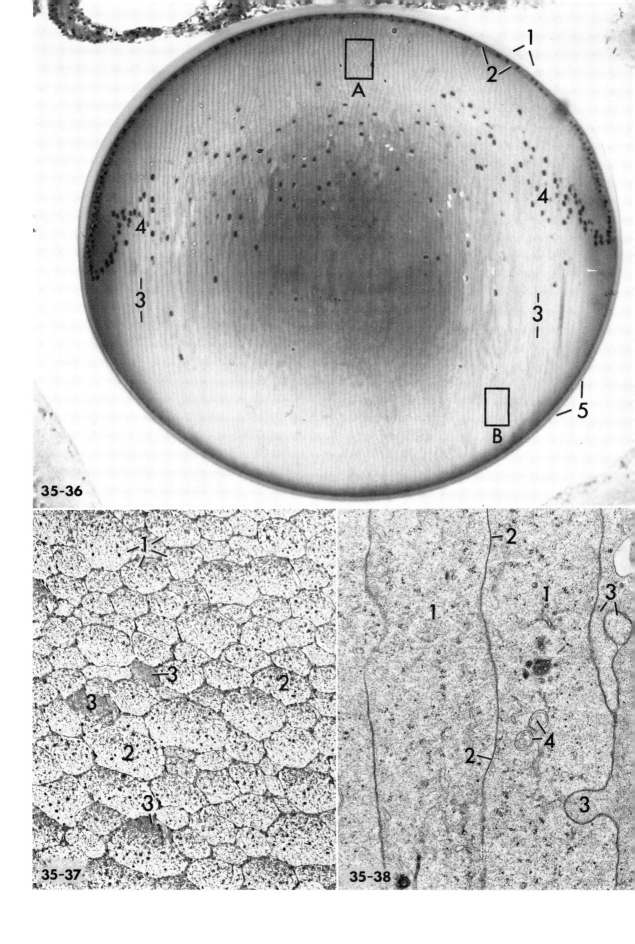

35-36

35-37

35-38

cate filaments and minute particles of unknown nature. The limited number of mitochondria and ribosomes present in the superficial lens fibers also disappear in the condensing cytoplasm of older and more central lens fibers. Finally, the central lens fibers become extremely dense and hard, and in some instances, their transparency can be lost in the process referred to as cataract.

ZONULES

The lens is attached to the ciliary processes via the suspensory ligament consisting of zonular fibers (zonules). These fibers consist of 100-Å thick collagenous fibrils with an axial periodicity of 125 Å. They are attached to the lens capsule and their tension is controlled by the ciliary muscle. A relaxation of this muscle increases the tension of the zonules and flattens the lens, thus reducing its refracting power.

CONJUNCTIVA AND ASSOCIATED STRUCTURES

The **conjunctiva** is a mucous membrane which lines the posterior surface of the eyelids and the anterior surface of the eyeball to the sclerocorneal junction. The conjunctiva consists of a stratified squamous, non-keratinized epithelium which may contain some mucous goblet cells, particularly near the **fornix** where the conjunctiva of the eyelid folds back on itself to cover the surface of the sclera. (Fig. 35-43) The epithelial basal cells often possess melanin granules, and melanocytes occur in the subepithelial connective tissue stroma, which is rich in connective tissue cells such as fibroblasts, macrophages, mast cells, plasma cells, stray granular leukocytes, and diffuse lymphocyte infiltrations.

The **lacrimal glands** are compound tubulo-acinar serous glands located in the orbit above the superior eyelid. The gland opens onto the upper fornix of the conjunctiva by 10 to 20 separate ducts. The constant secretion of tears keeps the con-

junctiva and the cornea moist. The secretion is collected by the **lacrimal canaliculi** near the nasal ends of the eyelid margins. The canaliculi are also lined by a stratified squamous, non-keratinized epithelium. They empty into the **lacrimal sacs** which in turn are drained by the **nasolacrimal duct,** which is lined by a double layer of epithelial cells and conducts the lacrimal secretion to the nasal cavity.

The **eyelids** are folds of skin containing a dense fibrous connective tissue support, the **tarsal plate;** skeletal muscle fibers of the **orbicularis oculi** muscle; smooth muscle cells above the tarsal plate of the upper eyelid, the **tarsal muscle;** and modified sebaceous glands, the **tarsal glands** (of Meibom), which open onto the margins of the eyelid. (Fig. 35-39) Eyelashes **(cilia)**

Fig. 35-39. Upper eyelid. Enlarged from Fig. 35-1. Monkey. L.M. X 28. **1.** Epidermis. **2.** Orbicularis oculi muscle. **3.** Tarsal plate. **4.** Conjunctiva. **5.** Cornea. **6.** Tarsal glands. **7.** Eyelashes (cilia).

Fig. 35-40. Upper eyelid. Enlargement of rectangle (A) in Fig. 35-39. L.M. X 130. **1.** Orbicularis oculi muscle. **2.** Connective tissue. **3.** Tarsal plate. **4.** Tarsal glands. **5.** Conjunctiva.

Fig. 35-41. Upper eyelid. Enlargement of rectangle (B) in Fig. 35-39. L.M. X 120. **1.** Ciliary sweat glands of Moll. **2.** Hair follicles. **3.** Sebaceous glands of Zeiss.

Fig. 35-42. Lower eyelid. Tarsal glands of Meibom. Monkey. L.M. X 110. **1.** Saccules of modified sebaceous gland cells. **2.** Excretory duct. **3.** Dense connective tissue.

Fig. 35-43. Area of upper fornix of conjunctival sac. Direct continuation of Fig. 35-39 and enlarged from Fig. 35-1. Monkey. L.M. X 52. **1.** Fornix of conjunctival sac. **2.** Bulbar conjunctiva. **3.** Sclera. **4.** Limbus (corneoscleral junction). **5.** Cornea. **6.** Ciliary body. **7.** Iris. **8.** Anterior chamber. **9.** Posterior chamber. **10.** Ciliary processes.

Fig. 35-44. Conjunctival sac. Enlargement of rectangle in Fig. 35-43. L.M. X 185. **1.** Connective tissue of upper eyelid. **2.** Conjunctival epithelium with numerous mucous (goblet) cells lining posterior surface of upper eyelid. **3.** Stratified squamous, non-keratinized epithelium of bulbar conjunctiva.

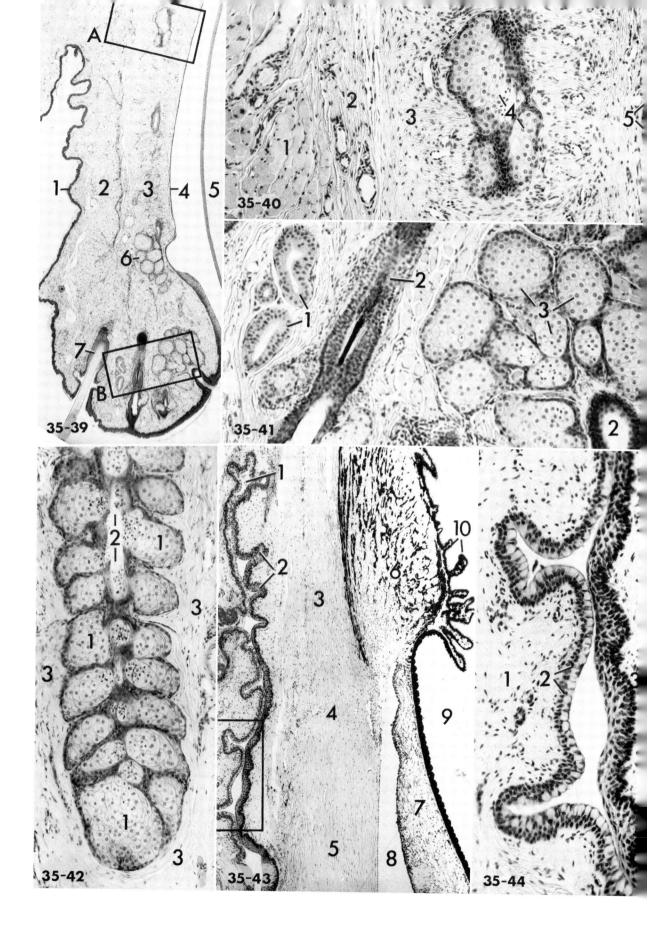

35-39

35-40

35-41

35-42

35-43

35-44

border the edges of the eyelids and originate from deeply located hair follicles associated with ordinary **sebaceous glands** (of Zeiss) and several modified sweat glands, the **ciliary glands** (of Moll).

References

EYE

Cohen, A. I. Vertebrate retinal cells and their organization. Biol. Rev. *8*: 427–459 (1963).

Davson, H. (Ed.). The Eye. Vols. 1–4. Academic Press, New York, 1962.

Dowling, J. E. Organization of vertebrate retinas. Invest. Ophthal. *9*: 665–680 (1970).

Fine, B. S. and Yanoff, M. Ocular Histology. Harper & Row, New York, 1972.

Hogan, M. J., Alvarado, J. A., and Weddell, J. E. Histology of the Human Eye. Saunders, Philadelphia, 1971.

Orzalesi, N., Riva, A. and Testa, F. Fine structure of human lacrimal gland. I. The normal gland. J. Submicroscop. Cytol. *3*: 283–296 (1971).

Rohen, J. W. Das Auge und seine Hilfsorgane. Handbuch mikr. Anat. Menschen. W. Möllendorff and W. Bargmann (Eds.), Vol. 3, Part 4. Springer-Verlag, Berlin, 1964.

Smelser, G. K. (Ed.). The Structure of the Eye. Academic Press, New York, 1961.

Villegas, G. M. Ultrastructure of the human retina. J. Anat. *98*: 501–513 (1964).

36 Ear

The ear consists of the external ear, middle ear, and inner ear. The epithelial cells which serve as receptors and transducers for hearing and for the perception of head position and movement are situated within fluid-filled spaces in the inner ear, transmitting generator impulses to endings of nerve fibers (vestibular and cochlear nerves) which enter the inner ear from the cranial cavity through the internal auditory meatus. The external ear and the middle ear serve to pick up sound waves, to transmit them to the inner ear, and to convert them into vibrations which are propagated by the fluid of the inner ear.

panic membrane, the umbo, where the manubrium of the malleus (one of the ossicles) is attached to the tympanic membrane. The collagenous fibers also occur in circular strata. The fibers form a fibrocartilaginous ring that connects the circumference of the ear drum with the bone. The **flaccid** upper sector of the tympanic membrane does not contain collagenous fibers. The outer surface of the tympanic membrane is covered with the same stratified squamous epithelium present in the meatus. The inner surface is lined by a simple squamous, non-ciliated epithelium. The same type of epithelium lines the rest of the middle ear and is often referred to as the mucous layer.

External Ear

The external ear consists of the auricle (pinna), the lobule, and the external auditory meatus. (Fig. 36-1) An irregularly shaped elastic cartilage forms the framework of the **auricle**; there is none in the **lobule**. Both the auricle and the lobule are covered by epidermis and connective tissue. The lobule contains adipose tissue also. The skin of the external ear is thin and rich in large sebaceous glands. Hairs are often associated with these glands. Ordinary sweat glands are present on the posterior surface of the external ear. The **external auditory meatus** is lined by a thin skin with small hairs and ceruminous (wax) glands, which are modified apocrine sweat glands. The auditory canal is slightly S-shaped, and supported by elastic cartilage (outer part) and by bone (inner part). The **tympanic membrane** (ear drum) is the semitransparent, inner (medial) wall of the auditory canal. It separates the external auditory meatus from the tympanic cavity of the middle ear. The **tense** portion of the membrane consists of a central plate of dense connective tissue in which the collagenous fibers radiate from that part of the tym-

Fig. 36-1. Greatly schematized representation of the outer, middle, and inner ear to assist in forming a concept of the general topography of this region. **1.** Auricle of external ear. **2.** Lobule. **3.** Cartilage. **4.** External auditory meatus. **5.** Tympanic membrane. **6.** Tympanic cavity. **7.** Malleus. **8.** Incus. **9.** Stapes. **10.** Oval window. **11.** Facial nerve (cross-sectioned). **12.** Vestibule. **13.** Saccule with macula. **14.** Lateral (horizontal) semicircular canal and duct with ampulla and crista. **15.** Anterior (vertical) semicircular canal and duct with ampulla and crista. **16.** Posterior (vertical) semicircular canal and duct with ampulla and crista. **17.** Endolymphatic duct. **18.** Endolymphatic sac. **19.** Utricle with macula. **20.** Ductus reuniens. **21.** Cochlea. **22.** Cochlear aqueduct. **23.** Round window. **24.** Internal auditory meatus. **25.** Dura mater. **26.** Cranial cavity. **27.** Auditory (Eustachian) tube. **28.** Parotid gland. **29.** Temporal bone.

Fig. 36-2. Cochlea. Axial section. Guinea pig. L.M. X 29. **1.** Modiolus. **2.** Space in modiolus for the cochlear nerve. **3.** Bony shell of guinea pig cochlea. **4.** Scala tympani. **5.** Cochlear duct. **6.** Scala vestibuli. **7.** Helicotrema.

Fig. 36-3. Cochlea. Enlargement of area similar to rectangle in Fig. 36-2. L.M. X 52. **1.** Scala vestibuli. **2.** Cochlear duct. **3.** Scala tympani. **4.** Spiral ligament. **5.** Organ of Corti; rectangle enlarged in Fig. 36-4. **6.** Bony spiral lamina. **7.** Spiral ganglion. **8.** Cochlear nerve. **9.** Temporal bone.

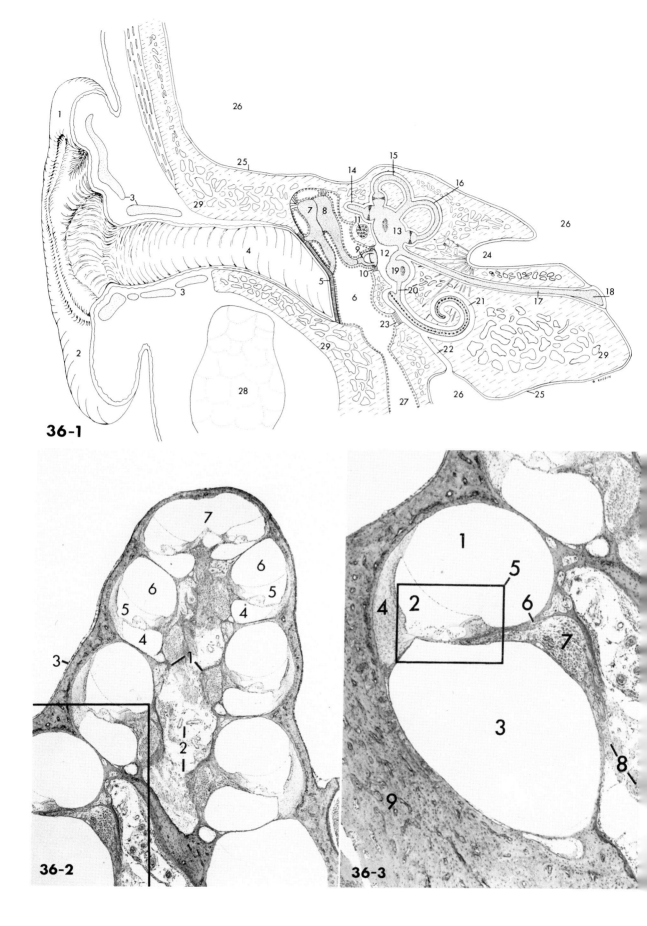

36-1

36-2

36-3

Middle Ear

The middle ear is located in the temporal bone and consists of the tympanic cavity and auditory ossicles. The **tympanic cavity** is an air-filled narrow chamber which communicates with the nasopharynx via the auditory (eustachian) tube, and with the air spaces of the bony mastoid process through the tympanic antrum. The medial wall of the cavity shows several structural peculiarities of which the oval and the round windows are the most prominent. For a detailed review of the topography of the tympanic cavity, consult textbooks of anatomy. The auditory ossicles form a chain of small bones strung across the tympanic cavity between the tympanic membrane on the lateral wall and the oval window on the medial wall. (Fig. 36-1) The manubrium of the **malleus** is attached to the tympanic membrane, and vibrations in the membrane are transmitted by regular joints via the **incus** to the footplate (base) of the **stapes,** which is fixed firmly to the border of the **oval window** (fenestra vestibuli) by an annular ligament. The base of the stapes separates the tympanic cavity from the perilymphatic space of the inner ear. The **round window** (fenestra cochleae), situated below the oval window, is closed by a connective tissue membrane, the secondary tympanic membrane, which is rich in elastic fibrils.

The walls of the tympanic cavity and the surface of the auditory ossicles are covered with a fibrous connective tissue and a simple **epithelium** that is mostly squamous. Areas may be present which have a cuboidal, columnar, or even pseudostratified columnar epithelium, in which occur both ciliated cells and mucous (goblet) cells. There is a rich subepithelial capillary network.

The epithelium that lines the **auditory** (Eustachian) **tube** is usually of the ciliated low columnar type near the tympanic cavity, where the tube is surrounded by a bony wall. The epithelium is pseudostratified ciliated columnar near the nasopharynx, where the tube is supported by a cartilage plate and fibrous membrane. The subepithelial connective tissue of this part contains abundant lymphocytes and mixed glands.

Inner Ear

The inner ear is a labyrinth of cavities and channels located in the pars petrosa of the temporal bone and lined by fibrous connective tissue and a simple squamous epithelium (endosteum). Collectively, the cavities and channels are referred to as the **bony labyrinth.** This labyrinth is filled with **perilymph** and communicates with the arachnoid space of the brain cavity via a narrow channel, the **perilymphatic aqueduct.** (Fig. 36-1) Suspended in the perilymph is the **membranous labyrinth,** a closed system of interconnected tubes and vesicles which contains the **vestibular** and **auditory** sensory receptors. The membranous layrinth is somewhat smaller than the bony labyrinth (Fig. 36-18), but follows rather faithfully the contours of the bony labyrinth. The wall of the membranous labyrinth consists of dense fibrous connective tissue, lined with simple squamous epithelium, except for certain, restricted areas which are provided with a special neuroepithelium. The membranous labyrinth is filled with endolymph

Fig. 36-4. Organ of Corti. Guinea pig. L.M. X 300.
Fig. 36-5. Organ of Corti. Guinea pig. E.M. X 600.
  1. Scala vestibuli (containing perilymph).
  2. Vestibular (Reissner's) membrane.
  3. Cochlear duct (containing endolymph).
  4. Tectorial membrane. **5.** Limbus. **6.** Osseus spiral lamina. **7.** Cochlear nerve. **8.** Basilar membrane. **9.** Capillaries. **10.** Scala tympani (containing perilymph). **11.** Inner hair cells. **12.** Inner tunnel (of Corti) between inner and outer pillar cells. **13.** Outer hair cells. **14.** Supporting cells. **15.** Spiral ligament. **16.** Spiral prominence. **17.** Stria vascularis. **18.** Epithelial cells. **19.** Cells of Claudius.

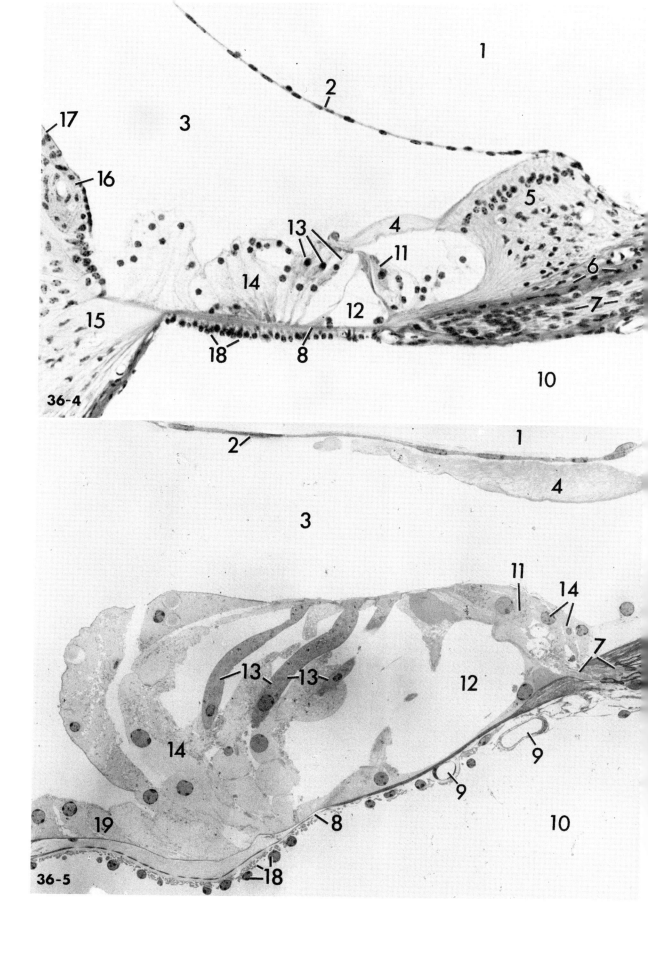

36-4

36-5

and consists of the following major parts: 1) cochlear duct; 2) saccule; 3) utricle; 4) three semicircular ducts; and 5) endolymphatic duct and sac. The microanatomy of the various parts of the bony and membranous labyrinths will now be described.

COCHLEA

The cochlea is the auditory part of the inner ear, innervated by the cochlear nerve of the eighth cranial nerve. Its bony labyrinth forms a spiral channel, which in man makes two and a half turns, whereas in the guinea pig it makes five turns. (Fig. 36-2) There is a central bony stalk, the **modiolus,** from which projects a spiral bony shelf, the **osseus spiral lamina,** which winds around the modiolus. Numerous bipolar ganglion cells are located in a spiral canal within the modiolus, forming the **spiral ganglion.** The spiral bony channel is lined by fibrous connective tissue and simple squamous epithelium, the periosteum. On the outer wall of the spiral bony channel the periosteum is particularly thick, forming the **spiral ligament.** (Fig. 36-3) This ligament is spongy and highly vascular. The **cochlear duct** is the spiral membranous labyrinth of the cochlea which terminates as a blind end at the apex of the cochlea. The basal turn of the cochlear duct communicates with the sacculus of the vestibular labyrinth via the **ductus reuniens.**

Cochlear duct. The cochlear duct is fused laterally with the spiral ligament of the bony channel, whereas the side of the cochlear duct which faces the modiolus is fused with the spiral bony shelf. By these fusions, the cochlear duct divides the perilymphatic space of the bony cochlea into two "staircases," the upper termed **scala vestibuli** and the lower, **scala tympani.** (Fig. 36-4) The scala vestibuli originates near the oval window of the vestibule; the scala tympani near the round window with its secondary tympanic membrane. The perilymph present in both scalae passes over from one to the other at the

apex of the cochlea via the **helicotrema,** the communicating opening. (Fig. 36-2)

The cochlear duct has an unevenly trapezoid cross-sectional profile. (Fig. 36-3) The roof of the cochlear duct, bordering on the scala vestibuli, is referred to as the **vestibular membrane** (of Reissner). It is a thin, delicate membrane consisting of two apposed layers of squamous epithelial cells. (Fig. 36-14) The floor of the cochlear duct is formed by the **basilar membrane,** which consists of compact bundles of minute collagenous fibrils disposed radially and embedded in an amorphous substance. (Fig. 36-11) The striations of the membrane are often referred to as **auditory strings.** The width of the basilar membrane is about 0.21 mm in the basal turn of the cochlear duct. It gradually increases to about 0.36 mm in the apical turn. The specific auditory receptor cells rest on the basilar membrane, forming the spiral **organ of Corti.** The under surface of the basilar membrane facing the perilymph of the scala tympani is lined by squamous or cuboidal epithelial cells (Fig. 36-5), enclosing a narrow connective tissue space in which blood capillaries form a discontinuous looped border beneath the organ of Corti. The outer wall of the cochlear duct, connected to the spiral ligament, is lined by the **stria vascularis,** a stratified, cuboidal epithelium which carries num-

Fig. 36-6. Organ of Corti. Guinea pig. E.M. X 2300. 1. Cochlear duct. 2. Stereocilia. 3. Outer hair cells. 4. Outer phalangeal cells. 5. Nuclei.

Fig. 36-7. Apical part of outer hair cell. Enlargement of area similar to rectangle (A) in Fig. 36-6. Guinea pig. E.M. X 9000. 1. Stereocilia of outer hair cell. 2. Cuticular cell plate. 3. Outer phalangeal cells. 4. Junctional complexes. 5. Mitochondria.

Fig. 36-8. Basal end of outer hair cell. Enlargement of area similar to rectangle (B) in Fig. 36-6. Guinea pig. E.M. X 15,000. 1. Part of nucleus of inner hair cell. 2. Mitochondria. 3. Afferent nerve endings. 4. Efferent nerve endings with numerous synaptic vesicles. 5. Nerve processes. 6. Phalangeal cells.

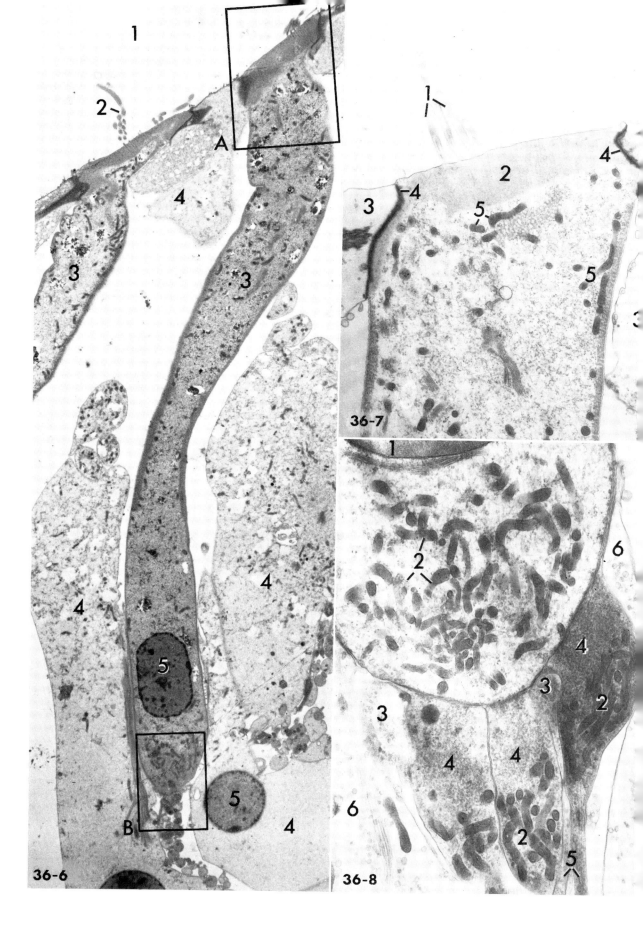

36-6

36-7

36-8

erous intraepithelial capillaries. (Fig. 36-9) The component epithelial cells vary in cytoplasmic electron density. It is believed that the more electron-dense cells, which contain numerous mitochondria, are actively transporting ions into the endolymph (Fig. 36-10), because the stria vascularis is generally considered to be the source of endolymph production. The medial wall of the cochlear duct is small and characterized by the **limbus,** a collection of peculiar connective tissue cells which synthesizes an extracellular fibrillar material, the **tectorial membrane,** which hovers over the epithelial cells of the organ of Corti. (Figs. 36-13, 36-14)

Organ of Corti. The spiral organ of Corti is the auditory receptor organ of the inner ear. It is an avascular epithelium consisting of sensory hair cells, supporting cells, and spaces communicating with the endolymphatic space of the cochlear duct and filled with endolymph. (Figs. 36-4, 36-5)

The **sensory hair cells** are distributed in two groups along the spiral organ of Corti. The **inner hair cells** form a single row of teardrop-shaped cells. Their basal ends do not reach the basilar membrane but are surrounded by the **inner phalangeal** supporting cells, which also reach the epithelial surface surrounding the apex of each hair cell. From the free surface of the inner hair cells project stereocilia arranged in straight rows. The **outer hair cells** form three to four rows of cylindrical cells; they are surrounded by **outer phalangeal** supporting cells. About 100 stereocilia, inserted into a cuticular cell plate, project from the surface of each outer hair cell into the endolymph (Fig. 36-7); they are arranged in bundles to form a W-pattern. The bases of the hair cells are contacted by both afferent and efferent **nerve endings.** The efferent nerve endings contain numerous synaptic vesicles. (Fig. 36-8) The bipolar ganglion cells in the spiral ganglion, located in the spiral canal of the modiolus (Fig. 36-15), send out peripheral processes through small canals in the osseus spiral lamina. (Fig. 36-13) The nerve processes travel via the basilar membrane and spaces between supporting cells of the organ of Corti, and make membranous contacts with the base of the hair cells. Central processes of the bipolar neurons form the cochlear nerve of the eighth cranial nerve, and reach the cochlear nuclei of the medulla oblongata.

There are several **supporting cells** other than the inner and outer phalangeal cells already mentioned. The outer phalangeal cells border outwardly on the columnar **Hensen's** cells with their highly lucent cytoplasm. These cells, in turn, border on the cuboidal cells of Claudius (Fig. 36-5), which laterally join the epithelial cells of the stria vascularis. In the center of the organ of Corti, **inner** and **outer pillar cells** form a triangular **tunnel** of Corti which contains endolymph. The pillar cells contain bundles of cytoskeletal filaments and microtubules, and their apices are occu-

Fig. 36-9. Topography of the external (lateral) wall of the cochlear duct. Guinea pig. E.M. X 500. **1.** Scala vestibuli. **2.** Vestibular (Reissner's) membrane. **3.** Cochlear duct. **4.** Attachment of basilar membrane to the spiral ligament. **5.** Spiral ligament. **6.** Cells of Claudius. **7.** Spiral prominence. **8.** Epithelium of stria vascularis. **9.** Intraepithelial capillaries.

Fig. 36-10. Survey of epithelium of stria vascularis. Guinea pig. E.M. X 1900. **1.** Lumen of cochlear duct. **2.** Nuclei of epithelial cells. **3.** Numerous mitochondria and an intricate system of interlocking cell membranes. **4.** Lumina of intraepithelial capillaries. **5.** Epithelial cells of scala tympani.

Fig. 36-11. Survey of basilar membrane, peripheral to the organ of Corti. Guinea pig. E.M. X 1900. **1.** Lumen of cochlear duct. **2.** Nuclei of Claudius' cells. **3.** Amorphous substance of basilar membrane. **4.** Auditory strings. **5.** Epithelial cells of scala tympani. **6.** Lumen of scala tympani.

Fig. 36-12. Auditory string. Longitudinal section of basilar membrane. Enlargement of area similar to rectangle in Fig. 36-11. Guinea pig. E.M. X 64,000. **1.** Amorphous substance of basilar membrane. **2.** Filaments of auditory strings.

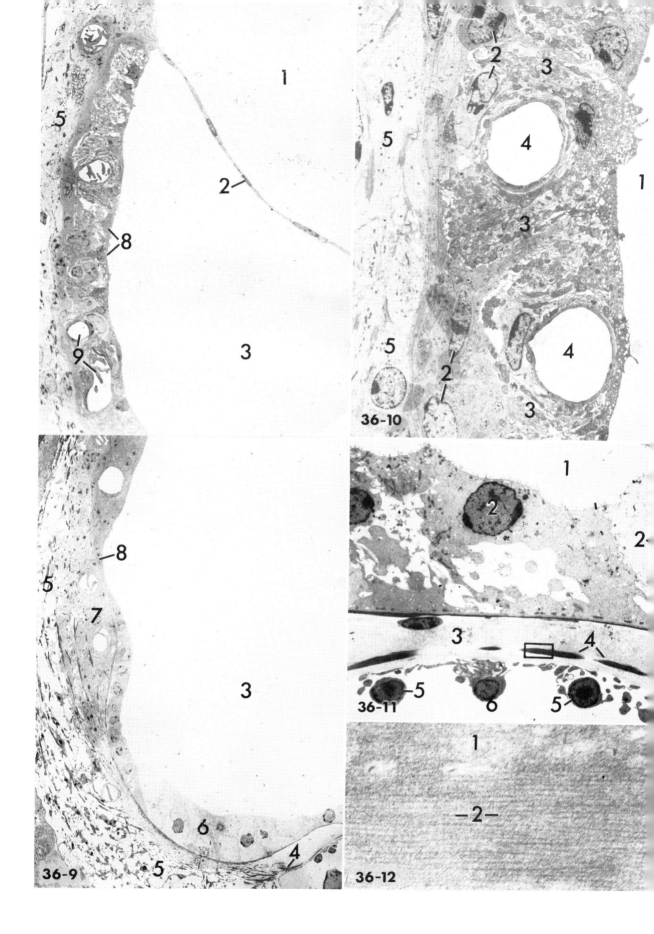

36-9

36-10

36-11

36-12

pied by a cytoplasmic cuticular plate. The apposing apical ends of the pillar cells are united by junctional complexes, interlocking to form the **reticular membrane** which supports the uppermost ends of the hair cells.

Functional considerations. The sound waves are picked up by the external ear and converted to vibrations by the tympanic membrane. These vibrations are transmitted to the perilymph via the auditory ossicles of the middle ear and the base plate of the stapes, which is in contact with the perilymph of the vestibule. A pressure wave is set up in the perilymph and a shift in fluid occurs in both the scala vestibuli and scala tympani. This shift is counterbalanced by the free movement of the secondary tympanic membrane in the round window. The shift in fluid also displaces slightly the cochlear duct, including the basilar membrane, and shearing forces develop between the stereocilia of the hair cells and the tectorial membrane. A generator potential arises in the nerve endings through a stimulation of the hair cells, probably through the mechanical distortion of the stereocilia. This is brought about either via the tectorial membrane touching the stereocilia, or via vibrations in the basilar membrane, since this membrane may record vibrations selectively, depending on the length of its component auditory strings. At the base of the cochlea, the basilar membrane is sensitive to high frequency sounds, whereas it seems to be responsive to low frequency sounds elsewhere throughout the entire cochlear duct.

VESTIBULAR LABYRINTH

The vestibular membranous labyrinth consists of the saccule, the utricle, three semicircular ducts, and the endolymphatic duct and sac. It serves as a receptor organ for equilibrium (balance and orientation).

The saccule and the utricle together occupy the one bony **vestibule,** whereas the semicircular membranous ducts are lodged in similarly shaped **semicircular bony ca-** nals. (Fig. 36-1) The **saccule** is a cone-shaped membranous bag, which is interposed between the cochlear duct and the utricle. It is connected to the cochlear duct via ductus reuniens, and to the utricle via a Y-shaped tube, the fork giving rise to the **endolymphatic duct.** The latter terminates as the **endolymphatic sac** in the subdural space of the cranial cavity. The **utricle** is irregularly oblong in shape and larger than the saccule. There are three semicircular ducts. The **anterior semicircular duct** is oriented vertically and placed transversely to the long axis of the pars petrosa of the temporal bone. The duct connects with the utricle via a widening, the **ampulla,** and it joins the posterior semicircular duct to form the **crus commune,** which in turn opens into the utricle. The **posterior semicircular duct** is also vertical and positioned at right angle to the superior duct. It con-

Fig. 36-13. Topography of the inner (medial) wall of the cochlear duct. Guinea pig. E.M. X 5000. **1.** Lumen of scala vestibuli. **2.** Vestibular membrane. **3.** Origin of tectorial membrane. **4.** Limbus. **5.** Osseus spiral lamina. **6.** Myelinated cochlear nerve fibers in bony canal. **7.** Lumen of scala tympani. **8.** Arrow indicates continuity with structures in Fig. 36-16.

Fig. 36-14. Tectorial membrane. Enlargement of area similar to rectangle in Fig. 36-13. Guinea pig. E.M. X 4500. **1.** Scala vestibuli. **2.** Vestibular membrane consists of two squamous epithelia. **3.** Bundles of delicate filaments embedded in an amorphous substance form the tectorial membrane. **4.** Lumen of cochlear duct.

Fig. 36-15. Spiral ganglion. Cochlea. Guinea pig. L.M. X 220. **1.** Scala tympani. **2.** Osseus spiral lamina. **3.** Peripheral nerve processes of bipolar ganglion cells. **4.** Bipolar nerve cells of spiral ganglion. **5.** Central nerve processes of bipolar ganglion cells. **6.** Bony frame of modiolus. **7.** Hollow center of modiolus.

Fig. 36-16. Survey of bipolar ganglion cells of spiral ganglion. Cochlea. Enlargement of area similar to rectangle in Fig. 36-15. Guinea pig. E.M. X 620. **1.** Bipolar ganglion cells. **2.** Arrow. Peripheral myelinated nerve fibers are directly continuous with those seen at arrow in Fig. 36-13. **3.** Blood capillaries. **4.** Loose connective tissue. **5.** Bone matrix.

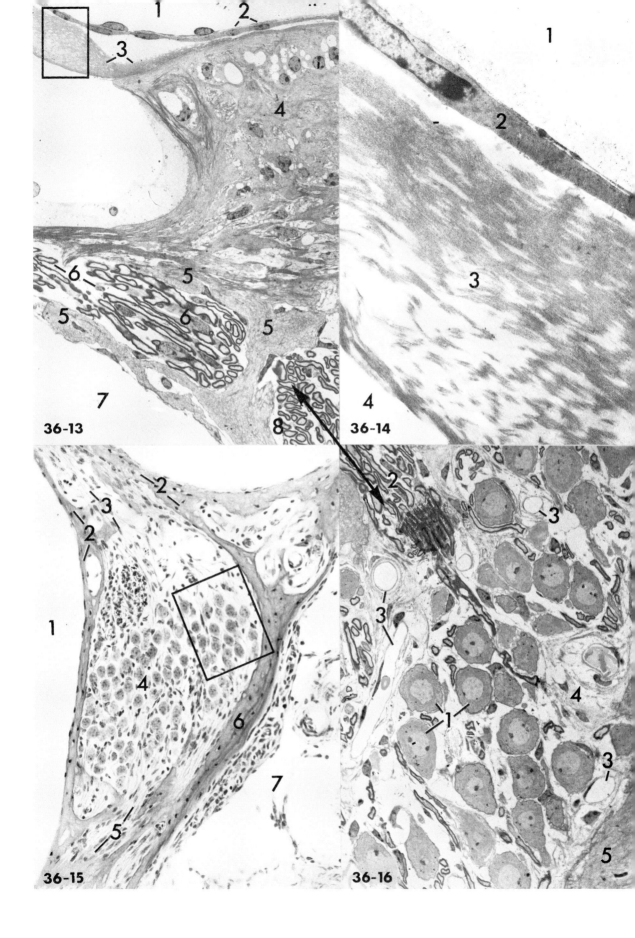

36-13

36-14

36-15

36-16

nects with the utricle via an ampulla and the crus commune. The **lateral semicircular duct** is horizontal. It does not merge with another semicircular duct, and connects with the utricle via an ampulla and the opposite end of the duct. The saccule and the utricle, each has areas of specialized neuroepithelial cells, the crista ampullaris.

Crista ampullaris. In each ampulla of the semicircular ducts, the lining epithelium becomes tall columnar, to form a small 8-shaped ridge which projects into the lumen of the ampulla and is arranged transversely to the long axis of the duct. (Fig. 36-17) The epithelium consists of two types of sensory hair cells, supporting cells, and a cupula. (Fig. 36-21) The **type I hair cell** is piriform with a rounded base and a short neck. The nucleus is located near the base of the cell and surrounded by many mitochondria and numerous smooth, light-core vesicles. This type of hair cell is most frequent near the apex of the crista. The **type II hair cell** is cylindrical and its cytoplasm contains many more smooth vesicles than Type I hair cell does. The apical free surfaces of both cell types are provided with up to 100 **stereocilia** arranged in regular hexagonal array, and one so-called **kinocilium,** always located in the same position in relation to the stereocilia. All hair cells in a crista face in the same direction. They face the utricle in the horizontal crista, and away from the utricle in the vertical crista. The kinocilium contains nine doublets of microtubules which form a basal body in the apical cytoplasm. The central two microtubules present in cilia of other tissues may be missing in the kinocilium.

Tall **supporting cells** surround the hair cells. (Fig. 36-22) They rest on a basal lamina which separates the epithelium of the vestibular membranous labyrinth from the surrounding fibrous connective tissue and periosteum of the bony vestibule and bony semicircular canals. The supporting cells are provided with microvilli and contain granules that could represent secretory

granules. The microvilli of the supporting cells, the stereocilia and kinocilia of the hair cells are embedded in the **cupula,** a dome-shaped mass of gelatinous protein and polysaccharides. (Fig. 36-21)

Maculae. The epithelial cells of the utricle become taller within an area approximately 2 mm × 3 mm in size which is referred to as the macula. Similarly in the saccule, tall epithelial cells aggregate to form an oval area of the same size, the macula of the saccule. (Fig. 36-19) Both maculae consist of two types of hair cells and supporting cells. The structure of these hair cells and the supporting cells is similar to that described for the crista ampullaris. The maculae are covered by an **otolithic membrane** (Fig. 36-20), which is a gelatinous mass with many small crystalline bodies, the otoliths (otoconia).

Fig. 36-17. Inner ear. Vestibular labyrinth. Guinea pig. L.M. X 29. **1.** Vestibule. **2.** Saccule with macula. **3.** Ampulla of semicircular canal with crista ampullaris. **4.** Semicircular duct. **5.** Semicircular canal. **6.** Temporal bone. **7.** Cranial cavity.

Fig. 36-18. Cross section of semicircular canal and duct. Guinea pig. L.M. X 171. **1.** Semicircular duct (containing endolymph). **2.** Wall of duct. **3.** Semicircular canal (containing perilymph). **4.** Endosteum. **5.** Temporal bone.

Fig. 36-19. Part of saccule. Vestibular labyrinth. Guinea pig. L.M. X 115. **1.** Cavity of saccule (containing endolymph). **2.** Wall of saccule. **3.** Macula. **4.** Vestibular nerve fibers.

Fig. 36-20. Part of macula of saccule. Enlargement of rectangle in Fig. 36-19. L.M. X 460. **1.** Otolithic membrane with otoconia. **2.** Stereocilia. **3.** Hair cells and supporting cells. **4.** Vestibular nerve fibers. **5.** Capillaries.

Fig. 36-21. Crista ampullaris. Semicircular duct. Guinea pig. L.M. X 220. **1.** Lumen of semicircular duct (containing endolymph). **2.** Cupula. **3.** Hair cells. **4.** Connective tissue of crista. **5.** Edge of bone, marking the extent of the bony ampulla.

Fig. 36-22. Crista ampullaris. Enlargement of area similar to rectangle in Fig. 36-21. L.M. X 506. **1.** Part of cupula. **2.** Stereocilia. **3.** Hair cells and supporting cells. **4.** Nerve fibers. **5.** Level of basal lamina.

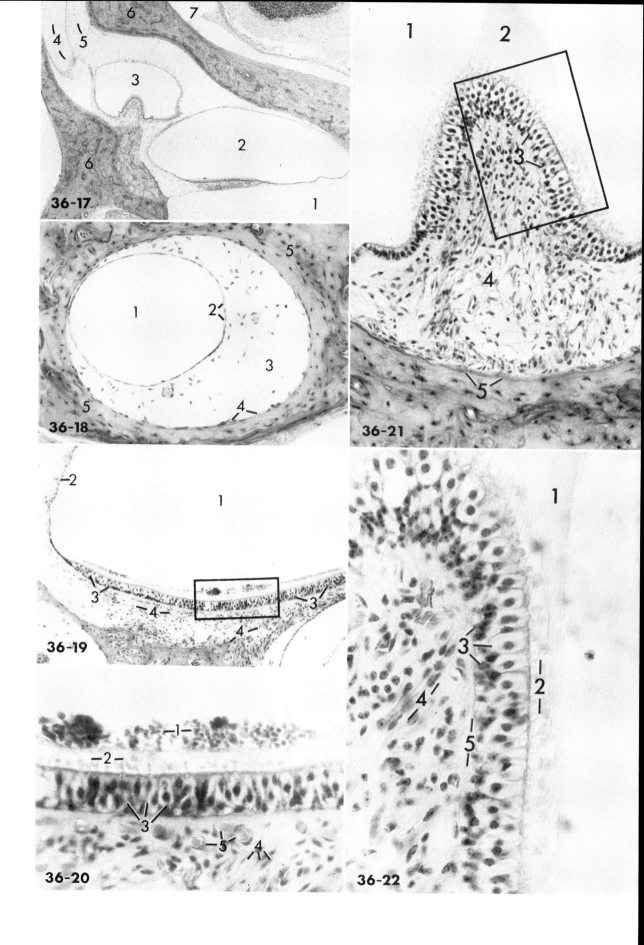

36-17

36-18

36-19

36-20

36-21

36-22

Nerves of vestibular labyrinth. The vestibular ganglion (of Scarpa) lies in the internal auditory meatus. The peripheral processes of the bipolar ganglion cells reach the bases of the hair cells in the maculae and cristae ampullaris via narrow bony channels. Both types of hair cells receive afferent and efferent **nerve endings.** The peripheral processes of the bipolar cells are afferent in nature, forming goblet-shaped chalices around type I hair cells, and bud-like synaptic boutons in relation to type II hair cells. These nerve endings contain light-core (non-granulated) vesicles. Junctional specializations similar to gap-junctions or modifications thereof are often present between hair cell and nerve ending. Efferent nerve endings contact both types of hair cells. They contain dense-core (granulated) vesicles. The central processes of the vestibular bipolar ganglion cells form the vestibular portion of the eighth cranial nerve. They end in the vestibular nuclei of the medulla oblongata near the fourth ventricle.

Functional considerations. The hair cells of the ampullary crests and the maculae of the utricle and the saccule register changes in position of head and body. In the ampullary crests, hair cells are stimulated by movement or pressure changes in the endolymph, caused by angular acceleration of the head, resulting in a deviation of the stereocilia and the kinocilium. The hair cells of the macula of the utricle are stimulated by an increase or a decrease of the pressure exerted upon them by the otolithic membrane caused by change of the position of the head in space. In some lower forms the hair cells of the macula of the saccule may be stimulated by low frequency vibrations, and this part of the membranous labyrinth may therefore respond to auditory stimuli. Its function in man is not established unequivocally.

The function of the efferent nerve endings present in relation to hair cells throughout the neuroepithelial cells of the inner ear is not completely understood. It has been postulated that they modify the effective cellular threshold to sensory stimuli.

References

EAR

Davis, H. Biophysics and physiology of the inner ear. Physiol. Rev. *37*: 1–49 (1957).

de Lorento, A. J. D. (Ed.). Vascular Disorders and Hearing Defects. University Park Press, Baltimore, 1973.

Engström, H. and Wersäll, J. Structure and innervation of the inner ear sensory epithelia. Int. Rev. Cytol. *7*: 535–585 (1958).

Engström, H. and Ades, H. W. (Eds.). Inner ear studies. Acta Otolaryng. Suppl. 301 (1973).

Engström, H., Ades, H. and Anderson, A. Structural Pattern of the Organ of Corti. Almquist and Wiksell, Stockholm, 1966.

Flock, Å. Structure of the macula utriculi with special reference to directional interplay of sensory response as revealed by morphological polarization. J. Cell Biol. *22*: 413–431 (1964).

Hinojosa, R. and Rodriquez-Echandia, E. L. The fine structure of the stria vascularis of the cat inner ear. Am. J. Anat. *118*: 631–664 (1966).

Iurato, S. (Ed.). Submicroscopic Structure of the Inner Ear. Pergamon Press, New York, 1967.

Johnson, F. R., McMinn, R. M. H. and Atfield, G. N. Ultrastructural and biochemical observations on the tympanic membrane. J. Anat. *103*: 297–310 (1968).

Kawabata, I. and Paparella, M. M. Ultrastructure of normal human middle ear mucosa. Ann. Otol. Rhin. Laryngol. *78*: 125–137 (1968).

Kimura, R. S., Schuknecht, H. F. and Sando, I. Fine morphology of the sensory cells in the organ of Corti of man. Acta Otolaryngol. *58*: 390–408 (1965).

Lundquist, P.-G. The endolymphatic duct and sac in the guinea pig. An electron microscopic and experimental investigation. Acta Otolaryngol. Suppl. 201 (1965).

Nakai, Y. and Hilding, D. Vestibular and endolymph-producing epithelium. Electron microscopic study of the development and histochemistry of the dark cells of the crista ampullaris. Acta Otolaryngol. *66*: 120–128 (1968).

Smith, C. A. Electron microscopy of the inner ear. Ann. Otol. Rhin. Laryngol. *77*: 629–643 (1968).

Smith, C. A. and Sjöstrand, F. S. Structure of the nerve endings on the external hair cells of the guinea pig cochlea as studied by serial sections. J. Ultrastruct. Res. *5*: 523–556 (1961).

Spoendlin, H. H. Organization of the sensory hairs in the gravity receptors in utricle and saccule of the squirrel monkey. Z. Zellforsch. *62*: 701–716 (1964).

Spoendlin, H. H. The organization of the cochlear receptor. *In* Advances in Oto-Rhino-Laryngology, Vol. 13, S. Karger, Basel, 1966.

Wersäll, J. Studies on the structure and innervation of the sensory epithelium of the cristae ampullares in the guinea pig. Acta Otolaryngol. Suppl. 126 (1956).

Index

Main entry indicated by boldface type.

of retina, 764
sensory, 264
Gap-junction, 14
Gastric gland proper, 542
Gastrin, 548
Gene, 54
Generator potential, 288
Genetic code, 24, 54
Genital corpuscle, 302
Germinal center, of lymphatic nodule, 384
Germinal epithelium, of ovary, 704
Glands
adrenal, 456
cytology of secretion, 84
endocrine, 78
exocrine, 80
gastric, 540
general considerations, 78
hypophysis, 428
intestinal, 560
lacrimal, 770
liver, 580
mammary, 738
organization of compound glands, 82
pancreas, 594
parathyroid, 450
pineal body, 468
salivary, 520
sebaceous, 494
sweat, 496
thyroid, 442
uterine, 722
Glassy membrane
of hair follicle, 492
of ovarian follicle, 708, 712
Glial (neuroglial) cell, 314
Glomerular filtration membrane, 654
Glomerulus (renal corpuscle), 652
Glomus cell, 304
Glomus pulmonale, 302
Glucagon, 602
Glucocorticoids, 460
Gluconeogenesis, 40
Glycocalyx, **10**, 30, 558
Glycogen, **46**, 590
Glycoprotein, 88
Goblet cell, 80, 556, 620
Golgi apparatus (zone, region), 28
Golgi tendon organ, 296
Golgi type I neuron, 280
Golgi type II neuron, 282
Gonadotroph, 432
Graafian follicle, 708
Granular endoplasmic reticulum, 24
Granular leukocyte, 98
Granule
alpha, 108
azurophilic, 100, 104, 106
chromatin, 50
dense, 238

endothelial, 40
hemosiderin, 36
lipofuscin, 38
matrix, 32
melanin, 46
pigment, 46
secretory, 46
specific, 100
very dense, 108
Granule of
cartilage matrix, 176
leukocytes, 98
lymphocytes, 104
mast cells, 154
platelets, 108
Granulomere, 106
Granulosa lutein cell, 714
Ground substance
cartilage, 176
connective tissue, 148
Growth hormone, 420
Grumose body, 468
Gustatory cell, 512

Hair, 486
Hair cell, of inner ear, 780, 784
Hair follicle, 490
Half-desmosome, **14**, 478
Haploid, 56
Hassall's corpuscle, 420
Haversian canal, 188
Headcap, 686
Heart
blood and lymphatic vessels, 338
connective tissue, 336
endocardium, 332
epicardium, 334
impulse-conducting system, 336
myocardium, 334
nerves, 338
Heat receptor, 300
Helicine artery, 344, 347, 700, 716
Helicotrema, 778
Hematocrit, 94
Heme, 130
Hemocytoblast, 118
Hemoglobin, **96**, 130
Hemopoiesis, 112
Hemosiderin, 130
Henle, loop of, 656
Henle's layer, 490
Heparin, 154, 102
Hepatic cell, 588
Hepatic lobule, 586
Hepatic sinusoid, 584
Hering's nerve, 302
Herring bodies, 436
Heterochromatin, 50
His, bundle of, 336
Histamine, 102, 154, 548